WORLD HEALTH ORGANIZATION
INTERNATIONAL AGENCY FOR RESEARCH ON CANCER

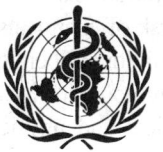

IARC Monographs on the Evaluation of Carcinogenic Risks to Humans

VOLUME 83

Tobacco Smoke and Involuntary Smoking

This publication represents the views and expert opinions
of an IARC Working Group on the
Evaluation of Carcinogenic Risks to Humans,
which met in Lyon,

11–18 June 2002

DISCARD

2004

IARC MONOGRAPHS

In 1969, the International Agency for Research on Cancer (IARC) initiated a programme on the evaluation of the carcinogenic risk of chemicals to humans involving the production of critically evaluated monographs on individual chemicals. The programme was subsequently expanded to include evaluations of carcinogenic risks associated with exposures to complex mixtures, life-style factors and biological and physical agents, as well as those in specific occupations.

The objective of the programme is to elaborate and publish in the form of monographs critical reviews of data on carcinogenicity for agents to which humans are known to be exposed and on specific exposure situations; to evaluate these data in terms of human risk with the help of international working groups of experts in chemical carcinogenesis and related fields; and to indicate where additional research efforts are needed.

The lists of IARC evaluations are regularly updated and are available on Internet: http://monographs.iarc.fr/

This project was supported by Cooperative Agreement 5 UO1 CA33193 awarded by the United States National Cancer Institute, Department of Health and Human Services. Additional support has been provided since 1993 by the United States National Institute of Environmental Health Sciences.

This project was funded in part by the European Commission, Directorate-General EMPL (Employment and Social Affairs), Health, Safety and Hygiene at Work Unit.

IARC Library Cataloguing in Publication Data

Tobacco smoke and involuntary smoking /
IARC Working Group on the Evaluation of Carcinogenic Risks to Humans
(2004 : Lyon, France)

(IARC monographs on the evaluation of carcinogenic risks to humans ; 83)

1. Carcinogens – congresses 2. Tobacco smoke – congresses 3. Involuntary
smoking – congresses I. IARC Working Group on the Evaluation of Carcinogenic
Risks to Humans II. Series

ISBN 92 832 1283 5   (NLM Classification: W1)
ISSN 1017-1606

PRINTED IN FRANCE

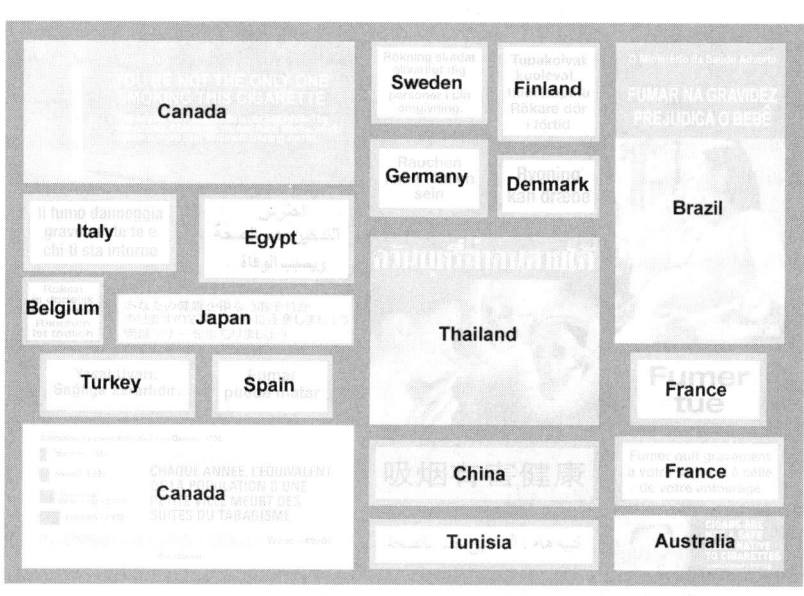

Canada	Warning: You're not the only one smoking this cigarette.
Italy	Smoking is seriously harmful to you and whoever is around you.
Egypt	Smoking harms health and causes death.
Belgium	Smoking kills (*Dutch, French and German*).
Japan	Because smoking can be harmful to your health, be careful not to smoke too much, observe smoking etiquette.
Turkey	Legal warning: Harmful to health.
Spain	Smoking can kill.
Canada	Warning: Each year, the equivalent of a small city dies from tobacco.

Sweden	Smoking seriously harms you and the people around you.
Finland	Smokers die prematurely (*Finnish and Swedish*).
Germany	Smoking can be deadly.
Denmark	Smoking can kill.
Thailand	Tobacco smoke kills (*warning to become compulsory in March 2005*).
China	Smoking harms health.
Tunisia	Important warning: Smoking is harmful to health.

Brazil	Smoking during pregnancy harms the baby.
France	Smoking kills.
France	Smoking seriously harms your health and that of those around you.
Australia	Cigars are not a safe alternative to cigarettes (*warning proposed by the Department of Health and Ageing, image provided by Dr Christopher Hughes, Sydney*).

Cover design by Georges Mollon, IARC

... And for the vanities committed in this filthy custom, is it not both great vanity and uncleanness, that at the table, a place of respect, of cleanliness, of modesty, men should not be ashamed, to sit tossing of tobacco pipes, and puffing of the smoke of tobacco one to another, making the filthy smoke and stink thereof, to exhale across the dishes, and infect the air, when very often men that abhor it are at their repast? ... It makes a kitchen also often-times in the inward parts of men, soiling and infecting them, with an ... oily kind of soot, as has been found in some great tobacco takers, that after their death were opened .... Have you not reason then to be ashamed and to forbear this filthy novelty ... a custom loathsome to the eye, hateful to the nose, harmful to the brain, dangerous to the lungs, and in the black stinking fume thereof, nearest resembling the horrible Stygian smoke of the Pit that is bottomless ?

From '*A Counterblaste to Tobacco*'
by *King James I of England* (1566–1625)
Published by R. Barker, London, 1604

CONTENTS

NOTE TO THE READER

The term 'carcinogenic risk' in the *IARC Monographs* series is taken to mean the probability that exposure to an agent will lead to cancer in humans.

Inclusion of an agent in the *Monographs* does not imply that it is a carcinogen, only that the published data have been examined. Equally, the fact that an agent has not yet been evaluated in a monograph does not mean that it is not carcinogenic.

The evaluations of carcinogenic risk are made by international working groups of independent scientists and are qualitative in nature. No recommendation is given for regulation or legislation.

Anyone who is aware of published data that may alter the evaluation of the carcinogenic risk of an agent to humans is encouraged to make this information available to the Unit of Carcinogen Identification and Evaluation, International Agency for Research on Cancer, 150 cours Albert Thomas, 69372 Lyon Cedex 08, France, in order that the agent may be considered for re-evaluation by a future Working Group.

Although every effort is made to prepare the monographs as accurately as possible, mistakes may occur. Readers are requested to communicate any errors to the Unit of Carcinogen Identification and Evaluation, so that corrections can be reported in future volumes.

IARC WORKING GROUP ON THE EVALUATION
OF CARCINOGENIC RISKS TO HUMANS:
TOBACCO SMOKE AND INVOLUNTARY SMOKING

Lyon, 11–18 June 2002

LIST OF PARTICIPANTS

Members[1]

Michael Alavanja, Division of Cancer Epidemiology & Genetics, National Cancer Institute, 6120 Executive Boulevard, Room 8000, Rockville, MD 20892, USA

John A. Baron, Biostatistics/Epidemiology, Evergreen Center, 46 Centerra Parkway, Lebanon, NH 03756, USA

Ross C. Brownson, Saint Louis University School of Public Health, Salus Center Room 469, 3545 Lafayette Avenue, St Louis, MO 63104, USA

Patricia A. Buffler, School of Public Health, University of California at Berkeley, 140 Earl Warren Hall, Berkeley, CA 94720-7360, USA

David M. DeMarini, Environmental Carcinogenesis Division (MD-68), US Environmental Protection Agency, 86 Alexander Drive, Research Triangle Park, NC 27711, USA

Mirjana V. Djordjevic, Tobacco Control Research Branch, Division of Cancer Control & Population Sciences, National Cancer Institute, 6130 Executive Boulevard, EPN 4044, MSC 7337, Bethesda, MD 20852-7337, USA

Richard Doll, Clinical Trial Service Unit & Epidemiological Studies Unit, Nuffield Department of Clinical Medicine, University of Oxford, Harkness Building, Radcliffe Infirmary, Oxford OX2 6HE, United Kingdom

Elizabeth T.H. Fontham, Department of Public Health & Preventive Medicine, Louisiana State University Health Sciences Center, 1600 Canal Street, 8th Floor, New Orleans, LA 70112, USA

Yu-Tang Gao, Department of Epidemiology, Shanghai Cancer Institute, 2200/25 Xie Tu Road, Shanghai 200032, People's Republic of China

---

[1] Unable to attend: Freddy Sitas, National Cancer Registry, Cancer Epidemiology Research Group, 4th Floor, James Murray Building, South African Institute for Medical Research, de Korte Street, Corner Hospital Street, Braamfontein, PO Box 1038, Johannesburg 2000, South Africa

Nigel Gray[1], 112 Robinson Road, Hawthorn, Victoria 3122, Australia

Prakash C. Gupta, Tata Institute of Fundamental Research, Homi Bhabha Road, Mumbai 400 005, India

Allan Hackshaw, Epidemiology & Medical Statistics, Wolfson Institute of Environmental & Preventive Medicine, Barts & The Royal London School of Medicine & Dentistry, Queen Mary College, University of London, Charterhouse Square, London EC1M 6BQ, United Kingdom

Stephen S. Hecht, University of Minnesota Cancer Center, Mayo Mail Code 806, 420 Delaware St, SE, Minneapolis, MN 55455, USA

Kirsti Husgafvel-Pursiainen, Department of Industrial Hygiene & Toxicology, Finnish Institute of Occupational Health, Topeliuksenkatu 41 aA, 02500 Helsinki, Finland

Elena Matos, Research Department, Oncology Institute, Angel H. Roffo Faculty of Medicine, University of Buenos Aires, Avenida San Martin 5481, 1417 Buenos Aires, Argentina

Richard Peto, Clinical Trial Service Unit & Epidemiological Studies Unit, Nuffield Department of Clinical Medicine, University of Oxford, Harkness Building, Radcliffe Infirmary, Oxford OX2 6HE, United Kingdom

David H. Phillips, Section of Molecular Carcinogenesis, Institute of Cancer Research, The Haddow Laboratories, 15 Cotswold Road, Sutton, Surrey SM2 5NG, United Kingdom

Jonathan M. Samet, Department of Epidemiology, Johns Hopkins University, Bloomberg School of Public Health, 615 North Wolfe Street/Suite W6041, Baltimore, MD 21205-2179, USA (*Chairman*)

Gary Stoner, Division of Environmental Health Sciences, School of Public Health, Ohio State University, 1148 CHRI, 300 W. 10th Avenue, Columbus, OH 43210-1240, USA

Michael J. Thun, Epidemiology & Surveillance Research, American Cancer Society, 1599 Clifton Road NE, Atlanta, GA 30329-4251, USA

Jean Trédaniel, Unit of Thoracic Carcinogenesis, Saint-Louis Hospital, 1 avenue Claude Vellefaux, 75475 Paris cedex 10, France

Paolo Vineis, Unit of Cancer Epidemiology, Department of Biomedical Science & Human Oncology, University of Turin, Via Santena 7, 10126 Torino, Italy

H.-Erich Wichmann, GSF – Institute of Epidemiology, Ingolstädter Landstrasse 1, 85764 Neuherberg, Germany

Anna H. Wu, Department of Preventive Medicine, Norris Comprehensive Cancer Center, University of Southern California, 1441 Eastlake Avenue, MC9175, Los Angeles, CA 90089, USA

David Zaridze, Institute of Carcinogenesis, N.N. Blokhin Russian Cancer Research Centre, Academy of Medical Sciences, 24 Kashirskoye Shosse, 115478 Moscow, Russia

---

[1] Present address: Division of Epidemiology & Biostatistics, European Institute of Oncology, Via Ripamonti 435, 20141 Milan, Italy

Representatives/Observers

Observer
Hiroshi Nakajima, BP 10, 86300 Chauvigny, France

Observer, representing the US Centers for Disease Control & Prevention
Patricia Richter, Office on Smoking and Health (K-50), Centers for Disease Control & Prevention, 4770 Buford Highway N.E., Atlanta, GA 30341, USA

Representative of WHO Tobacco Free Initiative
Michael Eriksen, Tobacco Free Initiative, Noncommunicable Diseases & Mental Health, World Health Organization, Avenue Appia 20, 1211 Geneva 27, Switzerland

IARC Secretariat
Robert Baan, Unit of Carcinogen Identification and Evaluation
Paolo Boffetta, Unit of Environmental Cancer Epidemiology
Paul Brennan, Unit of Environmental Cancer Epidemiology
Silvia Franceschi, Unit of Field and Intervention Studies
Marlin Friesen, Unit of Nutrition and Cancer
Yann Grosse, Unit of Carcinogen Identification and Evaluation
Pierre Hainaut, Unit of Molecular Carcinogenesis
Rayjean J. Hung, Unit of Environmental Cancer Epidemiology
Susan Kaplan, Berne, Switzerland (*Editor*)
Sarah Lewis, Unit of Environmental Cancer Epidemiology
Andrea 't Mannetje, Unit of Environmental Cancer Epidemiology
Nikolai Napalkov[1]
Hiroko Ohgaki, Unit of Molecular Pathology
Hiroshi Ohshima, Unit of Endogenous Cancer Risk Factors
Christiane Partensky, Unit of Carcinogen Identification and Evaluation
Jerry Rice, Unit of Carcinogen Identification and Evaluation (*Head of Programme, Co-responsible Officer*)
Annie Sasco, Unit of Epidemiology for Cancer Prevention
Jennifer Smith, Unit of Field and Intervention Studies
Leslie Stayner[2], Unit of Carcinogen Identification and Evaluation (*Visiting Scientist*)
Kurt Straif, Unit of Carcinogen Identification and Evaluation (*Co-Responsible Officer*)
Eero Suonio, Unit of Carcinogen Identification and Evaluation

---

[1] Present address: Director Emeritus, Petrov Institute of Oncology, Pesochny-2, 197758 St Petersburg, Russia
[2] Present address: NIOSH, Robert Taft Laboratories, Risk Evaluation Branch, REB C15, 4676 Columbia Parkway, Cincinnati, OH 45157

Jerzy E. Tyczynski, Unit of Descriptive Epidemiology
Harri Vainio, Unit of Chemoprevention

Post-meeting scientific assistance
Vincent James Cogliano
Catherine Cohet
Fatiha El Ghissassi
Heidi Mattock
Béatrice Secretan

Technical assistance
Sandrine Egraz
Brigitte Kajo
Martine Lézère
Jane Mitchell
Elspeth Perez
Annick Rivoire

PREAMBLE

IARC MONOGRAPHS PROGRAMME ON THE EVALUATION OF CARCINOGENIC RISKS TO HUMANS

PREAMBLE

1. BACKGROUND

In 1969, the International Agency for Research on Cancer (IARC) initiated a programme to evaluate the carcinogenic risk of chemicals to humans and to produce monographs on individual chemicals. The *Monographs* programme has since been expanded to include consideration of exposures to complex mixtures of chemicals (which occur, for example, in some occupations and as a result of human habits) and of exposures to other agents, such as radiation and viruses. With Supplement 6 (IARC, 1987a), the title of the series was modified from *IARC Monographs on the Evaluation of the Carcinogenic Risk of Chemicals to Humans* to *IARC Monographs on the Evaluation of Carcinogenic Risks to Humans*, in order to reflect the widened scope of the programme.

The criteria established in 1971 to evaluate carcinogenic risk to humans were adopted by the working groups whose deliberations resulted in the first 16 volumes of the *IARC Monographs series*. Those criteria were subsequently updated by further ad-hoc working groups (IARC, 1977, 1978, 1979, 1982, 1983, 1987b, 1988, 1991a; Vainio *et al.*, 1992).

2. OBJECTIVE AND SCOPE

The objective of the programme is to prepare, with the help of international working groups of experts, and to publish in the form of monographs, critical reviews and evaluations of evidence on the carcinogenicity of a wide range of human exposures. The *Monographs* may also indicate where additional research efforts are needed.

The *Monographs* represent the first step in carcinogenic risk assessment, which involves examination of all relevant information in order to assess the strength of the available evidence that certain exposures could alter the incidence of cancer in humans. The second step is quantitative risk estimation. Detailed, quantitative evaluations of epidemiological data may be made in the *Monographs*, but without extrapolation beyond the range of the data available. Quantitative extrapolation from experimental data to the human situation is not undertaken.

The term 'carcinogen' is used in these monographs to denote an exposure that is capable of increasing the incidence of malignant neoplasms; the induction of benign neoplasms may in some circumstances (see p. 19) contribute to the judgement that the exposure is carcinogenic. The terms 'neoplasm' and 'tumour' are used interchangeably.

Some epidemiological and experimental studies indicate that different agents may act at different stages in the carcinogenic process, and several mechanisms may be involved. The aim of the *Monographs* has been, from their inception, to evaluate evidence of carcinogenicity at any stage in the carcinogenesis process, independently of the underlying mechanisms. Information on mechanisms may, however, be used in making the overall evaluation (IARC, 1991a; Vainio *et al.*, 1992; see also pp. 25–27).

The *Monographs* may assist national and international authorities in making risk assessments and in formulating decisions concerning any necessary preventive measures. The evaluations of IARC working groups are scientific, qualitative judgements about the evidence for or against carcinogenicity provided by the available data. These evaluations represent only one part of the body of information on which regulatory measures may be based. Other components of regulatory decisions vary from one situation to another and from country to country, responding to different socioeconomic and national priorities. **Therefore, no recommendation is given with regard to regulation or legislation, which are the responsibility of individual governments and/or other international organizations.**

The *IARC Monographs* are recognized as an authoritative source of information on the carcinogenicity of a wide range of human exposures. A survey of users in 1988 indicated that the *Monographs* are consulted by various agencies in 57 countries. About 2500 copies of each volume are printed, for distribution to governments, regulatory bodies and interested scientists. The Monographs are also available from IARC*Press* in Lyon and via the Marketing and Dissemination (MDI) of the World Health Organization in Geneva.

3.   SELECTION OF TOPICS FOR MONOGRAPHS

Topics are selected on the basis of two main criteria: (a) there is evidence of human exposure, and (b) there is some evidence or suspicion of carcinogenicity. The term 'agent' is used to include individual chemical compounds, groups of related chemical compounds, physical agents (such as radiation) and biological factors (such as viruses). Exposures to mixtures of agents may occur in occupational exposures and as a result of personal and cultural habits (like smoking and dietary practices). Chemical analogues and compounds with biological or physical characteristics similar to those of suspected carcinogens may also be considered, even in the absence of data on a possible carcinogenic effect in humans or experimental animals.

The scientific literature is surveyed for published data relevant to an assessment of carcinogenicity. The IARC information bulletins on agents being tested for carcinogenicity (IARC, 1973–1996) and directories of on-going research in cancer epidemiology (IARC, 1976–1996) often indicate exposures that may be scheduled for future meetings. Ad-hoc working groups convened by IARC in 1984, 1989, 1991, 1993 and

1998 gave recommendations as to which agents should be evaluated in the IARC Mono-graphs series (IARC, 1984, 1989, 1991b, 1993, 1998a,b).

As significant new data on subjects on which monographs have already been prepared become available, re-evaluations are made at subsequent meetings, and revised mono-graphs are published.

4.   DATA FOR MONOGRAPHS

The *Monographs* do not necessarily cite all the literature concerning the subject of an evaluation. Only those data considered by the Working Group to be relevant to making the evaluation are included.

With regard to biological and epidemiological data, only reports that have been published or accepted for publication in the openly available scientific literature are reviewed by the working groups. In certain instances, government agency reports that have undergone peer review and are widely available are considered. Exceptions may be made on an ad-hoc basis to include unpublished reports that are in their final form and publicly available, if their inclusion is considered pertinent to making a final evaluation (see pp. 25–27). In the sections on chemical and physical properties, on analysis, on production and use and on occurrence, unpublished sources of information may be used.

5.   THE WORKING GROUP

Reviews and evaluations are formulated by a working group of experts. The tasks of the group are: (i) to ascertain that all appropriate data have been collected; (ii) to select the data relevant for the evaluation on the basis of scientific merit; (iii) to prepare accurate summaries of the data to enable the reader to follow the reasoning of the Working Group; (iv) to evaluate the results of epidemiological and experimental studies on cancer; (v) to evaluate data relevant to the understanding of mechanism of action; and (vi) to make an overall evaluation of the carcinogenicity of the exposure to humans.

Working Group participants who contributed to the considerations and evaluations within a particular volume are listed, with their addresses, at the beginning of each publi-cation. Each participant who is a member of a working group serves as an individual scientist and not as a representative of any organization, government or industry. In addition, nominees of national and international agencies and industrial associations may be invited as observers.

6.   WORKING PROCEDURES

Approximately one year in advance of a meeting of a working group, the topics of the monographs are announced and participants are selected by IARC staff in consul-tation with other experts. Subsequently, relevant biological and epidemiological data are collected by the Carcinogen Identification and Evaluation Unit of IARC from recognized sources of information on carcinogenesis, including data storage and retrieval systems such as MEDLINE and TOXLINE.

For chemicals and some complex mixtures, the major collection of data and the preparation of first drafts of the sections on chemical and physical properties, on analysis, on production and use and on occurrence are carried out under a separate contract funded by the United States National Cancer Institute. Representatives from industrial associations may assist in the preparation of sections on production and use. Information on production and trade is obtained from governmental and trade publications and, in some cases, by direct contact with industries. Separate production data on some agents may not be available because their publication could disclose confidential information. Information on uses may be obtained from published sources but is often complemented by direct contact with manufacturers. Efforts are made to supplement this information with data from other national and international sources.

Six months before the meeting, the material obtained is sent to meeting participants, or is used by IARC staff, to prepare sections for the first drafts of monographs. The first drafts are compiled by IARC staff and sent before the meeting to all participants of the Working Group for review.

The Working Group meets in Lyon for seven to eight days to discuss and finalize the texts of the monographs and to formulate the evaluations. After the meeting, the master copy of each monograph is verified by consulting the original literature, edited and prepared for publication. The aim is to publish monographs within six months of the Working Group meeting.

The available studies are summarized by the Working Group, with particular regard to the qualitative aspects discussed below. In general, numerical findings are indicated as they appear in the original report; units are converted when necessary for easier comparison. The Working Group may conduct additional analyses of the published data and use them in their assessment of the evidence; the results of such supplementary analyses are given in square brackets. When an important aspect of a study, directly impinging on its interpretation, should be brought to the attention of the reader, a comment is given in square brackets.

7.   EXPOSURE DATA

Sections that indicate the extent of past and present human exposure, the sources of exposure, the people most likely to be exposed and the factors that contribute to the exposure are included at the beginning of each monograph.

Most monographs on individual chemicals, groups of chemicals or complex mixtures include sections on chemical and physical data, on analysis, on production and use and on occurrence. In monographs on, for example, physical agents, occupational exposures and cultural habits, other sections may be included, such as: historical perspectives, description of an industry or habit, chemistry of the complex mixture or taxonomy. Monographs on biological agents have sections on structure and biology, methods of detection, epidemiology of infection and clinical disease other than cancer.

For chemical exposures, the Chemical Abstracts Services Registry Number, the latest Chemical Abstracts primary name and the IUPAC systematic name are recorded; other synonyms are given, but the list is not necessarily comprehensive. For biological agents, taxonomy and structure are described, and the degree of variability is given, when applicable.

Information on chemical and physical properties and, in particular, data relevant to identification, occurrence and biological activity are included. For biological agents, mode of replication, life cycle, target cells, persistence and latency and host response are given. A description of technical products of chemicals includes trade names, relevant specifications and available information on composition and impurities. Some of the trade names given may be those of mixtures in which the agent being evaluated is only one of the ingredients.

The purpose of the section on analysis or detection is to give the reader an overview of current methods, with emphasis on those widely used for regulatory purposes. Methods for monitoring human exposure are also given, when available. No critical evaluation or recommendation of any of the methods is meant or implied. The IARC published a series of volumes, *Environmental Carcinogens: Methods of Analysis and Exposure Measurement* (IARC, 1978–93), that describe validated methods for analysing a wide variety of chemicals and mixtures. For biological agents, methods of detection and exposure assessment are described, including their sensitivity, specificity and reproducibility.

The dates of first synthesis and of first commercial production of a chemical or mixture are provided; for agents which do not occur naturally, this information may allow a reasonable estimate to be made of the date before which no human exposure to the agent could have occurred. The dates of first reported occurrence of an exposure are also provided. In addition, methods of synthesis used in past and present commercial production and different methods of production which may give rise to different impurities are described.

Data on production, international trade and uses are obtained for representative regions, which usually include Europe, Japan and the United States of America. It should not, however, be inferred that those areas or nations are necessarily the sole or major sources or users of the agent. Some identified uses may not be current or major applications, and the coverage is not necessarily comprehensive. In the case of drugs, mention of their therapeutic uses does not necessarily represent current practice, nor does it imply judgement as to their therapeutic efficacy.

Information on the occurrence of an agent or mixture in the environment is obtained from data derived from the monitoring and surveillance of levels in occupational environments, air, water, soil, foods and animal and human tissues. When available, data on the generation, persistence and bioaccumulation of the agent are also included. In the case of mixtures, industries, occupations or processes, information is given about all agents present. For processes, industries and occupations, a historical description is also given, noting variations in chemical composition, physical properties and levels of occupational exposure with time and place. For biological agents, the epidemiology of infection is described.

Statements concerning regulations and guidelines (e.g., pesticide registrations, maximal levels permitted in foods, occupational exposure limits) are included for some countries as indications of potential exposures, but they may not reflect the most recent situation, since such limits are continuously reviewed and modified. The absence of information on regulatory status for a country should not be taken to imply that that country does not have regulations with regard to the exposure. For biological agents, legislation and control, including vaccines and therapy, are described.

8.   STUDIES OF CANCER IN HUMANS

(a)   Types of studies considered

Three types of epidemiological studies of cancer contribute to the assessment of carcinogenicity in humans — cohort studies, case–control studies and correlation (or ecological) studies. Rarely, results from randomized trials may be available. Case series and case reports of cancer in humans may also be reviewed.

Cohort and case–control studies relate the exposures under study to the occurrence of cancer in individuals and provide an estimate of relative risk (ratio of incidence or mortality in those exposed to incidence or mortality in those not exposed) as the main measure of association.

In correlation studies, the units of investigation are usually whole populations (e.g. in particular geographical areas or at particular times), and cancer frequency is related to a summary measure of the exposure of the population to the agent, mixture or exposure circumstance under study. Because individual exposure is not documented, however, a causal relationship is less easy to infer from correlation studies than from cohort and case–control studies. Case reports generally arise from a suspicion, based on clinical experience, that the concurrence of two events — that is, a particular exposure and occurrence of a cancer — has happened rather more frequently than would be expected by chance. Case reports usually lack complete ascertainment of cases in any population, definition or enumeration of the population at risk and estimation of the expected number of cases in the absence of exposure. The uncertainties surrounding interpretation of case reports and correlation studies make them inadequate, except in rare instances, to form the sole basis for inferring a causal relationship. When taken together with case–control and cohort studies, however, relevant case reports or correlation studies may add materially to the judgement that a causal relationship is present.

Epidemiological studies of benign neoplasms, presumed preneoplastic lesions and other end-points thought to be relevant to cancer are also reviewed by working groups. They may, in some instances, strengthen inferences drawn from studies of cancer itself.

(b)   *Quality of studies considered*

The Monographs are not intended to summarize all published studies. Those that are judged to be inadequate or irrelevant to the evaluation are generally omitted. They may be mentioned briefly, particularly when the information is considered to be a useful supplement to that in other reports or when they provide the only data available. Their inclusion does not imply acceptance of the adequacy of the study design or of the analysis and interpretation of the results, and limitations are clearly outlined in square brackets at the end of the study description.

It is necessary to take into account the possible roles of bias, confounding and chance in the interpretation of epidemiological studies. By 'bias' is meant the operation of factors in study design or execution that lead erroneously to a stronger or weaker association than in fact exists between disease and an agent, mixture or exposure circumstance. By 'confounding' is meant a situation in which the relationship with disease is made to appear stronger or weaker than it truly is as a result of an association between the apparent causal factor and another factor that is associated with either an increase or decrease in the incidence of the disease. In evaluating the extent to which these factors have been minimized in an individual study, working groups consider a number of aspects of design and analysis as described in the report of the study. Most of these considerations apply equally to case–control, cohort and correlation studies. Lack of clarity of any of these aspects in the reporting of a study can decrease its credibility and the weight given to it in the final evaluation of the exposure.

Firstly, the study population, disease (or diseases) and exposure should have been well defined by the authors. Cases of disease in the study population should have been identified in a way that was independent of the exposure of interest, and exposure should have been assessed in a way that was not related to disease status.

Secondly, the authors should have taken account in the study design and analysis of other variables that can influence the risk of disease and may have been related to the exposure of interest. Potential confounding by such variables should have been dealt with either in the design of the study, such as by matching, or in the analysis, by statistical adjustment. In cohort studies, comparisons with local rates of disease may be more appropriate than those with national rates. Internal comparisons of disease frequency among individuals at different levels of exposure should also have been made in the study.

Thirdly, the authors should have reported the basic data on which the conclusions are founded, even if sophisticated statistical analyses were employed. At the very least, they should have given the numbers of exposed and unexposed cases and controls in a case–control study and the numbers of cases observed and expected in a cohort study. Further tabulations by time since exposure began and other temporal factors are also important. In a cohort study, data on all cancer sites and all causes of death should have been given, to reveal the possibility of reporting bias. In a case–control study, the effects of investigated factors other than the exposure of interest should have been reported.

Finally, the statistical methods used to obtain estimates of relative risk, absolute rates of cancer, confidence intervals and significance tests, and to adjust for confounding should have been clearly stated by the authors. The methods used should preferably have been the generally accepted techniques that have been refined since the mid-1970s. These methods have been reviewed for case–control studies (Breslow & Day, 1980) and for cohort studies (Breslow & Day, 1987).

(c)   Inferences about mechanism of action

Detailed analyses of both relative and absolute risks in relation to temporal variables, such as age at first exposure, time since first exposure, duration of exposure, cumulative exposure and time since exposure ceased, are reviewed and summarized when available. The analysis of temporal relationships can be useful in formulating models of carcino-genesis. In particular, such analyses may suggest whether a carcinogen acts early or late in the process of carcinogenesis, although at best they allow only indirect inferences about the mechanism of action. Special attention is given to measurements of biological markers of carcinogen exposure or action, such as DNA or protein adducts, as well as markers of early steps in the carcinogenic process, such as proto-oncogene mutation, when these are incorporated into epidemiological studies focused on cancer incidence or mortality. Such measurements may allow inferences to be made about putative mecha-nisms of action (IARC, 1991a; Vainio et al., 1992).

(d)   Criteria for causality

After the individual epidemiological studies of cancer have been summarized and the quality assessed, a judgement is made concerning the strength of evidence that the agent, mixture or exposure circumstance in question is carcinogenic for humans. In making its judgement, the Working Group considers several criteria for causality. A strong asso-ciation (a large relative risk) is more likely to indicate causality than a weak association, although it is recognized that relative risks of small magnitude do not imply lack of causality and may be important if the disease is common. Associations that are replicated in several studies of the same design or using different epidemiological approaches or under different circumstances of exposure are more likely to represent a causal relation-ship than isolated observations from single studies. If there are inconsistent results among investigations, possible reasons are sought (such as differences in amount of exposure), and results of studies judged to be of high quality are given more weight than those of studies judged to be methodologically less sound. When suspicion of carcino-genicity arises largely from a single study, these data are not combined with those from later studies in any subsequent reassessment of the strength of the evidence.

If the risk of the disease in question increases with the amount of exposure, this is considered to be a strong indication of causality, although absence of a graded response is not necessarily evidence against a causal relationship. Demonstration of a decline in risk after cessation of or reduction in exposure in individuals or in whole populations also supports a causal interpretation of the findings.

Although a carcinogen may act upon more than one target, the specificity of an association (an increased occurrence of cancer at one anatomical site or of one morphological type) adds plausibility to a causal relationship, particularly when excess cancer occurrence is limited to one morphological type within the same organ.

Although rarely available, results from randomized trials showing different rates among exposed and unexposed individuals provide particularly strong evidence for causality.

When several epidemiological studies show little or no indication of an association between an exposure and cancer, the judgement may be made that, in the aggregate, they show evidence of lack of carcinogenicity. Such a judgement requires first of all that the studies giving rise to it meet, to a sufficient degree, the standards of design and analysis described above. Specifically, the possibility that bias, confounding or misclassification of exposure or outcome could explain the observed results should be considered and excluded with reasonable certainty. In addition, all studies that are judged to be methodologically sound should be consistent with a relative risk of unity for any observed level of exposure and, when considered together, should provide a pooled estimate of relative risk which is at or near unity and has a narrow confidence interval, due to sufficient population size. Moreover, no individual study nor the pooled results of all the studies should show any consistent tendency for the relative risk of cancer to increase with increasing level of exposure. It is important to note that evidence of lack of carcinogenicity obtained in this way from several epidemiological studies can apply only to the type(s) of cancer studied and to dose levels and intervals between first exposure and observation of disease that are the same as or less than those observed in all the studies. Experience with human cancer indicates that, in some cases, the period from first exposure to the development of clinical cancer is seldom less than 20 years; studies with latent periods substantially shorter than 30 years cannot provide evidence for lack of carcinogenicity.

9.   STUDIES OF CANCER IN EXPERIMENTAL ANIMALS

All known human carcinogens that have been studied adequately in experimental animals have produced positive results in one or more animal species (Wilbourn *et al.*, 1986; Tomatis *et al.*, 1989). For several agents (aflatoxins, 4-aminobiphenyl, azathioprine, betel quid with tobacco, bischloromethyl ether and chloromethyl methyl ether (technical grade), chlorambucil, chlornaphazine, ciclosporin, coal-tar pitches, coal-tars, combined oral contraceptives, cyclophosphamide, diethylstilboestrol, melphalan, 8-methoxypsoralen plus ultraviolet A radiation, mustard gas, myleran, 2-naphthylamine, nonsteroidal estrogens, estrogen replacement therapy/steroidal estrogens, solar radiation, thiotepa and vinyl chloride), carcinogenicity in experimental animals was established or highly suspected before epidemiological studies confirmed their carcinogenicity in humans (Vainio *et al.*, 1995). Although this association cannot establish that all agents and mixtures that cause cancer in experimental animals also cause cancer in humans, nevertheless, **in the absence of adequate data on humans, it is biologically plausible and prudent to regard agents and mixtures for which there is *sufficient evidence* (see p. 24) of carcinogenicity in experimental animals as if they presented a carcinogenic risk to humans**. The possibility that a given agent may cause cancer through a species-specific mechanism which does not operate in humans (see p. 27) should also be taken into consideration.

The nature and extent of impurities or contaminants present in the chemical or mixture being evaluated are given when available. Animal strain, sex, numbers per group, age at start of treatment and survival are reported.

Other types of studies summarized include: experiments in which the agent or mixture was administered in conjunction with known carcinogens or factors that modify carcinogenic effects; studies in which the end-point was not cancer but a defined precancerous lesion; and experiments on the carcinogenicity of known metabolites and derivatives.

For experimental studies of mixtures, consideration is given to the possibility of changes in the physicochemical properties of the test substance during collection, storage, extraction, concentration and delivery. Chemical and toxicological interactions of the components of mixtures may result in nonlinear dose–response relationships.

An assessment is made as to the relevance to human exposure of samples tested in experimental animals, which may involve consideration of: (i) physical and chemical characteristics, (ii) constituent substances that indicate the presence of a class of substances, (iii) the results of tests for genetic and related effects, including studies on DNA adduct formation, proto-oncogene mutation and expression and suppressor gene inactivation. The relevance of results obtained, for example, with animal viruses analogous to the virus being evaluated in the monograph must also be considered. They may provide biological and mechanistic information relevant to the understanding of the process of carcinogenesis in humans and may strengthen the plausibility of a conclusion that the biological agent under evaluation is carcinogenic in humans.

(a)   Qualitative aspects

An assessment of carcinogenicity involves several considerations of qualitative importance, including (i) the experimental conditions under which the test was per-formed, including route and schedule of exposure, species, strain, sex, age, duration of follow-up; (ii) the consistency of the results, for example, across species and target organ(s); (iii) the spectrum of neoplastic response, from preneoplastic lesions and benign tumours to malignant neoplasms; and (iv) the possible role of modifying factors.

As mentioned earlier (p. 11), the *Monographs* are not intended to summarize all published studies. Those studies in experimental animals that are inadequate (e.g., too short a duration, too few animals, poor survival; see below) or are judged irrelevant to the evaluation are generally omitted. Guidelines for conducting adequate long-term carcinogenicity experiments have been outlined (e.g. Montesano *et al.*, 1986).

Considerations of importance to the Working Group in the interpretation and eva-luation of a particular study include: (i) how clearly the agent was defined and, in the case of mixtures, how adequately the sample characterization was reported; (ii) whether the dose was adequately monitored, particularly in inhalation experiments; (iii) whether the doses and duration of treatment were appropriate and whether the survival of treated animals was similar to that of controls; (iv) whether there were adequate numbers of animals per group; (v) whether animals of each sex were used; (vi) whether animals were allocated randomly to groups; (vii) whether the duration of observation was adequate; and (viii) whether the data were adequately reported. If available, recent data on the incidence of specific tumours in historical controls, as well as in concurrent controls, should be taken into account in the evaluation of tumour response.

When benign tumours occur together with and originate from the same cell type in an organ or tissue as malignant tumours in a particular study and appear to represent a stage in the progression to malignancy, it may be valid to combine them in assessing tumour incidence (Huff *et al.*, 1989). The occurrence of lesions presumed to be pre-neoplastic may in certain instances aid in assessing the biological plausibility of any neo-plastic response observed. If an agent or mixture induces only benign neoplasms that appear to be end-points that do not readily progress to malignancy, it should nevertheless be suspected of being a carcinogen and requires further investigation.

(b)   Quantitative aspects

The probability that tumours will occur may depend on the species, sex, strain and age of the animal, the dose of the carcinogen and the route and length of exposure. Evidence of an increased incidence of neoplasms with increased level of exposure strengthens the inference of a causal association between the exposure and the develop-ment of neoplasms.

The form of the dose–response relationship can vary widely, depending on the particular agent under study and the target organ. Both DNA damage and increased cell division are important aspects of carcinogenesis, and cell proliferation is a strong deter-minant of dose–response relationships for some carcinogens (Cohen & Ellwein, 1990). Since many chemicals require metabolic activation before being converted into their reactive intermediates, both metabolic and pharmacokinetic aspects are important in determining the dose–response pattern. Saturation of steps such as absorption, activation, inactivation and elimination may produce nonlinearity in the dose–response relationship, as could saturation of processes such as DNA repair (Hoel *et al.*, 1983; Gart *et al.*, 1986).

(c)   *Statistical analysis of long-term experiments in animals*

Factors considered by the Working Group include the adequacy of the information given for each treatment group: (i) the number of animals studied and the number examined histologically, (ii) the number of animals with a given tumour type and (iii) length of survival. The statistical methods used should be clearly stated and should be the generally accepted techniques refined for this purpose (Peto *et al.*, 1980; Gart *et al.*, 1986). When there is no difference in survival between control and treatment groups, the Working Group usually compares the proportions of animals developing each tumour type in each of the groups. Otherwise, consideration is given as to whether or not appropriate adjustments have been made for differences in survival. These adjustments can include: comparisons of the proportions of tumour-bearing animals among the effective number of animals (alive at the time the first tumour is discovered), in the case where most differences in survival occur before tumours appear; life-table methods, when tumours are visible or when they may be considered 'fatal' because mortality rapidly follows tumour development; and the Mantel-Haenszel test or logistic regression, when occult tumours do not affect the animals' risk of dying but are 'incidental' findings at autopsy.

In practice, classifying tumours as fatal or incidental may be difficult. Several survival-adjusted methods have been developed that do not require this distinction (Gart *et al.*, 1986), although they have not been fully evaluated.

10.   OTHER DATA RELEVANT TO AN EVALUATION OF CARCINOGENICITY AND ITS MECHANISMS

In coming to an overall evaluation of carcinogenicity in humans (see pp. 25–27), the Working Group also considers related data. The nature of the information selected for the summary depends on the agent being considered.

For chemicals and complex mixtures of chemicals such as those in some occupational situations or involving cultural habits (e.g. tobacco smoking), the other data considered to be relevant are divided into those on absorption, distribution, metabolism and excretion; toxic effects; reproductive and developmental effects; and genetic and related effects.

Concise information is given on absorption, distribution (including placental transfer) and excretion in both humans and experimental animals. Kinetic factors that may affect the dose–response relationship, such as saturation of uptake, protein binding, metabolic activation, detoxification and DNA repair processes, are mentioned. Studies that indicate the metabolic fate of the agent in humans and in experimental animals are summarized briefly, and comparisons of data on humans and on animals are made when possible. Comparative information on the relationship between exposure and the dose that reaches the target site may be of particular importance for extrapolation between species. Data are given on acute and chronic toxic effects (other than cancer), such as organ toxicity, increased cell proliferation, immunotoxicity and endocrine effects. The presence and toxicological significance of cellular receptors is described. Effects on reproduction, teratogenicity, fetotoxicity and embryotoxicity are also summarized briefly.

Tests of genetic and related effects are described in view of the relevance of gene mutation and chromosomal damage to carcinogenesis (Vainio *et al.*, 1992; McGregor *et al.*, 1999). The adequacy of the reporting of sample characterization is considered and, where necessary, commented upon; with regard to complex mixtures, such comments are similar to those described for animal carcinogenicity tests on p. 18. The available data are interpreted critically by phylogenetic group according to the end-points detected, which may include DNA damage, gene mutation, sister chromatid exchange, micro-nucleus formation, chromosomal aberrations, aneuploidy and cell transformation. The concentrations employed are given, and mention is made of whether use of an exogenous metabolic system *in vitro* affected the test result. These data are given as listings of test systems, data and references. The data on genetic and related effects presented in the *Monographs* are also available in the form of genetic activity profiles (GAP) prepared in collaboration with the United States Environmental Protection Agency (EPA) (see also Waters *et al.*, 1987) using software for personal computers that are Microsoft Windows® compatible. The EPA/IARC GAP software and database may be downloaded free of charge from *www.epa.gov/gapdb*.

Positive results in tests using prokaryotes, lower eukaryotes, plants, insects and cultured mammalian cells suggest that genetic and related effects could occur in mammals. Results from such tests may also give information about the types of genetic effect produced and about the involvement of metabolic activation. Some end-points described are clearly genetic in nature (e.g., gene mutations and chromosomal aberra-tions), while others are to a greater or lesser degree associated with genetic effects (e.g. unscheduled DNA synthesis). In-vitro tests for tumour-promoting activity and for cell transformation may be sensitive to changes that are not necessarily the result of genetic alterations but that may have specific relevance to the process of carcinogenesis. A critical appraisal of these tests has been published (Montesano *et al.*, 1986).

Genetic or other activity detected in experimental mammals and humans is regarded as being of greater relevance than that in other organisms. The demonstration that an agent or mixture can induce gene and chromosomal mutations in whole mammals indi-cates that it may have carcinogenic activity, although this activity may not be detectably expressed in any or all species. Relative potency in tests for mutagenicity and related effects is not a reliable indicator of carcinogenic potency. Negative results in tests for mutagenicity in selected tissues from animals treated *in vivo* provide less weight, partly because they do not exclude the possibility of an effect in tissues other than those examined. Moreover, negative results in short-term tests with genetic end-points cannot be considered to provide evidence to rule out carcinogenicity of agents or mixtures that act through other mechanisms (e.g. receptor-mediated effects, cellular toxicity with regenerative proliferation, peroxisome proliferation) (Vainio *et al.*, 1992). Factors that may lead to misleading results in short-term tests have been discussed in detail elsewhere (Montesano *et al.*, 1986).

When available, data relevant to mechanisms of carcinogenesis that do not involve structural changes at the level of the gene are also described.

The adequacy of epidemiological studies of reproductive outcome and genetic and related effects in humans is evaluated by the same criteria as are applied to epidemiological studies of cancer.

Structure–activity relationships that may be relevant to an evaluation of the carcinogenicity of an agent are also described.

For biological agents — viruses, bacteria and parasites — other data relevant to carcinogenicity include descriptions of the pathology of infection, molecular biology (integration and expression of viruses, and any genetic alterations seen in human tumours) and other observations, which might include cellular and tissue responses to infection, immune response and the presence of tumour markers.

11.   SUMMARY OF DATA REPORTED

In this section, the relevant epidemiological and experimental data are summarized. Only reports, other than in abstract form, that meet the criteria outlined on p. 11 are considered for evaluating carcinogenicity. Inadequate studies are generally not summarized: such studies are usually identified by a square-bracketed comment in the preceding text.

(*a*)   *Exposure*

Human exposure to chemicals and complex mixtures is summarized on the basis of elements such as production, use, occurrence in the environment and determinations in human tissues and body fluids. Quantitative data are given when available. Exposure to biological agents is described in terms of transmission and prevalence of infection.

(*b*)   *Carcinogenicity in humans*

Results of epidemiological studies that are considered to be pertinent to an assessment of human carcinogenicity are summarized. When relevant, case reports and correlation studies are also summarized.

(*c*)   *Carcinogenicity in experimental animals*

Data relevant to an evaluation of carcinogenicity in animals are summarized. For each animal species and route of administration, it is stated whether an increased incidence of neoplasms or preneoplastic lesions was observed, and the tumour sites are indicated. If the agent or mixture produced tumours after prenatal exposure or in single-dose experiments, this is also indicated. Negative findings are also summarized. Dose–response and other quantitative data may be given when available.

(*d*)   *Other data relevant to an evaluation of carcinogenicity and its mechanisms*

Data on biological effects in humans that are of particular relevance are summarized. These may include toxicological, kinetic and metabolic considerations and evidence of DNA binding, persistence of DNA lesions or genetic damage in exposed humans. Toxicological information, such as that on cytotoxicity and regeneration, receptor binding and hormonal and immunological effects, and data on kinetics and metabolism in experimental animals are given when considered relevant to the possible mechanism of the carcinogenic action of the agent. The results of tests for genetic and related effects are summarized for whole mammals, cultured mammalian cells and nonmammalian systems.

When available, comparisons of such data for humans and for animals, and particularly animals that have developed cancer, are described.

Structure–activity relationships are mentioned when relevant.

For the agent, mixture or exposure circumstance being evaluated, the available data on end-points or other phenomena relevant to mechanisms of carcinogenesis from studies in humans, experimental animals and tissue and cell test systems are summarized within one or more of the following descriptive dimensions:

(i) Evidence of genotoxicity (structural changes at the level of the gene): for example, structure–activity considerations, adduct formation, mutagenicity (effect on specific genes), chromosomal mutation/aneuploidy

(ii) Evidence of effects on the expression of relevant genes (functional changes at the intracellular level): for example, alterations to the structure or quantity of the product of a proto-oncogene or tumour-suppressor gene, alterations to metabolic activation/inactivation/DNA repair

(iii) Evidence of relevant effects on cell behaviour (morphological or behavioural changes at the cellular or tissue level): for example, induction of mitogenesis, compensatory cell proliferation, preneoplasia and hyperplasia, survival of premalignant or malignant cells (immortalization, immunosuppression), effects on metastatic potential

(iv) Evidence from dose and time relationships of carcinogenic effects and interactions between agents: for example, early/late stage, as inferred from epidemiological studies; initiation/promotion/progression/malignant conversion, as defined in animal carcinogenicity experiments; toxicokinetics

These dimensions are not mutually exclusive, and an agent may fall within more than one of them. Thus, for example, the action of an agent on the expression of relevant genes could be summarized under both the first and second dimensions, even if it were known with reasonable certainty that those effects resulted from genotoxicity.

12.   EVALUATION

Evaluations of the strength of the evidence for carcinogenicity arising from human and experimental animal data are made, using standard terms.

It is recognized that the criteria for these evaluations, described below, cannot encompass all of the factors that may be relevant to an evaluation of carcinogenicity. In considering all of the relevant scientific data, the Working Group may assign the agent, mixture or exposure circumstance to a higher or lower category than a strict inter-pretation of these criteria would indicate.

(a) Degrees of evidence for carcinogenicity in humans and in experimental animals and supporting evidence

These categories refer only to the strength of the evidence that an exposure is carcino-genic and not to the extent of its carcinogenic activity (potency) nor to the mechanisms involved. A classification may change as new information becomes available.

An evaluation of degree of evidence, whether for a single agent or a mixture, is limited to the materials tested, as defined physically, chemically or biologically. When the agents evaluated are considered by the Working Group to be sufficiently closely related, they may be grouped together for the purpose of a single evaluation of degree of evidence.

(i) Carcinogenicity in humans

The applicability of an evaluation of the carcinogenicity of a mixture, process, occu-pation or industry on the basis of evidence from epidemiological studies depends on the variability over time and place of the mixtures, processes, occupations and industries. The Working Group seeks to identify the specific exposure, process or activity which is considered most likely to be responsible for any excess risk. The evaluation is focused as narrowly as the available data on exposure and other aspects permit.

The evidence relevant to carcinogenicity from studies in humans is classified into one of the following categories:

Sufficient evidence of carcinogenicity: The Working Group considers that a causal relationship has been established between exposure to the agent, mixture or exposure circumstance and human cancer. That is, a positive relationship has been observed between the exposure and cancer in studies in which chance, bias and confounding could be ruled out with reasonable confidence.

Limited evidence of carcinogenicity: A positive association has been observed between exposure to the agent, mixture or exposure circumstance and cancer for which a causal interpretation is considered by the Working Group to be credible, but chance, bias or confounding could not be ruled out with reasonable confidence.

Inadequate evidence of carcinogenicity: The available studies are of insufficient quality, consistency or statistical power to permit a conclusion regarding the presence or absence of a causal association between exposure and cancer, or no data on cancer in humans are available.

Evidence suggesting lack of carcinogenicity: There are several adequate studies covering the full range of levels of exposure that human beings are known to encounter, which are mutually consistent in not showing a positive association between exposure to the agent, mixture or exposure circumstance and any studied cancer at any observed level of exposure. A conclusion of 'evidence suggesting lack of carcinogenicity' is inevitably limited to the cancer sites, conditions and levels of exposure and length of observation covered by the available studies. In addition, the possibility of a very small risk at the levels of exposure studied can never be excluded.

In some instances, the above categories may be used to classify the degree of evidence related to carcinogenicity in specific organs or tissues.

(ii) *Carcinogenicity in experimental animals*

The evidence relevant to carcinogenicity in experimental animals is classified into one of the following categories:

Sufficient evidence of carcinogenicity: The Working Group considers that a causal relationship has been established between the agent or mixture and an increased incidence of malignant neoplasms or of an appropriate combination of benign and malignant neoplasms in (a) two or more species of animals or (b) in two or more independent studies in one species carried out at different times or in different laboratories or under different protocols.

Exceptionally, a single study in one species might be considered to provide sufficient evidence of carcinogenicity when malignant neoplasms occur to an unusual degree with regard to incidence, site, type of tumour or age at onset.

Limited evidence of carcinogenicity: The data suggest a carcinogenic effect but are limited for making a definitive evaluation because, e.g. (a) the evidence of carcinogenicity is restricted to a single experiment; or (b) there are unresolved questions regarding the adequacy of the design, conduct or interpretation of the study; or (c) the agent or mixture increases the incidence only of benign neoplasms or lesions of uncertain neoplastic potential, or of certain neoplasms which may occur spontaneously in high incidences in certain strains.

Inadequate evidence of carcinogenicity: The studies cannot be interpreted as showing either the presence or absence of a carcinogenic effect because of major qualitative or quantitative limitations, or no data on cancer in experimental animals are available.

Evidence suggesting lack of carcinogenicity: Adequate studies involving at least two species are available which show that, within the limits of the tests used, the agent or mixture is not carcinogenic. A conclusion of evidence suggesting lack of carcinogenicity is inevitably limited to the species, tumour sites and levels of exposure studied.

(b) *Other data relevant to the evaluation of carcinogenicity and its mechanisms*

Other evidence judged to be relevant to an evaluation of carcinogenicity and of sufficient importance to affect the overall evaluation is then described. This may include data on preneoplastic lesions, tumour pathology, genetic and related effects, structure–activity relationships, metabolism and pharmacokinetics, physicochemical parameters and analogous biological agents.

Data relevant to mechanisms of the carcinogenic action are also evaluated. The strength of the evidence that any carcinogenic effect observed is due to a particular mechanism is assessed, using terms such as weak, moderate or strong. Then, the Working Group assesses if that particular mechanism is likely to be operative in humans. The strongest indications that a particular mechanism operates in humans come from data on humans or biological specimens obtained from exposed humans. The data may be considered to be especially relevant if they show that the agent in question has caused changes in exposed humans that are on the causal pathway to carcinogenesis. Such data may, however, never become available, because it is at least conceivable that certain compounds may be kept from human use solely on the basis of evidence of their toxicity and/or carcinogenicity in experimental systems.

For complex exposures, including occupational and industrial exposures, the chemical composition and the potential contribution of carcinogens known to be present are considered by the Working Group in its overall evaluation of human carcinogenicity. The Working Group also determines the extent to which the materials tested in experimental systems are related to those to which humans are exposed.

(c)   Overall evaluation

Finally, the body of evidence is considered as a whole, in order to reach an overall evaluation of the carcinogenicity to humans of an agent, mixture or circumstance of exposure.

An evaluation may be made for a group of chemical compounds that have been evaluated by the Working Group. In addition, when supporting data indicate that other, related compounds for which there is no direct evidence of capacity to induce cancer in humans or in animals may also be carcinogenic, a statement describing the rationale for this conclusion is added to the evaluation narrative; an additional evaluation may be made for this broader group of compounds if the strength of the evidence warrants it.

The agent, mixture or exposure circumstance is described according to the wording of one of the following categories, and the designated group is given. The categorization of an agent, mixture or exposure circumstance is a matter of scientific judgement, reflecting the strength of the evidence derived from studies in humans and in experimental animals and from other relevant data.

Group 1 — The agent (mixture) is carcinogenic to humans.
The exposure circumstance entails exposures that are carcinogenic to humans.

This category is used when there is *sufficient evidence* of carcinogenicity in humans. Exceptionally, an agent (mixture) may be placed in this category when evidence of carcinogenicity in humans is less than sufficient but there is *sufficient evidence* of carcinogenicity in experimental animals and strong evidence in exposed humans that the agent (mixture) acts through a relevant mechanism of carcinogenicity.

Group 2

This category includes agents, mixtures and exposure circumstances for which, at one extreme, the degree of evidence of carcinogenicity in humans is almost sufficient, as well as those for which, at the other extreme, there are no human data but for which there is evidence of carcinogenicity in experimental animals. Agents, mixtures and exposure circumstances are assigned to either group 2A (probably carcinogenic to humans) or group 2B (possibly carcinogenic to humans) on the basis of epidemiological and experimental evidence of carcinogenicity and other relevant data.

Group 2A — The agent (mixture) is probably carcinogenic to humans.
The exposure circumstance entails exposures that are probably carcinogenic to humans.

This category is used when there is *limited evidence* of carcinogenicity in humans and *sufficient evidence* of carcinogenicity in experimental animals. In some cases, an agent (mixture) may be classified in this category when there is *inadequate evidence* of carcinogenicity in humans, *sufficient evidence* of carcinogenicity in experimental animals and strong evidence that the carcinogenesis is mediated by a mechanism that also operates in humans. Exceptionally, an agent, mixture or exposure circumstance may be classified in this category solely on the basis of *limited evidence* of carcinogenicity in humans.

Group 2B — The agent (mixture) is possibly carcinogenic to humans.
The exposure circumstance entails exposures that are possibly carcinogenic to humans.

This category is used for agents, mixtures and exposure circumstances for which there is *limited evidence* of carcinogenicity in humans and less than *sufficient evidence* of carcinogenicity in experimental animals. It may also be used when there is *inadequate evidence* of carcinogenicity in humans but there is *sufficient evidence* of carcinogenicity in experimental animals. In some instances, an agent, mixture or exposure circumstance for which there is *inadequate evidence* of carcinogenicity in humans but *limited evidence* of carcinogenicity in experimental animals together with supporting evidence from other relevant data may be placed in this group.

Group 3 — The agent (mixture or exposure circumstance) is not classifiable as to its carcinogenicity to humans.

This category is used most commonly for agents, mixtures and exposure circumstances for which the *evidence of carcinogenicity* is *inadequate* in humans and *inadequate* or *limited* in experimental animals.

Exceptionally, agents (mixtures) for which the *evidence of carcinogenicity* is *inadequate* in humans but *sufficient* in experimental animals may be placed in this category when there is strong evidence that the mechanism of carcinogenicity in experimental animals does not operate in humans.

Agents, mixtures and exposure circumstances that do not fall into any other group are also placed in this category.

Group 4 — The agent (mixture) is probably not carcinogenic to humans.

This category is used for agents or mixtures for which there is *evidence suggesting lack of carcinogenicity* in humans and in experimental animals. In some instances, agents or mixtures for which there is *inadequate evidence* of carcinogenicity in humans but *evidence suggesting lack of carcinogenicity* in experimental animals, consistently and strongly supported by a broad range of other relevant data, may be classified in this group.

13. REFERENCES

Breslow, N.E. & Day, N.E. (1980) *Statistical Methods in Cancer Research*, Vol. 1, *The Analysis of Case–Control Studies* (IARC Scientific Publications No. 32), Lyon, IARC*Press*

Breslow, N.E. & Day, N.E. (1987) *Statistical Methods in Cancer Research*, Vol. 2, *The Design and Analysis of Cohort Studies* (IARC Scientific Publications No. 82), Lyon, IARC*Press*

Cohen, S.M. & Ellwein, L.B. (1990) Cell proliferation in carcinogenesis. *Science*, **249**, 1007–1011

Gart, J.J., Krewski, D., Lee, P.N., Tarone, R.E. & Wahrendorf, J. (1986) *Statistical Methods in Cancer Research*, Vol. 3, *The Design and Analysis of Long-term Animal Experiments* (IARC Scientific Publications No. 79), Lyon, IARC*Press*

Hoel, D.G., Kaplan, N.L. & Anderson, M.W. (1983) Implication of nonlinear kinetics on risk estimation in carcinogenesis. *Science*, **219**, 1032–1037

Huff, J.E., Eustis, S.L. & Haseman, J.K. (1989) Occurrence and relevance of chemically induced benign neoplasms in long-term carcinogenicity studies. *Cancer Metastasis Rev.*, **8**, 1–21

IARC (1973–1996) *Information Bulletin on the Survey of Chemicals Being Tested for Carcinogenicity/Directory of Agents Being Tested for Carcinogenicity*, Numbers 1–17, Lyon, IARC*Press*

IARC (1976–1996), Lyon, IARC*Press*

    Directory of On-going Research in Cancer Epidemiology 1976. Edited by C.S. Muir & G. Wagner

    Directory of On-going Research in Cancer Epidemiology 1977 (IARC Scientific Publications No. 17). Edited by C.S. Muir & G. Wagner

    Directory of On-going Research in Cancer Epidemiology 1978 (IARC Scientific Publications No. 26). Edited by C.S. Muir & G. Wagner

    Directory of On-going Research in Cancer Epidemiology 1979 (IARC Scientific Publications No. 28). Edited by C.S. Muir & G. Wagner

    Directory of On-going Research in Cancer Epidemiology 1980 (IARC Scientific Publications No. 35). Edited by C.S. Muir & G. Wagner

    Directory of On-going Research in Cancer Epidemiology 1981 (IARC Scientific Publications No. 38). Edited by C.S. Muir & G. Wagner

Directory of On-going Research in Cancer Epidemiology 1982 (IARC Scientific Publications No. 46). Edited by C.S. Muir & G. Wagner

Directory of On-going Research in Cancer Epidemiology 1983 (IARC Scientific Publications No. 50). Edited by C.S. Muir & G. Wagner

Directory of On-going Research in Cancer Epidemiology 1984 (IARC Scientific Publications No. 62). Edited by C.S. Muir & G. Wagner

Directory of On-going Research in Cancer Epidemiology 1985 (IARC Scientific Publications No. 69). Edited by C.S. Muir & G. Wagner

Directory of On-going Research in Cancer Epidemiology 1986 (IARC Scientific Publications No. 80). Edited by C.S. Muir & G. Wagner

Directory of On-going Research in Cancer Epidemiology 1987 (IARC Scientific Publications No. 86). Edited by D.M. Parkin & J. Wahrendorf

Directory of On-going Research in Cancer Epidemiology 1988 (IARC Scientific Publications No. 93). Edited by M. Coleman & J. Wahrendorf

Directory of On-going Research in Cancer Epidemiology 1989/90 (IARC Scientific Publications No. 101). Edited by M. Coleman & J. Wahrendorf

Directory of On-going Research in Cancer Epidemiology 1991 (IARC Scientific Publications No.110). Edited by M. Coleman & J. Wahrendorf

Directory of On-going Research in Cancer Epidemiology 1992 (IARC Scientific Publications No. 117). Edited by M. Coleman, J. Wahrendorf & E. Démaret

Directory of On-going Research in Cancer Epidemiology 1994 (IARC Scientific Publications No. 130). Edited by R. Sankaranarayanan, J. Wahrendorf & E. Démaret

Directory of On-going Research in Cancer Epidemiology 1996 (IARC Scientific Publications No. 137). Edited by R. Sankaranarayanan, J. Wahrendorf & E. Démaret

IARC (1977) *IARC Monographs Programme on the Evaluation of the Carcinogenic Risk of Chemicals to Humans*. Preamble (IARC intern. tech. Rep. No. 77/002)

IARC (1978) *Chemicals with* Sufficient Evidence *of Carcinogenicity in Experimental Animals —* IARC Monographs *Volumes 1–17* (IARC intern. tech. Rep. No. 78/003)

IARC (1978–1993) *Environmental Carcinogens. Methods of Analysis and Exposure Measurement*, Lyon, IARC*Press*

Vol. 1. Analysis of Volatile Nitrosamines in Food (IARC Scientific Publications No. 18). Edited by R. Preussmann, M. Castegnaro, E.A. Walker & A.E. Wasserman (1978)

Vol. 2. Methods for the Measurement of Vinyl Chloride in Poly(vinyl chloride), Air, Water and Foodstuffs (IARC Scientific Publications No. 22). Edited by D.C.M. Squirrell & W. Thain (1978)

Vol. 3. Analysis of Polycyclic Aromatic Hydrocarbons in Environmental Samples (IARC Scientific Publications No. 29). Edited by M. Castegnaro, P. Bogovski, H. Kunte & E.A. Walker (1979)

Vol. 4. Some Aromatic Amines and Azo Dyes in the General and Industrial Environment (IARC Scientific Publications No. 40). Edited by L. Fishbein, M. Castegnaro, I.K. O'Neill & H. Bartsch (1981)

Vol. 5. Some Mycotoxins (IARC Scientific Publications No. 44). Edited by L. Stoloff, M. Castegnaro, P. Scott, I.K. O'Neill & H. Bartsch (1983)

Vol. 6. N-Nitroso Compounds (IARC Scientific Publications No. 45). Edited by R. Preussmann, I.K. O'Neill, G. Eisenbrand, B. Spiegelhalder & H. Bartsch (1983)

Vol. 7. Some Volatile Halogenated Hydrocarbons (IARC Scientific Publications No. 68). Edited by L. Fishbein & I.K. O'Neill (1985)

Vol. 8. Some Metals: As, Be, Cd, Cr, Ni, Pb, Se, Zn (IARC Scientific Publications No. 71). Edited by I.K. O'Neill, P. Schuller & L. Fishbein (1986)

Vol. 9. Passive Smoking (IARC Scientific Publications No. 81). Edited by I.K. O'Neill, K.D. Brunnemann, B. Dodet & D. Hoffmann (1987)

*Vol. 10. Benzene and Alkylated Benzenes (*IARC Scientific Publications No. 85). Edited by L. Fishbein & I.K. O'Neill (1988)

Vol. 11. Polychlorinated Dioxins and Dibenzofurans (IARC Scientific Publications No. 108). Edited by C. Rappe, H.R. Buser, B. Dodet & I.K. O'Neill (1991)

Vol. 12. Indoor Air (IARC Scientific Publications No. 109). Edited by B. Seifert, H. van de Wiel, B. Dodet & I.K. O'Neill (1993)

IARC (1979) *Criteria to Select Chemicals for* IARC Monographs (IARC intern. tech. Rep. No. 79/003)

IARC (1982) *IARC Monographs on the Evaluation of the Carcinogenic Risk of Chemicals to Humans*, Supplement 4, *Chemicals, Industrial Processes and Industries Associated with Cancer in Humans* (IARC Monographs, Volumes 1 to 29), Lyon, IARC*Press*

IARC (1983) *Approaches to Classifying Chemical Carcinogens According to Mechanism of Action* (IARC intern. tech. Rep. No. 83/001)

IARC (1984) *Chemicals and Exposures to Complex Mixtures Recommended for Evaluation in IARC Monographs and Chemicals and Complex Mixtures Recommended for Long-term Carcinogenicity Testing* (IARC intern. tech. Rep. No. 84/002)

IARC (1987a) *IARC Monographs on the Evaluation of Carcinogenic Risks to Humans*, Supplement 6, *Genetic and Related Effects: An Updating of Selected* IARC Monographs *from Volumes 1 to 42*, Lyon, IARC*Press*

IARC (1987b) *IARC Monographs on the Evaluation of Carcinogenic Risks to Humans*, Supplement 7, *Overall Evaluations of Carcinogenicity: An Updating of* IARC Monographs *Volumes 1 to 42*, Lyon, IARC*Press*

IARC (1988) *Report of an IARC Working Group to Review the Approaches and Processes Used to Evaluate the Carcinogenicity of Mixtures and Groups of Chemicals* (IARC intern. tech. Rep. No. 88/002)

IARC (1989) *Chemicals, Groups of Chemicals, Mixtures and Exposure Circumstances to be Evaluated in Future IARC Monographs, Report of an ad hoc Working Group* (IARC intern. tech. Rep. No. 89/004)

IARC (1991a) *A Consensus Report of an IARC Monographs Working Group on the Use of Mechanisms of Carcinogenesis in Risk Identification* (IARC intern. tech. Rep. No. 91/002)

IARC (1991b) *Report of an ad-hoc* IARC Monographs *Advisory Group on Viruses and Other Biological Agents Such as Parasites* (IARC intern. tech. Rep. No. 91/001)

IARC (1993) *Chemicals, Groups of Chemicals, Complex Mixtures, Physical and Biological Agents and Exposure Circumstances to be Evaluated in Future* IARC Monographs, *Report of an ad-hoc Working Group* (IARC intern. Rep. No. 93/005)

IARC (1998a) *Report of an ad-hoc* IARC Monographs *Advisory Group on Physical Agents* (IARC Internal Report No. 98/002)

IARC (1998b) *Report of an ad-hoc* IARC Monographs *Advisory Group on Priorities for Future Evaluations* (IARC Internal Report No. 98/004)

McGregor, D.B., Rice, J.M. & Venitt, S., eds (1999) *The Use of Short and Medium-term Tests for Carcinogens and Data on Genetic Effects in Carcinogenic Hazard Evaluation* (IARC Scientific Publications No. 146), Lyon, IARC*Press*

Montesano, R., Bartsch, H., Vainio, H., Wilbourn, J. & Yamasaki, H., eds (1986) *Long-term and Short-term Assays for Carcinogenesis — A Critical Appraisal* (IARC Scientific Publications No. 83), Lyon, IARC*Press*

Peto, R., Pike, M.C., Day, N.E., Gray, R.G., Lee, P.N., Parish, S., Peto, J., Richards, S. & Wahrendorf, J. (1980) Guidelines for simple, sensitive significance tests for carcinogenic effects in long-term animal experiments. In: *IARC Monographs on the Evaluation of the Carcinogenic Risk of Chemicals to Humans*, Supplement 2, *Long-term and Short-term Screening Assays for Carcinogens: A Critical Appraisal*, Lyon, IARC*Press*, pp. 311–426

Tomatis, L., Aitio, A., Wilbourn, J. & Shuker, L. (1989) Human carcinogens so far identified. *Jpn. J. Cancer Res.*, **80**, 795–807

Vainio, H., Magee, P.N., McGregor, D.B. & McMichael, A.J., eds (1992) *Mechanisms of Carcinogenesis in Risk Identification* (IARC Scientific Publications No. 116), Lyon, IARC*Press*

Vainio, H., Wilbourn, J.D., Sasco, A.J., Partensky, C., Gaudin, N., Heseltine, E. & Eragne, I. (1995) Identification of human carcinogenic risk in IARC Monographs. *Bull. Cancer,* **82**, 339–348 (in French)

Waters, M.D., Stack, H.F., Brady, A.L., Lohman, P.H.M., Haroun, L. & Vainio, H. (1987) Appendix 1. Activity profiles for genetic and related tests. In: *IARC Monographs on the Evaluation of Carcinogenic Risks to Humans*, Suppl. 6, *Genetic and Related Effects: An Updating of Selected IARC Monographs from Volumes 1 to 42*, Lyon, IARC*Press*, pp. 687–696

Wilbourn, J., Haroun, L., Heseltine, E., Kaldor, J., Partensky, C. & Vainio, H. (1986) Response of experimental animals to human carcinogens: an analysis based upon the IARC Monographs Programme. *Carcinogenesis*, **7**, 1853–1863

GENERAL REMARKS

Future worldwide health effects of current smoking patterns

As a cause of human cancer, tobacco smoke is uniquely important. In some populations it has, in recent decades, caused about half of all cancer deaths in men, plus a smaller, but increasing proportion of cancer deaths in women. Worldwide, it causes more cancer deaths than can be attributed to all other known causes of the disease and, in addition, it causes even more deaths from vascular and respiratory diseases than from cancer (US DHHS, 1989; Peto et al., 1994; Parkin et al., 2000).

The fact that prolonged cigarette smoking is a cause — and the major cause — of lung cancer was reliably established during the 1950s, as was the fact that it can also cause several other types of cancer and various other diseases (for a historical review, see Doll, 1998). In the previous IARC *Monograph* on tobacco smoking (IARC, 1986), it was concluded that there was *sufficient evidence* that the habit could cause not only lung cancer, but also cancers of the upper aerodigestive tract, pancreas and lower urinary tract. Section 2 of the present monograph on tobacco smoke reviews and confirms these qualitative conclusions about particular types of cancer. It also reviews epidemiological studies on other types of cancer, which provide good evidence for some cancers (e.g. of the breast, endometrium and prostate) that smoking is of little or no causal relevance. Findings for other cancers (of the stomach, liver and cervix, renal-cell carcinoma and myeloid leukaemia) provide *sufficient evidence* that they can be caused by smoking, i.e. that smoking can increase their age-specific incidence rates. Other sections review the changing patterns of exposure, and the experimental evidence that tobacco smoke contains many chemicals that can, under certain circumstances, induce DNA damage or cancer in experimental animals. These qualitative conclusions about the many different chemicals in smoke and the many different types of cancer caused in humans do not, however, adequately reflect the real magnitude of the overall effects of smoking on mortality. This general introduction therefore summarizes the net effects of smoking on mortality from all cancers and overall mortality (for individuals and for populations), and indicates the extent to which individuals or populations who have already smoked for some years or decades can still limit these risks by cessation of the habit. Smoking lowers the risk for a few diseases and for one cancer (endometrial carcinoma), but this reduced risk is inconsequential, when compared with the net detriment of smoking to health.

Persistent cigarette smoking throughout adult life

Two observations are of particular relevance to assessing the current and future hazards of smoking. First, cigarettes, as commonly smoked during the twentieth century, have proved to be substantially more hazardous than other forms of tobacco that were commonly smoked in the nineteenth century. Second, the earlier in life that cigarette smoking is fully established, the greater are the hazards among persistent smokers in middle and old age. These differences in hazard can be substantial: for example, a difference of only a few years in the age at which smoking was established may lead to an approximately twofold difference in hazard many years later (Doll & Peto, 1981). Thus, national rates for lung cancer in people of around 70 years of age depend strongly on the intensity of pulmonary exposure to cigarette smoke half a century ago, when they were about 20 years of age. Retrospective assessment of smoking behaviour in previous decades, however, is subject to error; this limits the ability of epidemiological data to identify the ensuing consequences of earlier smoking. Current disease rates also depend strongly on current smoking patterns; even after a few decades of smoking, people who stop smoking before they develop lung cancer (or some other serious disease) decrease their risk of death from the habit: see Figure 1.

This dependence of current disease rates (not only on current smoking patterns but also on cigarette smoking patterns many decades earlier) implies a delay of about half a century between an upsurge in cigarette use by young adults in a particular population and the main upsurge in cases of lung cancer, and of some of the other smoking-related diseases, that eventually results. In contrast with this extremely long delay between increases in smoking and increases in risk, population-wide decreases in tobacco smoking can produce substantial benefits within just one or two decades.

Emerging hazards

Tobacco has been used for many centuries, originally in America, then in the sixteenth and seventeenth centuries in Europe, and subsequently throughout the world. The reasons for its widespread use are still imperfectly understood, but there are both psychosocial and pharmacological factors involved. Nicotine is addictive for many smokers, but other components of the smoke from tobacco, or from flavourants or other chemicals added to tobacco, may also be important. At first tobacco was smoked in pipes or as cigars: later, 'bidis', consisting of a small amount of tobacco wrapped in the leaf of another plant, began to be smoked in South Asia. Cigarettes, which would eventually cause much greater harm than did pipe or cigar smoking in the nineteenth century, only began to be manufactured in the second half of the nineteenth century; even in the early years of the twentieth century, cigarette consumption still remained low. Thereafter, however, cigarette consumption by men increased rapidly in the United Kingdom, the USA and several other industrialized countries, followed (decades later) by increased cigarette consumption by women in developed countries and also by men in developing countries.

Figure 1. Cumulative risk (%) of death from lung cancer (in the absence of other causes of death) in men at ages 45–75 years: in continuing cigarette smokers, ex-cigarette smokers who stopped at age 50 or at age 30 and lifelong nonsmokers, based on lung cancer death rates for men in the United Kingdom in 1990

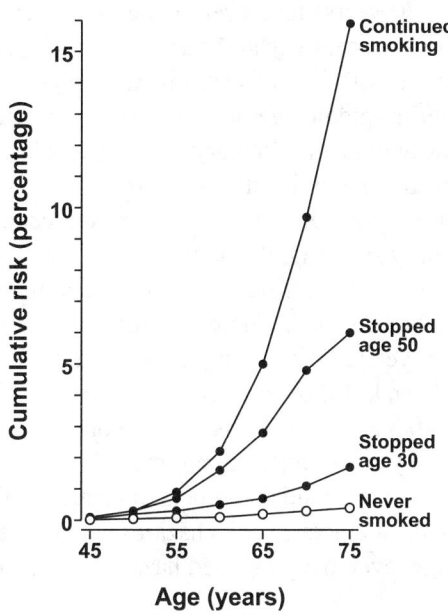

From Peto *et al.* (2000)
[a] Nonsmoker risks are taken from a US prospective study of mortality

(For example, although the main increase in cigarette consumption by men was eventually about as great in China as in the United Kingdom or the USA, it took place about 50 years later, i.e. in the last quarter of the twentieth century, and its full effects on the mortality rates for Chinese men may take several more decades to emerge.) At present, cigarette consumption by women in developing countries is still relatively low.

In some countries, the spread of cigarette smoking during the twentieth century was driven or maintained by extensive advertising and promotion by tobacco companies. More recently, substantial efforts have been made in some countries to discourage smoking, and over the past few decades, cigarette consumption has been halved in a few countries such as the USA and the United Kingdom. Worldwide, however, about a thousand million men and a quarter of a thousand million women now smoke, consuming 5.5 million million cigarettes a year (plus many other tobacco products), and about 30 million young adults take up the habit each year (see Section 1). The emergence of increasingly large multinational tobacco companies with global reach could result in even more tobacco use in the future.

Because the main hazards of cigarette smoking in middle age (35–69 years) take several decades to become substantial, it was not until the 1950s (several decades after cigarette smoking became widespread) that clear medical evidence emerged, particularly from the USA and the United Kingdom, that smoking was a major cause of many fatal diseases, and was responsible for almost half of all male mortality in middle age. The main hazards in old age (≥ 70 years) take even longer — at least half a century — to become substantial, so only in recent decades has it become apparent that, for men in developed countries, about half of all persistent cigarette smokers would eventually be killed by the habit (a quarter in middle age plus a quarter in old age) (Doll *et al.*, 1994). In addition, during the past quarter of a century, it has become increasingly clear that, although the main hazard is to the individual who smokes, there is some cancer hazard to nonsmokers (including former smokers) from exposure to secondhand tobacco smoke (see monograph on involuntary smoking, this volume).

Figure 2 illustrates the effects of persistent cigarette smoking on mortality throughout adult life in male doctors in the United Kingdom: the difference in survival at age 70 years (i.e. 83% among nonsmokers versus 60% among smokers) reflects the fact that about one-quarter of the smokers had been killed by tobacco in middle age (35–69 years). Moreover, of those still alive at age 70 years, two-fifths of the nonsmokers and one-fifth of the smokers were still alive at 85 years of age. Among male doctors in the United Kingdom, many of those who had smoked substantial numbers of cigarettes for a long time gave up the habit permanently when clear evidence of its hazards emerged, and the extent to which cessation, even in middle age, eventually avoided hazard is illustrated in Figure 3.

Trends in tobacco-attributed mortality in the United Kingdom and the USA, 1950–99

Cigarette smoking first became widespread among both men and women in the United Kingdom and the USA, and large epidemiological studies by the American Cancer Society yield indirect estimates of the overall cancer mortality attributed (and, by subtraction, that not attributed) to smoking over the past half century (1950–99) in those two countries (Figures 4 and 5). In the 1960s, men in the United Kingdom were probably the worst-affected major population in the world, but in recent decades male mortality from tobacco has declined substantially in the United Kingdom (Figure 4). In the USA, however, the mortality rate among men is only just beginning to decline substantially, whereas that among women in the USA has increased. In 1990, 34% of all cancer deaths in the USA were attributed to smoking (90% of the lung cancer deaths and 13% of the deaths from other, or unspecified, types of cancer; Table 1). Of the cancer deaths in the USA in 1990 that were attributed to smoking, three-quarters involved lung cancer (72% specified as such, plus one-third of the few deaths from cancer of an unspecified site). In people aged 35–69 years, the proportion of all cancer deaths in the USA in 1990 that were attributed to smoking was 40% (52% male, 27% female); at older ages, it was 31%. Relatively few deaths from cancer occur at younger ages. The rise in tobacco-attributed cancer mortality in the USA during the second half of the twentieth century, first among men and then among women, is chiefly the inevitable but delayed effect of the rise in cigarette consumption during the first half of the twentieth century.

Figure 2. Effects of persistent cigarette smoking on the probability of surviving from 35 years to various ages

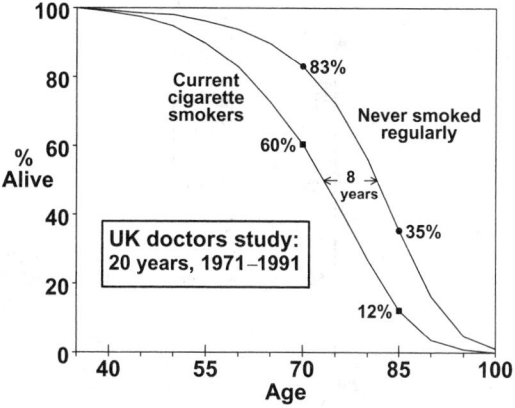

From Doll *et al.* (1994)

Figure 3. Effects of smoking cessation at ages 35–44 (broken line) on survival from age 35

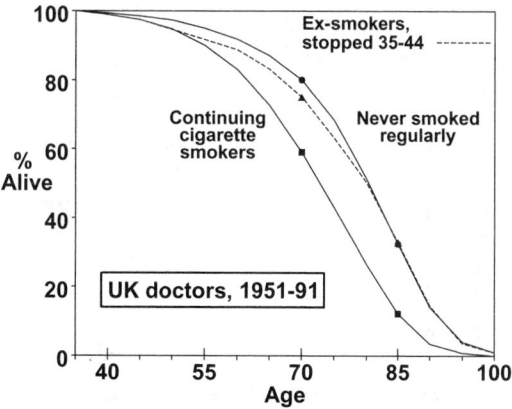

From Doll *et al.* (1994)
Even in middle age, those who stop before they have incurable cancer, or some other serious disease, avoid most of their subsequent risk of death from tobacco; stopping earlier is even more effective.

Figure 4. Cancer mortality rates in the United Kingdom, 1950–2000, subdivided into the parts attributed, and not attributed to smoking

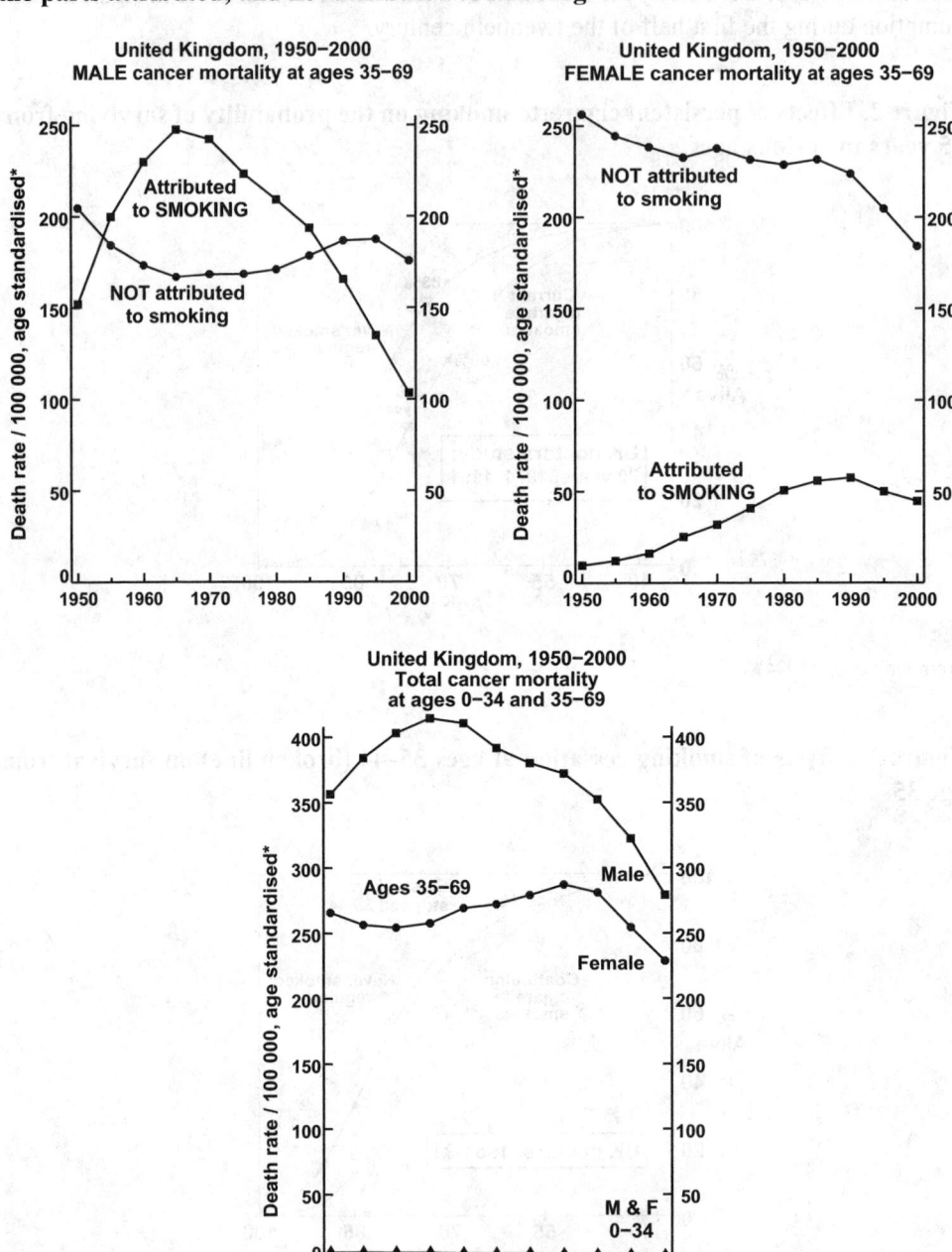

From Peto *et al.* (1994)

*Mean of annual rates per 100 000 in component 5-year age groups

Figure 5. Cancer mortality rates in the USA, 1950–2000, subdivided into the parts attributed, and not attributed to smoking

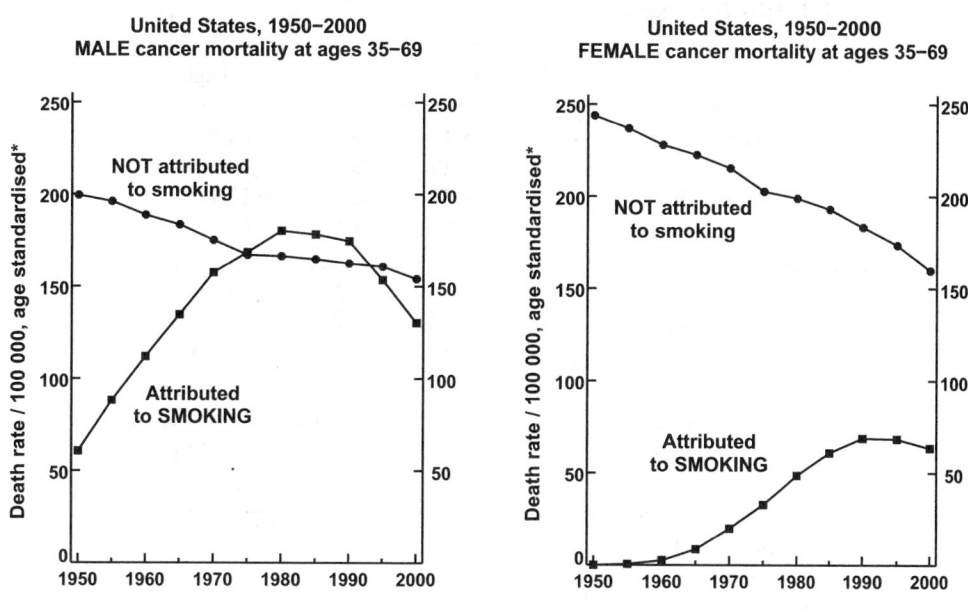

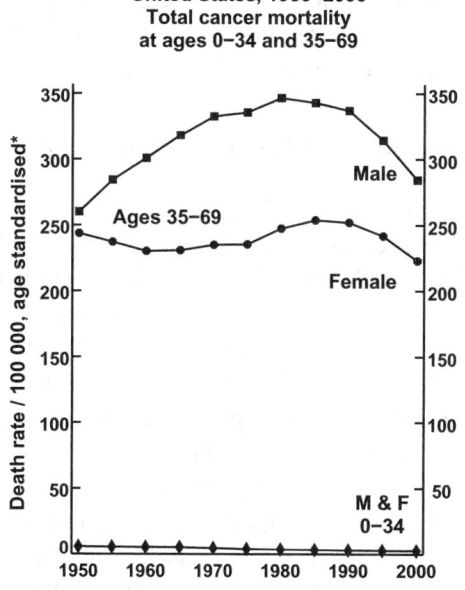

From Peto *et al.* (1994)

*Mean of annual rates per 100 000 in component 5-year age groups

Table 1. Deaths in the USA based on the Cancer Prevention Study II in 1990 attributed to smoking/total number of deaths (thousands)

		0–34	35–69	≥ 70	All ages
Lung cancer	Male	–	45/48	39/43	84/91
	Female	–	22/26	20/24	43/50
	Both	–	68/75	59/66	127/141
			(91%)	(89%)	(90%)
All cancers	Male	–/5	64/123	56/140	120/268
	Female	–/4	28/104	26/129	54/237
	Both	–/9	92/228	83/269	174/505
			(40%)	(31%)	(34%)
All causes	Male	–/103	150/415	136/595	286/1113
	Female	–/48	73/257	102/730	175/1035
	Both	–/151	223/672	238/1325	461/2148
			(33%)	(18%)	(21%)

From Peto *et al.* (1994)
–, not available

Table 1 also indicates that tobacco smoking caused substantially more deaths from vascular, respiratory and other non-neoplastic causes than from cancer. The proportion of all deaths in the USA (neoplastic, vascular, respiratory or other causes) at ages 35–69 years that were attributed to tobacco was 33% in 1990, compared with only 12% in 1950.

Trends in tobacco-attributed mortality in developed and developing countries

In the aggregate of all developed countries, the epidemic of death from tobacco of men in middle age may have reached its peak by about 1990, and was by then almost as great as that in the USA (Table 2). In 1990, the epidemic in women, however, although still increasing, was less than half as great in the aggregate of all developed countries as it was in the USA. If current smoking patterns persist, the main increases in tobacco deaths over the next few decades are likely to be among women in developed countries and, in particular, among men in developing countries. In some of the developing countries, the populations are large and cigarette consumption by men in these countries has increased substantially in recent decades (Table 3).

Worldwide, the only major causes of mortality that are currently increasing rapidly are HIV, tobacco and, probably, obesity (Doll *et al.*, 1994; Peto *et al.*, 1994; Ad Hoc Committee on Health Research, 1996; Murray & Lopez, 1996; WHO, 1997; Peto *et al.*, 1999). If current smoking patterns persist, there will be about one thousand million deaths from tobacco during the twenty-first century, as against 'only' about 0.1 thousand million

Table 2. All developed countries: deaths based on the Cancer Prevention Study II in 1990 attributed to smoking/total number of deaths (thousands)

		0–34	35–69	≥ 70	All ages
Lung cancer	Male	–/1	231/246	141/156	372/402
	Female	–/1	44/64	42/61	86/125
	Both	–/2	275/310	183/217	458/529
			(89%)	(84%)	(87%)
All cancers	Male	–/27	360/736	212/600	572/1362
	Female	–/23	56/500	56/564	112/1087
	Both	–/50	416/1236	268/1164	684/2449
			(34%)	(23%)	(28%)
All causes	Male	–/504	865/2458	554/2851	1419/5813
	Female	–/244	160/1376	236/3998	396/5618
	Both	–/748	1025/3834	790/6849	1815/11431
			(27%)	(12%)	(16%)

From Peto *et al.* (1994)
–, not available

(100 million) during the whole of the twentieth century (Table 4). About half of these deaths will be of people in middle age (35–69 years) rather than old age — and those killed by tobacco in middle age lose, on average, more than 20 years of life expectancy when compared with nonsmokers.

There are two main reasons for expecting this large increase in tobacco deaths. First, the population of middle-aged and old people worldwide is expected to increase. Second, the proportion of deaths in middle and old age that are caused by tobacco is expected to increase over the next few decades as a result of the delayed effects of the large increase in cigarette smoking among young adults over the past few decades (Doll *et al.*, 1994; Peto *et al.*, 1994; Ad Hoc Committee on Health Research, 1996; Murray & Lopez, 1996; WHO, 1997; Peto *et al.*, 1999). Among persistent cigarette smokers, the risk of death from tobacco-related diseases in middle or old age is particularly great (about 1 in 2) only for those who start smoking in early adult life (Doll & Peto, 1981; Peto, 1986; Doll *et al.*, 1994; Peto *et al.*, 1994). Hence, the numbers of deaths from tobacco around the year 2000 were strongly influenced by the numbers of young adults who took up smoking around 1950, whereas the numbers of young adults who took up smoking around the year 2000 will strongly influence the numbers of deaths from tobacco around and beyond the year 2050.

In China, which is the largest and best studied of the developing countries (Liu *et al.*, 1998; Niu *et al.*, 1998; Peto *et al.*, 1999), the increase in cigarette consumption by men and the increase in tobacco-related deaths both lag almost exactly 40 years behind the

Table 3. Forty-year delay between cigarette smoking and mortality from tobacco-related diseases in US adults and Chinese men

Cigarettes per day, by year

US adults		Chinese men	
1910	1	1952	1
1930	4	1972	4
1950	10	1992	10

Proportion of overall mortality at ages 35–69 years attributed to tobacco

US adults		Chinese men	
1950	12%	1990	12%
1990	33%	2030	33%[a]

From Peto et al. (1999)

[a] Projection if current smoking patterns persist, i.e. two-thirds of the young men in mainland China start smoking cigarettes, and few give up the habit. In Hong Kong, where cigarette consumption by men reached its peak in the early 1970s, the proportion of deaths that was attributed to tobacco in men aged 35–69 years was one-third in 1998 (Lam et al., 2001).

Table 4. Projected numbers of deaths from tobacco during the twenty-first century, if current smoking patterns persist[a]

Period	Tobacco deaths (millions)
2000–24	~150
2025–49	~300
2050–99	> 500
Total, twenty-first century	~1000
(Twentieth century: for comparison)	(~100)

[a] Of 100 million people per year now reaching adulthood, ~30 million become smokers. If most persist, and about half of those who do are eventually killed by smoking, then the annual number of tobacco-related deaths will eventually be 10–15 million.

USA (Table 3). At present, few young women in China become smokers (Liu *et al.*, 1998). Cigarette consumption by Chinese men averaged 1, 4 and 10 per day in 1952, 1972 and 1992, respectively, with no further increase occurring during the past few years. The proportion of deaths attributed to tobacco in Chinese men at ages 35–69 years was measured to be 12% in 1990, and is projected to be about 33% in 2030 (Liu *et al.*, 1998; Niu *et al.*, 1998). Two-thirds of the young men become persistent smokers, and about half of those who do so will eventually be killed by the habit: therefore, about one-third of all the young men in China will eventually be killed by tobacco if current smoking patterns persist. China, which has 20% of the world's population, produces and consumes about 30% of the world's cigarettes, and a large nationwide study has shown that China already suffers almost a million deaths a year from tobacco-related diseases, a figure that is likely to double at least by 2025.

Worldwide, about 4 million deaths a year are currently caused by tobacco; 2 million of these occur in developed and 2 million in developing countries. However, these current numbers reflect smoking patterns decades ago, and worldwide cigarette consumption has increased substantially over the past half century (WHO, 1997). At present, about 30% of young adults become persistent smokers and relatively few quit (except in selected populations, such as educated adults living in parts of western Europe and North America). The main diseases by which smoking kills people differ substantially between different populations, but there is no good reason to expect the overall 50% risk of death from persistent cigarette smoking to differ greatly between different populations.

There are already well over one thousand million smokers, and by the 2030s about another thousand million young adults will, at current uptake rates, have started to smoke. Based on current smoking patterns, worldwide annual mortality from tobacco is likely to rise from about 4 million around the year 2000 to about 10 million around the year 2030 (i.e. 100 million per decade) (Peto *et al.*, 1994), and will rise somewhat further in later decades. Tobacco is therefore expected to cause about 150 million deaths in the first quarter of the twenty-first century and 300 million in the second quarter. Predictions for the third and, particularly, the fourth quarter of the century are inevitably more speculative. However, if over the next few decades about 20–30 million young adults a year become persistent smokers and about half are eventually killed by their habit, then about 10–15% of adult mortality in the second half of the century will be due to tobacco smoking (probably implying more than 500 million deaths due to tobacco for 2050–99; Table 4).

The numbers of tobacco deaths predicted to occur before 2050 cannot be greatly reduced unless a substantial proportion of the adults who have already been smoking for some time give up the habit. A decrease over the next decade or two in the proportion of children who become smokers will not have its main effects on mortality until the third quarter of this century.

The effects on tobacco deaths of adult smokers quitting before 2050 and of young people not starting to smoke after 2050 will probably be as follows:

- *Quitting*: If many of the adults who now smoke were to give up over the next decade or two, thus halving global cigarette consumption per adult by the year 2020, this would prevent about one-third of tobacco-related deaths in 2020 and would almost halve tobacco-related deaths in the second quarter of the century. Such changes would avoid about 20 or 30 million tobacco-related deaths in the first quarter of the century and would avoid about 100 or 150 million in the second quarter.

- *Not starting*: If, by progressive reduction over the next decade or two in the global uptake rate of smoking by young people, the proportion of young adults who become smokers were to be halved by 2020, this would avoid hundreds of millions of deaths from tobacco after 2050. It would, however, avoid almost none of the 150 million deaths from tobacco in the first quarter of the century, and would probably avoid 'only' about 10 or 20 million of the 300 million deaths from tobacco in the second quarter of the century.

Thus, using widely practicable ways of helping large numbers of young people not to become smokers could avoid hundreds of millions of tobacco-related deaths in the middle and second half of the twenty-first century, but not before. In contrast, widely practicable ways of helping large numbers of adult smokers to quit (preferably before middle age, but also in middle age) might avoid one or two hundred million tobacco-related deaths in the first half of this century. Large numbers of deaths during the second half of the century could also be avoided if many of those who, despite warnings, still start to smoke in future years could be helped to stop before they are killed by the habit. Such calculations suggest that the effects of quitting could be more rapidly appreciated on a population scale than the effects of prevention of starting smoking. However, a more thorough evaluation of different strategies, in particular on a worldwide scale, and consideration of the specificities of developed and developing countries, respectively, is outside the scope of the present monograph.

Methodological considerations in interpreting epidemiological evidence on smoking and disease

The epidemiological evidence on smoking and risk for disease comes largely from observational studies that compare the risk for disease in smokers with that in people who have never smoked. Evidence from such studies may be affected by bias and confounding, and chance may also explain the observed associations of smoking with risk for disease. Most of the evidence comes from case–control and cohort studies; both types of study are potentially subject to particular forms of bias. For case–control studies, comparability of cases and controls and success in their recruitment are particularly critical. For cohort studies, the degree of success in recruiting and retaining participants are important considerations in interpreting data.

In studies of smoking, as for studies of any agent, information bias and confounding are of concern. Information bias may affect the classification of both active and involuntary smoking and extend to the classification of disease. The potential for error in classifying active and involuntary smoking is well recognized and the potential magnitude of any resulting bias has been considered both qualitatively and quantitatively. The Working Group does not regard information bias as an important consideration in interpreting the evidence on active smoking. For involuntary smoking, several analyses on information bias were considered by the Working Group. This is discussed in detail in the monograph on involuntary smoking.

Confounding arises when the effect of active or involuntary smoking is artificially increased or decreased by a factor that is associated with exposure to smoke in a particular data set and is a risk factor on its own. Confounding becomes more plausible as an alternative to causality as the magnitude of risk decreases. There are various causes, other than smoking, of the cancers considered in this monograph and hence there is potential for confounding. However, these other agents produce confounding only if associated with smoking in specific data sets. Control may be incomplete, leaving the possibility of residual confounding. The Working Group considered the potential for confounding and noted the approach used to control for such.

Active smoking and involuntary smoking have been reported to be associated with the development of many forms of cancer, with a wide range of relative risks ranging from about 1.2 to 20 and higher. When the apparent relative risk is high (for example 10), confounding is unlikely to explain all the excess risk; it has seldom been difficult to recognize such an association and, in most instances, to deduce that it is causal. However, if the apparent relative risk approaches unity, the data need to be interpreted more carefully and subtle sources of bias and confounding must be taken into account. Under these circumstances, the findings from case–control studies may be difficult to interpret, because they may be distorted by the inclusion of controls who are not truly representative of the population from which the cases are drawn. When controls are selected from hospital patients, care has to be taken to exclude those with tobacco-related diseases because the relative risk of the condition being studied will be underestimated. When controls are drawn from the general population, it is important to know what proportion of the selected controls responded. Even if the proportion is known and the compliance rate is reasonably high, ensuring that the results are not biased to some extent by the inclusion of a disproportionate number of people who are interested in questions of health and are therefore unusually health conscious may be difficult. Such people may be less likely to smoke, causing the relative risk to be overestimated.

Cohort studies have their own problems and their results also require careful interpretation. One problem is that the reports do not always cover the same types of cancers. The findings for common cancers (e.g. cancers of the lung, stomach and large bowel) are nearly always reported, but those for rare cancers (e.g. cancers of the nasal sinuses and testis and leukaemia) may be reported only when the numbers observed are unexpectedly high. It may be necessary to limit the data used to those from cohort studies that have reported on many types of cancer (say 20 or more), although selection bias in reporting may still not be excluded for some of the less common cancers.

A second problem, which particularly affects cancers that may grow slowly, such as prostate cancer, is that many patients may die with the disease and not necessarily because of it. This, however, may not be adequately reflected on death certificates because death may be attributed to the cancer when the patient had actually died of an independent broncho-pneumonia, myocardial infarction or another of the many conditions that are made more common by cigarette smoking, thus creating an artefactual positive relationship between smoking and the cancer (Adami et al., 1996).

A third problem is that observations may continue to be made for many years after the characteristics of the individual members of the cohort have been recorded and, during this period, these characteristics may have changed. Some smokers may have stopped smoking and, as benefit is commonly obtained within a few years of stopping, this may result in an underestimation of the harmful effects of smoking.

Although cohort studies allow repeated assessments of smoking behaviour to capture any changes, in some studies (e.g. CPS-II, US Veterans), smoking was assessed only at the start of follow-up and cessation after enrolment was not recorded.

During their evaluation of smoking and disease, the Working Group had substantial evidence available for many cancer sites. These data were summarized in tables for qualitative evaluation as to the consistency of findings, strength of association and dose–response. Such evaluation of large bodies of data can also be accomplished through a collaborative, combined analysis of the original data from multiple studies or by pooling the summary results of individual studies, an approach referred to as meta-analysis.

In a collaborative re-analysis, the relevant investigators contribute the raw data for a pooled analysis and give detailed accounts of their procedures for reconciliation of differences. It is often possible to check the results obtained in case–control studies by comparing them with those obtained in cohort studies. Under these circumstances, the data from all the different types of study may prove sufficiently comparable to allow them to be combined.

When collaborative re-analyses are not possible or feasible, the next best approach to interpreting the data from multiple studies is to perform a meta-analysis of the results reported in the published literature. However, aspects of study design and other issues that may affect the results may not be fully allowed for because only summary findings are used. Meta-analysis can be used to evaluate heterogeneity between study findings. It is particularly informative when the results of individual studies lack precision.

An example of a collaborative re-analysis of data is the one relating the risk for breast cancer and active smoking described in Section 2 of this monograph. This type of analysis has not been undertaken in the study of cancers weakly related to smoking and, under these circumstances, reliable estimates of risk are most likely to be obtained from the results of cohort studies. Consequently, in considering such diseases as prostate cancer and leukaemia, which are certainly not strongly related to smoking and for which many sets of data are available, the results of case–control studies are less important.

References

Adami, H.O., Bergström, R., Engholm, G., Nyren, O., Wolk, A., Ekbom, A., Englund, A. & Baron, J. (1996) A prospective study of smoking and risk of prostate cancer. *Int. J. Cancer*, **67**, 764–768

Ad Hoc Committee on Health Research (1996) *Investing in Health Research and Development*, Geneva, World Health Organization

Doll, R. (1998) Uncovering the effects of smoking: Historical perspective. *Stat. Meth. med. Res.*, **7**, 87–117

Doll, R. & Peto, R. (1981) The causes of cancer: Quantitative estimates of avoidable risks of cancer in the United States today. *J. natl Cancer Inst.*, **66**, 1193–1308

Doll, R., Peto, R., Wheatley, K., Gray, R. & Sutherland, I. (1994) Mortality in relation to smoking: 40 years' observations on male British doctors. *Br. med. J.*, **309**, 901–911

IARC (1986) *IARC Monographs on the Evaluation of the Carcinogenic Risks of Chemicals to Humans*, Vol. 38, *Tobacco Smoking*, Lyon, IARC*Press*

Lam, T.H., Ho, S.Y., Hedley, A.J., Mak, K.H. & Peto, R. (2001) Mortality and smoking in Hong Kong: Case–control study of all adult deaths in 1998. *Br. med. J.*, **323**, 361

Liu, B.Q., Peto, R., Chen, Z.M., Boreham, J., Wu, Y.P., Li, J.Y., Campbell, T.C. & Chen, J.S. (1998) Emerging tobacco hazards in China: 1. Retrospective proportional mortality study of one million deaths. *Br. med. J.*, **317**, 1411–1422

Murray, C.J.L. & Lopez, A.D. (1996) *The Global Burden of Disease and Injury Series*, Vol. I, *The Global Burden of Disease, A Comprehensive Assessment of Mortality and Disability from Diseases, Injuries, and Risk Factors in 1990 and Projected to 2020*, Cambridge, MA, Harvard University Press

Niu, S.R., Yang, G.H., Chen, Z.M., Wang, J.L., Wang, G.H., He, X.Z., Schoepff, H., Boreham, J., Pan, H.C. & Peto, R. (1998) Emerging tobacco hazards in China: 2. Early mortality results from a prospective study. *Br. med. J.*, **317**, 1423–1424

Parkin, D.M., Pisani, P. & Masuyer, E. (2000) Tobacco-attributable cancer burden: A global review. In: Lu, R., Mackay, J., Niu, S. & Peto, R., eds, *Tobacco: The Growing Epidemic*, London, Springer-Verlag, pp. 81–84

Peto, R. (1986) Influence of dose and duration of smoking on lung cancer rates. In: Zaridze, D. & Peto, R., eds, *Tobacco: A Growing International Health Hazard* (IARC Scientific Publications No. 74), Lyon, IARC*Press*, pp. 23–33

Peto, R., Lopez, A.D., Boreham, J., Thun, M. & Heath, C., Jr (1994) *Mortality from Smoking in Developed Countries 1950–2000: Indirect Estimates from National Vital Statistics*, Oxford, Oxford University Press

Peto, R., Chen, Z.M. & Boreham, J. (1999) Tobacco — The growing epidemic. *Nat. Med.*, **5**, 15–17

Peto, R., Darby, S., Deo, H., Silcocks, P., Whitley, E. & Doll, R. (2000) Smoking, smoking cessation, and lung cancer in the US since 1950: Combination of national statistics with two case–control studies. *Br. med. J.*, **321**, 323–329

US DHHS (1989) *Reducing the Health Consequences of Smoking: 25 Years of Progress. A Report of the Surgeon General* (DHHS Publication No. (CDC) 89-8411), Rockville, MD, US Department of Health and Human Services

WHO (1997) *Tobacco or Health: A Global Status Report*, World Health Organization, Geneva

THE MONOGRAPHS

TOBACCO SMOKE

1. Production, Composition, Use and Regulations

1.1 Production and trade

1.1.1 *History*

The common tobacco plants of commerce had apparently been used for millenia by the peoples of the Western hemisphere before contact with Europeans began in 1492. The plants were cultivated by native Americans in Central and South America. Tobacco often had religious uses as depicted in Mayan temple carvings (Slade, 1997).

The start of the spread of tobacco from the Americas to the rest of the world invariably seems to date back to 11 October 1492, when Columbus was offered dried tobacco leaves at the House of the Arawaks, and took the plant back with him to Europe (IARC, 1986a). Presumably, the technique of smoking was picked up at the same time. The plant was named 'nicotiana' after the French ambassador to Portugal, who is said to have introduced it to the French court. The tobacco grown in France and Spain was *Nicotiana tabacum*, which came from seed that originated in Brazil and Mexico. The species first grown in Portugal and England was *Nicotiana rustica*, the seed coming from Florida and Virginia, respectively (IARC, 1986a).

Although claims were made that tobacco had been used earlier in China, no convincing documentation for this exists, but it is clear from Table 1.1 (IARC, 1986a) that tobacco was used widely and that a number of early societies discovered the effects of a self-administered dose of nicotine independently of each other, which implies that the plant was widely distributed, at least throughout the Americas.

Tobacco was grown, smoked and chewed by numerous peoples and eventually became ubiquitous; it certainly featured as an important tradeable source of income from the time of its discovery by Columbus until the present day.

The modern history of tobacco really starts with the design of the cigarette machine in the middle of the nineteenth century; a machine was patented in 1880 by James Bonsack (Bonsack, 1881). Another factor that contributed to the rise of cigarette smoking was concern over the spread of tuberculosis by spitting of smokeless tobacco (Glover & Glover, 1992). Since the 1920s, most tobacco has been smoked in cigarettes, with cigars, pipes and chewing tobacco declining to relatively small proportions of the global consumption. This does not mean that these other forms of use are trivial, as fashions have

Table 1.1. Chronicle of early tobacco cultivation and use

Date	Event
1492 (11 October)	Columbus sighted the home of the Arawaks and was offered 'dried' tobacco leaves.
1499	Amerigo Vespucci recorded the use of chewing tobacco on an island off Venezuela.
1545	Iroquois Indians near Montreal, Canada, were found to have smoking habits.
1556	Tobacco was first grown or became known in France.
1558	Tobacco was used in Brazil and Portugal.
1559	Tobacco was used in Spain.
1560	*Nicotiana rustica* was used in Central Africa.
1565	Tobacco was used in England.
1600	Tobacco was introduced to Italy, Germany, Norway, Sweden, Russia, Persia, India, Indochina, Japan, China and the west coast of Africa.
1612	John Rolfe, at Jamestown, Virginia, was the first man known to grow tobacco commercially for export.
1631	Tobacco production extended to Maryland and then gradually to other areas.
1650s	Portuguese took tobacco to South Africa and other countries. Spaniards distributed tobacco to the Philippines, Guatemala and other Central and South American countries and to the West Indies. Tobacco cultivation was begun in Indonesia. Tobacco cultivation was extended in Europe.

From IARC (1986a)

been started for the use of chewing tobacco and cigars as deliberate marketing ploys within the last two decades (Glover & Glover, 1992; Gupta, 1992; Gerlach *et al.*, 1998).

1.1.2 *World production and trade*

World tobacco production is currently declining. It peaked in 1997 at 7 975 360 tonnes (US Department of Agriculture, 2001a) and by 2001 had fallen to 5 883 324 (US Department of Agriculture, 2002a; see Table 1.2). It is a little early to interpret the significance of these figures, and certainly too early to conclude that they reflect the beginning of a long-term downward trend.

The pattern of production has shifted significantly in recent decades. Whereas exports from the USA have fallen slightly, those from Brazil, China and Zimbabwe have increased substantially.

Table 1.2. World tobacco production

Crop year	Hectares	Tonnes
1976/77	4 127 740	5 892 000
1980	3 823 340	5 575 000
1985	4 519 600	6 433 300
1990	4 612 420	7 096 730
1996	4 544 060	7 349 480
1997	4 893 810	7 975 360
1998	4 658 040	7 473 000
1999	3 755 130	6 341 430
2000[a]	NA	5 923 797
2001[a]	NA	5 883 324
2002[a]	NA	5 678 753

From US Department of Agriculture (2001b)
[a] From US Department of Agriculture (2002a)
NA, not available

Table 1.3. Tobacco leaf imports and exports in selected countries between 1970 and 1998 (tonnes)

Country	1970		1998	
	Import	Export	Import	Export
Brazil	9	54 468	14 726	300 513
China	10 337	19 055	20 687	106 355
Malawi	3 602	19 801	1 100	81 000
Turkey	–	74 014	42 174	155 058
USA	99 241	234 262	246 763	215 222
Zimbabwe	–	40 000	9 573	194 141

From Corrao *et al.* (2000)

Table 1.3 gives examples of some of the substantial shifts in tobacco production over the past three decades. Complex reasons lie behind the change in pattern. Economic pressures, often following political decisions, dictate who grows what and where. In developed areas, e.g. in the USA and the European Union, where farmers have, and still do, receive subsidies to grow tobacco, specific measures and programmes have also been initiated to pay farmers to stop growing tobacco or to switch to other crops (Council of the European Union, 2002; US Congress, 2002a,b; Womack, 2002). In developing countries, the cigarette manufacturers may provide seed and expertise as well as an assured market for the tobacco type they need (Time Asia, 2000). In other countries, cigarette manufacturers are compelled to purchase a proportion of their tobacco locally. Furthermore, consolidation of cigarette manufacturing followed the opening up of central and eastern Europe with the purchase by transnational corporations of antiquated tobacco monopolies (Griffin-Pustay, 1999, 2002). This affected the pattern of leaf production, import and export. The downward trend in tar and nicotine yields of cigarettes sold in developing countries during the 1990s meant that manufacturers' requirements were changed. The move towards tobacco with a low nitrosamine yield in the USA led to the export of substantial amounts of existing leaf.

The trend towards a smaller number of global brands was accompanied by the trend to global advertising. The complex trading situation is aggravated by the fact that a reported one-third (355 billion cigarettes) of annual global exports are smuggled (Joossens & Raw, 1998). Many smuggled cigarettes may be exported and imported several times.

1.1.3   What is produced

There is a wide variety of smoking tobacco products on the world market to chose from, including cigarettes, cigars, cigarillos, bidis, chuttas and kreteks (Table 1.4). Cigarettes and cigars use blended tobaccos and the type of tobacco used in these products has

Table 1.4. Smoking tobacco products

Cigarette	Any roll of tobacco wrapped in paper or other non-tobacco material; filter-tipped or untipped; approximately 8 mm in diameter, 70–120 mm in length
Cigar	Any roll of tobacco wrapped in leaf tobacco or in any other substance containing tobacco Types: little cigars, small cigars ('cigarillos'), regular cigars, premium cigars Some little cigars are filter tipped and are shaped like cigarettes. Regular cigars are up to 17 mm in diameter, 110–150 mm in length.
Bidi	Hand-rolled Indian cigarette; sun-dried temburni leaf rolled into a conical shape together with flaked tobacco and secured with a thread
Chutta[a]	Hand-rolled cigarette used for reverse smoking primarily by women in India
Kretek	Small cigar containing tobacco (approximately 60%[b]), cloves and cocoa. The burning blend gives a characteristic flavour and 'honey' taste to the smoke.

From Stratton et al. (2001)
[a] From Narayan et al. (1996)
[b] From Clark (1989)

a decisive influence on the physicochemical nature of the smoke they produce. The chemical composition of the tobacco leaf is determined by plant genetics, cultivation practices, weather conditions and curing methods (Tso, 1991). The classification of the leaf tobacco commonly used in cigarettes is primarily based on curing methods and tobacco types. For example, a standard system of classification by the US Department of Agriculture designates six major classes of US tobacco (Table 1.5). Each class comprises two or more different types. Individual types of flue-cured tobacco are no longer easily identified, and the type designation usually refers only to a marketing area. Different countries may use different classification terms, but the general principle is the same.

Table 1.5. Classification of US tobacco types

Tobacco type	Class	Characteristics	Main use	Growing regions
Flue-cured	1	Yellow, blond bright	95% in cigarettes	Alabama, Florida, Georgia, North Carolina, South Carolina, Virginia
Fire-cured	2	Light to dark brown; cured over open fires	'Roll-your-own' cigarettes, chewing tobacco, cigars and smoking tobacco	Kentucky, Tennessee, Virginia
Light air-cured	3A	Burley: cured without supplementary heat	> 90% in cigarettes	Indiana, Kentucky, Missouri, North Carolina, Ohio, Tennessee, Virginia, West Virginia
		Maryland	Almost all in cigarettes	Maryland
Dark air-cured	3B	Light to medium brown	For chewing tobacco and snuff	Kentucky, Tennessee, Virginia
Cigar filler	4	–	Tobacco types for use as cigar fillers, binders and wrappers; used for cigars	Indiana, Ohio, Pennsylvania, Puerto Rico
Cigar binder	5	–	Tobacco types for use as cigar fillers, binders and wrappers; used for cigars	Connecticut, Massachusetts, Minnesota, New York, Pennsylvania, Wisconsin
Cigar wrapper	6	–	Tobacco types for use as cigar fillers, binders and wrappers; used for cigars	Connecticut, Florida, Georgia, Massachusetts
Miscella-neous	7	–		Louisiana

From Tso (1991); US Department of Agriculture (2001c)

The major components of American blend cigarettes are flue-cured tobaccos (often called Virginia, blond or bright tobaccos), air-cured (burley) and Maryland tobaccos, sun-cured (Oriental) tobaccos and reconstituted or homogenized sheet tobacco which is made from tobacco dust, fines and particles, and leaf ribs and stems (Beauman *et al.*, 1996; Hoffmann & Hoffmann, 1997). The American blend cigarette has been the predominant type in the USA, and the Virginia blend cigarette has been the most predominant type in Australia, Canada, China, Japan and the United Kingdom (Hoffmann & Hoffmann, 2001).

Blending is done to achieve specific pH, taste, burning characteristics and nicotine content and the type of tobacco blend significantly affects the pH, nicotine content and toxicity of the smoke. The pH strongly influences the concentration of free nicotine in tobacco smoke, whereas the nitrate content influences the carcinogenic potential of smoke. There is a choice of 60 *Nicotiana* species and 100 varieties of tobacco that can be blended. However, almost all commercial tobacco products use *Nicotiana tabacum* species and small amount of *N. rustica*. Cured tobacco lines can contain between 0.2 and 4.75% nicotine by weight, depending on plant genetics, growing conditions, degree of ripening, fertilizer treatment and position of leaf on the stalk (Tso, 1991; Stratton *et al.*, 2001).

The actual recipes for blending are closely kept trade secrets and the consolidation of the manufacturing industry worldwide seems to be leading towards a relatively homo-geneous cigarette with relatively modest differences in tar and nicotine yield, but consi-derable diversity in nitrosamine yield (Gray *et al.*, 2000).

Roll-your-own (RYO) cigarettes are a cheaper substitute for commercially manu-factured brands and are gaining in popularity worldwide. In Europe, two of the major markets for RYO are Germany and the Netherlands (Dymond, 1996). In Canada, they became so popular that, by the end of 1989, sales of RYO accounted for approximately 14% of the Canadian cigarette market (Kaiserman & Rickert, 1992a). In the United Kingdom in 1994, more than 20% of male smokers used RYO products as compared with less than 4% of female smokers (Darrall & Figgins, 1998). In the USA, 3.4 billion RYO cigarettes were smoked in 1994 (Maxwell Tobacco Fact Book, 2000).

A cigar is any roll of tobacco wrapped in leaf tobacco or any other substance con-taining tobacco. There are four main types of cigar: little cigars, small cigars ('cigarillos'), regular cigars and premium cigars. Little cigars contain air-cured and fermented tobacco and are wrapped either in reconstituted tobacco or in cigarette paper that contains tobacco and/or tobacco extract. Some little cigars have cellulose acetate filter tips and are shaped like cigarettes. Cigarillos are small, narrow cigars with no cigarette paper or acetate filter. Regular and premium cigars are available in various shapes and sizes and are rolled to a tip at one end. The dimensions of regular cigars are from 110 to 150 mm in length and up to 17 mm in diameter. Regular cigars weigh between 5 and 17 g. Premium cigars (hand-made from natural, long filler tobacco) vary in size, ranging from 12 to 23 mm in diameter and 127 to 214 mm in length (Stratton *et al.*, 2001). Although the use of cigarettes declined in the USA throughout the 1990s, consumption of large cigars and cigarillos increased by 64% during the same period (from 2.34 billion to 3.85 billion pieces; US Department of Agriculture, 2002b).

In certain countries, considerable quantities of tobacco are consumed in forms other than cigarette smoking. Kreteks are a type of small cigarette that contain tobacco (approximately 60%), ground clove buds (40%) and cocoa, which gives a characteristic flavour and 'honey' taste to the smoke (Clark, 1989; Stratton *et al.*, 2001). Kreteks are indigenous to Indonesia, but are also available in the USA. In India, about seven times more bidis are consumed than cigarettes. Bidis are used extensively in India and in the rural areas of several south-east Asian countries (Stratton *et al.*, 2001). They are also becoming increasingly popular among teenagers in the USA (Malson & Pickworth, 2002). A bidi is made by rolling a rectangular piece of a dried temburni leaf around approximately 0.2–0.3 g of sun-dried, oriental tobacco and securing the roll with a thread. These cigarettes are perceived by some as a better-tasting, cheaper, safer or more natural alternative to conventional cigarettes (Malson *et al.*, 2001; Stanfill *et al.*, 2003). Chutta is an Indian home-made cigar, 5–9 cm long, prepared by rolling local tobacco inside a sun-dried tobacco leaf. Reverse smoking of chutta (with the burning end inside the mouth) is prevalent among women in the rural communities of Andhra Pradesh (van der Eb *et al.*, 1993). Chutta is also smoked in the usual way. Additionally, about 40% of total tobacco consumption in India is in the form of smokeless or chewing tobacco (WHO, 1997). Two nicotine-delivery devices which mimic the cigarette, but heat the tobacco rather than burn it, have been developed and test-marketed under the names of Eclipse™ (deBethizy *et al.*, 1990; Borgerding *et al.*, 1998) and Accord™ (Buchhalter & Eissenberg, 2000).

Reliable figures for the proportion of tobacco that is used for pipes, hand-rolled cigarettes, chewing and snuff (including oral snuff) are not readily available for most countries. Nor is there any good record of the types and amounts of tobacco used as smokeless products.

Tobacco that is grown and used locally is not necessarily taxed or included in national statistics.

1.2   Composition

Both tobacco and tobacco smoke are very complex matrices consisting of thousands of compounds. A total of 3044 constituents have been isolated from tobacco and 3996 from the mainstream smoke of cigarettes (Roberts, 1988). Mainstream smoke is the smoke that is released at the mouth end of the cigarette during puffing whereas sidestream smoke is the smoke released from the burning cone and through the cigarette paper, mostly between puffs. Some 4000 mainstream smoke compounds have been identified to date, and account for more than 95% of the weight of mainstream smoke (Green & Rodgman, 1996; Jenkins *et al.*, 2000). A total of 1172 constituents are present both in tobacco and tobacco smoke (Roberts, 1988). 'Tobacco smoke constituents' refers to all substances present in smoke, regardless of their origin, i.e. whether they come from the tobacco itself, or from the tobacco additives, the paper, the filter or from the air drawn into the cigarette.

The qualitative composition of smoke components is mainly identical in mainstream smoke, sidestream smoke and secondhand tobacco smoke, sometimes referred to as 'environmental' tobacco smoke (an air-diluted mixture of sidestream smoke and exhaled mainstream smoke). The quantitative composition of these different smoke matrices may, however, vary considerably.

Advances in chemical analytical techniques and an increased knowledge of the genotoxic environmental agents brought the number of carcinogens identified in tobacco smoke to 69 by the year 2000. These carcinogens include 10 species of polynuclear aromatic hydrocarbons (PAHs), six heterocyclic hydrocarbons, four volatile hydrocarbons, three nitrohydrocarbons, four aromatic amines, eight N-heterocyclic amines, 10 N-nitrosamines, two aldehydes, 10 miscellaneous organic compounds, nine inorganic compounds and three phenolic compounds (Hoffmann et al., 2001).

Eleven compounds (2-naphthylamine, 4-aminobiphenyl, benzene, vinyl chloride, ethylene oxide, arsenic, beryllium, nickel compounds, chromium, cadmium and polonium-210) classified as IARC Group 1 human carcinogens have been reported as present in mainstream smoke (IARC, 1987, 1990, 1993a, 1994; Hoffmann et al., 2001; IARC, 2001).

Since the last IARC Monograph on tobacco smoking (IARC, 1986a), the focus of research on carcinogens in tobacco and tobacco smoke has predominantly been on benzo-[a]pyrene (a surrogate for all PAHs), tobacco-specific N-nitrosamines (TSNA), especially N'-nitrosonornicotine (NNN) and 4-(N-nitrosomethylamino)-1-(3-pyridyl)-1-butanone (NNK) and aromatic amines, especially 4-aminobiphenyl (4-ABP), because of their established carcinogenic potency (Vineis & Pirastu, 1997; Hecht, 1998, 1999; Castelao et al., 2001; Hecht, 2002).

1.2.1   Cigarette tobacco

The types of tobacco used in smoking products are listed in Table 1.5. The most common tobacco product in developed countries is the manufactured cigarette. A cigarette is defined as any roll of tobacco wrapped in paper or other non-tobacco material. Cigarettes can be either commercially manufactured or individually made (roll-your-own). Cigarettes are lit, and the burning process produces smoke that is inhaled through the unlit end. Cigarettes are approximately 8 mm in diameter and 70–120 mm in length (Borgerding et al., 2000; Stratton et al., 2001).

(a)   Occurrence of tobacco-specific carcinogens and their precursors in tobacco

Unlike cigarette smoke, measurements of nicotine content and other constituents of tobacco have not been made or reported as a part of official tests of commercial cigarettes, although the smoke composition is directly dependent (both qualitatively and quantitatively) on the profile of tobacco smoke precursors.

Table 1.6 shows an international comparison of the concentrations of two carci-nogenic tobacco-specific *N*-nitrosamines, NNN and NNK, and their putative precursors, nicotine and nitrate in the tobacco from commercial cigarettes. The assays of a large number of cigarette brands from Canada, the United Kingdom, the USA and other countries around the world, have demonstrated that there is a very wide variation in con-centrations of nicotine (from 7.2 to 18.3 mg/cigarette) in the tobacco filler, of nitrate (from 0.3 to 20.6 mg/cigarette), NNN (from 45 to 58 000 ng/g tobacco) and NNK (from not detected to 10 745 ng/cigarette; detection limit < 50 ng/cigarette) (Fischer *et al.*, 1989a; Nair *et al.*, 1989; Djordjevic *et al.*, 1990; Fischer *et al.*, 1990b,c; Djordjevic *et al.*, 1991b; Tricker *et al.*, 1991; Atawodi *et al.*, 1995; Kozlowski *et al.*, 1998; Djordjevic *et al.*, 2000b,c). The country of origin plays a profound role in the chemical composition of the product (e.g. cigarettes from India and Italy contained extremely high levels of tobacco-specific carcinogens, namely, up to 58 000 ng/g NNN and 10 745 ng/cigarette NNK).

The higher TSNA concentrations were usually measured in the tobacco from untipped cigarettes, especially those made of dark tobacco. Among the 55 brands sold in Germany in 1987, the lowest amounts of nitrate, NNN and NNK were measured in Oriental-type cigarettes, followed by Virginia and American blend cigarettes (Table 1.7). The highest levels were reported in the dark tobacco cigarettes (Djordjevic *et al.*, 1989a; Fischer *et al.*, 1989a,b; Tricker *et al.*, 1991). Typically, the levels of NNK are lower than those of NNN in cigarettes except in those made from Virginia flue-cured tobacco, in which higher levels of NNK were reported (Fischer *et al.*, 1989a,b, 1990b).

Despite the large variation in the amount of the components measured in various ciga-rettes by Fischer *et al.* (1989a), the correlations between TSNA and nitrate were high to moderate (NNN: $r^2 = 0.61$; NNK: $r^2 = 0.4$). NNN concentrations increased with increased nitrate concentrations and did not depend on the tobacco type. Oriental and Virginia type cigarettes were very low in nitrate and also had the lowest NNN concentrations. The highest NNN concentrations were found in cigarettes made of dark tobaccos, which also had the highest nitrate levels. The correlation between NNK and nitrate was not as strong as for NNN suggesting that other factors such as the tobacco type may have an influence on the formation of NNK. Although both nitrate and nicotine are precursors for NNN and NNK, only nitrate seems to play a predominant role in their formation. Table 1.7 also shows that NNN, NNK and nitrate levels in tobacco from unfiltered and filtered cigarettes in the same blend category were of the same order of magnitude, although somewhat higher values were reported for unfiltered brands (Tricker *et al.*, 1991).

Different types of cigarette are manufactured to deliver different smoke yields under machine-smoking conditions. The terms 'ultra low-', 'low-', 'medium-' and 'high-yield ci-garettes' are not official government-designated terms but are part of the trademarked names of products that provide information on the smoke yields obtained by machine-smoking using standardized protocols. In general, ultra low-yield products deliver less than 6 mg tar per cigarette, low-yield products between 6 and 15 mg tar and regular 'full-flavoured' ciga-rettes deliver more than 15 mg of tar, although different research groups have made their

Table 1.6. International comparison of the concentration ranges for nitrate, nicotine and preformed tobacco-specific *N*-nitrosamines in tobacco from commercial cigarettes

Country	NO$_3^-$ (nitrate) (mg/cigarette)	Nicotine (mg/g)	NNN (ng/cigarette)	NNK (ng/cigarette)	Reference
Austria	4.2–8.0	NA	306–1122	92–310	Fischer *et al.* (1990c)
Belgium	1.8–10.8	NA	504–1939	219–594	Fischer *et al.* (1990c)
Canada	0.3–3.3	8.0–18.3[a]	259–982	447–884	Fischer *et al.* (1990b); Kozlowski *et al.* (1998)
Germany	0.6–20.6	NA	45–5340	ND[b]–1120	Fischer *et al.* (1989a, 1990c); Tricker *et al.* (1991)
France	1.5–19.4	10.7	120–6019	57–990	Fischer *et al.* (1990c); Djordjevic *et al.* (1989a)
India	NA	14–16.2	1300–58 000[c]	40–4800[c]	Nair *et al.* (1989); Pakhale & Maru (1998)
Italy	6.2–13.3	NA	632 –12 454	153–10 745	Fischer *et al.* (1990c)
Japan	3.7–13.1 mg/g	NA	360–1110[c]	190–330[c]	Djordjevic *et al.* (2000c)
Moldova	NA	NA	93–2090[c]	104–484[c]	Stepanov *et al.* (2002)
Netherlands	1.5–8.8	NA	58–1647	105–587	Fischer *et al.* (1990c)
Poland	4.4–12.8	NA	870–2760	140–450	Fischer *et al.* (1990c)
			670–4870[c]	70–660[c]	Djordjevic *et al.* (2000b)
Sweden	2.4–8.6	NA	544–1511	192–569	Fischer *et al.* (1990c)
Switzerland	6.4–7.8	NA	1280–2208	450–554	Fischer *et al.* (1990c)
United Kingdom	1.4–8.0	9.0–17.5[a]	140–1218	92–433	Fischer *et al.* (1990c); Kozlowski *et al.* (1998)
USA	6.2–13.5	7.2–13.4[a]	993–1947	433–733	Fischer *et al.* (1990c); Kozlowski *et al.* (1998)
	7.8–15.9 mg/g	16.9–17.9	1290–3050[c]	420–920[c]	Djordjevic *et al.* (1990, 2000c)
Former USSR	1.7–9.1	NA	60–850	ND–150[b]	Fischer *et al.* (1990c)
	4.2–17.2 mg/g	7.6–9.4	360–850[c]	ND–70[c,d]	Djordjevic *et al.* (1991b)

NA, not available

[a] Total nicotine (mg/cigarette; Kozlowski *et al.*, 1998)

[b] ND, not detected (NNK detection limit < 50 ng/cigarette; Fischer *et al.*, 1989a, 1990c)

[c] ng/g tobacco

[d] ND, not detected (NNK detection limit < 10 ng/g; Djordjevic *et al.*, 1991b)

Table 1.7. Comparison of the ranges for nitrate, nicotine and preformed tobacco-specific-*N*-nitrosamines in tobacco from commercial cigarettes with a wide range of nicotine and 'tar' yields

Country (total no. of cigarette brands in the study)	Tobacco filler	F/NF	NO$_3^-$ (nitrate) (mg/cigarette)	Nicotine (mg/g)	NNN (ng/cigarette)	NNK (ng/cigarette)	Reference
Canada (n = 25)	Ultra-low yield (V)[a]	F	0.3–3.3[b]	11.2–14.4[b]	288–982	447–785	Fischer et al. (1990b); Kozlowski et al. (1998)
	Low yield (V)	F	0.4–0.6[b]	11.9–16.7[b]	292–527	510–884	
	Moderate yield (V)	F	0.4–0.8[b]	11.9–18.6[b]	337–407	569–705	
	High yield (V)	F	0.3–1.0[b]	8.0–15.4[b]	259–381	495–663	
Germany (n = 20)	Blend	F	2.2–7.8	NA	400–1390	100–410	Tricker et al. (1991)
	Blend	NF	5.4–12.3	NA	660–2670	270–500	
(n = 55)	Dark	NF	14.2–20.6	NA	4500–5340	800–960	Fischer et al. (1989a,c)
	Oriental	F + NF	0.6–2.7	NA	45–432	ND–177	
	Virginia	F + NF	0.7–3.3	NA	133–330	170–580	
	American blend	F	1.8–6.3	NA	500–2534	160–696	
	Dark	NF	10.9–14.4	NA	3660–5316	370–1120	
Japan (n = 6)	Low yield	F	5.7–13.1 mg/g	NA	810–1110[c]	190–330[c]	Djordjevic et al. (2000c)[d]
	Medium yield	F	3.7–7.5 mg/g	NA	360–1040[c]	200–320[c]	
USA (n = 13)	Ultra-low yield (AB)	F	13.6–14.0 mg/g	17.6–17.9	1750–1980[c]	500–580[c]	Djordjevic et al. (1990, 2000c)[d]
	Low yield (AB)	F	9.0–12.3 mg/g	17.9	1900–3050[c]	490–800[c]	
	Moderate yield (AB)	F	7.8–10.8 mg/g	16.9	1780–2890[c]	420–890[c]	
	High yield (AB)	NF	11.7–15.9 mg/g	17.9	1290–2160[c]	770–920[c]	

F, filter-tipped cigarettes; NF, non-filtered cigarettes; V, Virginia type cigarettes; AB, American blend cigarettes; NA, not available; ND, not detected
[a] Definite data on the composition of three cigarette brands not available
[b] 23 Canadian cigarette brands; total nicotine (mg/cigarette)
[c] ng/g tobacco
[d] Cigarettes were designated into classes according to nicotine concentrations in mainstream smoke as follows: ultra-low, delivering < 0.5 mg FTC (Federal Trade Commission) nicotine/cigarette; low, delivering 0.5–< 0.85 mg FTC nicotine/cigarette; medium, delivering 0.85–1.2 mg FTC nicotine/cigarette; high, delivering > 1.2 mg FTC nicotine/cigarette. [In Djordjevic et al. (2000c), the authors only report the mean nicotine concentration in mainstream smoke of the six brands analysed, and do not specify which brand is unfiltered; the Working Group assumed that it corresponded to a high-yield brand.]

own classifications (Stratton *et al.*, 2001). Tobacco from ultra low-, low-, medium- and high-yield cigarettes contain similar amounts of preformed TSNA and their precursors (Table 1.7) within the brand type regardless the country of origin (Djordjevic *et al.*, 1990; Fischer *et al.*, 1990b; Kozlowski *et al.*, 1998; Djordjevic *et al.*, 2000c). The tobacco from Canadian brands had the least preformed NNN (up to 982 ng/cigarette) and brands in the USA the highest amounts (up to 3050 ng/cigarette). NNK content was of the same order of magnitude between countries (up to 884 ng/cigarette in Canadian cigarettes and up to 920 ng/cigarette in cigarettes in the USA). Japanese cigarettes contained the lowest concentrations of pre-formed NNK in tobacco (up to 330 ng/g tobacco).

The separate analysis of blend ingredients showed that pure Oriental and flue-cured, pure Virginia tobaccos contain the least nitrate (mean, 1.73 mg/g and 1.54 mg/g, res-pectively) and preformed tobacco-specific *N*-nitrosamines (mean, 34 ng/g tobacco and 216 ng/g tobacco NNK, respectively) (Table 1.8). The highest nitrate and NNK levels were measured in air-cured pure burley tobaccos (mean, 22.5 mg/g nitrate and 477 ng/g tobacco NNK) (Fischer *et al.*, 1989a). Similar data were reported for flue-cured and sun-dried tobaccos from the former USSR (Djordjevic *et al.*, 1991b).

Table 1.8. Nitrate and tobacco-specific *N*-nitrosamine concentrations in different cured tobaccos produced worldwide

Tobacco type	Nitrate (mg/g)	NNN (ng/g)	NNK (ng/g)
Oriental	0.2–6.0	20–460	ND–70
Virginia	< 0.05–16.0	10–600	30–1100
Burley	8.0–41.0	1300–8850	162–1400

From Fischer *et al.* (1989a); Djordjevic *et al.* (1991b)
ND, not detected (NNK < 50 ppb)

An international comparison of nicotine content in blended cigarettes (Kozlowski *et al.*, 1998) showed a similar spread across the whole range of smoke yields (0.1–1.3 mg nicotine and 1–17 mg tar per cigarette). Tobacco from American blended cigarettes (n = 32) contained an average of 10.2 mg nicotine/cigarette (range, 7.2–13.4 mg). The tobacco from Canadian Virginia blend cigarettes (n = 23) contained an average of 13.5 mg nicotine/cigarette (range, 8.0–18.3 mg), and that from British Virginia blend cigarettes (n = 37), 12.5 mg nicotine/cigarette (range, 9.0–17.5 mg).

(*b*)   *The significance of the content of preformed TSNA precursors in tobacco*

The TSNA are formed predominantly during the curing process (Bush *et al.*, 2001; Peele *et al.*, 2001) although small quantities of TSNA have also been found in freshly harvested (green) leaves. The mean concentrations of NNN and NNK in green leaves harvested from all stalk positions of the NC-95 flue-cured tobacco plant were 260 ppb and 280 ppb, respectively (Djordjevic *et al.*, 1989b). These concentrations were six times higher in cured tobacco (1560 ppb and 1810 ppb, respectively). Bhide *et al.* (1987) reported on the presence of TSNA in green leaves of *N. tabacum* and *N. rustica* species grown in India in two different seasons. In one season, at one location, mature green leaves of *N. rustica* contained as much as 46 100 ppb NNN and 2340 ppb NNK. One year later, tobacco harvested at the same location contained 5730 ppb NNN and 352 ppb NNK. These levels were elevated to 15 000 ppb NNN and 25 800 ppb NNK in sun-cured tobacco. The extremely high potential of *N. rustica* to form carcinogenic TSNA is important because this tobacco species is still commercially grown in Russia, and several other former republics of the former USSR, and in Poland, South America and, to a limited extent, in India (Hoffmann & Hoffmann, 1997). The data shown in Table 1.6 suggest that *N. rustica* may have been used as a component of the blend in Indian (Nair *et al.*, 1989), but not in Polish cigarettes or those from the former USSR.

(c)   *TSNA-reduced tobacco*

In recent years, it has been demonstrated that the use of new curing technologies can considerably reduce the levels of TSNA, especially NNK, or even completely eliminate them (Djordjevic *et al.*, 1999; Wahlberg *et al.*, 1999; Peele *et al.*, 2001). Inhibition of the microbial reduction of nitrate to nitrite that reacts with tobacco alkaloids to form TSNA is one method to reduce the levels of these carcinogens in tobacco. The second method was described by Peele *et al.* (2001). It is common practice to flue-cure Virginia tobacco in bulk barns that have forced air ventilation and temperature control. Nitrogen oxides (NOx) are a combustion by-product of the liquid propane gas commonly used for curing; they react with naturally occurring tobacco alkaloids to form TSNA. The newly developed heat-exchange curing method precludes exposure of the tobacco to combustion gases and by-products, thereby eliminating this significant source of TSNA formation.

The flue-cured lamina that were used to produce test cigarettes for the evaluation of smoke composition contained from undetectable levels of NNK to 22 ng/g tobacco (detection limit for NNK, 0.11 ng/g tobacco; Djordjevic *et al.*, 1999). The concentration of nitrogen in the form of nitrite in 'TSNA-reduced' tobacco was similar, however, to that determined for a commercial American blend cigarette (1.8 versus 1.9 μg/g tobacco). The concentration of nitrogen in the form of nitrate was somewhat lower (1.5 versus 2.0 mg/g tobacco) and the nicotine content was higher (22.2 versus 15.9 mg/g tobacco). The levels of NNK in mainstream smoke as determined using the Federal Trade Commission (FTC) method in the test cigarette made with 'TSNA-reduced' tobacco were 6.5 ng/cigarette compared with 130 ng in a commercial American blend cigarette tested under the same experimental conditions (30% and 25% of the levels measured in tobacco, respectively).

(d)   *The origin of TSNA in tobacco smoke*

The question of the origin of TSNA in the mainstream smoke has been also the subject of investigation since the previous *IARC Monograph* on tobacco smoking (IARC,

1986a). The studies have reported different results. In one study, the tobacco column was spiked with [carbonyl-^{14}C]NNK to determine the recovery of unchanged NNK in the smoke, and with [methyl-^{14}C]nicotine, to determine the extent of nicotine nitrosation during smoking. The researchers found that most of the NNK in cigarette smoke (63–74%) is pyrosynthesized from nicotine and nitric oxides during combustion and that the NNK yield in the smoke is independent of the nitrate content in the tobacco (Adams et al., 1983). Similarly, based on the 11.3% transfer rate of [^{14}C]-labelled NNN, it was concluded that 46% of NNN in the mainstream smoke of US blended cigarettes is due to the transfer from tobacco and that the remainder is synthesized during smoking (Hoffmann et al., 1977). More recent studies, however, have demonstrated that the levels of preformed TSNA in tobacco determine yields in smoke. The addition of the nitrosamine precursors nitrate and nicotine to the tobacco before the machine-smoking of cigarettes did not change the levels of NNN and NNK in mainstream smoke (Fischer et al., 1990a). The mainstream smoke/tobacco ratios for NNN and NNK for the commercial German cigarettes, even when corrected for the ventilation and cigarette length, remained constant and were dependent neither on the nicotine nor the nitrate content of the tobacco with the exception of NNK in the cigarettes made from nitrate-rich dark tobacco (Fischer et al., 1990a). The calculated transfer rates for NNN and NNK from tobacco in the mainstream smoke were 23% and 34%, respectively, for untipped cigarettes and 13% and 23%, respectively, for filter-tipped cigarettes. Based on these results, Fischer et al. (1990a) concluded that pyrosynthesis of NNN and NNK is not likely, at least for cigarettes containing Virginia, American blend and Oriental type tobacco.

The addition of increasing amounts of potassium nitrate (0.22%, 0.53%, 1.12% and 1.78% in the tobacco filler) in experimental blend cigarettes (50% Virginia, 15% Oriental, 10% Burley and 25% reconstituted tobacco sheets) resulted in a linear increase in the concentrations of oxides of nitrogen and N-nitrosopyrrolidine (NPYR), a volatile N-nitrosamine. NNK was not influenced by the nitrate concentrations in the tobacco filler whereas NNN and N'-nitrosoanatabine increased slightly with increased nitrate concentrations (Tricker et al., 1993a).

When an American blend unfiltered cigarette was spiked with 10 mg nicotine prior to machine-smoking, no detectable NNN or NNK was formed (Djordjevic et al., 1991a). The addition of 1 mg of the secondary tobacco alkaloid nornicotine, however, increased the concentration of NNN in mainstream smoke by 27%. The spiking of a French dark tobacco, untipped cigarette with 10 mg nicotine increased the NNK level in mainstream smoke by 40%. Brunnemann et al. (1996) concluded, based on the analysis of a variety of commercial Thai cigarettes, across a wide range of yields in smoke, that the concentration of TSNA in mainstream smoke, as well as the tar and nicotine yields, depend on tobacco composition.

The preformed TSNAs in tobacco appear to be determinants of the TSNA yields in the mainstream smoke of certain types of cigarette, although some formation may also occur under certain conditions during smoking.

However, there are other (qualitative) factors to be considered. Of particular note is the trend, at least in the USA, towards tobaccos higher in nitrate that lead to an increase in carcinogenic TSNAs in smoke and a reduction in carcinogenic PAHs (Hoffmann & Hoffmann, 1997). A major US cigarette manufacturer was awarded a patent in 1978 for developing a process that reduces the nitrate content of the reconstituted tobacco made from ribs and stems by more than 90%. It is unclear to what extent this patented method has been applied to the manufacture of cigarettes (Hoffmann & Hoffmann, 2001).

(e)   *The occurrence of volatile* N-*nitrosamines and non-volatile*
N-*nitrosamino acids and other toxic compounds in tobacco*

In addition to TSNA, the presence of several carcinogenic volatile *N*-nitrosamines, including *N*-nitrosodimethylamine (NDMA), *N*-nitrosoethylmethylamine (NEMA) and NPYR has been reported in cigarette tobacco (Tricker *et al.*, 1991). The levels of volatile *N*-nitrosamines in tobaccos from 20 commercial German cigarettes were: NDMA, from 0.4 to 5.0 ng/cigarette; NEMA, from not detected (limit of detection, 0.1 ng/cigarette) to 1.5 ng; and NPYR, from 0.6 to 5.2 ng/cigarette. The levels of NEMA and NPYR were 87% and 53% higher in untipped than in filter-tipped cigarettes of the same blend type. The highest levels were measured in unfiltered brands made of dark tobacco.

The presence of several non-volatile *N*-nitrosamino acids, such as 4-(*N*-nitroso-*N*-methylamino)butyric acid (NMBA), *N*-nitrosopipecolic acid (NPIC), *N*-nitrososarcosine (NSAR), 3-(*N*-nitroso-*N*-methylamino)propionic acid (NMPA), *N*-nitrosoproline (NPRO), *N*-nitrosodiethanolamine (NDELA) and 4-(*N*-nitrosomethylamino)-4-(3-pyridyl)butyric acid (*iso*-NNAC), have also been reported in cigarette tobaccos (Djordjevic *et al.*, 1989a, 1990; Tricker *et al.*, 1991). Some of them, such as NSAR (IARC, 1978), NMPA and NMBA, are carcinogenic *per se* (Hoffmann *et al.*, 1992), whereas others may undergo thermal decarboxylation during the pyrolysis of cigarette tobacco (Brunnemann *et al.*, 1991) to yield their corresponding volatile *N*-nitroso analogues; for example, pyrolytic decarboxylation of NPRO gives rise to NPYR, whereas NMPA gives rise to NEMA. The levels of *N*-nitrososarcosine in cigarette tobacco range from 22 to 460 ng per cigarette, NMPA from 110 to 4990 ng/cigarette, and NMBA from not detected (limit of detection, 1.0 ng/cigarette) to 200 ng/cigarette. The upper values were usually found in untipped cigarettes made from dark tobacco (Tricker *et al.*, 1991).

In 1989, the nicotine derived *N*-nitroso acid *iso*-NNAC was identified (Djordjevic *et al.*, 1989a) and its concentration measured in both French dark tobacco and American blend cigarettes (Djordjevic *et al.*, 1989a, 1990, 1991a). The *iso*-NNAC levels in tobacco ranged from not detected to 50 ppb, being higher in French dark tobacco cigarettes. *iso*-NNAC was not detected in the mainstream smoke of American blend cigarettes and was formed in minute amounts when the filler was spiked with the putative precursors cotinine and cotinine acid 4-(methylamino)-4-(3-pyridyl)butyric acid (COTAC) prior to machine smoking (Djordjevic *et al.*, 1991a).

The minute amounts of preformed *iso*-NNAC in blended tobacco (other than dark tobacco), its very low transfer rate in mainstream smoke (1.1%), and the possibility that this compound can also be formed endogenously, could make it a suitable candidate bio-marker for the assessment of the levels of endogenously formed tobacco-derived N–nitrosamines. However, in one study, *iso*-NNAC was detected in the urine of four of 20 cigarette smokers (at levels of 44, 65, 74 and 163 ng/day) (Tricker *et al.*, 1993b). The oral administration of nicotine and cotinine to abstaining smokers did not result in *iso*-NNAC excretion even after supplementation with 150 mg oral nitrate. The authors concluded that the occasional presence of *iso*-NNAC in smokers' urine resulted from exogenous expo-sure to the preformed compounds in mainstream smoke and not from the endogenous nitrosation of nicotine and its metabolites. It was not clear whether there were any smokers of dark tobacco cigarettes among the 20 volunteers in this study.

Stanfill and Ashley (1999) quantified 12 flavour-related compounds in cigarette tobacco: coumarin, pulegone, piperonal and nine alkenylbenzenes, including *trans*-ane-thole, safrole, methyleugenol and myristicin. In 62% of 68 brands analysed, one or more of these flavour-related compounds were detected (concentrations ranged from 0.0018 to 43 µg/g tobacco). The toxic properties and in some cases carcinogenic properties (e.g. of coumarin and safrole) (IARC, 1976) of these flavour-related compounds may constitute an additional health risk related to cigarette smoking.

1.2.2   *Mainstream cigarette smoke*

Cigarette mainstream smoke aerosol can be broadly categorized as consisting of CO, other vapour-phase components, particulate matter (tar) and nicotine. These four major components of smoke are simultaneously delivered to the active smoker as a complex and dynamic aerosol containing thousands of chemical constituents composed of several billion electrically-charged semi-liquid particles per cm^3 (aerodynamic diameter, 0.1–0.3 µm; 5×10^9 particles per cm^3) within the mixture of combustion gases (Smith & Fischer, 2001). The chemicals in the mainstream smoke aerosol are distributed between the particulate and vapour phase depending on their physical properties (e.g. volatility and stability) and their chemical properties as well as the characteristics of the environment (Jenkins *et al.*, 2000).

According to Hoffmann and Hoffmann (1997, 2001) and Kozlowski *et al.* (2001), the composition of cigarettes and of cigarette smoke has changed dramatically since the first large-scale epidemiological studies linking smoking and lung cancer were conducted in the 1950s (Doll & Hill, 1950; Wynder & Graham, 1950) and the subsequent reports of the Royal College of Physicians (1962), US Department of Health and Human Services (1964) and IARC (1986a). During that period, numerous carcinogens in tobacco smoke were identified and quantified and their biological activities and relevance to cancer have also been studied. The major focus, though, has been on PAHs such as benzo[*a*]pyrene and TSNAs such as NNK, which are considered to be major lung carcinogens (Hecht, 1998, 1999). 4-ABP and other aromatic amines have also been studied intensively because of their role in bladder carcinogenesis (Castelao *et al.*, 2001). The carcinogenic heterocyclic amines such as 2-amino-1-methyl-6-phenylimidazo(4,5-*b*)pyridine (PhIP), frequently found in cooked foods, and 2-amino-6-methyldipyrido[1,2-*a*:3′,2′-*d*]imidazole (Glu-P-1) and 2-aminodipyridol[1,2-*a*:3′,2′-*d*]imidazole (Glu-P-2), the pyrolysis products of glutamic acid, have also been quantified in the smoke of filtered cigarettes from Japan, the United Kingdom and the USA (Kanai *et al.*, 1990; Manabe *et al.*, 1991).

(*a*)   *Nicotine, tar and CO yields and other components in cigarette smoke*

(i)   *Machine-smoking method — ISO/FTC parameters*

In 1998, there were 1294 brands of cigarette on the market in the USA for which the emissions of tar, nicotine and carbon monoxide (CO) had been measured (Federal Trade Commission, 2000). The reported emissions were based on a standardized machine-smoking procedure, introduced in 1936 by Bradford *et al.*, and adopted with some modifications by the Federal Trade Commission (Federal Trade Commission, 1967; Pillsbury *et al.*, 1969). This method sets up the smoking machine to draw 35-mL puffs of 2 sec duration once per minute until the predetermined butt length of 23 mm for unfiltered cigarettes — or the length of filter over wrapping paper plus 3 mm for filtered cigarettes — has been reached. Ventilation holes (when present) are not blocked during smoking.

The FTC machine-smoking method, which is used in the USA, is very similar to that of the International Organization for Standardization (ISO), which is used widely throughout the rest of the world (Eberhardt & Scherer, 1995). The key parameters of these and of the other machine-smoking protocols referred to in this monograph are summarized in Table 1.9.

Table 1.9. Machine-smoking protocols for measuring smoke yields of tobacco products

Protocol	Puff duration (sec)	Puff interval (sec)	Puff volume (mL)	Butt length (mm)	Filter ventilation holes
Tobacco Research Council	2	60	35	25	NA
Federal Trade Commission	2	60	35	23[a]	Open
International Standards Organization	2	60	35	23[a]	Open
Massachusetts	2	30	45	23[a]	50% blocked
Health Canada 1998–99	2	26	56	23[a]	Fully blocked
Health Canada 2000	2	30	55	23[a]	Fully blocked
International Committee for Cigar Smoke Study	1.5	40	20	33	Open

NA, not applicable
[a] Cigarettes smoked to a 23-mm butt length or, if in excess of 23 mm, to the length of the filter and overwrap plus 3 mm

Tar yields in mainstream smoke are influenced primarily by filtration, ventilation (filter tip ventilation and paper porosity) and the choice of tobacco type and blending recipe. As with any agricultural product, there is natural variation in tobacco composition from year to year. In order to manufacture a consistent product, tobacco blends are made using the crops from previous years. The length of cigarettes and their burning rate also influence smoke yields. A faster rate of burning results in a lower tar yield in mainstream smoke per cigarette, because the burn time determines the number of puffs and the total tar delivery increases with each puff (Kozlowski et al., 1980; Darby et al., 1984; Kozlowski et al., 1998).

The tar and nicotine yields of cigarettes marketed in the USA have been systematically reported by the FTC since 1967, and the carbon monoxide (CO) ratings since 1980. The mainstream smoke of cigarettes currently marketed in the USA yields from < 0.05 mg to 2 mg nicotine, < 0.5 mg to 27 mg tar and < 0.5 mg to 22 mg CO per cigarette. The sales-weighted average yields of nicotine and 'tar' in smoke are now 0.9 mg and 12 mg per cigarette, compared with 1.4 mg and 21.6 mg, respectively, in 1968, a decrease of about 40% (Federal Trade Commission, 2000).

The reduction in tar has been achieved by several methods including reduced tobacco weight, improved filtration, dilution with air through ventilation holes on the filter wrapping paper, the use of reconstituted and expanded tobacco, the use of chemical additives to control the combustion rate and changes in agronomic practices. These modifications have also significantly reduced the yields of constituents associated with the vapour phase (Hoffmann & Hoffmann, 2001; Kozlowski et al., 2001). For example, in comparison with an untipped cigarette with a yield of vinyl chloride of 15.3 ng/cigarette, charcoal filtration reduced vinyl chloride in mainstream smoke to 5.1 ng/cigarette. The yield of benzene in mainstream smoke was correlated with the amount of tobacco burned and with the tar level. Agronomic factors such as production practices and soil characteristics, and environmental conditions such as rainfall, reportedly influence the accumulation of metals, including cadmium, beryllium, chromium, nickel and arsenic in the leaf. The use of fertilizers low in nitrates and heavy metals could reduce the yields of specific constituents in mainstream smoke (Smith et al., 1997).

In the USA, the FTC-rated yields of tar and nicotine in smoke decreased by at least 60% between 1950 and 1993 due largely to the introduction of filters (Stellman et al., 1997). However, smokers responded to low-yield cigarettes by changing their smoking behaviour so that they still obtained the desired amount of nicotine. Nicotine concentration in mainstream smoke is highly correlated with that of tar ($r = 0.97$ [0.93–0.99]; Kozlowski et al., 1998). The subject of changes in lung cancer mortality or incidence subsequent to changes in cigarette composition is discussed in Section 2.1.

In the United Kingdom, sales-weighted average tar yields have declined steadily. For example, in 1999, tar yield was 9.6 mg per cigarette, less than half the level in 1972. Over the same period, nicotine yields have decreased from 1.33 mg to 0.8 mg per cigarette; CO yields have shown smaller declines. At the same time as the absolute yields have declined, there have also been changes in tar to nicotine ratios. Smokers in the United Kingdom in

1999 were exposed to 22% less tar per unit of nicotine than in 1973. In the United Kingdom, cigarettes have been tested according to ISO standards since 1991. Before 1991, the Laboratory of the Government Chemist used a UK-specific definition of butt length, which resulted in slightly higher yields than the ISO method. There were also changes to the way nicotine was measured in 1991 which resulted in a decline of about 5% in values measured, or 0.05 mg/cigarette for a mean yield of 1 mg (Jarvis, 2001). During 1983–90, a series of special studies investigated the yields and range of additional analytes (e.g. hydrogen cyanide, aldehydes, acrolein, nitric oxide (NO), low-molecular weight phenols and PAHs) and their inter-relationship with the routinely monitored components. With the exception of NO, which is strongly dependent on tobacco type, and the delivery of some phenols and PAHs, the routinely monitored tar, nicotine and CO provided an adequate guide to the yields of other analytes in mainstream smoke of cigarettes available in the United Kingdom in the 1980s. Standard machine smoking conditions in terms of the duration (2 sec), volume (35 mL) and interval (58 sec) between puffs were applied (Phillips & Waller, 1991).

(ii)   *ISO–FTC machine-smoking method — human smoking parameters*

When standard international smoking conditions (cigarettes were machine-smoked to a fixed butt length of 30 mm or filter-plus-overwrap plus 3 mm, when this length was greater than 27 mm; FTC puff volume, duration and frequency were applied) were compared with 26 different nonstandard conditions (variable puff volume, puff duration and interval between puffs), it was revealed that up to 95% of the variation in tar yield per cigarette could be explained by variation in the total volume of smoke produced per cigarette (Rickert *et al.*, 1986).

When the influence of smoking parameters (puff profile including duration, volume and frequency of puffs) on the delivery of TSNAs into mainstream smoke was investigated, the total volume drawn through the cigarette was found to be the main factor responsible for the amount of TSNA delivery in mainstream smoke (Fischer *et al.*, 1989c).

To obtain realistic estimates of smokers' exposure to components of cigarette smoke, the puffing characteristics of 133 adult smokers of cigarettes rated by the FTC as having yields of 1.2 mg of nicotine or less (56 smokers of low-yield cigarettes (≤ 0.8 mg nicotine/cigarette) and 77 smokers of medium-yield cigarettes (0.9–1.2 mg nicotine per cigarette)) were assessed by a pressure transducer system. The smoking profiles for a randomly chosen subset of 72 smokers were then programmed into a piston-type machine to generate smoke from each smoker's usual brand of cigarettes for assays of nicotine, tar, carbon monoxide, benzo[*a*]pyrene and NNK. The FTC protocol was used in parallel to assess levels of benzo[*a*]pyrene and NNK in the 11 brands most frequently smoked by study subjects. Comparison with the FTC protocol values showed that smokers of low- and medium-yield brands took statistically significantly larger puffs (48.6-mL and 44.1-mL puffs, respectively) at statistically significantly shorter intervals (21.3 and

18.5 sec, respectively) and they drew larger total smoke volumes than those specified in the FTC parameters. Consequently, smokers of low- and medium-yield brands received 2.5 and 2.2 times more nicotine and 2.6 and 1.9 times more tar, respectively, than FTC-derived amounts, as well as about approximately twice as much benzo[*a*]pyrene and NNK. Smokers of medium-yield cigarettes received higher doses of all components than did smokers of low-yield cigarettes. The major conclusion of this study was that the FTC protocol underestimates doses of nicotine and carcinogens received by smokers and over-estimates the proportional benefit of low-yield cigarettes (Djordjevic *et al.*, 2000a).

(iii)   *Machine-smoking method — Massachusetts parameters*

The most comprehensive data on the profile of the biologically active mainstream and sidestream smoke constituents of contemporary cigarettes, based on standardized machine-smoking methods, were compiled in 'The 1999 Massachusetts Benchmark Study. Final Report' (Borgerding *et al.*, 2000). Eighteen leading brands from the USA (26 brand styles with between 0.05 and 9% of market share by brand style), delivering from 1 to 26 mg tar per cigarette (by FTC parameters) were screened. All were American blend cigarettes made by mixing different tobacco types and grades, including reconstituted tobacco sheets, expanded tobacco and additives. Cigarette smoke was generated for the assay of 44 constituents (Table 1.10) both in vapour and particulate phase using both the FTC method and the Massachusetts machine-smoking method (45-mL puffs of 2 sec duration drawn twice a minute until the predetermined butt length of 23 mm for untipped cigarettes (or the length of filter over wrapping paper plus 3 mm) was reached: when applicable, the ventilation holes were 50% blocked) (Borgerding *et al.*, 2000). The 'more intense' Massachusetts method was developed in response to the debate on the validity of the FTC method for the assessment of smokers' exposure (Shopland, 2001).

The yields of selected toxic and carcinogenic mainstream smoke constituents obtained by machine-smoking of the 26 brand styles of cigarettes using the Massachusetts method are shown in Table 1.10 (these data were also summarized by Gray & Boyle, 2002). The average nicotine yields of the 26 brands tested ranged from 0.50 mg to 3.32 mg/cigarette. The results are representative of the nature of mainstream smoke, as they illustrate the variety of constituents present and their variations in yield even within a narrow range of products. Relatively few constituents (e.g. tar, nicotine and CO) are delivered in milligram-per-cigarette quantities. Twenty-four of the 44 constituents assayed (including benzene, formaldehyde, 1,3-butadiene and acetaldehyde) are delivered in microgram-per-cigarette quantities and the remainder in nanogram-per-cigarette quantities. For some compounds, the data presented in Table 1.10 compare well with those published earlier by the National Research Council (1986). However the emission of others (e.g. acetone, acrolein and benzene) exceeds the levels reported in 1986. The explanation for these discrepancies is that the NRC values described the range of deliveries measured by the machine-smoking of commercial untipped cigarettes using the FTC method, whereas the data from the Massachusetts Benchmark Study describe the mainstream smoke emissions from filtered cigarettes measured using the more intense smoking method.

Table 1.10. Yields of 44 smoke constituents in the mainstream smoke of cigarettes assayed for the 1999 Massachusetts Benchmark Study

Constituent	Median yield/ cigarette	Range/cigarette	Unit
Tar	25.8	6.1–48.7	mg
Carbon monoxide	22.5	11.0–40.7	mg
Nicotine	1.70	0.50–3.32	mg
Acetaldehyde	1618.1	596.2–2133.4	µg
Isoprene	713.2	288.1–1192.8	µg
Acetone	627.9	258.5–828.9	µg
Nitric oxide	457.3	202.8–607.1	µg
Hydrogen cyanide	380.8	98.7–567.5	µg
Methyl ethyl ketone	170.3	72.5–230.2	µg
Acrolein	162.9	51.2–223.4	µg
Toluene	124.2	48.3–173.7	µg
Propionaldehyde	110.2	46.8–144.7	µg
Hydroquinone	103.9	27.7–203.4	µg
Catechol	92.1	28.1–222.8	µg
Benzene	75.9	28.0–105.9	µg
1,3-Butadiene	75.2	23.6–122.5	µg
Butyraldehyde	70.0	28.8–95.6	µg
Formaldehyde	49.5	12.2–105.8	µg
Crotonaldehyde	44.1	11.6–66.2	µg
Ammonia	36.6	9.8–87.7	µg
Phenol	25.1	7.0–142.2	µg
Acrylonitrile	23.2	7.8–39.1	µg
meta-Cresol + *para*-cresol	19.4	7.3–77.3	µg
Pyridine	14.9	2.8–27.7	µg
Styrene	11.7	4.5–19.3	µg
ortho-Cresol	8.0	ND–33.9	µg
Quinoline	1.0	0.3–2.7	µg
Resorcinol	NQ	NQ	µg
NNN	199.1	99.9–317.3	ng
N-Acetyltransferase	186.3	95.2–298.6	ng
NNK	147.3	53.5–220.7	ng
Cadmium	131.8	31.0–221.8	ng
Lead	52.1	11.0–92.1	ng
1-Aminonaphthalene	30.7	13.4–64.5	ng
N-Nitrosoanabasine	26.2	14.2–45.3	ng
Benzo[*a*]pyrene	22.5	5.6–41.5	ng
2-Aminonaphthalene	15.5	5.7–28.6	ng
Arsenic	10.7	1.6–24.9	ng
Mercury	4.8	2.5–14.2	ng

Table 1.10 (contd)

Constituent	Median yield/ cigarette	Range/cigarette	Unit
4-Aminobiphenyl	4.5	1.8–7.8	ng
3-Aminobiphenyl	2.9	1.3–4.8	ng
Nickel	NQ	ND	ng
Chromium	NQ	ND	ng
Selenium	NQ	ND	ng

From Borgerding *at al.* (2000)
ND, not detected (limit of detection for nickel, 8.4 ng/cigarette; for chromium, 3 ng/ cigarette; for selenium, 11.4 ng/cigarette; and for *ortho*-cresol, 1.3 µg/cigarette); NQ, not quantifiable (limit of quantification for resorcinol, 3 µg/cigarette); NNN, N'-nitrosonornico- tine; NNK, 4-(N-nitrosomethylamino)-1-(3-pyridyl)-1-butanone

The functional relationships established by the Massachusetts Benchmark Study can be used to predict the yields of certain individual mainstream smoke constituents for other brand styles that have not yet been tested, but for which data on nicotine, tar and CO yields measured using the FTC parameters are available. The example brand of cigarette illustrated in Table 1.11 is a full-flavour brand style that delivers 1.1 mg nicotine and 14.5 mg tar according to the FTC method. By using the data on nicotine obtained by the FTC method for the example brand, the yields of mainstream smoke constituents found in the particulate phase can be predicted (these values are shown in the 'mean' column). Similarly, the CO yield for the example brand provides the basis for predicting main- stream smoke vapour-phase constituents. The highlighted constituents in Table 1.11 are predicted based on the CO yield. In addition to the mean values interpolated from the mainstream smoke functional relationships, lower and upper prediction interval values are provided. For nicotine, the predicted upper yield for the example brand was 2.4 mg per cigarette and that for tar 34 mg per cigarette. Therefore, the established functional relationships provide both tentative predictions of the yields of some individual consti- tuents, given standard nicotine and CO yields, and the expected range of yields of some constituents.

The drawback of this approach is that cigarettes with different tar and nicotine yields as measured by the FTC method are designed in ways that lead smokers to smoke them differently. Therefore, no single set of machine-smoking parameters will adequately reflect individual smoking behaviours and the resulting exposure to smoke carcinogens. Moreover, a very large inter-individual variation in smoking topography[1] for each brand needs to be taken into consideration during the exposure assessment. To demonstrate this,

---

[1]Smoking topography is a method of assessing exposure, e.g. how much smoke enters the lung as estimated by measuring puff volume, the number of puffs per cigarette, puff duration, total inhalation time, flow rate and interval between puffs.

Table 1.11. Application of mainstream functional relationships to estimate yield values for a hypothetical brand style: Massachusetts smoke constituent form

Brand name.. Example brand
Sub brand... Full flavour
FTC Nicotine yield (mg/cigarette)................ 1.10
FTC Carbon monoxide yield (mg/cigarette)..... 14.5

Constituents	Units	Massachusetts yields predicted from 1999 Benchmark Study		
		Mainstream smoke		
		Mean	Lower[a]	Upper[a]
Nicotine	mg/cigarette	2.2	1.9	2.4
'Tar'	mg/cigarette	31	28	34
CO	mg/cigarette	27	19	34
Ammonia	µg/cigarette	50	32	67
2-Aminonaphthalene	ng/cigarette	18	13	23
1-Aminonaphthalene	ng/cigarette	37	29	44
4-Aminobiphenyl	ng/cigarette	5	4	6
Benzo[a]pyrene	ng/cigarette	27	24	31
Formaldehyde	µg/cigarette	69	43	95
Acetaldehyde	µg/cigarette	1796	1488	2104
Acetone	µg/cigarette	696	566	825
Acrolein	µg/cigarette	184	150	218
Propionaldehyde	µg/cigarette	125	100	150
Crotonaldehyde	µg/cigarette	55	42	67
Methyl ethyl ketone	µg/cigarette	196	154	238
Butyraldehyde	µg/cigarette	81	64	98
Hydrogen cyanide	µg/cigarette	436	373	500
Mercury	ng/cigarette	6	2	10
Nickel	ng/cigarette	< 12	NA	NA
Lead	ng/cigarette	63	44	82
Cadmium	ng/cigarette	151	110	192
Chromium	ng/cigarette	< 12	NA	NA
Arsenic	ng/cigarette	14	< 12	19
Selenium	ng/cigarette	< 12	NA	NA
Nitric oxide	µg/cigarette	514	409	618
N'-Nitrosonornicotine	ng/cigarette	250	158	342
4-(N-Nitrosomethylamino)-1-(3-pyridyl)-1-butanone	ng/cigarette	176	140	213
N-Nitrosoanatabine	ng/cigarette	231	154	308
N-Nitrosoanabasine	ng/cigarette	33	21	46
Pyridine	µg/cigarette	19	13	24

Table 1.11 (contd)

Constituents	Units	Massachusetts yields predicted from 1999 Benchmark Study		
		Mainstream smoke		
		Mean	Lower[a]	Upper[a]
Quinoline	µgcigarette	1	1	2
Hydroquinone	µg/cigarette	125	89	160
Resorcinol	µg/cigarette	< 3	NA	NA
Catechol	µgcigarette	121	80	161
Phenol	µg/cigarette	37	10	64
meta + *para*-Cresol	µg/cigarette	26	12	41
ortho-Cresol	µg/cigarette	9	< 5	19
1,3-Butadiene	µg/cigarette	89	60	119
Isoprene	µg/cigarette	846	594	1099
Acrylonitrile	µg/cigarette	30	16	43
Benzene	µg/cigarette	87	62	113
Toluene	µg/cigarette	143	102	184
Styrene	µg/cigarette	14	9	19

From Borgerding *et al.* (2000)
[a] 'Lower' and 'upper' values calculated from 95% prediction intervals
NA, not applicable

the smoke yields measured by the Massachusetts method for the two leading full flavour regular and mentholated cigarettes in the USA were compared with the values obtained by mimicking the puffing patterns of two individuals who smoked those particular ciga-rettes (Table 1.12). The smoker of the mentholated brand drew in 5.6 mg nicotine per cigarette and the smoker of the non-mentholated brand drew in 4.1 mg nicotine. These amounts were twice those estimated by the Massachusetts method. Moreover, the smoker of non-mentholated brand took in four times more carcinogenic TSNAs (Djordjevic *et al.*, 2000a) than determined by the 'intense' Massachusetts method or by the FTC method.

When hand-rolled Thai cigarettes made with local-brand tobacco were machine-smoked at a rate of two puffs per minute, an average of 5.8 mg nicotine per cigarette was measured in the mainstream smoke by the FTC method (Mitacek *et al.*, 1990). Indian cigarettes delivered up to 34 mg total particulate matter and up to 2.6 mg nicotine per cigarette when machine-smoked under the same conditions (Pakhale & Maru, 1998).

The delivered doses of some gaseous carcinogens could be higher than those shown in Table 1.10 if smokers completely blocked the filter air vents during puffing. Brunnemann *et al.* (1990) found that the levels of 1,3-butadiene, acrolein, isoprene, benzene and toluene were 3.3–8.8 times higher than the levels obtained by not blocking the ventilation holes. Stanfill and Ashley (2000) also reported that complete blocking of

Table 1.12. The yields of four components in the mainstream smoke of the two leading full-flavour filter-tipped cigarettes from the USA smoked by two individuals

	Full-flavour, non-mentholated				Full-flavour, mentholated			
	FTC[a]	Mass.[b]	HSC[c]	HSC/ Mass.	FTC	Mass.	HSC[d]	HSC/ Mass
Nicotine (mg/cigarette)	1.1	2.1	4.1	2.0	1.2	2.6	5.6	2.2
BaP (ng/cigarette)	12.5	27.8	34.6	1.2	15.4	31.2	34.3	1.1
NNN (ng/cigarette)	270	202.0	794.0	3.9	302	243.1	537.0	2.2
NNK (ng/cigarette)	156	184.0	714.0	3.9	164	198.4	239.0	1.2

From Borgerding *et al.* (2000); Djordjevic *et al.* (2000a)

[a] Federal Trade Commission machine-smoking parameters: a 35-mL, 2-sec puff once per minute

[b] Massachusetts machine-smoking parameters: a 45-mL, 2-sec puff every 30 sec, 50% of the ventilation holes blocked

[c] Human Smoking Conditions: smoking machine programmed to imitate the puffing behaviour of a smoker of full-flavour, non-mentholated cigarettes

[d] Human Smoking Conditions: smoking machine programmed to imitate the puffing behaviour of a smoker of full-flavour, mentholated cigarettes

BaP, benzo[*a*]pyrene; NNN, *N'*-nitrosonornicotine; NNK, 4-(*N*-nitrosomethylamino)-1-(3-pyridyl)-1-butanone

ventilation holes in a cigarette's filter increased the percentage transfer of flavour-related alkenylbenzenes (eugenol, isoeugenol, methyleugenol, myristicin and elemicin) from tobacco to the particulate fraction of mainstream smoke by twofold to sevenfold.

(iv)   *Machine-smoking method — Health Canada parameters*

The Tobacco Sales Act (1998) of British Columbia, Canada, mandates a machine-smoking method for cigarette testing that utilizes even more intense settings (puff volume, 55 mL; puff interval, 30 sec; puff duration, 2 sec; and 100% of the ventilation holes must be blocked during smoking). (For the reporting years 1998 and 1999, puff volume was 56 mL, puff interval 26 sec and the other parameters were the same as those currently in use).

The British Columbia Ministry of Health web site provides information on both in mainstream and sidestream smoke deliveries of 44 constituents in commercial leading Canadian cigarettes (the top 22 brands in British Columbia account for 70–80% of the market) under both standard (FTC/ISO methods) and modified, more intense smoking conditions, known as Health Canada smoking parameters (http://www.healthplanning. gov.bc.ca/ttdr/index.html). In 1999, 'regular', 'light', 'extra light' and 'ultra light' varieties of a leading Canadian cigarette brand sold in British Columbia were reported to deliver into mainstream smoke an average of 0.8–1.1 mg nicotine as measured by ISO smoking parameters and 2.5–2.9 mg nicotine per cigarette when measured by Health Canada

Table 1.13. Yields of IARC carcinogens in the mainstream smoke of Canadian regular size cigarettes — Comparison of ISO and Health Canada machine-smoking parameters

Compound	ISO smoking parameters[a]						
	Regular	Light	Extra light	Ultra light	Regular/ light	Regular/ extra light	Regular/ ultra light
Tar (mg/cig)	13.4	11.1	8.6	5.7	1.2	1.6	2.3
Nicotine (mg/cig)	1.1	1.1	1.1	0.8	1.0	1.0	1.3
IARC Group 1							
Benzene (μg/cig)	56.3	51.8	40.6	27.2	1.1	1.4	2.1
Cadmium (ng/cig)	114.0	108.0	80.2	32.4	1.1	1.4	3.5
2-Aminonapththalene (ng/cig)	11.8	7.5	9.5	6.7	1.6	1.2	1.8
Nickel (ng/cig)	4.0	5.1	3.8	3.9	0.8	1.1	1.0
Chromium (ng/cig)	5.0	2.1	3.3	2.8	2.4	1.5	1.8
Arsenic (ng/cig)	BDL	NQ	BDL	BDL			
4-Aminobiphenyl (ng/cig)	1.4	1.2	1.4	1.1	1.2	1.0	1.3
IARC Group 2A							
Formaldehyde (μg/cig)	60.8	25.8	20.5	9.7	2.4	3.0	6.3
1,3-Butadiene (μg/cig)	46.6	26.4	26.9	15.3	1.8	1.7	3.0
Benzo[a]pyrene (ng/cig)	11.3	10.6	8.7	6.2	1.1	1.3	1.8
IARC Group 2B							
Acetaldehyde (μg/cig)	703.0	565.0	439.0	260.0	1.2	1.6	2.7
Isoprene (μg/cig)	222.0	173.0	131.0	78.8	1.3	1.7	2.8
Catechol (μg/cig)	74.5	74.7	69.0	50.9	1.0	1.1	1.5
Acrylonitrile (μg/cig)	11.9	11.3	7.2	4.4	1.1	1.6	2.7
Styrene (μg/cig)	10.9	5.7	3.5	2.9	1.9	3.1	3.8
NNK (ng/cig)	84.4	58.0	73.1	56.9	1.5	1.2	1.5
NNN (ng/cig)	42.0	23.3	35.2	26.4	1.8	1.2	1.6
Lead (ng/cig)	15.2	13.4	8.7	5.2	1.1	1.7	2.9

BDL, below detection level; NQ, not quantifiable; NNK, 4-(*N*-nitrosomethylamino)-1-(3-pyridyl)-1-buta-none; NNN, *N*′-nitrosonornicotine

[a] International Standards Organization/United States Federal Trade Commssion test conditions: puff vo-lume, 35 mL; puff interval, 60 sec; puff duration, 2 sec; ventilation holes not blocked

[b] Modified ISO test conditions: puff volume, 56 mL; puff interval, 26 sec; puff duration, 2 sec; ventilation holes full blocked

smoking parameters. The tar deliveries into mainstream smoke were 5.7–13.4 mg per ciga-rette under ISO, and 28.2–36.1 mg per cigarette, under the Health Canada smoking con-ditions (Table 1.13).

The yields of six IARC Group 1 carcinogens (benzene, cadmium, 2-aminonaphthalene, nickel, chromium and 4-aminobiphenyl) in the mainstream smoke from the above-men-tioned Canadian cigarettes were an average of 2–4 times higher when measured by Health Canada than when measured by ISO smoking parameters. For example, using the ISO para-meters, the mean yields of benzene were 27–56 μg/cigarette and using Health Canada para-meters, 82–121 μg/cigarette. Similar 2–4-fold differences were seen in mainstream smoke

Table 1.13 (contd)

Health Canada (HC) smoking parameters[b]							HC/ ISO Regular	HC/ ISO Light	HC/ ISO Extra light	HC/ ISO Ultra light
Regular	Light	Extra light	Ultra light	Regular/ light	Regular/ extra light	Regular/ ultra light				
36.1	34.2	28.3	28.2	1.1	1.3	1.3	2.7	3.1	3.3	4.9
2.5	2.9	2.6	2.6	0.9	1.0	1.0	2.4	2.7	2.3	3.3
81.9	121.0	97.0	92.0	0.7	0.8	0.9	1.5	2.3	2.4	3.4
258.0	216.0	263.0	244.0	1.2	1.0	1.1	2.3	2.0	3.3	7.5
18.1	6.2	18.3	16.8	2.9	1.0	1.1	1.5	0.8	1.9	2.5
7.2	23.5	9.4	11.5	0.3	0.8	0.6	1.8	4.6	2.5	2.9
11.8	13.1	15.1	15.5	0.9	0.8	0.8	2.4	6.4	4.6	5.5
NQ	NQ	NQ	NQ							
3.0	1.3	3.2	3.0	2.3	0.9	1.0	2.2	1.1	2.3	2.8
140.0	81.6	79.9	100.0	1.7	1.8	1.4	2.3	3.2	3.9	10.3
76.3	71.9	66.2	66.2	1.1	1.2	1.2	1.6	2.7	2.5	4.3
29.3	21.6	26.8	24.7	1.4	1.1	1.2	2.6	2.0	3.1	4.0
1372.0	1354.0	1133.0	1098.0	1.0	1.2	1.2	2.0	2.4	2.6	4.2
357.0	428.0	356.0	344.0	0.8	1.0	1.0	1.6	2.5	2.7	4.4
144.0	144.0	163.0	168.0	1.0	0.9	0.9	1.9	1.9	2.4	3.3
21.2	34.0	23.5	22.0	0.6	0.9	1.0	1.8	3.0	3.2	5.0
26.5	29.5	26.0	25.4	0.9	1.0	1.0	2.4	5.2	7.4	8.8
174.0	115.0	184.0	166.0	1.5	0.9	1.0	2.1	2.0	2.5	2.9
82.3	52.5	90.6	76.5	1.6	0.9	1.1	2.0	2.3	2.6	2.9
32.1	27.5	25.2	27.0	1.2	1.3	1.2	2.1	2.1	2.9	5.2

yields of 11 IARC Group 2 carcinogens (formaldehyde, 1,3-butadiene, benzo[a]pyrene, acetaldehyde, isoprene, catechol, acrylonitrile, styrene, NNN, NNK and lead) between the results obtained using the ISO and Health Canada methods. Whereas the yields of most of the 17 IARC carcinogens measured in mainstream smoke are significantly lower in the 'ultra light' cigarette than in the 'regular' cigarette, there was practically no difference in yields for most IARC carcinogens between the 'ultra light' cigarette and the 'regular' cigarette when measured by the Health Canada method. For example, in the 'regular' and 'ultra light' cigarettes, benzene yields were 56 and 27 μg/cigarette using ISO parameters compared with 82 and 92 μg/cigarette using the Health Canada parameters (Table 1.13).

(*b*)   *The emissions of nicotine and carcinogens in mainstream smoke:
international comparison*

Regardless of the designation of the cigarettes as low-yield and high-yield, the presence of a large pool of nicotine in tobacco enables the smoker, driven by a physiological need, to titrate his or her own dose by engaging in compensatory (more intense) smoking behaviours (i.e. more and longer puffs) (Henningfield *et al.*, 1994; Kozlowski *et al.*, 1998; Djordjevic *et al.*, 2000a). As a consequence, the more intense smoking will not only drive up the nicotine yield in smoke, but carcinogen yields as well. Therefore, both the qualitative and quantitative composition of a cigarette blend need to be considered when evaluating the addictive and carcinogenic potential of a specific product.

Table 1.14 lists the tobacco smoke carcinogens that have been evaluated previously in the *IARC Monographs* series and for which there is at least sufficient evidence of carcinogenicity in laboratory animals. Among these, there are 11 human carcinogens. The compounds listed here are those primarily responsible for the cancer-causing effects of tobacco smoke. There are also other compounds in tobacco smoke that may be carcinogenic, but have not been evaluated by IARC. Tobacco smoke also contains tumour promoters (phenolics), co-carcinogens (catechol and related compounds), toxic agents (acrolein and other aldehydes) and free radical species (nitric oxide and others). Most of the compounds listed in Table 1.14 are thought to exert their carcinogenic effects through classical genotoxic mechanisms, e.g. the formation and persistence of DNA adducts with consequent miscoding. Non-genotoxic (epigenetic) mechanisms such as cytotoxicity through means other than DNA damage, changes in gene expression via hypermethylation and genomic instability are other mechanisms of carcinogenesis that could operate after exposure to compounds in tobacco smoke.

Data on the carcinogenicity of the specific compounds in animals and humans in Table 1.14 are not discussed in this monograph, which focuses on the effects of tobacco smoke as a mixture. All the data on the carcinogenicity of these compounds are given in the appropriate *IARC Monographs*. The carcinogenic properties of some of these compounds are described briefly below.

PAHs are a diverse group of carcinogens formed during the incomplete combustion of organic material such as tobacco. They are found in tobacco smoke, broiled foods and polluted environments. Workers in iron and steel foundries and aluminium production plants are exposed to PAHs and these exposures are thought to be the cause of excess cancers in these settings (IARC, 1983a, 1984). Benzo[*a*]pyrene is the best known member of this class of compounds. PAHs are potent locally acting carcinogens in laboratory animals. They induce tumours of the upper respiratory tract and lung when administered by inhalation, instillation in the trachea or implantation in the lung (IARC, 1973, 1983a).

N-Nitrosamines are a large group of carcinogens that induce tumours in a wide variety of animal species and tissues. There is no reason to assume that humans might be resistant to the effects of these carcinogens. They are present in small amounts in foods and can be formed endogenously, but tobacco products are the most widespread and largest source of

Table 1.14. Carcinogens in cigarette smoke

Agent	Amount in mainstream cigarette smoke	IARC Monographs evaluation of carcinogenicity			Monograph volume, year
		In animals	In humans	IARC Group	
Polynuclear aromatic hydrocarbons					
Benz[a]anthracene	20–70 ng	Sufficient		2A	32, 1983a; S7, 1987
Benzo[b]fluoranthene	4–22 ng	Sufficient		2B	32, 1983a; S7, 1987
Benzo[j]fluoranthene	6–21 ng	Sufficient		2B	32, 1983a; S7, 1987
Benzo[k]fluoranthene	6–12 ng	Sufficient		2B	32, 1983a; S7, 1987
Benzo[a]pyrene	8.5–11.6 ng[a]	Sufficient		2A	32, 1983a; S7, 1987
Dibenz[a,h]anthracene	4 ng	Sufficient		2A	32, 1983a; S7, 1987
Dibenzo[a,i]pyrene	1.7–3.2 ng	Sufficient		2B	32, 1983a; S7, 1987
Dibenzo[a,e]pyrene	Present	Sufficient		2B	32, 1983a; S7, 1987
Indeno[1,2,3-cd]pyrene	4–20 ng	Sufficient		2B	32, 1983a; S7, 1987
5-Methylchrysene	ND–0.6 ng	Sufficient		2B	32, 1983a; S7, 1987
Heterocyclic hydrocarbons					
Furan	20–40 µg[b]	Sufficient		2B	63, 1995b
Dibenz(a,h)acridine	ND– 0.1 ng	Sufficient		2B	32, 1983a; S7, 1987
Dibenz(a,j)acridine	ND–10 ng	Sufficient		2B	32, 1983a; S7, 1987
Dibenzo(c,g)carbazole	ND– 0.7 ng	Sufficient		2B	32, 1983a; S7, 1987
Benzo(b)furan	present	Sufficient		2B	63, 1995b
N-Nitrosamines					
N-Nitrosodimethylamine	0.1–180 ng[b]	Sufficient		2A	17, 1978; S7, 1987
N-Nitrosoethylmethylamine	ND–13 ng	Sufficient		2B	17, 1978; S7, 1987
N-Nitrosodiethylamine	ND–25 ng[b]	Sufficient		2A	17, 1978; S7, 1987
N-Nitrosopyrrolidine	1.5–110 ng[b]	Sufficient		2B	17, 1978; S7, 1987
N-Nitrosopiperidine	ND–9 ng	Sufficient		2B	17, 1978; S7, 1987
N-Nitrosodiethanolamine	ND–36 ng[b]	Sufficient		2B	17, 1978; 77, 2000
N'-Nitrosonornicotine	154–196 ng[a]	Sufficient		2B[c]	37, 1985b; S7, 1987
4-(Methylnitrosamino)-1-(3-pyridyl)-1-butanone	110–133 ng[a]	Sufficient		2B[c]	37, 1985b; S7, 1987
Aromatic amines					
2-Toluidine	30–200 ng[b]	Sufficient	Limited	2A	S7, 1987; 77, 2000
2,6-Dimethylaniline	4–50 ng	Sufficient		2B	57, 1993
2-Naphthylamine	1–22 ng[b]	Sufficient	Sufficient	1	4, 1974; S7, 1987
4-Aminobiphenyl	2–5 ng[b]	Sufficient	Sufficient	1	1, 1972; S7, 1987
N-Heterocyclic amines					
A-α-C	25–260 ng	Sufficient		2B	40, 1986b; S7, 1987
MeA-α-C	2–37 ng	Sufficient		2B	40, 1986b; S7, 1987
IQ	0.3 ng	Sufficient		2A	S7, 1987; 56, 1993

Table 1.14 (contd)

Agent	Amount in mainstream cigarette smoke	*IARC Monographs* evaluation of carcinogenicity			Monograph volume, year
		In animals	In humans	IARC Group	
Trp-P-1	0.3–0.5 ng	Sufficient		2B	*31*, 1983b; *S7*, 1987
Trp-P-2	0.8–1.1 ng	Sufficient		2B	*31*, 1983b; *S7*, 1987
Glu-P-1	0.37–0.89 ng	Sufficient		2B	*40*, 1986b; *S7*, 1987
Glu-P-2	0.25–0.88 ng	Sufficient		2B	*40*, 1986b; *S7*, 1987
PhIP	11–23 ng	Sufficient		2B	*56*, 1993b
Aldehydes					
Formaldehyde	10.3–25 µg[a]	Sufficient	Limited	2A	*S7*, 1987; *62*, 1995a
Acetaldehyde	770–864 µg[a]	Sufficient		2B	*S7*, 1987; *71*, 1999
Phenolic compounds					
Catechol	59–81 µg[a]	Sufficient		2B	*S7*, 1987; *71*, 1999
Caffeic acid	< 3 µg	Sufficient		2B	*56*, 1993b
Volatile hydrocarbons					
1,3-Butadiene	20–40 µg[b]	Sufficient	Limited	2A	*S7*, 1987; *71*, 1999
Isoprene	450–1000 µg	Sufficient		2B	*60*, 1994; *71*, 1999
Benzene	12–50 µg[b]	Sufficient	Sufficient	1	*29*, 1982; *S7*, 1987
Nitrohydrocarbons					
Nitromethane	0.5–0.6 µg	Sufficient		2B	*77*, 2000
2-Nitropropane	0.7–1.2 ng[c]	Sufficient		2B	*S7*, 1987; *71*, 1999
Nitrobenzene	25 µg	Sufficient		2B	*65*, 1996
Miscellaneous organic compounds					
Acetamide	38–56 µg	Sufficient		2B	*S7*, 1987; *71*, 1999
Acrylamide	present	Sufficient		2A	*S7*, 1987; *60*, 1994
Acrylonitrile	3–15 µg	Sufficient		2B	*S7*, 1987; *71*, 1999
Vinyl chloride	11–15 ng	Sufficient	Sufficient	1	*19*, 1979; *S7*, 1987
1,1-Dimethylhydrazine	present	Sufficient		2B	*4*, 1974; *71*, 1999
Ethylene oxide	7 µg	Sufficient	Limited	1	*60*, 1994; *S7*, 1987
Propylene oxide	0–100 ng	Sufficient		2B	*60*, 1994; *S7*, 1987
Hydrazine	24–43 ng	Sufficient		2B	*S7*, 1987; *71*, 1999
Urethane	20–38 ng[b]	Sufficient		2B	*7*, 1974; *S7*, 1987
Metals and metal compounds					
Arsenic	40–120 ng[b]	Sufficient	Sufficient	1	*84*, 2004a
Beryllium	0.5 ng	Sufficient	Sufficient	1	*S7*, 1987; *58*, 1993a
Nickel	ND–600 ng	Sufficient	Sufficient	1	*S7*, 1987; *49*, 1990
Chromium (hexavalent)	4–70 ng	Sufficient	Sufficient	1	*S7*, 1987; *49*, 1990
Cadmium	41–62 ng[b]	Sufficient	Sufficient	1	*S7*, 1987; *58*, 1993a
Cobalt	0.13–0.20 ng	Sufficient		2B	*52*, 1991

Table 1.14 (contd)

Agent	Amount in mainstream cigarette smoke	IARC Monographs evaluation of carcinogenicity			Monograph volume, year
		In animals	In humans	IARC Group	
Lead (inorganic)	34–85 ng	Sufficient	Limited	2A	*23*, 1980; *S7*, 1987; *87*, 2004b
Radio-isotope Polonium-210	0.03–1.0 pCi	Sufficient		1	*78*, 2001

This table (modified from Hoffmann *et al.*, 2001) shows components of unfiltered mainstream cigarette smoke, with amounts given per cigarette. Virtually all these compounds are known carcinogens in experimental animals. In combination with data on cancer in humans and – in some cases – other relevant data (see *Preamble*), IARC Monographs classifications for these agents have been established as Group 2B (possibly carcinogenic to humans), Group 2A (probably carcinogenic to humans) or Group 1 (carcinogenic to humans). When IARC evaluations were made more than twice, only the two most recent Monographs are listed, with volume number and year of publication. No entry in the column 'humans' indicates inadequate evidence or no data.

Abbreviations: *S7*, Supplement 7 of the *IARC Monographs*; ND, not detected; A-α-C, 2-amino-9*H*-pyrido[2,3-*b*]indole; MeA-α-C, 2-amino-3-methyl-9*H*-pyrido[2,3-*b*]indole; IQ, 2-amino-3-methylimidazo-[4,5-*b*]quinoline; Trp-P-1,3-amino-1,4-dimethyl-5*H*-pyrido[4,3-*b*]indole; Trp-P-2, 3-amino-1-methyl-5*H*-pyrido[4,3-*b*]indole; Glu-P-1,2-amino-6-methyl[1,2-*a*:3′,2″-*d*]imidazole; Glu-P-2,2-aminodipyrido[1,2-*a*:3′,2″-*d*]imidazole; PhIP, 2-amino-1-methyl-6-phenylimidazo[4,5-*b*]pyridine; pCi, picoCurie.

[a] Data from Swauger *et al.* (2002) (for 'full-flavour' cigarettes)
[b] Data from US Department of Health and Human Services (1989)
[c] Corrected value (see Fowler & Bates, 2000)

exposure to these carcinogens. Tobacco smoke contains volatile *N*-nitrosamines such as NDMA and NPYR as well as TSNAs such as NNN and NNK. TSNAs are chemically related to nicotine and other tobacco alkaloids and are therefore found only in tobacco products or related materials. Many *N*-nitrosamines are powerful carcinogens in laboratory animals, displaying striking organospecificity. For example, NNN causes tumours of the oesophagus and nasal cavity in rats, whereas the principal target of NNK in rodents is the lung. NNK is the only tobacco smoke carcinogen that induces lung tumours systemically in all three commonly used rodent models (i.e. rat, mouse and hamster) (IARC, 1978; Hecht, 1998).

Aromatic amines were first identified as carcinogens as a result of the exposure of workers in the dye industry. Of these, 4-aminobiphenyl and 2-naphthylamine are well-established human bladder carcinogens (IARC, 1972, 1974). Aromatic amines cause tumours at a variety of sites in laboratory animals. Some members of this class such as *ortho*-toluidine are only weakly carcinogenic. Heterocyclic aromatic amines are protein pyrolysate products found in broiled foods as well as in tobacco smoke. They are moderately carcinogenic in various tissues including breast and colon (IARC, 1983b, 1986b, 1987, 1993b).

Formaldehyde and acetaldehyde induce respiratory tract tumours in rodents when administered by inhalation (IARC, 1987, 1995, 1999). They are weaker carcinogens than PAHs, N-nitrosamines and aromatic amines, but their concentrations in tobacco smoke are thousands of times higher. Butadiene and benzene are volatile hydrocarbons that also occur in considerable quantities in tobacco smoke. Butadiene is a multi-organ carcinogen, with particular potency in mice, whereas benzene causes leukaemia in humans (IARC, 1982, 1987, 1999). Metals such as nickel, chromium and cadmium are human carcinogens that are also present in tobacco smoke (IARC, 1987, 1990, 1993a).

Of the carcinogens discussed here, only NNK and NNN are specific to tobacco products. This is important when considering biomarkers of human carcinogen uptake. Carcinogen uptake in humans exposed to tobacco smoke can thus be specifically monitored by measurement of NNK metabolites (Hecht, 2003).

The total yields of carcinogens per cigarette are often several times higher than their yields in mainstream smoke. For example, total yields (mainstream smoke + sidestream smoke) of four popular Canadian cigarette brands including 'regular', 'light', 'extra light' and 'ultra light' cigarettes measured in nanograms per cigarette were: benzene, 278 000–548 000; cadmium, 115–592; arsenic, below detection level; nickel, 38–631; chromium, 64–78; 2-naphthylamine, 155–193; and 4-aminobiphenyl, 21–24 (Government of British Columbia, 2002).

The data presented in Table 1.15 on the composition of mainstream smoke generated by machine-smoking according to the FTC standard of cigarettes sold globally point to a wide range of emissions of nicotine, 'tar' and TSNA. The highest concentrations of TSNA were measured in unfiltered cigarettes sold in France and Italy (up to 1353 ng NNN and up to 1749 ng NNK per cigarette). The same brands contained the highest amounts of pre-formed TSNA (Fischer et al., 1990c). The lowest emissions were measured in blended cigarettes sold in Canada, Japan, the Netherlands, Sweden and the United Kingdom, with upper values of 66–103 ng NNK. Surprisingly, the NNN and NNK levels in the mainstream smoke of two cigarette brands from India were very low given the extremely high levels of preformed TSNA in the tobacco (Nair et al., 1989). The concentrations of benzo-[a]pyrene in mainstream smoke ranged from 2.2 ng/cigarette to 28.4 ng/cigarette, except in Indian brands, in which the concentrations were 85–114 ng/cigarette (Table 1.15).

The comparative assessment of the composition of mainstream smoke of three popular brands of filter-tipped cigarette from the USA purchased on the open market in 29 countries worldwide showed little remarkable variation in the amounts of tar and nicotine, but substantial differences in the yields of NNN and NNK within each brand (Table 1.16). While the maximal variation in 'tar' levels in mainstream smoke ranged from 1.5-to twofold, the yields of NNK varied from three- to ninefold. NNK and NNN yields were highly correlated ($r = 0.88$; Gray et al., 2000).

To determine what governs the nitric oxide yields of cigarettes, 17 British, 14 American, eight French and one Turkish brand with a mean tar yield of 14.4 mg/cigarette in

Table 1.15. International comparison of the ranges of mainstream smoke yields of selected constituents of commercial cigarettes[a]

Country	Tar (mg/cig)	Nicotine (mg/cig)	Carbon monoxide (mg/cig)	Benzo[a]-pyrene (ng/cig)	NNN (ng/cig)	NNK (ng/cig)	Reference
Austria	9–15[b]	0.7–0.9[b]	NA	NA	42–172	12–100	Fischer et al. (1990c)
Belgium	13–16[b]	1.0–1.3[b]	NA	NA	38–203	29–150	Fischer et al. (1990c)
Canada	0.7–19[b]	0.1–1.4[b]	1–21[b]	3.4–28.4	4–37	6–97	Rickert et al. (1985); Fischer et al. (1990b); Kaiserman & Rickert (1992a); Kozlowski et al. (1998)
Germany	1–28[b]	0.1–2.0[b]	NA	NA	5–855	ND–470	Fischer et al. (1989c, 1990c); Tricker et al. (1991)
France	6–44[b]	0.3–2.7[b]	NA	NA	11–1000	19–498	Djordjevic et al. (1989a); Fischer et al. (1990c)
India	18.3–28.3[c]	0.94–1.79	NA	85–114	6–401	ND–34.4	Pakhale et al. (1988); Nair et al. (1989); Pakhale et al. (1989, 1990); Pakhale & Maru (1998)
Italy	NA	NA	NA	NA	21–1353	8–1749	Fischer et al. (1990c)
Japan	6–16	0.6–1.6	6–19	5.1–13.3	36–129	37–66	Djordjevic et al. (1996)
Netherlands	1–18[b]	0.2–1.5[b]	NA	NA	9–163	5–102	Fischer et al. (1990c)
Poland	19[b]	1.4[b]	NA	NA	68–347	36–105	Fischer et al. (1990c); Djordjevic et al. (2000b)
Sweden	9–23[b]	0.8–1.8[b]	NA	NA	44–141	27–84	Fischer et al. (1990c)
Switzerland	12–15[b]	0.9–1.2[b]	NA	NA	121–226	69–124	Fischer et al. (1990c)

Table 1.15 (contd)

Country	Tar (mg/cig)	Nicotine (mg/cig)	Carbon monoxide (mg/cig)	Benzo[a]-pyrene (ng/cig)	NNN (ng/cig)	NNK (ng/cig)	Reference
Thailand	5–28	0.2–2.4	15–19	NA	28–730	16–369	Mitacek et al. (1990); Brunnemann et al. (1996)
United Kingdom	1–24	0.2–2.4	0.5–17.5	NA	17–123	18–103	Borland & Higenbottam (1987); Fischer et al. (1990c); Kozlowski et al. (1998)
USA	< 0.5–27	0.04–2.0	< 0.5–22	2.2–26.2	14–1007	6–425	Adams et al. (1987); Fischer et al. (1990c); Djordjevic et al. (1990, 1996); Brunnemann et al. (1994); Kozlowski et al. (1998); Federal Trade Commission (2000)
Former USSR	21.6–29.2	0.9–1.4	NA	16.1–27.3	23–389	4–55	Fischer et al. (1990c); Djordjevic et al. (1991b)

[a] Obtained by FTC method
[b] From cigarette package declaration
[c] Total particulate matter
NA, not available; ND, not detected, limit < 4 ng/cigarette; NNN, N'-nitrosonornicotine; NNK, 4-(N-nitrosomethylamino)-1-(3-pyridyl)-1-butanone

Table 1.16. The chemical composition of the three cigarette brands sold in 29 countries worldwide

	Brand I (Camel)	Brand II (Lucky Strike)	Brand III (Marlboro)
Tar (mg/cig)	10.6–15.7	11.8–20.4	8.4–15.9
Nicotine (mg/cig)	0.85–1.3	0.85–1.3	0.68–1.25
NNK (ng/cig)	40–150	50–240	35–325

From Gray *et al.* (2000)
NNK, 4-(*N*-nitrosomethylamino)-1-(3-pyridyl)-1-butanone

mainstream smoke were analysed under standard machine-smoking conditions (Borland & Higenbottam, 1987). The country of origin appeared to be the major factor affecting NO yield. The mean values for American and French brands exceeded those for British brands by three- to fivefold. The NO yields in the mainstream smoke of British cigarettes ranged from 10 to 222 µg/cigarette, those in American cigarettes from 230 to 384 µg and those in French cigarettes from 320 to 409 µg/cigarette. These international differences in NO yields reflect differences in the nitrate content of tobaccos traditionally used in the manufacture of cigarettes in those countries. In 1996, the yields of tar and NO in the mainstream smoke of 33 cigarette brands from the British market were determined to ascertain if the formulations that reduced FTC tar yields when compared with those measured in the 1980s had an effect on NO yields. The mean tar yield was 10.8 mg/cigarette and the mean NO yield 141.4 µg/cigarette (range, 22–279 µg/cigarette). For the 11 cigarette brands for which samples manufactured in the 1980s were available for comparison, the median NO yields in 1996 were higher: 145 versus 110 µg/cigarette, with corresponding ranges of 70–279 and 40–450 µg/cigarette (Laboratory of the Government Chemist, 1998).

The yields of volatile *N*-nitrosamines in mainstream smoke are one or two orders of magnitude lower than those of TSNA. In Germany and the USA, NDMA yields ranged from 4.1 ng to 15.2 ng/cigarette in filter-tipped cigarettes and from 9.4 ng to 76 ng in untipped cigarettes. NPYR levels ranged from 3.9 to 32.7 and from 6.9 to 64.5 ng/cigarette for filter-tipped and untipped cigarettes, respectively (Adams *et al.*, 1987; Tricker *et al.*, 1991; Brunnemann *et al.*, 1994). In Thai cigarettes, NDMA yields ranged from 8.5 to 31.9 ng/cigarette and NPYR from 8.8 to 49.6 ng/cigarette (Mitacek *et al.*, 1999).

The concentrations of benzene and associated volatile compounds were determined in the mainstream smoke of 26 cigarette brands on the British market by the ISO smoking parameters. The average benzene yield was 40 µg/cigarette (range from 3.2 to 61.7 µg per cigarette) in British brands, in comparison with an average yield of 55 µg/cigarette in the USA (Darrall *et al.*, 1998).

In the six major brands of Thai filter-tipped and untipped cigarettes with tar yields of 4.98–34.8 mg, the levels of benzene were 25.5–40 µg/cigarette and the levels of 1,3-butadiene were 44.6–78.7 µg/cigarette. The amount of acrolein ranged from 79.9 to 181 µg/cigarette and that of isoprene from 313 to 694 µg/cigarette. The yields of these substances showed no correlation with tar deliveries in mainstream smoke (Mitacek *et al.*, 2002).

Smoking fewer cigarettes may erroneously be expected to reduce exposure to toxins even if the smoker smokes more intensely to compensate for the reduced number of cigarettes. In a controlled experiment in which the average number of cigarettes smoked was reduced from an average of 37 to 5 cigarettes per day, the resulting urinary mutagenic activity per cigarette increased roughly threefold and daily exposure to nicotine and CO declined by only 60 and 50%, respectively (Benowitz *et al.*, 1986). The reduction of the number of cigarettes smoked from 40 per day to 20 per day was not followed by a consistent reduction in the concentration of biomarkers of exposure to tobacco carcinogens (Hurt *et al.*, 2000).

(c)   *Other constituents of cigarette smoke*

Polychlorodibenzodioxins (PCDDs) and polychlorodibenzofurans (PCDFs) have been quantified in the 10 best-selling brands of German cigarettes. None of the cigarettes were found to contain 2,3,7,8-tetrachlorodibenzodioxin (TCDD). The total delivery of tetra-octachlorodibenzodioxins in mainstream smoke expressed as TCDD equivalents ranged from 0.05 to 0.17 pg/cigarette. The total PCDD deliveries were 4.4–10.3 pg/cigarette, and PCDF deliveries were 1.4–5.2 pg/cigarette (Ball *et al.*, 1990). 2,3,7,8-TCDD concentrations were also below the limit of detection (0.5 pg/g) in cigarettes and cigarette smoke analysed in Japan, but the toxic equivalent value for total PCDDs in smoke was 1.81 ng/m^3. Daily intake of PCDDs by smoking 20 cigarettes was estimated to be approximately 4.3 pg/kg bw per day (Muto & Takizawa, 1989).

The levels of organochlorinated pesticides were assessed in cigarettes from Japan, the USA and the former USSR. The major organochlorinated pesticides identified in tobacco and in the mainstream smoke of commercial cigarette brands in the USA that were manufactured between 1961 and 1979 were: *p,p′*-isomers of DDD (1540–20 220 ng/g tobacco), DDT (720–13 390 ng/g tobacco) and DDE (58–730 ng/tobacco). Since 1970, the concentrations of individual organochlorinated pesticides in tobacco have gradually decreased by over 98%. The transfer rates from tobacco into mainstream smoke were 22% for DDD, 19% for DDT and 27% for DDE. In 1995, the concentrations of organochlorinated pesticides in tobacco from the USA were below the maximum permissible limits set by the US Environmental Protection Agency. Until 1970, the organochlorinated pesticides in tobacco and mainstream tobacco smoke contributed significantly to the bioaccumulation of these pesticides in smokers. Currently, tobacco and mainstream cigarette smoke are minor sources of human exposure to organochlorinated pesticides (Djordjevic *et al.*, 1995).

During the smoking of cigarettes with charcoal filters, toxin-coated charcoal granules and other components of the filter are released in the mainstream smoke and inhaled or ingested by the smoker. An average of 3.3 charcoal granules per cigarette were observed on the filter tips of 80% of the 400 cigarettes examined. An increased health risk may result from the inhalation of tar-coated particles (cellulose acetate fibres, paper and tobacco fibres, glass fibres and charcoal granules) released from the filter (Pauly et al., 1995, 1997, 1998).

The free radical and hydrophobicity-related toxicity of 203 of the 253 different substituted phenols present in cigarette smoke was considered. Of these, 162 that have electron-releasing groups may form potentially toxic phenoxyl-free radicals. In contrast, 41 substituted phenols with electron-withdrawing groups do not form phenoxyl-free radicals, but exert their toxic action primarily through lipophilicity. According to quantitative studies of the structure–activity relationship and evaluations of in-vitro cytotoxicity, the most toxic phenols in mainstream smoke included in descending order of toxicity: 2-(dimethylamino)-phenol, 2-ethyl-6-methyl-1,4-benzenediol, 2-methoxy-1,4-benzenediol and 4-ethyl-2-methoxy-6-methylphenol (Smith et al., 2002).

1.2.3   Roll-your-own cigarettes

In a study by Darrall and Figgins (1998), 57% of cigarettes rolled by smokers for their own consumption produced higher levels of tar than the 15 mg/cigarette that was the maximum allowed for manufactured cigarettes in the United Kingdom until 1998. Seventy-seven per cent of smokers of roll-your-own (RYO) cigarettes made cigarettes with smoke nicotine yields greater than 1.1 mg/cigarette. Dutch consumers make RYO cigarettes that deliver, on average, 13.2 mg tar and 1.2 mg nicotine per cigarette (Dymond, 1996). These findings are comparable with the smoke yields for 31 brands of RYO tobaccos tested in Canada (15.5 mg tar and 1.1 mg nicotine per cigarette; Kaiserman & Rickert, 1992b). In another study, the same authors (1992a) reported even higher levels of tar and nicotine (19.4 mg and 1.6 mg per cigarette, respectively). Similar smoke yields were reported by Rickert et al. (1985) for fine-cut tobacco (21 mg tar and 1.3 mg nicotine per cigarette). Five of six brands handmade from fine-cut tobacco delivered significantly more tar, nicotine and CO both per cigarette and per litre of smoke than did the identically named manufactured brand. According to Kaiserman and Rickert (1992b), in addition to tobacco, it is the combination of the tube and filter that determines the delivery of toxic constituents to smokers. The mainstream smoke of three brands of hand-rolled cigarettes from Thailand was reported to yield 28.5–40.8 mg tar and 1.1–5.5 mg nicotine per cigarette (Mitacek et al., 1991).

The amount of benzo[a]pyrene in RYO cigarettes was reported to be 22.9–25.93 ng/cigarette in the particulate matter of the mainstream smoke of Canadian cigarettes (Kaiserman & Rickert, 1992a) and 48 ng/g tobacco for RYO cigarettes in the USA (Appel et al., 1990). Benzene and associated volatile components (toluene, ethylbenzene, xylene, styrene, isoprene and acrylonitrile) were measured in the vapour phase of the mainstream smoke of commercial and RYO cigarettes in the United Kingdom. The mean quantities of the above-mentioned compounds in the mainstream smoke of RYO cigarettes that had been made using 0.5 g of tobacco per cigarette were of the same order of magnitude or up to 2.6 times higher than the mean values reported for 26 commercial brands of cigarette sold in the United Kingdom (Darrall *et al.*, 1998). Based on a representative sample of 110 cigarette brands available on the United Kingdom market in 1999, the average weight of tobacco in a single cigarette was reported to be 0.76 g (Laboratory of the Government Chemist, 2001). The highest concentrations of benzene (an average of 68 µg/g tobacco) in the mainstream smoke of RYO cigarettes were reported by Appel *et al.* (1990). Appel *et al.* (1990) also tried to measure the lead content in the mainstream smoke of RYO cigarettes, but the concentrations were below the limit of reliable quantitation. No data are presently available on the levels of other carcinogens in the smoke of RYO cigarettes or on smoking topography and the true deliveries of smoke constituents as the result of specific smoking behaviours.

1.2.4   *De-nicotinized cigarettes*

Tobacco-based de-nicotinized cigarettes have been used in smoking research to distinguish the effects of smoking related to the delivery of nicotine or other components of tobacco smoke, from those related to the sensory process of smoking (Robinson *et al.*, 1992, 2000). For research purposes, four types of cigarettes were developed with FTC mainstream smoke yields ranging from 10 to 17.3 mg tar and from 0.07 mg to 1.0 mg nicotine per cigarette (Pickworth *et al.*, 1999). The commercial de-nicotinized brand that was briefly test-marketed in the 1990s had similar mainstream smoke nicotine and tar yields as measured by the FTC criteria (0.04 and 10.2 mg, respectively) and detectable quantities of nicotine in tobacco (0.4 mg/g). However, despite being de-nicotinized, the commercial brand still contained amounts of preformed carcinogenic NNK in the tobacco comparable to five other commercial cigarettes (650 ng/g versus 500–890 ng/g tobacco; Djordjevic *et al.*, 1990). This observation is very significant because it indicates that manipulation of tobacco composition, such as removing a single compound or group of compounds from tobacco, would not necessarily result in a reduction in the overall toxicity of the product.

1.2.5   *Cigars*

Concentrations of benzene, benzo[*a*]pyrene and lead were measured in the mainstream smoke of six brands of cigar following the Tobacco Research Council (TRC) recommended machine-smoking parameters (puff duration, 2 sec; puff volume, 35 mL; butt length, 25 mm), with the puff frequency altered to two per minute. The mean yields per gram of tobacco burned were 156 µg (range, 92–246 µg) for benzene and 42 ng (range, 35–49 ng) for benzo[*a*]pyrene. The quantities of lead were below the limit of reliable quantification (0.2 µg/cigar) (Appel *et al.*, 1990).

In 1997 in the USA, the leading brands of little, large and premium cigars (ranging in length from 7.3 to 17.6 cm and in weight from 1.24 to 8.1 g) were analysed and the levels of nicotine and selected carcinogens (e.g. benzo[*a*]pyrene, NNN and NNK) measured in the mainstream smoke (Table 1.17; Djordjevic *et al.*, 1997). The results were obtained by

Table 1.17. Smoke yields of leading cigarette brands and little, large and premium cigars in the USA

	Medium-yield cigarettes (0.9–1.2 mg FTC nicotine)[a,b]	Cigars[c,d]		
		Little[e]	Large	Premium
Nicotine (mg/unit)	1.11	1.5	1.4	3.4
Tar (mg/unit)	15.4	24	37	44
Carbon monoxide (mg/unit)	14.6	38	98	133
Benzo[a]pyrene (ng/unit)	14.0	26.2	96	97.4
NNK (ng/unit)	146.2	290	805	2490

[a] From Djordjevic *et al.* (2000a)

[b] The cigarettes were smoked under FTC conditions: 1 puff/min, 35-mL volume, 2-sec puff duration, butt length; length of filter overwrap plus 3 mm (Pillsbury *et al.*, 1969).

[c] From Djordjevic *et al.* (1997)

[d] The cigars were smoked under the ICCSS (International Committee for Cigar Smoke Study, 1974) conditions: 1 puff/40 sec, 20-mL volume, 1.5-sec puff duration, butt length 33 mm.

[e] Little cigars had filter tips

FTC, Federal Trade Commission; NNK, 4-(*N*-nitrosomethylamino)-1-(3-pyridyl)-1-butanone

machine-smoking the cigars under standard smoking conditions as defined by the International Committee for Cigar Smoke Study (ICCSS 1974; i.e. 20-mL puffs of 1.5 sec duration drawn once every 40 sec to the predetermined butt length of 33 mm). The delivered dosages of nicotine, tar and CO were higher in premium cigars than in cigarettes. The levels of nicotine, benzo[a]pyrene and NNK were higher by three, seven and 17 times, respectively, in the mainstream smoke of premium cigars. The NNN levels were reported to be 22.4 times higher in cigar smoke (Rickert & Kaiserman, 1999). Another study compared mainstream smoke yields of tar, nicotine, CO and PAHs from 30 cigarette brands with those of 10 small cigar brands, using the ISO/FTC machine-smoking parameters. It was expected that the mainstream smoke yields of those cigars that were heavier than cigarettes would be significantly higher than the yields from cigarettes. However the yields from cigarette-size cigars (length, 74–99 mm; weight, 0.65–1.14 g) are also well above the corresponding cigarette yields: mean tar yield, 10.6 mg/cigarette versus 29 mg/cigar and mean benzo[a]pyrene yield, 11 ng/cigarette versus 21 ng/cigar. This is undoubtedly because cigars do not have the physical characteristics that are used to modify yields in cigarettes, such as filter retention, ventilation and paper porosity. It is evident, therefore, that yields of cigars are approximately proportional to the weight of tobacco burnt (Laboratory of the Government Chemist, 2002).

When little filter-tipped cigars were machine-smoked in a way that stimulated the puffing characteristics of smokers (larger puff volume, more frequent puffs), the emissions of total TSNA were twice as high (Djordjevic *et al.*, 1997) as those determined using the standard ICCSS method. A similar 2.2-fold difference in the level of all smoke constituents due to more 'intense smoking' was reported by Rickert and Kaiserman (1999).

Under standard ISO conditions, the yields of certain mainstream smoke constituents generated from three brands of cigarette and one brand of cigar were substantially different (ammonia, 12.7 versus 327 µg/unit; nitric oxide, 48 µg versus 1.08 mg/unit; NNN, 41.5 versus 931 ng/unit) (Rickert & Kaiserman, 1999).

To control for variations in the total volumes of smoke delivered from cigarettes and cigars, standardized comparisons in milligrams of toxic substance per litre of smoke were made by Rickert *et al.* (1985). The mean deliveries of tar, nicotine and CO per litre of smoke were highest for small cigars, followed by hand-rolled and manufactured cigarettes. Large cigars had the lowest deliveries.

Henningfield *et al.* (1999) analysed 17 brands of cigar ranging in weight from 0.53 to 21.5 g. There was considerable variation in the total nicotine content of the tobacco, which ranged from 5.9 to 335.2 mg per cigar, as well as in the aqueous pH of the tobacco from the cigars (range, 5.7–7.8). The smoke pH values of the smallest cigars were generally acidic, changed little across the puffs and more closely resembled the profiles previously reported for typical cigarettes. The smoke pH of smaller cigars and cigarillos only became acidic after the first third of the rod had been smoked and remained acidic thereafter. The smoke pH of larger cigars was acidic during the smoking of the first third of the rod and became quite alkaline during the smoking of the last third. This phenomenon needs to be taken into consideration when the bio-availability and addictive potential of cigars is being evaluated.

Using the FTC smoking conditions, but with the puff frequency altered to two per minute, the average benzene and benzo[a]pyrene levels in the mainstream smoke of six brands of cigar sold on the US market reported by Appel *et al.* (1990) were 156 µg/g tobacco and 42 ng/g, respectively.

When tested in a similar manner, Thai cigars delivered 7.95–11.4 mg nicotine per cigar, 91–201 mg tar and 111–819 mg CO in mainstream smoke (Mitacek *et al.*, 1991). The tobacco from an Indian cigar brand contained 25 000 ng preformed NNN and 8900 ng NNK per g tobacco (Nair *et al.*, 1989).

It has been suggested that switching from smoking cigarettes to cigars, or smoking both products intermittently, may increase the exposure of smokers to toxic and carcinogenic compounds. In contrast with 'only cigar smokers' who relatively seldom inhale smoke into the lung, former cigarette smokers and concurrent cigar and cigarette smokers have a tendency to maintain their cigarette smoke inhalation pattern when they smoke cigars (Fant & Henningfield, 1998).

1.2.6   *Pipe tobacco*

Five brands of pipe tobacco were evaluated by machine-smoking in a pre-conditioned wooden pipe (bowl dimensions: 20 mm internal diameter, depth at centre 39 mm, stem length 60 mm from centre of bowl). The pipe required 3–4 g of tobacco for filling as follows: the pipe was filled loosely with tobacco to the top of the bowl, the tobacco was compressed by half, the bowl refilled and the tobacco compressed to fill about three-quarters of the bowl. The amount of tobacco consumed was approximated from the difference in weight of the pipe plus tobacco before and after smoking (Appel *et al.*, 1990). The mean yield of benzene in mainstream smoke from smoking the pipe was 344 µg/g tobacco (range, 253–473 µg/g tobacco). (The FTC machine-smoking guidelines for puff duration and puff volume were applied, but puff frequency was increased to 12/min to keep the tobacco burning.)

1.2.7   *Other products*

Bidis: American versions of bidis were shown to have a lower percentage of tobacco by weight than US and Indian untipped commercial cigarettes (42.4% versus 94%, respectively) (Malson *et al.*, 2001).

The concentration of nicotine in the tobacco of bidi cigarettes (21.2 mg/g) is greater than that in the tobacco from commercial filter-tipped (mean: 16 mg/g; Malson *et al.*, 2001; mean: 17.6 mg/g; Djordjevic *et al.*, 1990; mean: 10.2 mg/g; Kozlowski *et al.*, 1998) and untipped American and Indian commercial brands of cigarette (13.5 mg/g; Malson *et al.*, 2001).

The levels of preformed NNN and NNK in bidi tobacco range from 6200 to 12 000 ng/g and from 400 to 1400 ng/g tobacco, respectively (Nair *et al.*, 1989). When the concentrations of flavour-related compounds — nine alkenylbenzenes, coumarin, piperonal and pulegone — in Indian bidi cigarette tobacco sold in the USA were measured, two alkenylbenzene compounds, *trans*-anethole and eugenol, were found in more than 90% of the 23 brands analysed. Methyleugenol, pulegone and estragole were each detected in 30% or more of the brands, whereas safrole and elemicin were not detected in any of the brands. The flavour-related compounds with the highest concentrations in tobacco were eugenol (12 000 µg/g tobacco) and *trans*-anethole (2200 µg/g tobacco) — that is about 70 000 and 7500 times more, respectively, than the highest levels previously found in US cigarette brands (Stanfill *et al.*, 2003).

Ten volunteers smoked longer and took more puffs to consume bidis (354–452 sec, 14 puffs) than to smoke their usual cigarette brand (297 sec, 10 puffs) (Malson *et al.*, 2002). In smokers who switched to Irie bidi (strawberry-flavoured) cigarettes, plasma nicotine levels increased above the levels recorded when they smoked regular filter-tipped cigarettes (26 ng/mL versus 18.5 ng/mL) (Malson *et al.*, 2002).

The amount of nicotine in Indian bidi tobacco was higher than that in Indian filter-tipped cigarettes (38 mg/g versus 14 mg/g). The mainstream smoke of Indian bidis delivered less nicotine than Indian cigarettes (1.86 mg versus 2.58 mg/cigarette). The NNN levels in the mainstream smoke of bidis ranged from 11.6 ng to 250 ng per cigarette and the NNK levels from not detected to 40 ng per cigarette. These concentrations were comparable with those measured in the mainstream smoke of Indian cigarettes (Pakhale & Maru, 1998).

In conclusion, because of their higher content of nicotine than in cigarette tobacco, and their similar or higher nicotine and TSNA deliveries in the mainstream smoke, bidis cannot be considered less harmful to health than regular cigarettes.

Kreteks: Eugenol, a natural compound found in high concentrations in clove buds, is the active ingredient that distinguishes kreteks from conventional cigarettes (Guidotti, 1989). In addition to eugenol, other constituents of clove and clove cigarette smoke include eugenol acetate, β-caryophyllene and α-humulene (LaVoie *et al.*, 1986).

Chuttas: The nicotine content of chutta tobacco is comparable with that of bidi tobacco — 35 mg/g versus 38 mg/g. However, the nicotine level in mainstream smoke from chutta is higher (7 mg/product) than that from bidis (1.9 mg/product) (Pakhale & Maru, 1998). The quantities of NNN and NNK in chutta tobacco were reported to be extremely high (from 21 100 ng to 296 000 ng and from 12 600 ng to 210 000 ng/g, respectively). The reverse smoker inhales both the mainstream and sidestream smoke. The NNN and NNK levels in the mainstream smoke of chutta ranged from 289 ng to 1260 ng per chutta and from 150 ng to 2651 ng per chutta, respectively (Nair *et al.*, 1989).

1.2.8   *Novel potentially reduced-exposure products*

There are currently two categories of potentially reduced-exposure smoking tobacco products that are being test-marketed worldwide:

- cigarettes made with modified tobacco containing reduced levels of carcinogens such as tobacco-specific nitrosamines (particularly NNK), or using technologies that reduce PAHs (particularly benzo[*a*]pyrene) and genetically modified tobacco containing no nicotine; and
- cigarette-like nicotine delivery devices (e.g. Eclipse™ and Accord™) engineered to reduce exposure to tobacco toxins using advanced technologies (Fisher, 2001; Stratton *et al.*, 2001; Womack, 2002).

The cigarette test-marketed as a reduced-nitrosamine product is, according to the FTC ranking, a low-yield American blend cigarette. The chemical composition of the mainstream smoke as assessed by both the FTC and Massachusetts machine-smoking methods does not differ greatly from that of a normal cigarette except that there is a significant reduction in the amount of NNN and NNK in the smoke (Stratton *et al.*, 2001).

No epidemiological data are available for these products and they are therefore not considered further in this monograph.

1.3 Use of tobacco

The forms of tobacco use are as diverse as the cultures and countries in which it is used and the people who use it. It is therefore difficult to compare different populations, as behaviours vary greatly. Although differences in smoking behaviour between one person and another within countries abound, there is some uniformity within national practices, e.g. almost all Japanese smokers use cigarettes. Figures for total consumption provide only a rough, albeit useful, measure of global dose and trends need to be observed over a reasonable period of time before acceptance of their significance (Table 1.18).

With regard to dose, using cigarettes as an example, the indices bearing on it are:
— numbers of cigarettes smoked;
— amount of carcinogen delivered per cigarette (discussed in detail in Section 1.2);
— duration of the behaviour and inhalation practice.

The components of dose are different and less measurable for other practices such as tobacco chewing and pipe smoking.

At present, exposure to tobacco components in most countries is almost entirely through smoke. The products used are mainly cigarettes, although pipes and cigars accounted for proportionally more of the exposure in earlier population cohorts. Several measures bear on the ways in which some populations are exposed to tobacco. These include estimates of national tobacco consumption and surveys of smoking behaviours (which are not always available in developing countries). This section mainly describes global patterns in adult cigarette smoking. Per-capita cigarette consumption appears to have risen in developing countries from 1970 to 2000 (Figure 1.1). The effects of tobacco on health are directly related to the dose consumed and the duration of use. In this context the trends in production and consumption might be expected to give an approximate indication of the trends in risk likely to be seen in the future.

Information on trends in per-capita consumption for most countries is collected by the World Health Organization and, in a general way, reflects actual consumption patterns, with the caveat that they are subject to many of the same economic factors that affect production estimates. The available world data on total cigarette consumption are shown in Table 1.18 (Mackay & Eriksen, 2002).

Selected comparative data from Australia, China, Japan, the United Kingdom and the USA (Corrao et al., 2000) offer a picture of the trend in cigarette consumption in those countries (Figure 1.2). The data from Australia show a persistent decline since 1980, those

Table 1.18. Global consumption of cigarettes (in thousand millions)

Year	1950	1960	1070	1980	1990	2000
Cigarettes consumed	1686	2150	3112	4388	5419	5500

From Mackay & Eriksen (2002)

Figure 1.1. Trends in per-capita cigarette consumption by level of development of countries[a]

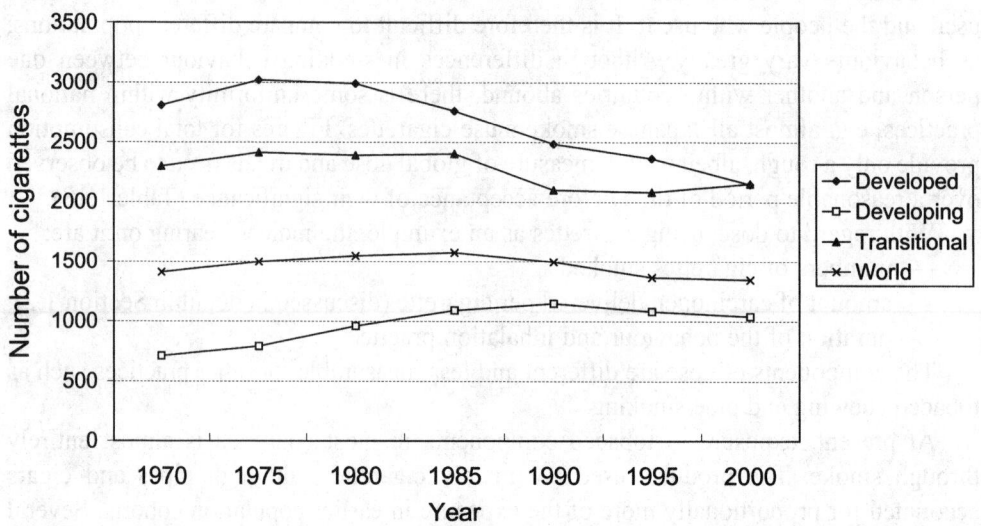

From Guindon & Boisclair (2003)

[a] Australia, Canada, Japan, New Zealand, USA and western Europe are considered 'developed countries'. Countries in transition from centrally planned to marked economies are labelled 'transitional'. All other countries fall into the 'developing category'.

Figure 1.2. Trends in per-capita cigarette consumption in selected countries

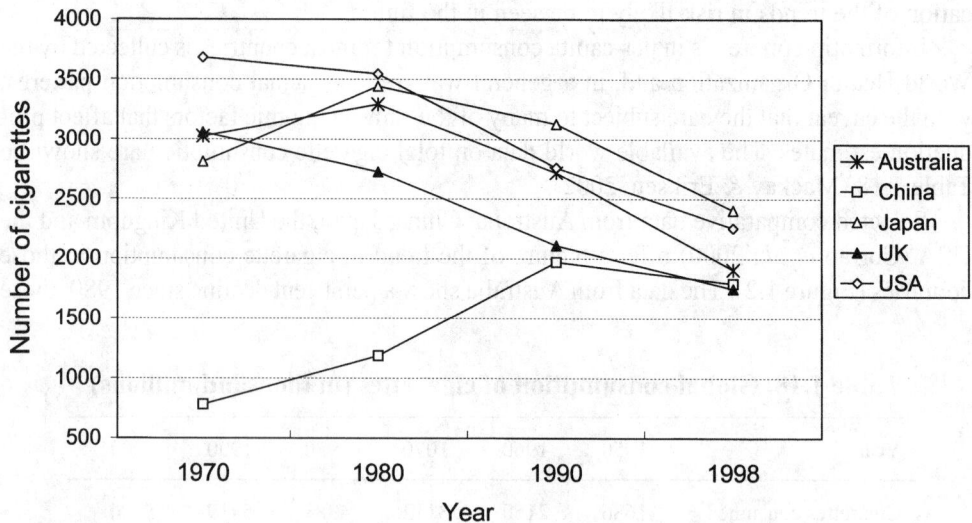

From Corrao *et al.* (2000)

from Japan show a less steep decline also since 1980 and in China, there has been a substantial increase up to the 1990s from a low base in the 1970s.

(a)   Surveys of smoking behaviour

The only means by which it can be ascertained who is smoking, what is smoked, how much, for how long and (sometimes) in what way is through surveys. Regular surveys provide useful public health information, as they may identify populations at risk and some of the reasons they are at risk. Reliable random-sample surveys (using both telephone and in-person interviews) are carried out routinely in most developed countries and, if similar definitions are used, allow useful international comparisons. Table 1.19 shows smoking prevalence rates among adults in the WHO Regions. Since the methods used to collect information vary across these studies, small differences should be interpreted with caution. Nonetheless, smoking rates vary widely across regions. There is about a 1.5-fold difference in total smoking rates between the African or Eastern Mediterranean Regions and the Western Pacific Region. Similarly, smoking rates for women in the Western Pacific Region (5.8%) are much lower than in the European Region (23.4%). A nearly twofold difference in smoking rates is seen in men across the WHO Regions, with the lowest levels in the Eastern Mediterranean Region (34.2%) and the

Table 1.19. Prevalence of tobacco use and number of smokers by WHO Region and level of development in 2000

	Prevalence (% of the population ≥ 15 years of age)			No. of tobacco users (≥ 15 years) (millions)		
	Men	Women	Total	Men	Women	Total
WHO Region						
African Region	29.4	7.4	18.4	51.967	13.420	65.387
Region of the Americas	32.0	20.9	26.3	94.035	64.072	158.107
Eastern Mediterranean Region	35.3	6.1	21.0	52.543	8.670	61.213
European Region	44.9	18.7	31.2	150.628	68.545	219.173
South-East Asian Region	48.1	5.3	27.3	251.699	26.484	278.183
Western Pacific Region	61.2	5.7	33.8	390.632	35.784	426.416
Levels of development						
Developed	33.9	21.2	27.4	114.783	75.891	190.674
Developing	49.8	7.2	28.9	809.725	114.718	924.443
Transitional	54.1	13.9	32.7	82.837	24.153	106.990
World	57.4	10.3	28.9	1005.927	217.755	1223.682

From Guindon & Boisclair (2003)

highest in the Western Pacific Region (62.3%). Based on these weighted prevalence estimates, there are estimated to be over 1.2 billion smokers across the six WHO Regions.

Table 1.20 illustrates the variation in smoking prevalence rates by country (Corrao *et al.*, 2000). Even with the limitations in these data, some striking differences are evident. Women in China, Egypt, India, Republic of Korea, Singapore, Thailand and the United Arab Emirates smoke infrequently, whereas up to one-third of women smoke in other countries, such as Brazil, Denmark, Germany, Kenya, Norway and the United Kingdom.

Table 1.20. Smoking prevalence rates for men and women in selected countries[a]

Country	Year	Age group (years)	Men (%)	Women (%)
Argentina	1999	16–64	46.8	34
Australia	1995	≥ 16	27.1	23.2
Brazil	1995	≥ 15	38.2	29.3
Canada	1999	≥ 15	27	23
China	1996	15–69	63	3.8
Denmark	1998	≥ 14	32	30
Egypt	1997	≥ 18	43.6	4.8
Finland	1999	15–64	27	20
France	1997	≥ 18	39	27
Germany	1997	18–59	43.2	30
Hungary	1998–99	≥ 18	44	27
India	1985–86	25–64	45	7
Israel	1999	≥ 18	33	25
Italy	1998	≥ 14	32.2	17.3
Japan	1998	≥ 15	52.8	13.4
Kenya	1995	≥ 20	66.8	31.9
Mexico	1998	18–65	51.2	18.4
Norway	1998	16–74	33.7	32.3
Peru	1998	12–50	41.5	15.7
Poland	1998	–	39	19
Republic of Korea	1996	≥ 18	64.8	5.5
Russian Federation	1996	≥ 18	63	14
Singapore	1998	18–64	26.9	3.1
South Africa	1998	≥ 15	42	11
Spain	1997	≥ 16	42.1	24.7
Sweden	1998	16–84	17.1	22.3
Thailand	1999	≥ 11	38.9	2.4
United Arab Emirates	1995	≥ 15	24	1
United Kingdom	1996	≥ 16	29	28
USA	1997	≥ 18	27.6	22.1

From Corrao *et al.* (2000)

[a] These data are not age-adjusted or weighted.

The highest prevalences of male smokers are found in Japan, Kenya, Republic of Korea and Russia. In general, more men tend to smoke than women, except in Sweden. The differences between the numbers of men and women smokers are also near zero in other countries such as Denmark, Norway and the United Kingdom.

The data in Tables 1.19 and 1.20 represent only a snapshot of current smoking at one point in time. A more comprehensive set of behavioural endpoints (e.g. time trends in current and former smoking rates) is needed to give a robust explanation of the causes of present and future morbidity and mortality attributable to smoking. As an example, Figure 1.3 illustrates current and former smoking rates since 1950 in the United Kingdom (Peto *et al.*, 2000). Between 1948 and 1952, the prevalence of smoking in men aged 25–34 years was 80% and for women of the same age, 53%. In 1998, however, the prevalence was 39% for men and 33% for women.

The prevalence of smoking in adolescents, although of considerable public health importance as an indication of future cancer trends and patterns, is extremely difficult to measure accurately and, consequently, to compare with other countries. It is usual for smoking habits to become established during adolescence, and smoking rates of young people in their late teens may approximate those of adults.

Figure 1.3. Trends in prevalence of smoking at ages 35–59 (left) and ≥ 60 (right) in men and women in the United Kingdom, 1950–98

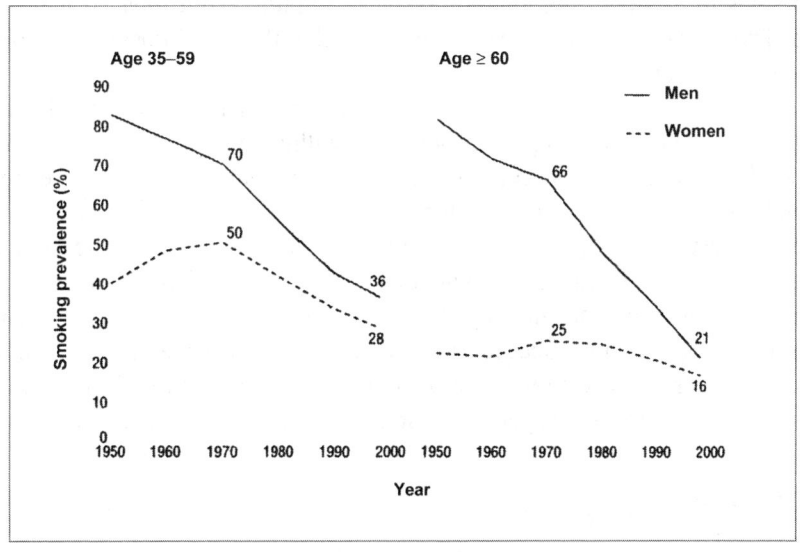

From Peto *et al.* (2000)

(b)   Other indices of dose in developing countries and future surveillance needs

Although the relationship between tobacco smoke and lung cancer in developed countries may be the most researched subject in epidemiological history, there remains a paucity of precise information concerning smoking behaviours in developing countries.

It is already clear that there is a worldwide trend towards the sale of machine-made cigarettes. On one hand, the manufacture of bidis and the various other home-grown, home-made products cannot be quantified readily because it is based on village culti-vation or small industry. These products are generally cheap, vary widely in size and com-position from district to district, and may or may not be subject to taxation. Conversely, cigarettes are mass produced or imported, easy to count and are almost invariably taxed before sale. For this reason, increases in sales can be measured, and taxation figures can be used to monitor sales trends. What cannot be seen is the effect of the market expansion of manufactured cigarettes on the use of other tobacco products. In addition, cigarette smuggling is a significant problem in several regions, e.g. southern Europe, North America and South America (Pagano et al., 1996; Galbraith & Kaiserman, 1997; Square, 1998; Yurekli & Zhang, 2000; Shafey et al., 2002) and a high rate of smuggling will make taxation figures inaccurate. Almost a third of global cigarette exports are estimated to go to the contraband market (Joossens & Raw, 1998).

In some areas (e.g. South-east Asia and India), it is not clear how far the behaviour of cigarette smoking is becoming a substitute for bidi smoking or for chewing, or whether cigarette smoking is becoming an additional behaviour. Mixed tobacco habits are also common. There is no way of estimating precisely the lifetime exposure to smoking pro-ducts such as bidis or chuttas.

The detailed patterns and trends in national smoking behaviours can be identified only by regular measures of smoking rates operating within surveillance systems. There are considerable limitations to the current measures of prevalence. Data are expensive to collect and are incomplete or non-existent in many regions. In many cases, prevalence rates are underestimated because of the limitations in surveillance systems (e.g. fewer members of the lower income groups who tend to smoke more have telephones). Data on smoking by young people are incomplete and inaccurate for most countries. To address these issues, information is needed on initiation, prevalence and cessation. Routine surveillance data are needed to track smoking behaviours over time. In the future, much better methods for systematic reporting of smoking rates need to be applied worldwide.

1.4   Regulations

This section reviews the scope and potential impacts of tobacco control regulations. Because the focus of this monograph is on the risks of tobacco smoking, the preventive implications of regulation are covered only briefly with references to the literature for key studies and reviews of regulatory effects and effectiveness. Increasing the cost of cigarettes through taxation and restrictions on smoking in the workplace are two public policy changes for which substantial bodies of information exist to define their effectiveness (Burns, 2000).

In recent years, researchers have increasingly recognized the role of regulation in influencing the use of tobacco. Policy or regulatory measures alter or control the legal, social, economic and physical environment (Brownson *et al.*, 1995). Policies are 'those laws, regulations, formal, and informal rules and understandings that are adopted on a collective basis to guide individual and collective behaviour' (Schmid *et al.*, 1995). Smokers frequently respond to environmental cues, such as a work break or entering a restaurant, when deciding whether or not to smoke. Regulatory interventions are based on the knowledge that individuals are strongly influenced by the sociopolitical and cultural environment in which they act (US Department of Health and Human Services, 2000).

Roemer (1988) clearly listed a set of purposes for tobacco regulation:
- to set forth governmental policy on the production, promotion and use of tobacco, and to protect the right of nonsmokers to breathe clean air;
- to reduce to some extent the harmful substances in cigarettes;
- to contribute to the development of a social climate in which smoking is unacceptable;
- to provide the basis of allocating resources to support effective programmes to combat smoking; and
- to encourage smokers to stop smoking and to dissuade potential smokers, particularly young persons, from starting to smoke.

The place of legislation in tobacco control was very clearly defined by a World Health Organization Expert Committee in 1983. It stated: 'It may be tempting to try to introduce smoking control programmes without a legislative component, in the hope that relatively inoffensive activity of this nature will placate those concerned with public health, while generating no real opposition from cigarette manufacturers. This approach, however, is not likely to succeed. A genuine broadly defined education programme, aimed at reducing smoking must be complemented by legislation and restrictive measures' (WHO, 1983).

In 2003, the 192 Member States of the World Health Organization unanimously adopted the Global Framework Convention on Tobacco Control (FCTC, 2003), the world's first international tobacco control treaty [added in print after the meeting]. The FCTC was prepared over four years by participants from a wide range of sectors and included representatives of WHO Member States representing 95% of the world's population. The FCTC is intended to provide a comprehensive regulatory structure, which when ratified and enacted as proposed, will lay the legal foundations for the regulation of tobacco and tobacco smoking in a range of situations (e.g. protecting children from tobacco use and exposure, promoting smoke-free environments and promoting healthy tobacco-free lifestyles).

As one example from a developed country, Figure 1.4 shows the correlation between per capita consumption of cigarettes in the USA and historical events since 1900. These events, such as the first US Surgeon General's report, the ban on tobacco advertising in

Figure 1.4. Annual adult per-capita consumption of cigarettes and major smoking and health events, USA, 1900–1998

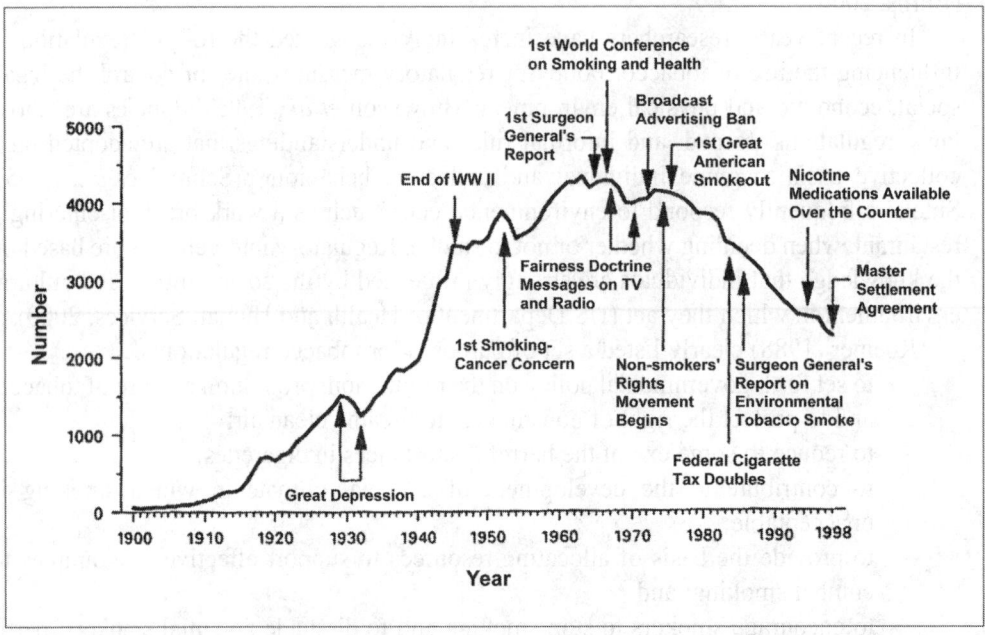

From US Department of Agriculture; US Department of Health and Human Services (1986)
WWII, Second World War

the broadcast media and increases in the federal cigarette tax were followed by a decrease in tobacco consumption. Similar tracking of regulatory events, such as restrictions on tobacco advertising, may be used by any country wishing to monitor changes in tobacco consumption.

Although most of the regulatory interventions discussed below focus on the passage of a law or ordinance, many others can be implemented through an executive order or regulatory action. An example of an executive order is a ban on tobacco advertising on all city-owned buses. An example of a regulatory action is the adoption of an accrediting standard prohibiting smoking in hospital buildings (Longo et al., 1995).

Regulations regarding clean indoor air are described in detail in the monograph on involuntary smoking (Section 1.3). There has been a dramatic increase in the fraction of the working population protected by total bans on smoking in the workplace, which increased from 3% in 1986 to 64% in 1996. The implementation of these restrictions has had two effects on smokers: they have increased the rate at which smokers attempt to quit, and have reduced the number of cigarettes smoked per day (Burns et al., 2000). To estimate the impact of smoking bans on cigarette use, Chapman et al. (1999) estimated the contributions of smoke-free workplaces to the recent declines in cigarette consumption noted in Australia and the USA. In Australia, smoke-free workplaces are considered to be responsible for 22.3% of the 2.7 thousand million decrease in the number of cigarettes smoked between 1988 and 1995. Similarly in the USA, it was estimated that workplace bans are responsible for 12.7% of the 76.5 thousand million decrease in the number of cigarettes smoked between 1988 and 1994.

(a)   Price/excise taxes

A substantial increase in tobacco excise taxes may be the single most effective measure at the national, state and local level for decreasing tobacco consumption (Sweanor et al., 1992; Jha & Chaloupka, 2000). Youths and young adults may be more sensitive to increases in tobacco price than adults (Chaloupka & Warner, 2000). Excise taxes on tobacco products vary widely between the developed countries and in many cases the increases in taxes have been much smaller than the price increases imposed by cigarette manufacturers. The 'earmarking' (allocation of a portion) of tobacco price increases for prevention efforts has proved to be an effective strategy in California, USA (Elder et al., 1996; Fichtenberg & Glantz, 2000), Victoria, Australia (Chapman & Wakefield, 2001) and other places.

Numerous studies have quantified the effects of increases in excise tax on smoking rates. A recent systematic review that looked at the median estimates from a number of studies found that a 10% increase in the price of tobacco products resulted in a 3.7% decrease in the number of adolescents and young adults who used tobacco and 4.1% decrease in the amount of tobacco used by the general population (Hopkins et al., 2001).

One of the main arguments raised against increases in tobacco tax involves the regressivity of such taxes — that is, a tax where the proportion of an individual's income consumed by the tax is inversely related to income. Health advocates argue that the concern over regressivity is outweighed by the lives saved from unnecessary cancer and heart disease due to the reduced prevalence of smoking (Jacobs, 2001). Smoking and mortality rates from these diseases are disproportionately higher among individuals in lower income groups. Therefore, greater decreases in smoking-related disease and death rates in these groups would be expected to follow a tax increase.

(b)   Restricting tobacco advertising and promotion

Cigarettes are possibly the most heavily advertised and promoted consumer product in the world (Mackay & Eriksen, 2002). In 2000, the six major US tobacco companies spent US$ 9.57 thousand million on cigarette advertising and promotion in the USA — more than US$ 26 million each day (Federal Trade Commission, 2002). The advertising and promotion of tobacco products leads to increased use of tobacco products, particularly by youths (Pierce et al., 1991). Advertising and promotion affect cigarette consumption by conveying to children and young adults that smoking has social benefits and that it is far more common than it really is; by creating attitudes and images that reinforce the desirability of smoking, and by suppressing full disclosure by the media of the health hazards of smoking. Numerous institutions involved in cultural events, minority causes and sports are financed by contributions from the tobacco industry. This situation undermines an institution's ability to enact policies and practices to reduce tobacco use (Kaufman & Nichter, 2001).

Numerous governments have enacted laws banning tobacco advertising by cinemas, posters, press, radio, television and at points of sale. Giving samples and sponsorship are also banned in some countries (European Union, 2000). Governmental entities have banned advertising on public transport, in sports stadiums or on property owned by local government. These actions are based upon the conclusion reached by many localities that national laws do not preempt them from restricting advertising on their own property or within their jurisdiction.

Governments also can support legislative, regulatory and non-legislative policies to reduce tax deductions for tobacco advertising, to restrict tobacco promotions like the Marlboro Adventure Team incentives, to prohibit the exhibition of a cigarette brand name, to restrict product placement and ultimately to eliminate tobacco advertising. Recent evidence has also demonstrated that most of the current warning labels on cigarette packets are neither effective in transferring knowledge regarding the health hazards associated with tobacco use, nor likely to have a positive impact on the health behaviour of people using these products. The experiences in countries such as Canada and Poland where the warning labels and package inserts are larger, more visible and simpler should be examined in detail to determine their effects on public health (Canada ASH; Health Promotion Foundation, 2002). Despite mixed findings on the effectiveness of these warning labels, they are viewed as a cost-effecive anti-smoking measure by their mere presence and are considered to be an important part of larger anti-smoking efforts (Guttman & Peleg, 2003).

(c)   Restricting the uptake of tobacco use by young people

In most countries, adult smokers began their smoking behaviour as young teenagers (National Cancer Institute, 2001). In several developed countries, there has been virtually no decline in smoking rates among all teenagers over the past decade. Because smoking begins at a young age, the most important potential actions for affecting the overall rates of tobacco use should emphasize prevention of tobacco use in youth. As yet, the effects of many of the regulatory actions intended to prevent smoking by young people have not been established by research studies.

For example, in most parts of the world, there are laws prohibiting the sale of cigarettes to persons under 18 years of age. Many researchers and public health practitioners have concluded that the only way to limit minors' access to cigarettes is to ban vending machines, raise tobacco prices and excise taxes and enforce laws governing the access of young people to tobacco. Yet the enforcement of comprehensive laws on the access of minors to tobacco has been the subject of considerable debate and the existing literature on the effectiveness of specific types of enforcement efforts is limited and inconsistent (Forster & Wolfson, 1998; Stead & Lancaster, 2000).

Other approaches that may be used to protect young people from becoming smokers include educational programmes, which in some countries have been made compulsory by law, and specific prohibitions against smoking in places where young people congregate, such as schools and recreational facilities.

(d)   Regulation and litigation

Litigation efforts include four main categories: individual cases, class actions, public interest lawsuits and health care cost recovery actions. Within the final category, several cases have been brought by several states of the USA to attempt to recover the costs of medical care attributable to cigarette smoking as product liability suits. In general, these actions are based on the fact that taxpayers pay for medical care for smoking-related illnesses through Medicaid and other state-supported systems. The states had no choice as to whether the taxpayers should pay for damages caused by a dangerous product; therefore, the suits claim a need for the recovery of costs on behalf of all state taxpayers. As data on state-specific costs became available, specific damages were calculated that permitted substantial cost recovery from the tobacco companies. As an example, state attorneys general in the USA agreed to a US$ 206 thousand million settlement with the tobacco industry in November 1998, the so-called 'Master Settlement Agreement' (National Association of Attorneys General, 1998). Results to date from this settlement have been less successful than anticipated because much of the funding from the Master Settlement that was originally intended for smoking prevention activities is being diverted to other governmental programmes. Of particular relevance to this monograph, is that one important outcome of the recent tobacco litigation has been the public release of numerous tobacco industry documents (CDC, 2002) (close to 40 million pages) showing what the industry knew about the carcinogenic potential of tobacco and when they knew it.

(e)   Regulation of tobacco smoke constituents

Worldwide, only minimal regulation applies to the constituents of cigarettes and tobacco smoke, as for example in Europe. The maximum tar yield of cigarettes marketed in the European Union was set at 15 mg/cigarette in 1992, 12 mg/cigarette in 1997 (European Commission, 1999) and 10 mg/cigarette in 2001. In addition to tar, the new Directive lays down the maximum permitted nicotine and CO yields for cigarettes released for free circulation, marketed or manufactured in the Member States, i.e. 1 mg/cigarette for nicotine and 10 mg/cigarette for CO. In 2003, it was prohibited to describe one product as less harmful than another (by using names, symbols). Moreover, manufacturers and importers are now required to submit to the Member States, on a yearly basis since 2002, a list of all ingredients used in the manufacture of tobacco products and their quantities, together with toxicological data on their effects on health and any addictive effects. This list must be accompanied by a statement setting out the reasons for the inclusion of the ingredients. It must also be made public and be submitted to the Commission (European Parliament, 2001). For example, currently over 600 additives to tobacco products are permitted in the United Kingdom (Department of Health, 2000).

In the future, it is likely that upper limits for carcinogens and toxins will be set for cigarette smoke as they have already been for car exhausts and other ambient pollutants. This is dependent on the acquisition of appropriate legal powers by regulatory agencies.

References

Adams, J.D., Lee, S.J., Vinchoski, N., Castonguay, A. & Hoffmann, D. (1983) On the formation of the tobacco-specific carcinogen 4-(methylnitrosamino)-1-(3-pyridyl)-1-butanone during smoking. *Cancer Lett.*, **17**, 339–346

Adams, J.D., O'Mara-Adams, K.J. & Hoffmann, D. (1987) Toxic and carcinogenic agents in undiluted mainstream smoke and sidestream smoke of different types of cigarettes. *Carcinogenesis*, **8**, 729–731

Appel, B.R., Guirguis, G., Kim, I.S., Garbin, O., Fracchia, M., Flessel, C.P., Kizer, K.W., Book, S.A. & Warriner, T.E. (1990) Benzene, benzo(a)pyrene, and lead in smoke from tobacco products other than cigarettes. *Am. J. public Health*, **80**, 560–564

Atawodi, S.E., Preussmann, R. & Spiegelhalder, B. (1995) Tobacco-specific nitrosamines in some Nigerian cigarettes. *Cancer Lett.*, **97**, 1–6

Ball, M., Päpke, O. & Lis, A. (1990) Polychlorinated dibenzodioxins and dibenzofurans in cigarette smoke. *Beitr. Tabakforsch. int.*, **14**, 393–402

Beauman, E., Cowling, P., Leister, D.L. & Roope, R.H. (1996) *Reconstituted Tobacco Material and Method for its Production* (Patent No. 5584306 dated 17 December 1996), United States Patent Office

Benowitz, N.L., Jacob, P., III, Kozlowski, L.T. & Yu, L. (1986) Influence of smoking fewer cigarettes on exposure to tar, nicotine, and carbon monoxide. *New Engl. J. Med.*, **315**, 1310–1313

deBethizy, J.D., Borgerding, M.F., Doolittle, D.J., Robinson, J.H., McManus, K.T., Rahn, C.A., Davis, R.A., Burger, G.T., Hayes, J.R., Reynolds, J.H., IV & Hayes, A.W. (1990) Chemical and biological studies of a cigarette that heats rather than burns tobacco. *J. clin. Pharmacol.*, **30**, 755–763

Bhide, S.V., Nair, J., Maru, G.B., Nair, U.J., Rao, B.V.K., Chakraborty, M.K. & Brunnemann, K.D. (1987) Tobacco-specific N-nitrosamines [TSNA] in green mature and processed tobacco leaves from India. *Beitr. Tabakforsch. int.*, **14**, 29–32

Bonsack, J.A. (1881) *Cigarette-Machine* (Patent No. 238640 dated 8 March 1881), United States Patent Office [http://www.uspto.gov/patft/index.html]

Borgerding, M.F., Bodnar, J.A., Chung, H.L., Mangan, P.P., Morrison, C.C., Risner, C.H., Rogers, J.C., Simmons, D.F., Uhrig, M.S., Wendelboe, F.N., Wingate, D.E. & Winkler, L.S. (1998) Chemical and biological studies of a new cigarette that primarily heats tobacco. Part I. Chemical composition of mainstream smoke. *Food chem. Toxicol.*, **36**, 169–182

Borgerding, M.F., Bodnar, J.A. & Wingate, D.E. (2000) *The 1999 Massachusetts Benchmark Study — Final Report. A Research Study Conducted after Consultation with the Massachusetts Department of Public Health* [http://www.brownandwilliamson.com/APPS/PDF/Final_ Report_1999_Mass_Benchmark_Study.pdf]

Borland, C. & Higenbottam, T. (1987) Nitric oxide yields of contemporary UK, US and French cigarettes. *Int. J. Epidemiol.*, **16**, 31–34

Bradford, J.A., Harlan, W.R. & Hanmer, H.R. (1936) Nature of cigaret smoke. Technic of experimental smoking. *Ind. Eng. Chem.*, **28**, 836–839

Brownson, R.C., Koffman, D.M., Novotny, T.E., Hughes, R.G. & Eriksen, M.P. (1995) Environmental and policy interventions to control tobacco use and prevent cardiovascular disease. *Health Educ. Q.*, **22**, 478–498

Brunnemann, K.D., Kagan, M.R., Cox, J.E. & Hoffmann, D. (1990) Analysis of 1,3-butadiene and other selected gas-phase components in cigarette mainstream and sidestream smoke by gas chromatography–mass selective detection. *Carcinogenesis*, **11**, 1863–1868

Brunnemann, K.D., Djordjevic, M.V., Feng, R. & Hoffmann, D. (1991) Analysis and pyrolisis of some *N*-nitrosamino acids in tobacco and tobacco smoke. In: O'Neill, I.K., Chen, J. & Bartsch, H., *Relevance to Human Cancer of N-Nitroso Compounds, Tobacco and Mycotoxins* (IARC Scientific Publications No. 105), Lyon, IARC*Press*, pp. 477–481

Brunnemann, K.D., Hoffmann, D., Gairola, C.G. & Lee, B.C. (1994) Low ignition propensity cigarettes: Smoke analysis for carcinogens and testing for mutagenic activity of the smoke particulate matter. *Food chem. Toxicol.*, **32**, 917–922

Brunnemann, K.D., Mitacek, E.J., Liu, Y., Limsila, T. & Suttajit, M. (1996) Assessment of major carcinogenic tobacco-specific *N*-nitrosamines in Thai cigarettes. *Cancer Detect. Prev.*, **20**, 114–121

Buchhalter, A.R. & Eissenberg, T. (2000) Preliminary evaluation of a novel smoking system: Effects on subjective and physiological measures and on smoking behavior. *Nicotine Tob. Res.*, **2**, 39–43

Burns, D.M. (2000) Smoking cessation: Recent indicators of what's working at a population level. In: *Population Based Smoking Cessation: Proceedings of a Conference on What Works to Influence Cessation in the General Population* (Smoking and Tobacco Control Monograph No. 12; NIH Publ. No. 00-4892), Bethesda, MD, National Cancer Institute

Burns, D.M., Shanks, T.G., Major, J.M., Gower, K.B. & Shopland, D.R. (2000) Restrictions on smoking in the workplace. In: *Population Based Smoking Cessation: Proceedings of a Conference on What Works to Influence Cessation in the General Population* (Smoking and Tobacco Control Monograph No. 12; NIH Publ. No. 00-4892), Bethesda, MD, National Cancer Institute

Bush, L.P., Cui, M., Shi, H., Burton, H.R., Fannin, F.F., Lei, L. & Dye, N. (2001) Formation of tobacco-specific nitrosamines in air-cured tobacco. *Recent Adv. Tob. Sci.*, **27**, 23–46

Canada ASH (Action on Smoking and Health) website [http://ash.org/Canada-health-warnings.html]

Castelao, J.E., Yuan, J.-M., Skipper, P.L., Tannenbaum, S.R., Gago-Dominez, M., Crowder, J.S., Ross, R.K. & Yu, M.C. (2001) Gender- and smoking-related bladder cancer risk. *J. natl Cancer Inst.*, **93**, 538–545

Centers for Disease Control and Prevention (CDC) (2002) *Tobacco Industry Documents* [http://www.cdc.gov/tobacco/industrydocs/index.htm]

Chaloupka, F.J. & Warner, K.E. (2000) The economics of smoking. In: Culyer, A.J. & Newhouse, J.P., eds, *The Handbook of Health Economics*, Vol. 1B, Amsterdam, North Holland

Chapman, S. & Wakefield, M. (2001) Tobacco control advocacy in Australia: Reflections on 30 years of progress. *Health Educ. Behav.*, **28**, 274–289

Chapman, S., Borland, R., Scollo, M., Brownson, R.C., Dominello, A. & Woodward, S. (1999) The impact of smoke-free workplaces on declining cigarette consumption in Australia and the United States. *Am. J. public Health*, **89**, 1018–1023

Clark, G.C. (1989) Comparison of the inhalation toxicity of kretek (clove cigarette) smoke with that of American cigarette smoke. I. One day exposure. *Arch. Toxicol.*, **63**, 1–6

Council of the European Union (2002) Council Regulation (EC) No. 546/2002 of 25 March 2002 fixing the premiums and guarantee thresholds for leaf tobacco by variety group and Member State for the 2002, 2003 and 2004 harvests and amending Regulation (EEC) No. 2075/92. *Off. J. Eur. Commun.*, **L84/4–7**

Corrao, M.A., Guindon, G.E., Sharma, N. & Shokoohi, D.F., eds (2000) *Tobacco Control Country Profiles. The 11th World Conference on Tobacco and Health*, Atlanta, GA, American Cancer Society

Darby, T.D., McNamee, J.E. & van Rossum, J.M. (1984) Cigarette smoking pharmacokinetics and its relationship to smoking behaviour. *Clin. Pharmacokinet.*, **9**, 435–449

Darrall, K.G. & Figgins, J.A. (1998) Roll-your-own smoke yields: Theoretical and practical aspects. *Tob. Control*, **7**, 168–175

Darrall, K.G., Figgins, J.A., Brown, R.D. & Phillips, G.F. (1998) Determination of benzene and associated volatile compounds in mainstream cigarette smoke. *Analyst*, **123**, 1095–1101

Department of Health (2000) *Permitted Additives to Tobacco Products in the United Kingdom*, London

Djordjevic, M.V., Brunnemann, K.D. & Hoffmann, D. (1989a) Identification and analysis of a nicotine-derived N-nitrosamino acid and other nitrosamino acids in tobacco. *Carcinogenesis*, **10**, 1725–1731

Djordjevic, M.V., Gay, S.L., Bush, L.P. & Chaplin, J.F. (1989b) Tobacco-specific nitrosamine accumulation and distribution in flue-cured tobacco alkaloid isolines. *J. agric. Food Chem.*, **37**, 752–756

Djordjevic, M.V., Sigountos, C.W., Brunnemann, K.D. & Hoffmann, D. (1990) Tobacco-specific nitrosamine delivery in the mainstream smoke of high- and low-yield cigarettes smoked with varying puff volume. In: *CORESTA Symposium Proceedings, Smoke Study Group, Kallithea, Greece*, pp. 54–62

Djordjevic, M.V., Sigountos, C.W., Brunnemann, K.D. & Hoffmann, D. (1991a) Formation of 4-(methylnitrosamino)-4-(3-pyridyl)butyric acid in vitro and in mainstream cigarette smoke. *J. agric. Food Chem.*, **39**, 209–213

Djordjevic, M.V., Sigountos, C.W., Hoffmann, D., Brunnemann, K.D., Kagan, M.R., Bush, L.P., Safaev, R., Belitsky, G. & Zaridze, D. (1991b) Assessment of major carcinogens and alkaloids in the tobacco and mainstream smoke of USSR cigarettes. *Int. J. Cancer*, **47**, 348–351

Djordjevic, M.V., Fan, J. & Hoffmann, D. (1995) Assessment of chlorinated pesticide residues in cigarette tobacco based on supercritical fluid extraction and GC-ECD. *Carcinogenesis*, **16**, 2627–2632

Djordjevic, M.V., Eixarch, L., Bush, L.P. & Hoffmann, D. (1996) A comparison of the yields of selected components in the mainstream smoke of the leading US and Japanese cigarettes. In: *CORESTA Congress Proceedings, Joint Smoke and Technology Groups, Yokohama, Japan*, pp. 200–217

Djordjevic, M.V., Eixarch, L. & Hoffmann, D. (1997) Self-administered and effective dose of cigar smoke constituents. In: *Proceedings of the 51st Tobacco Chemists' Research Conference, Winston-Salem, NC, September 14–17, 1997*

Djordjevic, M.V., Barr, W.H., Branciforte, S., Burton, H.R. & Jaffe, J.H. (1999) Reduced levels of 4-(methylnitrosamino)-1-(3-pyridyl)-1-butanol in smokers of cigarettes produced from nitrosamine-free tobacco. In: *Proceedings of CORESTA Meeting of the Smoke and Technology Study Groups, Innsbruck, Austria, September 5–9, 1999*

Djordjevic, M.V., Stellman, S.D. & Zang, E. (2000a) Doses of nicotine and lung carcinogens delivered to cigarette smokers. *J. natl Cancer Inst.*, **92**, 106–111

Djordjevic, M.V., Prokopczyk, B. & Zatonski, W. (2000b) Tobacco-specific *N*-nitrosamines (TSNA) in tobacco and mainstream smoke of the leading Polish cigarettes: A comparison with the US and Japanese brands. In: *Proceedings of the CORESTA Congress, Smoke Study Group, ST1, Lisbon, Portugal, October 2000*

Djordjevic, M.V., Stellman, S.D., Takezaki, T. & Tajima, K. (2000c) Cigarette composition as a possible explanation of US-Japan differences in lung cancer rates (Abstract No. 5120). In: *Proceedings of the 91st Annual Meeting of the American Association for Cancer Research, Vol. 41, San Francisco, CA, April 1–5, 2000*

Doll, R. & Hill, A.B. (1950) Smoking and carcinoma of the lung: Preliminary report. *Br. med. J.*, **ii**, 739–748

Dymond, H.F. (1996) Making habits of roll-your-own smokers in the Netherlands and tar and nicotine yields from the resultant products. *Tob. Sci.*, **40**, 87–91

van der Eb, M.M., Leyten, E.M., Gavarasana, S., Vandenbroucke, J.P., Kahn, P.M. & Cleton, F.J. (1993) Reverse smoking as a risk factor for palatal cancer: A cross-sectional study in rural Andhra Pradesh, India. *Int. J. Cancer*, **54**, 754–758

Eberhardt, H.-J. & Scherer, G. (1995) Human smoking behavior in comparison with machine smoking methods: A summary of the five papers presented at the 1995 meeting of the CORESTA Smoke and Technology groups in Vienna. *Beitr. Tabakforsch. int.*, **16**, 131–140

Elder, J.P., Edwards, C.C., Conway, T.L., Kenney, E., Johnson, C.A. & Bennett, E.D. (1996) Independent evaluation of the California tobacco education program. *Public Health Rep.*, **111**, 353–358

European Commission (1999) *Progress Achieved in Relation to Public Health Protection from the Harmful Effects of Tobacco Consumption. Commission Report to the European Parliament, the Council, the Economic and Social Committee and the Committee for the Regions* (COM 99), Brussels

European Parliament (2001) Directive 2001/37/CE of the European Parliament and of the Council of 5 June 2001 on the approximation of the laws, regulations and administrative provisions of the Member States concerning the manufacture, presentation and sale of tobacco products. *Off. J.*, **L194**, 18.07.2001

European Union (2000) *What is the Current Legislative Situation in the EU on Tobacco Products?* (Press Release 5 October 2000), Brussels, Health and Consumer Protection Directorate-General

Fant, R.B. & Henningfield, J.E. (1998) Pharmacology and abuse potential of cigars. In: *Cigars: Health Effects and Trends* (Smoking and Tobacco Control Monograph No. 9), Bethesda, MD, National Cancer Institute

Federal Trade Commission (FTC) (1967) *FTC to Begin Cigarette Testing* (Federal Trade Commission Press Release 1 August 1967), Washington DC

Federal Trade Commission (FTC) (2000) *'Tar', Nicotine, and Carbon Monoxide of the Smoke of 1294 Varieties of Domestic Cigarettes for the Year 1998*, Washington DC

Federal Trade Commission (FTC) (2002) *Cigarette Report for 2000*, Washington DC

Fichtenberg, C.M. & Glantz, S.A. (2000) Association of the California Tobacco Control Program with declines in cigarette consumption and mortality from heart disease. *New Engl. J. Med.*, **343**, 1772–1777

Fischer, S., Spiegelhalder, B. & Preussmann, R. (1989a) Preformed tobacco-specific nitrosamines in tobacco — Role of nitrate and influence of tobacco type. *Carcinogenesis*, **10**, 1511–1517

Fischer, S., Spiegelhalder, B. & Preussmann, R. (1989b) Influence of smoking parameters on the delivery of tobacco-specific nitrosamines in cigarette smoke — A contribution to relative risk evaluation. *Carcinogenesis*, **10**, 1059–1066

Fischer, S., Spiegelhalder, B. & Preussmann, R. (1989c) Tobacco-specific nitrosamines in main-stream smoke of West German cigarettes — Tar alone is not a sufficient index for the carcino-genic potential of cigarette smoke. *Carcinogenesis*, **10**, 169–173

Fischer, S., Spiegelhalder, B., Eisenbarth, J. & Preussmann, R. (1990a) Investigations on the origin of tobacco-specific nitrosamines in mainstream smoke of cigarettes. *Carcinogenesis*, **11**, 723–730

Fischer, S., Castonguay, A., Kaiserman, M., Spiegelhalder, B. & Preussmann, R. (1990b) Tobacco-specific nitrosamines in Canadian cigarettes. *J. Cancer Res. clin. Oncol.*, **116**, 563–568

Fischer, S., Spiegelhalder, B. & Preussmann, R. (1990c) Tobacco-specific nitrosamines in Euro-pean and USA cigarettes. *Arch. Geschwulstforsch.*, **60**, 169–177

Fisher, B. (2001) Safeguarding smokers. Vector Tobacco will employ new methods to reduce carcinogenic compounds in smoke and to eliminate nicotine. *Tob. Rep.*, **March**

Forster, J.L. & Wolfson, M. (1998) Youth access to tobacco: Policies and politics. *Annu. Rev. public Health*, **19**, 203–235

Fowler, J. & Bates, M. (2000) *The Chemical Constituents in Cigarettes and Cigarette Smoke: Prio-rities for Harm Reduction. Report to the New Zealand Ministry of Health. Epidemiology and Toxicology Group*, Porirua, ESR, Kenepuru Science Centre

Framework Convention on Tobacco Control (FCTC) (2003) [http://www5.who.int/tobacco/page.cfm?pid=40]

Gajalakshmi, C.K., Jha, P., Ranson, K. & Nguyen, S. (2000) Global patterns of smoking and smo-king-attributable mortality. In: Jha, P. & Chaloupka, F., eds, *Tobacco Control in Developing Countries*, Oxford, Oxford University Press

Galbraith, J.W. & Kaiserman, M. (1997) Taxation, smuggling and demand for cigarettes in Canada: Evidence from time-series data. *J. Health Econ.*, **16**, 287–301

Gerlach, K.K., Cummings, K.M., Hyland, A., Gilpin, E.A., Johnson, M.D. & Pierce, J.P. (1998) Trends in cigar consumption and smoking prevalence. In: *Cigars: Health Effects and Trends* (Smoking and Tobacco Control Monograph No. 9), Bethesda, MD, National Cancer Institute, pp. 21–53

Glover, E.D. & Glover, P.N. (1992) The smokeless tobacco problem: Risk groups in North America. In: *Smokeless Tobacco or Health: An International Perspective* (Smoking and Tobacco Control Monograph No. 2), Bethesda, MD, National Cancer Institute, pp. 3–10

Government of British Columbia (2002) *What Is in Cigarettes? Mainstream Smoke and Sidestream Smoke Chemical Constituents by Cigarette Brand*. [http://www.healthplanning.gov.bc.ca/ttdr/index.html]

Gray, N. & Boyle, P. (2002) Regulation of cigarette emissions. Editorial. *Ann. Oncol.*, **13**, 19–21

Gray, N., Zaridze, D., Robertson, C., Krivosheeva, L., Sigacheva, N., Boyle, P. & the International Cigarette Variation Group (2000) Variation within global cigarette brands in tar, nicotine, and certain nitrosamines: Analytic study. *Tob. Control*, **9**, 351

Green, C.R. & Rodgman, A. (1996) The tobacco chemists' research conference; A half century of advances in analytical methodology of tobacco and its products. *Recent Adv. Tob. Sci.*, **22**, 131–304

Griffin, R.W. & Pustay, M.W. (1999) *International Business. A Managerial Perspective*, 2nd Ed., London, Addison-Wesley, pp. 774–777

Griffin, R.W. & Pustay, M.W. (2002) *International Business. A Managerial Perspective*, 3rd Ed., London, Prentice-Hall International, pp. 116–118

Guidotti, T.L. (1989) Critique of available studies on the toxicology of kretek smoke and its constituents by routes of entry involving the respiratory tarct. *Arch. Toxicol.*, **63**, 7–12

Guindon, G.E. & Boisclair, D. (2003) *Past, Current and Future Trends in Tobacco Use, HNP Discussion Paper* (Economics of Tobacco Control Paper No. 6), Washington DC, World Bank

Gupta, P.C. (1992) Smokeless tobacco use in India. In: *Smokeless Tobacco or Health: An International Perspective* (Smoking and Tobacco Control Monograph No. 2), Bethesda, MD, National Cancer Institute, pp. 19–25

Guttman, N. & Peleg, H. (2003) Public preferences for an attribution to government or to medical research versus unattributed messages in cigarette warning labels in Israel. *Health Commun.*, **15**, 1–25

Health Promotion Foundation (2002) *Law on the Protection of Public Health Against the Effects of Tobacco Use* [http://www.promocjazdrowia.pl/ustawa.htm]

Hecht, S.S. (1998) Biochemistry, biology, and carcinogenicity of tobacco-specific N-nitrosamines. *Chem. Res. Toxicol.*, **11**, 559–603

Hecht, S.S. (1999) Tobacco smoke carcinogens and lung cancer. *J. natl Cancer Inst.*, **91**, 1194–1210

Hecht, S.S. (2002) Tobacco smoke carcinogens and breast cancer. *Environ. mol. Mutag.*, **39**, 119–126

Hecht, S.S. (2003) Tobacco carcinogens, their biomarkers and tobacco-induced cancer. *Nat. Rev. Cancer*, **3**, 733–744

Henningfield, J.E., Kozlowski, L.T. & Benowitz, N.L. (1994) A proposal to develop meaningful labeling for cigarettes. *J. Am. med. Assoc.*, **272**, 312–314

Henningfield, J.E., Fant, R.V., Radzius, A. & Frost, S. (1999) Nicotine concentration, smoke pH and whole tobacco aqueous pH of some cigar brands and types popular in the United Sates. *Nicotine Tob. Res.*, **1**, 163–168

Hoffmann, D. & Hoffmann, I. (1997) The changing cigarette, 1950–1995. *J. Toxicol. environ. Health*, **50**, 307–364

Hoffmann, D. & Hoffmann, I. (2001) The changing cigarette: Chemical studies and bioassays. In: *Risks Associated with Smoking Cigarettes with Low Machine-Measured Yields of Tar and Nicotine* (Smoking and Tobacco Control Monograph No. 13; NIH Publ. No. 02-5074), Bethesda, MD, National Cancer Institute, pp. 159–191

Hoffmann, D., Dong, M. & Hecht, S.S. (1977) Origin in tobacco smoke of *N'*-nitrosonornicotine, a tobacco-specific carcinogen: Brief communication. *J. natl Cancer Inst.*, **58**, 1841–1844

Hoffmann, D., Rivenson, A. & Hecht, S.S. (1992) Carcinogens of smokeless tobacco. In: *Smokeless Tobacco or Health: An International Perspective* (Smoking and Tobacco Control Monograph No. 2), Bethesda, MD, National Cancer Institute, pp. 109–117

Hoffmann, D., Hoffmann, I. & El-Bayoumy, K. (2001) The less harmful cigarette: A controversial issue. A tribute to Ernst L. Wynder. *Chem. Res. Toxicol.*, **14**, 767–790

Hopkins, D.P., Briss, P.A., Ricard, C.J., Husten, C.G., Carande-Kulis, V.G., Fielding, J.E., Alao, M.O., McKenna, J.W., Sharp, D.J., Harris, J.R., Woollery, T.A., Harris, K.W. & the Task Force on Community Preventive Services (2001) Reviews of evidence regarding interventions to reduce tobacco use and exposure to environmental tobacco smoke. *Am. J. prev. Med.*, **20**, 16–66

Hurt, R.D., Croghan, G.A., Wolter, T.D., Croghan, I.T., Offord, K.P., Williams, G.M., Djordjevic, M.V., Richie, J.P., Jr & Jeffrey, A.M. (2000) Does smoking reduction result in reduction of biomarkers associated with harm. A pilot study using a nicotine inhaler. *Nicotine Tob. Res.*, **2**, 327–336

IARC (1972) *IARC Monographs on the Evaluation of Carcinogenic Risk of Chemicals to Man*, Vol. 1, *Some Inorganic Substances, Chlorinated Hydrocarbons, Aromatic Amines, N-Nitroso Compounds, and Natural Products*, Lyon, IARCPress

IARC (1973) *IARC Monographs on the Evaluation of Carcinogenic Risk of Chemicals to Man*, Vol. 3, *Certain Polycyclic Aromatic Hydrocarbons and Heterocyclic Compounds*, Lyon, IARCPress

IARC (1974a) *IARC Monographs on the Evaluation of Carcinogenic Risk of Chemicals to Man*, Vol. 4, *Some Aromatic Amines, Hydrazine and Related Substances, N-Nitroso Compounds and Miscellaneous Alkylating Agents*, Lyon, IARCPress

IARC (1974b) *IARC Monographs on the Evaluation of Carcinogenic Risk of Chemicals to Man*, Vol. 7, *Some Anti-Thyroid and Related Substances, Nitrofurans and Industrial Chemicals*, Lyon, IARCPress

IARC (1976) *IARC Monographs on the Evaluation of Carcinogenic Risk of Chemicals to Man*, Vol. 10, *Some Naturally Occurring Substances*, Lyon, IARCPress

IARC (1978) *IARC Monographs on the Evaluation of the Carcinogenic Risk of Chemicals to Humans*, Vol. 17, *Some N-Nitroso Compounds*, Lyon, IARCPress

IARC (1979) *IARC Monographs on the Evaluation of the Carcinogenic Risk of Chemicals to Humans*, Vol. 19, *Some Monomers, Plastics and Synthetic Elastomers, and Acrolein*, Lyon, IARCPress

IARC (1980) *IARC Monographs on the Evaluation of the Carcinogenic Risk of Chemicals to Humans*, Vol. 23, *Some Metals and Metallic Compounds*, Lyon, IARCPress

IARC (1982) *IARC Monographs on the Evaluation of the Carcinogenic Risk of Chemicals to Humans*, Vol. 29, *Some Industrial Chemicals and Dyestuffs*, Lyon, IARCPress

IARC (1983a) *IARC Monographs on the Evaluation of the Carcinogenic Risk of Chemicals to Humans*, Vol. 32, *Polynuclear Aromatic Compounds, Part 1: Chemical, Environmental and Experimental Data*, Lyon, IARCPress

IARC (1983b) *IARC Monographs on the Evaluation of the Carcinogenic Risk of Chemicals to Humans*, Vol. 31, *Some Food Additives, Feed Additives and Naturally Occurring Substances*, Lyon, IARCPress

IARC (1985a) *IARC Monographs on the Evaluation of the Carcinogenic Risk of Chemicals to Humans*, Vol. 36, *Allyl Compounds, Aldehydes, Epoxides and Peroxides*, Lyon, IARCPress

IARC (1985b) *IARC Monographs on the Evaluation of the Carcinogenic Risk of Chemicals to Humans*, Vol. 37, *Tobacco Habits Other than Smoking; Betel-Quid and Areca-Nut Chewing; and Some Related Nitrosamines*, Lyon, IARCPress

IARC (1986a) *IARC Monographs on the Evaluation of the Carcinogenic Risk of Chemicals to Humans*, Vol. 38, *Tobacco Smoking*, Lyon, IARC*Press*

IARC (1986b) *IARC Monographs on the Evaluation of the Carcinogenic Risk of Chemicals to Humans*, Vol. 40, *Some Naturally Occurring and Synthetic Food Components, Furocoumarins and Ultraviolet Radiation*, Lyon, IARC*Press*

IARC (1987) *IARC Monographs on the Evaluation of Carcinogenic Risks to Humans*, Suppl. 7, *Overall Evaluations of Carcinogenicity: An Updating of* IARC Monographs *Volumes 1 to 42*, Lyon, IARC*Press*

IARC (1990) *IARC Monographs on the Evaluation of Carcinogenic Risks to Humans*, Vol. 49, *Chromium, Nickel and Welding*, Lyon, IARC*Press*

IARC (1991) *IARC Monographs on the Evaluation of Carcinogenic Risks to Humans*, Vol. 52, *Chlorinated Drinking-Water; Chlorination By-products; Some Other Halogenated Compounds; Cobalt and Cobalt Compounds*, Lyon, IARC*Press*

IARC (1993a) *IARC Monographs on the Evaluation of Carcinogenic Risks to Humans*, Vol. 58, *Beryllium, Cadmium, Mercury and Exposures in the Glass Manufacturing Industry*, Lyon, IARC*Press*

IARC (1993b) *IARC Monographs on the Evaluation of Carcinogenic Risks to Humans*, Vol. 56, *Some Naturally Occurring Substances: Food Items and Constituents, Heterocyclic Aromatic Amines and Mycotoxins*, Lyon, IARC*Press*

IARC (1993c) *IARC Monographs on the Evaluation of Carcinogenic Risks to Humans*, Vol. 57, *Occupational Exposures of Hairdressers and Barbers and Personal Use of Hair Colourants; Some Hair Dyes, Cosmetic Colourants, Industrial Dyestuffs and Aromatic Amines*, Lyon, IARC*Press*

IARC (1994) *IARC Monographs on the Evaluation of Carcinogenic Risks to Humans*, Vol. 60, *Some Industrial Chemicals*, Lyon, IARC*Press*

IARC (1995a) *IARC Monographs on the Evaluation of Carcinogenic Risks to Humans*, Vol. 62, *Wood Dust and Formaldehyde*, Lyon, IARC*Press*

IARC (1995b) *IARC Monographs on the Evaluation of Carcinogenic Risks to Humans*, Vol. 63, *Dry Cleaning, Some Chlorinated Solvents and Other Industrial Chemicals*, Lyon, IARC*Press*

IARC (1996) *IARC Monographs on the Evaluation of Carcinogenic Risks to Humans*, Vol. 65, *Printing Processes and Printing Inks, Carbon Black and Some Nitro Compounds*, Lyon, IARC*Press*

IARC (1999) *IARC Monographs on the Evaluation of Carcinogenic Risks to Humans*, Vol. 71, *Re-evaluation of Some Organic Chemicals, Hydrazine and Hydrogen Peroxide*, Lyon, IARC*Press*

IARC (2000) *IARC Monographs on the Evaluation of Carcinogenic Risks to Humans*, Vol. 77, *Some Industrial Chemicals*, Lyon, IARC*Press*

IARC (2001) *IARC Monographs on the Evaluation of Carcinogenic Risks to Humans*, Vol. 78, *Ionizing Radiation, Part 2: Some Internally Deposited Radionuclides*, Lyon, IARC*Press*

IARC (2004a) *IARC Monographs on the Evaluation of Carcinogenic Risks to Humans*, Vol. 84, *Some Drinking-water Disinfectants and Contaminants, including Arsenic*, Lyon (in press)

IARC (2004b) *IARC Monographs on the Evaluation of Carcinogenic Risks to Humans*, Vol. 87, *Lead and Lead Compounds*, Lyon (in press)

International Committee for Cigar Smoke Study (1974) Machine smoking of cigars. *CORESTA Inform. Bull.*, **1**, 31–34

Jacobs, R. (2001) Economic policies, taxation and fiscal measures. In: Samet, J. & Yoon, S.-Y., eds, *Women and the Tobacco Epidemic: Challenges for the 21st Century*, Geneva, World Health Organization, pp. 177–200

Jarvis, M.J. (2001) Trends in sales weighted tar, nicotine, and carbon monoxide yields of UK cigarettes. *Thorax*, **56**, 960–963

Jenkins, R.A., Guerin, M.R. & Tomkins, B.A. (2000) Mainstream and sidestream smoke. In: *The Chemistry of Environmental Tobacco Smoke: Composition and Measurement*, 2nd Ed., Boca Raton, FL, Lewis Publishers, pp. 49–75

Jha, P. & Chaloupka, F.J. (2000) The economics of global tobacco control. *Br. med. J.*, **321**, 358–361

Joossens, L. & Raw, M. (1998) Cigarette smuggling in Europe: Who really benefits. *Tob. Control*, **7**, 66–71

Kaiserman, M.J. & Rickert, W.S. (1992a) Carcinogens in tobacco smoke: Benzo(a)pyrene from Canadian cigarettes and cigarette tobacco. *Am. J. public Health*, **82**, 1023–1026

Kaiserman, M.J. & Rickert, W.S. (1992b) Hand made cigarettes. It's the tube that counts. *Am. J. public Health*, **82**, 107–109

Kanai, Y., Wada, O. & Manabe, S. (1990) Detection of carcinogenic glutamic acid pyrolysis products in cigarette smoke condensate. *Carcinogenesis*, **11**, 1001–1003

Kaufman, N. & Nichter, M. (2001) The marketing of tobacco to women: Global perspectives. In: Samet, J. & Yoon, S.-Y., eds, *Women and the Tobacco Epidemic: Challenges for the 21st Century*, Geneva, World Health Organization, pp. 69–98

Kozlowski, L.T., Rickert, W.S., Robinson, J.C. & Grunberg, N.E. (1980) Have tar and nicotine yields of cigarettes changed? *Science*, **209**, 1550–1551

Kozlowski, L.T., Mehta, N.Y., Sweeney, C.T., Schwartz, S.S., Vogler, G.P., Jarvis, M.J. & West, R.J. (1998) Filter ventilation and nicotine content of tobacco in cigarettes from Canada, the United Kingdom, and the United States. *Tob. Control*, **7**, 369–375

Kozlowski, L.T., O'Connor, R.J. & Sweeney, C.T. (2001) Cigarette design. In: *Risks Associated with Smoking Cigarettes with Low Machine-Measured Yields of Tar and Nicotine* (Smoking and Tobacco Control Monograph No. 13), Bethesda, MD, National Cancer Institute, pp. 13–37

Laboratory of the Government Chemist (LGC) (1998) *Nitric Oxide Yields of Cigarettes. Results for Cigarettes Sampled in 1996 (LGC Report EH40/M016/98)*, London, Department of Health

Laboratory of the Government Chemist (LGC) (2001) *Determination of the Fate of Nicotine When a Cigarette is Smoked (LGC Report FN40/M24/01)*, London, Department of Health [http://www.doh.gov.uk/scoth/technicaladvisorygroup/nicotfate.pdf Accessed 14.03.2003]

Laboratory of the Government Chemist (LGC) (2002) Comparison of Mainstream Smoke Yields of Tar, Nicotine, Carbon Monoxide and Polycyclic Aromatic Hydrocarbons from Cigarettes and Small Cigars (LGC Report GC15/M09/02), London, Department of Health [http://www.doh.gov.uk/scoth/pdfs/cigarcigarettepah.pdf Accessed 17.03.2003]

LaVoie, E.J., Adams, J.D., Reinhardt, J., Rivenson, A. & Hoffmann, D. (1986) Toxicity studies on clove cigarette smoke and constituents of clove: Determination of the LD50 of eugenol by intratracheal instillation in rats and hamsters. *Arch. Toxicol.*, **59**, 78–81

Longo, D.R., Brownson, R.C. & Kruse, R.L. (1995) Smoking bans in US hospitals. Results of a national survey. *J. Am. med. Assoc.*, **274**, 488–491

Mackay, J. & Eriksen, M. (2002) *The Tobacco Atlas*, Geneva, World Health Organization

Malson, J.L. & Pickworth, W.B. (2002) Bidis — Hand-rolled, Indian cigarettes: Effects on physiological, biochemical and subjective measures. *Pharmacol. Biochem. Behav.*, **72**, 443–447

Malson, J.L., Sims, K., Murty, R. & Pickworth, W.B. (2001) Comparison of the nicotine content of tobacco used in bidis and conventional cigarettes. *Tob. Control*, **10**, 181–183

Malson, J.L., Lee, E.M., Moolchan, E.T. & Pickworth, W.B. (2002) Nicotine delivery from smoking bidis and an additive-free cigarette. *Nicotine Tob. Res.*, **4**, 485–490

Manabe, S., Tohyama, K., Wada, O. & Aramaki, T. (1991) Detection of carcinogen, 2-amino-1-methyl-6-phenylimidazo(4,5-b)pyridine (PhIP), in cigarette smoke condensate. *Carcinogenesis*, **12**, 1945–1947

Maxwell Tobacco Fact Book (2000) (Table 3, cigarettes; Table 9, cigars; Table 15, RYO)

Mitacek, E.J., Brunnemann, K.D. & Polednak, A.P. (1990) 'Tar', nicotine, and carbon monoxide content of Thai cigarettes, and implications for cancer prevention in Thailand. *Cancer Detect. Prev.*, **14**, 515–520

Mitacek, E.J., Brunnemann, K.D., Polednak, A.P., Hoffmann, D. & Suttajit, M. (1991) Composition of popular tobacco products in Thailand and its relevance to disease prevention. *Prev. Med.*, **20**, 764–773

Mitacek, E.J., Brunnemann, K.D., Hoffmann, D., Limsila, T., Suttajit, M., Martin, N. & Caplan, L.S. (1999) Volatile nitrosamines and tobacco-specific nitrosamines in the smoke of Thai cigarettes: A risk factor for lung cancer and a suspected risk factor for liver cancer in Thailand. *Carcinogenesis*, **20**, 133–137

Mitacek, E.J., Brunnemann, K.D., Polednak, A.P., Limsila, T., Bhothisuwan, K. & Hummel, C.F. (2002) Rising leukemia rates in Thailand: The possible role of benzene and related compounds in cigarette smoke. *Oncol. Rep.*, **9**, 1399–1403

Muto, H. & Takizawa, Y. (1989) Dioxins in cigarette smoke. *Arch. environ. Health*, **44**, 171–174

Nair, J., Pakhale, S.S. & Bhide, S.V. (1989) Carcinogenic tobacco-specific nitrosamines in Indian tobacco products. *Food chem. Toxicol.*, **27**, 751–753

Narayan, K.M., Chadha, S.L., Hanson, R.L., Tandon, R., Shekhawat, S., Fernandes, R.J. & Gopinath, N. (1996) Prevalence and patterns of smoking in Delhi: Cross sectional study. *Br. med. J.*, **312**, 1576–1579

National Association of Attorneys General (1998) *Master Settlement Agreement and Amendments* [http://www.naag.org/issues/tobacco/index.php]

National Cancer Institute (2001) *Changing Adolescent Smoking Prevalence* (Smoking and Tobacco Control Monograph No. 14), Bethesda, MD

National Research Council (NRC) (1986) *Environmental Tobacco Smoke. Measuring Exposures and Assessing Health Effects*, Washington DC, National Academy Press

Pagano, R., La Vecchia, C. & Decarli, A. (1996) Smoking in Italy, 1994. *Tumori*, **82**, 309–313

Pakhale, S.S. & Maru, G.B. (1998) Distribution of major and minor alkaloids in tobacco, mainstream and sidestream smoke of popular Indian smoking products. *Food chem. Toxicol.*, **36**, 1131–1138

Pakhale, S.S., Sarkar, S., Jayant, K. & Bhide, S.V. (1988) Carcinogenicity of Indian bidi and cigarette smoke condensate in Swiss albino mice. *J. Cancer Res. clin. Oncol.*, **114**, 647–649

Pakhale, S.S., Jayant, K. & Bhide, S.V. (1989) Total particulate matter and nicotine in Indian bidis and cigarettes: A comparative study of standard machine estimates and exposure levels in smokers in Bombay. *Indian J. Cancer*, **26**, 227–232

Pakhale, S.S., Jayant, K. & Bhide, S.V. (1990) Chemical analysis of smoke of Indian cigarettes, bidis and other indigenous forms of smoking — Levels of steam-volatile phenol, hydrogen cyanide and benzo(a)pyrene. *Indian J. Chest Dis. All Sci.*, **32**, 75–81

Pauly, J.L., Allaart, H.A., Rodriguez, M.I. & Streck, R.J. (1995) Fibers released from cigarette filters: An additional health risk to the smoker? *Cancer Res.*, **55**, 253–258

Pauly, J.L., Stegmeier, S.J., Mayer, A.G., Lesses, J.D. & Streck, R.J. (1997) Release of carbon granules from cigarettes with charcoal filters. *Tob. Control*, **6**, 33–40

Pauly, J.L., Lee, H.J., Hurley, E.L., Cummings, K.M., Lesses, J.D. & Streck, R.J. (1998) Glass fiber contamination of cigarette filters: An additional health risk to the smoker? *Cancer Epidemiol. Biomarkers Prev.*, **7**, 967–979

Peele, D.M., Riddick, M.G. & Edwards, M.E. (2001) Formation of tobacco-specific nitrosamines in flue-cured tobacco. *Recent Adv. Tob. Sci.*, **27**, 3–12

Peto, R., Darby, S., Deo, H., Silcocks, P., Whitley, E. & Doll, R. (2000) Smoking, smoking cessation, and lung cancer in the UK since 1950: Combination of national statistics with two case–control studies. *Br. med. J.*, **321**, 323–329

Phillips, G.F. & Waller, R.E. (1991) Yields of tar and other smoke components from UK cigarettes. *Food chem. Toxicol.*, **29**, 469–474

Pickworth, W.B., Fant, R.V., Nelson, R.A., Rohrer, M.S. & Henningfield, J.E. (1999) Pharmacodynamic effects of new de-nicotinized cigarettes. *Nicotine Tob. Res.*, **1**, 357–364

Pierce, J.P., Gilpin, E., Burns, D.M., Whalen, E., Rosbrook, B., Shopland, D. & Johnson, M. (1991) Does tobacco advertising target young people to start smoking? Evidence from California. *J. Am. med. Assoc.*, **266**, 3154–3158

Pillsbury, H.C., Bright, C.C., O'Connor, K.J. & Irish, F.W. (1969) Tar and nicotine in cigarette smoke. *J. Assoc. off. anal. Chem.*, **52**, 458–462

Rickert, W.S. & Kaiserman, M.J. (1999) Application of proposed Canadian test methods to the analysis of cigarette filler, fine cut tobacco, and tobacco smoke (Abstract No. 16). In: *Proceedings of the 53rd Tobacco Science Research Conference, Montreal, Canada, September 12–15, 1999*

Rickert, W.S., Robinson, J.C., Bray, D.F., Rogers, B. & Collishaw, N.E. (1985) Characterization of tobacco products: Comparative study of the tar, nicotine, and carbon monoxide yields of cigars, manufactured cigarettes, and cigarettes made from fine-cut tobacco. *Prev. Med.*, **14**, 226–233

Rickert, W.S., Collishaw, N.E., Bray, D.F. & Robinson, J.C. (1986) Estimates of maximum or average cigarette tar, nicotine, and carbon monoxide yields can be obtained from yields under standard conditions. *Prev. Med.*, **15**, 82–91

Roberts, D.L. (1988) Natural tobacco flavor. *Recent Adv. Tob. Sci.*, **14**, 49–81

Robertson, A.S., Burge, P.S. & Cockrill, B.L. (1987) A study of serum thiocyanate concentrations in office workers as a means of validating smoking histories and assessing passive exposure to cigarette smoke. *Br. J. ind. Med.*, **44**, 351–354

Robinson, J.H., Pritchard, W.S. & Davis, R.A. (1992) Psychopharmacological effects of smoking a cigarette with typical 'tar' and carbon monoxide yields but minimal nicotine. *Psychopharmacology*, **108**, 466–472

Robinson, M.L., Houtsmuller, E.J., Moolchan, E.T. & Pickworth, W.B. (2000) Placebo cigarettes in smoking research. *Exp. clin. Psychopharmacol.*, **8**, 326–332

Roemer, R. (1988) *Legislative Strategies for a Smoke-free Europe*, Copenhagen, World Health Organization Regional Committee for Europe and the Commission of the European Community

Royal College of Physicians (1962) *Smoking and Health. A Report of the Royal College of Physicians on Smoking in Relation to Cancer of the Lung and Other Diseases*, London, Pitman Medical

Russell, M.A., Jarvis, M.J., Feyerabend, C. & Saloojee, Y. (1986) Reduction of tar, nicotine and carbon monoxide intake in low tar smokers. *J. Epidemiol. Community Health*, **40**, 80–85

Scherer, G., Conze, C., von Meyerinck, L., Sorsa, M. & Adlkofer, F. (1990) Importance of exposure to gaseous and particulate phase components of tobacco smoke in active and passive smokers. *Int. Arch. occup. environ. Health*, **62**, 459–466

Schmid, T.L., Pratt, M. & Howze, E. (1995) Policy as intervention: Environmental and policy approaches to the prevention of cardiovascular disease. *Am. J. public Health*, **85**, 1207–1211

Shafey, O., Cokkinides, V., Cavalcante, T.M., Teixeira, M., Vianna, C. & Thun, M. (2002) Case studies in international tobacco surveillance: Cigarette smuggling in Brazil. *Tob. Control*, **11**, 215–219

Shopland, D.R. (2001) Historical perspective: The low tar lie. *Tob. Control*, **10** (Suppl. I), i1–i3

Slade, J. (1997) Historical notes on tobacco. *Prog. respir. Res.*, **28**, 1–11

Smith, C.J. & Fischer, T.H. (2001) Particulate and vapor phase constituents of cigarette mainstream smoke and risk of myocardial infarction. *Atherosclerosis*, **158**, 257–267

Smith, C.J., Livingston, S.D. & Doolittle, D.J. (1997) An international literature survey of 'IARC Group I Carcinogens' reported in mainstream cigarette smoke. *Food chem. Toxicol.*, **35**, 1107–1130

Smith, C.J., Perfetti, T.A., Morton, M.J., Rodgman, A., Garg, R., Selassie, C.D. & Hansch, C. (2002) The relative toxicity of substituted phenols reported in cigarette mainstream smoke. *Toxicol. Sci.*, **69**, 265–278

Square, D. (1998) Cigarette smuggling finds a home in the West. *Can. med. Assoc. J.*, **158**, 95–97

Stanfill, S.B. & Ashley, D.L. (1999) Solid phase microextraction of alkenylbenzenes and other flavor-related compounds from tobacco for analysis by selected ion monitoring gas chromatography–mass spectrometry. *J. Chromatogr.*, **858**, 79–89

Stanfill, S.B. & Ashley, D.L. (2000) Quantitation of flavor-related alkenylbenzenes in tobacco smoke particulate by selected ion monitoring gas chromatography-mass spectrometry. *J. agric. Food Chem.*, **48**, 1298–1306

Stanfill, S.B., Calafat, A.M., Brown, C.R., Polzin, G.M., Chiang, J.M., Watson, C.H. & Ashley, D.L. (2003) Concentrations of nine alkenylbenzenes, coumarin, piperonal and pulegone in Indian bidi cigarette tobacco. *Food chem. Toxicol.*, **41**, 303–317

Stead, L.F. & Lancaster, T. (2000) A systematic review of interventions for preventing tobacco sales to minors. *Tob. Control*, **9**, 169–176

Stellman, S.D., Muscat, J.E., Hoffmann, D. & Wynder, E.L. (1997) Impact of filter cigarette smoking on lung cancer histology. *Prev. Med.*, **26**, 451–456

Stepanov, I., Carmella, S.G., Hecht, S.S. & Duca, G. (2002) Analysis of tobacco-specific nitrosamines in Moldovan cigarette tobacco. *J. agric. Food Chem.*, **50**, 2793–2797

Stratton, K., Shetty, P., Wallace, R. & Bondurant, S., eds (2001) Products for tobacco exposure reduction. In: *Clearing the Smoke. Assessing the Science Base for Tobacco Harm Reduction*, Washington DC, National Academy Press, pp. 82–92

Swauger, J.E., Steichen, T.J., Murphy, P.A. & Kinsler, S. (2002) An analysis of the mainstream smoke chemistry of samples of the US cigarette market acquired between 1995 and 2000. *Regul. Toxicol. Pharmacol.*, **35**, 142–156

Sweanor, D., Ballin, S., Corcoran, R.D., Davis, A., Deasy, K., Ferrence, R.G., Lahey, R., Lucido, S., Nethery, W.J. & Wasserman, J. (1992) Report of the Tobacco Policy Research Study Group on tobacco pricing and taxation in the United States. *Tob. Control*, **1** (Suppl.), S31–S36

Time Asia (2000) Thank you for smoking in destitute Cambodia. Big Tobacco is showing that cigarettes can be healthy, if only for the economy. *Time Asia*, **10**, July

Tobacco Sales Act (1998) *Tobacco Testing and Disclosure Regulation* [British Columbia Reg. 282/98; O.C. 1107/98 includes amendments up to B.C. Reg.93/2001]

Tricker, A.R., Ditrich, C. & Preussmann, R. (1991) N-Nitroso compounds in cigarette tobacco and their occurrence in mainstream tobacco smoke. *Carcinogenesis*, **12**, 257–261

Tricker, A.R., Scherer, G. & Adlkofer, F. (1993a) Influence of tobacco nitrate on the yields of selected mainstream smoke components. In: *Proceedings of the 47th Tobacco Chemists' Research Conference, Gatlinburg, TN, October 18–21, 1993*

Tricker, A.R, Scherer, G., Conze, C., Adlkofer, F., Pachinger, A. & Klus, H. (1993b) Evaluation of 4-(N-methylnitrosamino)-4-(3-pyridyl)butyric acid as a potential monitor of endogenous nitrosation of nicotine and its metabolites. *Carcinogenesis*, **14**, 1409–1414

Tso, T.C. (1991) The production of tobacco. In: *Production, Physiology, and Biochemistry of Tobacco Plant*, Beltsville, MD, Ideals, pp. 55–64

US Congress (2002a) *Tobacco Equity Elimination Act of June 27 2002, 107th Congress, 2nd session* (H.R. 5035), Washington DC, Government Printing Office

US Congress (2002b) *Tobacco-dependent Communities Assistance Act of September 24 2002, 107th Congress, 2nd session* (S. 2995), Washington DC, Government Printing Office

US Department of Agriculture (2001a) *Tobacco World Markets and Trade*, Washington DC [http://www.fas.usda.gov/tobacco/circular/2001/0109/index.htm]

US Department of Agriculture (2001b) *World Tobacco Production*, Washington DC, [http://Afubra.com.br/engl/link11.html]

US Department of Agriculture (2001c) *Tobacco, Background*, Washington DC, *Economic Research Service, Briefing Room* [http://www.ers.usda.gov/Briefing/Tobacco/background.htm]

US Department of Agriculture (2002a) *Tobacco: World Markets and Trade* (Circular Series FT-08-02), Washington DC, Foreign Agricultural Service

US Department of Agriculture (2002b) *Tobacco Outlook* (TBS-252), Washington DC, Economic Research Service

US Department of Health and Human Services (DHHS) (1964) *Smoking and Health. Report of the Advisory Committee to the Surgeon General of the Public Health Service* (Public Health Service Publ. No. 1103), Washington DC, US Government Printing Office

US Department of Health and Human Services (DHHS) (1986) *Smoking and Health, A National Status Report: A Report to Congress*, Rockville, MD, Centers for Disease Control

US Department of Health and Human Services (DHHS) (1989) *Reducing the Health Consequences of Smoking: 25 Years of Progress. A Report of the Surgeon General* (DHHS Publ. No. (CDC) 89-8411), Washington DC, US Government Printing Office

US Department of Health and Human Services (DHHS) (2000) *Reducing Tobacco Use: A Report of the Surgeon General*, Atlanta, GA, Centers for Diseases Control and Prevention

Vineis, P. & Pirastu, R. (1997) Aromatic amines and cancer. *Cancer Causes Control*, **8**, 346–355

Wahlberg, I., Long, R.C., Brandt, P. & Wiernik, A. (1999) The development of low TSNA air-cured tobaccos. I. Effects of tobacco genotype and fertilization on the formation of TSNA. In: *Pro-*

ceedings of the CORESTA Meeting of the Smoke and Technology Study Groups, Innsbruck, Austria, September 5–9, 1999

WHO (1983) *Smoking Control Strategies in Developing Countries. Report of a WHO Expert Committee* (Technical Report Series No. 695), Geneva, p. 43

WHO (1997) *Tobacco or Health: A Global Status Report*, Geneva

WHO (2001) *Confronting the Tobacco Epidemic in an Era of Trade Liberalization* (WHO/NMH/TFI/01.4), Geneva

Womack, R. (2002) The concern over commingling. Editorial. *Tob. Farmer*, **May**

Woodward, M. & Tunstall-Pedoe, H. (1992) Do smokers of lower tar cigarettes consume lower amounts of smoke components ? Results from the Scottish Heart Health Study. *Br. J. Addict.*, **87**, 921–928

Wynder, E.L. & Graham, E.A. (1950) Tobacco smoking as a possible etiologic factor in bronchiogenic carcinoma. A study of six hundred and eighty-four proved cases. *J. Am. med. Assoc.*, **143**, 329–336

Yurekli, A.A. & Zhang, P. (2000) The impact of clean indoor-air laws and cigarette smuggling on demand for cigarettes: An empirical model. *Health Econ.*, **9**, 159–170

2. Studies of Cancer in Humans

The available knowledge on the relationship between tobacco usage and a variety of human cancers is based primarily on epidemiological evidence. An immense amount of such evidence has been obtained, and, of necessity, only a small proportion can be referred to here. The cancers considered to be causally related to tobacco smoking in the previous *IARC Monograph* on tobacco smoking (IARC, 1986) included those of the lung, upper aerodigestive tract (oral cancer and cancer of the oropharynx, hypopharynx, larynx and oesophagus), urinary bladder and renal pelvis and pancreas. Since 1986, there have been numerous additional cohort and case–control studies on the relationship of cigarette smoking and other forms of tobacco use to these and other cancers in many different countries. The most comprehensive evidence, although often not the first or most detailed, has been obtained from several large cohort studies that are referred to repeatedly in this monograph with respect to different cancer sites and types of tobacco product. These cohort studies are described briefly below and in Table 2.1, listed by country. The case–control studies are described in the sections pertaining to particular cancer sites.

Description of cohort studies

(a)   Europe

(i)   United Kingdom

British Doctors' Study

In 1951, a questionnaire on smoking habits was sent to all British doctors included in the Medical Register; 34 440 men and 6194 women responded, representing 69% and 60%, respectively, of those doctors not known to have died at the time of the inquiry. [The exact number of men and women included in the study varies between publications as a number of women were misclassified as men in early reports.] Further questionnaires about changes in smoking habits were sent in 1957, 1966, 1972, 1978 and 1990 to men and in 1961 and 1973 to women; on each occasion, at least 94% of those alive responded. Reports were published on cause-specific deaths after 10, 20 and 40 years for men and after 10 and 22 years for women; more than 99% of the subjects had been traced. Information on causes of death was obtained principally from the Registrars General of the United Kingdom and, otherwise, from the records of the general Medical Council, the

Bristish Medical Association, relatives or friends. Because the subjects in the study were themselves physicians, they were a reasonably uniform socioeconomic group and the causes of death were certified more accurately than might have been the case among a sample of the general population. For the first 20 years of the study, confirmation of all deaths attributed to lung cancer was obtained from a chest physician who was unaware of the patient's smoking history (Doll & Hill, 1964a,b; Doll & Peto, 1976; Doll et al., 1980, 1994).

Whitehall Study

A total of 19 018 men aged 40–69 years from the British Civil Service were clinically examined between 1967 and 1969, and followed up for vital status until 1987 through the National Health Service Central Registry. Information on exposure was collected only at baseline. The study concentrated on residual risk after smoking cessation as well as comparing risk associated with different tobacco products (Ben-Shlomo et al., 1994).

British United Provident Association (BUPA) Study

Wald and Watt (1997) studied a cohort of 21 520 professional and businessmen with a National Health Service identification number who attended a routine health examination between 1975 and 1982 at a British United Provident Association (BUPA) Medical Centre in London. At this examination, a detailed smoking history was obtained, including self-reported level of inhalation (rated as nil, slight, moderate or deep). In addition, a blood sample was collected and carboxyhaemoglobin saturation and cholesterol levels were measured. Causes of death of cohort members were obtained from records of the National Health Service and the Office of Population Censuses and Surveys records. The risks of mortality from three causes (i.e. ischaemic heart disease, lung cancer and chronic obstructive lung disease) were computed using Cox's proportional hazard analysis.

(ii)   Sweden

Swedish Twin Registry Study

A cohort of 10 945 twin pairs of the same sex, identified using the Swedish Twin registry, was asked to complete a questionnaire in 1961. Zygosity was based on questions of childhood similarity. Mortality in twins was followed up by record linkage with the central registry of causes of death through 1997. The information from death certificates, hospital records and other data was collected for the period up until 1981 and was reviewed without prior knowledge of smoking status; the underlying cause of death was determined according to the ICD 8th revision. For the period after 1981, the underlying cause of death as stated in the death certificate was used (Floderus et al., 1988; Steineck et al., 1988; Grönberg et al., 1996; Terry et al., 1998, 1999, 2001).

Swedish Census Study

A sample of the Swedish population drawn from the 1960 census was stratified by sex, year of birth and residence (urban or rural). The objective was to determine the smoking habits of the Swedish population by means of postal questionnaires, telephone interviews and home visits. A questionnaire was posted in 1963, and, of 55 074 eligible subjects, 89% responded. Information was collected by telephone or personal interview for another 5.3%. A sub-sample of 20% was sent a second questionnaire in 1969, with the aim of validating the accuracy of the replies and collecting information about changes in smoking patterns. Mortality in the cohort was ascertained through death certificates. In addition, cancer incidence was ascertained through the nationwide Swedish Cancer Registry, which recorded an estimated 95.5% of all cancers. The follow-up period extended from 1964 until 1989. Cancer outcomes were reported after 10 and 26 years for men and women combined (Cederlöf et al., 1975; Nordlund et al., 1999) and after 16 years for men only (Carstensen et al., 1987) and after 26 years for women only (Nordlund et al., 1997). Cox proportional hazards regression models were used to compute odds ratios stratified by age and place of residence.

Swedish Construction Workers' Study

A cohort of male Swedish construction workers was identified in 1971, when workers filled out a questionnaire, the answers to which included a detailed smoking history. The cohort included about 135 000 men recruited between 1971 and 1975 or 350 000 men recruited between 1971 and 1992. Each cohort member contributed person–years of observation from the date of first registration visit until the date of diagnosis, death, migration or end of follow-up (Adami et al., 1996; Nyrén et al., 1996; Adami et al., 1998; Chow et al., 2000). Data on cancer incidence were obtained through linkage with the population-based national cancer registry established in 1958. Each cohort member was identified by his national registration number, a unique personal identifier assigned to all residents in Sweden.

(iii)   Norway

Norwegian Cohort Study

Heuch et al. (1983), Engeland et al. (1996a,b) and Kjaerheim et al. (1998) reported the cancer incidence of a cohort of 26 000 Norwegians who completed a self-administered questionnaire in 1964–1965. The target population was drawn from three sources: approximately 19 000 persons were randomly drawn from lists of residents of Norway from the 1960 population census, approximately 5200 were drawn from four selected counties, and approximately 13 000 were drawn from a cohort of Norwegians living in Norway who had siblings living in the USA. The final study population comprised 26 126 persons, contributing approximately 540 000 person–years for analysis (230 000 for men and 310 000 for women). At the initial assessment, 17% of the men reported never having been a smoker, whereas 68% of the women had never smoked. Information on cancer incidence was obtained through the population-based Norwegian Cancer Registry, which has been operational through the mandatory reporting of cancer cases by physicians since 1953. All cohort members were followed up from 1966 to the date of the first diagnosis of the cancer being considered, the date of emigration, the date of death, or until 31 December 1993. The only exception was for cancers of the upper aerodigestive tract, where more than one diagnosis per person was allowed. Questionnaire data were not updated during the follow-up period. Analyses were performed using the Cox proportional hazards regression models.

Norwegian Screening Study

The Norwegian Screening study followed the cancer incidence in a random sample of adults from two cities and three counties in Norway who were screened for coronary heart disease between different time periods (see Table 2.1). Participants were followed until death or emigration up to 1988. The officially coded underlying cause of death was used as the end-point. Mortality rates were adjusted for age and area of residence and analysed with Cox proportional hazards models (Vatten & Kvinnsland, 1990; Tverdal *et al.*, 1993; Thune & Lund, 1994; Veierød *et al.*, 1997).

(iv)   *Finland*

Finnish Men's Study

A cohort of 4604 Finnish–Norwegian men was interviewed in 1962 about their smoking habits and cardiorespiratory symptoms. The study subjects were selected from three urban areas in western and central Finland, and three rural areas in western and eastern Finland (Pedersen *et al.*, 1969). One hundred and thirty-two men who died or were diagnosed with lung cancer before 1964, and 20 who had not given details of their smoking habits at the interview, were excluded, leaving an effective cohort size of 4452 men. The follow-up period for analysis covered 1964–80. Lung cancer cases were identified through the population-based cancer registry in Finland, by use of the Finnish personal identification number. The effect of smoking and different respiratory symptoms on lung cancer incidence was assessed by a log-linear modelling technique (Tenkanen *et al.*, 1987; Hakulinen *et al.*, 1997).

Finnish Mobile Clinic Health Examination Study

Between 1966 and 1972, the Finnish Mobile Clinic Health Examination Survey performed multiphasic health examinations in rural, semiurban and industrial municipalities in different parts of Finland. A total of 62 440 white adults aged $\geq$ 15 years were invited to participate, and the participation rate was 83%. All participants completed a questionnaire that had been sent in advance and checked at baseline examination. Participants were followed up until 1991 (Knekt *et al.*, 1998; Heikkilä *et al.*, 1999).

(v)   *Iceland*

Reykjavík Study

Tulinius *et al.* (1997) assembled a cohort of 22 946 adult Icelanders in five stages for a study on risk factors for cardiovascular disease. The first stage took place from 1967 to 1969, the second from 1970 to 1972, the third from 1974 to 1979, the fourth from 1979 to 1984 and the fifth from 1985 to 1991. The initial enrolment interview took place at a clinic visit at which the completion of a comprehensive questionnaire concerning various risk factors was followed by a series of anthropometric and biochemical measurements. Although interviews were conducted at each stage, this study used only data from each subject's first interview. Overall, 73% of the initial target population was successfully recruited into the study. The cohort was linked with the Icelandic Cancer Registry, a population-based registry of the entire country that was begun in 1954. Linking to the registry was facilitated by the unique identification number assigned to all residents in Iceland. Cox's regression was used to analyse the predictive power of a number of variables on the incidence of first cancer after enrolment into the study.

(vi)   *Netherlands*

Dutch Study

A cohort of 26 697 women from the city of Utrecht in the Netherlands answered a questionnaire and provided a 12-h urine sample at the beginning of the follow-up period. Follow-up continued from entry to the study for up to 15 years. The full cohort was drawn from two previously established screening programmes. The first was a population-based screening programme for the early detection of breast cancer in women aged 40–64 years, called the DOM project. This portion of the cohort had 14 697 women who were enrolled from early 1975 until mid-1977, 72% of whom participated. One year later, 81% of this group participated in a follow-up effort in which a second 12-h urine sample was collected. The second breast cancer screening programme (Lutine study) was undertaken in 1982–83 and included more than 12 000 women 40–49 years of age [exact number not stated by the author]. For this second screening programme, 12-h urine samples were taken on days 21–23 of three consecutive menstrual cycles. Participation in the second screening programme was only 44%, probably because of the demanding study protocol. An all-cause-of-death register was established for this study to which all medical practitioners in the city of Utrecht who saw cohort members in their practices reported. In 1987, a regional cancer register was established, making it possible to follow the entire study cohort for cancer incidence. There were three distinct follow-up periods (Ellard *et al.*, 1995; de Waard *et al.*, 1995; van Wayenburg *et al.*, 2000).

(vii)   *Denmark*

Copenhagen City Heart Study

In 1976, a prospective epidemiological study was initiated in which participants were selected from 90 000 persons living in a defined area around the University Hospital of Copenhagen. An age-stratified sample of subjects aged 20 years or more was selected at random. Seventy-four per cent of those invited to participate (14 223 subjects) attended. The subjects were followed up until 1989. Notification of deaths and causes of death were obtained from the Central Death Registry of the National Board of Health (Lange *et al.*, 1992).

(b)   North America

(i)   USA

Framingham Heart Study

The Framingham Heart Study included 5209 subjects who were first examined between 1948 and 1952, and were aged 45–84 years at baseline examination. Participants were routinely examined every two years for 24 or 34 years. At these examinations, information on smoking status and other risk factors was updated. A tumour registry was set up for this cohort (Williams *et al.*, 1981; Freund *et al.*, 1993).

American Cancer Society (nine-state) Study

In 1952, more than 22 000 volunteers for the American Cancer Society each distributed a questionnaire to 10 white men aged 50–69 years whom the volunteer knew well. Smoking histories were collected from 204 547 men in nine states. After exclusion of unsuitable subjects, a cohort of 187 783 men was followed by the volunteers from 1952 through 1955 (average duration, 44 months). A total of 11 870 deaths (6.2%) and 1.1% losses to follow-up were recorded. Death certificates were obtained for all reported deaths and further information was sought from the physician, hospital or tumour registry whenever cancer was mentioned in the certificate (Hammond & Horn, 1958a,b). The distribution of smoking habits in the study population was in close agreement with that reported in a large survey on smoking habits in a sample of the US population (Haenszel *et al.*, 1956).

US Veterans' Study

Beginning in January 1954, 293 958 holders of US government Life Insurance policies who had served in the armed forces at any time between 1917 and 1940 were sent a questionnaire on smoking habits; 198 834 (68%) responded and 49 361 additional replies were obtained by a subsequent mailing in 1957 (total response rate, 85%). Policy holders were almost exclusively white men of the middle and upper social classes. Subjects were followed up from 1954 until 1980 during which time there were 192 756 deaths. Whenever a claim was filed for payment of a policy, a copy of the death certificate was sent by the Veterans' Administration to the National Institutes of Health study office. 'Terminated' policies were also checked annually to ascertain if termination was due to death or to other reasons. Additional information on policy holders who had died was requested from a certifying physician or hospital. The 26-year follow-up was considered to be almost complete by Chow *et al.* (1995), with 95% of the death certificates of cohort members who had died having been obtained (Kahn, 1966; Rogot & Murray, 1980; Kinlen & Rogot, 1988; McLaughlin *et al.*, 1989; Hsing *et al.*, 1990a; McLaughlin *et al.*, 1990a,b; Hsing *et al.*, 1991; Heineman *et al.*, 1992; Zahm *et al.*, 1992; Chow *et al.*, 1993; Heineman *et al.*, 1994; Chow *et al.*, 1995; McLaughlin *et al.*, 1995; Chow *et al.*, 1996).

Californian Study

Information on occupational exposures and smoking history was collected from self-administered questionnaires in 1954–57 from 68 153 male labour union members, aged 35–64 years, in California. Subjects were followed up for mortality up to December 1962 (average follow-up time, 7.1 years) through California death records. A total of 4706 deaths occurred in the cohort, 936 of which were from cancer (Weir & Dunn, 1970). [The Working Group noted that the data available on smoking habits were less extensive than those obtained in other studies.]

Cancer Prevention Study I (CPS-I)

Between October 1959 and February 1960, volunteers for the American Cancer Society in 25 states recruited more than one million subjects from among their friends, neighbours and acquaintances. Families were enrolled, with the condition that there be at least one person aged over 45 years in the family. All family members over 30 years of age were requested to fill out a detailed four-page questionnaire. Participants were predominantly white (97%), married (82%) and college-educated. For the 1 051 038 subjects enrolled, vital status was monitored by the volunteers, originally to September 1965 (Thun & Heath, 1997). Each subject was traced annually and every 2 years was requested to fill out a brief follow-up questionnaire. Of the subjects originally enrolled, 1% could not be traced in the follow-up, and 2% of the questionnaires were unusable. Death certificates were obtained from state or local authorities and, when cancer was mentioned, further information was sought from physicians. The underlying cause of death was coded according to the ICD 7th revision. During the first 6 years of follow-up, 76 888 subjects died and 14 029 (1.4%) were lost to follow-up; 483 519 white women and 358 422 white men alive at the end of 1966 were further followed up for mortality until 1972 with a success rate for follow-up of 99%. This is the largest of the early cohort studies on tobacco and mortality (Hammond & Garfinkel, 1961; Hammond, 1966; Garfinkel, 1980; Hammond & Seidman, 1980; Garfinkel, 1985; Stellman & Garfinkel, 1986, 1989a,b; Garfinkel & Boffetta, 1990; Thun et al., 1995; Thun & Heath, 1997; Thun et al., 1997a; Shanks & Burns, 1998).

Harvard Alumni Study

A cohort of undergraduates who had entered the University of Harvard between the years of 1916 and 1950 was identified when they responded to a health questionnaire sent out in 1962 or 1966. Updated information was obtained from 13 905 cohort members from periodic surveys that assessed lifestyle habits and medical history. The questions asked for information on daily amount of cigarette smoking, age at start and cessation of cigarette smoking, weight, height and physical activity. In surveys conducted in 1988 and 1993, participants were asked whether a cancer had been diagnosed by a physician. Deaths that occurred up to 1992 were traced using information from the alumni office to obtain death certificates. The authors claimed that mortality follow-up was virtually complete (Paffenbarger et al., 1977, 1978).

Tecumseh Community Health Study

The Tecumseh Community Health Study involved subjects who participated in one or more rounds of physical examinations offered to 9794 persons from a semi-rural community in 1959–60, 1962–65 and 1967–69. Cigarette smoking history was taken at each examination cycle. A retrospective cohort was created from those participants aged 25 years and older and who were free of cancer (except for non-melanoma skin cancer) at baseline or within 1 year of entering the study. These criteria resulted in a fixed cohort of 3956 subjects, for whom complete follow-up data were available. In 1986–87, a comprehensive cancer incidence survey was conducted by means of a questionnaire sent to the participants or their next-of-kin. An estimated completeness of 95% was achieved. The reported cancer cases were verified, with the permission of the participant, by requesting abstracts of hospital records. A Cox proportional hazards model was used to examine lung cancer incidence in relation to smoking habits (Islam & Schottenfeld, 1994).

Kaiser Permanente Medical Care Program Study

The first cohort included approximately 175 000 subjects aged 15–94 years who underwent at least one multi-phasic health check-up between 1964 and 1973 within the Kaiser Permanente Medical Care Program. Cancer incidence was ascertained from the first health examination until 1988 through the San Francisco-Oakland Surveillance, Epidemiology and End Result (SEER) programme and the Northern California Kaiser Permanente Medical Care Program. Approximately 4.4% of the cohort were lost to the study (Hiatt & Bawol, 1984; Hiatt & Fireman, 1986; Friedman, 1993; Friedman & van den Eeden, 1993; Herrinton & Friedman, 1998; Iribarren et al., 2001). Between 1978 and 1985, a similar cohort was established, which included a maximum of 120 000 subjects aged 30–89 years. In one study, the cohort was further followed up until 1987 (Sidney et al., 1993). Cancer cases were ascertained as for the first cohort (Hiatt et al., 1988; Klatsky et al., 1988; Sidney et al., 1993; Hiatt et al., 1994; Herrinton & Friedman, 1998).

American Men of Japanese Ancestry Study

A cohort of 8006 American men of Japanese ancestry, born during the years 1900–19 and who resided on the Hawaiian island of Oahu, were interviewed and examined clinically from 1965 to 1968. Information obtained at the interview included age, smoking history, usual occupation, type of housing, education and religion. A 24-h dietary recall questionnaire was also administered. Newly diagnosed cases of cancer were identified through continuous surveillance of Oahu hospitals and linkage with the Hawaii Tumor Registry (Stemmermann et al., 1988; Severson et al., 1989; Nomura et al., 1990a,b; Chyou et al., 1992, 1993a,b, 1995; Nomura et al., 1995; Chyou et al., 1996).

Lutheran Brotherhood Insurance Study

A cohort of 17 633 white male life insurance policy holders of the Lutheran Brotherhood Insurance Society was identified in 1966. A response rate of 68.5% was achieved and little difference was observed between responders and non-responders to the questionnaire with regard to age, urban or rural residence, policy status and cancer mortality at 11.5 years of follow-up. The questionnaire included questions on tobacco use in the form of cigarettes, cigars, pipes and smokeless tobacco. Other questions asked for details of the longest held occupation, frequency of consumption of 35 food items and the consumption of coffee, beer and spirits. Death certificates were coded for underlying and contributory causes of death. Person–years were accumulated up to death, loss to follow-up or the end of the study in 1986. The age-adjusted relative risks for cancer mortality resulting from exposure to tobacco, occupation and dietary variables were computed using Poisson regression. Statistical interaction between smoking and other risk factors was also examined. About 23% of the cohort members were lost to follow-up (Hsing *et al.*, 1990b; Kneller *et al.*, 1991; Linet *et al.*, 1991; Chow *et al.*, 1992; Linet *et al.*, 1992; Zheng *et al.*, 1993; Hsing *et al.*, 1998).

MRFIT Study

The MRFIT study was conducted on a cohort of 361 662 men who were seen at an initial screening visit at 22 clinical centres throughout the USA and were thereby enrolled into the cohort in 1975. At the initial visit, 37% ($n = 133\ 117$) were current smokers, consuming an average of 26 cigarettes per day. A total of 12 866 participants were selected for an intervention trial based on a high risk score for coronary heart disease assigned at the baseline physical examination. High risk for coronary heart disease was determined by a combination of factors, using a logistic regression function derived from men in the same age group in the Framingham Heart Study, including cigarette smoking habits, diastolic blood pressure and serum cholesterol at the first screening visit (Kuller *et al.*, 1991).

Nurses' Health Study

In 1976, a cohort of 121 700 female registered nurses was assembled in the USA. At enrolment, the nurses completed a mailed questionnaire on risk factors for cancer and heart disease. Responses to food-frequency questionnaires were also collected in 1980, 1984, 1986 and 1990. The response rate to follow-up questionnaires was almost 96% through to 1990. Family members were the main source of vital status information for non-respondents but the National Death Index was also used. Multiple logistic regression models were used to compute odds ratios, after controlling for age, total energy intake and other potentially confounding variables (Willett *et al.*, 1987; Hunter *et al.*, 1990; Chute *et al.*, 1991; Giovannucci *et al.*, 1994a; Grodstein *et al.*, 1995; Kearney *et al.*, 1995; Fuchs *et al.*, 1996; Egan *et al.*, 2002).

Using the same cohort, Speizer *et al.* (1999) collected and updated information on smoking status and health status by means of a follow-up questionnaire distributed every 2 years from baseline until 1992.

Adventists' Health Study

A cohort of 34 198 non-Hispanic white Seventh-day Adventists in California (mean age, 55.4 years) was formed in 1976 when they completed a questionnaire concerning lifestyle. During the period of follow-up from enrolment until December 1982, newly diagnosed cancers were ascertained by various means. First, a record linkage of the cohort members was made with two population-based cancer registries, the Cancer Surveillance Program in Los Angeles and the Resource for Cancer Epidemiology in San Francisco. Second, annual contact was maintained with every member of the cohort by means of a mailed questionnaire in which the study subject was asked to report whether he or she had been hospitalized in the previous 12 months. Study staff reviewed all medical records for evidence of cancer diagnoses. The authors stated that follow-up was 99% complete. Relative risks adjusted for permanent covariates were computed by use of the Cox proportional hazards model (Mills *et al.*, 1988, 1989a,b, 1990, 1991; Singh & Fraser, 1998).

Leisure World Study

A detailed health questionnaire was sent to all residents of a retirement community in California in 1981, and to new residents in 1982, 1983 and 1985. A response rate of 61% was achieved overall. Almost all of the residents were Caucasians of the upper-middle class; about two-thirds were women; and 80% were aged 65–86 years. Histological diagnosis of cancer was obtained from local hospitals. All participants were sent a follow-up questionnaire every 2 years (Wu *et al.*, 1987; Ross *et al.*, 1990; Shibata *et al.*, 1994).

Cancer Prevention Study II (CPS-II)

The Cancer Prevention Study II (CPS-II) is a nationwide prospective mortality cohort study of nearly 1.2 million adults enrolled by volunteers of the American Cancer Society in 1982. As in CPS-I, enrolment was based on families and excluded persons in institutions and military service and others who would be difficult to trace (Garfinkel, 1985). Each participant completed a confidential four-page postal questionnaire on tobacco and alcohol use, diet and other factors potentially related to cancer. Deaths were ascertained from month of enrolment until 31 December 1996 through personal enquiries made by the volunteers in 1984, 1986 and 1988 and later through linkage with the National Death Index. Most of the smoking-related analyses were based on follow-up through 1986, 1988 or 1989 to minimize misclassification of exposure of those smokers who quit during follow-up. By 1988, 1.8% of the cohort were lost to follow-up and 79 802 (6.7%) had died (Thun & Heath, 1997). The ninth revision (ICD-9) of the International Classification of Diseases was used to code the underlying cause of death. Participants in CPS-II were more likely to be white (93%), married (81%) and educated (high school graduates or above, 85.6%) than the general population of the USA. The analyses excluded former cigarette smokers and persons with incomplete or unclassifiable data on smoking status or on the frequency or duration of cigarette smoking; men who ever smoked a pipe or a cigar or for whom pipe or cigar smoking status was unclear, were also excluded (Garfinkel, 1985; Stellman & Garfinkel, 1986; Garfinkel & Stellman, 1988; Stellman & Garfinkel, 1989a; Garfinkel & Boffetta, 1990; Calle *et al.*, 1994; Thun *et al.*, 1995; Heath *et al.*, 1997; Thun & Heath, 1997; Thun *et al.*, 1997a,b; Kahn *et al.*, 1998; Chao *et al.*, 2000; Shapiro *et al.*, 2000; Chao *et al.*, 2002).

Iowa Women's Health Study

The Iowa Women's Health Study was conducted on a cohort of 41 837 women who completed a postal questionnaire (response rate, 42.7%) sent in 1986 to a random sample of women from the Iowa driver's licence list (Potter *et al.*, 1992). The questionnaire covered information on age, smoking history, physical activity, level of education and alcohol consumption. Cigarette consumption was analysed as pack–years for both current and former smokers. Physical activity was ascertained by questionnaire and translated into a three-level physical activity score (low, medium and high). Incident cases of cancer were ascertained by the Health Registry of Iowa, which is a population-based cancer registry in the SEER Program of the National Cancer Institute (Bostick *et al.*, 1994; Harnack *et al.*, 1997; Parker *et al.*, 2000).

Health Professionals' Follow-up Study

In 1986, a cohort of 51 529 male dentists, optometrists, osteopaths, podiatrists, pharmacists and veterinarians in the USA were asked to respond to a postal questionnaire. The questionnaire included questions on age, current and past tobacco use, marital status, height and weight, ancestry, medications, disease history, physical activity and diet. Only men who completed the diet questionnaire adequately at baseline and who reported no cancer other than non-melanoma skin cancer were included in the analysis. After all base-line exclusions, 47 781 men comprised the analysis cohort. Follow-up questionnaires were sent in 1988, 1990, 1992 and 1994 to ascertain new cancer cases and to update smoking status. Family members and the National Death Index were the main source of information on vital status of non-respondents. After repeated mailings, the follow-up response rate was 94% up to 1994 and ascertainment of death was estimated to be 98%. Pooled logistic regression was used in analysis, which accounts for varying time to the outcome event and which is asymptotically equivalent to a Cox regression model with time-dependent covariate, given the short intervals and low probability of outcomes (Giovannuci *et al.*, 1994b; Kearney *et al.*, 1995; Fuchs *et al.*, 1996; van Dam *et al.*, 1999; Giovannuci *et al.*, 1999).

(ii) *Canada*

Canadian War Veterans' Study

After a pilot study to validate the questionnaire in 1955–56, 207 397 war veterans listed by the Canadian Pension Commission were sent a questionnaire on smoking habits, principal occupations and residence history. Approximately 118 000 forms (57%) were returned; after removal of duplicates and unusable forms some 92 000 (44%) (78 000 men and 14 000 women) remained. Follow-up was conducted from 1956 to 1962 through quarterly lists of deaths made available by the Department of Veterans Affairs. There were 9491 deaths among men and 1794 deaths among women; in most cases the cause of death was confirmed by autopsy (Best *et al.*, 1961; Lossing *et al.*, 1966).

National Breast Screening Study

The National Breast Screening Study is a multicentre, randomized controlled trial of mammography screening for breast cancer. Between 1980 and 1985, 89 835 women aged 40–59 years were recruited. In 1982, a second questionnaire was distributed to new attendees and previously enrolled women returning to the screening centres for further screening. A total of 56 837 women returned the questionnaires. Analyses are based mainly on respondents to the second questionnaire (Friedenreich *et al.*, 1993; Terry *et al.*, 2002).

       (*c*)   *Asia*

         (i)   *China*

Shanghai Factory Study

Chen *et al.* (1997) studied a cohort of 9351 adults from 11 factories in urban Shanghai. This cohort was identified in two stages: one during 1972–73 and the other during 1977–78, when members completed an interview based on a structured questionnaire. The questionnaire included questions on smoking, alcohol consumption, occupation, medical history and physical exercise. Vital status of the cohort members was monitored using factory records until 1 January 1993, with only 4% of subjects lost to follow-up. Cause of death was ascertained by examination of death certificates and the underlying cause of death was determined by two nosologists blinded to the smoking status of the individual. The Cox proportional hazards model was used for comparing a gradient of smoking categories with nonsmokers, while simultaneously adjusting for relevant covariates. At baseline, 61% of men and 7% of women smoked. Of the men, 46% consumed more than 20 cigarettes per day whereas only 11% of the female smokers consumed this number. Thirty-eight per cent of male smokers had started smoking prior to their twenty-fifth birthday, whereas among women, this figure was 25%.

Xi'an Factory Study

A cohort of 1696 persons was identified for a cross-sectional survey of coronary heart disease among employees of a machinery factory in Xi'an in May 1976. Employees were monitored for cause-specific mortality until 1996. Approximately 7% of the cohort members were subjected to occupationally hazardous exposures according to factory physicians. Vital status was ascertained from personnel and union records and confirmed through interviews of co-workers or relatives. The Cox regression model was used, adjusting for potential confounding factors including age, marital status, occupation, education, diastolic blood pressure and triglycerides and total cholesterol levels. During the 20 years of follow-up, 173 men and 45 women died (Lam *et al.*, 1997).

Shanghai Residential Study

A cohort of 213 800 residents from urban, suburban and surrounding rural areas of Shanghai were surveyed for smoking status. Subjects in urban areas were followed up annually for 12 years (January 1983 to December 1994) and subjects in suburban areas and rural counties for 11 years (January 1984 to December 1994). The cause of deaths during the follow-up period was ascertained by medical professionals. Only data on subjects aged 40 years and over at enrolment were analysed. Because the prevalence of smoking among women aged 40 years and over in suburban and rural areas was very low (3.1% and 1.5%, respectively), data on women in these areas were excluded from the analysis. Person–years observed were calculated by sex, age, smoking status and area of residence. A Poisson regression model was used to estimate age-adjusted relative risks with 95% confidence limits for each cause of death (Gao *et al.*, 1999).

Linxian Intervention Trial Study

In the frame of an intervention trial for micronutrients, approximately 30 000 residents of the Linxian region were interviewed to obtain information on usual dietary intake, tobacco use, alcohol drinking, family history of cancer and other factors. The cohort was followed up from 1986 until 1991, with little loss to follow-up. Information on cause of death and incidence of cancer was collected from local hospitals or a study medical team. Relative risks were adjusted for potential confounders as well as the vitamin/mineral intervention group (Guo *et al.*, 1994).

Shanghai Men's Study

Ross *et al.* (1992) and Yuan *et al.* (1996) studied a cohort of 18 244 male residents of Shanghai, enrolled between 1986 and 1989 (80% of eligible subjects). A structured questionnaire was completed at a face-to-face interview. The information obtained included level of education, history of tobacco and alcohol use, current diet and medical history. At recruitment, 50% of study subjects were current smokers, half of whom smoked 20 or more cigarettes per day. Former smokers represented 7% of the cohort while 43% of cohort members had never smoked cigarettes regularly. Cancer incidence was ascertained through the population-based Shanghai Cancer Registry and vital status was ascertained by inspection of the Shanghai death certificate records. Only 50 subjects were lost to follow-up which continued until 1993.

Taiwanese Study

A cohort of 14 397 residents of metropolitan, urban and rural areas in Taiwan, China were recruited between 1982 and 1986. Information on sociodemographic characteristics, smoking status, alcohol drinking and food habits was collected at interview using a structured questionnaire. The cohort was followed up until 1994 by linkage with the death certification system in Taiwan. Causes of death were classified according to ICD-9. Cox proportional hazards regression models were used to derive relative risks for mortality and to examine dose–responses (Liaw & Chen, 1998).

(ii)   *Japan*

Life Span Study

The Life Span Study cohort originally consisted of 100 000 survivors [sex distribution not reported] of the atomic bomb blasts in Hiroshima and Nagasaki. The cohort was expanded in 1968 and 1985 by adding approximately 10 000 survivors each time. The total cohort included approximately 120 000 individuals, of whom approximately 27 000 were non-exposed controls. Information on smoking was obtained from three interview surveys conducted on a subgroup of the entire cohort in 1963–64, 1964–68 and 1968–70, and four postal surveys conducted on various subgroups in 1965, 1969, 1979 and 1980. The cancer incidence in 61 505 survivors for whom smoking data were available was reported. For 42% of this group, information on smoking was available from at least two surveys. Information on cancer incidence and mortality was obtained from the Radiation Effects Research Foundation tumour registry and mortality database. Poisson regression models were used to fit log-linear relative risk and linear excess relative risk models (Akiba, 1994; Land *et al.*, 1994; Goodman *et al.*, 1995).

Japanese Physicians' Study

A survey of smoking and drinking habits among physicians in western Japan was carried out using self-administered questionnaires in 1965. From 6815 male respondents in nine prefectures (51% response rate), a cohort of 5477 male physicians was established. Vital status was followed until 1983 and confirmed by various medical associations. Copies of death certificates were obtained from the District Legal Affairs Bureau and the cause of death coded with the ICD-8. After exclusions, the analysis was done on 5130 men. Statistical analysis was performed using the Cox proportional hazards model (Kono *et al.*, 1987).

Six-prefecture Study

In 1965, 122 261 men and 142 857 women aged ≥ 40 years (95% of the census population) in 29 health centre districts from six prefectures in Japan were interviewed. The six prefectures were selected as being representative of the entire country. The questionnaire included questions on smoking, alcohol consumption and dietary habits, occupation, and marital status. A record linkage system was established for the annual follow-up. During the 16-year follow-up period, 8% of the cohort migrated from the original health districts. Deaths among cohort members were monitored by linkage to vital statistics kept at each public health centre. Cause of death was coded using the 7th revision of the International Classification of Diseases (Hirayama, 1967, 1975a,b, 1977a,b, 1978, 1981, 1982, 1985, 1989a,b,c; Mizuno *et al.*, 1989; Akiba & Hirayama, 1990; Hirayama, 1990; Kinjo *et al.*, 1998).

Regular male smokers who had started smoking between 18 and 22 years of age, and who were, at that time, between the ages of 40 and 79 years, were selected from the cohort for further analysis, resulting in a subcohort of 49 013 men (Mizuno *et al.*, 1989). [This study was large and unique in that it involved a non-Caucasian population and was based on interviews rather than self-completed questionnaires.]

Chiba Center Association Study

The Chiba Center Association Study was a nested case–control study based on a cohort population of 17 200 male participants in a mass screening for gastric cancer by the Chiba Cancer Association in Japan in 1984. Cancer cases in cohort members were detected by record linkage to the Chiba Cancer Registry. The participants were followed from 1984 until 1993. For each cancer case, two controls were selected from the cohort population by matching on sex, birth year and area of residence (Murata *et al.*, 1996).

Fukuoka Study

A baseline survey was conducted from 1986 until 1989 among the general population of Fukuoka, the region with the highest liver cancer mortality in Japan. All inhabitants aged > 30 years were asked to answer a questionnaire, to which the response rate was 84.3%. A follow-up survey was conducted annually to verify the vital status of participants. For study subjects who had died, the cause of death was determined from the health certificate and classified according to ICD-9. The participants were followed up until 1996.

Women were excluded from this survey because of the small numbers of deaths and current smokers. After exclusions, 4050 men were included in the analysis. Cox proportional hazards regression analysis was employed to estimate relative risks and 95% confidence intervals (Mizoue *et al.*, 2000).

(*d*)   *Others*

Seven-country Study

Jacobs *et al.* (1999) studied a cohort of 12 763 men in seven countries between 1957 and 1964, after administration of a standardized questionnaire. The questionnaire included questions about daily cigarette consumption at entry, years of smoking cessation for former smokers, age, weight and height. A physical examination at baseline included a comprehensive history of cardiovascular and cerebral vascular health. Information on vital status and cause of death was obtained during the 25 years of follow-up, by examining death certificates, collecting medical records from hospitals and from interviews with physicians and relatives. A Cox proportional hazards model was used to compute relative risk.

Israel Civil Service Centre Study

In 1963, Kark *et al.* (1995) studied a cohort of 9975 male civil servants between the ages of 40 and 69 years living in Haifa, Jerusalem and Tel Aviv, Israel. The initial examination included a physical examination, measurement of blood pressure, weight and height, electrocardiography and venipuncture. A questionnaire, which included questions on sociodemography, health behaviour, diet and psychosocial factors, was administered by a trained interviewer. Further examinations were carried out in 1965 and 1968. The follow-up period ended on 31 December 1986 and included 198 298 person–years of cancer surveillance by linking the cohort list to both the National Cancer Registry and the National Death Registry. A total of 153 cases of lung cancer were identified. The Cox proportional hazards model was used to compute relative risk by including age as a continuous variable, and city of employment, cigarette smoking and body-mass index as dummy variables. The reference categories were never-smokers, resident in Haifa and Tel Aviv, and the upper fifth of the body-mass index frequency distribution.

Table 2.1. Cohort studies of cancer and cigarette smoking

Country Name of study	Date of cohort sampling	References	Maximum years of follow-up	Cohort sample and age at beginning of follow-up	Collection of information	Cases/ deaths	Neoplasms analysed	Comments
United Kingdom								
British Doctors' Study	1951	Doll & Hill (1964a,b); Doll & Peto (1976); Doll et al. (1980, 1994)	1951–91	40 634 (34 440 men, 6194 women) British doctors [age not reported]	Postal questionnaire	Deaths	Lung, urinary bladder, kidney, upper aerodigestive tract (oesophagus, mixed), pancreas, stomach, colon, rectum, liver, leukaemia, ovary, non-Hodgkin lymphoma, multiple myelomas	Information on pipe and cigars
Whitehall Study	1967–69	Ben-Shlomo et al. (1994)	1967–87	19 018 men from the British Civil Service, clinically examined, aged 40–69 years	Interview	Deaths	Lung	Information on pipe and cigars
British United Provident Association (BUPA) Study	1975–82	Wald & Watt (1997)	1975–93	21 520 professional and businessmen, aged 35–64 years	Interview	Deaths	Lung	Information on pipe and cigars
Sweden								
Swedish Twin Registry Study	1961	Floderus et al. (1988); Steineck et al. (1988); Grönberg et al. (1996); Terry et al. (1998, 1999, 2001)	1961–97	10 942 same-sex twin pairs, born 1886–1925	Postal questionnaire	Deaths	Lung, urinary bladder, stomach, colon, rectum, endometrium, prostate	Information on pipe and cigars Floderus et al. mentioned 10 945 pairs.

Table 2.1 (contd)

Country Name of study	Date of cohort sampling	References	Maximum years of follow-up	Cohort sample and age at beginning of follow-up	Collection of information	Cases/deaths	Neoplasms analysed	Comments
Swedish Census Study	1963	I: Cederlöf et al. (1975); Carstensen et al. (1987)	1963–72	Adults selected from the 1960 census population, aged 18–69 years I: 51 911 (25 444 men, 26 467 women)	Postal questionnaire (94%), telephone, interview	Deaths	Lung, urinary bladder, pancreas, colon, rectum, liver, endometrium, cervix	Information on pipe and cigars Stratified by urban-rural residence
		II: Nordlund et al. (1997, 1999)	1964–89	II: 41 710 (15 881 men, 25 829 women)	Postal questionnaire (87%), telephone, home visits	Cases	Lung, urinary bladder, kidney, upper aerodigestive tract (oral cavity, pharynx, oesophagus, mixed), pancreas, stomach, colon/rectum, liver, breast, endometrium, cervix, leukaemia	Stratified by place of residence
Swedish Construction Workers' Study	1971–75 (I) 1971–91 (II) 1971–92 (III)	I: Adami et al. (1996); Nyrén et al. (1996) II: Adami et al. (1998) III: Chow et al. (2000)	1971–92	Male construction workers, aged ≥ 35 years I: 143 998 II: 334 957 III: 363 992	Self-administered questionnaire/interview	Cases	Kidney, colon, rectum, prostate, leukaemia, non-Hodgkin lymphoma, Hodgkin lymphoma, multiple myelomas	

Table 2.1 (contd)

Country Name of study	Date of cohort sampling	References	Maximum years of follow-up	Cohort sample and age at beginning of follow-up	Collection of information	Cases/ deaths	Neoplasms analysed	Comments
Norway								
Norwegian Cohort Study	1964–65	Heuch et al. (1983); Engeland et al. (1996a,b); Kjaerheim et al. (1998)	1966–93	26 132 subjects (11 863 men, 14 269 women) including a sample of the 1960 census population, a random sample from 4 selected counties and a sample of siblings living in Norway with a sibling living in the USA, aged 33–72 years	Postal questionnaire	Cases	Lung, urinary bladder, kidney, upper aerodigestive tract (mixed), pancreas, stomach, colon, rectum, breast, endometrium, cervix, prostate, leukaemia, ovary	·
Norwegian Screening Study	1974–78 (I) 1972–78 (II) 1977–83 (III)	I: Vatten & Kvinnsland (1990) II: Tverdal et al. (1993); Thune & Lund (1994) III: Veierød et al. (1997)	1972–88	Participants in a health screening programme, aged 35–49 years I: 24 329 women II: 44 290 men, 24 535 women; 53 242 men III: 26 119 men	Interview	Deaths	Lung, pancreas, stomach, colon, rectum, breast, cervix, prostate	Information on pipe and cigars
Finland								
Finnish Men's Study	1962	Pedersen et al. (1969); Tenkanen et al. (1987); Hakulinen et al. (1997)	1964–80	4452 men from 3 urban and 3 rural areas, born 1898–1917	Interview	Cases	Lung, prostate	Hakulinen et al. (1997) also included subjects from another survey in 1972–77

Table 2.1 (contd)

Country Name of study	Date of cohort sampling	References	Maximum years of follow-up	Cohort sample and age at beginning of follow-up	Collection of information	Cases/ deaths	Neoplasms analysed	Comments
Finnish Mobile Clinic Health Examination Study	1966–72	Knekt et al. (1998); Heikkilä et al. (1999)	1966–91	56 973 subjects having received multiphasic health examination from the Mobile Clinic [sex distribution not reported]	Postal questionnaire, checked by interview	Cases	Colon, rectum, prostate	
Iceland								
Reykjavik Study	1967–91	Tulinius et al. (1997)	1968–95	22 946 (11 366 men, 11 580 women) residents of Reykjavik, born 1907–1954, aged 31–61 years	Self-administered questionnaire	Cases	Lung, urinary bladder, oesophagus, pancreas, stomach, colon, endometrium, cervix, prostate, leukaemia	
The Netherlands								
Dutch Study	1975–77, 1982–83	Ellard et al. (1995); de Waard et al. (1995); van Wayenburg et al. (2000)	1975–90	26 697 women from 2 breast cancer screening programmes (DOM project and Lutine Study) in Utrecht, aged 40–64 years	Self-administered questionnaire	Cases	Lung, colon/rectum	

Table 2.1 (contd)

Country Name of study	Date of cohort sampling	References	Maximum years of follow-up	Cohort sample and age at beginning of follow-up	Collection of information	Cases/ deaths	Neoplasms analysed	Comments
Denmark								
Copenhagen City Heart Study	1976–78, 1981–83	Lange et al. (1992); Prescott et al. (1999)	1976–89	14 223 subjects (6511 men, 7703 women) randomly selected among 90 000 persons living in a defined area of Copenhagen, aged ≥ 20 years	Self-administered questionnaire	Deaths	Lung	The study by Prescott et al. (1999) was based on data from three cohorts, including the Copenhagen City Heart Study, the Centre of Preventive Medicine and the Copenhagen Male Study.
USA								
Framingham Heart Study	1948–52	Williams et al. (1981); Freund et al. (1993)	1948–82	5209 subjects receiving routine examinations at the Framingham Heart Study Clinic, MA	Interview	Cases	Lung, colon	
American Cancer Society (nine-state) Study	1952	Hammond & Horn (1958a,b)	1952–55	187 783 men from 9 states, aged 50–69 years	Self-administered questionnaire	Deaths	Lung, urinary bladder, upper aerodigestive tract (mixed), pancreas, colon, rectum	Information on pipe and cigars

Table 2.1 (contd)

Country Name of study	Date of cohort sampling	References	Maximum years of follow-up	Cohort sample and age at beginning of follow-up	Collection of information	Cases/ deaths	Neoplasms analysed	Comments
US Veterans' Study	1954, 1957	Kahn (1966); Rogot & Murray (1980); Kinlen & Rogot (1988); McLaughlin et al. (1989); Hsing et al. (1990a); McLaughlin et al. (1990a,b); Hsing et al. (1991); Heineman et al. (1992); Zahm et al. (1992); Chow et al. (1993); Heineman et al. (1994); Chow et al. (1995); Heineman et al. (1995); McLaughlin et al. (1995); Chow et al. (1996)	1954–80	293 958 male holders of a US Government Life Insurance, aged 31–84 years	Postal questionnaire	Deaths	Lung, urinary bladder, kidney, upper aerodigestive tract (oral cavity, nasopharynx, larynx, pharynx, oesophagus), pancreas, stomach, colon, rectum, liver, leukaemia, soft-tissue sarcoma, brain, biliary ducts, adrenals, non-Hodgkin lymphoma, Hodgkin's lymphoma, multiple myelomas	Information on pipe and cigars
Californian Study	1954–57	Weir & Dunn (1970)	1954–62	68 153 male labour union members, aged 35–64 years	Postal questionnaire	Deaths	Lung, urinary bladder, upper aerodigestive tract (oral cavity, larynx, pharynx, oesophagus), pancreas	

Table 2.1 (contd)

Country Name of study	Date of cohort sampling	References	Maximum years of follow-up	Cohort sample and age at beginning of follow-up	Collection of information	Cases/ deaths	Neoplasms analysed	Comments
Cancer Prevention Study I (CPS-I)	1959–60	Hammond & Garfinkel (1961); Hammond (1966); Garfinkel (1980); Hammond & Seidman (1980); Garfinkel (1985); Stellman & Garfinkel (1986, 1989a,b); Garfinkel & Boffetta (1990); Thun et al. (1995); Thun & Heath (1997); Thun et al. (1997a); Shanks & Burns (1998)	1959–72	1 051 038 adults from 25 states, aged > 30 years	Postal questionnaire	Deaths	Lung, urinary bladder, upper aerodigestive tract (oesophagus, mixed), pancreas, stomach, colon/rectum, liver, endometrium, cervix, leukaemia, biliary ducts	Information on pipe and cigars For women, all sites of the aerodigestive tract and all cancers of the haematopoietic system were grouped.
Harvard Alumni Study	1962, 1966	Paffenbarger et al. (1977, 1978)	1962–92	13 905 male Harvard alumni; mean age, 58.3 years	Postal questionnaire	Cases/ deaths	Leukaemia, Hodgkin lymphoma	
Tecumseh Community Health Study (I/II/III)	1962–69	Islam & Schottenfeld, 1994	1962–87	3956 residents (1857 men, 2099 women) of Tecumseh, MI, aged > 25 years	Interview	Cases	Lung	

Table 2.1 (contd)

Country Name of study	Date of cohort sampling	References	Maximum years of follow-up	Cohort sample and age at beginning of follow-up	Collection of information	Cases/ deaths	Neoplasms analysed	Comments
Kaiser Permanente Medical Care Program Study	1964–73 (I) 1978–85 (II) 1964–91 (I+II)	I: Hiatt & Bawol (1984); Hiatt & Fireman (1986); Friedman (1993); Friedman & van den Eeden (1993); Iribarren et al. (1999, 2001) II: Hiatt et al. (1988); Klatsky et al. (1988); Sidney et al. (1993); Hiatt et al. (1994) I+II: Herrinton & Friedman (1998)	I: 1964–97 II: 1978–87 I + II: 1973–93	Members of the Kaiser Permanente Medical Care Program I: approx. 175 000 members aged 15–94 years II: approx. 80 000 members aged 30–89 years I+II: 252 836 members aged 16–84 years	Interview	Cases	Lung, pancreas, colon, rectum, breast, prostate, leukaemia, thyroid, non-Hodgkin lymphoma, multiple myelomas	Information on pipe and cigars Period of collection and age range of participants at baseline vary slightly between studies, leading to different cohort sizes
American Men of Japanese Ancestry Study	1965–68	Stemmermann et al. (1988); Severson et al. (1989); Nomura et al. (1990a,b); Chyou et al. (1992, 1993a,b, 1995); Nomura et al. (1995); Chyou et al. (1996)	1965–95	8 006 American men of Japanese ancestry residing in Hawaii, born 1900–19	Interview	Cases	Lung, urinary bladder, upper aerodigestive tract (mixed), stomach, colon, rectum, colorectal polyps, prostate	
Lutheran Brotherhood Insurance Study	1966	Hsing et al. (1990b); Kneller et al. (1991); Linet et al. (1991); Chow et al. (1992); Linet et al. (1992); Zheng et al. (1993); Hsing et al. (1998)	1966–86	17 633 male holders of a Lutheran Brotherhood Insurance policy, largely of Swedish, Norwegian or German descent, aged ≥ 35 years	Postal questionnaire	Deaths	Lung, pancreas, stomach, colon/rectum, leukaemia, non-Hodgkin lymphoma, multiple myelomas	Information on pipe and cigars
MRFIT Study	1975	Kuller et al. (1991)	1975–85	12 866 randomized participants initially selected for the MRFIT, aged 35–57 years	Interview	Deaths	Lung, urinary bladder, kidney, upper aerodigestive tract (oesophagus, mixed), pancreas	

Table 2.1 (contd)

Country Name of study	Date of cohort sampling	References	Maximum years of follow-up	Cohort sample and age at beginning of follow-up	Collection of information	Cases/ deaths	Neoplasms analysed	Comments
Nurses' Health Study	1976	Willett et al. (1987); Hunter et al. (1990); Chute et al. (1991); Giovannucci et al. (1994a); Kearney et al. (1995); Grodstein et al. (1995); Fuchs et al. (1996); Speizer et al. (1999); Egan et al. (2002)	1976–92	121 700 female nurses from 11 states, aged 30–55 years	Postal questionnaire	Cases	Lung, colon, rectum, colorectal polyps, pancreas, breast, skin	
Adventists' Health Study	1976	Mills et al. (1988, 1989a,b, 1990, 1991); Singh & Fraser (1998)	1976–82	34 198 male and female Adventists, aged > 25 years	Postal questionnaire	Cases	Urinary bladder, breast, pancreas, colon, prostate, leukaemia, multiple myeloma	
Leisure World Study	1981–82 (I) 1981–85 (II)	I: Wu et al. (1987) II: Ross et al. (1990); Shibata et al. (1994)	1981–85	Retirees living in a retirement community I: 11888 II: 13 976 [sex distribution not reported]	Postal questionnaire	Cases	Pancreas, colon/rectum, prostate	

Table 2.1 (contd)

Country Name of study	Date of cohort sampling	References	Maximum years of follow-up	Cohort sample and age at beginning of follow-up	Collection of information	Cases/ deaths	Neoplasms analysed	Comments
Cancer Prevention Study II (CPS-II)	1982	Garfinkel (1985); Stellman & Garfinkel (1986); Garfinkel & Stellman (1988); Stellman & Garfinkel (1989a); Garfinkel & Boffetta (1990); Calle et al. (1994); Thun et al. (1995); Heath et al. (1997); Thun & Heath (1997); Thun et al. (1997a,b); Kahn et al. (1998); Chao et al. (2000); Shapiro et al. (2000); Chao et al. (2002)	1982–96	1 185 106 adults from 25 states, aged > 30 years	Postal questionnaire	Deaths	Lung, kidney, stomach, colon/rectum, colorectal polyps, breast, leukaemia	Information on pipe and cigars
Iowa Women's Health Study	1986	Potter et al. (1992); Gapstur et al. (1992); Bostick et al. (1994); Harnack et al. (1997); Parker et al. (2000)	1986–98	41 837 women randomly selected from the Iowa driver's licence list, aged 55–69 years	Postal questionnaire	Cases	Lung, pancreas, colon, breast, non-Hodgkin lymphoma	
Health Professionals' Follow-up Study	1986	Giovannucci et al. (1994b); Kearney et al. (1995); Fuchs et al. (1996); van Dam et al. (1999); Giovannucci et al. (1999)	1986–94	47 781 male health professionals, aged 40–75 years	Postal questionnaire	Cases	Pancreas, colon/rectum, colorectal polyps, prostate, skin	

Table 2.1 (contd)

Country Name of study	Date of cohort sampling	References	Maximum years of follow-up	Cohort sample and age at beginning of follow-up	Collection of information	Cases/ deaths	Neoplasms analysed	Comments
Canada								
Canadian War Veterans' Study	1956	Best et al. (1961); Lossing et al. (1966)	1956–62	92 000 war veterans (78 000 men, 14 000 women), aged 55–79 years	Postal questionnaire	Deaths	Lung, urinary bladder, pancreas	
National Breast Screening Study (NBSS)	1980–85	Friedenreich et al. (1993); Terry et al. (2002)	1980–93	Multicentre randomized controlled trial of mammography screening for breast cancer in almost 90 000 women, aged 40–59 years	Self-administered questionnaire	Cases	Breast, endometrium	Friedenreich et al. (1993) conducted a nested case–control study.
China								
Shanghai Factory Study	1972–73, 1977–78	Chen et al. (1997)	1972–93	9351 factory employees (6494 men, 2857 women) aged 35–64 years	Interview	Deaths	Lung, upper aerodigestive tract (oesophagus), stomach, colon/rectum, liver	Site-specific analyses conducted for men only
Xi'an Factory Study	1976	Lam et al. (1997	1976–96	1696 factory employees (1124 men, 572 women) aged ≥ 35 years	Interview	Deaths	Lung, upper aerodigestive tract (oesophagus), liver	

Table 2.1 (contd)

Country Name of study	Date of cohort sampling	References	Maximum years of follow-up	Cohort sample and age at beginning of follow-up	Collection of information	Cases/ deaths	Neoplasms analysed	Comments
Shanghai Residential Study	1983–84	Gao et al. (1999)	1983–94	213 800 residents of urban, suburban and rural areas of Shanghai, aged > 20 years [sex distribution not reported]	Interview	Deaths	Lung, upper aerodigestive tract (oesophagus), stomach, liver	
Linxian Intervention Trial Study	1985	Guo et al. (1994)	1985–91	Approx. 30 000 residents of 4 communes in Linxian, aged 40–69 years [sex distribution not reported]	Interview	Cases	Upper aerodigestive tract (oesophagus), stomach	Nested case–control study
Shanghai Men's Study	1986–89	Ross et al. (1992); Yuan et al. (1996)	1986–93	18 244 male residents of 4 communities in Shanghai, aged 45–64 years	Interview	Cases	Lung, urinary bladder, upper aerodigestive tract (oesophagus, mixed), pancreas, stomach, colon, rectum, liver	Ross et al. (1992) conducted a nested case–control study on smoking and risk of colorectal adenomatous polyps.
China, Province of Taiwan								
Taiwanese Study	1982–86	Liaw & Chen (1998)	1982–94	14 397 residents (11 096 men, 3301 women) of Taiwan, aged > 41 years	Interview	Deaths	Lung, urinary bladder, upper aerodigestive tract (nasopharynx, oesophagus, mixed), stomach, colon/rectum, liver, pancreas, cervix	

Table 2.1 (contd)

Country Name of study	Date of cohort sampling	References	Maximum years of follow-up	Cohort sample and age at beginning of follow-up	Collection of information	Cases/ deaths	Neoplasms analysed	Comments
Japan								
Life Span Study	1963, 1968, 1985	Akiba (1994); Land et al. (1994); Goodman et al. (1995)	1963–87	93 000 exposed survivors of the atomic blasts and 27 000 non-exposed controls [sex distribution not reported]	Postal questionnaire, interview	Cases	Lung, upper aerodigestive tract (nasal cavity and sinuses, larynx, oesophagus, mixed), colon, rectum, liver, breast	
Japanese Physicians' Study	1965	Kono et al. (1987	1965–83	5477 male physicians, aged 27–89 years	Self-administered questionnaire	Deaths	Lung, upper aerodigestive tract (oesophagus, mixed), stomach, colon/rectum, liver	
Six-prefecture Study	1965	Hirayama (1967, 1975a,b, 1977a,b, 1978, 1981, 1982, 1985, 1989a,b,c); Mizuno et al. (1989); Akiba & Hirayama (1990); Hirayama (1990); Kinjo et al. (1998)	1965–81	265 118 subjects (122 261 men, 142 857 women) covering > 90% of the census population from 29 districts, aged > 40 years	Interview	Deaths	Lung, urinary bladder, upper aerodigestive tract (larynx, oesophagus, mixed), pancreas, stomach, colon, rectum, liver, cervix	
Chiba Center Association Study	1984	Murata et al. (1996)	1984–93	17 200 male participants in a mass screening for gastric cancer	Self-administered questionnaire	Cases	Lung, urinary bladder, upper aerodigestive tract (mixed), pancreas, stomach, colon, rectum, liver	
Fukuoka Study	1986–89	Mizoue et al. (2000)	1986–96	13 270 residents of 4 towns in Fukuoka, aged ≥ 30 years [sex distribution not reported]	Self-administered questionnaire	Deaths	Stomach, liver	Results reported include only men because of the low prevalence of site-specific cancer deaths in women.

Table 2.1 (contd)

Country Name of study	Date of cohort sampling	References	Maximum years of follow-up	Cohort sample and age at beginning of follow-up	Collection of information	Cases/ Deaths	Neoplasms analysed	Comments
Others								
Seven-Country Study	1957–64	Jacobs et al. (1999)	25 years	12 763 men from 16 cohorts in Croatia, Finland, Greece, Italy, Japan, the Netherlands, Serbia and the USA, aged 40–59 years	Self-administered questionnaire	Deaths	Lung	
Israel Civil Service Centre Study	1963	Kark et al. (1995)	1963–86	9975 male civil servants in Israel, aged 40–69 years	Interview	Cases	Lung	

References

Adami, H.O., Bergström, R., Engholm, G., Nyrén, O., Wolk, A., Ekbom, A., Englund, A. & Baron, J. (1996) A prospective study of smoking and risk of prostate cancer. *Int. J. Cancer*, **67**, 764–768

Adami, J., Nyrén, O., Bergström, R., Ekbom, A., Engholm, G., Englund, A. & Glimelius, B. (1998) Smoking and the risk of leukemia, lymphoma, and multiple myeloma (Sweden). *Cancer Causes Control*, **9**, 49–56

Akiba, S. (1994) Analysis of cancer risk related to longitudinal information on smoking habits. *Environ. Health Perspect.*, **102** (Suppl 8), 15–20

Akiba, S. & Hirayama, T. (1990) Cigarette smoking and cancer mortality risk in Japanese men and women — Results from reanalysis of the six-prefecture cohort study data. *Environ. Health Perspect.*, **87**, 19–26

Ben-Shlomo, Y., Smith, G., Shipley, M. & Marmot, M. (1994) What determines mortality risk in male former cigarette smokers? *Am. J. public Health*, **84**, 1235–1242

Best, E.W.R., Josie, G.H. & Walker, C.B. (1961) A Canadian study of mortality in relation to smoking habits. A preliminary report. *Can. J. public Health*, **52**, 99–106

Bostick, R.M., Potter, J.D., Kushi, L.H., Sellers, T.A., Steinmetz, K.A., McKenzie, D.R., Gapstur, S.M. & Folsom, A.R. (1994) Sugar, meat, and fat intake, and non-dietary risk factors for colon cancer incidence in Iowa women (United States). *Cancer Causes Control*, **5**, 38–52

Calle, E.E., Miracle-McHill, H.L., Thun, M.J. & Heath, C.W. (1994) Cigarette smoking and risk of fatal breast cancer. *Am. J. Epidemiol.*, **139**, 1001–1007

Carstensen, J.M., Pershagen, G. & Eklund, G. (1987) Mortality in relation to cigarette and pipe smoking: 16 years' observation of 25,000 Swedish men. *J. Epidemiol. Community Health*, **41**, 166–172

Cederlöf, R., Friberg, L., Hrubec, Z. & Lorich, U. (1975) *The Relationship of Smoking and Some Social Covariables to Mortality and Cancer Morbidity. A Ten Year Follow-up in a Probability Sample of 55 000 Swedish Subjects, Age 18–69, Part 1 and Part 2*, Stockholm, The Karolinska Institute, Department of Environmental Hygiene

Chao, A., Thun, M.J., Jacobs, E.J., Henley, S.J., Rodriguez, C. & Calle, E.E. (2000) Cigarette smoking and colorectal cancer mortality in the Cancer Prevention Study II. *J. natl Cancer Inst.*, **92**, 1888–1896

Chao, A., Thun, M.J., Henley, S.J., Jacobs, E.J., McCullough, M.L. & Calle, E.E. (2002) Cigarette smoking, use of other tobacco products and stomach cancer mortality in US adults: The Cancer Prevention Study II. *Int. J. Cancer*, **101**, 380–389

Chen, Z.M., Xu, Z., Collins, R., Li, W.X. & Peto, R. (1997) Early health effects of the emerging tobacco epidemic in China. A 16-year prospective study. *J. Am. med. Assoc.*, **278**, 1500–1504

Chow, W.H., Schuman, L.M., McLaughlin, J.K., Bjelke, E., Gridley, G., Wacholder, S., Co Chien, H.T. & Blot, W.J. (1992) A cohort study of tobacco use, diet, occupation, and lung cancer mortality. *Cancer Causes Control*, **3**, 247–254

Chow, W.H., McLaughlin, J.K., Hrubec, Z., Nam, J.M. & Blot, W.J. (1993) Tobacco use and nasopharyngeal carcinoma in a cohort of US veterans. *Int. J. Cancer*, **55**, 538–540

Chow, W.H., McLaughlin, J.K., Hrubec, Z. & Fraumeni, J.F., Jr (1995) Smoking and biliary tract cancers in a cohort of US veterans. *Br. J. Cancer*, **72**, 1556–1558

Chow, W.H., Hsing, A.W., McLaughlin, J.K. & Fraumeni, J.F., Jr (1996) Smoking and adrenal cancer mortality among United States veterans. *Cancer Epidemiol. Biomarkers Prev.*, **5**, 79–80

Chow, W.H., Gridley, G., Fraumeni, J.F., Jr & Jarvholm, B. (2000) Obesity, hypertension, and the risk of kidney cancer in men. *New Engl. J. Med.*, **343**, 1305–1311

Chute, C.G., Willett, W.C., Colditz, G.A., Stampfer, M.J., Baron, J.A., Rosner, B. & Speizer, F.E. (1991) A prospective study of body mass, height, and smoking on the risk of colorectal cancer in women. *Cancer Causes Control*, **2**, 117–124

Chyou, P.H., Nomura, A.M.Y. & Stemmermann, G.N. (1992) A prospective study of the attributable risk of cancer due to cigarette smoking. *Am. J. public Health*, **82**, 37–40

Chyou, P.H., Normura, A.M.Y., Stemmermann, G.N. & Kato, I. (1993a) Lung cancer: A prospective study of smoking, occupation, and nutrient intake. *Arch. environ. Health*, **48**, 69–72

Chyou, P.H., Nomura, A.M.Y. & Stemmermann, G.N. (1993b) A prospective study of diet, smoking, and lower urinary tract cancer. *Ann. Epidemiol.*, **3**, 211–216

Chyou, P.H., Nomura, A.M.Y. & Stemmermann, G.N. (1995) Diet, alcohol, smoking and cancer of the upper aerodigestive tract: A prospective study among Hawaii Japanese men. *Int. J. Cancer*, **60**, 616–621

Chyou, P.H., Nomura, A.M.Y. & Stemmermann, G.N. (1996) A prospective study of colon and rectal cancer among Hawaii Japanese men. *Ann. Epidemiol.*, **6**, 276–282

van Dam, R.M., Huang, Z., Rimm, E.B., Weinstock, M.A., Spiegelman, D., Colditz, G.A., Willett, W.C. & Giovannucci, E. (1999) Risk factors for basal cell carcinoma of the skin in men: Results from the Health Professionals Follow-up Study. *Am. J. Epidemiol.*, **150**, 459–468

Doll, R. & Hill, A.B. (1964a) Mortality in relation to smoking: Ten years' observations of British doctors. *Br. med. J.*, **i**, 1399–1410

Doll, R. & Hill, A.B. (1964b) Mortality in relation to smoking. Ten years' observations of British doctors. *Br. med. J.*, **i**, 1460–1467

Doll, R. & Peto, R. (1976) Mortality in relation to smoking: 20 years' observations on male British doctors. *Br. med. J.*, **ii**, 1525–1536

Doll, R., Gray, R., Hafner, B. & Peto, R. (1980) Mortality in relation to smoking: 22 years' observations on female British doctors. *Br. med. J.*, **280**, 967–971

Doll, R., Peto, R., Wheatley, K., Gray, R. & Sutherland, I. (1994) Mortality in relation to smoking: 40 years' observations on male British doctors. *Br. med. J.*, **309**, 901–911

Egan, K.M., Stampfer, M.J., Hunter, D., Hankinson, S., Rosner, B.A., Holmes, M., Willett, W.C. & Colditz, G.A. (2002) Active and passive smoking in breast cancer: Prospective results from the Nurses' Health Study. *Epidemiology*, **13**, 138–145

Ellard, G.A., de Waard, F. & Kemmeren, J.M. (1995) Urinary nicotine metabolite excretion and lung cancer risk in a female cohort. *Br. J. Cancer*, **72**, 788–791

Engeland, A., Haldorsen, T., Andersen, A. & Tretli, S. (1996a) The impact of smoking habits on lung cancer risk: 28 years' observation of 26,000 Norwegian men and women. *Cancer Causes Control*, **7**, 366–376

Engeland, A., Andersen, A., Haldorsen, T. & Tretli, S. (1996b) Smoking habits and risk of cancers other than lung cancer: 28 years' follow-up of 26,000 Norwegian men and women. *Cancer Causes Control*, **7**, 497–506

Floderus, B., Cederlöf, R. & Friberg, L. (1988) Smoking and mortality: A 21-year follow-up based on the Swedish Twin Registry. *Int. J. Epidemiol.*, **17**, 332–340

Freund, K.M., Belanger, A.J., D'Agostino, R.B. & Kannel, W.B. (1993) The health risks of smoking: The Framingham Study: 34 years of follow-up. *Ann. Epidemiol.*, **3**, 417–424

Friedenreich, C.M., Howe, G.R. & Miller, A.B. (1993) A cohort study of alcohol consumption and risk of breast cancer. *Am. J. Epidemiol.*, **137**, 512–520

Friedman, G.D. (1993) Cigarette smoking, leukemia, and multiple myeloma. *Ann. Epidemiol.*, **3**, 425–428

Friedman, G.D. & van den Eeden, S.K. (1993) Risk factors for pancreatic cancer: An exploratory study. *Int. J. Epidemiol.*, **22**, 30–37

Fuchs, C.S., Colditz, G.A., Stampfer, M.J., Giovannucci, E.L., Hunter, D.J., Rimm, E.G., Willett, W.C. & Speizer, F.E. (1996) A prospective study of cigarette smoking and the risk of pancreatic cancer. *Arch. intern. Med.*, **156**, 2255–2260

Gao, Y.T., Den, J., Xiang, Y., Ruan, Z., Wang, Z., Hu, B., Guo, M., Teng, W., Han, J. & Zhang, Y. (1999) [Smoking, related cancers, and other diseases in Shanghai: A 10-year prospective study.] *Chin. J. Prev. Med.*, **33**, 5–8 (in Chinese)

Gapstur, S.M., Potter, J.D., Sellers, T.A. & Folsom, A.R. (1992) Increased risk of breast cancer with alcohol consumption in postmenopausal women. *Am. J. Epidemiol.*, **136**, 1221–1231

Garfinkel, L. (1980) Cancer mortality in nonsmokers: Prospective study by the American Cancer Society. *J. natl Cancer Inst.*, **65**, 1169–1173

Garfinkel, L. (1985) Selection, follow-up, and analysis in the American Cancer Society prospective studies. *Natl Cancer Inst. Monogr.*, **67**, 49–52

Garfinkel, L. & Boffetta, P. (1990) Association between smoking and leukemia in two American Cancer Society prospective studies. *Cancer*, **65**, 2356–2360

Garfinkel, L. & Stellman, S.D. (1988) Smoking and lung cancer in women: Findings in a prospective study. *Cancer Res.*, **48**, 6951–6955

Giovannucci, E., Colditz, G.A., Stampfer, M.J., Hunter, D., Rosner, B.A., Willett, W.C. & Speizer, F.E. (1994a) A prospective study of cigarette smoking and risk of colorectal adenoma and colorectal cancer in US women. *J. natl Cancer Inst.*, **86**, 192–199

Giovannucci, E., Rimm, E.B., Stampfer, M.J., Colditz, G.A., Ascherio, A., Kearney, J. & Willett, W.C. (1994b) A prospective study of cigarette smoking and risk of colorectal adenoma and colorectal cancer in US men. *J. natl Cancer Inst.*, **86**, 183–191

Giovannucci, E., Rimm, E.B., Ascherio, A., Colditz, G.A., Spiegelman, D., Stampfer, M.J. & Willett, W.C. (1999) Smoking and risk of total and fatal prostate cancer in United States health professionals. *Cancer Epidemiol. Biomarkers Prev.*, **8**, 277–282

Goodman, M.T., Moriwaki, H., Vaeth, M., Akiba, S., Hayabuchi, H. & Mabuchi, K. (1995) Prospective cohort study of risk factors for primary liver cancer in Hiroshima and Nagasaki, Japan. *Epidemiology*, **6**, 36–41

Grodstein, F., Speizer, F.E. & Hunter, D.J. (1995) A prospective study of incident squamous cell carcinoma of the skin in the Nurses' Health Study. *J. natl Cancer Inst.*, **87**, 1061–1066

Grönberg, H., Damber, L. & Damber, J.E. (1996) Total food consumption and body mass index in relation to prostate cancer risks. A case–control study in Sweden with prospectively collected exposure data. *J. Urol.*, **155**, 969–974

Guo, W., Blot, W.J., Li, J.Y., Taylor, P.R., Liu, B.Q., Wang, W., Wu, Y.P., Zheng, W., Dawsey, S.M., Li, B. & Fraumeni, J.F., Jr (1994) A nested case–control study of oesophageal and stomach cancers in the Linxian nutrition intervention trial. *Int. J. Epidemiol.*, **23**, 444–450

Haenszel, W., Marcus, S.C. & Zimmerer, E.G. (1956) *Cancer Morbidity in Urban and Rural Iowa* (Public Health Monograph No. 37; Public Health Series Publication No. 426), Washington DC, US Government Printing Office

Hakulinen, T., Pukkala, E., Puska, P., Tuomilehto, J. & Vartiainen, E. (1997) Various measures of smoking as predictors of cancer of different types in two Finnish cohorts. In: Colditz, G.A., ed., *Proceedings of the RMA Consensus Conference on Smoking and Prostate Cancer, Brisbane, February 12–14, 1996*, Canberra, Repatriation Medical Authority

Hammond, E.C. (1966) Smoking in relation to the death rates of one million men and women. *Natl. Cancer Inst. Monogr.*, **19**, 127–204

Hammond, E.C. & Garfinkel, L. (1961) Smoking habits of men and women. *J. natl Cancer Inst.*, **27**, 419–442

Hammond, E.C. & Horn, D. (1958a) Smoking and death rates — Report on forty-four months of follow-up of 187 783 men. I. Total mortality. *J. Am. med. Assoc.*, **166**, 1159–1172

Hammond, E.C. & Horn, D. (1958b) Smoking and death rates — Report on forty-four months of follow-up of 187 783 men. II. Death rates by cause. *J. Am. med. Assoc.*, **166**, 1294–1308

Hammond, E.C. & Seidman, H. (1980) Smoking and cancer in the United States. *Prev. Med.*, **9**, 169–173

Harnack, L.J., Anderson, K.E., Zheng, W., Folsom, A.R., Sellers, T.A. & Kushi, L.H. (1997) Smoking, alcohol, coffee, and tea intake and incidence of cancer of the exocrine pancreas: The Iowa Women's Health Study. *Cancer Epidemiol. Biomarkers Prev.*, **6**, 1081–1086

Heath, C.W., Jr, Lally, C.A., Calle, E.E., McLaughlin, J.K. & Thun, M.J. (1997) Hypertension, diuretics, and antihypertensive medications as possible risk factors for renal cell cancer. *Am. J. Epidemiol.*, **145**, 607–613

Heikkilä, R., Aho, K., Heliövaara, M., Hakama, M., Marniemi, H., Reunanen, A. & Knekt, P. (1999) Serum testosterone and sex hormone-binding globulin concentrations and the risk of prostate cancer. *Cancer*, **86**, 312–315

Heineman, E.F., Zahm, S.H., McLaughlin, J.K., Vaught, J.B. & Hrubec, Z. (1992) A prospective study of tobacco use and multiple myeloma: Evidence against an association. *Cancer Causes Control*, **3**, 31–36

Heineman, E.F., Zahm, S.H., McLaughlin, J.K. & Vaught, J.B. (1994) Increased risk of colorectal cancer among smokers: Results of a 26-year follow-up of US veterans and a review. *Int. J. Cancer*, **59**, 728–738

Herrinton, L.J. & Friedman, G.D. (1998) Cigarette smoking and risk of non-Hodgkin's lymphoma subtypes. *Cancer Epidemiol. Biomarkers Prev.*, **7**, 25–28

Heuch, I., Kvåle, G., Jacobsen, B.K. & Bjelke, E. (1983) Use of alcohol, tobacco and coffee, and risk of pancreatic cancer. *Br. J. Cancer*, **48**, 637–643

Hiatt, R.A. & Bawol, R.D. (1984) Alcoholic beverage consumption and breast cancer incidence. *Am. J. Epidemiol.*, **120**, 676–683

Hiatt, R.A. & Fireman, B.H. (1986) Smoking, menopause, and breast cancer. *J. natl Cancer Inst.*, **76**, 833–838

Hiatt, R.A., Klatsky, A.L. & Armstrong, M.A. (1988) Pancreatic cancer, blood glucose and beverage consumption. *Int. J. Cancer*, **41**, 794–797

Hiatt, R.A., Armstrong, M.A., Klatsky, A.L. & Sidney, S. (1994) Alcohol consumption, smoking, and other risk factors and prostate cancer in a large health plan cohort in California (United States). *Cancer Causes Control*, **5**, 66–72

Hirayama, T. (1967) *Smoking in Relation to the Death Rates of 265 118 Men and Women in Japan*, Tokyo, National Cancer Center, Research Institute

Hirayama, T. (1975a) Smoking and cancer: A prospective study on cancer epidemiology based on a census population in Japan. In: Steinfeld, J., Griffiths, W., Ball, K. *et al.*, eds, *Proceedings of the 3rd World Conference on Smoking and Health*, Vol. II, Washington DC, US Department of Health, Education, and Welfare, pp. 65–72

Hirayama, T. (1975b) Prospective studies on cancer epidemiology based on census population in Japan. In: Bucalossi, P., Veronesi, U. & Cascinelli, N., eds, *Proceedings of the XIth International Cancer Congress, Florence, 1974*, Vol. 3, *Cancer Epidemiology, Environmental Factors*, Amsterdam, Excerpta Medica, pp. 26–35

Hirayama, T. (1977a) Epidemiology of lung cancer based on population studies. In: National Cancer Center Library, ed., *Collected Papers from the National Cancer Center Research Institute*, Vol. 12, Tokyo, National Cancer Center, pp. 452–461

Hirayama, T. (1977b) Changing patterns of cancer in Japan with special reference to the decrease in stomach cancer mortality. In: Hiatt, H.H., Watson, J.D. & Winsten, J.A., eds, *Origins of Human Cancer*, Book A, *Incidence of Cancer in Humans*, Cold Spring Harbor, NY, Cold Spring Harbor Laboratory, pp. 55–75

Hirayama, T. (1978) Prospective studies on cancer epidemiology based on census population in Japan. In: Nieburgs, H.E., ed., *Prevention and Detection of Cancer*, Vol. 1, *Etiology*, New York, Marcel Dekker, pp. 1139–1147

Hirayama, T. (1981) A large-scale cohort study on the relationship between diet and selected cancers of digestive organs. In: Bruce, W.R., Correa, P., Lipkin, M., Tannenbaum, S.R. & Wilkins, T.D., eds, *Gastrointestinal Cancer: Endogenous Factors* (Banbury Report 7), Cold Spring Harbor, NY, Cold Spring Harbor Laboratory, pp. 409–426

Hirayama, T. (1982) Smoking and cancer in Japan. A prospective study on cancer epidemiology based on census population in Japan. Results of 13 years follow up. In: Tominaga, S. & Aoki, K., eds, *The UICC Smoking Control Workshop, Nagoya, Japan, August 24–25, 1981*, Nagoya, The University of Nagoya Press, pp. 2–8

Hirayama, T. (1985) A cohort study on cancer in Japan. In: Blot, W.J., Hirayama, T. & Hoel, D.G., eds, *Statistical Methods in Cancer Epidemiology*, Hiroshima, Radiation Effects Research Foundation, pp. 73–91

Hirayama, T. (1989a) Epidemiology of pancreatic cancer in Japan. *Jpn. J. clin. Oncol.*, **19**, 208–215

Hirayama, T. (1989b) Association between alcohol consumption and cancer of the sigmoid colon: Observations from a Japanese cohort study. *Lancet*, **ii**, 725–727

Hirayama, T. (1989c) A large-scale cohort study on risk factors for primary liver cancer, with special reference to the role of cigarette smoking. *Cancer Chemother. Pharmacol.*, **23** (Suppl.), 114–117

Hirayama, T. (1990) [A large-scale cohort study on the effect of life style on the risk of cancer by each site.] *Gan No Rinsho*, **36**, 233 (in Japanese)

Hsing, A.W., McLaughlin, J.K., Hrubec, Z., Blot, W.J. & Fraumeni, J.F., Jr (1990a) Cigarette smoking and liver cancer among US veterans. *Cancer Causes Control*, **1**, 217–221

Hsing, A.W., McLaughlin, J.K., Schuman, L.M., Bjelke, E., Gridley, G., Wacholder, S., Co Chien, H.T. & Blot, W.J. (1990b) Diet, tobacco use, and fatal prostate cancer: Results from the Lutheran Brotherhood Cohort Study. *Cancer Res.*, **50**, 6836–6840

Hsing, A.W., McLaughlin, J.K., Hrubec, Z., Blot, W.J. & Fraumeni, J.F., Jr (1991) Tobacco use and prostate cancer: 26-year follow-up of US veterans. *Am. J. Epidemiol.*, **133**, 437–441

Hsing, A.W., McLaughlin, J.K., Chow, W.H., Schuman, L.M., Co Chien, H.T., Gridley, G., Bjelke, E., Wacholder, S. & Blot, W.J. (1998) Risk factors for colorectal cancer in a prospective study among US white men. *Int. J. Cancer.*, **77**, 549–553

Hunter, D.J., Colditz, G.A., Stampfer, M.J., Rosner, B., Willett, W.C. & Speizer, F.E. (1990) Risk factors for basal cell carcinoma in a prospective cohort of women. *Ann. Epidemiol.*, **1**, 13–23

IARC (1986) *IARC Monographs on the Evaluation of the Carcinogenic Risk of Chemicals to Humans*, Vol. 38, *Tobacco Smoking*, Lyon, IARCPress

Iribarren, C., Tekawa, I., Sidney, S. & Friedman, G. (1999) Effect of cigar smoking on the risk of cardiovascular disease, chronic obstructive pulmonary disease, and cancer in men. *New Engl. J. Med.*, **340**, 1773–1780

Iribarren, C., Haselkorn, T., Tekawa, I.S. & Friedman, G.D. (2001) Cohort study of thyroid cancer in a San Francisco Bay area population. *Int. J. Cancer*, **93**, 745–750

Islam, S.S. & Schottenfeld, D. (1994) Declining FEV_1 and chronic productive cough in cigarette smokers: A 25-year prospective study of lung cancer incidence in Tecumseh, Michigan. *Cancer Epidemiol. Biomarkers Prev.*, **3**, 289–298

Jacobs, D.R., Adachi, H., Mulder, I., Kromhout, D., Menotti, A., Nissinen, A. & Blackburn, H. (1999) Cigarette smoking and mortality risk: Twenty-five year follow-up of the seven countries study. *Arch. intern. Med.*, **159**, 733–740

Kahn, H.A. (1966) The Dorn study of smoking and mortality among US veterans: Report on eight and one-half years of observation. *Natl. Cancer Inst. Monogr.*, **19**, 1–125

Kahn, H.S., Tatham, L.M., Thun, M.J. & Heath, C.W., Jr (1998) Risk factors for self-reported colon polyps. *J. gen. intern. Med.*, **13**, 303–310

Kark, J.D., Yaari, S., Rasooly, I. & Goldbourt, U. (1995) Are lean smokers at increased risk of lung cancer? The Israel Civil Servant Cancer Study. *Arch. intern. Med.*, **155**, 2409–2416

Kearney, J., Giovannucci, E., Rimm, E.B., Stampfer, M.J., Colditz, G.A., Ascherio, A., Bleday, R. & Willett, W.C. (1995) Diet, alcohol, and smoking and the occurrence of hyperplastic polyps of the colon and rectum (United States). *Cancer Causes Control*, **6**, 45–56

Kinjo, Y., Cui, Y., Akiba, S., Watanabe, S., Yamaguchi, N., Sobue, T., Mizuno, S. & Beral, V. (1998) Mortality risks of oesophageal cancer associated with hot tea, alcohol, tobacco and diet in Japan. *J. Epidemiol.*, **8**, 235–243

Kinlen, L.J. & Rogot, E. (1988) Leukaemia and smoking habits among United States veterans. *Br. med. J.*, **297**, 657–659

Kjaerheim, K., Gaard, M. & Andersen, A. (1998) The role of alcohol, tobacco, and dietary factors in upper aerogastric tract cancers: A prospective study of 10 900 Norwegian men. *Cancer Causes Control*, **9**, 99–108

Klatsky, A.L., Armstrong, M.A., Friedman, G.D. & Hiatt, R.A. (1988) The relations of alcoholic beverage use to colon and rectal cancer. *Am. J. Epidemiol.*, **128**, 1007–1015

Knekt, P., Hakama, M., Jarvinen, R., Pukkala, E. & Heliovaara, M. (1998) Smoking and risk of colorectal cancer. *Br. J. Cancer*, **78**, 136–139

Kneller, R.W., McLaughlin, J.K., Bjelke, E., Schuman, L.M., Blot, W.J., Wacholder, S., Gridley, G., Co Chien, H.T. & Fraumeni, J.F., Jr (1991) A cohort study of stomach cancer in a high-risk American population. *Cancer*, **68**, 672–678

Kono, S., Ikeda, M., Tokudome, S., Nishizumi, M. & Kuratsune, M. (1987) Cigarette smoking, alcohol and cancer mortality: A cohort study of male Japanese physicians. *Jpn. J. Cancer Res.*, **78**, 1323–1328

Kuller, L.H., Ockene, J.K., Meilahn, E., Wentworth, D.N., Svendsen, K.H. & Neaton, J.D. for the MRFIT Research Group (1991) Cigarette smoking and mortality. *Prev. Med.*, **20**, 638–654

Lam, T.H., He, Y., Li, L.S., Li, L.S., He, S.F. & Liang, B.Q. (1997) Mortality attributable to cigarette smoking in China. *J. Am. med. Assoc.*, **278**, 1505–1508

Land, C.E., Hayakawa, N., Machado, S.G., Yamada, Y., Pike, M.C., Akiba, S. & Tokunaga, M. (1994) A case–control interview study of breast cancer among Japanese A-bomb survivors. Interactions with radiation dose. *Cancer Causes Control*, **5**, 167–176

Lange, P., Nyboe, J., Appleyard, M., Jensen, G. & Schnohr, P. (1992) Relationship of the type of tobacco and inhalation pattern to pulmonary and total mortality. *Eur. respir. J.*, **5**, 1111–1117

Liaw, K.M. & Chen, C.J. (1998) Mortality attributable to cigarette smoking in Taiwan: A 12-year follow-up study. *Tob. Control*, **7**, 141–148

Linet, M.S., McLaughlin, J.K., Hsing, A.W., Wacholder, S., Co Chien, H.T., Schuman, L.M., Bjelke, E. & Blot, W.J. (1991) Cigarette smoking and leukaemia: Results from the Lutheran Brotherhood Cohort Study. *Cancer Causes Control*, **2**, 413–417

Linet, M.S., McLaughlin, J.K., Hsing, A.W., Wacholder, S., Co Chien, H.T., Schuman, L.M., Bjelke, E. & Blot, W.J. (1992) Is cigarette smoking a risk factor for non-Hodgkin's lymphoma or multiple myeloma? Results from the Lutheran Brotherhood Cohort Study. *Leuk. Res.*, **16**, 621–624

Lossing, E.H., Best, E.W.R., McGregor, J.T., Josie, G.H., Walker, C.B., Delaquis, F.M., Baker, P.M. & McKenzie, A.C. (1966) *A Canadian Study of Smoking and Health*, Ottawa, Department of National Health and Welfare

McLaughlin, J.K., Hrubec, Z., Linet, M.S., Heineman, E.F., Blot, W.J. & Fraumeni, J.F., Jr (1989) Cigarette smoking and leukemia. *J. natl Cancer Inst.*, **81**, 1262–1263

McLaughlin, J.K., Hrubec, Z., Blot, W.J. & Fraumeni, J.F., Jr (1990a) Stomach cancer and cigarette smoking among US veterans, 1954–1980. *Cancer Res.*, **50**, 3804

McLaughlin, J.K., Hrubec, Z., Heineman, E.F., Blot, W.J. & Fraumeni, J.F., Jr (1990b) Renal cancer and cigarette smoking in a 26-year followup of US veterans. *Public Health Rep.*, **105**, 535–537

McLaughlin, J.K., Hrubec, Z., Blot, W.J. & Fraumeni, J.F., Jr (1995) Smoking and cancer mortality among US veterans: A 26-year follow-up. *Int. J. Cancer.*, **60**, 190–193

Mills, P.K., Beeson, W.L., Abbey, D.E., Fraser, G.E. & Phillips, R.L. (1988) Dietary habits and past medical history as related to fatal pancreas cancer risk among Adventists. *Cancer*, **61**, 2578–2585

Mills, P.K., Beeson, W.L., Phillips, R.L. & Fraser, G.E. (1989a) Cohort study of diet, lifestyle, and prostate cancer in Adventist men. *Cancer*, **64**, 598–604

Mills, P.K., Beeson, W.L., Phillips, R.L. & Fraser, G.E. (1989b) Prospective study of exogenous hormone use and breast cancer in Seventh-day Adventists. *Cancer*, **64**, 591–597

Mills, P.K., Newell, G.R., Beeson, W.L., Fraser, G.E. & Phillips, R.L. (1990) History of cigarette smoking and risk of leukemia and myeloma: Results from the Adventist Health Study. *J. natl Cancer Inst.*, **82**, 1832–1836

Mills, P.K., Beeson, W.L., Phillips, R.L. & Fraser, G.E. (1991) Bladder cancer in a low risk population: Results from the Adventist Health Study. *Am. J. Epidemiol.*, **133**, 230–239

Mizoue, T., Tokui, N., Nishisaka, K., Nishisaka, S., Ogimoto, I., Ikeda, M. & Yoshimura, T. (2000) Prospective study on the relation of cigarette smoking with cancer of the liver and stomach in an endemic region. *Int. J. Epidemiol.*, **29**, 232–237

Mizuno, S., Akiba, S. & Hirayama, T. (1989) Lung cancer risk comparison among male smokers between the 'Six-prefecture Cohort' in Japan and the British physicians' cohort. *Jpn. J. Cancer Res.*, **80**, 1165–1170

Murata, M., Takayama, K., Choi, B.C.K. & Pak, A.W.P. (1996) A nested case–control study on alcohol drinking, tobacco smoking, and cancer. *Cancer Detect. Prev.*, **20**, 557–565

Nomura, A., Grove, J.S., Stemmermann, G.N. & Severson, R.K. (1990a) A prospective study of stomach cancer and its relation to diet, cigarettes, and alcohol consumption. *Cancer Res.*, **50**, 627–631

Nomura, A., Grove, J.S., Stemmermann, G.N. & Severson, R.K. (1990b) Cigarette smoking and stomach cancer. *Cancer Res.*, **50**, 7084

Nomura, A.M.Y., Stemmermann, G.N. & Chyou, P.H. (1995) Gastric cancer among the Japanese in Hawaii. *Jpn. J. Cancer Res.*, **86**, 916–923

Nordlund, L.A., Carstensen, J.M. & Pershagen, G. (1997) Cancer incidence in female smokers: A 26-year follow-up. *Int. J. Cancer*, **73**, 625–628

Nordlund, L.A., Carstensen, J.M. & Pershagen, G. (1999) Are male and female smokers at equal risk of smoking-related cancer: Evidence from a Swedish prospective study. *Scand. J. public Health*, **27**, 56–62

Nyrén, O., Bergström, R., Nystrom, L., Engholm, G., Ekbom, A., Adami, H.O., Knutsson, A. & Stjernberg, N. (1996) Smoking and colorectal cancer: A 20-year follow-up study of Swedish construction workers. *J. natl Cancer Inst.*, **88**, 1302–1307

Paffenbarger, R.S., Jr, Wing, A.L. & Hyde, R.T. (1977) Characteristics in youth indicative of adult-onset Hodgkin's disease. *J. natl Cancer Inst.*, **58**, 1489–1491

Paffenbarger, R.S., Jr, Wing, A.L. & Hyde, R.T. (1978) Characteristics in youth predictive of adult-onset malignant lymphomas, melanomas, and leukaemias: Brief communication. *J. natl Cancer Inst.*, **60**, 89–92

Parker, A.S., Cerhan, J.R., Dick, F., Kemp, J., Habermann, T.M., Wallace, R.B., Sellers, T.A. & Folsom, A.R. (2000) Smoking and risk of non-Hodgkin lymphoma subtypes in a cohort of older women. *Leuk. Lymphoma*, **37**, 341–349

Pedersen, E., Magnus, K., Mork, T., Hougen, A., Bjelke, E., Hakama, M. & Saxén, E. (1969) Lung cancer in Finland and Norway. An epidemiological study. *Acta pathol. microbiol. scand.*, **Suppl. 199**

Potter, J.D., Sellers, T.A., Folsom, A.R. & McGovern, P.G. (1992) Alcohol, beer, and lung cancer in postmenopausal women. The Iowa Women's Health Study. *Ann. Epidemiol.*, **2**, 587–595

Prescott, E., Grobaek, M., Becker, U. & Sorensen, T.I.A. (1999) Alcohol intake and the risk of lung cancer: Influence of type of alcoholic beverage. *Am. J. Epidemiol.*, **149**, 463–470

Rogot, E. & Murray, J.L. (1980) Smoking and causes of death among US veterans: 16 years of observation. *Public Health Rep.*, **95**, 213–222

Ross, R.K., Bernstein, L., Paganini-Hill, A. & Henderson, B.E. (1990) Effects of cigarette smoking on 'hormone-related' diseases in a southern Californian retirement community. In: Wald, N. & Baron, J., eds, *Smoking and Hormone-related Disorders*, Oxford, Oxford University Press, pp. 32–54

Ross, R.K., Yuan, J.M., Yu, M.C., Wogan, G.N., Qian, G.S., Tu, J.T., Groopman, J.D., Gao, Y.T. & Henderson, B.E. (1992) Urinary aflatoxin biomarkers and risk of hepatocellular carcinoma. *Lancet*, **339**, 943–946

Severson, R.K., Numura, A.M.Y., Grove, J.S. & Stemmermann, G.M. (1989) A prospective study of demographics, diet, and prostate cancer among men of Japanese ancestry in Hawaii. *Cancer Res.*, **49**, 1857–1860

Shanks, T. & Burns, D. (1998) Disease consequences of cigar smoking. In: *Cigars — Health Effects and Trends* (Smoking and Tobacco Control Monograph No. 9; NIH Publication No. 98-4302), Washington DC, US Department of Health and Human Services, National Institutes of Health, pp. 105–160

Shapiro, J., Jacobs, E. & Thun, M. (2000) Cigar smoking in men and risk of death from tobacco-related cancers. *J. natl Cancer Inst.*, **92**, 333–337

Shibata, A., Mack, T.M., Paganini-Hill, A., Ross, R.K. & Henderson, B.E. (1994) A prospective study of pancreatic cancer in the elderly. *Int. J. Cancer*, **58**, 46–49

Sidney, S., Tekawa, I.S. & Friedman, G.D. (1993) A prospective study of cigarette tar yield and lung cancer. *Cancer Causes Control*, **4**, 3–10

Singh, P.N. & Fraser, G.E. (1998) Dietary risk factors for colon cancer in a low-risk population. *Am. J. Epidemiol.*, **148**, 761–774

Speizer, F.E., Colditz, G.A., Hunter, D.J., Rosner, B. & Hennekens, C. (1999) Prospective study of smoking, antioxidant intake, and lung cancer in middle-aged women (USA). *Cancer Causes Control*, **10**, 475–482

Steineck, G., Norell, S.E. & Feychting, M. (1988) Diet, tobacco and urothelial cancer. A 14-year follow-up of 16 477 subjects. *Acta oncol.*, **27**, 323–327

Stellman, S.D. & Garfinkel, L. (1986) Smoking habits and tar levels in a new American Cancer Society prospective study of 1.2 million men and women. *J. natl Cancer Inst.*, **76**, 1057–1063

Stellman, S.D. & Garfinkel, L. (1989a) Proportions of cancer deaths attributable to cigarette smoking in women. *Women Health*, **15**, 19–28

Stellman, S.D. & Garfinkel, L. (1989b) Lung cancer risk is proportional to cigarette tar yield: Evidence from a prospective study. *Prev. Med.*, **18**, 518–525

Stemmermann, G.N., Heilbrun, L.K. & Nomura, A.M.Y. (1988) Association of diet and other factors with adenomatous polyps of the large bowel: A prospective autopsy study. *Am. J. clin. Nutr.*, **47**, 312–317

Tenkanen, L., Hakulinen, T. & Teppo, L. (1987) The joint effect of smoking and respiratory symptoms on risk of lung cancer. *Int. J. Epidemiol.*, **16**, 509–515

Terry, P., Nyrén, O. & Yuen, J. (1998) Protective effect of fruits and vegetables on stomach cancer in a cohort of Swedish twins. *Int. J. Cancer*, **76**, 35–37

Terry, P., Baron, J.A., Weiderpass, E., Yuen, J., Lichtenstein, P. & Nyrén, O. (1999) Lifestyle and endometrial cancer risk: A cohort study from the Swedish Twin Registry. *Int. J. Cancer*, **82**, 38–42

Terry, P., Ekbom, A., Lichtenstein, P., Feychting, M. & Wolk, A. (2001) Long-term tobacco smoking and colorectal cancer in a prospective cohort study. *Int. J. Cancer*, **91**, 585–587

Terry, P., Miller, A.B. & Rohan, T.E. (2002) A prospective cohort study of cigarette smoking and the risk of endometrial cancer. *Br. J. Cancer*, **86**, 1430–1435

Thun, M.J. & Heath, C.W., Jr (1997) Changes in mortality from smoking in two American Cancer Society prospective studies since 1959. *Prev. Med.*, **26**, 422–426

Thun, M.J., Day-Lally, C.A., Calle, E.E., Flanders, W.D. & Heath, C.W. (1995) Excess mortality among cigarette smokers: Changes in a 20-year interval. *Am. J. public Health*, **85**, 1223–1230

Thun, M.J., Lally, C.A., Flannery, J.T., Calle, E.E., Flanders, W.D. & Heath, C.W., Jr (1997a) Cigarette smoking and changes in the histopathology of lung cancer. *J. natl Cancer Inst.*, **89**, 1580–1586

Thun, M.J., Peto, R., Lopez, A.D., Monaco, J.H., Henley, S.J., Heath, C.W. & Doll, R. (1997b) Alcohol consumption and mortality among middle-aged and elderly US adults. *New Engl. J. Med.*, **337**, 1705–1714

Thune, I. & Lund, E. (1994) Physical activity and the risk of prostate and testicular cancer: A cohort study of 53,000 Norwegian men. *Cancer Causes Control*, **5**, 549–556

Tulinius, H., Sigfússon, N., Sigvaldason, H., Bjarnadóttir, K. & Tryggvadóttir, L. (1997) Risk factors for malignant diseases: A cohort study on a population of 22,946 Icelanders. *Cancer Epidemiol. Biomarkers Prev.*, **6**, 863–873

Tverdal, A., Thelle, D., Stensvold, I., Leren, P. & Bjartveit, K. (1993) Mortality in relation to smoking history: 13 years' follow-up of 68 000 Norwegian men and women 35–49 years. *J. clin. Epidemiol.*, **46**, 475–487

Vatten, L.J. & Kvinnsland, S. (1990) Cigarette smoking and risk of breast cancer: A prospective study of 24,329 Norwegian women. *Eur. J. Cancer*, **26**, 830–833

Veierød, M.B., Laake, P. & Thelle, D.S. (1997) Dietary fat intake and risk of prostate cancer: A prospective study of 25,708 Norwegian men. *Int. J. Cancer*, **73**, 634–638

de Waard, F., Kemmeren, J.M., van Ginkel, L.A. & Stolker, A.A.M. (1995) Urinary cotinine and lung cancer risk in a female cohort. *Br. J. Cancer*, **72**, 784–787

Wald, N.J. & Watt, H.C. (1997) Prospective study of effect of switching from cigarettes to pipes or cigars on mortality from three smoking related diseases. *Br. med. J.*, **314**, 1860–1863

van Wayenburg, C.A., van der Schouw, Y.T., van Noord, P.A. & Peeters, P.H. (2000) Age at menopause, body mass index, and the risk of colorectal cancer mortality in the Dutch Diagnostich Onderzoek Mammacarcinoom (DOM) cohort. *Epidemiology*, **11**, 304–308

Weir, J.M. & Dunn, J.E., Jr (1970) Smoking and mortality: A prospective study. *Cancer*, **25**, 105–112

Willett, W.C., Stampfer, M.J., Colditz, G.A., Rosner, B.A., Hennekens, C.H. & Speizer, F.E. (1987) Moderate alcohol consumption and the risk of breast cancer. *New Engl. J. Med.*, **316**, 1174–1180

Williams, R.R., Sorlic, P.D., Feinleib, M., McNamara, P.M., Kannel, W.D. & Dawber, T.R. (1981) Cancer incidence by levels of cholesterol. *J. Am. med. Assoc.*, **245**, 247–252

Wu, A.H., Paganini-Hill, A., Ross, R.K. & Henderson, B.E. (1987) Alcohol, physical activity and other risk factors for colorectal cancer: A prospective study. *Br J Cancer*, **55**, 687–694

Yuan, J.M., Ross, R.K., Wang, X.L., Gao, Y.T., Henderson, B.E. & Yu, M.C. (1996) Morbidity and mortality in relation to cigarette smoking in Shanghai, China. A prospective male cohort study. *J. Am. med. Assoc.*, **275**, 1646–1650

Zahm, S.H., Heineman, E.F. & Vaught, J.B. (1992) Soft tissue sarcoma and tobacco use: Data from a prospective study of United States veterans. *Cancer Causes Control*, **3**, 371–376

Zheng, W., McLaughlin, J.K., Gridley, G., Bjelke, E., Schuman, L.M., Silverman, D.T., Wacholder, S., Co Chien, H.T., Blot, W.J. & Fraumeni, J.F., Jr (1993) A cohort study of smoking, alcohol consumption, and dietary factors for pancreatic cancer (United States). *Cancer Causes Control*, **4**, 477–482

2.1 Cigarette smoking

2.1.1 *Lung cancer*

Lung cancer is now the most common type of cancer in the world, and the total number of cases that occur annually is estimated to be 1.2 million (Parkin *et al.*, 2000).

The causal relationship between tobacco smoking and lung cancer was established during the 1950s (Medical Research Council, 1957; Doll, 1998).

Tobacco smoking was considered to be causally related to cancer of the lung in the *IARC Monograph* on tobacco smoking based on the findings of the studies available at that time (IARC, 1986). Since 1986, much further evidence has accumulated on the magnitude of the increase in lung cancer risk associated with prolonged smoking, the progressive increase in smoking rates in women as well as in men, the decrease in risk that occurs among smokers after cessation compared with smokers who continue smoking, and the increase in the risk for adenocarcinoma of the lung in smokers in recent years. The current epidemiological evidence comes from many more countries and geographical regions than were considered in 1986. The following section summarizes the epidemiological evidence on how the relationship between smoking and lung cancer varies with duration and intensity of smoking, cessation of smoking, type of cigarette, histological type of lung cancer and population characteristics. The main characteristics and the results of the cohort studies are presented in Tables 2.1 and Tables 2.1.1.1–2.1.1.3, respectively. For the case–control studies, the study designs are summarized in Table 2.1.1.4 while results are presented in Tables 2.1.1.5–2.1.1.13.

(*a*) *Factors affecting risk*

(i) *Duration and intensity of smoking*

The results of cohort and case–control studies that reported on duration and intensity of smoking in association with lung cancer risk are presented in Tables 2.1.1.1 and Tables 2.1.1.5–2.1.1.7, respectively. In smokers, the most important parameter of smoking that affects lung cancer risk is the duration of regular smoking, although risk also increases with the number of cigarettes smoked per day. The stronger association of lung cancer risk with the duration than with the intensity of smoking may in part reflect the accuracy with which these two parameters are measured. Duration is determined by the age at initiation and attained age in current smokers or by age at smoking cessation. These parameters can be estimated reasonably accurately in epidemiological studies. The intensity of smoking is influenced not only by the number of cigarettes smoked per day, which can be estimated from self-reporting, but also by depth of inhalation, number of puffs taken per cigarette and retention time in the lung. Misclassification of smoking intensity may occur because of the necessity for a smoker to maintain his or her accustomed level of nicotine intake. Smokers therefore compensate for reductions in the number of cigarettes smoked per day by smoking each cigarette more intensively. The studies that are most informative about the relative importance of duration of smoking versus number of cigarettes smoked per day are large cohort studies where age-specific lung cancer rates can be compared across a broad range of ages and durations of smoking within narrow strata of numbers of cigarettes smoked per day.

For example, Figure 2.1.1.1 presents the annual death rate from lung cancer (per 100 000) among men and women enrolled in the American Cancer Society cohort (CPS-II) during the first 6 years of follow-up (1982–88) (see Table 2.1 for cohort description). Age-specific death rates are presented for lifelong nonsmokers and for participants who reported that they smoked 20 cigarettes per day or 40 cigarettes per day at the time of enrolment in the study. For men and women, the death rate from lung cancer increased approximately 30-fold from age 45–49 years to age 75–79 years among those who reported currently smoking either 20 cigarettes per day or 40 cigarettes per day at enrolment. This age interval corresponds to an average increase in the duration of smoking from 22–26 years to 62–66 years among current smokers in this population. There is a much smaller increase in the age-specific death rates between participants who smoked 40 cigarettes per day and those who smoked 20 cigarettes per day.

The critical relationship between the duration of smoking and risk for lung cancer was demonstrated by Peto and Doll (1984) based on a 20-year follow-up of the British Doctors' Study (Doll & Peto, 1976). Using a statistical model fitted to data from the men

Figure 2.1.1.1. Lung cancer mortality rates by age and amount currently smoked

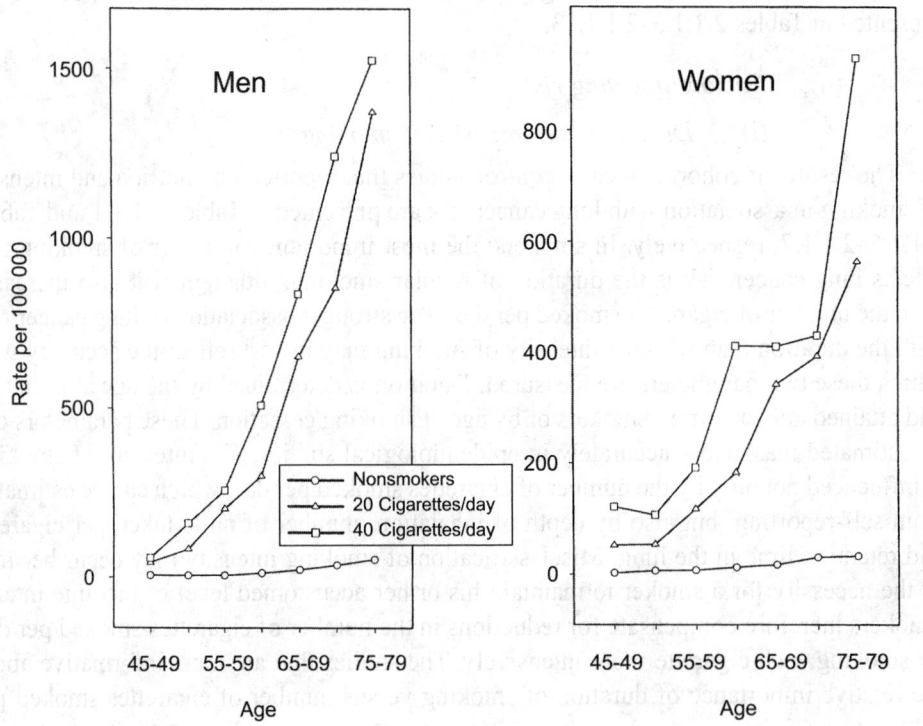

in the British Doctors' Study, Doll and Peto (1978) estimated that the annual excess incidence of lung cancer increased approximately 100-fold when men who had smoked for 45 years were compared with those who had smoked for 15 years (see Table 2.1.1.14). This 100-fold increase with duration of smoking is seen for both moderate and heavy smokers. Case–control studies that have examined risk in relation to both duration of smoking and number of cigarettes smoked per day have demonstrated a stronger association with duration (see Table 2.1.1.7).

The effects of duration of smoking are so strong, and so closely correlated with age, that it is difficult to determine whether ageing itself has any independent effect on excess lung cancer rates among people of different ages who have similar smoking histories. Lung cancer risk was found to increase exponentially with age among male current smokers in both the British Doctors' Study (Figure 2.1.1.2) and in CPS-II (Figure 2.1.1.3). Death rates from lung cancer also increased exponentially with age among female current smokers in CPS-II during the 1982–88 follow-up, except in women aged $\geq$ 80, who represented birth cohorts of women who started smoking 4–15 years later than the average age of starting smoking among women aged 40 in 1982 (Thun *et al.*, 1997a).

The close correspondence between the age of starting smoking and the duration of cigarette smoking among current smokers results in higher age-specific cancer death rates in smokers who began smoking at earlier ages. This is illustrated in Figure 2.1.1.4, based on 8.5 years of follow-up of the US Veterans cohort (Kahn, 1966). In both 'moderate'

Figure 2.1.1.2. Lung cancer mortality rates among male nonsmokers and regular cigarette smokers

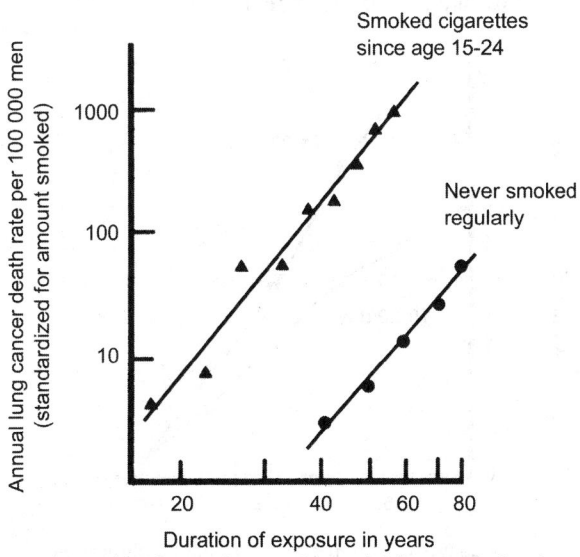

From Doll (1971) and Peto and Doll (1984)

Figure 2.1.1.3. Lung cancer mortality rates by cigarette smoking status and age in men and women from the CPS-II cohort, 1982–88

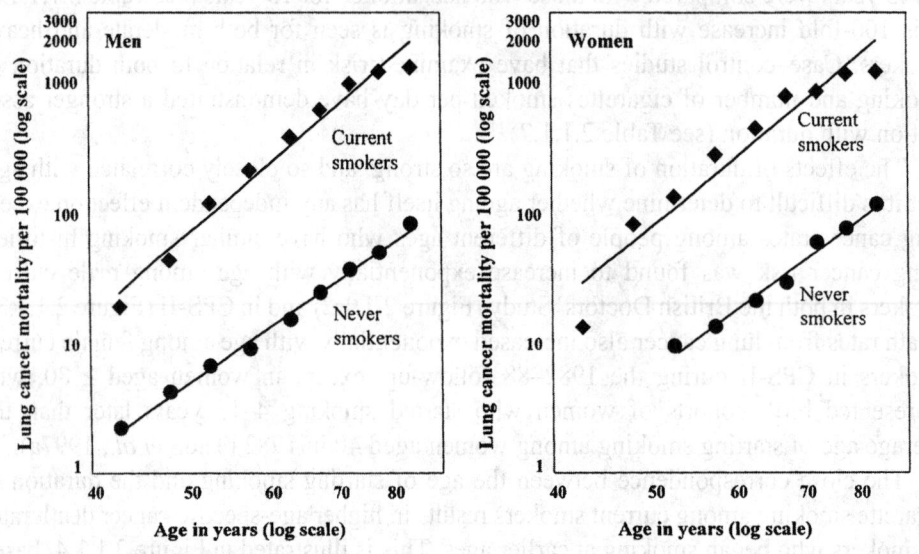

Adapted from Thun *et al.* (1997a)

Figure 2.1.1.4. Relationship between age at starting regular cigarette smoking and lung cancer death rates at age 55–64 years in US men

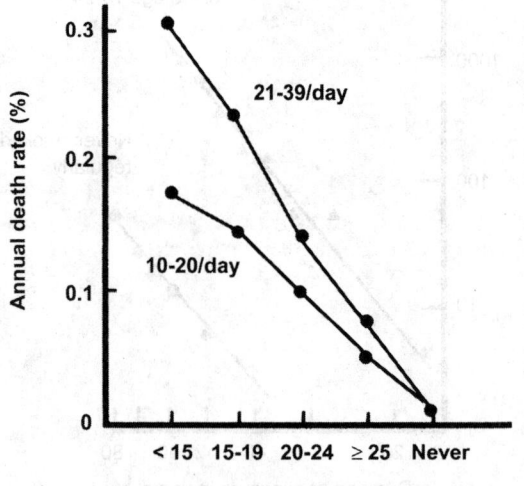

From Doll and Peto (1981)

smokers (10–20 cigarettes per day) and 'heavy' smokers (21–39 cigarettes per day), the annual death rate from lung cancer at age 55–64 was higher the younger the age at which the men had started to smoke. Age at starting smoking cannot be separated from the duration of smoking in analyses of current smoking by attained age.

A consequence of the strong relationship between prolonged smoking and lung cancer risk is that the full effect of smoking in a population is not seen in national rates of lung cancer until regular smoking has been entrenched in that population for at least 50 years. The consequences of smoking on lung cancer may also be underestimated in epidemio-logical studies that do not include long-term smokers. Differences in the distribution of the age groups of the smokers being studied and in the duration of regular heavy smoking contribute to the quantitative variations in the age-specific absolute lung cancer rates and in the relative risks associated with current smoking. The maturation of the smoking epidemic is evident in temporal changes in age-specific death rates for lung cancer in countries where cigarette smoking has been common for many decades. The age-specific lung cancer rates reflect the ageing of successive birth cohorts of smokers. For example, Figure 2.1.1.5 depicts the changes in age-specific death rates from lung cancer in white and non-white men and women in the USA from 1930 to 1996. Within each age group, the death rate from lung cancer has first increased and then decreased, with the downturn in the age-specific death rate from lung cancer beginning earlier at younger than at older ages. These temporal patterns in lung cancer reflect historical patterns in cigarette smoking over the previous 10–60 years. Successive birth cohorts (generations) of men and women smoked progressively more than the previous generation over the first half of the twentieth century, and then progressively less until intensified marketing to ado-lescents began in the 1990s.

(ii)   Smoking cessation

The effect of smoking cessation on relative risk for lung cancer has been evaluated by a large number of analytical studies. In many case–control studies (Table 2.1.1.8) and in cohort studies (Table 2.1.1.2) that examined the lung cancer risk among people who quit smoking cigarettes, a significant reduction in the relative risk of lung cancer was observed. This reduction in relative risk was observed in both men and women, among light (i.e. < 20 cigarettes/day) and moderate to heavy cigarette smokers (i.e. ≥ 20 ciga-rettes/day), and among those who typically smoked manufactured cigarettes as well as who rolled their own cigarettes. The reduction in risk was observed within 1–4 years of smoking cessation, and the magnitude of the reduction in relative risk increased with increased time since cessation.

However, comparisons between smokers and former smokers in particular popu-lations were often made when the hazards among the continuing smokers in those popu-lations were still far from maximal; therefore, the comparisons seriously underestimated the magnitude of the long-term benefits of stopping. The most accurate estimate of the benefit of smoking cessation comes from studies conducted in populations, like the United Kingdom, where the full hazards of continued smoking were already apparent and

Figure 2.1.1.5. Lung cancer mortality rates in US white and non-white men and women, 1930–1996

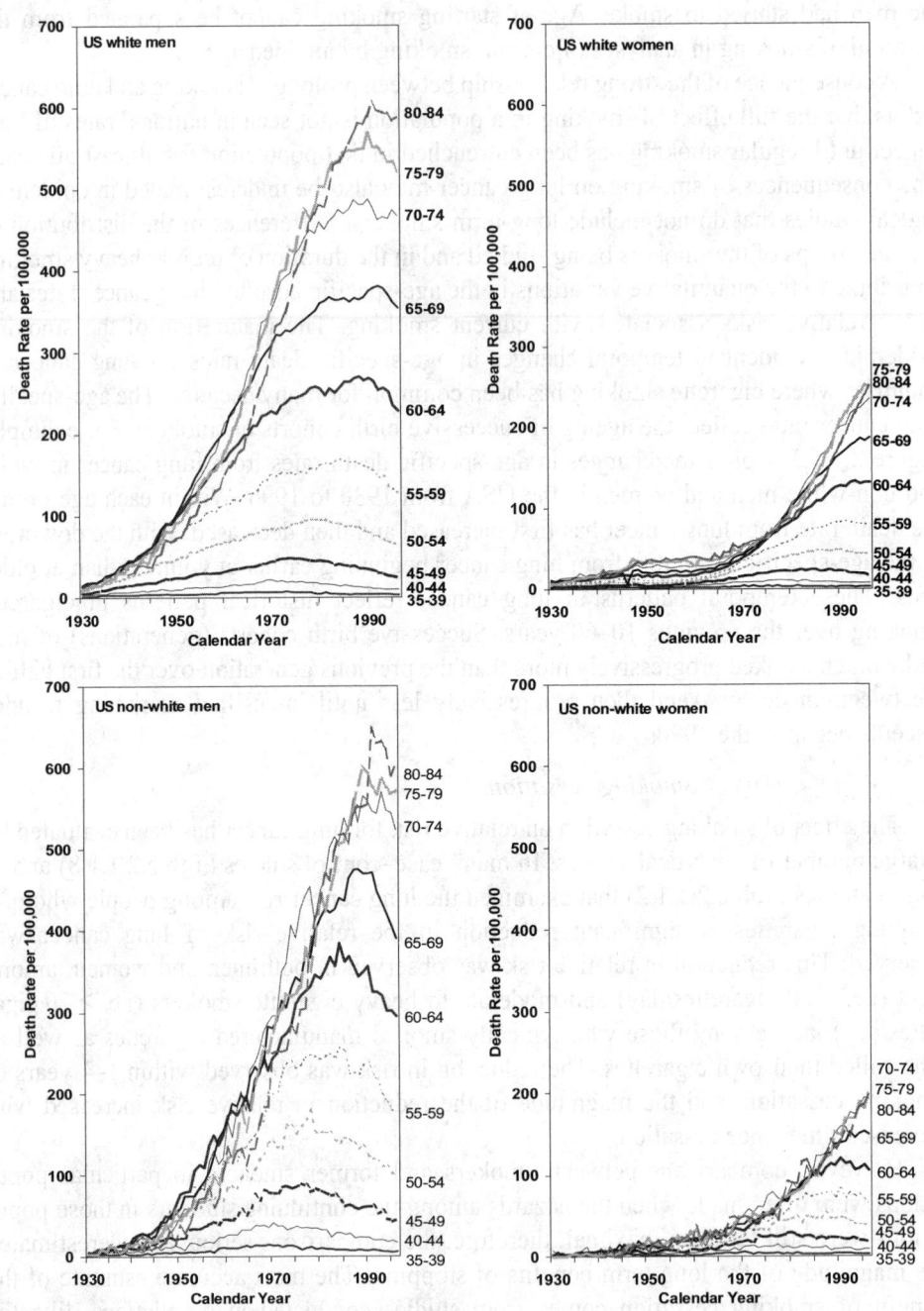

Source: US Vital Statistics

Figure 2.1.1.6. Cumulative lung cancer risk by smoking status and age at quitting smoking in men in the United Kingdom

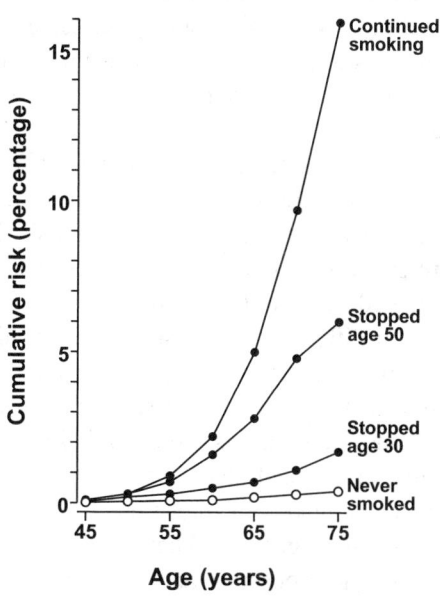

From Peto *et al.* (2000)

where there were many long-term former smokers. For men in the United Kingdom, where the worst affected generation of smokers was that born around 1900, a study conducted in 1990 (and published 10 years later — Peto *et al.*, 2000) found a high lifelong risk of lung cancer among continuing smokers and substantially lower lifelong risks among those who stopped at 50 or, particularly, at 30 years of age (see Figure 2.1.1.6). Former smokers had significantly higher risks than men who had never smoked, but they also had very substantially lower lifelong risks than those who continued, with most of the benefit accruing not in the first decade after stopping, but in subsequent decades (see Figure 2.1.1.6).

(iii)   *Type of cigarette and inhalation*

The *IARC Monograph* on tobacco smoking (IARC, 1986) concluded that case–control and cohort studies available at that time suggested that prolonged use of 'high-tar' and untipped cigarettes is associated with greater risks than prolonged use of filter-tipped and 'low-tar' cigarettes. The results of cohort and case–control studies on the type of cigarette, tar level in cigarettes, type of tobacco and inhalation are summarized in Table 2.1.1.3 and Tables 2.1.1.9, 2.1.1.10, 2.1.1.11 and 2.1.1.12, respectively.

As discussed in Section 1.1, cigarette composition changed substantially during the second half of the twentieth century with the introduction of blended tobacco, filter-tipped cigarettes and other changes intended to modify the nicotine and tar yield of these cigarettes as measured by machine smoking. The actual impact of these changes on the exposure of an individual smoker to carcinogens is difficult to assesss because of the large increase in tobacco-specific nitrosamines from the introduction of blended tobacco, variability in curing processes over time and in different countries, and compensatory changes in smoking behaviour by smokers to maintain their accustomed level of nicotine intake. Most importantly, the majority of smokers have used several different products at different stages of their life as a smoker.

In the absence of large populations of smokers who have consumed a single tobacco product for many decades, epidemiologists have relied on three lines of evidence to examine the relationship between cigarette design and cancer risk. The first involves analytical studies that compare smoking histories (particularly the switch from unfiltered, high-tar cigarettes to filter-tipped medium-tar cigarettes) in relation to lung cancer; the second involves comparisons of different time periods of the epidemic in cohort studies of long duration; the third examines trends in age-specific death rates from lung cancer in different countries in relation to the types of cigarettes being smoked. Each of these approaches has its strengths and limitations, as discussed below.

Many case–control studies conducted since the 1960s have reported a somewhat lower risk for lung cancer among smokers of filter-tipped 'reduced yield' cigarettes than in smokers of untipped 'high-yield' cigarettes. These studies are summarized in Tables 2.1.1.3 and 2.1.1.9–2.1.1.10. A similar observation was made in an analysis of the CPS-I cohort by Hammond et al. (1976). The majority of case–control studies (Kaufman et al., 1989; Zang & Wynder, 1992; Harris et al., 1993; Benhamou et al., 1994; Kabat, 1996; Zang & Wynder, 1996) show a dose–response relationship between the tar content of the cigarette smoked and the relative risk for lung cancer. The greater risk associated with higher tar level has been shown in both sexes in both Kreyberg I and Kreyberg II histological types and in both squamous-cell carcinoma and in adenocarcinoma.

In cohort studies, the reported magnitude of the risk reduction associated with low-tar cigarettes ranged from 25–50% in the CPS-I cohort (Hammond et al., 1976; Stellman & Garfinkel, 1989b) to 14% in the MRFIT cohort (Kuller et al., 1991) and to no reduction in the Kaiser Permanente cohort (Sidney et al., 1993). The studies comparing 'high-yield' and 'reduced yield' cigarettes have had limited ability to control for all the factors that affect smoking behaviour, compensatory changes or selection of type of cigarettes. Furthermore, since the quantification of the tar content of cigarettes varied somewhat from study to study, the measures of the magnitude of risk reduction are not directly comparable. In all of these studies, the risk for lung cancer in smokers greatly exceeded that in never-smokers and former smokers irrespective of the type of cigarette.

Several cohort studies have examined changes in risk for lung cancer among cigarette smokers in the United Kingdom and the USA during the mid-twentieth century, when most of the cigarettes smoked were untipped, high-tar types, and during the late twentieth century, when the majority of smokers used filter-tipped, intermediate yield cigarettes. These cohort studies have indicated that the relative and absolute risks for lung cancer associated with smoking continued to increase among older smokers, despite a dramatic decrease in machine-measured tar delivery over the same time period. The increase in risk associated with smoking has been interpreted as evidence against the efficacy of lower yield products in reducing risk for lung cancer (Burns et al., 2001). However, the interpretation of the trend in risk from CPS-I to CPS-II is difficult because these cohorts represent time intervals in which there were major increases in the intensity of smoking by young people (Peto & Doll, 1984; IARC, 1986). A similar comparison was made for male smokers in the British Doctors' Study in which the first 20 years of follow-up (1951–70) were compared with the second 20 years (1971–90). Although the age-specific comparisons are based on a much smaller number of deaths in the British Doctors' Study than in the American Cancer Society cohorts, this study also showed higher age-standardized death rates from lung cancer during the second than during the first follow-up interval. A strength of these cohort studies is that they indicate that the introduction of filter-tipped cigarettes did not result in the expected rapid reduction in risk for lung cancer, especially among older smokers, for whom risk actually continued to increase. The principal limitation of these studies is that they cannot distinguish between potential changes in the pathogenicity of cigarettes and unmeasured differences in lifetime smoking, particularly differences in the intensity of smoking by young people.

Another line of evidence involves ecological comparisons of changes in age- and sex-specific death rates from lung cancer in various countries in relation to the type of cigarette being smoked. These national trends highlight major differences in lung cancer rates between men and women and across countries. In the United Kingdom, the lung cancer death rate in men aged 35–44 years decreased by more than 75% between the early 1960s and 2000, whereas the rate in women remained approximately stable. The decrease in lung cancer mortality among men in this age group exceeded the 48% decrease in smoking prevalence in British men aged 25–34 years over the same interval. In contrast, the decrease in death rates from lung cancer among men aged 35–44 years in the USA (Figure 2.1.1.7a) began later and has been smaller than that in the United Kingdom (Figure 2.1.1.7b), consistent with the later uptake of widespread cigarette smoking in the USA. The 54% decrease in death rates from lung cancer in this age range in the USA roughly equals the 51% decrease in age-specific smoking prevalence (Thun & Burns, 2001). Among men in France (Figure 2.1.1.7c), death rates from lung cancer have increased precipitously in men aged 35–44 years since 1950 and in women since 1985. It is plausible that the continued use of high-tar cigarettes may have influenced these patterns, but it is not possible to separate the effects of changing cigarette consumption from the effects of changing cigarette composition. A final example is that of Hungary, where death rates from lung cancer increased precipitously from 1960 to 1980 to levels exceeding the highest rates reported in the USA, and have subsequently declined (Figure 2.1.1.7d). A strength of the ecological data is that they suggest that the shift from very high-tar cigarettes to medium yield products may attenuate the lung cancer risk, as can be seen, for example, in men in the United Kingdom where this trend is not obscured by rapidly increasing lung cancer rates from increasing cigarette consumption. Limitations

Figure 2.1.1.7. Trends in lung cancer mortality rates in men and women, 35–44 years in a) USA, b) United Kingdom, c) France and d) Hungary

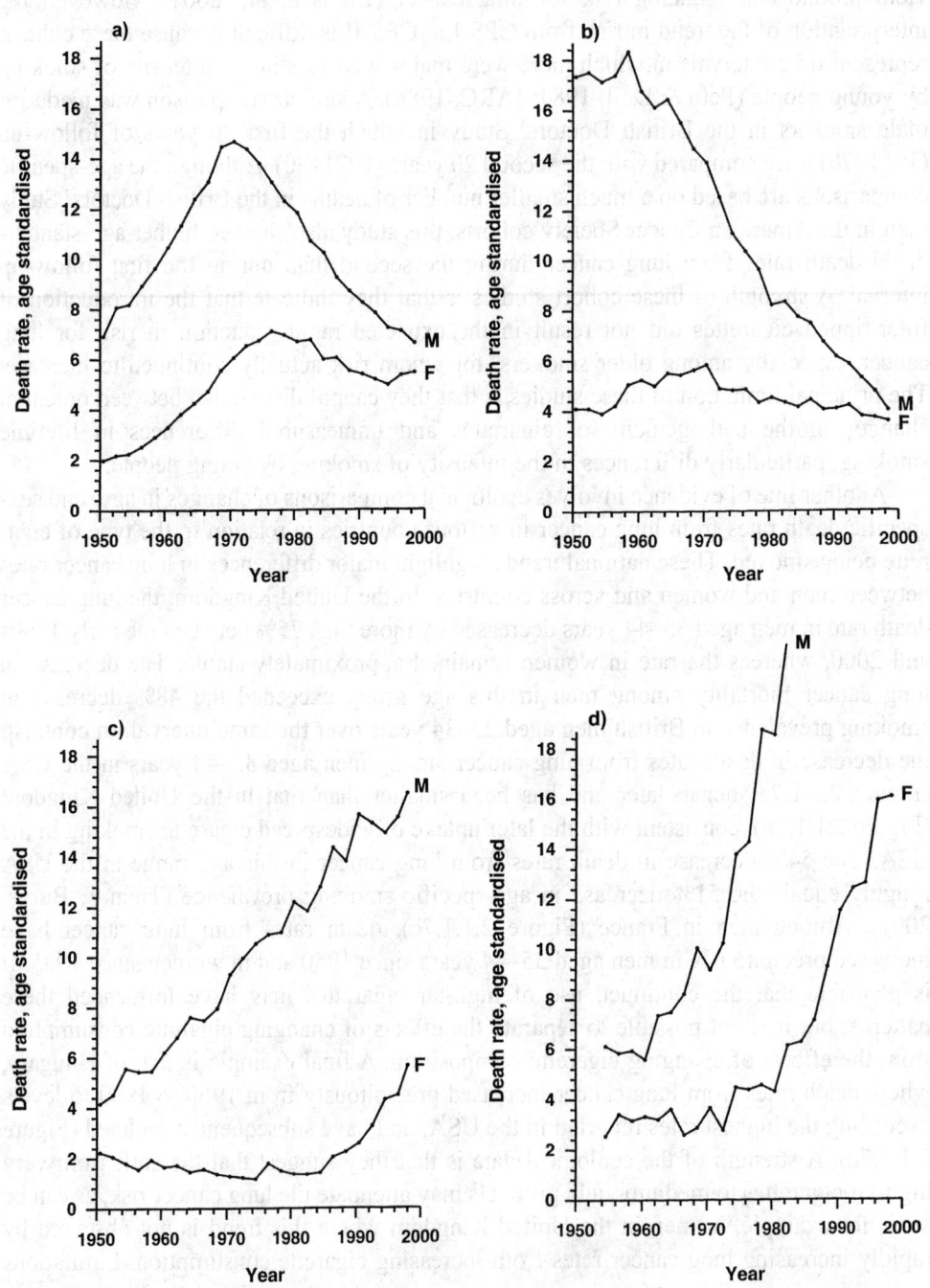

of the ecological studies are that such analyses lack data on individual exposure and out-comes and cannot control for potentially relevant covariates such as diet and air pollution.

The Working Group considered each of the lines of observational evidence that contribute to the assessment of the consequences of changes in cigarettes. Each has serious limitations that reflect the inherent difficulties of tracking the consequences of a single aspect of smoking that has varied over time concomitantly with other aspects of smoking, including intensity of smoking, particularly at younger ages. Successive birth cohorts have had differing profiles of exposure to cigarettes of differing characteristics. These patterns have varied between countries.

Nevertheless, after considering the limitations of the evidence, the Working Group concluded that changes in cigarettes since the 1950s have probably tended to reduce the risk for lung cancer associated with the smoking of particular numbers of cigarettes at particular ages. Supporting evidence for this conclusion came from the limited data from case–control and cohort studies on cigarette type and from the patterns of declining mortality rates from lung cancer among men in early middle age, particularly in the United Kingdom. However, the introduction of cigarettes that can be misperceived as 'safe' may well have adversely affected smoking uptake rates, cessation rates and con-sumption per smoker. Hence, the Working Group could not estimate the net impact of changes in cigarettes on national mortality rates. Moreover, there are still massive epi-demics of lung cancer and other diseases caused by cigarette smoking in the United Kingdom, the USA and many other countries.

Differences in risk associated with type of tobacco, i.e. blond versus black, have been examined in case–control studies as summarized in Table 2.1.1.11. Relative risks are consistently higher among smokers of black tobacco than smokers of blond or mixed types.

(iv)   *Histological type*

The major histological types of lung cancer are squamous-cell carcinoma, adeno-carcinoma (including bronchioloalveolar), large-cell carcinoma and small-cell undifferen-tiated carcinoma. In the 1950s and 1960s, Doll *et al.* (1957) and Kreyberg (1962) found little or no relationship between tobacco smoking and adenocarcinoma. Similarly, early studies of bronchioloalveolar carcinoma reported no relation between tobacco smoking and this subtype of adenocarcinoma. Since that time a number of studies have examined this issue and are summarized in Table 2.1.1.13. In general, these more recent studies have demonstrated a statistically significant association and exposure–response relationship between tobacco smoke and all histological types of lung cancer. However, the asso-ciation has been weaker historically for adenocarcinoma than for the other histological types of lung cancer.

There have been notable shifts over time in the incidence rates of lung cancer by histological type. In the initial decades of the smoking-related epidemic of lung cancer, squamous-cell carcinoma was the most common type of lung cancer observed among smokers and small-cell carcinoma was the next most common. In the USA, incidence rates of adenocarcinoma increased steadily between 1973 and 1987, when adenocarcinoma supplanted squamous-cell carcinoma as the most frequent form of lung cancer (Travis *et al.*, 1995). Similar increases in adenocarcinoma have been observed in Asia (Lam *et al.*, 1987; Choi *et al.*, 1994; Sobue *et al.*, 1999) and in Europe (Levi *et al.*, 1997; Russo *et al.*, 1997).

A comparison of two large prospective cohort studies initiated by the American Cancer Society (CPS-I and CPS-II) in 1960 and 1980, respectively, indicates that the association between smoking and adenocarcinoma has strengthened in the most recent follow-up of these cohorts (Thun & Heath, 1997). The relative risk for adenocarcinoma increased for men from 4.6 (95% CI, 1.7–12.6) to 19.0 (95% CI, 8.3–47.7), and for women from 1.5 (95% CI, 0.3–7.7) to 8.1 (95% CI, 4.5–14.6) in CPS-I and CPS-II, respectively. The age-standardized rates for adenocarcinoma (44.2 for men and 18.1 for women per 100 000 person–years) were only slightly lower than the rates for squamous-cell carcinoma (60.2 for men and 21.7 for women) in the more recent study (CPS-II).

An association between cigarette smoking and bronchioloalveolar carcinoma has also been found (Morabia & Wynder, 1992; Falk *et al.*, 1992; Morabia & Wynder, 1993).

The reasons for the increase in the incidence rate of adenocarcinoma in the general population and among smokers are unclear. One possible contributory factor may be related to advances in methods to detect tumours in the distal airways. Since the late 1960s, there have been a number of innovations that have probably improved the diagnosis of adenocarcinoma, such as flexible bronchoscopy, fine-needle aspiration and computerized scans. The histological classification of lung cancer has also improved. [The Working Group noted that these diagnostic advances would contribute to the rise in adenocarcinoma, but seem inadequate to explain the full increase and cannot explain the increased association with smoking.] There are no known risk factors other than smoking for adenocarcinoma of the lung that might explain the increase in incidence.

The other explanation that has been proposed is that changes in the formulation of cigarettes could have led to a the shift in histological type. The introduction of filter cigarettes in the 1950s may have resulted in deeper inhalation of smoke, and thus higher doses to the distal airways from which adenocarcinomas most commonly arise. In addition, blended reconstituted tobacco, introduced in the 1950s, releases higher concentrations of nitrosamines, which are known to induce adenocarcinomas in rodents (Hoffman & Hoffmann, 1997). Thun *et al.* (1997b) observed in an analysis of the Connecticut cancer registry data that there was a relationship between adenocarcinoma rates and birth cohort that peaked among people born between 1930 and 1939, which might be consistent with changes that occurred in filter usage and tobacco composition in the 1950s.

   (b)   *Population characteristics*

      (i)   *Lung cancer risk in women versus men*

There is currently inconsistent and inadequate epidemiological evidence to support the proposal that women are more susceptible than men to developing lung cancer as a result of smoking. Several case–control (see Tables 2.1.1.5, 2.1.1.6, 2.1.1.8, 2.1.1.9, 2.1.1.10, 2.1.1.13) and cohort studies (Tables 2.1.1.1–2.1.1.3) have failed to show a greater relative risk in women (case–control studies: Higgins & Wynder, 1988; Lei *et al.*, 1996; Xu *et al.*, 1996; Yu & Zhao, 1996; Hu *et al.*, 1997; Muscat *et al.*, 1997; Jöckel *et al.*, 1998; Wunsch-Filho *et al.*, 1998; Kreuzer *et al.*, 2000; Mao *et al.*, 2001; Simonato *et al.*, 2001; Stellman *et al.*, 2001; cohort studies: Freund *et al.*, 1993; Sidney *et al.*, 1993; Islam *et al.*, 1994; Nordlund *et al.*, 1999), whereas several others have shown a greater relative risk among women (case–control studies: Gao *et al.*, 1988; Hebert & Kabat, 1991; Risch *et al.*, 1993; Yu & Zhao, 1996; Zang & Wynder, 1996; Pacella-Norman *et al.*, 2002; cohort studies: Engeland *et al.*, 1996a; Tulinius *et al.*, 1997). What is most relevant is the absolute risk rather than the relative risk. All of the studies that postulate greater risk in women than men are cohort or case–control studies that have estimated relative risk, but not absolute risk (Risch *et al.*, 1993; Hoover, 1994; McDuffie, 1994; Wilcox, 1994). In a large prospective study, women have been shown to have lower death rates from lung cancer than do men within equivalent strata of age and smoking (Thun *et al.*, 2000). Despite similar smoking characteristics among women and men up to and including early middle age in some countries in northern Europe, the lung cancer rates were the same in men and women (Nordlund *et al.*, 1999). Incidence rates for lung cancer in nonsmokers have generally been shown to be lower in women than men. This can result in large relative risks from an equivalent or even lower increase in absolute risk for lung cancer.

(ii)   *Ethnicity*

It has been postulated that susceptibility to lung cancer from tobacco smoking may differ by race and ethnicity. The best comparative data available are on risk in African Americans compared with risk in whites, and in Asian Americans compared with whites. Even for these groups, differences in nutritional and other factors between racial and ethnic groups complicate such comparisons.

African Americans versus Caucasians

Compared with white men, black men have a higher incidence of and death rate from lung cancer, younger age at diagnosis and shorter survival (Stewart, 2001). Furthermore, the racial and ethnic differences in smoking vary considerably depending on the parameter being measured. Black men and women begin smoking at a later age and consistently report smoking fewer cigarettes per day (Novotny *et al.*, 1988). However, smoking prevalence has been higher in black than white men since 1950 (Burns *et al.*, 1997) and the brands preferred by black smokers are more likely to be mentholated or to have higher machine-measured levels of nicotine and tar (King & Brunetta, 1999; Stellman *et al.*, 2003). However, studies that have compared the risk associated with mentholated and non-mentholated cigarettes have not found any difference (Carpenter *et al.*, 1999). Black smokers have higher blood levels of cotinine, the main metabolite of nicotine, than do whites who smoke a similar number of cigarettes per day (Caraballo *et al.*, 1998; King & Brunetta, 1999).

Several case–control studies have compared relative risks in whites with those in African Americans, especially in men (Harris *et al.*, 1993; Schwartz & Swanson, 1997; Stellman *et al.*, 2003). In a study that compared smokers of less than 41 pack–years with nonsmokers, African Americans had a higher relative risk than did whites aged 40–54 years (Schwartz & Swanson, 1997). In another study (Harris *et al.*, 1993), black smokers were at a higher risk only for Kreyberg II cancers. In the most recent study (Stellman *et al.*, 2003), similar risks for blacks and whites with similar smoking habits were reported.

Asians versus Caucasians

Comparisons of lung cancer risk in Caucasians with that in Chinese and Japanese populations are also perplexing. Absolute lung cancer rates were found to be high among nonsmoking women in certain areas of China, perhaps as a result of indoor cooking with poorly vented coal-fuelled stoves (Fraumeni & Mason, 1974; Law *et al.*, 1976; Gao *et al.*, 1988; Wu-Williams *et al.*, 1990). Because of the high background rate, the absolute increase in risk for lung cancer among women who smoke in some areas of China is actually larger than the absolute increase in lung cancer risk among women who smoke in the USA. Peto *et al.* (1999) have demonstrated that the absolute death rate from lung cancer among female smokers in these areas in China is substantially higher than the average death rates from lung cancer among women in the USA (Figure 2.1.1.8; Thun *et al.*, 1997c), despite a relative risk of approximately 2 associated with smoking in rural areas and a relative risk of 3 in urban areas.

The situation is substantially different in Japan, where lung cancer rates among men in the general population and among male smokers in large cohort studies (Wakai *et al.*, 2001) remain lower than in North America (Stellman *et al.*, 2001). Peto and others attribute this difference to the more recent initiation of regular heavy smoking, because consumption of cigarettes in Japan did not increase markedly until the 1970s, and the main increase in cigarette smoking prevalence occurred 40 years later in China than in the USA (Liu *et al.*, 1998; Niu *et al.*, 1998). However, the relative risk for lung cancer ranges between 3 and 5 among middle-aged women and men in the largely (95%) Chinese population of Hong Kong SAR, where cigarette smoking prevalence reached its peak about 20 years earlier than in mainland China (Lam *et al.*, 2001). There is some evidence that differences in nicotine metabolism may contribute to differences in intensity of smoking between Caucasians and Chinese and Japanese. Benowitz *et al.* (2002) reported slower clearance and reduced intake of nicotine from cigarette smoking in Chinese-Americans than whites; they postulated that this may cause Asian smokers to smoke fewer cigarettes per day. This issue has yet to be resolved.

(c)   Lifetime probability that a smoker will develop lung cancer

The lifetime probability that a smoker will develop lung cancer is conditional on lifetime smoking practices and competing causes of death. The frequently quoted axiom that 'only 10%' of cigarette smokers develop lung cancer (Mabry *et al.*, 1998) underestimated

Figure 2.1.1.8. Lung cancer mortality rates in male and female smokers and non-smokers aged 35–69 years in different parts of China, 1986–88

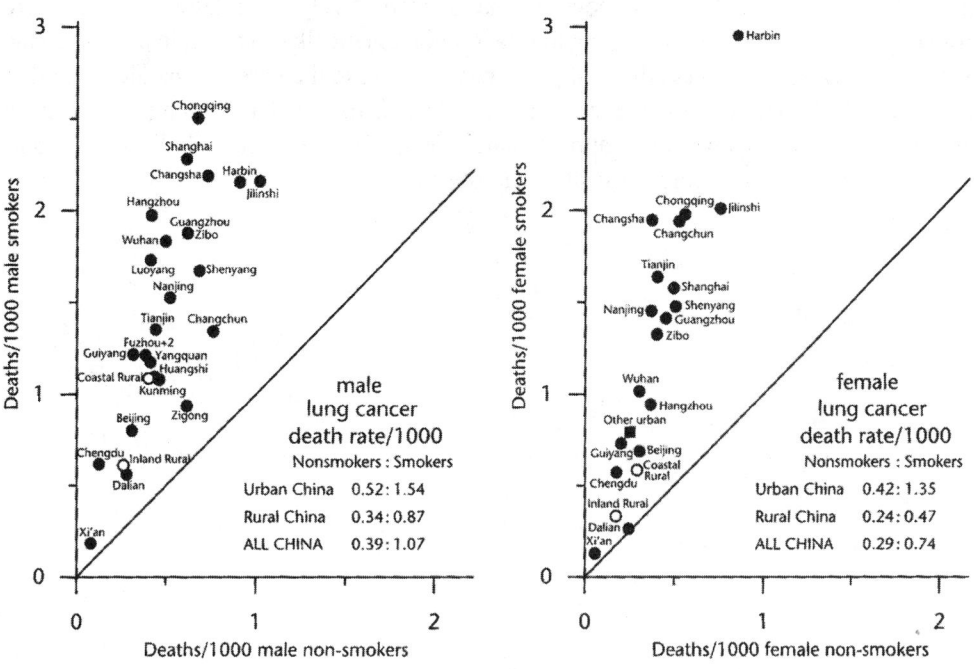

From Peto *et al.* (1999)

In comparison, the nationwide US lung cancer death rates in 1990, similarly standardized for age, were 1.4 per 1000 men and 0.6 per 1000 women, and 0.1 per 1000 male or female US nonsmokers.

the actual lifetime probability among smokers in the late twentieth century in countries such as the USA, where cigarette smoking has been entrenched for many decades and the death rates from competing conditions such as cardiovascular diseases have declined (Thun *et al.*, 2002).

Mattson *et al.* (1987) estimated the probability that a male smoker, aged 35 years, would develop lung cancer by the age of 85 years if he continued smoking. In analyses of over 293 000 US Veterans followed from 1954 to 1962 (Kahn, 1966), it was estimated that 9.3% of men who smoked < 25 cigarettes per day and 17.9% of those who smoked ≥ 25 cigarettes per day at age 35 would develop lung cancer by the age of 85 years. This led to the estimate that 'only 10%' of smokers develop lung cancer (Mabry *et al.*, 1998).

More recent studies indicate that the lifetime probability of a continuing cigarette smoker developing lung cancer has increased over time. Analyses of the American Cancer Society Cohort (CPS-II) have shown that the cumulative probability of death from lung cancer in male and female smokers aged ≥ 85 years, not conditioned on surviving other causes of death, reached 14.6% and 8.3%, respectively, compared with 1.1% among male and 0.9% among female lifelong nonsmokers of this age (Thun *et al.*, 2002). If the impact

of competing causes of death were excluded from the calculation, the lifetime probabilities would be 24.1% and 11.0% in male and female smokers, respectively, and 1.6%
and 1.1% in male and female never-smokers, respectively. The latter estimates are
probably more relevant for estimating the fraction of genetically susceptible persons in the
population than are the unconditional percentages, because they are independent of other
causes of death. These estimates reflect only the risk of developing lung cancer from
smoking; the estimates would be approximately 50% if they considered all of the conditions through which smoking causes premature death.

Table 2.1.1. Cohort studies on tobacco smoking and lung cancer

Reference Country and years of follow-up	Subjects	Number of cases	Smoking categories	Relative risk	95% CI	Comments
Hammond & Horn (1958a,b) USA, 1952–55	American Cancer Society (9-State) Study 187 783 men	8	Occasional smoker	1.5		
		249	Current smoker	9.9		
			Cigarettes/day			
		24	1–9	7.4		
		84	10–20	8.4		
		90	21–40	17.9		
		27	≥ 41	20.6		
Lossing et al. (1966) Canada 1956–62	Canadian War Veterans' study 78 000 men	18	Former smoker	6.1		
		325	Current smoker	14.9		
			Cigarettes/day			
		57	1–9	10.0		
		204	10–20	16.4		
		63	> 21	17.3		
Weir & Dunn (1970) USA 1954–62	Californian Study 68 153 men	368	Ever smoker			
			Cigarettes/day			
			1–14	3.7		
			15–24	9.1		
			≥ 25	9.6		
			Duration (years)			
			1–9	1.1		
			10–19	6.5		
			≥ 20	8.7		
Cederlöf et al. (1975) Sweden 1963–72	Swedish Census Study 25 444 men	12	Former smoker	6.1		
		28	Current smoker	7.0		
			Cigarettes/day			
		4	1–7	2.3		
		11	8–15	8.8		
		13	≥ 16	13.9		
			Duration (years)			
		5	1–29	1.8		
		23	≥ 30	7.4		

Table 2.1.1.1 (contd)

Reference Country and years of follow-up	Subjects	Number of cases	Smoking categories	Relative risk	95% CI	Comments
			Age at start (years)			Annual mortality rate per 100 000 women; adjusted for age and calendar period
		11	≥ 19	6.5		
		10	17–18	9.8		
		7	≤ 16	6.4		
Doll et al. (1980) United Kingdom 1951–73 (see also Doll et al., 1994)	British Doctors' Study 6194 women	27	Nonsmoker Former smoker	Mortality rate 7 23		
			Cigarettes/day			
		9	1–14	9		
		45	15–24	45		p for trend < 0.001
		208	≥ 25	208		
Kono et al. (1987) Japan 1965–83	Japanese Physicians Study 5130 men	74	Cigarettes/day 1–19 ≥ 20	3.2 8.2	1.6–6.5 4.1–16.1	Adjusted for age and alcohol consumption
Tenkanen et al. (1987) Finland 1963–80	Finnish Men's Study 4604 men		Tobacco/day (g) Cohort born 1908–17 Non/former smoker	Mortality rate		Annual incidence rate per 100 000 persons for the period 1972–80
		1		22		
		15	< 15	599		
		22	≥ 15	708		
			Cohort born 1898–1907 Non/former smoker			
		15		178		
		42	< 15	997		
		30	≥ 15	1094		
Floderus et al. (1988) Sweden 1961–97	Swedish Twin Registry Study 10 942 same-sex twin pairs	Men 14 78	Former smoker Current smoker	5.4 19.7	90% CI 2.3–12.9 9.1–42.7	
		33	Cigarettes/day ≤ 10	12.4	5.5–27.7	
		45	> 10	33.3	15.2–72.7	

Table 2.1.1.1 (contd)

Reference Country and years of follow-up	Subjects	Number of cases	Smoking categories	Relative risk	95% CI	Comments
		Women				
		19	Current smoker	5.1	3.0–8.7	
			Cigarettes/day			
		12	≤ 10	4.1	2.3–7.6	
		7	> 10	8.6	4.1–18.1	
Garfinkel &	Cancer Prevention	1006	Former smoker	SMR		Standardized mortality ratios based on
Stellman (1988);	Study II	262		4.8		age-specific rates in nonsmokers
Stellman &	619 925 women	570	Current smoker	12.7		within cohort; analysis by years of
Garfinkel (1989a)			Cigarettes/day			smoking restricted to women without
USA			for 21–30 years of smoking			history of chronic illness
1982–86		3	1–10	2.9		
		3	11–19	6.7		
		16	20	13.6		
		9	21–30	18.4		
		7	≥ 31	18.9		
			for 31–40 years of smoking			
		18	1–10	7.9		
		22	11–19	19.2		
		59	20	19.2		
		36	21–30	26.5		
		27	≥ 31	25.3		
			for 41–70 years of smoking			
		29	1–10	10.0		
		23	11–19	17.0		
		83	20	25.1		
		36	21–30	34.3		
		30	≥ 31	38.8		

Table 2.1.1.1 (contd)

Reference Country and years of follow-up	Subjects	Number of cases	Smoking categories	Relative risk	95% CI	Comments
Stellman & Garfinkel (1989b) USA 1959–72	Cancer Prevention Study I 222 830 men			SMR		Standardized mortality ratios based on age-specific rates in nonsmokers within cohort
		969	Never-smoker	1.0		
		51	Former smoker	2.7		
			Cigarettes/day			
			Low tar			
		20	1–19	5.2		
		32	20	9.2		
		25	21–39	10.9		
		16	≥40	11.0		
			Medium tar			
		87	1–19	7.7		
		131	20	10.5		
		95	21–39	14.1		
		66	≥40	18.2		
			High tar			
		62	1–19	7.2		
		140	20	12.8		
		88	21–39	15.6		
		60	≥40	19.3		
Akiba & Hirayama (1990) Japan 1965–81	Six-prefecture Study 122 261 men, 142 857 women	Men 1120	Current smoker	4.5	3.6–5.7	
			Cigarettes/day			
		14	1–4	2.5	1.4–4.3	
		361	5–14	3.3	2.6–4.3	
		629	15–24	5.4	4.3–6.9	
		76	25–34	7.1	5.1–9.7	
		40	≥35	8.4	5.7–12.3	p for trend < 0.001

Table 2.1.1.1 (contd)

Reference Country and years of follow-up	Subjects	Number of cases	Smoking categories	Relative risk	95% CI	Comments
		Women				
		91	Current smoker	2.5	2.0–3.2	
			Cigarettes/day			
		11	1–4	1.9	1.0–3.2	
		65	5–14	2.5	1.9–3.3	
		15	≥ 15	3.1	1.8–5.1	p for trend < 0.001
Kuller et al. (1991) USA 1975–85	MRFIT Study 12 866 men		Current smoker	6.7	p < 0.0001	Annual mortality rate per 10 000 persons; adjusted for age
		456	Nonsmoker	Mortality rate 19.2		
			Cigarettes/day			
		130	1–15	49.5		
		479	16–25	111.8		
		371	26–35	140.4		
		411	36–45	189.0		
		157	≥ 46	205.1		
Chow et al. (1992) USA 1966–86	Lutheran Brotherhood Insurance Study 17 818 men	63	Former + occasional smoker	6.3	2.5–15.6	Non-significant protective effect observed for higher dietary intake of vitamin A and β-carotene
			Cigarettes/day			
		38	1–19	15.1	5.9–38.4	
		60	20–29	23.8	9.5–59.5	
		40	≥ 30	48.4	19.0–123.7	
Chyou et al. (1992) USA 1965–95	American Men of Japanese Ancestry Study 8006 men		Pack–years			
		33	< 31	6.3	3.3–12.3	
		44	31–45	9.0	4.8–17.1	
		92	≥ 46	23.3	12.8–42.6	p for trend < 0.0001
Potter et al. (1992) USA 1986–88	Iowa Women's Health Study 41 843 women	126	Pack–years			Adjusted for alcohol consumption, education and physical activity
			< 20	2.9	1.2–7.0	
			20–39	9.4	4.8–18.4	
			≥ 40	17.6	9.5–32.3	

Table 2.1.1.1 (contd)

Reference Country and years of follow-up	Subjects	Number of cases	Smoking categories	Relative risk	95% CI	Comments
Chyou *et al.* (1993) USA 1965–90	American men of Japanese Ancestry Study 7961 men		Pack–years Current smoker[+]			Adjusted for age [+]Relative risk of 16.0 for squamous/ small-cell carcinoma and 6.8 for adenocarcinoma *p* for trend < 0.001
		16	< 25	4.3	2.1–9.0	
		83	25–49.9	9.8	5.5–17.6	
		82	≥ 50	23.3	12.9–41.8	
Freund *et al.* (1993) USA 1948–82	Framingham Heart Study 1916 men, 2587 women		Men	Incidence rate		Annual incidence rate per 1000 persons; adjusted for age The authors also reported relative risks for current smokers for each age group.
		31	45–64 years old Nonsmoker	0.0		
			Cigarettes/day			
			1–10	0.0		
			11–20	1.6		
			21–30	2.1		
			> 30	4.3		
		40	65–84 years old Nonsmoker	0.5		
			Cigarettes/day			
			1–10	4.2		
			11–20	4.7		
			21–30	4.7		
			> 30	13.1		

Table 2.1.1.1 (contd)

Reference Country and years of follow-up	Subjects	Number of cases	Smoking categories	Relative risk	95% CI	Comments
			Women			
			45–64 years old			
		10	Nonsmoker	0.2		
			Cigarettes/day			
			1–10	0.0		
			11–20	0.3		
			21–30	1.3		
			> 30	1.6		
			65–84 years old			
		13	Nonsmoker	0.4		
			Cigarettes/day			
			1–10	0.9		
			11–20	2.7		
			21–30	2.8		
Tverdal et al. (1993) Norway 1972–88	Norwegian Screening Study 44 290 men, 24 535 women	Men		Mortality rate		Annual mortality rate per 100 000 persons; adjusted for age and study area
		4	Nonsmoker	3.6		
		11	Former smoker	7.5		
		144	Current smoker	58.5		
			Cigarettes/day			
		18	1–9	32.4		
		68	10–19	50.3		
		57	≥ 20	99.4		
		Women				
		3	Nonsmoker	1.9		
		24	Current smoker	21.0		
			Cigarettes/day			
		5	1–9	8.6		
		19	≥ 10	34.2		

Table 2.1.1.1 (contd)

Reference Country and years of follow-up	Subjects	Number of cases	Smoking categories	Relative risk	95% CI	Comments
Akiba (1994) Japan 1968–87	Life Span Study 61 505 men and women	411	Men			†Upper 95% limit could not be obtained.
		48	Former smoker	2.5	1.5–4.3	
		345	Current smoker	5.1	3.3–?†	
			Cigarettes/day			
			1–14	3.5	2.2–6.0	
			15–24	6.1	3.9–?†	
			≥ 25	9.1	5.4–15.9	
		199	Women			
		9	Former smoker	1.4	0.7–2.6	
		74	Current smoker	3.9	2.9–5.3	
			Cigarettes/day			
			1–14	3.6	2.6–5.0	
			15–24	5.8	3.3–9.5	
Ben-Shlomo et al. (1994) United Kingdom 1967–87	Whitehall Study 19 018 men			Mortality rate		Annual mortality rate per 1000 persons; adjusted for age
		58	Nonsmoker	0.3		
			Former smoker	0.7		
		365	Current smoker	3.0		
Doll et al. (1994) United Kingdom 1957–91	British Doctor's Study 34 439 men	893		Mortality rate		Annual mortality rate per 100 000 men; adjusted for age and calendar period
			Nonsmoker	14		
			Former smoker	58		
			Current smoker	209		
			Cigarettes/day			
			1–14	105		
			15–24	208		
			≥ 25	355		p for trend < 0.001
Islam & Schottenfeld (1994) USA 1962–87	Tecumseh Community Health Study 1857 men, 2099 women	60	Men	Incidence rate		Annual incidence rate per 1000 persons; adjusted for age
			Nonsmoker	0.6		
			Current smoker	2.3		
			Cigarettes/day			
			1–19	1.3		
			20–39	2.0		

Table 2.1.1.1 (contd)

Reference Country and years of follow-up	Subjects	Number of cases	Smoking categories	Relative risk	95% CI	Comments
		17	Women			
			Nonsmoker	0.2		
			Current smoker	0.9		
			Cigarettes/day			
			1–19	0.4		
			20–39	1.3		
			> 40	2.0		
				Relative risk		
			Current smoker			
			Men	4.1	1.6–10.3	
			Women	5.3	1.7–16.4	
Ellard *et al.* (1995) The Netherlands 1974–88	Dutch Study over 26 000 women	47	Current smoker	6.3	3.5–11.4	
			Cigarettes/day			
		4	< 10	1.3	0.4–4.2	
		29	10–20	9.7	4.9–19.5	
		14	> 20	9.4	3.9–22.5	
Kark *et al.* (1995) Israel 1963–86	Israel Civil Service Centre Study 9975 men	153	Former smoker	1.5	0.7–3.2	Adjusted for age, city of employment and body mass index
			Cigarettes/day			
			1–10	1.6	0.8–3.4	
			11–20	5.1	2.8–9.3	
			> 20	10.0	5.7–17.5	
McLaughlin *et al.* (1995) USA 1954–80	US Veterans' Study 293 958 men	5097	Former smoker	3.6	3.1–4.1	
			Ever smoker	8.4	7.5–9.4	
			Current smoker	11.6	10.4–13.0	
			Cigarettes/day			
			1–9	3.7	3.1–4.5	
			10–20	9.9	8.8–11.2	
			31–39 [sic]	16.9	15.0–19.0	
			≥ 40	22.9	19.8–26.6	*p* for trend < 0.01

Table 2.1.1.1 (contd)

Reference Country and years of follow-up	Subjects	Number of cases	Smoking categories	Relative risk	95% CI	Comments
Engeland et al. (1996a) Norway 1966–93	Norwegian Cohort Study 11 857 men, 14 269 women	Men 48	Former smoker	1.3	0.8–2.2	Adjusted for age at start, cigarette type, pipe smoking and urban/rural status
			Cigarettes/day			
		28	1–4	1.4	0.6–3.7	
		49	5–9	4.1	1.7–10	
		97	10–14	7.0	2.9–17	
		27	15–19	11.0	4.2–28	
		57	≥ 20	15.0	6.1–37	
			Age at start (years)			
		173	< 20	1.0	–	
		50	20–29	0.5	0.4–0.7	
		17	≥ 30	0.6	0.3–0.9	
		Women 12	Cigarettes/day			
		12	1–4	12	4.5–32	
		20	5–9	12	4.4–30	
		24	10–14	24	9.5–59	
		9	≥ 15	26	9.2–73	
			Age at start (years)			
		18	< 20	1.0	–	Adjusted for daily number of cigarettes
		36	20–29	0.6	0.1–0.3	
		10	≥ 30	0.1	0.0–0.3	
Murata et al. (1996) Japan 1984–93	Chiba Centre Association Study 17 200 men		Cigarettes/day			Adjusted for age and county
		9	1–10	1.4		
		47	11–20	3.6	$p < 0.01$	
		20	≥ 21	4.6	$p < 0.01$	p for trend < 0.01
Yuan et al. (1996) China 1986–93	Shanghai Men's Study 18 244 men	142	Ever smoker	6.5		Adjusted for age
			Cigarettes/day			
			< 20	3.6		
			≥ 20	9.4		

Table 2.1.1.1 (contd)

Reference Country and years of follow-up	Subjects	Number of cases	Smoking categories	Relative risk	95% CI	Comments
Chen et al. (1997) China 1972–93	Shanghai Factory Study 9351 persons	97	Current smoker Cigarettes/day 1–19 ≥20	3.8 2.8 5.4	p < 0.001 p < 0.01 p < 0.001	Adjusted for age, systolic blood pressure, serum cholesterol, alcohol drinking (yes/no) and factory p for trend < 0.001
Lam et al. (1997) China 1976–96	Xi'an Factory Study 1124 men, 572 women	5	Women Ever smoker	1.8	0.1–18.1	Analysis for women only since none of the male cases were nonsmokers.
Liaw & Chen (1998) China, Province of Taiwan 1982–94	Taiwanese Study 11 096 men, 3301 women	105 22	Current smoker Men Women	3.7 3.6	2.1–6.6 1.0–12.2	Ajusted for age and sex
Tulinius et al. (1997) Iceland 1968–95	Reykjavik Study 11 366 men, 11 580 women	273 199	Men Former smoker Cigarettes/day 1–14 15–24 ≥25 Women Former smoker Cigarettes/day 1–14 15–24 ≥25	2.9 6.5 13.5 28.7 3.7 9.4 30.7 44.1	1.5–5.7 3.3–13.0 7.8–25.6 14.9–55.1 1.7–8.1 5.0–17.7 16.8–56.0 21.1–91.8	Adjusted for age
Wald & Watt (1997) United Kingdom 1975–93	British United Provident Association (BUPA) Study 21 520 men	77	Current smoker	16.4	7.55–44.2	Adjusted for age at entry

Table 2.1.1.1 (contd)

Reference Country and years of follow-up	Subjects	Number of cases	Smoking categories	Relative risk	95% CI	Comments
Gao et al. (1999) China 1983–94	Shanghai Residential Study 213 800 men and women		Men Urban Suburban Rural Women (urban)	5.6[†] 2.9[†] 3.3[†] 4.8[†]	[†]CI does not include 1.0	p for trend < 0.05 for intensity of smoking and age at start for men and women
Jacobs et al. (1999) 25 years	Seven-Country Study 12 763 men	24	Nonsmoker Current smoker Cigarettes/day 1–4 5–9 10–19 20–29 ≥ 30	Mortality rate 1.1 0.7 2.6 4.8 6.0 6.1	p < 0.05 p < 0.001 p < 0.001 p < 0.001	25-year mortality rate per 1000 men; adjusted for age and cohort
Nordlund et al. (1999) Sweden 1963–89	Swedish Census Study 15 881 men, 25 829 women	Men 16 18 135 5 25 33 72	Former smoker Occasional smoker Current smoker Pack–years ≤ 5 6–15 16–25 ≥ 26	1.3 1.6 8.4 1.6 4.4 14.2 17.9	0.7–2.3 0.8–2.9 5.5–12.9 0.6–4.3 2.5–7.7 8.3–24.3 11.1–28.8	p for trend < 0.001
		4 29 102	Age at start (years) > 24 20–23 < 19	1.0 2.2 3.1	– 0.7–6.3 1.1–8.7	p for trend = 0.005

Table 2.1.1.1 (contd)

Reference Country and years of follow-up	Subjects	Number of cases	Smoking categories	Relative risk	95% CI	Comments
		Women				
		3	Former smoker	1.1	0.3–3.4	
		5	Occasional smoker	0.6	0.3–1.6	
		59	Current smoker	4.7	3.3–6.8	
			Pack–years			
		15	≤ 5	2.1	1.2–3.8	
		27	6–15	6.3	4.0–10.0	
		11	16–25	10.3	5.3–19.8	
		6	≥ 26	16.5	7.0–38.5	*p* for trend < 0.001
			Age at start (years)			
		22	> 24	1.0	–	
		15	20–23	1.6	0.8–3.2	
		22	< 19	2.3	1.2–4.4	*p* for trend = 0.013
Prescott *et al.* (1999) Denmark 1964–94	Copenhagen City Heart Study 17 699 men, 13 525 women	480	Men			Adjusted for age
			Former smoker	5.4	2.4–12.3	
			Non-inhaling smoker	7.6	3.3–17.3	
			Tobacco/day (g)			
			1–14	12.1	5.3–27.4	
			15–24	20.9	9.3–47.0	
			> 24	25.9	11.4–59.0	
		194	Women			
			Former smoker	2.9	1.5–5.7	
			Non-inhaling smoker	3.3	1.8–6.3	
			Tobacco/day (g)			
			1–14	10.2	5.7–18.3	
			15–24	13.7	7.5–24.8	
			> 24	18.8	8.7–40.5	

Table 2.1.1.1 (contd)

Reference Country and years of follow-up	Subjects	Number of cases	Smoking categories	Relative risk	95% CI	Comments
Speizer *et al.* (1999) USA 1976–92	Nurses' Health Study 121 700 women		Age at start (years)			Adjusted for age and number of cigarettes per day *p* for trend < 0.0001 for number of cigarettes smoked per day (1–4, 5–14, 15–24, 25–34, ≥ 35 cigarettes/day) [categories for age at start are not comprehensive]
			> 21	0.8	0.6–1.1	
			18–19	1.0	–	
			< 18	1.1	0.9–1.5	

Table 2.1.1.2. Cohort studies on tobacco smoking and lung cancer: smoking cessation

Reference Country and years of follow-up	Subjects	Number of cases	Smoking categories	Relative risk	95% CI	Comments
Cederlöf et al. (1975) Sweden 1963–72	Swedish Census Study 25 444 men	7	Nonsmoker	1.0		
			Years since quitting			
		12	< 10	6.1		
		3	> 10	1.1		
Rogot & Murray (1980) USA, 1954–69	US Veterans' Study 293 958 men			SMR		Standardized mortality ratio, using nonsmokers as the reference group [†]Values estimated from graph
		2609	Years since quitting Current smoker	11.3		
		47	< 5	18.8		
		86	5–9	~7.5[†]		
		100	10–14	~5.0[†]		
		115	15–19	~5.0[†]		
		123	≥ 20	2.1		
Garfinkel & Stellman (1988) USA 1982–86	Cancer Prevention Study II 619 925 women			SMR		Standardized mortality ratios based on age-specific rates in nonsmokers within cohort; analysis for women stratified by history of heart disease, stroke or cancer
			Years since quitting Former smokers of 1–20 cigarettes/day			
		335	Current smoker	10.3		
		52	< 2	13.6		
		33	3–5	8.4		
		20	6–10	3.3		
		21	11–15	3.0		
		41	≥ 16	1.6		
			Former smokers of ≥ 21 cigarettes/day			
		195	Current smoker	21.2		
		39	< 2	32.4		
		23	3–5	20.3		
		17	6–10	11.4		
		6	11–15	4.1		
		9	≥ 16	4.0		

Table 2.1.1.2 (contd)

Reference Country and years of follow-up	Subjects	Number of cases	Smoking categories	Relative risk	95% CI	Comments
Chyou et al. (1993) USA 1965–90	American Men of Japanese Ancestry Study 7961 men		Former smoker (pack–years)			Adjusted for age
		14	< 25	2.2	1.1–4.8	
		10	25–49.9	3.1	1.4–7.1	p for trend = 0.0002
		8	≥ 50	6.3	2.6–15.3	
Tverdal et al. (1993) Norway 1972–88	Norwegian Screening Study 44 290 men, 24 535 women	Men	Years since quitting			Annual mortality rate per 100 000 persons; adjusted for age and area
		1	< 3 months	11.9		
		1	3–12 months	8.2		
		5	1–5 years	9.9		
		4	> 5 years	4.7		
Ben-Shlomo et al. (1994) United Kingdom 1967–87	Whitehall Study 19 018 men		Years since quitting			Rate ratios adjusted for age and civil service employment grade
		14	1–9	8.7	4.0–18.9	
		23	10–19	4.1	2.0–8.2	
		15	20–29	2.6	1.2–5.5	
		6	≥ 30	1.0	0.3–3.1	
			per 10 years	0.5	0.4–0.7	
			Cigarettes/day			
		3	1–9	0.8	0.2–2.8	
		10	10–19	1.5	0.6–3.6	
		26	20–29	4.6	2.2–9.5	
		19	≥ 30	6.7	3.1–14.4	
			per 10 cigarettes	1.4	1.2–1.6	
			Duration (years)			
		2	0–9	0.8	0.2–3.4	
		5	10–19	1.3	0.7–2.2	
		18	20–29	3.1	1.5–6.8	
		33	≥ 30	5.1	2.5–10.3	
			per 10 years	1.7	1.3–2.1	

Table 2.1.1.2 (contd)

Reference Country and years of follow-up	Subjects	Number of cases	Smoking categories	Relative risk	95% CI	Comments
Jacobs *et al.* (1999) 25 years	Seven-Country Study 12 763 men	11 19 5	Years since quitting < 1 1–9 > 10	3.4 1.6 0.2	*p* < 0.05	25-year mortality rate per 1000 men; adjusted for age and cohort
Speizer *et al.* (1999) USA 1976–92	Nurses' Health Study 121 700 women	391 24 34 41 17 28	Years since quitting Current smoker < 2 2–4.9 5–9.9 10–14.9 ≥ 15	1.0 0.4 0.6 0.6 0.1 0.1	– 0.2–0.7 0.4–1.0 0.4–0.9 0.1–0.3 0.1–0.2	Adjusted for age, 2-year follow-up interval and age at start

Table 2.1.1.3. Cohort studies on tobacco smoking and lung cancer: tobacco type

Reference Country and years of follow-up	Subjects	Number of cases	Smoking categories	Relative risk	95% CI	Comments
Garfinkel & Stellman (1988) USA 1982–86	Cancer Prevention Study II 619 925 women		Inhalation	SMR		Standardized mortality ratios based on age-specific rates in nonsmokers within cohort; analysis restricted to women with no history of chronic illness
		25	Non-inhaler	6.9		
		72	Slight	15.2		
		252	Moderate	18.5		
		84	Deep	31.9		
Sidney et al. (1993) USA 1979–87	Kaiser Permanente Medical Care Program Study II 34 975 men, 44 971 women	Men	Tar content (mg/cigarette)			Adjusted for age, race, education, cigarettes/day and duration of smoking
		14	< 11	1.0	–	
		39	11–18	1.3	0.7–2.4	
		29	> 18	1.3	0.7–2.4	
		Women				
		29	< 11	1.0	–	
		34	11–18	0.9	0.6–1.6	
		13	> 18	0.7	0.3–1.3	
Nordlund et al. (1999) Sweden 1963–89	Swedish Census Study 15 881 men, 25 829 women	Men	Inhalation			
		4	None/slight	1.0	–	
		131	Moderate/deep	1.6	0.6–4.4	
		Women	Inhalation			
		4	None/slight	1.0	–	
		55	Moderate/deep	2.1	0.7–5.9	

Table 2.1.1.4. Case–control studies on tobacco smoking and lung cancer: main characteristics of study design

Reference	Country	Study years	No. of cases/controls	No. of nonsmokers (cases/controls)	Source of cases and controls	Comments
Damber & Larsson (1986)	Sweden	1972–77	Men: 579 deceased/ 572 deceased/447 alive	42/208/171	Cases: P (deaths) Control 1: P (deaths) Control 2: P (alive)	Matched on sex, age, municipality, year of death or year of birth for living controls
Pathak et al. (1986)	USA, New Mexico	Jan. 1980– Aug. 1983	Men: 311/493 Women: 158/271	9/125 19/160	Cases: P Controls: P	Frequency-matched for sex, age and ethnicity
Benhamou et al. (1987)	France	1976–80	Women: 96/192	50/159	Cases: H Controls: H	Matched on age, sex, hospital and interviewer
Gao et al. (1988)	China, Shanghai	Feb. 1984– Feb. 1986	Men: 733/760 Women: 672/735	62/202 435/605	Cases: P Controls: P	Frequency-matched on age to the Cancer Registry distribution of lung cancer cases
Higgins & Wynder (1988)	USA, 6 cities	1977–84	Men: 2085/3948 Women: 1012/1891	64/918 125/991	Cases: H Controls: H	Crude odds ratios
Wilcox et al. (1988)	USA, New Jersey	1980–81	Men: 763/900	13/142	Cases: P Controls: P	Analysis includes 373 cases and 247 controls who smoked during 1973–80
Benhamou et al. (1989)	France	1976–80	Men: 1057/1503	Smokers only	Cases: H Controls: H	Further analysis of data already included in IARC (1986)
Kaufman et al. (1989)	USA, Canada	Nov. 1981– June 1986	Men: 534/998 Women: 347/1572	Sexes combined 35/925	Cases: H Controls: H	
Schoenberg et al. (1989)	USA, New Jersey	Aug. 1982– Sept. 1983	Women: 994/995	119/497	Cases: P Controls: P	Matched on race, age for living cases and date of death for deceased cases
Svensson et al. (1989)	Sweden, Stockholm	1983–86	Women: 210/209	38/120	Cases: multicentric H Controls: P	Matched on day of birth
Xu et al. (1989)	China, Shenyang, Liaoning	Sept. 1985– Sept. 1987	Men: 729/788 Women: 520/557	102/355 156/362	Cases: H Controls: P	Frequency-matched to expected age and sex distribution of cases

Table 2.1.1.4 (contd)

Reference	Country	Study years	No. of cases/controls	No. of nonsmokers (cases/controls)	Source of cases and controls	Comments
Jedrychowski et al. (1990)	Poland, Cracow	Jan. 1980–Dec. 1985	Men: 901/875 Women: 198/198	49/219 78/166	Cases: P Controls: P (death certificates)	Matched on age, date of death; controls excluding respiratory diseases
Wu-Williams et al. (1990)	China, Harbin and Shenyang	1985–87	Women: 964/959	415/601	Cases: 70 H Controls: P	Frequency-matched to the expected age distribution of the cases
Becher et al. (1991)	Germany	1985–86	Men: 146/146/146 Women: 48/48/48	3/32/22 10/31/21	Cases: H Control 1: H/control 2: P	Matched on sex and age
Hebert & Kabat (1991)	USA	Not stated	Men: 812/1719 Women: 568/1238	88/853 97/868	Cases: H Controls: H	Matched on sex, age, hospital and time of interview
Holowaty et al. (1991)	Canada, Ontario, Niagara	Jan. 1983–March 1985	Women: 51/45	5/27	Cases: H Controls: P	Matched on age and municipality
Kabat & Hebert (1991)	USA, 4 cities	1985–90	Men: 588/914 Women: 456/410	Current smokers only	Cases: H Controls: H	Matched on age, sex, race, hospital and date of interview
Katsouyanni et al. (1991)	Greece, Athens	18 mo. 1987–89	Women: 101/89	48/67	Cases: H Controls: H	
Liu et al. (1991)	China, Xuanwei	Nov. 1985–Dec. 1986	Men: 56/224 Women: 54/202	Both sexes combined: 4/52	Cases: H Controls: P	Restricted to farmers Matched on age, sex, occupation and residence
Morabia & Wynder (1991)	USA	1985–90	Men: 851/888 Women: 507/608	Not given	Cases: H Controls: H	Matched by age, hospital and date of admission
Osann (1991)	USA, California	1969–77	Women: 217/203	33/109	Cases: H Controls: H	Nested case–control study Matched on year of birth, race and date of first check-up

Table 2.1.1.4 (contd)

Reference	Country	Study years	No. of cases/controls	No. of nonsmokers (cases/controls)	Source of cases and controls	Comments
Alavanja et al. (1992)	USA, Missouri	June 1986–April 1991	Women: Never smoked 432/1169; Former smokers 186/234	Not applicable	Cases: P Controls: P	Excludes current smokers
Falk et al. (1992)	USA, Louisiana	1979–82	Both sexes combined: 21/101	3/31	Cases: H Controls: H	Only bronchioloalveolar carcinomas. Matched by hospital, race, sex and age (5:1)
Jedrychowski et al. (1992)	Poland, Cracow	Jan. 1980–Dec. 1987	Men: 627/1343	16/289	Cases: P Controls: P (death certificates)	Interviews with next-of-kin; matched on sex, age and date of death
Jöckel et al. (1992)	Germany, 5 cities, 7 hospitals	Not stated	Men: 146/146/146 Women: 48/48/48	3/32/22 10/31/21	Cases: H Controls: H/P	Matched by sex and age
Liu (1992)	China: Beijing, Shenyang, Harbin, Shanghai, Nanjing, Shengzou, Taiyuan, Nanchang	1984–89	Both sexes combined: 4081/4338	1151/1979	Cases: P (7 studies)/H (1 study) Controls: P (7 studies)/H (1 study)	Combined analysis of 8 studies; matched on age and sex
Lubin et al. (1992)	China, Yunnan, Gejiu	1984–88	Men: 427/1011	9/72	Cases: P Controls: P	Matched on age; city residents and Yunnan Tin Corporation workers
Morabia & Wynder (1992)	USA	1977–89	Both sexes combined: 87/286 non-cancer/ 297 cancer	15/97 non-cancer/122 cancer	Cases: H Controls: H	Only bronchioloalveolar carcinomas. Matched on sex, race, age, hospital, date of interview
Zang & Wynder (1992)	USA	1981–88	Men: 1380/2828 Women: 916/1839	51/820 83 /899	Cases: H Controls: H	Matched by age, sex, race and time of admission

Table 2.1.1.4 (contd)

Reference	Country	Study years	No. of cases/controls	No. of nonsmokers (cases/controls)	Source of cases and controls	Comments
Gao et al. (1993)	Japan, Nagoya	Jan. 1988– June 1991	Men: 282/282	13/56	Cases: H Controls: H	Matched by sex, age and date of first visit to the hospital
Ger et al. (1993)	China, Province of Taiwan	May 1990– July 1991	Men: 92/184/184 Women: 39/78/78	Both sexes combined: 48/111/118	Cases: H Controls: H/ neighbourhood	Matched on age, sex, date of interview and insurance status (H); age, sex and residence (neighbourhood)
Harris et al. (1993)	USA	1980–90	Men: white 2678/2445 black 238/169 Women: white 1394/1418 black 113/139	83/581 4/36 145/776 14/80	Cases: H Controls: H	Controls matched by sex, race, age and year of interview
Hegmann et al. (1993)	USA, Utah	Oct. 1989– May 1991	Men: 182/2195 Women: 100/1087	Both sexes combined: 27/2080	Cases: P (cancer registry) Controls: P	Frequency-matched on age and sex
Liu et al. (1993)	China	June 1983– June 1984	Men: 224/224 Women: 92/96	12/44 38/69	Cases: H Controls: H	Individually matched on age, sex, residence and date of diagnosis/hospital admission
Osann et al. (1993)	USA, Orange County	Jan. 1984– Dec. 1986	Men: 1153/1851 Women: 833/1656	45/833 96/1093	Cases: H Controls: H	Data extracted from medical records
Pezzotto et al. (1993)	Argentina, Rosario	1987–91	Men: 215/433	4/116	Cases: H Controls: H	Matched on age
Risch et al. (1993)	Canada	Jan. 1981– March 1985	Men: 403/362 Women : 442 /410	12/85 52/214	Cases: H Controls: P	Male cases matched to female cases; controls matched on sex, residence and age
Agudo et al. (1994)	Spain	1989–92	Women: 103/206	80/183	Cases: H Controls: H	Matched for age at diagnosis, hospital and interviewer

Table 2.1.1.4 (contd)

Reference	Country	Study years	No. of cases/controls	No. of nonsmokers (cases/controls)	Source of cases and controls	Comments
Benhamou & Benhamou (1994)	France	1976–80	Men: 1334/2409 Women: 96/192	36/650 50/159	Cases: H Controls: H	Matched on age, sex, hospital and interviewer
Benhamou et al. (1994)	France	1976–80	Men: 1114/1466	Only lifelong smokers	Cases: H Controls: H	
De Stefani et al. (1994)	Uruguay, Montevideo	Jan. 1989– Dec. 1992	Men: 476/561	Only former and current smokers	Cases: H Controls: H	
Miller et al. (1994)	USA, Erie County, PA	1972–76, 1979–84	Women: 168/5235	28/3638	Cases: P Controls: P (deaths)	Nested in a retrospective population study
Sankaranarayanan et al. (1994)	India, Trivandrum	1990	Men: 281/1207	28/767	Cases: H Controls: visitors and patients' bystanders	
Shimizu et al. (1994)	Japan, Tokyo	1973–91	Men: 413/82 Women: 192/101	37/65 43/21	Cases: H Controls: H	Information from hospital records; controls were patients with metastatic lung cancer
Sobue et al. (1994)	Japan, Osaka	Jan. 1986– Dec. 1988	Men: 1082/1141 Women: 294/1089	34/128 167/857	Cases: H Controls: H	Methods for selection of controls not stated
Suzuki et al. (1994)	Rio de Janeiro, Brazil	Aug. 1991– Feb. 1992	Men: 99/99 Women: 24/24	Both sexes combined: 11/55	Cases: H Controls: H	Matched on age, sex and race
Alavanja et al. (1995)	USA, Missouri	1986–92	Women: lifetime nonsmokers, 432/1168 long-term former smokers, 186/234	Not applicable	Cases: P Controls: P	Excludes current smokers A cancer group was also used as control, but data are not shown in tables
Siemiatycki et al. (1995)	Canada	Sept. 1979– June 1985	Men: 857/533	13/105	Cases: H Controls: P	Age-stratified, matched to age distribution of cases
De Stefani et al. (1996a)	Uruguay, Montevideo	May 1994– Dec. 1995	Men: 307/307 Women: 13/13	Both sexes combined: 20/108	Cases: H Controls: H	Frequency-matched on age and residence (urban/rural)

Table 2.1.1.4 (contd)

Reference	Country	Study years	No. of cases/controls	No. of nonsmokers (cases/controls)	Source of cases and controls	Comments
De Stefani et al. (1996b)	Uruguay, Montevideo	Jan. 1988– Dec. 1994	Men: 497/497	27/163	Cases: H Controls: H	Matched on sex, age and residence
Du et al. (1996)	China, Guangzhou	1985	Men: 566/566 Women: 283/283	Not given	Cases and controls: death registry	Review of published studies, with some updated data Matched on age, sex, race, hospital and date of admission
Kabat (1996)	USA	1969–91	Both sexes combined: 7553/17 992	Men: 2085/3951 Women: 1012/1891	Cases: H Controls: H	Matched on age, sex, race, hospital and date of admission
Lei et al. (1996)	China, Guangzhou	1986	Men: 563/563 Women: 229/229	41/123 85/147	Cases: P Controls: P	Matched on sex and closest birth date
Luo et al. (1996)	China, Fuzhou	1990–91 (1.5 years)	Both sexes combined: 102/306	37/160	Cases: H Controls: P	Frequency-matched by age and sex
Rylander et al. (1996)	Sweden	Jan. 1989– June 1993	Men: 308/644	16/160	Cases: H Controls: P	Matched by closest birth date, sex and residence
Shen et al. (1996)	China, Nanjing	1986–93	Both sexes combined: 163/163	No data	Cases: H Controls: P	Matched on age, sex, nationality and street of residence
Wang et al. (1996)	China, Guangzhou, Guangdong	1990–93	Men: 291/291 Women: 99/99	29/no data 82/no data	Cases: H Controls: H	Matched on sex, residence, education and age
Xu et al. (1996)	China, Shenyang, Liaoning	Sept. 1985– Sept. 1987	Men: 729/788 Women: 520/577	No data	Cases: P Controls: P	'Age and sex distribution of controls closely matched those of cases'
Yu & Zhao (1996)	China	1981–90	Both sexes combined: 5703/5669	1766/2644	Meta-analysis 15 studies	Matched on age, sex and residence

Table 2.1.1.4 (contd)

Reference	Country	Study years	No. of cases/controls	No. of nonsmokers (cases/controls)	Source of cases and controls	Comments
Zang & Wynder (1996)	USA	1981–94	Men: 1108/1122 Women: 781/948	*Men* SCC [2.3%†] AC [10.0%†] SCLC [0.0%†] Controls [52.6%†] *Women* SCC [7.3%†] AC [15.1%†] SCLC [2.1%†] Controls [71.0%†]	Cases: H Controls: H	Individually matched by age, sex, hospital and time of admission †% of nonsmokers for each histological type of lung cancer and % of nonsmoking controls
Barbone *et al.* (1997)	Italy, Trieste	1979–81; 1985–86	Men: 755/755	22/188	Cases and controls: autopsies	Matched on age and period of death
Dosemeci *et al.* (1997)	Turkey, Istanbul	1979–84	Men: 1210/829	142/293	Cases: H Controls: H	Matched by sex, age (within 5 years) and area of residence
Hu *et al.* (1997)	China, Heilongjiang	May 1985–April 1987	Men: 161/161 Women: 66/66	41/40 67/48	Cases: H Controls: H	Only large-cell cancer
Muscat *et al.* (1997)	USA	1980–95	Men: 228/2545 Women: 154/1715	7/650 13/936	Cases: H Controls: H	Only large-cell carcinoma Frequency-matched by age, sex, hospital and date of interview
Pawlega *et al.* (1997)	Poland, Cracow	Jan. 1992–Dec. 1994	Men: 176/341	4/92	Cases: P Controls: P	Matched by age
Pohlabeln *et al.* (1997)	Germany, Bremen, Frankfurt	1988–93	Men: 839/839	18/138	Cases: H Controls: P	Matched for age, sex and region
Rachtan & Sokolowski (1997)	Poland, Cracow	March 1991–June 1994	Women: 118/141	33/98	Cases: H Controls: H	Controls were next of kin of patients with diseases unrelated to smoking

Table 2.1.1.4 (contd)

Reference	Country	Study years	No. of cases/controls	No. of nonsmokers (cases/controls)	Source of cases and controls	Comments
Schwartz & Swanson (1997)	USA, Detroit, Michigan	Nov. 1984–June 1987	Men: white: 2767/1395 African American: 913/379 Women: white 1533/1492 African American: 375/426	119/376 50/104 182/855 40/247	Cases: P Controls: P	African Americans compared with whites
Stellman et al. (1997a)	USA	1997–95	Men: 1442/876 Women: 850/467	Only current smokers	Cases: H Controls: H	Frequency-matched on age, sex, hospital and date of admission
Stellman et al. (1997b)	USA	1997–95	Men: 1366 SCC/ 1332 AC/3442 controls Women: 431 SCC/982 AC/ 2190 controls	Men: SCC 2%[†] AC 5.4%[†] Women SCC 6%[†] AC 15%[†] Controls: No data	Cases: H Controls: H	Frequency-matched on age, sex, hospital and date of admission [†]% of nonsmokers for each histological type of lung cancer
Wakai et al. (1997)	Japan, Okinawa	Jan. 1998–Nov. 1991	Men: 245/490 Women: 88/176	10/65 50/145	Cases: H Controls: P	Matched by sex, region and age; nonsmokers included occasional smokers
Jöckel et al. (1998)	Germany, Bremen, Frankfurt	1989–93	Men: 839/839 Women: 165/165	18/138 53/98	Cases: H Controls: P	Adjusted for age, region and exposure to asbestos
Khuder et al. (1998)	USA, Philadelphia	1985–87	Men: 482/1094	23/309	Cases: H Controls: P	Matched by race and age
Kreuzer et al. (1998)	Germany	1990–96	Men: young: 183/200 older: 1709/1761 Women: young: 68/80 older: 300/278	6/54 22/403 7/38 95/177	Cases: H Controls: P	Cancer in young adults Frequency-matched on sex, age and region

Table 2.1.1.4 (contd)

Reference	Country	Study years	No. of cases/controls	No. of nonsmokers (cases/controls)	Source of cases and controls	Comments
Liu *et al.* (1998)	China, 24 urban, 74 rural areas	1989–91	Men, urban 16 317/30 709 Men, rural 38 82/22 046 Women, urban 7300/21 171 Women, rural 1530/13 389	13440/18544 3219/14208 3080/3124 325/1191	Cases: P Controls: P (deaths)	Proportional mortality study
Matos *et al.* (1998)	Argentina, Buenos Aires	March 1994–March 1996	Men: 200/397	11/110	Cases: H Controls: H	Matched for age, sex and hospital
Wunsch-Filho *et al.* (1998)	Brazil, São Paolo	July 1990–June 1991	Men: 307/546 Women: 91/314	14/99 29/208	Cases: H Controls: H	Matched on age, hospital and sex
Armadans-Gil *et al.* (1999)	Spain	1986–90	Men: 325/325	4/64	Cases: H Controls: H	Matched on age
Carpenter *et al.* (1999)	USA, Los Angeles County	Sept. 1990–Jan. 1994	Men: 202/349 Women: 135/129	Smokers only	Cases: H Controls: P	
Mzileni *et al.* (1999)	South Africa	1993–95	Men: 288/183 Women: 60/197	34/103 32/190	Cases: H Controls: H	Only 61% of the lung cancers diagnoses were confirmed
Tousey *et al.* (1999)	USA, Florida	1993–96	Men: 301/567 Women: 206/440	4/130 13/226	Cases: P Controls: P	Frequency-matched on age, race and sex distribution
Agudo *et al.* (2000)	Germany, France, Italy, Spain, United Kingdom	1988–94	Women: 1556/2450	441/1337	Cases: H Controls: P or H, according to centre	Data included in the study (multicentric) by Simonato *et al.* (2001)
Dikshit & Kanhere (2000)	India, Bhopal	Cases: 1986–92 Controls: 1989–92	Men: 163/260	17/146	Cases: P Controls: P	Selected randomly according to age distribution of cases
Kreuzer *et al.* (2000)	Germany, Italy	1988–94	Men: 3723/4075 Women: 900/1094	81/1043 286/715	Cases: H Controls: P or H (1 centre)	Frequency-matched on sex, age and area of residence or individually (1 centre)

Table 2.1.1.4 (contd)

Reference	Country	Study years	No. of cases/controls	No. of nonsmokers (cases/controls)	Source of cases and controls	Comments
Osann et al. (2000)	USA, Orange County, California	July 1990–June 1993	Women: 98/204	1/107	Cases: 28 H Controls: P	Only small-cell carcinoma Frequency-matched on age
Rauscher et al. (2000)	USA, New York	July 1982–Dec. 1984	Men: 206/206 Women: 206/206	Current smokers excluded	Cases: P Controls: P	Individually matched on smoking
Simonato et al. (2000)	Italy, Venice	Feb. 1992–Feb. 1994	Men: 178/277 Women: 41/52	Sexes combined: 20/135	Cases: H Controls: P	Stratified by Venice Islands and inland, frequency-matched by age and sex
Boffetta et al. (2001)	Germany, Spain, France	1991–94	Women < 45 years: 116/174	18/98	Cases: H Controls: H, Spain, France; P, Germany	Matched on age
Goldoni et al. (2001)	Italy, Ferrara	1988–93	Men: 249/500	4/77	Cases: P (deaths) Controls: P (alive)	Matched by age
Lam et al. (2001)	Hong Kong, SAR	Dec. 1997–Jan. 1999	Men 35–69 years 917/1480 ≥ 70 years 994/2425 Women 35–69 years 314/4930 ≥ 70 years 670/4183	789/841 887/1502 72/457 303/692	Cases: P (deaths) Controls: P (alive)	Living persons aged at least 60 years identified by the informant
Lee et al. (2001)	China, Province of Taiwan	1993–99	Men: 236/† Women: 291/†	42 cases of SCC, SCLC and AC, and 119 controls	Cases: H Controls: H	†Cases matched to 1 or 2 controls on age and sex; 805 controls in total. Data are presented separately for SCC + SCLC and AC.
Mao et al. (2001)	Canada, 8 provinces	1994–97	Men: 1722/2542 Women: 1558/2531	45/680 161/1271	Cases: P Controls: P	Frequency-matched to the age/sex distribution of all cancer cases

Table 2.1.1.4 (contd)

Reference	Country	Study years	No. of cases/controls	No. of nonsmokers (cases/controls)	Source of cases and controls	Comments
Simonato et al. (2001)	France, Germany, Italy, Spain, Sweden, United Kingdom	1988–94	Men: 6035/7967 Women: 1574/2464	120/1953 467/1601	Cases: H Controls: P or H, according to centre	Frequency-matched to the age and sex distribution of the cases
Stellman et al. (2001)	Japan, USA	USA: March 1992– Feb. 1997 Japan: June 1993– May 1998	Men: USA: 371/373 Japan: 410/252/411	USA: 16/153 Japan: 19/29/70	USA: Cases: H Controls: H Japan: Cases: H Controls: H/P	Hospital controls frequency-matched on age, hospital and date of interview; population controls matched on age, date of interview and residence
Bhurgri et al. (2002)	Karachi, Pakistan	Not given	Men: 282/561[†] Women: 38/79[†]	Men and women, 45/418	Cases: H Controls: 320 H; 320 V	[†]Men, 279 HC + 282 VC; women, 41 HC + 38 VC matched on age and sex
Kubik et al. (2001, 2002)	Prague, Czech Republic	1998–2000	Women: 269/1079	51/603	Cases: H Controls: H	Controls within the same age group and catchment area
Pacella-Norman et al. (2002)	Johannesburg, South Africa	March 1995– April 1999	Men: 105/804 Women: 41/1370	8/317 16/1143	Cases: H Controls: H	Only blacks; cancer controls
Petrauskaite et al. (2002)	Kedainiai, Lithuania	1981–91	Men: 226/886	4/80	Death certificates and cancer registry	Matched by age, year of death
Rachtan (2002)	Cracow, Poland	March 1991– Dec. 1997	Women: 242/352	54/251	Cases: H Controls: H	

Table 2.1.1.4 (contd)

Reference	Country	Study years	No. of cases/controls	No. of nonsmokers (cases/controls)	Source of cases and controls	Comments
Sasco et al. (2002)	Casablanca, Morocco	Jan. 1996–Jan. 1998	Men: 114/227 Women: 4/8	Both sexes: 5/94	Cases: H Controls: H	Matched on age, sex and residence
Stellman et al. (2003)	USA	1984–98	Men: white, 1710/4491 black, 254/440 Women: white, 1321/2862 black, 163/358	3.5%/29.8% 2.4%/25.5% 9.2%/50.5% 6.8%/49.7%	Cases: H Controls: H	Frequency-matched for sex, hospital and year of interview
Wang et al. (2002)	China, Gansu	Jan. 1994–April 1998	Men: 563/1232 Women: 205/427	28/110 181/385	Cases: P Controls: P	Matched on age, stratified on sex and prefecture

H, hospital; P, population; V, visitor; SCC, squamous-cell carcinoma; AC, adenocarcinoma; SCLC, small-cell carcinoma

Table 2.1.1.5. Case–control studies on tobacco smoking and lung cancer: intensity and cumulative amount

Reference	Subjects	Average no. of cigarettes/day[a]	Odds ratio	95% CI	Adjustments, comments
Damber & Larsson (1986)	Men/C1	1–7 8–15 ≥16	2.3 7.3 10.2	Numbers not stated [figure]	Reference level not stated; smoking includes any tobacco. C1 deceased, C2 alive; adjustment variables not stated
	Men/C2	1–7 8–15 ≥16	2.3 7.0 18.2		
Pathak et al. (1986)	Men < 65 years	1–15 16–20 21–30 ≥31	16.2 27.6 47.1 89.3		Reference level, never-smoker; adjusted for sex and ethnicity p < 0.001 for linear trend
	Men ≥ 65 years	1–15 16–20 21–30 ≥31	8.6 12.3 22.9 24.3		p < 0.001 for linear trend
Benhamou et al. (1987)	Women	< 10 10–19 ≥ 20	0.6 0.9 4.8	0.1–2.6 0.2–4.4 0.7–35.6	Reference level, nonsmoker; matched analysis, adjusted for filter, duration, inhalation, age at starting smoking and type of tobacco
Gao et al. (1988)	Men		Duration (years)	CI not provided	Reference level, lifelong nonsmoker; adjusted for age and education

Gao et al. (1988), Men:

Average no. of cigarettes/day	1–29	30–39	≥ 40
1–19	0.9	3.2	3.8
20–29	2.1	7.1	7.2
≥ 30	3.0	10.8	15.4

Gao et al. (1988), Women:

Average no. of cigarettes/day	< 30	≥ 30
< 10	1.4	2.4
10–19	2.6	3.2
≥ 20	8.9	14.2

Reference	Subjects	Average no. of cigarettes/day[a]	Odds ratio	95% CI	Adjustments, comments
Benhamou et al. (1989)	Men	1–9 10–19 ≥ 20	1.0 2.4 5.2	 1.6–3.6 3.5–7.6	Adjusted for age and duration of smoking

Table 2.1.1.5 (contd)

Reference	Subjects	Average no. of cigarettes/day[a]	Odds ratio	Duration (years) 1–29	30–39	≥40	95% CI	Adjustments, comments
Kaufman et al. (1989)	Men and women	<15	8.0				5–13	Adjusted for age, sex, ethnicity, region, education and date of interview
		15–24	15.0				10–23	
		25–34	28.0				17–44	
		35–44	43.0				27–68	
		≥45	60.0				35–102	
Schoenberg et al. (1989)	Women	<20/day < 35 years	3.2				2.3–4.4	Adjusted for age, race and respondent
		≥20/day < 35 years	6.5				4.5–9.4	
		<20/day ≥ 35 years	8.4				6.2–11.2	
		≥20/day ≥ 35 years	16.0				11.9–21.7	
Svensson et al. (1989)	Women	Former smoker						Reference level, never-smoker; ?, not given
		1–10	2.6				1.4–5.1	
		11–20	4.6				2.5–9.3	
		≥21	12.6				6.5–25.2	
			59.0				7.6–?	
Xu et al. (1989)	Men	1–19		1.8*	2.1	3.3*		Reference level, nonsmoker; adjusted for age and education
		20–29		1.5*	2.7*	6.0*		
		≥30		5.3*	4.9*	17.1*		
	Women	1–19		1.4	3.1	3.4*		
		≥20		2.1	3.4*	9.4*		
Jedrychowski et al. (1990)	Men	1–19	3.5				2.3–5.2	Reference level, never-smoker; adjusted for age
		20–29	6.2				4.2–8.9	
		≥30	7.7				5.1–11.5	
		Unknown	2.4				1.2–4.7	
	Women	1–19	6.4				2.7–15.2	
		20–29	2.4				1.2–6.9	
		≥30	7.4				2.2–24.7	
		Unknown	2.9				0.5–18.6	
Wu-Williams et al. (1990)	Women	1–19		1.3	2.6*	3.2*		†Only 9% of the cases and 4% of the controls in this category
		≥20†		1.8	3.3*	5.7*		

Table 2.1.1.5 (contd)

Reference	Subjects	Average no. of cigarettes/day[a]	Odds ratio	95% CI	Adjustments, comments
Hebert & Kabat (1991)	Men	1–19 20–29 ≥30	3.8 8.3 10.9	2.7–5.5 6.3–11.1 8.4–14.1	Reference level, never-smoker; adjustment not stated
	Women	1–19 20–29 ≥30	4.9 12.9 19.7	3.4–7.1 9.6–17.5 14.9–26.1	
Katsouyanni et al. (1991)	Women	Nonsmoker ≤20 ≥21	1.0 2.3 7.5	 1.1–4.8 2.4–23.2	Adjusted for age
Liu et al. (1991)	Men	Never-smoker ≤0.5 kg/month[†] 0.6–1 kg/month >1 kg/month	1.0 1.4 1.1 1.9	 0.3–6.1 0.2–4.8 0.3–11.4	Only 56 cases, restricted to farmers; adjusted on 'other risk factors' [†]kg/month of tobacco smoked [‡]Amount × years of smoking
		Smoking index[‡] <2 2–19 20–34 ≥35	 1.0 2.6 2.2 4.7	 0.7–9.8 0.5–8.6 1.03–21.4	
Osann (1991)	Women	<1 pack/day ≥1 pack/day	2.5 12.6	1.2–5.2 6.2–25.6	Adjusted on age
Jöckel et al. (1992)	Men	>0–20 pack–years >20–40 pack–years ≥41 pack–years	7.3 8.3 16.2	2.4–22.3 2.8–25.0 5.1–51.3	Reference level, nonsmoker; hospital and population controls combined
	Women	>0–20 pack–years ≥21 pack–years	5.7 20.0	1.3–24.7 5.0–80.2	
Liu (1992)	Men and women	<10 10–19 ≥20	1.0 2.0 3.3	0.8–1.3 1.7–2.5 2.7–4.2	Reference level, nonsmoker; combined analysis of 5 studies; Mantel-Haenzel summary odds ratios (each city = one stratum)

Table 2.1.1.5 (contd)

Reference	Subjects	Average no. of cigarettes/day[a]	Odds ratio	95% CI	Adjustments, comments
Lubin et al. (1992)	Men	1–6 7–14 15–19 ≥20	0.7 1.2 6.5 8.0		Reference level, nonsmoker; adjusted for age, source of subject, type of work underground and years of work underground p for trend < 0.01
Morabia & Wynder (1992)	Men and women	1–19 20–29 30–39 40–80	Non-cancer control / Cancer control 1.5 / 1.9 3.3* / 4.6* 4.1* / 6.7* 5.0* / 7.6*		Only bronchioalveolar carcinoma; reference level, never-smoker; adjusted for age and sex
Gao et al. (1993)	Men	1–19 20–29 ≥30	3.5 7.5 10.6	1.6–7.2 3.7–15.3 5.1–22.2	Reference level, nonsmoker; adjusted for age
Liu et al. (1993)	Men	Never-smoker 1–19 20–29 ≥30	1.0 1.2 7.1 21.4	0.4–3.5 2.6–19.5 7.1–64.0	Adjusted for education, occupation and living area; present and former smokers combined
	Women	Never-smoker 1–9 10–19 ≥20	1.0 1.8 3.5 17.9	0.6–5.9 1.2–9.8 4.0–80.6	
Pezzotto et al. (1993)	Men	< 21 21–40 > 40	1.0 8.2 11.6	$p < 0.0001$ $p < 0.0001$	Adjusted for age, hospital and duration of smoking
Risch et al. (1993)	Men	1–29 pack–years 30–59 pack–years ≥60 pack–years	5.2 11.0 22.6	2.4–11.5 5.4–22.3 10.0–51.2	Reference level, never-smoker; adjusted for sex, age, residence and years since cessation
	Women	1–29 pack–years 30–59 pack–years ≥60 pack–years	7.3 26.7 81.9	4.1–13.0 14.0–50.6 25.3–267	

Table 2.1.1.5 (contd)

Reference	Subjects	Average no. of cigarettes/day[a]	Odds ratio	95% CI	Adjustments, comments
Benhamou et al. (1994)	Men	1–14	1.0		Adjusted for age and other smoking variables
		15–20	1.7	1.4–2.1	
		> 20	3.2	2.5–4.0	
De Stefani et al. (1994)	Men	*Manufactured*			Smokers only; adjusted for age, residence, education and duration
		1–14	1.0		
		15–20	3.3	1.4–7.7	
		21–40	4.4	1.8–10.6	
		≥ 41	11.9	3.7–38.6	
		Hand rolled			
		1–14	1.0		
		15–20	1.9	1.2–3.0	
		21–40	2.4	1.5–3.9	
		≥ 41	4.1	2.4–6.8	
Sankanarayanan et al. (1994)	Men	*Pack–years*			Reference level, never-smoker; crude odds ratios
		1–5	1.7	0.8–3.8	
		6–10	3.7	1.8–7.5	
		11–15	7.7	3.9–15.2	
		16–20	9.3	4.8–17.9	
		21–25	21.7	11.0–42.8	
		26–30	35.8	16.8–76.2	
		31–40	44.2	23.9–81.8	
		41–50	57.5	25.2–131.0	
		51–60	71.6	29.3–174.5	
		≥ 61	113.6	35.2–303.3	
Sobue et al. (1994)	Men	1–19	1.0		Adjusted for duration, fraction smoked per cigarette, filter and inhalation
		20–29	1.3	1.0–1.8	
		≥ 30	1.7	1.2–2.3	
Suzuki et al. (1994)	Men and women	1–30[†]	1.0		Adjusted for age, sex and race, in a multivariate analysis excluding nonsmokers [†]overlapping intervals
		30–50[†]	2.2	0.9–5.0	
		> 50	7.4	3.1–17	

Table 2.1.1.5 (contd)

Reference	Subjects	Average no. of cigarettes/day[a]	Odds ratio	95% CI	Adjustments, comments
Siemiatycki et al. (1995)	Men	Nonsmoker	1.0		Adjusted by age, ethnic group, socioeconomic status, coffee consumption, and composite scores for consumption of alcohol and β-carotene
		1–500 cig–years	4.4	2.2–8.6	
		501–1000 cig–years	9.9	5.3–18.7	
		1001–1500 cig–years	16.1	8.5–30.8	
		≥ 1501 cig–years	28.0	14.5–54.0	
De Stefani et al. (1996a)	Men	1–10	2.9	1.6–5.0	Reference level, never-smoker; adjusted for age, residence, urban/rural status and education
		11–20	8.4	5.2–13.6	
		21–40	10.4	6.4–16.9	
		≥ 41	23.7	13.4–42.1	
		1–29 pack–years	3.8	2.3–6.3	
		30–50 pack–years	7.6	4.6–12.6	
		51–85 pack–years	12.7	7.7–21.1	
		≥ 86 pack–years	14.9	8.9–24.8	
De Stefani et al. (1996b)	Men and women	1–33 pack–years	1.9	1.0–3.8	Reference level, nonsmoker; adjusted for age, sex, residence, urban/rural, education, family history of cancer and body-mass index
		34–54 pack–years	6.5	3.5–12.1	
		55–84 pack–years	14.5	7.7–27.2	
		≥ 85 pack–years	16.1	8.6–30.4	
Lei et al. (1996)	Men	< 400 cig–years	1.8	1.2–3.3	[Adjustment not stated]
		400–799 cig–years	3.3	2.7–5.6	
		≥ 800 cig–years	5.4	3.6–7.9	
	Women	< 400 cig–years	1.9	1.7–3.0	
		400–799 cig–years	3.6	2.4–5.1	
		≥ 800 cig–years	5.5	3.2–7.2	

Rylander et al. (1996), Men:

Average no. of cigarettes/day[a]	Duration (years)					p trend	Adjustments, comments
	< 20	20–29	30–39	40–49	≥ 50		
< 10	0.9	1.4	4.3*	5.7*	17.6*	0.008	Reference level, nonsmoker; adjusted for age, marital status, job classification, 'other fruits and berries' and milk consumption.
10–19	2.6	2.3	6.0*	16.2*	22.6*	0.001	
≥ 20	1.3	2.8*	10.9*	12.6*	41.0*	0.001	

Table 2.1.5 (contd)

Reference	Subjects	Average no. of cigarettes/day[a]	Odds ratio	Duration (years) 1–29	30–39	≥40	95% CI	Adjustments, comments
Xu et al. (1996)	Men	1–19		1.8*	2.1*	3.3*		Reference level, nonsmoker; adjusted for age and education
		20–29		1.5*	2.7*	6.0*		
		≥30		5.3*	4.9*	17.1*		
	Women	1–19		1.4	3.1*	3.4*		
		≥20		2.1	3.4*	9.4*		
Yu & Zhao (1996)	Men and women	<10	1.2				0.9–1.8	Meta-analysis of 15 studies
		10–19	2.2				1.4–2.8	
		≥20	4.5				2.8–7.2	
	Women	<10	2.2				1.7–2.9	Meta-analysis of 12 studies
		10–19	6.1				4.6–8.1	
		≥20	12.2				8.8–16.8	
Barbone et al. (1997)	Men	1–9	2.7				1.5–5.1	Reference level, nonsmoker; adjusted for age
		10–19	9.8				5.9–16.3	
		20–29	10.9				6.7–17.8	
		30–39	13.6				8.1–23.0	
		≥40	17.7				10.7–29.2	
Dosemeci et al. (1997)	Men	1–10	2.2				1.4–3.3	Adjusted for age and alcohol consumption
		11–20	3.1				2.3–4.1	
		≥21	6.6				4.4–10.2	
Hu et al. (1997)	Men	Nonsmoker	1.0					Adjustment not stated †[Overlapping intervals]
		1–14†	1.6				0.8–3.0	
		14–24†	2.1				1.2–3.8	
		≥25	3.7				1.6–8.4	
	Women	Nonsmoker	1.0					‡Only 6 cases and 6 controls for 14–24 cigarettes/day and 1 case and 2 controls for ≥25 cigarettes/day
		1–14†	2.3				0.9–6.0	
		14–24†	1.2‡				0.3–4.6	
		≥25	0.6‡				0.3–9.7	

Table 2.1.1.5 (contd)

Reference	Subjects	Average no. of cigarettes/day[a]	Odds ratio				95% CI	Adjustments, comments
			Cig/day	1–19	20–39	≥40		
Muscat et al. (1997)	Men	Current smoker		8.3*	14.6*	37.0*		Analysis of large-cell carcinomas only; adjusted for age and education all p for trend < 0.01
		Former smoker		4.8*	7.4*	11.1*		
	Women	Current smoker		6.0*	21.0*	72.9*		
		Former smoker		4.2*	9.9*	10.5*		
Pawlega et al. (1997)	Men	1–20 pack–years	2.9				0.8–10.4	Adjusted for age, residence, education, years of occupational exposure and frequency of fruit and vegetable consumption
		21–40 pack–years	15.2				4.8–47.5	
		>40 pack–years	18.7				6.0–58.2	
Rachtan & Sokolowski (1997)	Women	<10	3.6				1.1–12.3	Reference level, never-smoker; adjusted for age
		10–19	3.5				1.7–7.2	
		≥20	13.8				6.5–29.2	
Schwartz & Swanson (1997)	Men	*40–54 years*						Risk for African Americans compared with whites in each category of smokers within each age group, for men and women separately; adjusted for age, education and number of years since cessation
		Nonsmoker	8.0				2–32.8	
		1–40 pack–years	3.1				1.9–5.4	
		≥41 pack–years	1.8				0.7–4.7	
		55–84 years						
		Nonsmoker	1.0				0.6–1.5	
		1–40 pack–years	0.8				0.6–1.1	
		≥41 pack–years	0.9				0.7–1.2	
	Women	*40–54 years*						
		Nonsmoker	0.8				0.2–3.4	
		1–40 pack–years	1.2				0.7–2.1	
		≥41 pack–years	–				–	
		55–84 years						
		Nonsmoker	0.8				0.5–1.1	
		1–40 pack–years	1.1				0.8–1.6	
		≥41 pack–years	0.8				0.5–1.2	

Table 2.1.1.5 (contd)

Reference	Subjects	Average no. of cigarettes/day[a]	Odds ratio	95% CI	Adjustments, comments
Wakai *et al.* (1997)	Men	1–19	1.8	0.8–4.0	Current smokers; reference level, nonsmoker; adjusted for age
		20–29	4.0	1.9–8.4	
		≥30	9.2	4.2–20.1	
Jöckel *et al.* (1998)	Men	Nonsmoker	1.0		Nonsmoker includes occasional smokers; matched for age, sex and region; no further adjustments
		0–20 pack–years	3.8	2.2–6.5	
		> 20–40 pack–years	9.7	5.7–16.5	
		> 40 pack–years	14.0	8.1–24.4	
	Women	Nonsmoker	1.0		
		0–20 pack–years	1.8	1.0–3.3	
		> 20–40 pack–years	5.2	2.6–10.4	
		> 40 pack–years	11.3	3.1–41.2	
Khuder *et al.* (1998)	Men	1–19	2.5	1.5–4.1	Reference level, nonsmoker Crude odds ratios
		20–39	10.4	6.6–16.5	
		≥40	32.8	19.6–55.0	
Kreuzer *et al.* (1998)	*≤45 years* Men	≤9	2.5	0.7–8.2	Adjusted for age, region and exposure to asbestos
		10–19	8.7	3.5–21.9	
		20–29	19.5	7.5–50.3	
		≥30	20.8	7.2–60.5	
	Women	≤9	5.7	1.6–16.6	
		10–19	11.8	3.5–29.0	
		20–29	12.1	3.0–48.0	
	55–69 years Men	≤9	8.2	5.2–13.0	
		10–19	25.1	16.2–38.7	
		20–29	32.8	20.9–51.4	
		≥30	33.3	20.5–54.0	
	Women	≤9	2.0	1.2–3.3	
		10–19	5.4	3.5–8.6	
		20–29	7.7	3.5–17.3	
		≥30	—	—	

Table 2.1.5 (contd)

Reference	Subjects	Average no. of cigarettes/day[a]	Odds ratio	95% CI	Adjustments, comments
Liu et al. (1998)	Men aged 35–69 years	*Urban*[†]			Proportional mortality study
		1–19	2.1	0.05[‡]	Reference level, nonsmoker
		20	3.6	0.06	[†]Most recent smoking habit
		>20	6.9	0.14	[‡]Standard error
		Rural[†]			Trends: $p < 0.0001$
		1–19	2.2	2.23	
		20	3.7	3.65	
		>20	7.3	7.26	
Matos et al. (1998)	Men	*Current smoker*			Reference level, nonsmoker;
		1–14	1.6	0.5–5.0	adjusted for age and hospital
		15–24	8.0	3.4–16.8	
		≥25	15.0	7.1–31.9	
		Former smoker			
		1–14	2.3	0.9–5.6	
		15–24	6.7	2.9–15.4	
		≥25	7.4	3.4–16.1	
Wunsch-Filho et al. (1998)	Men	<21 pack–years	1.3	0.7–2.8	Reference level, nonsmoker
		21–40 pack–years	4.2	2.2–8.1	
		41–60 pack–years	6.9	3.6–13.0	
		≥61 pack–years	7.7	4.1–14.6	
	Women	<21 pack–years	3.9	2.0–7.6	
		21–40 pack–years	9.0	3.6–22.5	
		41–60 pack–years	7.4	2.9–19.0	
		≥61 pack–years	3.6	1.1–11.4	
Armadans-Gil et al. (1999)	Men	1–14	3.3	1.4–7.4	Adjusted for age
		15–24	11.6	5.3–25.3	
		≥25	41.2	17.8–95.0	

Table 2.1.1.5 (contd)

Reference	Subjects	Average no. of cigarettes/day[a]	Odds ratio	95% CI	Adjustments, comments
Mzileni et al. (1999)	Men	Former smoker	2.2	1.0–4.6	Reference level, never-smoker; adjusted for age, dusty occupation and exposure to asbestos at birth
		Current smoker			
		<15 g/day	9.8	5.9–16.4	
		≥15 g/day	12.0	6.5–22.3	
	Women	Former smoker[†]	5.8	1.3–25.8	[†]Only 2 former and 5 current smokers among controls
		Current smoker[†]	5.5	2.6–11.3	
Agudo et al. (2000)	Women	<10	2.0	1.6–2.5	Reference level, never-smoker (includes smokers of less than 400 cig during lifetime) adjusted for age and centre
		10–19	5.9	4.8–7.3	
		20–29	9.5	7.0–12.8	
		≥30	15.4	9.6–24.7	
Dikshit & Kanhere (2000)	Men	1–10	1.5	0.3–6.7	Adjusted for age and bidi-smoking
		11–20	11.1	3.4–35.9	
		>20	26.8	6.0–120.2	
Kreuzer et al. (2000)	All[†]				Reference level, never-smoker
	Men	<15	8.6	6.7–10.9	Adjusted for age and centre [†]p for interaction gender/smoking < 0.0001
		15–29	21.7	17.2–27.4	
		≥30	25.4	19.4–33.3	
	Women	<15	2.9	2.4–3.6	[†]p for interaction gender/smoking = 0.8 Analysis restricted to ever-smokers, adjusted also for duration and time since cessation
		15–29	7.8	5.8–10.3	
		≥30	13.8	6.8–28.1	
	Age < 50[‡]				
	Men	<15	4.3	2.4–7.5	
		15–29	11.6	7.0–19.3	
		≥30	20.7	10.8–39.6	
	Women	<15	3.8	1.9–7.6	
		15–29	15.0	7.0–32.0	
		≥30	23.4	5.9–92.3	
	Ever-smoker				
	Men	<15	1.0		
		15–29	2.0	1.8–2.2	
		≥30	2.4	2.0–2.8	

Table 2.1.1.5 (contd)

Reference	Subjects	Average no. of cigarettes/day[a]	Odds ratio			95% CI	Adjustments, comments
	Women	<15	1.0				
		15–29	2.0			1.4–2.7	
		≥30	3.4			1.6–7.3	
Osann et al. (2000)	Women	Former smoker	31.5				Small-cell carcinoma only. Reference level, never-smoker (1 case/107 controls); adjusted for age and education
		Current smoker	278.9				[†] 1 case/146 controls; analysis by pack–years, also adjusted for years since cessation.
		<12 pack–years	1.0[†]				
		12.1–24.4 pack–years	27.0				
		≥24.5 pack–years	56.7				
Simonato et al. (2000)	Men and women	*Venice*					Reference level, never-smoker, includes former smokers with >20 years of cessation; adjusted for age, sex, education, duration, occupation and heating
		Former smoker	4.6			1.3–16.5	
		Current smoker	17.5			4.8–63.4	
		Mestre					
		Former smoker	4.9			2.3–10.5	
		Current smoker	9.7			4.7–19.9	
Boffetta et al. (2001)	Women		*< 35 years*	*35–39 years*	*40–44 years*		[†]Reference level, never-smoker, adjusted for center and age
		Current smoker[†]	3.4 (0.6–19)	5.4 (1.9–15)	18 (6.6–50)		[‡]Reference level, < 15 cigarettes/day, further adjusted for duration of smoking
		Former smoker[†]	4.9 (0.5–47)	2.2 (0.6–8.2)	5.3 (1.6–18)		
		1–9 pack–years[†]	3.6 (0.6–21)	1.0 (0.2–4.5)	3.9 (1.2–13)		
		10–14 pack–years[†]	3.7 (0.3–41)	6.6 (1.6–27)	18 (4.9–64)		
		≥15 pack–years[†]	4.4 (0.4–48)	6.9 (2.1–22)	33 (10–104)		
		15–24 cig/day[‡]	0.3 (0.1–2.6)	0.1 (0.02–1.0)	2.0 (0.7–5.4)		
		≥25 cig/day[‡]	—	0.4 (0.04–4.4)	5.7 (1.0–32)		

Table 2.1.1.5 (contd)

Reference	Subjects	Average no. of cigarettes/day[a]	Odds ratio	95% CI	Adjustments, comments
Goldoni et al. (2001)	Men	1–9	3.7	0.9–15.8	Reference level, nonsmoker; adjusted for passive smoking, age and diet
		10–19	9.9	3.3–29.5	
		≥ 20	44.9	14.5–139.3	
Lam et al. (2001)	35–69 years				Reference level, nonsmoker; adjusted for age and education all p for trend < 0.001
	Men	1–14	2.8*		
		15–24	5.6*		
		≥ 25	12.7*		
	Women	1–14	2.4*		
		15–24	4.2*		
		≥ 25	7.5*		
	≥ 70 years				
	Men	1–14	3.4*		
		15–24	6.5*		
		≥ 25	7.3*		
	Women	1–14	3.4*		
		15–24	6.2*		
		≥ 25	5.3*		
Mao et al. (2001)	Men	Former smoker	6.4	4.6–8.8	Reference level, never-smoker; adjusted for age group, province, years of exposure to passive smoking, total consumption of vegetables, vegetable juices and meat
		Current smoker	17.3	12.4–24.2	
		≤ 8 pack–years	2.1	1.4–3.2	
		9–18	3.6	2.4–5.2	
		19–32	12.7	9.0–17.9	
		≥ 33	27.9	19.8–39.4	
	Women	Former smoker	4.3	3.5–5.4	
		Current smoker	13.2	10.6–16.4	
		≤ 8 pack–years	1.5	1.2–2.1	
		9–18	4.1	3.1–5.4	
		19–32	13.0	10.2–16.6	
		≥ 33	29.0	22.1–38.0	

Table 2.1.1.5 (contd)

Reference	Subjects	Average no. of cigarettes/day[a]	Odds ratio	95% CI	Adjustments, comments
Simonato et al. (2001)	Men	<10	13.1	10.1–16.8	Reference level, nonsmoker; adjusted for age, education and centre. There is an increasing risk with duration for each category of average cigarettes/day. Only data for duration ≥ 40 years are shown.
		10–19	29.7	23.9–36.7	
		20–29	44.9	35.7–56.3	
		≥ 30	46.4	29.7–72.5	
	Women	<10	6.6	4.6–9.5	
		10–19	11.6	8.3–16.1	
		20–29	29.5	18.0–48.1	
		≥ 30	36.4	10.3–129.1	
Stellman et al. (2001)	Men USA (hospital controls)	<20	10.9	4.4–28.0	Reference level, nonsmoker; adjusted for age, education and hospital for hospital controls or residence for community controls
		20–29	53.4	23.1–135.2	
		≥ 30	73.3	32.5–181.6	
	Japan (hospital controls)	<20	1.6	0.7–3.9	
		20–29	3.5	1.5–8.4	
		≥ 30	6.2	2.6–15.0	
	Japan (community controls)	<20	2.6	1.4–4.9	
		20–29	4.3	2.4–7.6	
		≥ 30	9.3	5.2–16.7	
Bhurgi et al. (2002)	Men and women	Former smoker	16.7	9.8–28.4	Reference level, never-smoker; adjusted for age, sex, hospital [†] Also adjusted for years of smoking
		Current smoker	30.2	17.8–51.3	
		Cig-equivalents/day[†]			
		1–9	4.1	1.8–9.2	
		19–19	14.5	8.0–26.3	
		20–29	36.7	20.1–67.0	
		≥ 30	85.9	43.9–168.3	

Table 2.1.5 (contd)

Reference	Subjects	Average no. of cigarettes/day[a]	Odds ratio	95% CI	Adjustments, comments
Kubik et al. (2001, 2002)	Women	Former smoker	7.7	6.7–15.8	Reference level, never-smoker; adjusted for age, residence and education; information on duration and pack–years
		Current smoker	10.3	5.1–11.5	
		1–4	4.6	2.4–9.0	
		5–14	5.7	3.8–8.5	
		> 14	12.6	8.3–19.0	
Pacella-Norman et al. (2002)	Men	1–14 g/day[†]	6.3	2.6–15.0	Reference level, never-smoker; adjusted for age, place of birth, education, work category
		≥ 15 g/day[†]	23.9	9.5–60.3	[†] 1 cigarette = 1 pipe = 1 hand-rolled cigarette = 1 g
	Women	1–14 gday[†]	10.5	4.1–27.3	
		≥ 15 g/day[†]	50.9	12.6–204.6	
Petrauskaite (2002)	Men	Former smoker	14.0	4.9–40.3	Reference level, never-smoker; adjusted for age and year of death
		Current smoker	21.1	7.5–60.1	
		< 8	9.8	2.9–33.1	
		8–15	21.3	7.1–63.7	
		≥ 16	27.0	9.3–78.5	
Rachtan (2002)	Women	Former smoker	3.3	1.8–5.9	Reference level, never-smoker; adjusted for age
		Current smoker	14.0	9.0–21.7	
		< 11	4.0	2.3–7.0	
		11–20	11.2	7.1–17.6	
		21–30	23.0	8.2–64.3	
		≥ 30	45.8	10.3–204.1	
Sasco et al. (2002)	Men and women	Former light	1.8	0.5–6.8	Reference level, never-smoker; adjusted for use of hashish/kif, snuff; history of chronic bronchitis, passive smoking, occupational exposure, cooking and heat source, lighting sources, ventilation of the kitchen
		Former heavy	8.1	2.0–33.1	
		Current light	18.5	4.1–83.5	
		Current heavy	26.1	6.6–103.0	

IARC MONOGRAPHS VOLUME 83

Table 2.1.1.5 (contd)

Reference	Subjects		Average no. of cigarettes/day[a]	Odds ratio	95% CI	Adjustments, comments
Stellman et al. (2002)	Men	White	Former smoker	7.9	6.0–10.3	Reference level, never-smoker
			Current smoker	21.0	15.8–27.8	
			1–19	8.4	5.9–12.1	
			20	20.0	14.4–27.6	
			≥ 21	29.8	22.1–40.2	
		Black	Former smoker	8.1	3.4–19.4	
			Current smoker	18.2	7.6–43.4	
			1–19	7.5	3.0–18.7	
			20	34.2	13.3–88.3	
			≥ 21	42.2	15.9–111.9	
	Women	White	Former smoker	6.3	5.1–7.9	
			Current smoker	19.3	15.4–24.2	
			1–10	6.2	4.4–8.8	
			11–20	19.1	14.6–25.0	
			≥ 21	33.6	25.4–44.4	
		Black	Former smoker	9.3	4.5–19.2	
			Current smoker	17.2	8.7–33.7	
			1–10	8.3	3.8–18.2	
			11–20	21.3	10.0–45.2	
			≥ 21	42.9	17.0–108.4	
Wang et al. (2002)	Men and women		Light smoker	1.3	0.8–1.8	Reference level, never-smoker; adjusted for age, sex, prefecture and socioeconomic factors
			≥ 10 cig/day and ≥ 30 years	2.5	1.5–4.1	
			≥ 20 cig/day and ≥ 40 years	5.5	2.2–12.2	

*$p < 0.05$
[a] Unless otherwise specified

Table 2.1.1.6. Case–control studies on tobacco smoking and lung cancer: age at starting smoking

Reference	Subjects	Age at starting smoking (years)	Odds ratio	95% CI	Comments
Gao et al (1988)	Men	10–19	5.1	3.6–7.2	Reference level, lifelong nonsmoker; adjusted for age and education
		20–29	4.7	3.3–6.5	
		≥ 30	1.2	0.8–1.9	
	Women	10–19	5.6	3.4–9.0	
		20–29	3.8	2.6–5.8	
		≥ 30	2.0	1.4–3.0	
Jedrychowski et al. (1990)	Men	< 17	1.7	1.2–2.3	Reference level, never-smoker; adjusted for age
		17–18	1.3	1.0–1.7	
	Women	< 23	1.8	0.7–4.6	
Liu (1992)	Men and women	< 20	3.3	2.7–4.0	Reference level, nonsmoker; combined analysis of 3 studies; adjusted by city
		20–29	2.4	2.0–2.8	
		≥ 30	1.2	0.9–1.5	
Morabia & Wynder (1992)	Men and women		NCC		Only bronchioloalveolar carcinoma; reference level, never-smoker; adjusted for age and sex
		10–14	2.3	0.9–6.2	
		15–16	5.7	2.5–12.9	
		17–19	2.1	1.0–4.4	
		20–50	2.3	1.1–4.9	
			CC		
		10–14	6.0	2.1–17.3	
		15–16	5.2	2.3–11.3	
		17–19	4.1	1.9–8.7	
		20–50	2.4	1.2–5.1	

Table 2.1.1.6 (contd)

Reference	Subjects	Age at starting smoking (years)	Odds ratio	95% CI	Comments
Gao et al. (1993)	Men	<20	8.6	4.0–18.5	Reference level, nonsmoker; adjusted for age
		20–29	6.4	3.3–12.5	
		≥30	2.1	0.4–13.0	
Hegmann et al. (1993)	Men	≤19	12.7	6.4–25.2	Reference level, nonsmoker; adjusted for age and pack–years
		>19	6.0	2.8–12.9	
	Women	≤25	10.0	4.7–21.2	†Only 2 cases started > 25 years.
		>25†	2.6	0.5–12.4	
Pezzotto et al. (1993)	Men	<14	1.0		Adjusted for age, hospital and intensity of cigarette smoking
		14–18	1.4		
		>18	0.9		
Benhamou & Benhamou (1994)	Men	≤19	5.8	3.8–8.8	Reference level, nonsmoker; adjusted for age at diagnosis, hospital, interviewer and pack–years
		>19	5.9	3.9–8.9	
	Women	≤25	2.5	0.9–6.9	
		>25	1.2	0.4–3.5	
Suzuki et al. (1994)	Men and women	<12	2.4	0.8–7.3	Adjusted for age, sex, race and pack–years
		12–18	2.1	0.9–5.0	
		>18	1.0		
Yu & Zhao (1996)	Men and women	<20	3.3	2.4–3.6	Reference level, nonsmoker Meta-analysis of 15 studies
		20–29	2.4	1.9–3.1	
		≥30	1.3	0.9–1.9	
	Women	<20	3.2	2.4–4.3	Meta-analysis of 12 studies
		20–29	2.8	2.2–3.7	
		≥30	1.5	1.2–2.0	

Table 2.1.1.6 (contd)

Reference	Subjects	Age at starting smoking (years)	Odds ratio	95% CI	Comments
Barbone et al. (1997)	Men	< 15	50.8	27.2–95.0	Reference level, nonsmoker; adjusted for age
		15–19	9.9	6.2–15.8	
		≥ 20	8.2	5.0–13.3	
Rachtan & Sokolowski (1997)	Women	< 20	11.6	5.0–26.7	Reference level never-smoker; adjusted for age
		20–30	5.3	2.8–10.2	
		> 30	5.3	1.5–19.0	
Khuder et al. (1998)	Men	< 16	10.3	6.5–16.3	Reference level, nonsmoker; unadjusted odds ratios
		16–19	6.4	4.0–10.2	
		≥ 20	6.4	3.8–10.2	
Liu et al. (1998)	Men 35–69 years				Proportional mortality study
	Urban	< 20	4.11	0.07[†]	Reference level, nonsmoker
		20–24	2.94	0.05[†]	[†] standard error
		≥ 25	2.45	0.05[†]	trends: $p < 0.0001$
	Rural	< 20	3.07	0.11[†]	
		20–24	2.62	0.09[†]	
		≥ 25	2.26	0.09[†]	
Matos et al. (1998)	Men				Reference level, nonsmoker; adjusted for age and hospital
	Current smoker	< 15	11.3	5.3–24.3	
		15–19	8.6	4.1–18.4	
		≥ 20	5.3	2.3–12.5	
	Former smoker	< 15	4.9	2.2–11.0	
		15–19	7.5	3.5–16.0	
		≥ 20	2.6	1.0–6.7	

Table 2.1.1.6 (contd)

Reference	Subjects	Age at starting smoking (years)	Odds ratio	95% CI	Comments
Mao *et al.* (2001)	Men	≤ 15	11.5	8.3–16.0	Reference level, never-smoker; adjusted for age group, province, years of exposure to passive smoking, total consumption of vegetables, vegetable juices and meat
		16–19	9.1	5.5–12.7	
		≥ 20	6.3	4.4–9.1	
	Women	≤ 15	8.8	6.9–11.2	
		16–19	8.0	6.4–9.9	
		≥ 20	5.6	4.4–7.1	
Stellman *et al.* (2001)	Men	≤ 14	1.2	0.4–3.4	Adjusted for age, education and hospital for hospital controls or residence for community controls
	USA (community controls)	15–17	1.0	Reference	
		18–20	0.6	0.2–1.7	
		> 20	0.5	0.2–1.4	
	Japan (hospital controls)	15–17	1.0	Reference	No controls and only 2 cases started before 15 years in Japan.
		18–20	0.2	0.1–0.6	
		> 20	0.2	0.1–0.8	
	Japan (community controls)	15–17	1.0	Reference	
		18–20	0.8	0.5–1.3	
		> 20	0.5	0.3–0.9	
Petrauskaite *et al.* (2002)	Men	< 20	22.5	7.8–63.9	Reference level not clear; adjusted for age and year of death
		20–24	13.6	4.6–40.0	
		≥ 25	8.6	2.6–28.5	
Rachtan (2002)	Women	≤ 18	13.6	7.6–24.1	Reference level, never-smoker; adjusted for age
		> 18	8.2	5.4–12.4	

CI, confidence interval; NCC, non-cancer controls; CC, cancer controls

Table 2.1.1.7. Case–control studies on tobacco smoking and lung cancer: duration of smoking

Reference	Subjects	Duration (years)	Odds ratio	95% CI	Comments
Pathak et al. (1986)	Men < 65 years	1–29	12.9		Reference level, never-smoker; adjusted for sex and ethnicity
		30–39	37.3		p < 0.001 for linear trend
		40–49	57.3		
		50–59	91.4		
	≥ 65 years	1–29	22.9		p < 0.001 for linear trend
		30–39	6.6		
		40–49	11.7		
		50–59	16.1		
		≥ 60	11.9		
Benhamou et al. (1987)	Women	≤ 20	1.0		Matched analysis, adjusted for filter, inhalation, age at starting smoking and type of tobacco used
		21–40	2.1	0.5–9.0	
		> 40	3.3	0.4–24.1	
Benhamou et al. (1989)	Men	1–25	1.0		Adjusted for age and daily consumption of cigarettes
		26–35	1.6	1.2–2.3	
		≥ 36	2.1	1.5–2.9	
Katsouyanni et al. (1991)	Women	1–30	1.3	0.5–3.3	Reference level, nonsmoker; adjusted for age
		> 30	7.4	2.9–19.1	
Osann (1991)	Women	≤ 20	1.6	0.7–3.5	Reference level, never-smoker; adjusted for age
		> 20	11.6	5.8–23.3	
Liu (1992)	Men and women	< 30	1.0	0.8–1.3	Reference level, nonsmoker; combined analysis of 5 studies
		≥ 30	2.7	2.2–3.2	

Table 2.1.1.7 (contd)

Reference	Subjects	Duration (years)	Odds ratio		95% CI	Comments
Lubin *et al.* (1992)	Men	1–29 30–39 40–49 ≥ 50	1.3 2.3 4.4 9.6			Reference level, nonsmoker; adjusted for age, source of subject, type of respondent and years of work underground *p* for trend < 0.01
Morabia & Wynder (1992)	Men and women	1–19 20–29 30–39 40–49 50–80	NCC 1.2 2.2 2.7* 3.4* 5.1*	CC 1.4 2.5* 3.9* 5.6* 9.1*		Only bronchioloalveolar carcinoma Reference level, never-smoker; adjusted for age and sex
Pezzotto *et al.* (1993)	Men	< 31 31–40 > 40	1.0 3.6 6.0		 *p* < 0.0005 *p* < 0.005	Adjusted for age, hospital and intensity of cigarette smoking
Benhamou *et al.* (1994)	Men	1–25 26–35 36–45 ≥ 46	1.0 2.4 3.0 4.2		 1.8–3.1 2.2–4.2 2.7–6.5	Adjusted for age and smoking variables
De Stefani *et al.* (1994)	Men	*Manufactured* 1–31 32–43 44–52 ≥ 53	1.0 1.6 3.2 2.9		 0.6–4.0 0.6–7.4 0.9–17.0	Adjusted for age, residence, education and amount of smoking

Table 2.1.1.7 (contd)

Reference	Subjects	Duration (years)	Odds ratio	95% CI	Comments
		Hand-rolled			
Sobue *et al.* (1994)	Men	1–31	1.0		Adjusted for number of cigarettes/day, fraction smoked per cigarette, filter and inhalation
		32–43	2.9	1.7–5.2	
		44–52	5.0	2.8–8.9	
		≥53	7.6	4.1–14.0	
De Stefani *et al.* (1996a)	Men	1–29	1.0		Reference level, never-smoker; adjusted for age, residence, urban/rural status and education
		30–39	1.5	1.0–2.2	
		40–49	2.8	2.0–4.1	
		≥50	4.1	2.7–6.2	
		1–29	3.4	1.7–6.8	
		30–39	5.2	2.9–8.9	
		40–49	10.4	6.4–16.9	
		≥50	10.8	6.6–17.6	
Yu & Zhao (1996)	Men and women	0	1.0		Meta-analysis of 15 studies; †Illegible in original article
		<30	1.1	0.6–?†	
		≥30	2.5	1.7–3.6	
	Women	0	1.0		Meta-analysis of 12 studies
		<30	1.4	0.5–3.9	
		≥30	3.8	1.7–8.5	
Barbone *et al.* (1997)	Men	1–29	3.2	1.8–5.7	Reference level, nonsmoker; adjusted for age
		30–39	7.9	4.7–13.5	
		40–49	11.4	7.0–18.8	
		≥50	14.5	9.0–23.3	
Dosemeci *et al.* (1997)	Men	1–10	1.0	0.6–1.7	Adjusted for age and alcohol use
		11–20	3.8	2.6–5.7	
		≥21	4.9	3.5–7.0	

Table 2.1.1.7 (contd)

Reference	Subjects	Duration (years)	Odds ratio	95% CI	Comments
Hu et al. (1997)	Men	1–19	2.0	0.1–3.9	Reference level, nonsmoker; [variables of adjustment not stated]
		20–29	2.1	1.2–3.7	
		≥ 30	2.2	0.9–5.3	
	Women	1–19	1.7	0.6–5.0	
		20–29	1.9	0.6–6.0	
		≥ 30	1.6	0.3–9.7	
Muscat et al. (1997)	Men	1–19	2.9*	1.2–7.3	Large-cell carcinoma only; adjusted for age and education
		20–39	10.6*	4.9–22.9	All p for trends < 0.01
		≥ 40	23.1*	10.4–50.8	
	Women	1–19	2.9*	1.2–6.9	
		20–39	11.5*	6.3–21.1	
		≥ 40	30.1*	15.8–57.4	
Rachtan & Sokolowski (1997)	Women	1–20	2.0	0.9–4.7	Reference level, never-smoker; adjusted for age
		21–40	7.5	3.9–14.6	
		> 40	58.7	7.6–455.6	
Khuder et al. (1998)	Men	1–29	3.5	1.8–7.1	Reference level, nonsmoker; unadjusted odds ratios
		30–49	7.5	4.8–11.9	
		≥ 50	9.0	5.7–14.1	
Kreuzer et al. (1998)	≤ 45 years				Reference level, never-smoker; adjusted for age, region and exposure to asbestos
	Men	≤ 19	4.0	1.6–10.2	
		20–39	26.3	10.3–66.8	
	Women	≤ 19	4.9	1.7–14.2	
		20–39	47.5	13.2–173	
	55–69 years				
	Men	≤ 19	4.9	3.1–7.9	
		20–39	20.9	13.5–32.2	
		≥ 40	54.5	34.9–85.2	

Table 2.1.1.7 (contd)

Reference	Subjects	Duration (years)	Odds ratio	95% CI	Comments
	Women	≤ 19	0.9	0.5–1.6	
		20–39	4.9	3.1–7.6	
		≥ 40	8.3	4.7–14.5	
Matos et al. (1998)	Men	*Current smoker*			Reference level, nonsmoker; adjusted for the design variables, age and hospital
		1–24	5.2	1.7–16.4	
		25–39	7.4	3.3–16.6	
		≥ 40	10.2	4.7–22.1	
		Former smoker			
		1–24	1.5	0.6–3.9	
		25–39	7.5	3.4–16.8	
		≥ 40	15.4	6.2–37.9	
Dikshit & Kanhere (2000)	Men	1–20	2.5	1.1–5.6	Reference level, nonsmoker; adjusted for age
		21–30	12.0	5.9–24.0	
		> 30	52.0	24.0–112.8	
Armadans-Gil et al. (1999)	Men	1–24	2.6	1.0–6.6	Reference level, nonsmoker; adjusted for age
		25–49	11.9	5.5–25.5	
		≥ 50	26.8	11.0–65.1	
Agudo et al. (2000)	Women	< 20	1.3	1.0–1.6	Reference level, never-smoker and smokers who had smoked less than 400 cigarettes in their lifetime; adjusted for age and centre
		20–29	4.5	3.5–5.7	
		30–39	7.6	6.1–9.5	
		≥ 40	12.8	10.1–16.2	
Kreuzer et al. (2000)	*All*[†]				Reference level, nonsmoker; adjusted for age and centre
	Men	< 20	2.4	1.8–3.3	[†]p for interaction gender/smoking < 0.0001
		20–39	16.4	12.9–20.9	
		≥ 40	39.1	30.4–50.3	

Table 2.1.1.7 (contd)

Reference	Subjects	Duration (years)	Odds ratio	95% CI	Comments
	Women	<20	1.2	0.9–1.7	
		20–39	5.3	4.2–6.8	
		≥40	7.0	5.1–9.5	
	< 50 years‡				‡p for interaction gender/smoking = 1.0
	Men	<20	2.1	1.2–3.8	
		20–39	16.4	9.9–27.2	
	Women	<20	2.2	1.0–4.7	Also adjusted for average amount of smoking and time since cessation
		20–39	14.4	7.2–28.6	[There is probably an error in the original table; analysis by duration says adjusted for duration instead average amount of smoking.]
	Ever-smoker				
	Men	<20	1.0		
		20–39	3.2	2.5–4.0	
		≥40	4.1	3.1–5.6	
	Women	<20	1.0		
		20–39	2.7	1.7–4.1	
		≥40	3.3	1.9–5.8	
Simonato *et al.* (2000)	Men and women	*Venice*			Reference level, never-smoker and former smoker who quit more than 20 years ago; adjusted for age, sex, education, occupation and heating
		<20	4.4	0.3–67.4	
		20–40	6.0	1.7–21.9	
		≥40	16.9	4.5–63.3	
		Mestre			
		<20	0.6	0.1–6.0	
		20–40	7.6	3.5–16.4	
		≥40	9.3	4.4–19.7	

Table 2.1.1.7 (contd)

Reference	Subjects	Duration (years)	Odds ratio	95% CI	Comments
Boffetta *et al.* (2001)	Women				Reference level < 10 years of smoking; adjusted for centre, age, average number of cigarettes per day
	< 35 years	10–19	1.1	0.1–11	
		≥ 20	2.8	0.1–95	
	35–39 years	10–19	1.8	0.3–12	
		≥ 20	40.0	2.8–584	
	≥ 40 years	10–19	2.3	0.4–13	
		≥ 20	7.1	1.2–42	
Kubik *et al.* (2001)	Women	1–10	3.1	1.2–6.2	Reference level, never-smoker; adjusted for age, residence and education
		11–20	2.2	1.2–4.3	
		21–30	4.0	2.4–6.6	
		31–40	11.7	7.4–18.5	
		> 40	17.6	10.7–28.7	
Simonato *et al.* (2001)	Men	0–19	1.0	–	Adjusted for age, education, average number of cigarettes/day and centre
		20–29	5.0	4.3–5.8	
		30–39	11.0	9.6–12.7	
		≥ 40	21.6	18.6–24.9	
	Women	0–19	1.0	–	
		20–29	4.3	1.3–5.5	
		30–39	7.2	5.6–9.1	
		≥ 40	8.6	6.6–11.3	
Stellman *et al.* (2001)	Men				Reference level, nonsmoker; adjusted for age, education and hospital or residence for community controls
	USA (HC)	≤ 40	25.2	11.9–61.0	
		> 40	57.8	27.4–131.9	
	Japan (HC)	≤ 40	2.2	1.1–5.2	
		> 40	7.4	2.9–19.4	
	Japan (PC)	≤ 40	4.8	2.6–8.9	
		> 40	8.3	4.5–15.4	

Table 2.1.1.7 (contd)

Reference	Subjects	Duration (years)	Odds ratio		95% CI	Comments
Bhurgri et al. (2002)	Men and women	1–19	8.4 (3.8–18.5)	1.0†	Reference	Adjusted for age, sex and hospital †Also adjusted for average daily amount of smoking; study included all types of smoking.
		20–29	10.1 (5.0–20.1)	1.3	0.5–3.4	
		30–39	20.7 (11.5–37.2)	2.4	0.9–5.9	
		≥ 40	53.2 (29.4–96.2)	6.0	2.4–14.8	
Petrauskaite et al. (2002)	Men	< 41	13.0		4.5–37.7	Reference level not clear; adjusted for age and year of death
		≥ 41	22.2		7.7–63.6	
Rachtan (2002)	Women	< 26	3.0		1.8–5.0	Reference level, never- smoker; adjusted for age
		26–39	15.6		9.1–26.8	
		≥ 40	30.0		14.2–63.4	
Stellman et al. (2002)	Men White	< 40	15.8		11.5–21.8	Reference level, nonsmoker
		≥ 40	25.1		18.6–33.8	
	Black	< 40	16.1		6.7–45.7	
		≥40	20.1		8.7–54.7	
	Women White	< 40	13.4		10.2–17.6	
		≥ 40	24.7		19.1–32.0	
	Black	< 40	14.6		6.9–30.9	
		≥40	20.7		9.6–44.7	

CI, confidence interval; NCC, non-cancer control; CC, cancer control; HC, hospital control; PC, population control

$*p < 0.05$

Table 2.1.1.8. Case–control studies on tobacco smoking and lung cancer: smoking cessation

Reference	Subjects	Years since quitting	Odds ratio	95% CI	Comments
Gao et al. (1988)	Men	Current smoker	3.9	2.9–5.4	Reference level, lifelong nonsmoker; adjusted for age and education
		1–4	6.9	4.4–10.8	
		5–9	3.1	1.7–5.9	
		≥10	1.1	0.5–2.2	
	Women	Current smoker	2.9	2.2–3.8	
		1–4	7.2	3.4–15.1	
		5–9	3.9	1.5–9.9	
		≥10	2.2	1.0–4.6	
Higgins & Wynder (1988)	Men	1–4	17.4	12.5–24.1	Reference level, nonsmoker; odds ratios not adjusted
		5–9	7.2	5.1–10.3	
		10–19	6.1	4.5–8.4	
		20–29	3.7	2.5–5.5	
		≥30	1.9	1.1–3.1	
	Women	1–4	9.3	6.4–13.4	
		5–9	4.8	3.2–7.1	
		10–19	2.2	1.4–3.3	
		20–29	1.6	0.9–2.9	
		≥30	2.6	1.2–5.3	

Benhamou et al. (1989), Men

Years since quitting	Cigarettes/day				95% CI	Comments
	1–9[†]	10–19	≥20[†]	any[‡]		
Current smoker	1.0	2.4*	5.2*	1.0		[†]Adjusted for age and duration
1–4	3.3*	3.8*	5.8*	1.5	1.1–1.9[§]	[‡]Adjusted for duration and daily consumption of cigarettes
5–9	0.5	1.5	3.4*	0.7	0.5–1.0[§]	[§]95% CI for any number of cigarettes/day
10–19	0.9	1.0	1.9*	0.5	0.3–0.8[§]	
≥20	0.5	2.0	1.3	0.4	0.2–0.8[§]	

Table 2.1.1.8 (contd)

Reference	Subjects	Years since quitting	Odds ratio		95% CI	Comments
Jedrychowski et al. (1990)	Men	> 5–10	0.7		0.4–1.0	Reference level, never-smoker; adjusted for age
		> 10	0.4		0.3–0.6	
	Women	> 5	0.5		0.2–1.5	
Becher et al. (1991)	Men and women	0–1	1.0			Risks for both sexes and both groups of controls combined; adjusted for lifetime-cumulative cigarette consumption
		2–4	0.9		0.4–2.2	
		5–9	0.7		0.3–1.3	
		≥ 10	0.2		0.1–0.5	†Results based on 6 cases and 39 controls
		Nonsmoking interval (years)				
		0–< 1	1.0			
		1–< 3	0.8		0.4–1.9	
		≥ 3	0.2†		0.1–0.5	
Jöckel et al. (1992)	Men	0–5	1.0			Hospital controls and population controls combined
		> 5–10	0.9		0.4–1.8	
		> 10	0.4		0.2–0.7	
	Women	0–5	1.0			
		> 5	0.2		0.03–1.1	
Morabia & Wynder (1992)	Men and women		CC	NCC		Only bronchioloalveolar carcinoma; Reference level, never-smoker; adjusted for age and sex
		Current smoker	3.7*	2.3		
		1–9	2.9*	3.8*		
		10–19	2.6*	2.1		
		20–52	1.5	1.5		
Gao et al. (1993)	Men	1–4	5.1		2.3–11.4	Reference level, nonsmoker; adjusted for age
		5–9	3.5		1.1–8.0	
		10–14	3.8		1.5–9.5	

Table 2.1.1.8 (contd)

Reference	Subjects	Years since quitting	Odds ratio	95% CI	Comments
De Stefani et al. (1994)	Men	*Manufactured*			Adjusted for age, residence, education and amount of smoking
		Current smoker	1.0		
		1–4	0.5	0.2–1.4	
		5–9	0.7	0.2–1.9	
		≥10	0.5	0.2–1.5	
		Hand-rolled			
		Current smoker	1.0		
		1–4	0.9	0.5–1.4	
		5–9	0.5	0.3–1.0	
		≥10	0.2	0.1–0.3	
Suzuki et al. (1994)	Men and women	Current smoker	1.0		Adjusted for age, sex, race and pack–years; excluding nonsmokers
		1–5	0.5	0.2–1.4	
		5–10	0.5	0.2–1.5	
		>10	0.2	0.1–0.6	
De Stefani et al. (1996a)	Men	Current smoker	10.9	6.9–17.1	Reference level, never-smoker; adjusted for age, residence, urban/rural status and education
		1–4	9.0	5.2–15.9	
		5–9	6.2	3.2–12.2	
		≥10	2.8	1.4–5.7	
Barbone et al. (1997)	Men	Current smoker	13.8	8.7–21.9	Reference level, nonsmoker; adjusted for age
		1–4	13.9	6.8–28.5	
		5–14	9.1	5.3–15.5	
		15–24	6.8	3.6–12.8	
		>25	2.1	1.0–4.3	
Muscat et al. (1997)	Men	1–5	12.4	5.2–29.6	Only large-cell carcinoma Adjusted for age and education p for trend < 0.01
		6–10	12.9	5.3–31.1	
		>10	6.1	2.8–13.6	
		Never-smoker	1.0		

Table 2.1.1.8 (contd)

Reference	Subjects	Years since quitting	Odds ratio	95% CI	Comments
	Women	1–5	15.9	7.1–35.4	
		6–10	11.5	5.0–26.7	
		>10	4.2	3.0–9.0	
		Never-smoker	1.0		
Pohlabeln et al. (1997)	Men	Current smoker	1.0		Adjusted for age, region of residence and pack–years
		<1	20.3	9.8–42.3	
		1	6.9	3.3–14.2	
		2–5	1.6	1.0–2.3	
		6–10	1.0	0.6–1.4	
		11–20	0.5	0.4–0.8	
		>20	0.2	0.2–0.4	
		Never/occasional smoker	0.2	0.1–0.4	
Khuder et al. (1998)	Men	Current smoker	10.4	6.6–16.4	Reference level, nonsmoker; unadjusted odds ratios
		1–4	9.6	5.8–15.9	
		5–14	6.4	3.8–10.7	
		≥15	4.0	2.4–6.6	
Matos et al. (1998)	Men	1–5	1.4	0.8–2.6	Reference level, current smoker; adjusted for the design variables, age and hospital
		6–10	0.9	0.4–1.6	
		≥11	0.3	0.2–0.6	
		Nonsmoker	0.1	0.1–0.2	
Agudo et al. (2000)	Women	Current smoker	8.9	7.5–10.6	Adjusted for age and centre; never-smoker includes smokers who had smoked less than 400 cigarettes in their lifetime.
		<15	3.8	2.9–5.0	
		15–19	1.7	1.2–2.4	
		20–29	0.6	0.4–1.2	
		≥30	1.1	0.7–1.8	
		Never-smoker	1.0		

Table 2.1.1.8 (contd)

Reference	Subjects	Years since quitting	Odds ratio	95% CI	Comments
Kreuzer *et al.* (2000)	Men	Current smoker	1.0		Adjusted for age, centre and average amount of smoking
		2–9	0.7	0.6–0.8	
		10–19	0.2	0.2–0.3	
		≥ 20	0.1	0.1–0.1	
	Women	Current smoker	1.0		
		2–9	0.5	0.3–0.7	
		10–19	0.2	0.1–0.3	
		≥ 20	0.2	0.1–0.3	
Osann *et al.* (2000)	Women	Current smoker	14.8	4.3–51.4	Small-cell carcinoma only
		< 12	8.6	2.1–34.9	Adjusted for age, education and pack–years
		> 12	1.0		
Mao *et al.* (2001)	Men	≤ 10	14.5	10.2–20.6	Reference level, never-smoker; adjusted for age group, province, years of exposure to passive smoking, total consumption of vegetables, vegetable juices and meat
		11–19	7.3	5.0–10.5	
		20–28	3.5	2.4–5.2	
		≥ 29	1.5	1.0–2.4	
	Women	≤ 10	11.8	9.0–15.4	
		11–19	3.3	2.4–4.6	
		20–28	1.6	1.0–2.3	
		≥ 29	1.5	1.0–2.3	
Simonato *et al.* (2001)	Men	Current smoker	1.0		Adjusted for age, education and centre
		2–9	0.66	0.59–0.73	
		10–19	0.27	0.24–0.31	
		20–29	0.17	0.14–0.20	
		≥ 30	0.08	0.06–0.10	
		Nonsmoker	0.04	0.03–0.05	

Table 2.1.1.8 (contd)

Reference	Subjects		Years since quitting	Odds ratio	95% CI	Comments
	Women		Current smoker	1.00		
			2–9	0.41	0.31–0.55	
			10–19	0.19	0.14–0.27	
			20–29	0.08	0.05–0.14	
			≥ 30	0.13	0.08–0.21	
			Nonsmoker	0.11	0.10–0.14	
Stellman et al. (2001)	Men	USA (HC)	Current smoker	1.0		Adjusted for age, education and hospital or residence for community controls
			1–4	0.5	0.3–1.0	
			5–9	0.5	0.2–0.9	
			10–15	0.4	0.2–0.8	
			≥ 16	0.1	0.1–0.2	p for trend < 0.001
		Japan (HC)	Current smoker	1.0		
			1–4	0.9	0.3–2.9	
			5–9	0.8	0.3–1.8	
			10–15	0.2	0.1–0.5	
			≥ 16	0.2	0.1–0.4	
		Japan (PC)	Current smoker	1.0		
			1–4	0.9	0.5–1.7	
			5–9	0.8	0.5–1.4	
			10–15	0.2	0.1–0.4	
			≥ 16	0.2	0.1–0.3	

Table 2.1.1.8 (contd)

Reference	Subjects	Years since quitting	Odds ratio	95% CI	Comments
Bhurgri et al. (2002)	Men and women	Current smoker	1.0		Adjusted for age, sex and hospital
		2–4	1.7	0.9–3.4	
		5–9	0.9	0.4–1.8	
		10–14	0.3	0.1–0.7	
		15–19	0.2	0.1–0.5	
		≥ 20	0.2	0.1–0.3	
		Never-smoker	0.03	0.02–0.05	
Petrauskaite et al. (2002)	Men	Current smoker or	1.0		Adjusted for age and year of death
		< 2 years			
		2–4	1.2	0.6–2.0	
		5–9	0.6	0.3–1.3	
		10–19	0.4	0.2–0.9	
		≥ 20	0.4	0.2–0.9	
Stellman et al. (2002)	Men White	1–10	14.5	10.9–19.5	Reference level, nonsmoker
		11–20	7.8	5.8–10.6	
		≥ 21	3.7	2.8–5.1	
	Black	1–10	13.7	5.9–37.5	
		11–20	4.2	1.6–12.7	
		≥ 21	3.9	1.4–12.3	
	Women White	1–5	10.1	7.9–13.0	
		6–15	6.7	4.8–9.4	
		≥ 16	3.4	2.6–4.4	
	Black	1–5	11.0	5.0–24.2	
		6–15	6.5	2.0–20.7	
		≥ 16	7.2	2.9–17.5	

CI, confidence interval; HC, hospital controls; PC, population controls; CC, cancer controls; NCC, non-cancer controls
*$p < 0.05$

Table 2.1.1.9. Case–control studies on tobacco smoking and lung cancer: type of cigarettes

Reference	Subjects	Use of filter-tip	OR	95% CI	Comments
Pathak et al. (1986)	Men Non-Hispanic whites	Filter-tip only	0.8		Adjusted for age, sex and ethnic variables, ethnicity, amount and duration of smoking and age–duration interaction
		67–99% filter-tip	0.7		
		34–66% filter-tip	0.6		
		1–33% filter-tip	0.8		
		Untipped only	1.0		
	Hispanic	Filter-tip only	0.04*		
		67–99% filter-tip	0.3*		
		34–66% filter-tip	0.4		
		1–33% filter-tip	0.6		
		Untipped only	1.0		
Benhamou et al. (1987)	Women	≤ 50% untipped[†]	1		[†]Includes nonsmokers; adjusted for cigarettes/day, duration of smoking and inhalation
		> 50% untipped	1.3	0.3–6.0	
		100% untipped	3.6	0.7–19.2	
Benhamou et al. (1989)	Men	Filter-tipped	1.0		Only current smokers; adjustment not stated
		Mixed	1.8	1.3–2.5	
		Untipped	1.9	1.4–2.5	
Jöckel et al. (1992)	Men	Filter-tipped	1		Hospital and population controls combined
		Untipped (last 20 years)	2.4	1.2–4.8	
Pezzotto et al. (1993)	Men	Ever filter-tipped	1.0		Adjusted for age, hospital and years of cigarette smoking
		Untipped or both	3.5	$p < 0.0001$	
Sobue et al. (1994)	Men, current smokers	All histological types	1.5	0.9–2.6	Untipped versus filter-tipped cigarettes for each type; adjusted for duration, fraction smoked per cigarette, cigarettes/day, cigarette type, inhalation
		SCC	2.2	1.2–4.0	
		AC	1.2	0.6–2.5	
		Small-cell carcinoma	0.6	0.2–2.0	
		Large-cell carcinoma	1.3	0.4–4.5	
De Stefani et al. (1996a)	Men	Never-smoker	1.0		Adjusted for age, residence, urban/rural status and education
		Filter-tipped	7.3	4.6–11.8	
		Plain	10.1	6.4–15.6	
De Stefani et al. (1996b)	Men and women	Nonsmoker	1.0		Adjusted for age, sex, residence (urban/rural), education, family history of cancer and BMI
		Filter-tipped	7.4	4.2–13.2	
		Plain	10.1	5.7–17.8	

Table 2.1.1.9 (contd)

Reference	Subjects	Use of filter-tip	OR	95% CI	Comments
Kabat (1996)	Men[†]	**Kreyberg I**			[†]Current smokers; reference
		Switchers (1–9 years)	0.8	0.6–1.2	category untipped only;
		Switchers (≥ 10 years)	0.7	0.5–0.9	adjusted for cigarettes/day,
		Filter-tip only	0.7	0.4–1.3	age, inhalation and years of
		Kreyberg II			education
		Switchers (1–9 years)	1.0	0.6–1.5	[‡]Reference category;
		Switchers (≥ 10 years)	0.8	0.5–1.2	untipped and switchers
		Filter-tip only	0.9	0.4–1.5	1–9 years
	Women[†]	**Kreyberg I**			
		Switchers (1–9 years)	1.0	0.5–2.0	
		Switchers (≥ 10 years)	0.7	0.4–1.4	
		Filter-tip only	0.6	0.3–1.4	
		Kreyberg II			
		Switchers (≥ 10 years)[‡]	1.0	0.8–1.3	
		Filter-tip only	1.0	0.6–1.5	
Stellman et al. (1997a,b)	Men[†]	**SCC**			[†]Current smokers
		Switched	0.9	0.7–1.0	Reference level, lifetime
		Lifetime filter-tip	0.8	0.5–1.2	smoker of untipped
		AC		0.8–1.3	cigarettes; adjusted for age,
		Switched	1.0	0.7–1.5	education and number of
		Lifetime filter-tip	1.0		cigarettes/day
	Women[†]	**SCC**			
		Switched	0.6	0.3–0.99	
		Lifetime filter-tip	0.4	0.2–0.8	
		AC			
		Switched	1.2	0.7–2.0	
		Lifetime filter-tip	0.9	0.5–1.7	
Wakai et al. (1997)	Men[†]	With filter-tip	1.0		[†]Current smokers; adjusted
		Without filter-tip	1.0	0.3–3.2	for age, age at start, cigarettes/day, fraction smoked/cigarette, cigarette type and smoke inhalation
Khuder et al. (1998)	Men	Filter-tip yes	5.3	3.3–8.4	Reference level, nonsmoker
		Filter-tip no	11.4	7.3–18.0	
Armadans-Gil et al. (1999)	Men	Lifetime filter-tip			Adjusted for age and
		Never	1.0		cumulative cigarette
		Mixed	1.0	0.6–1.6	consumption
		Always	0.7	0.4–1.2	
Agudo et al. (2000)	Women	Never-smoker	1.0		Adjusted for age and centre;
		Only filter-tip	3.4	2.9–4.1	never-smoker included
		Untipped + mixed	7.5	6.0–9.3	smokers who had smoked < 400 cigarettes in their lifetime.

Table 2.1.1.9 (contd)

Reference	Subjects	Use of filter-tip	OR	95% CI	Comments
Simonato *et al.* (2001)	Men	Only filter-tip	1.0		Adjusted for age, education and centre
		Mixed	1.7	1.5–2.0	
		Only untipped	1.1	0.9–1.3	
	Women	Only filter-tip	1.0		
		Mixed	2.4	1.8–3.1	
		Only untipped	2.0	1.3–3.1	
Rachtan (2002)	Women	Nonsmoker	1.0		Adjusted for age
		Filter-tip	9.3	6.2–14.0	
		Untipped	9.8	4.7–20.5	

OR, odds ratio; H, hospital; P, population; SCC, squamous-cell carcinoma; AC, adenocarcinoma; BMI, body mass index; Kreyberg I, squamous-cell carcinoma, large-cell, oat-cell and small-cell carcinoma; Kreyberg II, adenocarcinoma, bronchiolar and alveolar-cell carcinoma

*$p < 0.05$

Table 2.1.1.10. Case–control studies on tobacco smoking and lung cancer: tar levels in cigarettes

Reference	Subjects	Histology/definition of smokers	Odds ratio				Comments
Wilcox et al. (1988)	Men	All histologies	Av. mg tar/cigarette (1973–80)				Adjusted for intensity and duration of smoking
			≤ 14	14.1–17.5	17.6–21.0	21.1–28.0	
			0.61	1.04	1.21	1.0	
Kaufman et al. (1989)	Men and women	All histologies	Av. mg tar/cigarette		< 22	22–28	≥ 29	Adjusted for age, sex, ethnicity, religion, education and interview
			All cigarettes		1	1.9	3.1*	
			Cigarettes smoked at least 10 years before admission		1	3.0*	4.0*	
Zang & Wynder (1992)	Men	*Kreyberg I*	Kg tar	1–2	3–5	6–8	≥ 9	Kg tar: cumulative measure for lifetime exposure
		Current smoker		17.3	29.7	38.7	60.2	Reference level, never-smoker; adjusted for age; no CI provided
		Former smoker		7.3	19.9	20.0	38.3	
		Kreyberg II						
		Current smoker		6.5	6.5	10.1	12.8	
		Former smoker		2.6	4.4	6.2	7.3	
	Women	*Kreyberg I*						
		Current smoker		23.1	47.6	58.9	102.9	
		Former smoker		7.9	15.3	33.2	22.9	
		Kreyberg II						
		Current smoker		8.3	15.1	11.6	16.3	
		Former smoker		3.2	4.8	8.5	6.8	

Table 2.1.1.10 (contd)

Reference	Subjects	Histology/defini-tion of smokers	Odds ratio Kg tar				Comments
			0	1–4	5–8	≥ 9	
Harris et al. (1993)	Men	Kreyberg I					All linear trends statistically significant at $p < 0.01$; adjustment not clear
		White					
		Current smoker	1.0	11.7*	24.5*	54.3*	
		Ever-smoker	1.0	6.8*	20.2*	42.6*	
		Black					
		Current smoker	1.0	12.8*	25.1*	55.4*	
		Ever-smoker	1.0	10.0*	23.6*	47.0*	
		Kreyberg II					
		White					
		Current smoker	1.0	5.7*	8.3*	13.1*	
		Ever-smoker	1.0	3.1*	6.5*	10.1*	
		Black					
		Current smoker	1.0	10.5*	18.6*	24.9*	
		Ever-smoker	1.0	8.3*	15.2*	24.0*	
	Women	Kreyberg I					
		White					
		Current smoker	1.0	13.8*	41.0*	108.7*	
		Ever-smoker	1.0	8.7*	34.9*	75.8*	
		Black					
		Current smoker	1.0	12.4*	72.3*	120.0*	
		Ever-smoker	1.0	11.2*	83.8*	146.7*	
		Kreyberg II					
		White					
		Current smoker	1.0	5.6*	11.4*	24.5*	
		Ever-smoker	1.0	3.9*	9.8*	17.9*	
		Black					
		Current smoker	1.0	3.0*	18.7*	29.1*	
		Ever-smoker	1.0	3.4*	20.8*	29.1*	

Table 2.1.1.10 (contd)

Reference	Subjects	Histology/definition of smokers	Odds ratio	Comments
Benhamou et al. (1994)	Men	Use of high-tar cigarettes (≥30 mg)	% years smoking cig. >30 mg tar: <51% = 2.4*; 51–75% = 3.0*; >75% = 3.0*	Reference level, lifelong smokers of light, imported cigarettes with unknown tar levels; adjusted for age, daily consumption and duration of smoking
Kabat (1996)	Men	White	Quartile tar intake (95% CI): 2 = 1.9 (1.6–2.2); 3 = 2.9 (2.5–3.5); 4 = 4.3 (3.6–5.2)	Reference level, never smoker and first quartile; adjusted for age, education, time period, hospital and smoking status
		Black	2 = 2.3 (1.4–3.7); 3 = 5.0 (2.9–8.5); 4 = 5.7 (3.0–10.9)	
	Women	White	2 = 2.3 (1.8–2.9); 3 = 4.5 (3.5–5.8); 4 = 5.3 (4.1–6.8)	
		Black	2 = 2.1 (1.0–4.2); 3 = 5.1 (2.4–11.5); 4 = 12.8 (4.3–38.7)	
Zang & Wynder (1996)	Men	SCC	Kg tar: 1–2 = 33.1*; 3–5 = 36.8*; 6–8 = 54.3*; ≥9 = 81.5*	Current smokers only; reference level, nonsmoker. All dose–response trends statistically significant. Dose–response for women was statistically significantly higher than for men.
		AC	7.1*; 6.8*; 12.4*; 14.7*	
	Women	SCC	24.5*; 38.5*; 56.2*; 129.3*	
		AC	11.6*; 13.9*; 25.4*; 33.3*	

CI, confidence interval; Kreyberg I, squamous-cell carcinoma, large-cell, oat-cell and small-cell carcinoma; Kreyberg II, adenocarcinoma and alveolar-cell carcinoma; SCC, squamous-cell carcinoma; AC, adenocarcinoma

$*p < 0.05$

Table 2.1.1.11. Case–control studies on tobacco smoking and lung cancer: type of tobacco

Reference	Subjects	Type	Odds ratio	95% CI	Comments
Benhamou et al. (1989)	Men	Light	1.0		Adjusted for age and duration of smoking
		Mixed	2.0	0.9–4.2	
		Dark	2.5	1.3–5.1	
		Manufactured	1.0		[Adjustment variables not stated]
		Mixed	1.2	0.9–1.6	
		Hand-rolled	1.2	0.8–1.7	
De Stefani et al. (1994)	Men	*Manufactured cigarettes*			Adjusted for age, residence, education, pack–years and cessation
		Blond	1.0		
		Black	2.1	1.1–3.9	
		Hand-rolled cigarettes			
		Blond	1.0		
		Black	1.2	0.9–1.7	
Suzuki et al. (1994)	Men and women	Cigarettes only	1.0		Adjusted for age, sex, race and pack–years, excluding nonsmokers; black tobacco smoked in the form of hand-rolled cigarettes
		Black tobacco and cigarettes	2.8	1.0–7.7	
De Stefani et al. (1996a)	Men	Blond	6.1	3.8–9.8	Reference level, never-smoker; adjusted for age, residence, urban/rural status and education
		Mixed	13.6	7.7–23.9	
		Black	10.9	6.8–17.4	
De Stefani et al. (1996b)	Men and women	Blond	4.7	2.6–8.6	Reference level, nonsmoker; adjusted for age, sex, residence, urban/rural, education, family history of cancer and body mass index
		Black	11.2	6.4–19.3	
Matos et al. (1998)	Men	*Only blond*			Reference level, nonsmoker; adjusted for the design variables, age and hospital
		1–14 cig/day	0.6	0.2–2.2	
		15–24 cig/day	8.4	3.7–18.9	
		≥ 25 cig/day	7.7	3.5–16.7	

Table 2.1.1.11 (contd)

Reference	Subjects	Type	Odds ratio	95% CI	Comments
		Duration			
		1–24 years	1.9	0.7–5.0	
		25–39 years	5.7	2.6–12.5	
		≥ 40 years	10.1	4.3–23.8	
		Only black			
		1–14 cig/day	2.7	0.6–11.5	
		15–24 cig/day	6.8	3.9–32.7	
		≥ 25 cig/day	12.9	5.2–45.0	
		Duration			
		1–24 years	1.2	0.2–6.3	
		25–39 years	11.3	3.9–32.7	
		≥ 40 years	15.5	5.2–45.0	
Armadans-Gil et al. (1999)	Men	Blond	1.0		Adjusted for age and cumulative cigarette consumption
		Both	4.9	1.7–13.7	
		Black	5.3	2.1–13.6	
Agudo et al. (2000)	Women	Only blond	3.1	2.5–3.7	Reference level, never-smoker and smokers who had smoked less than 400 cigarettes in their lifetime; adjusted for age and centre
		Dark + mixed	10.4	7.9–13.6	
Simonato et al. (2001)	Men	Only blond	1.0		Adjusted for age, education and centre
		Mixed	2.2	1.7–2.9	
		Only black	1.6	1.1–2.3	
	Women	Only blond	1.0		
		Mixed	3.9	2.6–5.8	
		Only black	4.8	3.1–7.4	

CI, confidence interval

Table 2.1.1.12. Case–control studies on tobacco smoking and lung cancer: degree of inhalation

Reference	Subjects	Inhalation	Odds ratio	95% CI	Comments
Osann (1991)	Women	No	1.0		Adjusted for age
		Yes	9.6	5.0–18.5	
Pezzotto et al. (1993)	Men	Slight or moderate	1.0		Adjusted for age, hospital, duration and intensity of cigarette smoking
		Deep	0.9		
Benhamou et al. (1994)	Men	No	1.0		Adjusted for age and smoking variables
		Moderate	1.2	0.9–1.6	
		Deep	1.5	1.2–1.8	
Sobue et al. (1994)	Men	All histological types	1.2	0.9–1.6	Reference level, no inhalation; adjusted for number of cigarettes/day, duration, fraction smoked per cigarette, filter
		SCC	1.0	0.7–1.6	
		AC	1.4	0.9–2.0	
		SCLC	1.4	0.8–2.6	
		Large-cell carcinoma	1.8	0.7–4.4	
Suzuki et al. (1994)	Men and women	No or slight	1.0		Adjusted for age, sex, race and pack–years, excluding nonsmokers
		Deep	2.6	1.3–5.4	
Rachtan & Sokolowski (1997)	Women	No	4.5	2.2–9.5	Reference level, never-smoker; adjusted for age
		Yes	8.7	4.5–16.7	
Wakai et al. (1997)	Men	*All histological types*			Reference level, no inhalation; adjusted for age, age at starting smoking, number of cigarettes per day, fraction of a cigarette smoked and cigarette type
		Moderate	1.1	0.6–2.0	
		Deep	2.1	1.1–3.8	
		SCC			
		Moderate	1.2	0.6–2.4	
		Deep	1.9	0.9–4.3	
		AC			
		Moderate	1.3	0.6–2.8	
		Deep	3.0	1.3–7.0	

Table 2.1.1.12 (contd)

Reference	Subjects	Inhalation	Odds ratio	95% CI	Comments
Khuder et al. (1998)	Men	No	1.4	0.8–2.4	Reference level, nonsmoker; unadjusted odds ratios
		Yes	15.4	9.8–24.0	
Agudo et al. (2000)	Women	Never inhaled	2.5	2.0–3.1	Reference level, never-smoker and smokers who had smoked less than 400 cigarettes during their lifetime; adjusted for age and center
		Ever inhaled	6.9	5.9–8.2	
Rachtan (2002)	Women	No	5.8	3.5–9.6	Reference level, nonsmoker; adjusted for age
		Yes	12.4	7.9–19.2	

CI, confidence interval; SCC, squamous-cell carcinoma; AC, adenocarcinoma; SCLC, small-cell carcinoma

Table 2.1.1.13. Case–control studies on tobacco smoking and lung cancer: histology

Reference	Subjects	Histology	Odds ratio (95% CI)				Comments
Damber & Larsson (1986)	Men		*Duration (years)*				Smoking includes any tobacco. Adjustment variables not stated.
			<30	31–40	41–50	≥51	
		SCC	4.4*	8.4*	13.8*	16.7*	
		SCLC	3.6	10.5*	19.6*	25.1*	
		AC, alveolar-cell carcinoma, bronchiolar carcinoma	1.8	1.2	3.4*	2.5	
Gao et al. (1988)	Men		*Duration (years)*				Reference level, lifelong nonsmoker; adjusted for age and education. Confidence interval or statistical significance not provided
			1–29	30–39	≥40		
		SCC					
		1–19 cig/day	1.1	5.2	7.0		
		20–29 cig/day	4.0	12.6	13.6		
		≥30 cig/day	6.1	22.1	25.0		
		AC					
		1–19 cig/day	0.8	1.6	1.9		
		20–29 cig/day	0.9	2.4	2.4		
		≥30 cig/day	0.7	4.2	5.5		
	Women		*Duration (years)*				
			1–29	≥30			
		SCC					
		1–19 cig/day	1.9	2.7			
		20–29 cig/day	4.7	7.0			
		≥30 cig/day	16.2	42.4			
		AC					
		1–19 cig/day	0.7	1.2			
		20–29 cig/day	1.3	1.4			
		≥30 cig/day	7.0	3.5			
Schoenberg et al. (1989)	Women		Cigarettes/day				All odds ratios statistically significant at 5% level. Adjusted for age, race and type of respondent
			< 20			≥ 20	
			Duration (years)				
			< 35	≥ 35			
		SCC	2.7	7.7	12.0	21.4	
		SCLC	19.0	40.6	62.5	140.0	
		AC	2.0	3.4	3.9	6.8	
Svensson et al. (1989)	Women		*Cigarettes/day*				Reference level, never-smoker; adjusted for age
			1–10	11–20	≥21		
		SCC	9.7*	36.2*	59.0*		
		SCLC	33.7*	72.1*	215.8*		
		AC	2.2	5.4*	19.7*		

Table 2.1.1.13 (contd)

Reference	Subjects	Histology	Odds ratio (95% CI)			Comments
Xu et al. (1989)	Men		*Duration (years)*			Reference level, nonsmoker; adjusted for age and education
			1–29	*30–39*	*≥40*	
		SCC/SCLC				
		1–19 cig/day	2.3*	2.9*	5.0*	
		20–29 cig/day	2.6*	3.9*	10.4*	
		≥30 cig/day	7.7*	8.3*	31.2*	
		AC				
		1–19 cig/day	1.4	2.2*	2.6*	
		20–29 cig/day	0.7	1.5	3.6*	
		≥30 cig/day	5.4*	3.2*	11.8*	
	Women	**SCC/SCLC**				
		1–19 cig/day	1.8*	4.2*	5.3*	
		≥20 cig/day	2.5	2.4	19.9*	
		AC				
		1–19 cig/day	0.9	2.2*	1.9*	
		≥20 cig/day	–	3.7*	6.8*	
Wu-Williams et al. (1990)	Women		*Duration (years)*			Reference not stated [probably nonsmokers]
			1–29	*30–39*	*≥40*	†Only 9% of the cases and 4% of the controls smoked more than 20 cigarettes per day.
		SCC/SCLC				
		1–19 cig/day	2.0*	3.9*	4.7*	
		≥20 cig/day†	2.0	3.8*	12.0*	
		AC				
		1–19 cig/day	0.8	1.7*	2.0*	
		≥20 cig/day†	0.8	3.8*	2.8*	
Morabia & Wynder (1991)	Men†		*Cigarettes/day*			Adjusted for age, race and state
			1–19	*20–29*	*≥30*	†Current smokers
		SCC	1.0	1.6	2.3*	
		SCLC	1.0	6.0*	5.5*	
		Large-cell	1.0	1.1	1.0	
		AC	1.0	1.7	1.9*	
	Women†	SCC	1.0	1.5	2.7*	
		SCLC	1.0	1.8	3.2*	
		Large-cell	1.0	1.9	1.4	
		AC	1.0	1.3	1.5	

Table 2.1.1.13 (contd)

Reference	Subjects	Histology	Odds ratio (95% CI)				Comments
Osann (1991)	Women		*Pack/day*				Reference level, never-smoker (7 cases and 58 controls for Kreyberg I); adjusted for age
			< 1		*≥ 1*		
		Kreyberg I	12.1 (1.5–96.3)		71.2 (8.3–609)		
		Kreyberg II	0.9 (0.3–2.7)		3.8 (1.6–8.8)		
			Duration (years)				
			≤ 20		*> 20*		
		Kreyberg I	4.9 (0.5–44.6)		101.1 (8.3–1230)		
		Kreyberg II	0.7 (0.2–1.9)		4.1 (1.8–9.4)		
			Inhalation				
			No		*Yes*		
		Kreyberg I	13.3 (1.7–106)		52.0 (6.6–408)		
		Kreyberg II	0.6 (0.2–1.9)		3.5 (1.5–8.0)		
Jedrychowski et al. (1992)	Men		*Cigarettes/day*				Adjusted for age, education and occupation
			1–19	*20–29*	*≥ 30*		
		SCC	7.5*	13.5*	21.4*		
		SCLC	7.8*	11.6*	16.8*		
		AC	2.2	4.4*	5.1*		
			Duration (years)				[Adjustments not clear]
			1–19	*20–39*	*≥ 40*		
		SCC	5.8*	12.4*	13.0*		
		SCLC	5.5*	11.4*	11.8*		
		AC	1.1	3.5*	4.4*		
Zang & Wynder (1992)	Men		*Cigarettes/day*				Odds ratios adjusted for age; no CI provided
			1–10	*11–20*	*21–40*	*≥ 41*	
		Kreyberg I					
		Current smoker	14.4	22.3	41.4	74.0	
		Former smoker	4.1	9.0	16.6	23.5	
		Kreyberg II					
		Current smoker	3.9	6.0	10.3	15.8	
		Former smoker	1.0	3.5	5.6	4.6	
	Women	**Kreyberg I**					
		Current smoker	7.5	33.6	76.0	153.9	
		Former smoker	1.2	13.8	14.2	12.4	
		Kreyberg II					
		Current smoker	3.6	9.3	20.5	30.5	
		Former smoker	2.2	5.0	5.4	1.8	

Table 2.1.1.13 (contd)

Reference	Subjects	Histology	Odds ratio (95% CI)			Comments
Ger et al. (1993)	Men and women		*Cigarettes/day*			Matched odds ratios (see Table 2.1.1.4)
			1–10	*11–20*	*≥21*	†Based on 19 cases/6 hospital and 7 neighbourhood controls nonsmokers
		AC (H)	0.8	1.04	0.7	
		AC (N)	0.8	1.7	1.05	
		SCC + small-cell (H)	1.8	3.6*	20.9*·†	
		SCC + small-cell (N)	2.3	2.9	19.8*·†	
			Duration (years)			
			1–30	*≥31*		
		AC (H)	1.4	0.6		
		AC (N)	1.4	1.06		
		SCC + small-cell (H)	1.9	6.0*		
		SCC + small-cell (N)	1.3	6.8*		
Osann et al. (1993)	Men		*Pack/day*			Adjusted for age and race
			<2		*≥2*	
		SCC	35.3 (17.0–73.3)		76.0 (36.8–157)	
		AC	16.5 (9.3–29.3)		37.5 (21.3–66.0)	
		SCLC	27.6 (9.8–77.4)		95.3 (34.7–262)	
	Women	SCC	24.0 (12.7–45.5)		72.3 (36.8–142)	
		AC	8.8 (6.1–12.8)		24.2 (15.8–37.2)	
		SCLC	76.7 (27.5–21.5)		316.1 (111–900)	
Pezzotto et al. (1993)	Men		*Cigarettes/day*			All odds ratios adjusted for age and hospital
			<21	*21–40*	*>40*	Cigarettes/day: also adjusted for years of cigarette smoking
		SCC	1.0	9.7*	15.4*	Duration: also adjusted for intensity of smoking
		AC	1.0	11.6*	11.6*	Years since cessation: reference level, current smoker; also adjusted for intensity of smoking
		SCLC	1.0	14.9*	54.2*	
			Duration (years)			
			<31	*31–40*	*>40*	
		SCC	1.0	9.7*	11.2*	
		AC	1.0	3.5*	4.7*	
		SCLC	1.0	1.2	3.5	
			Years since cessation			
			1–10	*>10*		
		SCC	0.8	0.05*		
		AC	0.2*	0.08*		
		SCLC	0.2*	0.007*		

Table 2.1.1.13 (contd)

Reference	Subjects	Histology	Odds ratio (95% CI)		Comments
			Filter		Filter: also adjusted for intensity and duration of smoking
			Yes	No or yes/no	
		SCC	1.0	4.9*	
		AC	1.0	2.6*	
		SCLC	1.0	4.0*	

Risch et al. (1993)

Subjects	Histology	Ever versus never	Current smokers at 40 pack-years versus non-smoker†	Comments
Men	AC	8.00*	5.44*	†Both cumulative cigarette consumption and duration since cessation were modelled as continuous variables and were included simultaneously in the models.
	SCC	18.00*	15.5*	
	SCLC/large-cell	6.33*	14.9*	
	Giant-cell carcinoma	6.00*	11.7*	
Women	AC	3.45*	8.75*	
	SCC	25.5*	101.0*	
	SCLC/large-cell	4.8*	87.3*	
	Giant-cell carcinoma	6.50*	18.0*	

De Stefani et al. (1994)

Subjects	Histology	Mixed cigarettes	Hand-rolled Life-time	Hand-rolled Ever	Comments
Men, smokers	AC	3.3	1.8	2.3*	Reference level, manufactured cigarettes; adjusted for age, residence, pack–years, cessation and type (black/blond); mixed: manufactured or hand-rolled.
	SCC	1.6	0.9	1.2	
	SCLC	5.3	4.1*	4.5*	
	Large-cell carcinoma	1.4*	0.6	0.8	

Sobue et al. (1994)

Subjects	Histology	Cigarettes/day 1–19	20–29	≥30	Comments
Men	AC	1.0	1.2	1.2	Adjusted for duration, fraction smoked per cigarette, filter-tip and inhalation
	SCC	1.0	1.5	1.9*	
	SCLC	1.0	0.8	2.3*	
	Large-cell carcinoma	1.0	2.1	2.6	

Histology	Duration (years) 1–29	30–39	40–49	≥50
AC	1.0	1.1	2.0*	2.1*
SCC	1.0	2.1*	4.3*	8.0*
SCLC	1.0	2.4	4.3*	7.6*
Large-cell carcinoma	1.0	1.3	2.1	1.6

Table 2.1.1.13 (contd)

Reference	Subjects	Histology	Odds ratio (95% CI)					Comments
Shimizu et al. (1994)	Men		*Cigarettes/day*	*1–20*	*≥21*			Reference level, nonsmoker; adjusted for age and education
		AC		1.1	2.1			
		Central SCC		5.0*	18.6*			
		Peripheral SCC		8.2*	15.5*			
			Duration (years)	*1–40*	*≥41*			
		AC		1.1	2.2			
		Central SCC		5.1*	16.5*			
		Peripheral SCC		6.0*	20.7*			
Kabat (1996)	Men†		*Cigarettes/day*	*1–10*	*11–20*	*21–30*	*31–40*	*≥41*	†Only current smokers; Reference category, never-smoker; [Adjustments not stated]
		Kreyberg I		13.3*	15.8*	29.6*	37.7*	64.1*	
		Kreyberg II		2.4*	8.4*	15.4*	11.1*	18.4*	
	Women†	Kreyberg I		6.6*	18.2*	26.5*	95.2*	88.7*	
		Kreyberg II		3.1*	4.5*	9.4*	13.4*	20.7*	
Xu et al. (1996)	Men		*Duration (years)*	*1–29*	*30–39*	*≥40*		Adjusted for age and education
		SCC						
		1–19 cig/day		2.3*	2.9*	5.0*		
		20–29 cig/day		2.6*	3.9*	10.4*		
		≥30 cig/day		7.7*	8.3*	31.2*		
		AC						
		1–19 cig/day		1.4	2.2*	2.6*		
		20–29 cig/day		0.7	1.5	3.6*		
		≥30 cig/day		5.4*	3.2*	11.8*		
	Women	**SCC**						
		1–19 cig/day		1.8*	4.2*	5.3*		
		≥20 cig/day		2.5	2.4	19.9*		
		AC						
		1–19 cig/day		0.9	2.2*	1.9*		
		≥20 cig/day		–	3.7*	6.8*		
Yu & Zhao (1996)	Men and women	AC	1.0 (0.9–1.2)					Meta-analysis of 15 studies
		SCC	4.8 (4.0–5.7)					
	Women	AC	1.1 (0.8–1.4)					Meta-analysis of 12 studies
		SCC	7.4 (4.2–10.7)					

Table 2.1.1.13 (contd)

Reference	Subjects	Histology	Odds ratio (95% CI)					Comments
Zang & Wynder (1996)	Men		*Pack–years*	*1–19*	*20–39*	*40–49*	*≥50*	Only current smokers; reference level, nonsmoker; odds ratios adjusted for age
		SCC		6.5*	24.1*	48.9*	82.1*	
		AC		2.4*	5.6*	11.6*	13.8*	
	Women	SCC		11.9*	26.4*	48.8*	95.2*	
		AC		6.8*	11.2*	21.4*	32.7*	
	Men		*Most recent no. of cigarettes smoked/day*	*1–10*	*11–20*	*21–40*	*≥41*	The dose-response relationships for women were statistically significantly higher than those for men.
		SCC		14.1*	16.0*	38.9*	66.8*	
		AC		4.4*	7.2*	12.1*	19.3*	
	Women	SCC		9.3*	33.0*	74.9*	85.3*	
		AC		4.5*	14.2*	27.2*	34.3*	
Barbone et al. (1997)	Men		*Cigarettes/day*	*1–9*	*10–19*	*20–29*	*30–39*	*≥40*	Reference level, nonsmoker; adjusted for age
		SCC		3.9*	13.2*	15.2*	18.5*	23.4*	
		SCLC		1.1	9.2*	11.8*	13.4*	19.8*	
		AC		2.2	7.4*	6.5*	9.7*	9.6*	
			Duration (years)	*1–29*	*30–39*	*40–49*	*≥50*	
		SCC		2.1	9.6*	14.6*	21.2*	
		SCLC		3.1*	8.8*	12.6*	15.5*	
		AC		3.7*	5.1*	8.2*	8.3*	
			Age at start (years)	*≥20*	*15–19*	*< 15*		
		SCC		9.4*	13.7*	71.3*		
		SCLC		8.8*	10.4*	47.5*		
		AC		5.7*	6.0*	33.4*		
			Years since cessation	*≥25*	*15–24*	*5–14*	*1–4*	*0*	
		SCC		1.9	8.1*	11.9*	18.7*	9.3*	
		SCLC		2.2	7.6*	7.7*	10.9*	14.5*	
		AC		1.8	4.6*	7.3*	9.4*	8.2*	

Table 2.1.1.13 (contd)

Reference	Subjects	Histology	Odds ratio (95% CI)	Comments
Dosemeci et al. (1997)	Men		*Cigarettes/day*	Adjusted for age and alcohol use; for all types p for trend < 0.001
				1–10	11–20	≥21	
		SCC	2.6*	3.2*	7.0*	
		SCLC	1.7	5.0*	13.5*	
		Other histology	1.8	2.7*	3.2*	
			Duration (years) 1–10 / 11–20 / ≥21	
		SCC	1.2 / 3.9* / 4.9*	
		SCLC	1.7 / 7.0* / 8.4*	
		Other histology	0.8 / 3.3* / 4.1*	
Pohlabeln et al. (1997)	Men		*Years since cessation* <1 / 1 / 2–5 / 6–10 / 11–20 / >20	Reference level, current smoker; adjusted for age, region of residence and pack–years
		SCLC	16.8* / 4.0* / 1.2 / 0.4 / 0.4* / 0.1*	
		SCC	19.9* / 6.8* / 1.6 / 1.0 / 0.3* / 0.1*	
		AC	24.1* / 10.2* / 1.8 / 1.0 / 0.8 / 0.5	
Schwartz & Swanson (1997)	African–American men		*Age 40–54 years* / *55–84 years*	Risk for African Americans compared with whites; odds ratios adjusted for age, education, number of cigarettes smoked, number of years of smoking and number of years since quitting
		All lung carcinoma	3.2 (2–5.1) / 0.9 (0.8–1.1)	
		AC	2.8 (1.6–5.1) / 0.9 (0.7–1.1)	
		SCC	4.0 (2.2–7.2) / 1.1. (0.9–1.4)	
		Large-cell carcinoma	2.1 (0.9–4.8) / 1.1 (0.7–1.6)	
		SCLC	2.5 (1.2–4.9) / 0.7 (0.5–1)	
	Women	All lung carcinoma	1.3 (0.8–2.1) / 1.0 (0.8–1.2)	
		AC	0.9 (0.5–1.8) / 0.9 (0.7–1.2)	
		SCC	3.7 (2.5–8.9) / 1.3 (1–1.9)	
		Large-cell carcinoma	1.6 (0.4–6.4) / 0.5 (0.2–1)	
		SCLC	2.7 (1.0–7.3) / 0.9 (0.6–1.3)	
Wakai et al. (1997)	Men		*Cigarettes/day* 1–19 / 20–29 / ≥30	Current smokers; reference level, nonsmoker; adjusted for age
		SCC	3.9* / 10.4* / 24.0*	
		AC	1.3 / 1.9 / 4.5*	
			Years since cessation 5–9 / 10–19 / ≥20	
		SCC	7.5* / 8.9* / 2.0	
		AC	1.2 / 2.5 / 0.5	

Table 2.1.1.13 (contd)

Reference	Subjects	Histology	Odds ratio (95% CI)				Comments
Khuder *et al.* (1998)	Men		*Cigarettes/day*	*1–39*	*≥40*		Adjusted for duration, number of cigarettes/day, age at start and whether or not subject had quit smoking
		SCC		1	8.7*		
		SCLC		1	11.5*		
		AC		1	3.5*		
			Duration (years)	*1–29*	*≥30*		
		SCC		1	1.9		
		SCLC		1	2.6		
		AC		1	2.7*		
			Age at start (years)	*≥20*	*16–19*	*<16*	
		SCC		1	0.8	1.0	
		SCLC		1	1.6	3.0*	
		AC		1	0.7	0.8	
			Cessation	*Yes*	*No*		
		SCC		1	0.6*		
		SCLC		1	1.1		
		AC		1	0.6*		
Matos *et al.* (1998)	Men		*Cigarettes/day*	*1–14*	*15–24*	*≥25*	Adjusted for age and hospital
		SCC		1.4	7.8*	9.7*	
		AC		2.8	7.0*	8.4*	
			Duration (years)	*1–24*	*25–39*	*≥40*	
		SCC		1.2	5.8*	18.5*	
		AC		1.7	7.3*	10.7*	
Kreuzer *et al.* (2000)	Men		*Cigarettes/day*	*<15*	*15–29*	*≥30*	Reference level, occasional smoker; 95% CI not provided; adjusted for age, centre and duration/average amount of smoking and time since quitting
		SCLC		1.0	2.2	2.6	
		SCC		1.0	2.2	3.0	
		AC		1.0	1.6	1.6	
	Women	SCLC		1.0	2.0	4.7	
		SCC		1.0	1.8	3.8	
		AC		1.0	2.1	4.6	

Table 2.1.1.13 (contd)

Reference	Subjects	Histology	Odds ratio (95% CI)				Comments
Kreuzer *et al.* (2000) (contd)			*Duration (years)*				
				< 20	*20–39*	*≥ 40*	
	Men	SCLC		1.0	3.3	3.8	
		SCC		1.0	3.2	4.1	
		AC		1.0	3.4	4.0	
	Women	SCLC		1.0	3.9	3.6	
		SCC		1.0	2.4	4.2	
		AC		1.0	2.2	2.3	
Lee *et al.* (2001)	Men and women		*Cigarettes/day*	*1–10*	*11–20*	*≥ 21*	Adjusted for education, residence, socioeconomic status
		SCC/SCLC		2.9*	3.1*	5.6*	
		AC		1.6	2.0	2.9*	
			Duration (years)	*1–30*	*31–40*	*≥ 41*	
		SCC/SCLC		2.8*	4.3*	5.0*	
		AC		1.7	1.8	3.0*	
			Age started (years)	*> 20*	*12–20*		
		SCC/SCLC		4.0*	4.3*		
		AC		1.6	2.8*		
			Inhalation	*Light†*	*Deep‡*	*Light* / *Deep*	†'Uncertain but light more' [sic] ‡'Uncertain but deep more' [sic]
		SCC/SCLC		1.6	5.0	3.4* / 6.8*	
		AC		1.6	0.7	1.9 / 2.5*	
Simonato *et al.* (2001)			*Former smoker*	*Current smoker*			Reference category, non-smoker; adjusted for age, education and centre
	Men	SCC/SCLC	16.2	57.9			
		AC	3.5	8.0			
	Women	SCC/SCLC	3.8	18.2			
		AC	1.1	4.1			

Table 2.1.1.13 (contd)

Reference	Subjects	Histology	Odds ratio (95% CI)				Comments
Stellman *et al.* (2001)	Men		*Cigarettes/day*				Adjusted for age and education and hospital for hospital controls (H)
	USA		*< 20*	*20–29*	*≥ 30*		
		AC	7.0*	37.3*	54.6*		
	Japan	AC (H)	0.6	2.2	3.3*		
		AC (CC)†	1.2	2.9*	5.5*		
		SCC (H)	7.4*	13.7*	31.8*		SCC could not be evaluated for USA (0 controls)
		SCC (CC)†	10.2*	14.1*	35.7*		†Community controls
			Duration (years)				
	USA		*≤ 40*	*> 40*			
		AC	15.1*	34.7*			
	Japan	AC (H)	1.1	3.9*			
		AC (CC)†	2.6*	4.1*			
		SCC (H)	6.3*	19.3*			
		SCC (CC)†	13.1*	22.8*			
Rachtan (2002)	Women		*Cigarettes/day*				Adjusted for age
			< 11	*11–20*	*21–30*	*> 30*	†Only 1 case
		SCC	3.3*	13.5*	30.2*	74.0*	
		AC	1.7	3.4	8.5*	5.3†	
		SCLC	12.9*	31.6*	43.5*	108.8*	
			Duration (years)				
			< 26	*26–39*	*≥ 40*		
		SCC	2.5*	18.2*	35.2*		
		AC	1.4	4.8*	9.6*		
		SCLC	7.7*	44.7*	98.5*		
			Age started (years)				
			> 18	*≤ 18*			
		SCC	8.4*	21.0*			
		AC	2.6*	4.2*			
		SCLC	25.1*	29.5*			
			Inhalation				
			No	*Yes*			
		SCC	6.4*	15.8*			
		AC	2.2	3.6*			
		SCLC	16.6*	34.6*			

SCC, squamous-cell carcinoma; SCLC, small-cell carcinoma; AC, adenocarcinoma; Kreyberg I, squamous-cell carcinoma; Kreyberg II, adenocarcinoma and alveolar-cell/bronchioalveolar carcinoma; H, hospital control; N, neighbourhood control

$*p < 0.05$

Table 2.1.1.14. Approximate[a] effects of various durations of cigarette smoking on annual excess incidence of lung cancer

Years of cigarette smoking	Annual excess incidence	
	Moderate smokers (%)	Heavy smokers (%)
15	0.005	0.01
30	0.1	0.2
45	0.5	1

[a] Estimated by Peto and Doll (1984) from the model reported by Doll and Peto (1978) fitted to incidence data for male UK doctors

References

Agudo, A., Barnadas, A., Pallares, C., Martinez, I., Fabregat, X., Rosello, J., Estape, J., Planas, J. & Gonzalez, C.A. (1994) Lung cancer and cigarette smoking in women: A case–control study in Barcelona (Spain). *Int. J. Cancer*, **59**, 165–169

Agudo, A., Ahrens, W., Benhamou, E., Benhamou, S., Boffetta, P., Darby, S.C., Forastiere, F., Fortes, C., Gaborieau, V. & Gonzalez, C.A. (2000) Lung cancer and cigarette smoking in women: A multicenter case–control study in Europe. *Int. J. Cancer*, **88**, 820–827

Akiba, S. (1994) Analysis of cancer risk related to longitudinal information on smoking habits. *Environ. Health Perspect.*, **102** (Suppl 8), 15–20

Akiba, S. & Hirayama, T. (1990) Cigarette smoking and cancer mortality risk in Japanese men and women — Results from reanalysis of the six-prefecture cohort study data. *Environ. Health Perspect.*, **87**, 19–26

Alavanja, M.C., Brownson, R.C., Boice, J.D. & Hock, E. (1992) Preexisting lung disease and lung cancer among nonsmoking women. *Am. J. Epidemiol.*, **136**, 623–632

Alavanja, M.C., Brownson, R.C., Benichou, J., Swanson, C. & Boice, J.D. (1995) Attributable risk of lung cancer in lifetime nonsmokers and long-term ex-smokers (Missouri, United States). *Cancer Causes Control*, **6**, 209–216

Armadans-Gil, L., Vaque-Rafart, J., Rossello, J., Olona, M. & Alseda, M. (1999) Cigarette smoking and male lung cancer risk with special regard to type of tobacco. *Int. J. Epidemiol.*, **28**, 614–619

Barbone, F., Bovenzi, M., Cavallieri, F. & Stanta, G. (1997) Cigarette smoking and histologic type of lung cancer in men. *Chest*, **112**, 1474–1479

Becher, H., Jöckel, K.H., Timm, J., Wichmann, H.E. & Drescher, K. (1991) Smoking cessation and nonsmoking intervals: Effect of different smoking patterns on lung cancer risk. *Cancer Causes Control*, **2**, 381–387

Benhamou, S. & Benhamou, E. (1994) The effect of age at smoking initiation on lung cancer risk. *Epidemiology*, **5**, 560

Benhamou, E., Benhamou, S. & Flamant, R. (1987) Lung cancer and women: Results of a French case–control study. *Br. J. Cancer*, **55**, 91–95

Benhamou, E., Benhamou, S., Auquier, A. & Flamant, R. (1989) Changes in patterns of cigarette smoking and lung cancer risk: Results of a case–control study. *Br. J. Cancer*, **60**, 601–604

Benhamou, S., Benhamou, E., Auquier, A. & Flamant, R. (1994) Differential effects of tar content, type of tobacco and use of a filter on lung cancer risk in male cigarette smokers. *Int. J. Epidemiol.*, **23**, 437–443

Benowitz, N.L., Perez-Stable, E.J., Herrera, B. & Jacob, P., III (2002) Slower metabolism and reduced intake of nicotine from cigarette smoking in Chinese–Americans. *J. natl Cancer Inst.*, **16**, 108–115

Ben-Shlomo, Y., Smith, G., Shipley, M. & Marmot, M. (1994) What determines mortality risk in male former cigarette smokers? *Am. J. public Health*, **84**, 1235–1242

Bhurgri, Y., Decullier, E., Bhurgri, A., Nassar, S., Usman, A., Brennan, P. & Boffetta, P. (2002) A case–control study of lung cancer in Karachi, Pakistan. *Int. J. Cancer*, **98**, 952–955

Boffetta, P., Kreuzer, M., Benhamou, S., Agudo, A., Wichmann, H.E., Gaborieau, V. & Simonato, L. (2001) Risk of lung cancer from tobacco smoking among young women from Europe. *Int. J. Cancer*, **91**, 745–746

Burns, D.M., Lee, L., Shen, L.Z., Gilpin, E., Tolley, H.D., Vaughn, J. & Shanks, T.G. (1997) Cigarette smoking behavior in the United States. In: *Changes in Cigarettes Related Disease Risks and Their Implication for Prevention and Control* (Smoking and Tobacco Control Monograph No. 8; NIH Publication No. 97-4213), Bethesda, MD, US Department of Health and Human Services, National Institutes of Health

Burns, D.M., Major, J.M., Shanks, T.G., Thun, M.J. & Samet, J.M. (2001) Smoking lower yield cigarettes and disease risks. In: *Risk Associated with Smoking Cigarettes with Low Machine-Measured Yields of Tar and Nicotine* (Smoking and Tobacco Control Monograph No. 13; NIH Publication No. 02-5074), Bethesda, MD, US Department of Health and Human Services, National Institutes of Health

Caraballo, R.S., Giovino, G.A., Pechacek, T.F., Mowery, P.D., Richter, P.A., Strauss, W.J., Sharp, D.J., Eriksen, M.P., Pirkle, J.L. & Maurer, K.R. (1998) Racial and ethnic differences in serum cotinine levels of cigarette smokers: Third National Health and Nutrition Examination Survey, 1988–1991. *J. Am. med. Assoc.*, **280**, 135–139

Carpenter, C.L., Jarvik, M.E., Morgenstern, H., McCarthy, W.J. & London, S.J. (1999) Mentholated cigarette smoking and lung-cancer risk. *Ann. Epidemiol.*, **9**, 114–120

Cederlöf, R., Friberg, L., Hrubec, Z. & Lorich, U. (1975) *The Relationship of Smoking and Some Social Covariables to Mortality and Cancer Morbidity. A Ten Year Follow-up in a Probability Sample of 55 000 Swedish Subjects, Age 18-69, Part 1 and Part 2*, Stockholm, The Karolinska Institute, Department of Environmental Hygiene

Chen, Z.M., Xu, Z., Collins, R., Li, W.X. & Peto, R. (1997) Early health effects of the emerging tobacco epidemic in China. A 16-year prospective study. *J. Am. med. Assoc.*, **278**, 1500–1504

Choi, J.H., Chung, H.C., Yoo, N.C., Lee, H.R., Lee, K.H., Choi, W., Lim, H.Y., Koh, E.H., Kim, J.H., Roh, J.K., Kim, S.K., Lee, W.Y. & Kim, B.S. (1994) Changing trends in histologic types of lung cancer during the last decade (1981–90) in Korea: A hospital-based study. *Lung Cancer*, **10**, 287–296

Chow, W.H., Schuman, L.M., McLaughlin, J.K., Bjelke, E., Gridley, G., Wacholder, S., Co Chien, H.T. & Blot, W.J. (1992) A cohort study of tobacco use, diet, occupation, and lung cancer mortality. *Cancer Causes Control*, **3**, 247–254

Chyou, P.H., Nomura, A.M.Y. & Stemmermann, G.N. (1992) A prospective study of the attributable risk of cancer due to cigarette smoking. *Am. J. public Health*, **82**, 37–40

Chyou, P.H., Normura, A.M.Y., Stemmermann, G.N. & Kato, I. (1993) Lung cancer: A prospective study of smoking, occupation, and nutrient intake. *Arch. environ. Health*, **48**, 69–72

Damber, L.A. & Larsson, L.G. (1986) Smoking and lung cancer with special regard to type of smoking and type of cancer. A case–control study in North Sweden. *Br. J. Cancer*, **53**, 673–681

De Stefani, E., Fierro, L., Larrinaga, M.T., Balbi, J.C., Ronco, A. & Mendilaharsu, M. (1994) Smoking of hand-rolled cigarettes as a risk factor for small cell lung cancer in men: A case–control study from Uruguay. *Lung Cancer*, **11**, 191–199

De Stefani, E., Fierro, L., Correa, P., Fontham, E., Ronco, A., Larrinaga, M., Balbi, J. & Mendilaharsu, M. (1996a) Mate drinking and risk of lung cancer in males: A case–control study from Uruguay. *Cancer Epidemiol. Biomarkers Prev.*, **5**, 515–519

De Stefani, E., Deneo-Pellegrini, H., Carzoglio, J.C., Ronco, A. & Mendilaharsu, M. (1996b) Dietary nitrosodimethylamine and the risk of lung cancer: A case–control study from Uruguay. *Cancer Epidemiol. Biomarkers Prev.*, **5**, 679–682

Dikshit, R.P. & Kanhere, S. (2000) Tobacco habits and risk of lung, oropharyngeal and oral cavity cancer: A population-based case–control study in Bhopal, India. *Int. J. Epidemiol.*, **29**, 609–614

Doll, R. (1971) The age distribution of cancer: Implications for models of carcinogenesis. *J. R. stat. Soc.*, **A134**, 133–155

Doll, R. (1998) The first reports on smoking and lung cancer. *Clio Med.*, **46**, 130–142

Doll, R. & Peto, R. (1976) Mortality in relation to smoking: 20 years' observations on male British doctors. *Br. med. J.*, **2**, 1525–1536

Doll, R. & Peto, R. (1978) Cigarette smoking and bronchial carcinoma: Dose and time relationships among regular smokers and lifelong non-smokers. *J. Epidemiol. Community Health*, **32**, 303–313

Doll, R. & Peto, R. (1981) The causes of cancer: Quantitative estimates of avoidable risks of cancer in the United States today. *J. natl Cancer Inst.*, **66**, 1191–1308

Doll, R., Hill, A.B. & Kreyberg, L. (1957) The significance of cell type in relation to the aetiology of lung cancer. *Br. J. Cancer*, **11**, 43–48

Doll, R., Gray, R., Hafner, B. & Peto, R. (1980) Mortality in relation to smoking: 22 years' observations on female British doctors. *Br. med. J.*, **280**, 967–971

Doll, R., Peto, R., Wheatley, K., Gray, R. & Sutherland, I. (1994) Mortality in relation to smoking: 40 years' observations on male British doctors. *Br. med. J.*, **309**, 901–911

Dosemeci, M., Gokmen, I., Unsal, M., Hayes, R.B. & Blair, A. (1997) Tobacco, alcohol use, and risks of laryngeal and lung cancer by subsite and histologic type in Turkey. *Cancer Causes Control*, **8**, 729–737

Du, Y.X., Cha, Q., Chen, X.W., Chen, Y.Z., Huang, L.F., Feng, Z.Z., Wu, X.F. & Wu, J.M. (1996) An epidemiological study of risk factors for lung cancer in Guangzhou, China. *Lung Cancer*, **14** (Suppl. 1), S9–S37

Ellard, G.A., de Waard, F. & Kemmeren, J.M. (1995) Urinary nicotine metabolite excretion and lung cancer risk in a female cohort. *Br. J. Cancer*, **72**, 788–791

Engeland, A., Haldorsen, T., Andersen, A. & Tretli, S. (1996a) The impact of smoking habits on lung cancer risk: 28 years' observation of 26 000 Norwegian men and women. *Cancer Causes Control*, **7**, 366–376

Falk, R.T., Pickle, L.W., Fontham, E.T., Greenberg, S.D., Jacobs, H.L., Correa, P. & Fraumeni, J.F. (1992) Epidemiology of bronchioloalveolar carcinoma. *Cancer Epidemiol. Biomarkers Prev.*, **1**, 339–344

Floderus, B., Cederlöf, R. & Friberg, L. (1988) Smoking and mortality: A 21-year follow-up based on the Swedish Twin Registry. *Int. J. Epidemiol.*, **17**, 332–340

Fraumeni, J.F., Jr & Mason, T.J. (1974) Cancer mortality among Chinese Americans, 1950–69. *J. natl Cancer Inst.*, **52**, 659–665

Freund, K.M., Belanger, A.J., D'Agostino, R.B. & Kannel, W.B. (1993) The health risks of smoking: The Framingham Study: 34 years of follow-up. *Ann. Epidemiol.*, **3**, 417–424

Gao, Y.T., Blot, W.J., Zheng, W., Fraumeni, J.F. & Hsu, C.W. (1988) Lung cancer and smoking in Shanghai. *Int. J. Epidemiol.*, **17**, 277–280

Gao, C.M., Tajima, K., Kuroishi, T., Hirose, K. & Inoue, M. (1993) Protective effects of raw vegetables and fruit against lung cancer among smokers and ex-smokers: A case–control study in the Tokai area of Japan. *Jpn. J. Cancer Res.*, **84**, 594–600

Gao, Y.T., Den, J., Xiang, Y., Ruan, Z.X., Wang, Z.X., Hu, B.Y., Guo, M.R., Teng, W.K., Han, J.J. & Zhang, Y.S. (1999) [Smoking, related cancers, and other diseases in Shanghai: A 10-year prospective study.] *Chin. J. prev. Med.*, **33**, 5–8 (in Chinese)

Garfinkel, L. & Stellman, S.D. (1988) Smoking and lung cancer in women: Findings in a prospective study. *Cancer Res.*, **48**, 6951–6955

Ger, L.P., Hsu, W.L., Chen, K.T. & Chen, C.J. (1993) Risk factors of lung cancer by histological category in Taiwan. *Anticancer Res.*, **13**, 1491–1500

Goldoni, C.A., Danielli, G., Turatti, C., Ranzi, A. & Lauriola, P. (2001) Case–control study in an area in the province of Ferrara showing a high death rate from lung cancer. *Epidemiol. Prev.*, **25**, 21–26

Hammond, E.C. & Horn, D. (1958a) Smoking and death rates — Report on forty-four months of follow-up of 187 783 men. I. Total mortality. *J. Am. med. Assoc.*, **166**, 1159–1172

Hammond, E.C. & Horn, D. (1958b) Smoking and death rates — Report on forty-four months of follow-up of 187 783 men. II. Death rates by cause. *J. Am. med. Assoc.*, **166**, 1294–1308

Hammond, E.C., Garfinkel, L., Seidman, H. & Lew, E.A. (1976) 'Tar' and nicotine content of cigarette smoke in relation to death rates. *Environ. Res.*, **12**, 263–274

Harris, R.E., Zang, E.A., Anderson, J.I. & Wynder, E.L. (1993) Race and sex differences in lung cancer risk associated with cigarette smoking. *Int. J. Epidemiol.*, **22**, 592–599

He, X.Z., Chen, W., Liu, Z.Y. & Chapman, R.S. (1991) An epidemiological study of lung cancer in Xuan Wei County, China: Current progress. Case–control study on lung cancer and cooking fuel. *Environ. Health Perspect.*, **94**, 9–13

Hebert, J.R. & Kabat, G.C. (1991) Distribution of smoking and its association with lung cancer: Implications for studies on the association of fat with cancer. *J. natl Cancer Inst.*, **83**, 872–874

Hegmann, K.T., Fraser, A.M., Keaney, R.P., Moser, S.E., Nilasena, D.S., Sedlars, M., Higham-Gren, L. & Lyon, J.L. (1993) The effect of age at smoking initiation on lung cancer risk. *Epidemiology*, **4**, 444–448

Higgins, I.T. & Wynder, E.L. (1988) Reduction in risk of lung cancer among ex-smokers with particular reference to histologic type. *Cancer*, **62**, 2397–2401

Hoffmann, D. & Hoffmann, I. (1997) The changing cigarette, 1950–95. *J. Toxicol. environ. Health*, **50**, 307–364

Holowaty, E.J., Risch, H.A., Miller, A.B. & Burch, J.D. (1991) Lung cancer in women in the Niagara Region, Ontario: A case–control study. *Can. J. public Health*, **82**, 304–309

Hoover, D.R. (1994) Re: "Are female smokers at higher risk for lung cancer than male smokers? A case–control analysis by histologic type". *Am. J. Epidemiol.*, **140**, 186–187

Hu, J., Johnson, K.C., Mao, Y., Xu, T., Lin, Q., Wang, C., Zhao, F., Wang, G., Chen, Y. & Yang, Y. (1997) A case–control study of diet and lung cancer in Northeast China. *Int. J. Cancer*, **71**, 924–931

IARC (1986) *IARC Monographs on the Evaluation of the Carcinogenic Risk of Chemicals to Humans*, Vol. 38, *Tobacco Smoking*, Lyon, IARC*Press*, p. 1

Islam, S.S. & Schottenfeld, D. (1994) Declining FEV_1 and chronic productive cough in cigarette smokers: A 25-year prospective study of lung cancer incidence in Tecumseh, Michigan. *Cancer Epidemiol. Biomarkers Prev.*, **3**, 289–298

Jacobs, D.R., Adachi, H., Mulder, I., Kromhout, D., Menotti, A., Nissinen, A. & Blackburn, H. (1999) Cigarette smoking and mortality risk: Twenty-five year follow-up of the Seven Countries Study. *Arch. intern. Med.*, **159**, 733–740

Jedrychowski, W., Becher, H., Wahrendorf, J. & Basa-Cierpialek, Z. (1990) A case–control study of lung cancer with special reference to the effect of air pollution in Poland. *J. Epidemiol. Community Health*, **44**, 114–120

Jedrychowski, W., Becher, H., Wahrendorf, J., Basa-Cierpialek, Z. & Gomola, K. (1992) Effect of tobacco smoking on various histological types of lung cancer. *J. Cancer Res. clin. Oncol.*, **118**, 276–282

Jöckel, K.H., Ahrens, W., Wichmann, H.E., Becher, H., Bolm-Audorff, U., Jahn, I., Molik, B., Briser, E. & Timm, J. (1992) Occupational and environmental hazards associated with lung cancer. *Int. J. Epidemiol.*, **21**, 202–213

Jöckel, K.H., Ahrens, W., Jahn, I., Pohlabeln, H. & Bolm-Audorff, U. (1998) Occupational risk factors for lung cancer: A case–control study in West Germany. *Int. J. Epidemiol.*, **27**, 549–560

Kabat, G.C. (1996) Aspects of the epidemiology of lung cancer in smokers and nonsmokers in the United States. *Lung Cancer*, **15**, 1–20

Kabat, G.C. & Hebert, J.R. (1991) Use of mentholated cigarettes and lung cancer risk. *Cancer Res.*, **51**, 6510–6513

Kahn, H.A. (1966) The Dorn study of smoking and mortality among US veterans: Report on eight and one-half years of observation. *Natl Cancer Inst. Monogr.*, **19**, 1–25

Kark, J.D., Yaari, S., Rasooly, I. & Goldbourt, U. (1995) Are lean smokers at increased risk of lung cancer? The Israel Civil Servant Cancer Study. *Arch. intern. Med.*, **155**, 2409–2416

Katsouyanni, K., Trichopoulos, D., Kalandidi, A., Tomos, P. & Riboli, E. (1991) A case–control study of air pollution and tobacco smoking in lung cancer among women in Athens. *Prev. Med.*, **20**, 271–278

Kaufman, D.W., Palmer, J.R., Rosenberg, L., Stolley, P., Warshauer, E. & Shapiro, S. (1989) Tar content of cigarettes in relation to lung cancer. *Am. J. Epidemiol.*, **129**, 703–711

Khuder, S.A., Dayal, H.H., Mutgi, A.B., Willey, J.C. & Dayal, G. (1998) Effect of cigarette smoking on major histological types of lung cancer in men. *Lung Cancer*, **22**, 15–21

King, T.E., Jr & Brunetta, P. (1999) Racial disparity in rates of surgery for lung cancer. *New Engl. J. Med.*, **341**, 1231–1233

Kono, S., Ikeda, M., Tokudome, S., Nishizumi, M. & Kuratsune, M. (1987) Cigarette smoking, alcohol and cancer mortality: A cohort study of male Japanese physicians. *Jpn. J. Cancer Res.*, **78**, 1323–1328

Kreuzer, M., Kreienbrock, L., Gerken, M., Heinrich, J., Brüske-Hohlfeld, I., Müller, K.M. & Wichmann, H.E. (1998) Risk factors for lung cancer in young adults. *Am. J. Epidemiol.*, **147**, 1028–1037

Kreuzer, M., Boffetta, P., Whitley, E., Ahrens, W., Gaborieau, V., Heinrich, J., Jockel, K.H., Kreienbrock, L., Mallone, S., Merletti, F., Roesch, F., Zambon, P. & Simonato, L. (2000) Gender differences in lung cancer risk by smoking: A multicentre case–control study in Germany and Italy. *Br. J. Cancer*, **82**, 227–233

Kreyberg, L. (1962) Histological lung cancer types. A morphological and biological correlation. *Acta pathol. microbiol. scand.*, **Suppl. 157**

Kubik, A., Zatloukal, P., Tomasek, L., Kriz, J., Petruzelka, L. & Plesko, I. (2001) Diet and the risk of lung cancer among women. A hospital-based case–control study. *Neoplasma*, **48**, 262–266

Kubik, A.K., Zatloukal, P., Tomasek, L. & Petruzelka, L. (2002) Lung cancer risk among Czech women: A case–control study. *Prev. Med.*, **34**, 436–444

Kuller, L.H., Ockene, J.K., Meilahn, E., Wentworth, D.N., Svendsen, K.H. & Neaton, J.D. for the MRFIT Research Group (1991) Cigarette smoking and mortality. *Prev. Med.*, **20**, 638–654

Lam, T.H., Kung, I.T., Wong, C.M., Lam, W.K., Kleevens, J.W., Saw, D., Hsu, C., Seneviratne, S., Lam, S.Y., Lo, K.K. & Chan, W.C. (1987) Smoking, passive smoking and histological types in lung cancer in Hong Kong Chinese women. *Br. J. Cancer*, **56**, 673–678

Lam, T.H., He, Y., Li, L.S., Li, L.S., He, S.F. & Liang, B.Q. (1997) Mortality attributable to cigarette smoking in China. *J. Am. med. Assoc.*, **278**, 1505–1508

Lam, T.H., Ho, S.Y., Hedley, A.J., Mak, K.H. & Peto, R. (2001) Mortality and smoking in Hong Kong: Case–control study of all adult deaths in 1998. *Br. med. J.*, **323**, 361

Law, C.H., Day, N.E. & Shanmugaratnam, K. (1976) Incidence rates of specific histological types of lung cancer in Singapore Chinese dialect groups, and their aetiological significance. *Int. J. Cancer*, **17**, 304–309

Lee, C.-H., Ko, Y.-C., Cheng, L.S.-C., Lin, Y.-C., Lin, H.-J., Huang, M.-S., Huang, J.-J., Kao, E.-L. & Wang, H.-Z. (2001) The heterogeneity in risk factors of lung cancer and the difference of histologic distribution between genders in Taiwan. *Cancer Causes Control*, **12**, 289–300

Lei, Y.X., Cai, W.C., Chen, Y.Z. & Du, Y.X. (1996) Some lifestyle factors in human lung cancer: A case–control study of 792 lung cancer cases. *Lung Cancer*, **14** (Suppl. 1), S121–S136

Levi, F., Franceschi, S., La Vecchia, C., Randimbison, L. & Te, V.C. (1997) Lung carcinoma trends by histologic type in Vaud and Neuchatel, Switzerland, 1974–1994. *Cancer*, **79**, 906–914

Liaw, K.M. & Chen, C.J. (1998) Mortality attributable to cigarette smoking in Taiwan: A 12-year follow-up study. *Tob. Control*, **7**, 141–148

Liu, Z. (1992) Smoking and lung cancer in China: Combined analysis of eight case–control studies. *Int. J. Epidemiol.*, **21**, 197–201

Liu, Z.Y., He, X.Z. & Chapman, R.S. (1991) Smoking and other risk factors for lung cancer in Xuanwei, China. *Int. J. Epidemiol.*, **20**, 26–31

Liu, Q., Sasco, A.J., Riboli, E. & Hu, M.X. (1993) Indoor air pollution and lung cancer in Guangzhou, People's Republic of China. *Am. J. Epidemiol.*, **137**, 145–154

Liu, B.Q., Peto, R., Chen, Z.M., Boreham, J., Wu, Y.P., Li, J.Y., Campbell, T.C. & Chen, J.S. (1998) Emerging tobacco hazards in China: 1. Retrospective proportional mortality study of one million deaths. *Br. med. J.*, **317**, 1411–1422

Lossing, E.H., Best, E.W.R., McGregor, J.T., Josie, G.H., Walker, C.B., Delaquis, F.M., Baker, P.M. & McKenzie, A.C. (1966) *A Canadian Study of Smoking and Health*, Ottawa, Department of National Health and Welfare

Lubin, J.H., Li, H.Y., Xuan, X.A., Cai, S.K., Luo, Q.S., Yang, L.F., Wang, J.Z., Yang, L. & Blot, W.J. (1992) Risk of lung cancer among cigarette and pipe smokers in southern China. *Int. J. Cancer*, **51**, 390–395

Luo, R.X., Wu, B., Yi, Y.N., Huang, Z.W. & Lin, R.T. (1996) Indoor burning coal air pollution and lung cancer — A case–control study in Fuzhou, China. *Lung Cancer*, **14** (Suppl. 1), S113–S119

Mabry, M., Nelkin, B. & Baylin, S. (1998) Lung cancer. In: Vogelstein, B. & Kinzler, K.W., eds, *The Genetic Basis of Human Cancer*, New York, McGraw-Hill, pp. 671–679

Mao, Y., Hu, J., Ugnat, A.M., Semenciw, R. & Fincham, S. (2001) Socioeconomic status and lung cancer risk in Canada. *Int. J. Epidemiol.*, **30**, 809–817

Matos, E., Vilensky, M., Boffetta, P. & Kogevinas, M. (1998) Lung cancer and smoking: A case–control study in Buenos Aires, Argentina. *Lung Cancer*, **21**, 155–163

Mattson, M.L., Pollack, E.S. & Cullen, J.W. (1987) What are the odds that smoking will kill you? *Am. J. public Health*, **77**, 425–431

McDuffie, H.H. (1994) Re: 'Are female smokers at higher risk for lung cancer than male smokers? A case–control analysis by histologic type'. *Am. J. Epidemiol.*, **140**, 185–186

McLaughlin, J.K., Hrubec, Z., Blot, W.J. & Fraumeni, J.F., Jr (1995) Smoking and cancer mortality among US veterans: A 26-year follow-up. *Int. J. Cancer.*, **60**, 190–193

Medical Research Council (1957) Tobacco smoking and cancer of the lung. *Br. med. J.*, **i**, 1523

Miller, G.H., Golish, J.A., Cox, C.E. & Chacko, D.C. (1994) Women and lung cancer: A comparison of active and passive smokers with nonexposed nonsmokers. *Cancer Detect. Prev.*, **18**, 421–430

Morabia, A. & Wynder, E.L. (1991) Cigarette smoking and lung cancer cell types. *Cancer*, **68**, 2074–2078

Morabia, A. & Wynder, E.L. (1992) Relation of bronchioloalveolar carcinoma to tobacco. *Br. med. J.*, **304**, 541–543

Morabia, A. & Wynder, E.L. (1993) Correspondence re: R. T. Falk et al. (1992) Epidemiology of bronchioloalveolar carcinoma. *Cancer Epidemiol. Biomarkers Prev.*, **1**, 339–344. *Cancer Epidemiol. Biomarkers Prev.*, **2**, 89–90

Murata, M., Takayama, K., Choi, B.C.K. & Pak, A.W.P. (1996) A nested case–control study on alcohol drinking, tobacco smoking, and cancer. *Cancer Detect. Prev.*, **20**, 557–565

Muscat, J.E., Stellman, S.D., Zhang, Z.F., Neugut, A.I. & Wynder, E.L. (1997) Cigarette smoking and large cell carcinoma of the lung. *Cancer Epidemiol. Biomarkers Prev.*, **6**, 477–480

Mzileni, O., Sitas, F., Steyn, K., Carrara, H. & Bekker, P. (1999) Lung cancer, tobacco, and environmental factors in the African population of the Northern Province, South Africa. *Tob. Control*, **8**, 398–401

Niu, S.R., Yang, G.H., Chen, Z.M., Wang, J.L., Wang, G.H., He, X.Z., Schoepff, H., Boreham, J., Pan, H.C. & Peto, R. (1998) Emerging tobacco hazards in China: 2. Early mortality results from a prospective study. *Br. med. J.*, **317**, 1423–1424

Nordlund, L.A., Carstensen, J.M. & Pershagen, G. (1999) Are male and female smokers at equal risk of smoking-related cancer: Evidence from a Swedish prospective study. *Scand. J. public Health*, **27**, 56–62

Novotny, T.E., Warner, K.E., Kendrick, J.S. & Remington, P.L. (1988) Smoking by blacks and whites: Socioeconomic and demographic differences. *Am. J. public Health*, **78**, 1187–1189

Osann, K.E. (1991) Lung cancer in women: The importance of smoking, family history of cancer, and medical history of respiratory disease. *Cancer Res.*, **51**, 4893–4897

Osann, K.E., Anton-Culver, H., Kurosaki, T. & Taylor, T. (1993) Sex differences in lung cancer risk associated with cigarette smoking. *Int. J. Cancer*, **54**, 44–48

Osann, K.E., Lowery, J.T. & Schell, M.J. (2000) Small cell lung cancer in women: Risk associated with smoking, prior respiratory disease, and occupation. *Lung Cancer*, **28**, 1–10

Pacella-Norman, R., Urban, M.I., Sitas, F., Carrara, H., Sur, R., Hale, M., Ruff Patel, M., Newton, R., Bull, D. & Beral, V. (2002) Risk factors for oesophageal, lung, oral and laryngeal cancers in black South Africans. *Br. J. Cancer*, **86**, 1751–1756

Parkin, D.M., Pisani, P. & Masuyer, E. (2000) Tobacco-attributable cancer burden: A global review. In: Lu, R., Mackay, J., Niu, S. & Peto, R., eds, *Tobacco: The Growing Epidemic*, London, Springer-Verlag, pp. 81–84

Pathak, D.R., Samet, J.M., Humble, C.G. & Skipper, B.J. (1986) Determinants of lung cancer risk in cigarette smokers in New Mexico. *J. natl Cancer Inst.*, **76**, 597–604

Pawlega, J., Rachtan, J. & Dyba, T. (1997) Evaluation of certain risk factors for lung cancer in Cracow (Poland) — A case–control study. *Acta oncol.*, **36**, 471–476

Peto, R. & Doll, R. (1984) Keynote address: The control of lung cancer. In: Mizell, M. & Correa, P., eds, *Lung Cancer: Causes and Prevention*, New York, Verlag Chemie International, pp. 1–19

Peto, R., Chen, Z.M. & Boreham, J. (1999) Tobacco — The growing epidemic. *Nat. Med.*, **5**, 15–17

Peto, R., Darby, S., Deo, H., Silcocks, P., Whitley, E. & Doll, R. (2000) Smoking, smoking cessation, and lung cancer in the UK since 1950: Combination of national statistics with two case–control studies. *Br. med. J.*, **321**, 323–329

Petrauskaite, R., Pershagen, G. & Gurevicius, R. (2002) Lung cancer near an industrial site in Lithuania with major emissions of airway irritants. *Int. J. Cancer*, **99**, 106–111

Pezzotto, S.M., Mahuad, R., Bay, M.L., Morini, J.C. & Poletto, L. (1993) Variation in smoking-related lung cancer risk factors by cell type among men in Argentina: A case–control study. *Cancer Causes Control*, **4**, 231–237

Pohlabeln, H., Jöckel, K.H. & Müller, K.M. (1997) The relation between various histological types of lung cancer and the number of years since cessation of smoking. *Lung Cancer*, **18**, 223–229

Potter, J.D., Sellers, T.A., Folsom, A.R. & McGovern, P.G. (1992) Alcohol, beer, and lung cancer in postmenopausal women. The Iowa Women's Health Study. *Ann. Epidemiol.*, **2**, 587–595

Prescott, E., Grobaek, M., Becker, U. & Sorensen, T.I.A. (1999) Alcohol intake and the risk of lung cancer: Influence of type of alcoholic beverage. *Am. J. Epidemiol.*, **149**, 463–470

Rachtan, J. (2002) Smoking, passive smoking and lung cancer cell types among women in Poland. *Lung Cancer*, **35**, 129–136

Rachtan, J. & Sokolowski, A. (1997) Risk factors for lung cancer among women in Poland. *Lung Cancer*, **18**, 137–145

Rauscher, G.H., Mayne, S.T. & Janerich, D.T. (2000) Relation between body mass index and lung cancer risk in men and women never and former smokers. *Am. J. Epidemiol.*, **152**, 506–513

Risch, H.A., Howe, G.R., Jain, M., Burch, J.D., Holowaty, E.J. & Miller, A.B. (1993) Are female smokers at higher risk for lung cancer than male smokers? A case–control analysis by histologic type. *Am. J. Epidemiol.*, **138**, 281–293

Rogot, E. & Murray, J.L. (1980) Smoking and causes of death among US veterans: 16 years of observation. *Public Health Rep.*, **95**, 213–222

Russo, A., Crosignani, P., Franceschi, S. & Berrino, F. (1997) Changes in lung cancer histological types in Varese Cancer Registry, Italy 1976–92. *Eur. J. Cancer*, **33**, 1643–1647

Rylander, R., Axelsson, G., Andersson, L., Liljequist, T. & Bergman, B. (1996) Lung cancer, smoking and diet among Swedish men. *Lung Cancer.*, **14** (Suppl. 1), S75–S83

Sankaranarayanan, R., Varghese, C., Duffy, S.W., Padmakumary, G., Day, N.E. & Nair, M.K. (1994) A case–control study of diet and lung cancer in Kerala, South India. *Int. J. Cancer*, **58**, 644–649

Sasco, A.J., Merrill, R.M., Dari, I., Benhaim-Luzon, V., Carriot, F., Cann, C.I. & Bartal, M. (2002) A case–control study of lung cancer in Casablanca, Morocco. *Cancer Causes Control*, **13**, 609–616

Schoenberg, J.B., Wilcox, H.B., Mason, T.J., Bill, J. & Stemhagen, A. (1989) Variation in smoking-related lung cancer risk among New Jersey women. *Am. J. Epidemiol.*, **130**, 688–695

Schwartz, A.G. & Swanson, G.M. (1997) Lung carcinoma in African Americans and whites. A population-based study in metropolitan Detroit, Michigan. *Cancer*, **79**, 45–52

Shen, X.B., Wang, G.X., Huang, Y.Z., Xiang, L.S. & Wang, X.H. (1996) Analysis and estimates of attributable risk factors for lung cancer in Nanjing, China. *Lung Cancer*, **14** (Suppl. 1), 107–112

Shimizu, H., Nagata, C., Tsuchiya, E., Nakagawa, K. & Weng, S.Y. (1994) Risk of lung cancer among cigarette smokers in relation to tumor location. *Jpn. J. Cancer Res.*, **85**, 1196–1199

Sidney, S., Tekawa, I.S. & Friedman, G.D. (1993) A prospective study of cigarette tar yield and lung cancer. *Cancer Causes Control*, **4**, 3–10

Siemiatycki, J., Kreski, D., Franco, E. & Kaiserman, M. (1995) Associations between cigarette smoking and each of 21 types of cancer: A multi-site case–control study. *Int. J. Epidemiol.*, **24**, 504–514

Simonato, L., Zambon, P., Ardit, S., Della-Sala, S., Fila, G., Gaborieau, V., Gallo, G., Magarotto, G., Mazzini, R., Pasini, L. & Stracca Pansa, V. (2000) Lung cancer risk in Venice: A population-based case–control study. *Eur. J. Cancer Prev.*, **9**, 35–39

Simonato, L., Agudo, A., Ahrens, W., Benhamou, E., Benhamou, S., Boffetta, P., Brennan, P., Darby, S.C., Forastiere, F., Fortes, C., Gaborieau, V., Gerken, M., Gonzales, C.A., Jöckel, K.H., Kreuzer, M., Merletti, F., Nyberg, F., Pershagen, G., Pohlabeln, H., Rosch, F., Whitley, E., Wichmann, H.E. & Zambon, P. (2001) Lung cancer and cigarette smoking in Europe: An update of risk estimates and an assessment of inter-country heterogeneity. *Int. J. Cancer*, **91**, 876–887

Sobue, T., Suzuki, T., Fujimoto, I., Matsuda, M., Doi, O., Mori, T., Furuse, K., Fukuoka, M., Yasumitsu, T., Kuwahara, O., Kono, K., Taki, T., Kuwabara, M., Nakahara, K., Endo, S., Sawamura, K., Kurata, M., Ichitani, M. & Hattori, S. (1994) Case–control study for lung cancer and cigarette smoking in Osaka, Japan: Comparison with the results from western Europe. *Jpn. J. Cancer Res.*, **85**, 464–473

Sobue, T., Tsukuma, H., Oshima, A., Genka, K., Tamori, H., Nishizawa, N. & Natsukawa, S. (1999) Lung cancer incidence rates by histologic type in high- and low-risk areas: A population-based study in Osaka, Okinawa, and Saku Nagano, Japan. *J. Epidemiol.*, **9**, 134–142

Speizer, F.E., Colditz, G.A., Hunter, D.J., Rosner, B. & Hennekens, C. (1999) Prospective study of smoking, antioxidant intake, and lung cancer in middle-aged women (USA). *Cancer Causes Control*, **10**, 475–482

Stellman, S.D. (1986) Cigarette yield and cancer risk: Evidence from case–control and prospective studies. In: Zaridze, D. & Peto, R., eds, *Tobacco: A Major International Health Hazard* (IARC Scientific Publications No. 74), Lyon, IARC*Press*, pp. 197–209

Stellman, S.D. & Garfinkel, L. (1989a) Proportions of cancer deaths attributable to cigarette smoking in women. *Women Health*, **15**, 19–28

Stellman, S.D. & Garfinkel, L. (1989b) Lung cancer risk is proportional to cigarette tar yield: Evidence from a prospective study. *Prev. Med.*, **18**, 518–525

Stellman, S.D., Muscat, J.E., Hoffmann, D. & Wynder, E.L. (1997a) Impact of filter cigarette smoking on lung cancer histology. *Prev. Med.*, **26**, 451–456

Stellman, S.D., Muscat, J.E., Thompson, S., Hoffmann, D. & Wynder, E.L. (1997b) Risk of squamous cell carcinoma and adenocarcinoma of the lung in relation to lifetime filter cigarette smoking. *Cancer*, **80**, 382–388

Stellman, S.D., Takezaki, T., Wang, L., Chen, Y., Citron, M.L., Djordjevic, M.V., Harlap, S., Muscat, J.E., Neugut, A.I., Wynder, E.L., Ogawa, H., Tajima, K. & Ao, K. (2001) Smoking and lung cancer risk in American and Japanese men: An international case–control study. *Cancer Epidemiol. Biomarkers Prev.*, **10**, 1193–1199

Stellman, S.D., Chen, Y., Muscat, J.E., Djordjevic, M.V., Richie, J.P., Jr, Laza Thompson, S., Altorki, N., Berwick, M., Citron, M.L., Harlap, S., Kaur, T.B., Neugut, A.I., Olson, S.,

Travaline, J.M., Witorsch, P. & Zhang, Z.F. (2003) Lung cancer risk in white and black Americans. *Ann. Epidemiol.*, **13**, 294–302

Stewart, J.H., IV (2001) Lung carcinoma in African Americans: A review of the current literature. *Cancer*, **91**, 2476–2482

Suzuki, I., Hamada, G.S., Zamboni, M.M., Cordeiro, P.D., Watanabe, S. & Tsugane, S. (1994) Risk factors for lung cancer in Rio de Janeiro, Brazil: A case–control study. *Lung Cancer*, **11**, 179–190

Svensson, C., Pershagen, G. & Klominek, J. (1989) Smoking and passive smoking in relation to lung cancer in women. *Acta oncol.*, **28**, 623–629

Tenkanen, L., Hakulinen, T. & Teppo, L. (1987) The joint effect of smoking and respiratory symptoms on risk of lung cancer. *Int. J. Epidemiol.*, **16**, 509–515

Thun, M.J. & Burns, D.M. (2001) Health impact of 'reduced yield' cigarettes: A critical assessment of the epidemiological evidence. *Tob. Control*, **10** (Suppl. 1), i4–i11

Thun, M.J. & Heath, C.W., Jr (1997) Changes in mortality from smoking in two American Cancer Society prospective studies since 1959. *Prev. Med.*, **26**, 422–426

Thun, M.J., Myers, D.G., Day-Lally, C., Namboodiri, M.M., Calle, E.E., Flanders, W.D., Adams, S.L. & Heath, C.W., Jr (1997a) Age and the exposure–response relationships between cigarette smoking and premature death in cancer prevention study II. In: *Changes in Cigarettes Related Disease Risks and Their Implication for Prevention and Control* (Smoking and Tobacco Control Monograph No. 8; NIH Publication No. 97-4213), Bethesda, MD, US Department of Health and Human Services, National Institutes of Health

Thun, M.J., Lally, C.A., Flannery, J.T., Calle, E.E., Flanders, W.D. & Heath, C.W., Jr (1997b) Cigarette smoking and changes in the histopathology of lung cancer. *J. natl Cancer Inst.*, **89**, 1580–1586

Thun, M.J., Day-Lally, C., Myers, D.G., Calle, E.E., Flanders, W.D., Zhu, B.-P., Namboodiri, M.M. & Heath, C.W., Jr (1997c) Trends in tobacco smoking and mortality from cigarette use in cancer prevention studies I (1959 through 1965) and II (1982 through 1988). In: *Changes in Cigarettes Related Disease Risks and Their Implication for Prevention and Control* (Smoking and Tobacco Control Monograph No. 8; NIH Publication No. 97-4213), Bethesda, MD, US Department of Health and Human Services, National Institutes of Health

Thun, M.J., Calle, E.E., Rodriguez, C. & Wingo, P.A. (2000) Epidemiological research at the American Cancer Society. *Cancer Epidemiol. Biomark. Prev.*, **9**, 861–868

Thun, M.J., Henley, S.J. & Calle, E.E. (2002) Tobacco use and cancer: An epidemiologic perspective for geneticists. *Oncogene*, **21**, 7307–7325

Tousey, P.M., Wolfe, K.W., Mozeleski, A., Mohr, D.L., Cantrell, B.B., O'Donnell, M., Heath, C.W. & Blot, W.J. (1999) Determinants of the excessive rates of lung cancer in northeast Florida. *South. med. J.*, **92**, 493–501

Travis, W.D., Travis, L.B. & Devesa, S.S. (1995) Lung cancer. *Cancer*, **75** (Suppl.), 191–202

Tulinius, H., Sigfússon, N., Sigvaldason, H., Bjarnadóttir, K. & Tryggvadóttir, L. (1997) Risk factors for malignant diseases: A cohort study on a population of 22 946 Icelanders. *Cancer Epidemiol. Biomarkers Prev.*, **6**, 863–873

Tverdal, A., Thelle, D., Stensvold, I., Leren, P. & Bjartveit, K. (1993) Mortality in relation to smoking history: 13 years' follow-up of 68 000 Norwegian men and women 35–49 years. *J clin. Epidemiol.*, **46**, 475–487

Wakai, K., Ohno, Y., Genka, K., Ohmine, K., Kawamura, T., Tamakoshi, A., Aoki, R., Kojima, M., Lin, Y., Aoki, K. & Fukuma, S. (1997) Smoking habits, local brand cigarettes and lung cancer risk in Okinawa, Japan. *J. Epidemiol.*, **7**, 99–105

Wakai, K., Seki, N., Tamakoshi, A., Kondo, T., Nishino, Y., Ito, Y., Suzuki, K., Ozasa, K., Watanabe, Y. & Ohno, Y. (2001) Decrease in risk of lung cancer death in males after smoking cessation by age at quitting: Findings from the JACC study. *Jpn. J. Cancer Res.*, **92**, 821–828

Wald, N.J. & Watt, H.C. (1997) Prospective study of effect of switching from cigarettes to pipes or cigars on mortality from three smoking related diseases. *Br. med. J.*, **314**, 1860–1863

Wang, S.Y., Hu, Y.L., Wu, Y.L., Li, X., Chi, G.B., Chen, Y. & Dai, W.S. (1996) A comparative study of the risk factors for lung cancer in Guangdong, China. *Lung Cancer*, **14** (Suppl. 1), S99–S105

Wang, Z., Lubin, J.H., Wang, L., Zhang, S,. Boice, J.D., Jr, Cui, H., Zhang, S., Conrath, S., Xia, Y., Shang, B., Brenner, A., Lei, S., Metayer, C., Cao, J., Chen, K.W., Lei, S. & Kleinerman, R.A. (2002) Residential radon and lung cancer risk in a high-exposure area of Gansu Province, China. *Am. J. Epidemiol.*, **155**, 554–564

Weir, J.M. & Dunn, J.E., Jr (1970) Smoking and mortality: A prospective study. *Cancer*, **25**, 105–112

Wilcox, A.J. (1994) Re: "Are female smokers at higher risk for lung cancer than male smokers? A case–control analysis by histologic type". *Am. J. Epidemiol.*, **140**, 186

Wilcox, H.B., Schoenberg, J.B., Mason, T.J., Bill, J.S. & Stemhagen, A. (1988) Smoking and lung cancer: Risk as a function of cigarette tar content. *Prev. Med.*, **17**, 263–272

Wunsch-Filho, V., Moncau, J.E., Mirabelli, D. & Boffetta, P. (1998) Occupational risk factors of lung cancer in Sao Paulo, Brazil. *Scand. J. Work Environ. Health*, **24**, 118–124

Wu-Williams, A.H., Dai, X.D., Blot, W., Xu, Z.Y., Sun, X.W., Xiao, H.P., Stone, B.J., Yu, S.F., Feng, Y.P., Ershow, A.G., Sun, J., Fraumeni, J.F., Jr & Henderson, B.E. (1990) Lung cancer among women in North-east China. *Br. J. Cancer*, **62**, 982–987

Xu, Z.Y., Blot, W.J., Xiao, H.P., Wu, A., Feng, Y.P., Stone, B.J., Sun, J., Ershow, A.G., Henderson, B.E. & Fraumeni, J.F. (1989) Smoking, air pollution, and the high rates of lung cancer in Shenyang, China. *J. natl Cancer Inst.*, **81**, 1800–1806

Xu, Z.Y., Brown, L., Pan, G.W., Li, G., Feng, Y.P., Guan, D.X., Liu, T.F., Liu, L.M., Chao, R.M., Sheng, J.H. & Gao, G.C. (1996) Lifestyle, environmental pollution and lung cancer in cities of Liaoning in northeastern China. *Lung Cancer*, **14** (Suppl. 1), S149–S160

Yu, S.Z. & Zhao, N. (1996) Combined analysis of case–control studies of smoking and lung cancer in China. *Lung Cancer*, **14** (Suppl. 1), 161–170

Yuan, J.M., Ross, R.K., Wang, X.L., Gao, Y.T., Henderson, B.E. & Yu, M.C. (1996) Morbidity and mortality in relation to cigarette smoking in Shanghai, China. A prospective male cohort study. *J. Am. med. Assoc.*, **275**, 1646–1650

Zang, E.A. & Wynder, E.L. (1992) Cumulative tar exposure. A new index for estimating lung cancer risk among cigarette smokers. *Cancer*, **70**, 69–76

Zang, E.A. & Wynder, E.L. (1996) Differences in lung cancer risk between men and women: Examination of the evidence. *J. natl Cancer Inst.*, **88**, 183–192

2.1.2 *Cancer of the lower urinary tract*

The 'lower urinary tract' comprises the renal pelvis, ureter, bladder and urethra. Cancers originating in the urothelium at these sites are mostly transitional-cell carcinomas or squamous-cell carcinomas. These cancers are discussed together, unless a particular distinction has been made in the studies that were considered.

In the previous *IARC Monograph* on tobacco smoking (IARC, 1986), cancer of the lower urinary tract was identified as being causally associated with cigarette smoking.

(*a*)   *Analytical studies*

Results in support of the association of cigarette smoking with cancer of the lower urinary tract have been reported from cohort studies conducted in the United Kingdom (British Doctors' Study), Sweden (Swedish Twin Registry Study, Swedish Census Study), Norway (Norwegian Cohort Study), Iceland (Reykjavík Study), the USA (American Cancer Society Study, US Veterans' Study, Californian Study, Cancer Prevention Study I, American Men of Japanese Ancestry Study, MRFIT Study, Adventists' Health Study), Canada (Canadian War Veterans' Study), China (Shanghai Men's Study), China, Province of Taiwan (Taiwanese Study), Japan (Life Span Study, Six-prefecture Study, Chiba Center Association Study). The design of these studies is described in the introduction to Section 2 and Table 2.1.

The designs of the available case–control studies are summarized in Table 2.1.2.1.

With the exception of the study by Anthony and Thomas (1970), in Leeds (United Kingdom) and the very small study of Liaw and Chen (1998) in China, Province of Taiwan, all the others have shown an association between cancer of the lower urinary tract and cigarette smoking. Irrespective of the design (cohort, hospital-based or population-based case–control), all other studies have found a positive association, and this overall result cannot be explained by bias. Potential confounders — in addition to age and gender — that may be considered are certain occupational exposures, particularly to aromatic amines, and schistosomiasis in developing countries.

However, Akiba and Hirayama (1990) and Momas *et al.* (1994a) reported estimates adjusted by occupation, which did not differ from other estimates. Two studies from Egypt (Makhyoun, 1974; Bedwani *et al.*, 1998) and one study from Zimbabwe (Vizcaino *et al.*, 1994) investigated smoking after stratification by bilharziasis (schistosomiasis); the risk of cancer of the lower urinary tract in smokers remained elevated after adjustment for urinary bilharziasis.

(i)   *Number of cigarettes smoked and duration of cigarette smoking*

Tables 2.1.2.2 and 2.1.2.3 give the relative risks according to average daily number of cigarettes smoked. One case–control study conducted in Leeds, United Kingdom (Cartwright *et al.*, 1983), failed to show a clear-cut dose–response relationship in men, although a statistically significant overall relative risk of 1.6 was found. [The Working

Group noted that the control group used in this study included patients with tobacco-related diseases, a choice that could have biased the result.] Considerable variations in the relationship between relative risks and average daily number of cigarettes smoked are evident. For male smokers of more than 20 cigarettes/day, the relative risks tend to be around 5.0 or higher in studies in Europe, and lower in studies in America and Japan. High estimates have been reported in particular from Uruguay (De Stefani *et al.*, 1991), France (Clavel *et al.*, 1989; Momas *et al.*, 1994b), Denmark (Lockwood, 1961) and Italy (Vineis *et al.*, 1984; Donato *et al.*, 1997).

Twelve of the 42 studies with a case–control design and 10/24 of those with a cohort design reported a levelling-off of the dose–response curve. This phenomenon can be interpreted either as an effect of bias (underestimation of consumption by heavy smokers) or as a genuine effect, due, for example, to the saturation of metabolic enzymes (Vineis *et al.*, 2000). [The Working Group noted that the wide variations in the dose–response relationship could be explained by a number of factors, namely, different study designs, different ways of smoking or different types of tobacco smoked. It was noted that the apparent levelling-off of the dose–response curve could reflect an artefact in data collection, due to under-reporting of levels of consumption by the interviewees.]

The 24 cohort studies have consistently shown an excess of deaths from bladder cancer among smokers; the relative risks were between 3.0 and 5.4 for smokers of 20 or more cigarettes/day (Table 2.1.2.2).

Duration of cigarette smoking showed a positive relationship with relative risks for bladder cancer in all the studies that have examined it (Table 2.1.2.4). Also, age at starting smoking (Table 2.1.2.4) has been found to be positively associated with risk; smokers who started smoking at an earlier age were at a higher risk for bladder cancer. However, duration, age at starting and age at stopping are closely correlated variables, and few studies have tried to disentangle them (Hartge *et al.*, 1993).

When cancers of the renal pelvis and of the ureter are considered separately, a dose–response relationship with daily or cumulative consumption of tobacco is found, and relative risks are similar to those reported for cancer of the bladder (McCredie *et al.*, 1982, 1983; McLaughlin *et al.*, 1983, 1992).

(ii)   *Effect of stopping cigarette smoking*

A lowering of risk after stopping cigarette smoking is seen in almost all the studies (Table 2.1.2.5), and it is particularly evident from studies conducted in the USA (Kahn, 1966; Wynder & Goldsmith, 1977; Rogot & Murray, 1980; Morrison *et al.*, 1984; Mills *et al.*, 1991), Canada (Howe *et al.*, 1980), France (Clavel *et al.*, 1989), Italy (Vineis *et al.*, 1984; D'Avanzo *et al.*, 1990; Donato *et al.*, 1997), Germany (Pommer *et al.*, 1999), the United Kingdom (Doll & Peto, 1976; Cartwright *et al.*, 1983; Morrison *et al.*, 1984), Japan (Morrison *et al.*, 1984) and Sweden (Steineck *et al.*, 1988).

(iii) *Type of cigarette and effect of inhaling*

In six studies (Vineis *et al.*, 1984; Clavel *et al.*, 1989; D'Avanzo *et al.*, 1990; De Stefani *et al.*, 1991; Lopez-Abente *et al.*, 1991; Momas *et al.*, 1994b) (Table 2.1.2.6), separate estimates were reported for the relative risks for lower urinary tract cancers for smokers of black (air-cured) and blond (flue-cured) tobacco. Relative risks for smokers of black tobacco were 1.5 to two times higher than those for smokers of blond tobacco, after adjustment for age, occupation, average daily consumption of cigarettes, years since stopping and use of a filter tip.

A strong effect of inhaling was shown in the studies by Clavel *et al.* (1989) and Lopez-Abente *et al.* (1991). A slight effect of inhaling was reported by Cole *et al.* (1971), Howe *et al.* (1980), Morrison *et al.* (1984) and Burch *et al.* (1989) but not by Lockwood (1961) (Table 2.1.2.6).

The effects of filter-tipped cigarettes have been analysed in several studies, with conflicting results (Table 2.1.2.7). A weak effect of filter-tipped cigarettes was reported by Howe *et al.* (1980), Cartwright *et al.* (1983), Vineis *et al.* (1984), López-Abente *et al.* (1991) and De Stefani *et al.* (1991), whereas no difference between the effects of smoking filter-tipped and untipped cigarettes was found in the studies by Wynder and Goldsmith (1977), Morrison *et al.* (1984) or Momas *et al.* (1994b).

(iv) *Histology*

Almost all of the cancers of the lower urinary tract encompassing bladder, renal pelvis and ureter are transitional-cell cancers in industrialized countries, but squamous-cell carcinomas are common in developing countries. One pooled analysis by Fortuny *et al.* (1999) (Table 2.1.2.3) considered non-transitional-cell bladder cancers, mainly epidermoid cancers, and found elevated relative risks in association with smoking and a positive dose–response relationship. A small study in Zimbabwe (Vizcaino *et al.*, 1994) found that the association with smoking was present (but not statistically significant) only in transitional-cell carcinomas.

(b) *Population characteristics*

(i) *Effect of gender*

Tables 2.1.2.2 and 2.1.2.3 show the relative risks according to the number of cigarettes smoked, by gender. There are only slight differences between men and women, and this holds true for subsequent tables. The differences seem to be attributable more to chance (specifically because there have been fewer studies among women) than to real differences in susceptibility to the effects of tobacco smoking.

A population-based study was conducted in Los Angeles, USA, with the aim of addressing the gender differences in susceptibility to bladder cancer (Castelao *et al.*, 2001). The risk for women was statistically significantly higher than that for men ($p = 0.016$ for interaction). Biochemical evidence was also provided: the slopes of the regression lines of 3-aminobiphenyl (3-ABP–) and 4-ABP–haemoglobin adducts by number of cigarettes smoked per day were statistically significantly steeper in women than in men ($p < 0.001$ and 0.006, respectively).

(ii)   *Effect of race/ethnicity*

Two studies considered the dose–response relationship in both whites and blacks living in the USA (Dunham *et al.*, 1968; Burns & Swanson, 1991). One study was conducted in Egypt (Makyoun, 1974), one in Iran (Sadeghi *et al.*, 1979), and several were conducted among Asians (e.g. Hirayama, 1977; Morrison *et al.*, 1984; Akiba & Hirayama, 1990; Yuan *et al.*, 1996). The differences between the various races and ethnic groups observed for the dose–response relationship are compatible with chance variation.

(c)   *Pooled analysis*

The original data from 11 of the case–control studies of bladder cancer together with those from one unpublished study have been analysed together as part of a pooled analysis consisting of 3285 cases of bladder cancer (2600 men, 685 women) and 7940 controls (5524 men, 2416 women) (Brennan *et al.*, 2000, 2001). These studies were selected as they were participating in a parallel reanalysis of data on occupational exposures and bladder cancer in Europe. Two case–control studies each were from France, Spain and Italy, three from Germany and one each from Denmark and Greece (Vineis *et al.*, 1985; Rebelakos *et al.*, 1985; Claude *et al.*, 1986; Jensen *et al.*, 1987; Lopez-Abente *et al.*, 1991; Clavel *et al.*, 1989; Bolm-Audorff *et al.*, 1993; Hours *et al.*, 1994; Greiser & Molzahn, 1997; Donato *et al.*, 1997; Serra *et al.*, 2000). All studies included both men and women.

(i)   *Duration of smoking*

An increasing risk of bladder cancer was observed with increasing duration of smoking. The relationship appeared to be approximately linear for both men and women. The relative increase in risk was approximately 100% after 10–19 years of smoking (odds ratio, 2.0; 95% CI, 1.5–2.6 for men; odds ratio, 2.2; 95% CI, 1.4–3.5 for women), 200% after 20–29 years of smoking (odds ratio, 3.1; 95% CI, 2.5–3.9 for men; odds ratio, 2.5; 95% CI, 1.7–3.8 for women) and 300% after 40 years of smoking (odds ratio, 3.8; 95% CI, 3.1–4.6 for men; odds ratio, 3.9; 95% CI, 2.8–5.4 for women).

(ii)   *Intensity of smoking*

A dose–relationship was observed between number of cigarettes smoked per day and bladder cancer up to an apparent threshold of 15–19 cigarettes per day (odds ratio, 4.5; 95% CI, 3.8–5.3 for men; odds ratio, 3.8; 95% CI, 2.7–5.4 for women), after which a plateau in the risk was observed for both male and female smokers of more than 20 cigarettes per day.

(iii)   *Smoking cessation*

An immediate decrease in risk of bladder cancer was observed among men who gave up smoking. Compared with current smokers, this fall was close to 40% for male smokers who had stopped smoking between 1 and 4 years prior to diagnosis (odds ratio, 0.65;

95% CI, 0.53–0.79) and reached 60% after 25 years of cessation (odds ratio, 0.37; 95% CI, 0.30–0.45). However, even after 25 years, the risk was not as low as that for non-smokers (odds ratio, 0.20; 95% CI, 0.17–0.24). Among women, the immediate decrease in risk was approximately 30% for smokers who stopped smoking between 1 and 4 years prior to diagnosis. The risk did not appear to decrease substantially after this and, even after 25 years of cessation, it remained considerably above the level found for never-smokers.

(iv)   *Attributable fraction*

The proportion of bladder cancer cases attributable to ever smoking, i.e. the population attributable risk (PAR), was calculated as 0.66 for men (95% CI, 0.61–0.70) and 0.30 (95% CI, 0.25–0.35) for women. Similarly, the PAR of bladder cancer cases attributable to current smoking was calculated as 0.32 (95% CI, 0.28–0.35) for men and 0.18 (95% CI, 0.14–0.22) for women. [The Working Group noted that the lower attributable proportions among women reflect the earlier stage of the smoking-related disease epidemic among women, and these attributable fractions may be expected to increase in the future as this epidemic becomes more widespread among women.]

Table 2.1.2.1. Case–control studies on tobacco smoking and lower urinary tract cancer: main characteristics of study design

Reference Country and years of study	Numbers of cases and controls	Criteria for eligibility and comments
Lilienfeld et al. (1956) USA 1945–55	Men: 321 cases and 663 controls; women: 118 cases and 1205 controls	Hospital-based study; controls: 287 men with prostate cancers, 39 men with benign bladder conditions and 337 healthy men; 776 women with breast cancers, 110 women with benign bladder conditions and 319 healthy women
Lockwood (1961) Denmark 1956–57	Men: 282 cases and 282 controls; women: 87 cases and 87 controls	Population-based study; living cases from the Danish Cancer Registry (1956–57); controls selected from Population Registry
Schwartz et al. (1961) France Study started in 1954	Men: 214 cases and 214 controls	Hospital-based study; age-matched controls were subjects admitted to hospitals for accidents
Wynder et al. (1963a) USA 1960–61	Men: 300 cases and 300 controls; women: 70 cases and 70 controls	Hospital-based study, papillomas excluded; sex- and age-matched controls: cancers of respiratory system, upper alimentary tract and myocardial infarction excluded
Cobb & Ansell (1965) USA 1951–61	Men and women: 136 cases and 342 controls	Hospital-based study; 120 colon cancer controls and 222 controls with 'pulmonary problems'; data on smoking available for 131 cases
Staszewski (1966) Poland 1958–64	Men: 150 cases and 750 controls	Hospital-based study; age-matched controls with cancer or other diseases
Dunham et al. (1968) USA 1958–64	Men: 334 cases and 350 controls; women: 159 cases and 177 controls	402 incident cases in New Orleans and 91 prevalent cases or cases not living in the city; hospital controls, including unspecified numbers of patients with bronchitis, emphysema, myocardial infarction; 162 (29%) of eligible cases not interviewed
Anthony & Thomas (1970) UK 1958–67	Men: 381 cases and 275 controls	Hospital-based study; surgical controls (excluding patients with chest, genitourinary and malignant disease) in 1955–58

Table 2.1.2.1 (contd)

Reference Country and years of study	Numbers of cases and controls	Criteria for eligibility and comments
Cole *et al.* (1971) USA 1967–68	Men: 360 cases and 381 controls; women: 108 cases and 117 controls	Cases randomly selected among all (668) eligible incident cases occurring in 1967–68 in 87 cities of the Boston area (20–89 years old); controls: random sample of 20–89-year-old residents, matched for sex and age; interviews of 140/470 cases and 78/500 controls conducted with spouse or next of kin
Tyrell *et al.* (1971) Ireland 1967–68	Men: 200 cases and 200 controls; women: 50 cases and 50 controls	Hospital-based study; age- and sex-matched urological controls
Makhyoun (1974) Egypt 1966–71	Men: 365 cases and 365 controls	Hospital-based study; age-matched non-cancer controls; 278 cases and 278 matched controls had previous urinary bilharziasis
Morgan & Jain (1974) Canada	Men: 158 cases and 158 controls; women: 74 cases and 74 controls	Hospital-based study; controls matched for sex and age; postal questionnaires: responses were 67% (cases) and 57% (controls) among men; 73% (cases) and 57% (controls) among women
Schmauz & Cole (1974) USA	Men: 18 cases and 376 controls	Population-based study of cancer of the renal pelvis and ureter (see Cole *et al.*, 1971, for design)
Wynder & Goldsmith (1977) USA 1969–74	Men: 574 cases and 574 controls; women: 158 cases and 158 controls	Hospital-based study on cases aged 40–80 years and controls matched for sex, ethnic group, hospital and age; controls had no 'tobacco-related condition'.
Miller *et al.* (1978) Canada	Men: 188 cases and 564 controls; women: 77 cases and 231 controls	Hospital-based study, using self-completed questionnaires of subjects over 40 years; two sex- and age-matched controls for each case
Sadeghi *et al.* (1979) Iran 1969–76	Men: 88 cases and 88 controls	Hospital-based study; sex- and age-matched hospital controls; patients with cancer, pulmonary and bladder disease excluded (23/122 cases excluded due to poor information)

Table 2.1.2.1 (contd)

Reference Country and years of study	Numbers of cases and controls	Criteria for eligibility and comments
Howe et al. (1980) Canada 1974–76	Men: 480 cases and 480 controls; women: 152 cases and 152 controls	Population-based study; eligible cases were all patients with newly diagnosed bladder cancer in 3 Canadian provinces (77% interviewed); controls matched for sex, age and neighbourhood (controls who refused were substituted); male cases had a higher level of education and income than controls.
Tola et al. (1980) Finland 1975–76	Men: 134 cases and 134 controls; women: 46 cases and 46 controls	Originally eligible cases were all those (274) reported to the Finnish Cancer Registry for 5 Finnish provinces; postal questionnaires sent to 269 cases and 271 sex- and age-matched hospital controls or their relatives; response rates were 80% (cases) and 81% (controls); source of information was a relative for 39% of cases and 12% of controls.
McCredie et al. (1982) Australia 1977–80	Men: 27 cases and 70 controls; women: 40 cases and 110 controls	Cancer registry and hospital-based study; renal pelvis cancer cases; first control group were friends or relatives of other patients; second control group were subjects attending a screening clinic; 24 cases interviewed by their doctors, remaining cases and all controls interviewed by researchers; higher socio-economic status among screening clinic controls
Najem et al. (1982) USA 1978	Men: 65 cases and 123 controls; women: 10 cases and 19 controls	Hospital-based study; prevalent cases only; 2 controls per case matched for sex, age, ethnic group, place of birth and place of residence (patients with cancer and tobacco-related heart disease excluded)
Cartwright et al. (1983) UK 1978–81	Men: 932 cases and 1402 controls; women: 327 cases and 579 controls	90% of incident cases in West Yorkshire (1978–81) and prevalent cases included; sex- and age-matched hospital controls (25% arterial disease; 60% accident, minor surgery; 10% chest conditions)

Table 2.1.2.1 (contd)

Reference Country and years of study	Numbers of cases and controls	Criteria for eligibility and comments
McCredie *et al.* (1983) Australia 1977–82 (ureter), 1980–82 (renal pelvis)	Men: 65 cases and 307 controls	Population-based (cancer registry) study; cancers of the ureter (36 cases) and renal pelvis (29 cases) only; controls were a random sample of the general population; questionnaires posted to cases and controls (no. of non-respondents not given); higher educational level among controls
McLaughlin *et al.* (1983) USA 1974–79	Men: 50 cases and 428 controls; women: 24 cases and 269 controls	Population-based study on cancer of the renal pelvis (71/74 were transitional-cell carcinomas); controls were (1) a random sample of the general population and (2) a group of deceased individuals matched to the deceased cases
Møller-Jensen *et al.* (1983) Denmark 1979–81	Men: 286 cases and 574 controls; women: 95 cases and 193 controls	Cases, two-thirds of all incident cases in Greater Copenhagen (under age 75 years); controls, a random sample of the general population (out of 1052 controls approached, 109 refused, 114 were not located and 39 were too ill)
Mommsen & Aagaard (1983) Denmark 1977–79 (men), 1977–80 (women)	Men: 165 cases and 165 controls; women: 47 cases and 94 controls	Population-based study; controls: random sample of general population; cases interviewed in hospital, controls by phone
Morrison *et al.* (1984) Japan and UK, 1976–78; USA, 1976–77	Men: Greater Manchester, 398 cases, 490 controls; Nagoya (Japan), 224 cases, 442 controls; Boston area, 427 cases, 391 controls Women: Greater Manchester, 155 cases, 241 controls; Nagoya, 66 cases, 146 controls; Boston area, 165 cases, 142 controls	Population-based study in Japan, UK and USA; 96% (Manchester), 84% (Nagoya) and 81% (Boston) of all incident cases (aged 21–89 years) were interviewed; controls were randomly selected from electoral registers; in Nagoya most cases were interviewed in hospital, all other groups at home; 95% of tumours were of the bladder.

Table 2.1.2.1 (contd)

Reference Country and years of study	Numbers of cases and controls	Criteria for eligibility and comments
Vineis *et al.* (1984) Italy 1978–83	Men: 512 cases and 596 controls	Hospital-based study; 210/512 prevalent cases; 225 age-matched controls (with urological disease); 287 cases and 371 unmatched controls from surgical departments (87 hernias, 41 peripheral arteriopathies and other diagnoses)
Rebekalos *et al.* (1985) Greece 1980–82	Men: 250 cases and controls; women: 50 cases and controls	Hospital-based study. Histologically confirmed cases of bladder cancer. Sex- and age-matched controls from accidents centre of another hospital (traumatic fractures, 185; other traumatic conditions, 30; osteoarthrosis, 32; rheumatoid arthritis, 28; other orthopaedic conditions, 24).
Claude *et al.* (1986) Germany 1977–82	Men: 340 cases and controls; women: 91 cases and controls	Hospital-based study; 21% of controls selected from homes for the elderly. Interviews carried out by medical students using a standardized questionnaire. 90% of cases had bladder tumours (remainder had cancers of renal pelvis, ureter or urethra or combinations of these). Male controls had prostate adenomas and infections (70%), urinary tract infections (20%). Female controls had urinary tract infections (68%) or no particular illness (24%).
Burch *et al.* (1989) Canada 1979–82	781 cases and 781 matched controls	Population-based study. Only 67% of eligible cases were interviewed. Response rate for controls, 53%.
Clavel *et al.* (1989) France 1984–87	477 cases and 477 matched controls	Hospital-based study using interview; 157 prevalent cases; controls: patients with tobacco-related conditions were excluded. Refusal rate not given
D'Avanzo *et al.* (1990) Italy 1985–89	337 cases and 392 controls	Hospital-based study using interviews. Refusals < 3%. Controls had trauma (30%), orthopaedic conditions (17%) and surgical conditions.

Table 2.1.2.1 (contd)

Reference Country and years of study	Numbers of cases and controls	Criteria for eligibility and comments
Harris *et al.* (1990) USA 1969 onwards	White men: 1114 cases, 3252 controls; black men, 84 cases, 271 controls; white women: 420 cases, 1289 controls; black women, 45 cases, 118 controls	Hospital-based study. Incident cases. Controls included gastrointestinal disease, infections, leukaemia, benign prostatic hypertrophy, benign neoplastic disease, other cancers and other causes. Controls were matched on sex, age, race, year of interview and hospital of diagnosis.
Burns & Swanson (1991) USA	White men: 1410 cases, 1615 controls; black men: 161 cases, 382 controls; white women: 504 cases, 1600 controls; black women, 85 cases, 382 controls	Population-based study; controls: incident cases of colorectal cancer. Telephone interviews. Response rates, 94% (cases) and 95% (controls)
De Stefani *et al.* (1991) Uruguay 1987–89	Men: 91 cases and 182 controls; women: 20 cases and 40 controls	Hospital-based study, only incident cases; 29% of controls had malignant tumours, 22% eye diseases. No refusals
López-Abente *et al.* (1991) Spain 1983–86	430 cases, 405 hospital controls and 386 population controls	Hospital and population-based study; 49% were prevalent cases. Controls matched by sex and age. Refusals: 5% of cases, 7% of hospital controls, 7% of population controls. Hospital controls: patients with tobacco-related diagnoses excluded
Kunze *et al.* (1992) Germany 1977–85	Men: 531 cases and 531 controls; women: 144 cases and 144 controls	Hospital-based study. Controls matched by sex and age; diagnoses included prostate hyperplasia (64% of men) or infection of urinary tract (73% of women)
McLaughlin *et al.* (1992) USA 1983–86	Men: 331 cases and 315 controls; women: 171 cases and 181 controls	Population-based study in New Jersey, Iowa and California. Incident cases of cancers of the renal pelvis and ureter, microscopically confirmed, aged 20–79 years, identified using the local population-based cancer registries; 58% of ascertained cases participated. Controls selected by random-digit dialling (< 65 years) or Health Care Financial Administration rosters (≥ 65 years), frequency-matched on age (5-year groups) and sex; response rate, 54–66%

Table 2.1.2.1 (contd)

Reference Country and years of study	Numbers of cases and controls	Criteria for eligibility and comments
Hartge et al. (1993) USA Study started in 1978	White men: 1925 cases, 3642 controls; black men: 88 cases, 277 controls; white women: 633 cases, 1295 controls; black women: 33 cases, 106 controls	Population-based study. Cases drawn from 5 states and 5 metropolitan areas in the SEER network of cancer registries in 1978; controls selected by random-digit dialling or Health Care Financing Administration files
Vena et al. (1993) USA 1979–85	White men: 351 cases and 855 controls	Population-based study. Only incident cases. Controls were matched on sex, age and neighbourhood. Response rates were 42% in controls and 76% in cases [sampling of controls not described].
Barbone et al. (1994) Italy 1986–90	273 cases and 573 controls	Hospital-based study using interviews. Controls had trauma (20%), orthopaedic conditions (35%), surgical conditions (26%).
Hours et al. (1994) France 1984–87	Men and women: 116 cases and 232 controls	Hospital-based study. Two groups of controls with diseases other than cancer, matched for sex, hospital, age and nationality, one from same hospital ward and one from another ward of same hospital as case; most frequent diagnoses among urological ward controls were benign adenoma of the prostate (48/116) and urinary lithiasis (22/116); most common among general hospital controls were cardiovascular (42/116), digestive system (10/116) and endocrine (11/116) diseases. Job/other histories obtained by interview. Papillomas of urinary bladder included; 30–75 years of age
Momas et al. (1994a,b) France 1987–89	219 cases and 794 controls	Population-based study. Controls sought from electoral rolls. Only incident cases. Cases and 558 controls interviewed by telephone, 236 controls by post. Response rate, 81% (telephone), 72% (postal) in controls and 219/272 (80.5%) cases
Sorahan et al. (1994) UK 1985–87	989 cases, 2059 population controls and 1599 patients of general practitioners	Mixed design (population controls and patients of general practitioners). Postal questionnaires. Response rate not given

Table 2.1.2.1 (contd)

Reference Country and years of study	Numbers of cases and controls	Criteria for eligibility and comments
Vizcaino *et al.* (1994) Zimbabwe 1963–77	Black men: 494 cases and 4412 controls; black women: 186 cases and 3789 controls	Analysis of data from Bulwayo cancer registry; controls comprised all other registered cancer cases excluding 'tobacco-related sites' (oesophagus, larynx and lung); interviews conducted either with subject at time of hospitalization or with relatives; individuals with current bilharzia or haematuria were excluded. Complete interview obtained for 72.2% of cases and 70.3% of controls
McCarthy *et al.* (1995) USA 1975–92	Men: 217 cases and 860 controls; women: 84 cases and 336 controls	Population-based study. Controls sampled from private census (covering 90% of residents), including information on smoking
Donato *et al.* (1997) Italy 1991–92	Men: 135 cases and 398 controls; women: 37 cases and 180 controls	Hospital-based study. Only incident cases. Controls had prostate adenoma (40%), urolithiasis (48%). Response rate not given.
Bedwani *et al.* (1998) Egypt 1994–96	Men: 151 cases and 157 controls	Hospital-based study; controls had traumatic and other orthopaedic conditions (35%), acute surgical diseases (27%), eye diseases (8%), miscellaneous (30%). Women were excluded due to low proportion of current smokers (1/39 cases); questionnaires completed by trained interviewers.
Pohlabeln *et al.* (1999) Germany 1989–92	Men: 239 matched pairs; women: 61 matched pairs (age and area of residence)	Hospital-based study. Incident cases. Response rate, 93% in cases and 98% in controls. Male controls had prostate adenoma (41%) or kidney stones (30%). Female controls had kidney stones (62%). Interviews
Pommer *et al.* (1999) Germany 1990–94	Men: 415 cases and 415 controls; women: 232 cases and 232 controls	Population-based study. Incident cases. Controls sought from municipality registry, matched on sex and age; 11% of cases and 29% of controls refused to participate.
Serra *et al.* (2000) Spain 1993–95	Men: 196 cases and 314 controls; women: 22 cases and 30 controls	Population-based study. Incidence cases, all histologically confirmed (93.6% transitional-cell carcinomas). Controls with no known benign or malignant tumour of the urinary tract, from the same county, selected using municipal-based census lists. Matched by sex, age and residence

Table 2.1.2.1 (contd)

Reference Country and years of study	Numbers of cases and controls	Criteria for eligibility and comments
Castelao *et al.* (2001) USA 1987–96	Men and women: 1514 cases and 1514 controls	Population-based study. Non-Asian patients with histologically confirmed bladder cancer. Controls matched by sex, age, race (non-Hispanic white, Hispanic, African American) and neighbourhood of residence. Structured questionnaires were completed at an interview in the participant's home. Peripheral blood samples collected to measure 3- and 4-aminobiphenyl–haemoglobin adducts.

Combined analyses

Fortuny *et al.* (1999) Europe 1983–95	Men and women: 146 cases and 292 controls	Combined analysis of 9 case–control studies (9/11 described in Brennan *et al.*, 2000). Non-transitional-cell carcinoma of the bladder only.
Brennan *et al.* (2000, 2001) Europe 1976–96	Men: 2600 cases and 5524 controls; women: 685 cases and 2416 controls	Combined analysis of 11 case–control studies. Recruitment of cases was hospital-based, that of controls either hospital-based (7 centres), population-based (3 centres) or both (1 centre). Diseases of hospital-based controls varied among centres, although all subjects were affected by diseases unrelated to smoking.

Table 2.1.2.2. Cohort studies on tobacco smoking and cancer of the lower urinary tract: intensity of smoking

Reference Country and years of study	Cohort study Subjects	Smoking categories	Relative risk (no. of cases or 95% CI)	Comments
Hammond & Horn (1958a,b) USA 1952–55	American Cancer Society (9-state) Study 187 783 men	Cig/day 1–9 10–20 > 21	2.0 (14) 2.0 (42) 3.4 (41)	Microscopically verified cancer of the genitourinary system
		Smoker	2.2 (59)	Microscopically verified bladder cancer only
Hammond (1966) USA 1959–63	Cancer Prevention Study (CPS) I 440 558 men	Ever-smoker aged 45–64 years aged 65–79 years	1.8 (59) 2.9 (56)	Relative risks calculated by the Working Group as ratios of age-adjusted annual death rates
Kahn (1966) USA 1954–62	US Veterans' Study 293 658 men	Cig/day < 10 10–20 21–39 ≥ 40	1.0 (11) 2.3 (71) 3.1 (51) 3.0 (9)	
Lossing et al. (1966) Canada 1956–62	Canadian War Veterans' Cohort 78 000 men	Cig/day < 10 10–20 > 20	1.3 (29) 1.4 (57) 1.4 (17)	Mortality ratios; genitourinary cancers
Weir & Dunn (1970) USA 1954–62	Californian Study 68 153 men	Cig/day 1–9 10–20 ≥ 21	1.5 2.8 5.4	
Cederlöf et al. (1975) Sweden 1963–72	Swedish Census Study 25 444 men, 26 467 women	Men Cig/day 1–7 8–15 ≥ 16	1.5 (6) 1.6 (6) 2.7 (6)	
		Women Cig/day 1–7 8–15 ≥ 16	1.2 (2) 2.1 (4) 0.8 (1)	
Doll & Peto (1976) UK 1951–71	British Doctors' Study 34 440 men	Cig/day 1–14 15–24 > 25	2.2 2.2 1.4	Relative risks, calculated by the Working Group, are ratios of age-adjusted annual death rates.
Hirayama (1977, 1985) Japan 1965–81	Six-prefecture Study 122 261 men	Current smoker	1.4 (59)	

Table 2.1.2.2 (contd)

Reference Country and years of study	Cohort study Subjects	Smoking categories	Relative risk (no. of cases or 95% CI)	Comments
Doll *et al.* (1980) UK 1951–1973	British Doctors' Study 6194 women	Current smoker	0.6 (5)	
Rogot & Murray (1980) USA 1954–69	US Veterans' Study 293 958 men	Current smoker	SMR 2.2 (326)	Standardized mortality ratio
Steineck *et al.* (1988) Sweden 1967–82 (14 years)	Swedish Twin Registry Study 16 477 persons	Men Cig/day 1–9 ≥ 10 Women Ever-smoker	4.5 (2.1–9.9) 4.7 (2.0–10.8) 1.6 (0.5–5.2)	Adjusted for age
Akiba & Hirayama (1990) Japan 1965–81	Six-prefecture Study 122 261 men, 142 857 women	Men Cig/day 1–4 5–14 15–24 25–34 ≥ 35 Women 1–4 5–14 ≥ 15	1.8 (0.4–5.0) 1.4 (0.9–2.3) 2.0 (1.3–3.3) 1.7 (0.6–4.1) 2.1 (0.5–6.1) 0.9 (0.1–4.0) 2.2 (1.1–4.1) 1.2 (0.1–5.7)	Adjusted for residence, age, occupation and observation period *p* for trend = 0.005
Kuller *et al.* (1991) USA 1975–85	MRFIT Study 12 866 men	Nonsmoker 1–15 16–25 26–35 36–45 > 45	Mortality rate 1.6 (39) 1.8 (5) 3.1 (13) 4.4 (12) 3.9 (9) 3.6 (3)	Annual mortality rates/10 000 men; adjusted for age, blood pressure, cholesterol and ethnicity
Mills *et al.* (1991) USA 1976–82	Adventists' Health Study 34 198 men and women	1–14 15–24 ≥ 25	1.6 (0.6–4.1) 4.3 (1.9–9.7) 3.3 (1.3–8.6)	Adjusted for age and sex
Chyou *et al.* (1993) USA 1954–80	American Men of Japanese Ancestry Study 8006 men	Pack–years > 0–30 > 30	2.1 (1.2–3.8) 2.3 (1.3–4.1)	Adjusted for relevant variables *p* for trend = 0.004
Doll *et al.* (1994) UK 1951–91	British Doctors'Study 34 439 men	Cig/day 0 1–14 15–24 ≥ 25	Mortality rate 13 29 29 37	Annual mortality rate per 100 000 men *p* for trend < 0.01

Table 2.1.2.2 (contd)

Reference Country and years of study	Cohort study Subjects	Smoking categories	Relative risk (no. of cases or 95% CI)	Comments
McLaughlin *et al.* (1995) USA 1954–80	US Veterans' Study 293 958 men	Cig/day 1–9 10–20 31–39 ≥ 40	1.1 (0.8–1.5) 2.3 (1.9–2.7) 2.7 (2.2–3.3) 2.2 (1.5–3.3)	Adjusted for age and calendar period *p* for trend ≤ 0.01
Engeland *et al.* (1996) Norway 1966–93	Norwegian Cohort Study 11 857 men, 14 269 women	Men Cig/day 1–4 5–9 10–14 ≥ 15 Women Cig/day 1–4 5–9 10–14 ≥ 15	2.5 (1.5–4.0) 2.7 (1.6–4.5) 3.4 (2.1–5.4) 5.1 (3.1–8.4) 1.5 (0.7–3.2) 2.2 (1.0–4.7) 5.4 (2.8–11) 7.9 (3.3–19)	Adjusted for age
Murata *et al.* (1996) Japan 1984–93	Chiba Center Association Study 17 200 men	1–10 11–20 ≥ 21	2.6 2.3 1.3	Adjusted for age and county
Yuan *et al.* (1996) China 1986–93	Shanghai Men's Study 18 244 men	Cig/day < 20 ≥ 20	2.1 1.7	Adjusted for age
Nordlund *et al.* (1997) Sweden 1963–89	Swedish Census Study 25 829 women	Cig/day 1–7 8–15 ≥ 16	1.9 (0.98–3.6) 2.9 (1.4–5.8) 3.4 (1.2–9.7)	
Tulinius *et al.* (1997) Iceland 1968–95	Reykjavík Study 11 366 men	Cig/day 1–14 15–24 ≥ 25	1.5 (0.7–3.0) 2.6 (1.4–4.7) 4.6 (2.4–6.9)	
Liaw & Chen (1998) China, Province of Taiwan 1982–94	Taiwanese Study 11 096 men	Smoker	0.5 (0.2–1.7)	Very small study

Table 2.1.2.3. Case–control studies on tobacco smoking and cancer of the lower urinary tract: intensity of smoking

Reference Country and years of study	Subjects	Smoking categories[a]	Relative risk (no. of cases/deaths or 95% CI)	Comments
Lilienfeld et al. (1956) USA 1945–55	Men	Nonsmoker	1.0 (51)	Crude risks calculated by the Working Group; unadjusted
		Smoker	2.1 (151)	
	Women	Nonsmoker	1.0 (108)	
		Smoker	0.4 (10)	
Lockwood (1961) Denmark 1956–57	Men	Nonsmoker	1.0 (24)	Crude risks calculated by the Working Group
		1–10 g tobacco/day	1.3 (16)	
		11–20 g tobacco/day	3.3 (40)	
		21–30 g tobacco/day	9.5 (18)	
		≥ 31 g tobacco/day	15.8 (10)	
	Women	Nonsmoker	1.0 (49)	
		1–10 g tobacco/day	0.9 (8)	
		11–20 g tobacco/day	4.6 (4)	
		≥ 21 g tobacco/day	–	No cases or controls
Schwartz et al. (1961) France 1954 onwards	Men	Nonsmoker	1.0 (24)	Crude risks calculated by the Working Group
		1–9	1.4 (31)	
		10–19	2.1 (69)	
		20–29	2.6 (63)	
		≥ 30	3.8 (15)	

Table 2.1.2.3 (contd)

Reference Country and years of study	Subjects	Smoking categories[a]	Relative risk (no. of cases/deaths or 95% CI)	Comments
Wynder et al. (1963a) USA 1960–61	Men	Nonsmoker	1.0 (21)	Crude risks calculated by the Working Group
		1–9	2.1 (12)	
		10–15	1.5 (15)	
		16–20	2.8 (86)	
		21–34	5.2 (63)	
		≥ 35	5.7 (78)	
	Women	Nonsmoker	1.0 (43)	
		1–9	3.1 (9)	
		10–20	3.3 (14)	
		≥ 21	–	4 cases, 0 controls
Cobb & Ansell (1965) USA 1951–61	Men and women	Nonsmoker	1.0 (6)	Hospital controls with colon cancer only; heavy smokers smoked > 1 pack of cigarettes/day for ≥ 30 years; age-adjusted relative risks calculated by the Working Group
		Light and medium smoker	3.0 (21)	
		Heavy smoker	10.3 (104)	
Staszewski (1966) Poland 1958–64	Men	Nonsmoker	1.0 (10)	Nonsmoker included smokers of < 1 g tobacco per day for < 1 year.
		Smoker	2.7 (140)	
Dunham et al. (1968) USA 1958–64	Men White	Nonsmoker	1.0 (55)	Crude risks calculated by the Working Group
		< 10	1.2 (19)	
		10–19	2.1 (76)	
		≥ 20	1.1 (114)	

Table 2.1.2.3 (contd)

Reference Country and years of study	Subjects	Smoking categories[a]	Relative risk (no. of cases/deaths or 95% CI)	Comments
	Black	Nonsmoker	1.0 (14)	
		< 10	0.9 (9)	
		10–19	2.7 (25)	
		≥ 20	1.9 (21)	
	Women White	Nonsmoker	1.0 (77)	
		< 10	0.7 (6)	
		10–19	1.0 (12)	
		≥ 20	1.9 (17)	
	Black	Nonsmoker	1.0 (28)	
		< 10	1.0 (8)	
		10–19	1.0 (5)	
		≥ 20	1.9 (6)	
Anthony & Thomas (1970) UK 1958–67	Men aged 40–69 years	Nonsmoker	1.0 (18)	Only controls with surgical conditions considered; age-adjusted relative risks calculated by the Working Group
		< 15 g/day	0.7 (81)	
		≥ 15 g/day	1.1 (104)	
Cole et al. (1971) USA 1967–68	Men aged 20–89 years	Nonsmoker	1.0 (70)	Smoker defined as smoking at least 100 cigarettes in lifetime; amount considered is maximum amount smoked per day during life
		≤ ½ pack/day	1.0 (36)	
		½–1½ packs/day	2.0 (140)	
		1½–2½ packs/day	2.2 (85)	
		> 2½ packs/day	1.8 (25)	

Table 2.1.2.3 (contd)

Reference Country and years of study	Subjects	Smoking categories[a]	Relative risk (no. of cases/deaths or 95% CI)	Comments
	Women aged 20–89 years	Nonsmoker	1.0 (50)	Crude relative risks calculated by the Working Group
		≤ ½ pack/day	1.5 (13)	
		½–1½ packs/day	2.0 (30)	
		> 1½ packs/day	3.8 (12)	
Tyrrell et al. (1971) Ireland 1967–68	Men	Nonsmoker	1.0 (7)	
		Smoker	3.7 (163)	
	Women	Nonsmoker	1.0 (31)	
		Smoker	0.8 (19)	
Makhyoun (1974) Egypt 1966–71	Men with urinary bilharziasis	Nonsmoker	1.0 (66)	Moderate smokers: (average number of cigarettes per day × duration of smoking) = 300–600; heavy smokers: > 600; crude relative risks calculated by the Working Group
		Moderate smoker	1.5 (42)	
		Heavy smoker	1.4 (21)	
	Men without urinary bilharziasis	Nonsmoker	0 (15)	
		Moderate smoker	2.3 (41)	
		Heavy smoker	3.3 (28)	
Morgan & Jain (1974) Canada	Men	Nonsmoker	1.0 (22)	
		1–14	2.6 (57)	
		15–24	2.7 (42)	
		≥ 25	6.4 (37)	
	Women	Nonsmoker	1.0 (45)	
		1–14	1.2 (16)	
		15–24	1.1 (9)	
		≥ 25	4.4 (4)	

Table 2.1.2.3 (contd)

Reference Country and years of study	Subjects	Smoking categories[a]	Relative risk (no. of cases/deaths or 95% CI)	Comments
Schmauz & Cole (1974) USA	Men	Nonsmoker ≤ ½ pack/day ½–1½ pack/day 1½–2½ packs/day > 2½ packs/day	1.0 (4) 1.2 (2) 1.3 (5) 1.1 (2) 10.0 (5)	Cancer of the renal pelvis and ureter
Wynder & Goldsmith (1977) USA 1969–74	Men	Nonsmoker 1–10 11–20 21–30 31–40 ≥ 41	1.0 (65) 1.4 (0.9–2.2) 2.4 (1.7–3.3) 2.7 (1.8–4.1) 2.3 (1.5–3.4) 3.3 (2.1–5.3)	
	Women	Nonsmoker 1–10 11–20 ≥ 21	1.0 (67) 1.7 (0.9–3.3) 2.3 (1.3–4.2) 2.4 (1.1–5.1)	
Miller et al. (1978) Canada	Men	Nonsmoker Ever-smoker	1.0 1.6	
	Women	Nonsmoker Ever-smoker	1.0 0.8	
Sadeghi et al. (1979) Iran 1969–76	Men	Nonsmoker Smoker	1.0 (17) 2.0 (27)	

Table 2.1.2.3 (contd)

Reference Country and years of study	Subjects	Smoking categories[a]	Relative risk (no. of cases/deaths or 95% CI)	Comments
Howe et al. (1980) Canada 1974–76	Men	Nonsmoker < 10 10–20 > 20	1.0 2.6 (1.7–4.4) 3.8 (2.6–6.0) 5.1 (3.5–8.6)	
	Women	Nonsmoker ≤ 15 > 15	1.0 2.3 (1.3–4.6) 2.6 (1.4–6.9)	
Tola et al. (1980) Finland 1975–76	Men	Nonsmoker Ever-smoker	1.0 (19) 1.9 (114)	Crude relative risks calculated by the Working Group
	Women	Nonsmoker Ever-smoker	1.0 (25) 5.4 (17)	
McCredie et al. (1982) Australia 1977–80	Men	Nonsmoker Smoker (contacts) Smoker (screening clinic)	1.0 1.0 (0.2–4.3) 2.8 (0.7–10.4)	Cancer of renal pelvis; first set of controls, 'contacts'; second set of controls, 'screening clinic'; relative risks adjusted for consumption of analgesics
	Women (cancer of renal pelvis)	Nonsmoker Smoker (contacts) Smokers (screening clinic)	1.0 2.2 (0.8–5.9) 7.0 (2.5–19.7)	

Table 2.1.2.3 (contd)

Reference Country and years of study	Subjects	Smoking categories[a]	Relative risk (no. of cases/deaths or 95% CI)	Comments
Mommsen et al. (1982); Mommsen & Aagaard (1983); Mommsen et al. (1983) Denmark 1977–80	Men	Nonsmoker	1.0	Crude odds ratios; Figure 1 in Mommsen & Aagaard (1983) suggests that relative risks are around 6.5 for smokers of 201–300 and 9.5 for smokers of 301–400 (years × no. of cigarettes/day) during lifetime
		Smoker	1.9 (1.2–3.0)	
	Women	Nonsmoker	1.0	
		Smoker	1.9 (0.9–3.9)	
Najem et al. (1982) USA 1978	Men and women	Nonsmoker	1.0	Data not given separately
		Smoker	2.0 (1.1–3.7)	

Cartwright et al. (1983) UK 1978–81

Comments: Incident and prevalent cases considered together; reference category included nonsmokers (< 1000 cigarettes in lifetime)

		Duration of cigarette smoking (years)					
		≤ 5	6–15	16–25	26–35	36–45	≥ 46
Men	< 10	1.0	0.85	1.3	1.6	1.3	1.9
	10–20	1.0	1.8	1.8	1.5	1.7	1.8
	≥ 21	1.0	1.4	1.1	1.3	1.5	0.85
Women	< 10	1.0	2.4	1.2	1.4	1.4	1.6
	10–20	1.0	1.0	2.0	1.5	1.6	1.5
	≥ 21	Insufficient data					

Table 2.1.2.3 (contd)

Reference Country and years of study	Subjects	Smoking categories[a]	Relative risk (no. of cases/deaths or 95% CI)	Comments
McCredie et al. (1983) Australia 1977–82	Men	Nonsmoker	1.0	Cancer of the ureter; relative risks adjusted for phenacetin consumption and age
		1–249 kg tobacco in lifetime	1.9	
		≥ 250 kg tobacco in lifetime	4.6	
		Nonsmoker	1.0	Cancer of renal pelvis
		1–249 kg tobacco in lifetime	1.3	
		≥ 250 kg tobacco in lifetime	4.2	
McLaughlin et al. (1983) USA 1974–79	Men	Nonsmoker	1.0 (3)	Cancer of renal pelvis; smoking categories: light, ≤ 32 pack–years of cigarettes; moderate, 33–57; heavy, ≥ 58; relative risks adjusted for age and type of respondent (living case/control or next of kin)
		Light smoker	5.5 (1.4–25.5)	
		Moderate smoker	9.6 (2.5–43.4)	
		Heavy smoker	10.7 (2.7–48.9)	
	Women	Nonsmoker	1.0 (8)	
		Light smoker	4.9 (1.2–20.2)	
		Moderate smoker	7.6 (1.9–31.3)	
		Heavy smoker	11.1 (1.8–68.7)	
Møller-Jensen et al. (1983) Denmark 1979–81	Men	Nonsmoker	1.0 (9)	Crude relative risks calculated by the Working Group
		1–14	4.2 (82)	
		15–24	4.9 (112)	
		≥ 25	4.3 (54)	
	Women	Nonsmoker	1.0 (23)	
		1–14	2.0 (30)	
		≥ 15	2.5 (42)	

Table 2.1.2.3 (contd)

Reference Country and years of study	Subjects	Smoking categories[a]	Relative risk (no. of cases/deaths or 95% CI)	Comments
Morrison et al. (1984) UK and Japan, 1976–78 USA, 1976–77	Boston area Men	Nonsmoker	1.0 (53)	
		Current smoker		
		< 1 pack/day	1.4 (25)	
		1 pack/day	3.2 (91)	
		≥ 2 packs/day	4.7 (67)	
		Former and current smoker	1.9 (1.3–2.8)	
	Women	Nonsmoker	1.0 (49)	
		Current smoker		
		< 1 pack/day	4.3 (18)	
		≥ 1 pack/day	6.2 (48)	
		Former and current smoker	4.2 (2.5–7.1)	
	Manchester area Men	Nonsmoker	1.0 (28)	
		Current smoker		
		< 1 pack/day	1.9 (85)	
		1 pack/day	3.2 (104)	
		≥ 2 packs/day	4.0 (31)	
		Former and current smoker	2.2 (1.4–3.5)	
	Women	Nonsmoker	1.0 (63)	
		Current smoker		
		< 1 pack/day	2.1 (40)	
		≥ 1 pack/day	2.2 (26)	
		Former and current smoker	1.3 (0.8–2.0)	

Table 2.1.2.3 (contd)

Reference Country and years of study	Subjects	Smoking categories[a]	Relative risk (no. of cases/deaths or 95% CI)	Comments
	Nagoya area			
	Men	Nonsmoker	1.0 (24)	
		Current smoker		
		< 1 pack/day	1.6 (47)	
		1 pack/day	2.1 (92)	
		≥ 2 packs/day	2.8 (33)	
		Former and current smoker	1.7 (1.1–2.9)	
	Women	Nonsmoker	1.0 (45)	
		Current smoker		
		< 1 pack/day	4.4 (11)	
		≥ 1 pack/day	4.2 (7)	
		Former and current smoker	4.3 (2.0–9.2)	
Vineis *et al.* (1984) Italy 1978–83	Men	Nonsmoker	1.0 (19)	
		1–14	4.0 (2.4–6.8)	
		15–29	5.7 (3.5–9.3)	
		≥ 30	10.1 (4.9–20.7)	
Rebekalos *et al.* (1985) Greece 1980–82	Men < 50–> 70 years	Never-smoker	1.0	
		1–10	1.6 (0.9–3.1)	
		11–20	2.9 (1.9–4.6)	
		21–30	4.4 (2.4–8.0)	
		≥ 31	4.4 (2.2–8.8)	

Table 2.1.2.3 (contd)

Reference Country and years of study	Subjects	Smoking categories[a]	Relative risk (no. of cases/deaths or 95% CI)	Comments
	Men and women <59–>70 years	Never-smoker	1.0	
		1–10	1.6 (0.9–2.9)	
		11–20	2.8 (1.8–4.4)	
		21–30	4.4 (2.4–8.0)	
		≥31	4.4 (2.2–8.8)	
Claude et al. (1986) Germany 1977–82	Men	Nonsmoker	1.0	
		1–10	1.7 (1.1–2.7)	$p < 0.05$
		11–20	2.4 (1.6–3.7)	$p < 0.01$
		>20	3.2 (1.9–5.0)	$p < 0.001$
	Women	Nonsmoker	1.0	
		1–10	2.4 (1.1–5.5)	$p < 0.05$
		>10	4.9 (1.3–18.8)	$p < 0.05$
Clavel et al. (1989) France 1984–87	Men	0	1.0	Adjusted for hospital, age and residence
		1–19	3.3 (2.1–5.1)	
		20–39	4.4 (2.8–6.9)	
		≥40	6.9 (3.7–12.9)	
D'Avanzo et al. (1990) Italy 1985–89	Men	<10	2.5 (1.1–6.0)	Adjusted for age
		10–19	2.3 (1.2–4.4)	
		≥20	4.0 (2.3–6.8)	

Table 2.1.2.3 (contd)

Reference Country and years of study	Subjects	Smoking categories[a]	Relative risk (no. of cases/deaths or 95% CI)	Comments
Harris et al. (1990) USA 1969 onwards	White men	Nonsmoker	1.0	Adjusted for age, education and years since quitting
		1–10	1.5 (1.1–2.2)	
		11–20	3.0 (2.5–3.7)	
		21–30	3.7 (3.0–4.5)	
		> 30	3.6 (3.0–4.4)	
	Black men	Nonsmoker	1.0	
		1–10	1.6 (0.7–3.6)	
		11–20	1.9 (0.9–3.9)	
		21–30	2.7 (1.1–6.6)	
		> 30	2.0 (0.7–5.9)	
	White women	Nonsmoker	1.0	
		1–10	1.7 (1.2–2.5)	
		11–20	3.3 (2.4–4.1)	
		21–30	4.7 (3.1–6.9)	
		> 30	2.3 (1.3–4.0)	
	Black women	Nonsmoker	1.0	
		Ever-smoker	3.9 (1.5–6.8)	
Burns & Swanson (1991) USA	White men	Nonsmoker	1.0	Adjusted for age
		1–19	1.7 (1.3–2.1)	
		20	2.4 (1.9–2.9)	
		> 20	2.6 (2.1–3.1)	

Table 2.1.2.3 (contd)

Reference Country and years of study	Subjects	Smoking categories[a]	Relative risk (no. of cases/deaths or 95% CI)	Comments
	Black men	Nonsmoker	1.0	
		1–19	2.3 (1.3–4.0)	
		20	3.6 (2.0–6.1)	
		> 20	4.3 (2.3–7.9)	
	White women	Nonsmoker	1.0	
		1–19	1.9 (1.4–2.5)	
		20	2.6 (2.0–3.4)	
		> 20	3.0 (2.1–4.1)	
	Black women	Nonsmoker	1.0	
		1–19	3.7 (2.0–6.7)	
		20	2.5 (1.1–5.6)	
		> 20	3.7 (1.4–9.5)	
De Stefani et al. (1991) Uruguay 1987–89	Men	Nonsmoker	1.0	Adjusted for age, residence, sex and hospital
		1–14	4.7 (1.3–16.9)	
		15–29	11.5 (3.3–40.6)	
		≥ 30	8.2 (2.2–30.2)	
Lopez-Abente et al. (1991) Spain 1983–86	Men	Nonsmoker	1.0	Adjusted for age and residence
		1–10	1.9 (1.1–3.2)	
		11–20	4.8 (3.0–7.8)	
		21–30	4.1 (2.4–7.1)	
		> 30	4.2 (2.1–8.4)	

Table 2.1.2.3 (contd)

Reference Country and years of study	Subjects	Smoking categories[a]	Relative risk (no. of cases/deaths or 95% CI)	Comments
Kunze et al. (1992) Germany 1977–85	Men	Nonsmoker	1.0	Adjusted for sex and age
		1–9	1.7 (1.1–2.5)	
		10–19	2.5 (1.7–3.6)	
		20–29	3.6 (2.4–5.4)	
		30–39	9.3 (4.3–20.0)	
		≥ 40	1.9 (1.1–3.5)	
	Women	Nonsmoker	1.0	
		1–9	2.2 (1.1–4.7)	
		10–19	3.3 (1.2–9.2)	
		≥ 20	6.3 (1.7–22.9)	
McLaughlin et al. (1992) USA 1983–86	Men (n = 193)	Ever-smoker	3.9 (2.1–7.3)	Adjusted for age and study area
		Current smoker	6.5 (1.2–12.7)	Renal pelvis
		< 20	3.2 (1.4–7.2)	
		20–39	3.8 (1.9–7.6)	
		≥ 40	5.1 (2.4–10.9)	
	Women (n = 115)	Ever-smoker	2.0 (1.2–3.5)	
		Current smoker	2.4 (1.3–4.3)	
		< 20	1.4 (0.7–3.0)	
		20–39	2.7 (1.4–5.2)	
		≥ 40	3.4 (0.9–13.4)	
	Men (n = 138)	Ever-smoker	5.2 (2.4–11.9)	Ureter
		Current smoker	11.4 (4.4–31.5)	
		< 20	5.6 (2.0–16.0)	
		20–39	5.4 (2.3–13.1)	
		≥ 40	7.7 (2.6–24.7)	

Table 2.1.2.3 (contd)

Reference Country and years of study	Subjects		Smoking categories[a]	Relative risk (no. of cases/deaths or 95% CI)	Comments
	Women (n = 56)		Ever-smoker	3.1 (1.4–7.0)	
			Current smoker	4.1 (1.7–10.2)	
			< 20	2.4 (0.9–6.4)	
			20–39	4.2 (1.6–11.3)	
			≥ 40	3.7 (0.4–38.9)	
Hartge et al. (1993) USA 1978 onwards	Men				Adjusted for age, geographical area, occupational risk and pipe or cigar use
		Black	Never-smoker	1.0	
			< 20	2.2 (1.0–4.8)	
			≥ 20	4.5 (2.1–9.3)	
		White	Never-smoker	1.0	
			< 20	2.1 (1.7–2.6)	
			≥ 20	3.0 (2.6–3.6)	
	Women				
		Black	Never-smoker	1.0	
			< 20	1.7 (0.6–4.7)	
			≥ 20	2.1 (1.4–10)	
		White	Never-smoker	1.0	
			< 20	2.0 (1.5–2.7)	
			≥ 20	3.1 (2.4–4.2)	
	Men		Former smoker		
		Black	< 20	1.6 (0.7–3.9)	
			≥ 20	1.8 (0.8–4.1)	
		White	< 20	1.3 (1.1–1.6)	
			≥ 20	1.9 (1.6–2.2)	

Table 2.1.2.3 (contd)

Reference Country and years of study	Subjects	Smoking categories[a]	Relative risk (no. of cases/deaths or 95% CI)	Comments
	Women			
	Black	< 20	3.6 (1.0–13)	
		≥ 20	5.0 (0.9–28)	
	White	< 20	2.0 (1.4–2.7)	
		≥ 20	1.3 (0.9–2.0)	
Vena et al. (1993) USA 1979–85	White men	0–2 pack–years	1.0	Adjusted for age, education and consumption of coffee, other liquids, carbonated drinks, carotene and calorie intake
		3–28 pack–years	1.7 (1.1–2.6)	
		29–48 pack–years	2.1 (1.4–3.1)	
		49–144 pack–years	2.7 (1.8–4.0)	p for trend < 0.001
Hours et al. (1994) France 1984–87	Men and women	≤ 10 pack–years	1.0	Ward controls
		11–30 pack–years	2.5 (1.2–5.4)	
		> 30 pack–years	3.6 (1.9–7.0)	
		≤ 10 pack–years	1.0	General controls
		11–30 pack–years	1.7 (0.8–3.6)	
		> 30 pack–years	2.3 (1.2–4.3)	
Momas et al. (1994a) France 1987–89	Men	Lifetime no. of cigarettes		
		< 365	1.0	
		365–146 000	3.4 (1.6–7.8)	
		146 000–320 000	5.0 (2.4–10.7)	
		> 320 000	8.7 (4.2–17.8)	

Table 2.1.2.3 (contd)

Reference Country and years of study	Subjects	Smoking categories[a]	Relative risk (no. of cases/deaths or 95% CI)	Comments
Momas et al. (1994b) France 1987–89	Men	1–10 11–30 > 30	3.6 (1.8–7.2) 5.9 (3.1–11.1) 8.4 (4.0–17.8)	Adjusted for age, occupation coffee intake, alcohol intake and diet
Sorahan et al. (1994) UK 1985–87	Men	< 10 10 20 30 ≥ 40	1.5 (1.0–2.1) 1.9 (1.4–2.6) 2.3 (1.8–3.0) 2.0 (1.4–2.8) 2.2 (1.5–3.3)	Adjusted for age
Vizcaino et al. (1994) Zimbabwe 1963–77	Men	Never-smoker Former smoker Current smoker < 15 g tobacco/day ≥ 15 g tobacco/day	1.0 0.3 (0.1–1.4) 1.1 (0.8–1.4) 1.0 (0.7–1.3) 1.4 (0.9–2.3)	Adjusted for age group, province, past history of bilharzia, education and drinking habits
	Women	Never-smoker Ever-smoker	1.0 1.4 (0.4–4.7)	Adjusted for age group, province, bilharzia and education
McCarthy et al.(1995) USA 1975–92	Men and women	< 14 15–24 > 24	1.5 (0.9–2.6) 1.6 (1.1–2.4) 2.0 (1.3–3.1)	Adjusted for sex and age

Table 2.1.2.3 (contd)

Reference Country and years of study	Subjects	Smoking categories[a]	Relative risk (no. of cases/deaths or 95% CI)	Comments
Donato et al. (1997) Italy 1991–92	Men	Lifetime no. of cigarettes 1000–99 000 100 000–199 000 200 000–299 000 ≥ 300 000	1.8 (0.6–4.9) 5.7 (2.4–13.7) 7.2 (2.9–17.8) 11.1 (4.7–26.4)	Adjusted for age, residence, education, date of interview, and coffee and alcohol intake
	Women	1000–99 000 100 000–199 000 ≥ 200 000	6.6 (1.8–24.7) 7.1 (1.4–36.9) 12.6 (2.0–77)	
Bedwani et al. (1998) Egypt 1994–96	Men	Never-smoker Current smoker < 20 ≥ 20	1.0 6.6 (3.1–13.9) 5.4 (2.4–12.1) 7.6 (3.4–16.8)	Adjusted for age, education, type of house, history of schistosomiasis and high-risk occupation; p for trend < 0.001
Pohlabeln et al. (1999) Germany 1989–92	Men	1–9 10–19 ≥ 20	2.5 (1.4–4.5) 2.6 1.4–4.9) 3.4 (1.8–6.2)	Adjusted for age, sex and residence
Pommer et al. (1999) Germany 1990–94	Men and women	Never/rare Former smoker Current smoker	1.0 1.6 (1.1–2.2) 3.2 (2.3–4.5)	Adjusted for age and sex [results for bladder; results also given for renal pelvis and renal pelvis or ureter]

Table 2.1.2.3 (contd)

Reference Country and years of study	Subjects	Smoking categories[a]	Relative risk (no. of cases/deaths or 95% CI)	Comments
Castelao et al. (2001) USA 1987–96	Men	< 10	1.2 (0.8–1.8)	Adjusted for age, occupation, diet and medical drugs
		10–< 20	1.4 (1.0–2.0)	
		20–< 30	2.2 (1.7–2.8)	
		30–< 40	3.1 (2.3–4.2)	
		≥ 40	4.0 (3.0–5.3)	
	Women	< 10	1.7 (1.0–3.0)	
		10–< 20	2.0 (1.2–3.3)	
		20–< 30	3.2 (2.1–4.9)	
		30–< 40	6.9 (2.8–16.9)	
		≥ 40	4.2 (2.2–7.7)	
Non-transitional-cell bladder cancer				
Fortuny et al. (1999) Europe 1983–95	Men and women	Former smoker		Pooled analysis; adjusted for age, gender and study centre
		0.06–21.51 pack–years	1.6 (0.8–3.0)	
		21.52–40.51 pack–years	1.4 (0.6–3.3)	
		≥ 40.52 pack–years	1.6 (0.7–3.9)	
		Current smoker		
		0.06–21.51 pack–years	2.2 (1.0–4.8)	
		21.52–40.51 pack–years	2.7 (1.3–5.6)	
		≥ 40.52 pack-years	7.0 (3.6–13.7)	

Table 2.1.2.3 (contd)

Reference Country and years of study	Subjects	Smoking categories[a]	Relative risk (no. of cases/deaths or 95% CI)	Comments
Combined analysis				
Brennan et al. (2000, 2001) Europe 1976–96	Men	1–2	1.0	Adjusted for age, centre and duration of smoking
		3–4	1.6 (0.9–2.8)	
		5–9	2.1 (1.3–3.5)	
		10–14	2.4 (1.5–4.0)	
		15–19	3.0 (1.8–5.0)	
		20–24	3.1 (1.8–5.3)	
		25–29	3.2 (1.9–5.5)	
		30–34	3.2 (1.8–5.8)	
		35–39	2.8 (1.6–5.8)	
		≥ 40	3.1 (1.7–5.5)	
	Women	1–4	1.0	
		5–9	1.4 (0.9–2.2)	
		10–14	1.6 (1.0–2.7)	
		15–19	1.6 (1.0–2.7)	
		20–24	1.6 (0.7–4.1)	
		25–29	1.8 (0.6–5.1)	
		≥ 30	1.6 (0.6–4.0)	

[a] Cigarettes/day, unless otherwise specified

Table 2.1.2.4. Studies on tobacco smoking and cancer of the bladder: duration of smoking and age at starting smoking

Reference Country and years of study	Subjects	Duration/age at starting smoking (years)	Relative risk (95% CI)	p for trend
Cohort studies				
Mills et al. (1991) USA 1976–82	Adventists' Health Study 34 198 men and women	Duration < 5 5–14 ≥ 15	1.9 (0.6–5.7) 0.9 (0.2–4.0) 4.2 (2.1–8.4)	0.0006
Nordlund et al. (1997) Sweden, Swedish Census Study II 1964–89	Swedish Census Study 25 829 women	Age at starting smoking 20–23 ≤ 19	3.3 (1.2–9.2) 3.4 (1.2–9.5)	0.018
Case–control studies				
Burch et al. (1989) Canada 1979–82	Men	Duration 1–10 11–20 21–30 ≥ 31	1.6 (0.9–2.7) 1.5 (0.9–2.5) 1.8 (1.2–2.9) 2.3 (1.6–3.4)	< 0.001
	Women	1–10 11–20 21–30 ≥ 31	0.8 (0.3–2.0) 1.1 (0.5–2.8) 3.4 (1.4–7.9) 2.2 (1.3–3.7)	< 0.001
	Men	Age at starting smoking ≥ 20 15–19 < 15	1.6 (1.1–2.4) 2.3 (1.6–3.3) 2.4 (1.6–3.6)	0.025
	Women	≥ 20 15–19 < 15	1.5 (0.9–2.5) 2.7 (1.4–5.0) 2.4 (0.9–6.4)	0.044
Claude et al. (1986) Germany 1977–82	Women	Duration 0 1–20 21–40 > 40	1.0 5.4 (1.4–21.0) 1.1 (0.4–3.1) 10.4 (1.9–56.0)	p < 0.05 p < 0.01

Table 2.1.2.4 (contd)

Reference Country and years of study	Subjects	Duration/age at starting smoking (years)	Relative risk (95% CI)	p for trend
Clavel et al. (1989) France 1984–87	Men	Duration		
		1–9	1.8 (0.9–3.6)	
		10–19	1.9 (1.0–3.5)	
		20–29	2.8 (1.7–4.8)	
		30–39	5.2 (3.22–8.39)	
		40–49	5.2 (3.2–8.5)	
		≥ 50	4.8 (2.6–8.9)	< 0.001
		Age at starting smoking		
		> 30	2.0 (0.8–5.0)	< 0.001
		25–30	1.5 (0.6–3.4)	
		21–24	3.5 (2.0–6.4)	
		18–20	4.0 (2.6–6.2)	
		≤ 17	4.9 (3.1–7.8)	
D'Avanzo et al. (1990) Italy 1985–89		Duration		
	Men	< 30	1.7 (0.9–3.1)	
		≥ 30	3.1 (1.9–4.9)	
	Women	< 30	1.5 (0.3–6.8)	
		≥ 30	4.6 (1.6–13.8)	
		Age at starting smoking		
	Men and women	> 20	1.8 (0.9–3.8)	
		≤ 20	2.7 (1.8–4.1)	
Burns & Swanson (1991) USA	Men White	Duration		
		1–10	1.1 (0.7–1.7)	
		11–20	1.3 (0.9–1.8)	
		21–30	2.0 (1.5–2.6)	
		31–40	2.3 (1.8–2.9)	
		> 40	2.9 (2.3–3.5)	
	Black	1–10	2.1 (0.7–6.4)	
		11–20	2.0 (0.7–5.5)	
		21–30	1.9 (0.9–4.0)	
		31–40	2.4 (1.2–4.6)	
		> 40	4.1 (2.4–6.8)	
	Women White	1–10	0.8 (0.4–1.6)	
		11–20	1.1 (0.6–2.0)	
		21–30	1.6 (0.9–2.8)	
		31–40	2.5 (1.9–3.5)	
		> 40	3.3 (2.5–4.3)	

Table 2.1.2.4 (contd)

Reference Country and years of study	Subjects	Duration/age at starting smoking (years)	Relative risk (95% CI)	p for trend
	Black	1–10	0.6 (0.1–4.5)	
		11–20	1.6 (0.3–8.1)	
		21–30	2.9 (1.1–7.5)	
		31–40	2.0 (0.8–4.8)	
		> 40	7.4 (3.8–14.2)	
De Stefani *et al.* (1991) Uruguay 1987–89	Men	Duration		
		1–29	2.7 (0.6–11.6)	
		30–39	9.5 (2.3–39.4)	
		40–49	9.4 (2.6–34.2)	
		≥ 50	8.7 (2.5–30.7)	< 0.001
		Age at starting smoking		
		≥ 20	1.0	
		15–19	2.1 (0.9–4.6)	
		≤ 14	1.8 (0.8–4.2)	0.24
Lopez-Abente *et al.* (1991) Spain 1983–86	Men	Duration		
		1–19	1.8 (0.9–3.5)	
		20–39	3.9 (2.4–6.5)	
		40–59	4.7 (2.9–7.5)	
		≥ 60	4.4 (2.0–9.8)	< 0.0001
Kunze *et al.* (1992) Germany 1977–85		Duration		
	Men	1–19	1.1 (0.7–1.7)	
		20–39	2.6 (1.6–3.3)	
		≥ 40	3.7 (2.6–5.3)	
	Women	1–19	3.8 (1.4–10.3)	
		20–39	1.3 (0.5–3.4)	
		≥ 40	5.6 (2.0–15.4)	
		Age at starting smoking		
	Men	≥ 21	2.2 (1.6–3.2)	
		16–20	2.6 (1.8–3.6)	
		≤ 15	6.2 (3.4–11.1)	
	Women	≥ 21	2.5 (1.3–5.0)	
		16–20	4.8 (1.7–13.3)	
		≤ 15	1.6 (0.2–12.2)	

Table 2.1.2.4 (contd)

Reference Country and years of study	Subjects	Duration/age at starting smoking (years)	Relative risk (95% CI)	*p* for trend
McLaughlin *et al.* (1992)[a] USA 1983–86	Men	Duration < 26 26–37 38–45 ≥ 46	 2.4 (1.1–5.5) 3.1 (1.5–6.7) 4.7 (2.1–10.7) 5.9 (2.6–13.7)	 < 0.001
	Women	< 26 26–37 38–45 ≥ 46	0.9 (0.3–2.2) 1.4 (0.6–3.4) 2.2 (1.0–4.9) 7.9 (2.8–22.6)	 < 0.001
	Men	Age at starting smoking ≥ 25 15–24 ≤ 14	 0.4 (0.7–6.6) 1.2 (2.3–8.4) 1.0	 0.10
	Women	≥ 25 15–24 ≤ 14	0.4 (0.0–7.2) 1.0 (0.1–7.4) 1.0	0.002
Momas *et al.* (1994b) France 1987–89	Men	Duration 1–39 40–55 > 55	 2.9 (1.2–6.8) 5.3 (2.8–9.9) 7.1 (3.3–15.2)	 < 0.0001
		Age at starting smoking ≥ 21 17–20 13–16 ≤ 12	 4.6 (2.0–10.4) 4.9 (2.6–9.2) 5.4 (2.8–10.6) 20.3 (6.9–59.8)	
Sorahan *et al.* (1994) UK 1985–87	Men	Duration 1–9 10–19 20–29 30–39 > 40	 0.9 (0.6–1.5) 1.4 (1.0–1.9) 1.8 (1.4–2.5) 2.5 (1.8–3.3) 2.9 (2.2–3.8)	 < 0.001
		Age at starting smoking ≥ 21 17–20 7–16	 2.0 (1.4–2.8) 1.9 (1.4–2.4) 2.3 (1.7–2.9)	 0.175

Table 2.1.2.4 (contd)

Reference Country and years of study	Subjects	Duration/age at starting smoking (years)	Relative risk (95% CI)	p for trend
Pohlabeln *et al.* (1999) Germany 1989–92	Men	Duration		
		1–19	1.8 (0.9–3.3)	
		20–39	2.8 (1.5–5.2)	
		≥ 40	5.0 (2.6–9.6)	
		Age at starting smoking		
		≥ 21	2.1 (1.1–3.9)	
		16–20	3.0 (1.7–5.4)	
		≤ 15	3.4 (1.6–7.2)	
	Women	Duration		
		1–19	5.2 (0.9–30.7)	
		20–39	5.7 (1.0–32.2)	
		≥ 40	5.2 (0.9–30.7)	
		Age at starting smoking		
		≥ 21	2.4 (0.6–9.9)	
		≤ 20	16.6 (2.0–136.7)	
Castelao *et al.* (2001) USA 1987–96	Men	Duration		Adjusted by age, medical drugs, occupation, diet
		Never-smoker	1.0	
		< 10	1.2 (0.8–1.7)	
		10–19	1.4 (1.1–1.9)	
		20–29	2.4 (1.8–3.2)	
		30–39	3.3 (2.5–4.3)	
		≥ 40	4.2 (3.1–5.6)	
	Women	Duration		
		Never-smoker	1.0	
		< 10	0.8 (0.4–1.7)	
		10–19	1.5 (0.9–2.8)	
		20–29	2.3 (1.4–3.9)	
		30–39	5.4 (3.2–9.2)	
		≥ 40	6.0 (3.1–11.7)	
Brennan *et al.* (2000, 2001) Europe 1976–96	Men	Duration	*1–9 cigarettes/day*	
		1–9	1.3 (0.8–1.9)	
		10–19	2.0 (1.4–2.8)	
		20–29	2.0 (1.4–2.7)	
		30–39	2.2 (1.7–2.9)	
		≥ 40	3.2 (2.6–4.1)	
			10–19 cigarettes/day	
		1–9	1.4 (0.7–2.5)	
		10–19	2.1 (1.5–2.9)	
		20–29	2.8 (2.1–3.6)	
		30–39	4.3 (3.5–5.2)	
		≥ 40	5.1 (4.3–6.1)	

Table 2.1.2.4 (contd)

Reference Country and years of study	Subjects	Duration/age at starting smoking (years)	Relative risk (95% CI)	*p* for trend
			20–29 cigarettes/day	
		1–9	0.9 (0.3–3.2)	
		10–19	1.5 (0.8–3.0)	
		20–29	3.6 (2.5–5.3)	
		30–39	5.8 (4.3–7.8)	
		≥ 40	5.7 (4.4–7.4)	
			≥ 30 cigarettes/day	
		1–9	0.4 (0.1–3.5)	
		10–19	2.2 (1.2–3.9)	
		20–29	4.2 (2.8–6.4)	
		30–39	4.3 (3.1–6.0)	
		≥ 40	5.2 (3.9–6.9)	
	Women	Duration		Adjusted for age,
		1–9	1.0	centre and
		10–19	1.2 (0.6–2.3)	number of
		20–29	1.3 (0.7–2.5)	cigarettes/day
		30–39	1.9 (1.1–3.5)	
		≥ 40	2.0 (1.1–3.5)	

CI, confidence interval

[a] Renal pelvis; similar data available for ureter

Table 2.1.2.5. Studies on tobacco smoking and cancer of the bladder: smoking cessation

Reference Country and years of study	Subjects	Years since cessation[a]	Relative risk (no. of cases or 95% CI)	p for trend/Comments
Cohort studies				
Kahn (1966) USA 1954–62	US Veterans' Study 293 958 men	Current smoker Former smoker	2.2 (82) 1.6 (51)	p for trend < 0.01
Doll & Peto (1976) UK 1957–71	British Doctors' Study 34 440 men	Current smoker Former smoker	Mortality ratio [2.1] (80) [1.2]	Ratios of annual mortality rates per 100 000 men
Rogot & Murray (1980) USA 1954–69	US Veterans Study 293 958 men	Current smoker Former smoker	SMR 2.2 (326) 1.4 (126)	Standardized mortality ratio
Steineck et al. (1988) Sweden 1967–82 (14 years)	Swedish Twin Registry Study 16 477 persons	Former smoker Ever-smoker	1.9 (0.8–4.7) 3.3 (1.7–6.7)	Analysis for men only
Mills et al. (1991) USA 1976–82	Adventist Health Study 34 198 men and women	Former smoker Current smoker	2.4 (1.3–4.7) 5.7 (1.7–18.6)	p for trend = 0.001
Chyou et al. (1993) USA 1965–95	American Men of Japanese Ancestry Study 8006 men	Former smoker Current smoker	1.4 (0.7–2.6) 2.9 (1.7–4.9)	
Doll et al. (1994) UK 1951–91	British Doctors' Study 34 439 men	Former smoker Current smoker	Mortality rate 13 21	Annual mortality rate per 100 000 men

Table 2.1.2.5 (contd)

Reference Country and years of study	Subjects	Years since cessation[a]	Relative risk (no. of cases or 95% CI)	p for trend/Comments
Mc Laughlin et al. (1995) USA 1954–80	US Veterans' Study 293 958 men	Former smoker Current smoker	1.3 (1.1–1.6) 2.2 (1.9–2.6)	
Engeland et al. (1996) Norway 1966–93	Norwegian Cohort Study 11 857 men, 14 269 women	Former smoker Men Women	2.1 (1.3–3.2) 1.5 (0.6–3.5)	Relative risks for current smoker by no. of cigarettes/day are given in Table 2.1.2.2.
Nordlund et al. (1997) Sweden 1963–89	Swedish Census Study 25 829 women	Former smoker Current smoker	2.5 (1.1–5.9) 2.3 (1.4–3.8)	
Tulinius et al. (1997) Iceland 1968–95	Reykjavik Study 11 580 men	Former smoker	2.3 (1.4–3.9)	Relative risks for current smoker by no. of cigarettes/day are given in Table 2.1.2.2.
Case–control studies				
Anthony & Thomas (1970) UK 1958–67	Men	Current smoker Fomer smoker	0.9 (185) 1.2 (43)	Age-adjusted relative risks calculated by the Working Group

Table 2.1.2.5 (contd)

Reference Country and years of study	Subjects	Years since cessation[a]	Relative risk (no. of cases or 95% CI)	p for trend/Comments
Tyrell et al. (1971) Ireland 1967–68	Men	0	3.9 (129)	Crude relative risks calculated by the Working Group
		0.1–3.9	1.5 3)	
		4.0–6.9	2.9 (5)	
		7.0–12.9	4.1 (6)	
		13.0–21.9	6.2 (9)	
		≥ 22.0	2.7 (11)	
Wynder & Goldsmith (1977) 1969–74	Men	1–3	2.6 (1.6–4.5)	
		4–6	2.9 (1.7–5.2)	
		7–9	1.5 (0.8–3.0)	
		10–12	1.6 (0.8–3.1)	
		13–15	1.2 (0.6–2.5)	
		≥ 16	1.1 (0.7–1.8)	
Howe et al. (1980) Canada 1974–76	Men	Current smoker	1.0	Relative risks calculated by the Working Group from logistic regression coefficients
		2–15	0.6 (0.4–0.9)	
		> 15	0.5 (0.4–0.8)	
	Women	Current smoker	1.0	
		Former smoker	0.2 (0.1–0.5)	
Cartwright et al. (1983) UK 1978–81	Men (current and former smokers)	≤ 5	1.7	
		6–15	1.0	
		16–25	1.1	
		26–35	0.9	
		> 35 and never-smoker	1.0 (reference)	

Table 2.1.2.5 (contd)

Reference Country and years of study	Subjects	Years since cessation[a]	Relative risk (no. of cases or 95% CI)	p for trend/Comments
McLaughlin et al. (1983)[b] USA 1974–79	Men	Current and former smokers ≥ 10	7.6 (47) 4.3	
	Women	Current and former smokers ≥ 10	5.8 (16) 3.9	
Morrison et al. (1984) Japan and UK, 1976–78 USA, 1976–77	Men, former smokers			Relative risks adjusted for intensity of smoking
	Boston area	Versus nonsmokers	1.5 (191)	
		Versus current smokers	0.5 (0.4–0.8)	
	Manchester area	Versus nonsmokers	1.8 (150)	
		Versus current smokers	0.7 (0.5–0.9)	
	Nagoya area	Versus nonsmokers	1.0 (28)	
		Versus current smokers	0.5 (0.3–0.8)	
	Women, former smokers			
	Boston	Versus nonsmokers	3.4 (50)	
	Manchester	Versus nonsmokers	0.7 (26)	
Vineis et al. (1984) Italy 1978–83	Men aged < 60	0–2	10.2 (5.0–21.2)	
		3–9	3.3 (1.2–9.2)	
		10–14	1.6 (0.3–8.2)	
		≥ 15	1.9 (0.5–7.9)	
	Men aged > 60	0–2	3.8 (2.0–7.2)	
		3–9	2.8 (1.2–6.6)	
		10–14	2.4 (0.9–6.3)	
		≥ 15	2.5 (1.0–5.8)	

Table 2.1.2.5 (contd)

Reference Country and years of study	Subjects	Years since cessation[a]	Relative risk (no. of cases or 95% CI)	p for trend/Comments
Clavel et al. (1989) France 1984–87	Men	0–2 (reference)	1.0	
		3–9	1.0 (0.6–1.3)	
		10–14	0.7 (0.4–1.2)	
		≥15	0.4 (0.3–0.6)	< 0.001
Burch et al. (1989) Canada 1979–82	Men	1–5	1.1 (0.6–1.9)	
		>5–10	0.8 (0.4–1.7)	
		>10	1.4 (0.7–2.8)	0.16
		Current	1.6 (0.8–3.0)	
	Women	1–5	0.4 (0.2–1.2)	
		>5–10	0.7 (0.1–4.1)	
		>10	0.8 (0.2–3.7)	0.09
		Current	1.0 (0.3–3.4)	
Harris et al. (1990) USA 1969 onwards	White men	Former	2.1 (1.7–2.6)	
		Current	3.2 (2.6–3.9)	
	Black men	Former	1.6 (0.8–3.4)	
		Current	2.0 (1.0–3.9)	
	White women	Former	1.3 (1.0–1.8)	
		Current	3.2 (2.4–4.1)	
	Black women	NA		
D'Avanzo et al. (1990) Italy 1985–89	Men and women	>15	1.2 (0.6–2.5)	
		5–14	1.8 (1.0–3.2)	
		2–14	3.1 (1.6–6.2)	< 0.01

Table 2.1.2.5 (contd)

Reference Country and years of study	Subjects	Years since cessation[a]	Relative risk (no. of cases or 95% CI)	p for trend/Comments
De Stefani et al. (1991) Uruguay 1987–89	Men	1–4 5–9 ≥ 10	0.5 (0.2–1.3) 0.5 (0.2–1.3) 0.4 (0.2–0.8)	0.009
López–Abente et al. (1991) Spain 1983–86	Men	0–5 6–15 ≥ 16	4.4 (2.8–7.0) 3.0 (1.7–5.2) 2.4 (1.3–4.3)	< 0.0001
Kunze et al. (1992) Germany 1977–85	Men Women	1–9 10–19 ≥ 20 1–9 10–19 ≥ 20	1.3 (0.9–1.8) 0.7 (0.5–1.0) 0.6 (0.4–0.9) 0.8 (0.3–2.7) 1.7 (0.4–7.0) 2.2 (0.8–6.3)	
Mc Laughlin et al. (1992)[b] USA 1983–86	Men Women	Current smoker (reference) < 10 10–24 ≥ 25 Current smoker (reference) < 10 10–24 ≥ 25	1.0 0.5 (0.1–1.6) 0.3 (0.2–0.6) 0.2 (0.1–0.6) 1.0 1.1 (0.3–4.2) 0.4 (0.1–1.2) 0.7 (0.1–4.7)	< 0.001 0.10

Table 2.1.2.5 (contd)

Reference Country and years of study	Subjects	Years since cessation[a]	Relative risk (no. of cases or 95% CI)	p for trend/Comments
Momas et al. (1994b) France 1987–89	Men	≤ 2 3–15 > 15	5.0 (2.6–9.7) 7.1 (3.6–13.9) 4.6 (2.3–9.1)	
Sorahan et al. (1994) UK 1985–87	Men	Current smoker 1–9 10–19 ≥ 20	3.1 (2.4–4.1) 1.9 (1.4–2.6) 1.5 (1.1–2.1) 1.2 (0.9–1.7)	
Mc Carthy et al. (1995) USA 1975–92	Men and women	Former smoker Current smoker	1.3 (1.0–1.7) 1.7 (1.2–2.3)	
Donato et al. (1997) Italy 1991–92	Men	Former smoker Current smoker	4.8 (2.2–10.7) 8.4 (3.7–19)	
Bedwani et al. (1998) Egypt 1994–96	Men	< 10 ≥ 10	5.8 (1.6–21.0) 3.4 (1.0–10.7)	Adjusted for age, education, type of house, history of schistosomiasis, high-risk occupation
Pohlabeln et al. (1999) Germany 1989–92	Men Women	Former smoker (1–9) Fomer smoker (> 10) Current smoker Former smoker Current smoker	3.4 (1.6–6.9) 1.7 (0.9–3.0) 5.2 (2.7–9.7) 5.2 (1.3–20.2) 5.6 (1.1–27.3)	

Table 2.1.2.5 (contd)

Reference Country and years of study	Subjects	Years since cessation[a]	Relative risk (no. of cases or 95% CI)	p for trend/Comments
Pommer et al. (1999) Germany 1990–94	Men women	Former smoker	1.6 (1.1–2.2)	
		Current smoker	3.2 (2.3–4.5)	
Castelao et al. (2001) USA 1987–96	Men	Never-smoker (reference)	1.0	
		Ever-smoker	2.5 (2.1–3.0)	
		Former smoker	1.7 (1.4–2.1)	
		< 10	2.3 (1.8–2.9)	
		10–19	1.9 (1.5–2.5)	
		≥ 20	1.1 (0.9–1.5)	< 0.001
		Current smoker	3.6 (2.8–4.6)	
	Women	Never-smoker (reference)	1.0	
		Ever-smoker	2.8 (2.0–4.0)	
		Former smoker	1.5 (1.0–2.4)	
		< 10	2.7 (1.5–4.8)	
		10–20	1.1 (0.6–2.1)	
		≥ 20	1.1 (0.6–2.0)	0.008
		Current smoker	4.6 (3.0–7.0)	
Combined analyses				
Fortuny et al. (1999) Europe 1983–85	Men and women	Nonsmoker	1.0	Adjusted for age, gender, study centre
		Former smoker	1.4 (0.8–2.5)	Non-cancer controls
		Current smoker	3.6 (2.1–6.3)	
		Former smoker	0.6 (0.3–1.3)	Cancer controls
		Current smoker	0.8 (0.4–1.4)	

Table 2.1.2.5 (contd)

Reference Country and years of study	Subjects	Years since cessation[a]	Relative risk (no. of cases or 95% CI) Average consumption (cigarettes/day)[c]			
			1–9	10–19	20–29	≥30
Brennan et al. (2000, 2001) Europe 1976–96	Men	Current smoker	1.0	1.0	1.0	1.0
		1–4	0.64 (0.53–0.79)	1.01 (0.36–2.82)	0.62 (0.43–0.89)	0.67 (0.52–0.86)
		5–9	0.67 (0.55–0.82)	0.21 (0.05–0.95)	0.63 (0.47–0.85)	0.87 (0.66–1.16)
		10–14	0.61 (0.50–0.75)	0.57 (0.25–1.28)	0.65 (0.49–0.86)	0.76 (0.54–1.08)
		15–19	0.46 (0.36–0.59)	0.61 (0.29–1.27)	0.57 (0.41–0.79)	0.33 (0.17–0.65)
		20–24	0.45 (0.35–0.58)	0.50 (0.25–1.01)	0.58 (0.39–0.78)	0.82 (0.27–2.47)
		>24	0.37 (0.30–0.45)	0.57 (0.34–0.97)	0.49 (0.34–0.70)	0.65 (0.24–1.78)
		Nonsmoker	0.20 (0.17–0.24)	0.34 (0.21–0.55)	0.21 (0.17–0.26)	0.20 (0.16–0.23)
	Women	Current smoker	1.0			
		<5	0.63 (0.28–1.1)			
		5–9	0.56 (0.28–1.1)			
		10–14	0.52 (0.26–1.0)			
		15–19	1.1 (0.53–2.2)			
		20–24	0.52 (0.23–1.2)			
		>24	0.84 (0.48–1.5)			
		All former smokers	0.67 (0.48–0.93)			

[a] The reference category is nonsmoker, unless otherwise specified.
[b] Cancer of the renal pelvis, similar results obtained for cancer of the ureter
[c] Adjusted for age, centre and number of cigarettes per day

Table 2.1.2.6. Case–control studies on tobacco smoking and cancer of the lower urinary tract: type of tobacco and inhalation

Reference Country and years of study	Subjects	Type of tobacco/type of inhalation	Relative risk[a] (95% CI or no. of cases/deaths)	Comments/p for trend
Lockwood (1961) Denmark 1956–57	Men	Non-inhalers (ref.) Inhalers	1.0 [0.7] (65)	Age-adjusted relative risks calculated by the Working Group
Cole et al. (1971) USA 1967–68	Men	Non-inhalers (ref.) Somewhat inhalers Deep inhalers	1.0 1.0 1.4	
	Women	Non-inhalers (ref.) Somewhat inhalers Deep inhalers	1.0 1.8 2.5	
Howe et al. (1980) Canada 1974–76	Men	Inhale untipped moderately Inhale untipped heavily Inhale filter-tipped moderately Inhale filter-tipped heavily	0.7 1.1 1.2 1.1	Calculated by the Working Group from regression coefficients; reference category is all other smokers of the same amount
	Women	Inhale untipped moderately Inhale untipped heavily Inhale filter-tipped moderately Inhale filter-tipped heavily	1.1 0.8 1.1 2.4	

Table 2.1.2.6 (contd)

Reference Country and years of study	Subjects	Type of tobacco/type of inhalation	Relative risk[a] (95% CI or no. of cases/deaths)	Comments/p for trend
Morrison et al. (1984) UK and Japan, 1976–78 USA, 1976–77	Men			Relative risks are for deep inhalers versus inhaling somewhat or not at all and adjusted for current intensity of smoking
	Boston area	Non-inhalers (ref.)	1.0	
		Inhalers	1.4 (0.8–2.3)	
	Manchester area	Non-inhalers (ref.)	1.0	
		Inhalers	1.3 (0.8–1.9)	
	Nagoya area	Non-inhalers (ref.)	1.0	
		Inhalers	1.4 (1.0–2.1)	
	Women			
	Boston area	Non-inhalers (ref.)	1.0	
		Inhalers	2.4 (0.7–7.8)	
	Manchester area	Non-inhalers (ref.)	1.0	
		Inhalers	0.7 (0.3–1.8)	
Burch et al. (1989) Canada 1979–82	Men	Non-inhalers	1.1 (0.7–2.0)	
		Somewhat inhalers	1.4 (0.9–2.2)	
		Deep inhalers	1.5 (0.9–2.4)	0.11
	Women	Non-inhalers	0.9 (0.4–2.2)	
		Somewhat inhalers	0.7 (0.3–1.6)	
		Deep inhalers	0.4 (0.1–1.0)	0.028
Clavel et al. (1989) France 1984–87	Men	Blond	1.9 (1.2–2.9)	
		Mixed	3.0 (1.6–5.7)	
		Black	4.4 (2.3–8.3)	
		Non-inhalers	2.1 (1.3–3.4)	
		Inhalers	5.7 (3.7–8.8)	

Table 2.1.2.6 (contd)

Reference Cuntry and years of study	Subjects	Type of tobacco/type of inhalation	Relative risk[a] (95% CI or no. of cases/deaths)	Comments/*p* for trend
D'Avanzo *et al.* (1990) Italy 1985–89	Men and women	Blond/mixed Black	2.7 (1.8–4.0) 3.8 (2.0–7.4)	
De Stefani *et al.* (1991) Uruguay 1987–89	Men	Blond Mixed Black	1.0 2.4 (1.0–5.6) 2.7 (1.3–5.4)	
López-Abente *et al.* (1991) Spain 1983–86	Men	No inhalation Moderate inhalation Deep inhalation Blond Black	1.5 (0.9–2.7) 3.7 (2.2–6.2) 4.9 (3.0–7.8) 3.2 (1.5–6.6) 3.7 (2.4–5.8)	
Momas *et al.* (1994b) France 1987–89	Men	Blond Black	3.1 (1.3–7.8) 6.7 (3.1–10.4)	
Castelao *et al.* (2001) USA 1987–86	Men and women	Light inhalation (ref.) Moderate inhalation Deep inhalation	1.0 1.2 (0.9–1.6) 1.1 (0.5–1.8)	

[a] Unless otherwise specified, the reference is nonsmoker.

Table 2.1.2.7. Case–control studies on tobacco smoking and cancer of the lower urinary tract: type of cigarette

Reference Country and years of study	Subjects	Use of filter-tipped cigarettes	Relative risk (95% CI or no. of cases/deaths)	Comments
Wynder & Goldsmith (1977) USA 1969–74	Men	Filter-tipped (> 10 years) Untipped (> 10 years)	3.0 (2.1–4.3) 3.1 (2.1–4.7)	
Howe et al. (1980) Canada 1974–76	Men Women	Filter-tipped Untipped Filter-tipped Untipped	1.0 1.1 1.0 1.1	Calculated by the Working Group from regression coefficients; reference category, all other smokers of the same amount
Cartwright et al. (1983) UK 1978–81	Men and women	Filter-tipped Untipped Both types	1.05 (0.7–1.5) 1.4 (1.1–1.7) 1.6 (1.3–2.0)	Adjusted for age and sex
Morrison et al. (1984) UK and Japan, 1976–78 USA, 1976–77	Men Boston area Manchester area Nagoya area	Filter-tipped Untipped (reference) Filter-tipped Untipped (reference) Filter-tipped Untipped (reference)	1.3 (0.7–2.3) 1.0 1.2 (0.8–1.8) 1.0 1.0 (0.5–1.9) 1.0	Adjusted for current intensity of smoking
Vineis et al. (1984) Italy 1978–83	Men	100% filter-tipped 75–99% filter-tipped 50–74% filter-tipped 50% filter-tipped	0.3 0.5 1.1 1.0	Relative risks adjusted for age, high-risk occupation, average daily amount of smoking, years since stopping and type of tobacco

Table 2.1.2.7 (contd)

Reference Country and years of study	Subjects	Use of filter-tipped cigarettes	Relative risk (95% CI or no. of cases/deaths)	Comments
Burch et al. (1989) Canada 1979–82	Men and women	Nonsmoker (reference)	1.0	
		Current smoker:		
		Filter-tipped only	1.4 (0.7–2.6)	
		Untipped only	1.0	
		Former smoker (quit < 10 years ago)		
		Filter-tipped only	1.4 (0.6–3.0)	
		Untipped only	0.9 (0.4–1.8)	
Clavel et al. (1989) France 1984–87	Men	Total life-long consumption		
		100% filter-tipped	3.1 (1.9–5.3)	
		75–99% filter-tipped	5.0 (2.5–10.4)	
		50–74% filter-tipped	4.8 (2.1–10.8)	
		< 50% filter-tipped	4.0 (2.6–6.2)	
De Stefani et al. (1991) Uruguay 1987–89	Men	Filter-tipped	0.7 (0.4–1.5)	
		Untipped (reference)	1.0	
López-Abente et al. (1991) Spain 1983–86	Men	Filter-tipped	0.6 (0.3–1.0)	
		Mixed use (reference)	1.0	
		Untipped	1.1 (0.6–2.5)	
Momas et al. (1994b) France 1987–89	Men	Nonsmoker (reference)	1.0	
		Filter-tipped	5.1 (2.6–10.0)	
		Untipped	5.5 (3.0–10.2)	

Table 2.1.2.7 (contd)

Reference Country and years of study	Subjects	Use of filter-tipped cigarettes	Relative risk (95% CI or no. of cases/deaths)	Comments
Sorahan et al. (1994) UK 1985–87	Men	Nonsmoker (reference) Filter-tipped Untipped	1.0 2.2 (1.7–2.8) 1.9 (1.4–2.4)	
Castelao et al. (2001) USA 1987–96	Men and women	Filter-tipped Untipped (reference)	1.2 (0.9–1.5) 1.0	

References

Akiba, S. & Hirayama, T. (1990) Cigarette smoking and cancer mortality risk in Japanese men and women — Results from reanalysis of the six-prefecture cohort study data. *Environ. Health Perspect.*, **87**, 19–26

Anthony, H.M. & Thomas, G.M. (1970) Bladder tumours and smoking. *Int. J. Cancer*, **5**, 266–272

Barbone, F., Franceschi, S., Talamini, R., Bidoli, E. & La Vecchia, C. (1994) Occupation and bladder cancer in Pordenone (North-east Italy): A case–control study. *Int. J. Epidemiol.*, **23**, 58–65

Bedwani, R., El-Khwsky, F., Renganathan, E., Braga, C., Abu Seif, H.H., Abul Azm, T., Zaki, A., Franceschi, S., Boffetta, P. & La Vecchia, C. (1997) Epidemiology of bladder cancer in Alexandria, Egypt: Tobacco smoking. *Int. J. Cancer*, **73**, 64–67

Bedwani, R., Renganathan, E., El Kwhsky, F., Braga, C., Abu Seif, H.H., Abul Azm, T., Zaki, A., Franceschi, S., Boffetta, P. & La Vecchia, C. (1998) Schistosomiasis and the risk of bladder cancer in Alexandria, Egypt. *Br. J. Cancer*, **77**, 1186–1189

Bolm-Audorff, U., Jöckel, K.H., Kilguss, B., Pohlabeln, H. & Siepenkothen, T. (1993) *Bösartige Tumoren der ableitenden Harnwege und Risiken am Arbeitsplatz,* Schriftenreihe der Bundesanstalt für Arbeitsschutz, Wirtschaftsverlag NW, Bremerhaven

Brennan, P., Bogillot, O., Cordier, S., Greiser, E., Schill, W., Vineis, P., Lopez-Abente, G., Tzonou, A., Chang-Claude, J., Bolm-Audorff, U., Jocke, K.H., Donato, F., Serra, C., Wahrendorf, J., Hours, M., 't Mannetje, A., Kogevinas, M. & Boffetta, P. (2000) Cigarette smoke and bladder cancer in men: A pooled analysis of 11 case–control studies. *Int. J. Cancer*, **86**, 289–294

Brennan, P., Bogillot, O., Greiser, E., Chang-Claude, J., Wahrendorf, J., Cordier, S., Jöckel, K.-H., Lopez-Abente, G., Tzonou, A., Vineis, P., Donato, F., Hours, M., Serra, C., Bolm-Audorff, U., Schill, W., Kogevinas, M. & Boffetta, P. (2001) The contribution of cigarette smoking to bladder cancer in women (pooled European data). *Cancer Causes Control*, **12**, 411–417

Burch, J.D., Rohan, T.E., Howe, G.R., Risch, H.A., Hill, G.B., Steele, R. & Miller, A.B. (1989) Risk of bladder cancer by source and type of tobacco exposure: A case–control study. *Int. J. Cancer*, **44**, 622–628

Burns, P.B. & Swanson, G.M. (1991) Risk of urinary bladder cancer among blacks and whites: The role of cigarette use and occupation. *Cancer Causes Control*, **2**, 371–379

Cartwright, R.A., Adib, R., Appleyard, I., Glashan, R.W., Gray, B., Hamilton-Stewart, P.A.., Robinson, M. & Barham-Hall, D. (1983) Cigarette smoking and bladder cancer: An epidemiological inquiry in West Yorkshire. *J. Epidemiol. Community Health*, **37**, 256–263

Castelao, J.E., Yuan, J.M., Skipper, P.L., Tannenbaum, S.R., Gago-Doming, M., Crowder, J.S., Ross, R.K. & Yu, M.C. (2001) Gender- and smoking-related bladder cancer risk. *J. natl Cancer Inst.*, **93**, 538–545

Cederlöf, R., Friberg, L., Hrubec, Z. & Lorich, U. (1975) *The Relationship of Smoking and Some Social Covariables to Mortality and Cancer Morbidity. A Ten Year Follow-Up in a Probability Sample of 55 000 Swedish Subjects, Age 18-69, Part 1 and Part 2*, Stockholm, The Karolinska Institute, Department of Environmental Hygiene

Chyou, P.H., Nomura, A.M. & Stemmermann, G.N. (1993) A prospective study of diet, smoking, and lower urinary tract cancer. *Ann. Epidemiol.*, **3**, 211–216

Claude, J., Kunze, E., Frentzel-Beyme, R., Paczkowski, K., Schneider, J. & Schubert, H. (1986) Life-style and occupational risk factors in cancer of the lower urinary tract. *Am. J. Epidemiol.*, **124**, 578–589

Clavel, J., Cordier, S., Boccon-Gibod, L. & Hemon, D. (1989) Tobacco and bladder cancer in males: Increased risk for inhalers and smokers of black tobacco. *Int. J. Cancer*, **44**, 605–610

Cobb, B.G. & Ansell, J.S. (1965) Cigarette smoking and cancer of the bladder. *J. Am. med. Assoc.*, **193**, 79–82

Cole, P., Monson, R.R., Haning, H. & Friedell, G.H. (1971) Smoking and cancer of the lower urinary tract. *New Engl. J. Med.*, **284**, 129–134

D'Avanzo, B., Negri, E., La Vecchia, C., Gramenzi, A., Bianchi, C., Franceschi, S. & Boyle, P. (1990) Cigarette smoking and bladder cancer. *Eur. J. Cancer*, **26**, 714–718

De Stefani, E., Correa, P., Fierro, L., Fontham, E., Chen, V. & Zavala, D. (1991) Black tobacco, mate, and bladder cancer. A case–control study from Uruguay. *Cancer*, **67**, 536–540

Doll, R. & Peto, R. (1976) Mortality in relation to smoking: 20 years' observations on male British doctors. *Br. med. J.*, **ii**, 1525–1536

Doll, R., Gray, R., Hafner, B. & Peto, R. (1980) Mortality in relation to smoking: 22 years' observations on female British doctors. *Br. med. J.*, **i**, 967–971

Doll, R., Peto, R., Wheatley, K., Gray, R. & Sutherland, I. (1994) Mortality in relation to smoking: 40 years' observations of male British doctors. *Br. med. J.*, **309**, 901–911

Donato, F., Boffetta, P., Fazioli, R., Aulenti, V., Gelatti, U. & Porru, S. (1997) Bladder cancer, tobacco smoking, coffee and alcohol drinking in Brescia, northern Italy. *Eur. J. Epidemiol.*, **13**, 795–800

Dunham, L.J., Rabson, A.S., Stewart, H.L., Frank, A.S. & Young, J.L. (1968) Rates, interview, and pathology study of cancer of the urinary bladder in New Orleans, Louisiana. *J. natl Cancer Inst.*, **41**, 683–709

Engeland, A., Anderson, A., Haldorsen, T. & Tretli, S. (1996) Smoking habits and risk of cancers other than lung cancer: 28 years' follow-up of 26,000 Norwegian men and women. *Cancer Causes Control*, **7**, 497–506

Fortuny, J., Kogevinas, M., Chang-Claude, J., Gonzalez, C.A., Hours, M., Jockel, K.H., Bolm-Audorff, U., Lynge, E., 't Mannetje, A., Porru, S., Ranft, U., Serra, C., Tzonou, A., Wahrendorf, J. & Boffetta, P. (1999) Tobacco, occupation and non-transitional-cell carcinoma of the bladder: An international case–control study. *Int. J. Cancer*, **80**, 44–46

Gao, Y., Den, J., Xiang, Y., Ruan, Z., Wang, Z., Hu, B., Guo, M., Teng, W., Han, J. & Zhang, Y. (1999) [Smoking, related cancers, and other diseases in Shanghai: A 10-year prospective study.] *Zhonghua Yu Gang Yi Xue Za Zhi*, **33**, 5–8 (in Chinese)

Greiser, E. & Molzahn, M., eds (1997) *Multizentrische Nieren- und Urothel-Carcinom-Studie (Abschlussbericht)*, Schriftenreihe der Bundesanstalt fur Arbeitsschutz und Arbeitsmedizin — Forschung — Fb780, Dortmund, Berlin

Hammond, E.C. (1966) Smoking in relation to the death rates of one million men and women. *Natl Cancer Inst. Monogr.*, **19**, 127–204

Hammond, E.C. & Horn, D. (1958a) Smoking and death rates — Report on forty-four months of follow-up of 187,783 men I. Total mortality. *J. Am. med. Assoc.*, **166**, 1159–1172

Hammond, E.C. & Horn, D. (1958b) Smoking and death rates — Report on forty-four months of follow-up of 187,783 men. II. Death rates by cause. *J. Am. med. Assoc.*, **166**, 1294–1308

Harris, R.E., Chen-Backlund, J.Y. & Wynder, E.L. (1990) Cancer of the urinary bladder in blacks and whites. A case–control study. *Cancer*, **66**, 2673–2680

Hartge, P., Silverman, D.T., Schairer, C. & Hoover, R.N. (1993) Smoking and bladder cancer risk in blacks and whites in the United States. *Cancer Causes Control*, **4**, 391–394

Hirayama,T. (1977) Changing patterns of cancer in Japan with special reference to the decrease in stomach cancer mortality. In: Hiatt, H.H., Watson, J.D. & Winsten, J.A., eds. *Origins of Human Cancer*, Book A, *Incidence of Cancer in Humans*, Cold Spring Harbor, NY, Cold Spring Harbor Laboratory, pp. 55–75

Hirayama, T. (1985) A cohort study on cancer in Japan. In: Blot, W.J., Hirayama, T. & Hoel, D.G., eds, *Statistical Methods in Cancer Epidemiology*, Hiroshima, Radiation Effects Research Foundation, pp. 73–91

Hours, M., Dananche, B., Fevotte, J,. Bergeret, A., Ayzac, L., Cardis, E., Etar, J.F., Pallen, C., Roy, P. & Fabry, J. (1994) Bladder cancer and occupational exposures. *Scand. J. Work Environ. Health*, **20**, 322–330

Howe, G.R., Burch, J.D., Miller, A.B., Cook, G.M., Esteve, J., Morrison, B., Gordon, P., Chambers, L.W., Fodor, G. & Winsor, G.M. (1980) Tobacco use, occupation, coffee, various nutrients, and bladder cancer. *J. natl Cancer Inst.*, **64**, 701–713

IARC (1986) IARC (1986) *IARC Monographs on the Evaluation of the Carcinogenic Risk of Chemicals to Humans*, Vol. 38, *Tobacco Smoking*, Lyon, IARCPress

Jensen, O.M., Wahrendorf, J., Blettner, M., Knudsen, J.B. & Sorensen, B.L. (1987) The Copenhagen case-control study of bladder cancer: role of smoking in invasive and non-invasive bladder tumours. *J. Epidemiol. Community Health*, **41**, 30–36

Kahn, H.A. (1966) The Dorn study of smoking and mortality among US veterans. Report on eight and one-half years of observation. *Natl Cancer Inst. Monogr.*, **19**, 1–125

Kuller, L.H., Ockene, J.K., Meilahn, E., Wentworth, D.H., Svendsen, K.H. & Neaton, J.D. (1991) Cigarette smoking and mortality. *Prev. Med.*, **20**, 638–654

Kunze, E., Chang-Claude, J. & Frentzel-Beyme, R. (1992) Life style and occupational risk factors for bladder cancer in Germany. A case–control study. *Cancer*, **69**, 1776–1790

Liaw, K.M. & Chen, C.J. (1998) Mortality attributable to cigarette smoking in Taiwan: A 12-year follow-up study. *Tob. Control*, **7**, 141–148

Lilienfeld, A.M., Levin, M.L. & Moore, G.E. (1956) The association of smoking with cancer of the urinary bladder in humans. *Arch. intern. Med.*, **98**, 129–135

Lockwood, K. (1961) On the etiology of bladder tumors in Kobenhavn-Frederiksberg. An inquiry of 369 patients and 369 controls. *Acta pathol. microbiol. scand.*, **51** (Suppl. 145)

López-Abente, G., Gonzalez, C.A., Errezola, M., Escolar, A., Izarzugaza, I., Nebot, M. & Riboli, E. (1991) Tobacco smoke inhalation pattern, tobacco type, and bladder cancer in Spain. *Am. J. Epidemiol.*, **134**, 830–839

Lossing, E.H., Best, E.W.R., McGregor, J.T., Josie, G.H., Walker, C.B., Delaquis, F.M., Baker, P.M. & McKenzie, A.C. (1966) *A Canadian Study of Smoking and Health*, Ottawa, Department of National Health and Welfare

Makhyoun, N.A. (1974) Smoking and bladder cancer in Egypt. *Br. J. Cancer*, **30**, 577–581

McCarthy, P.V., Bhatia, A.J., Saw, S.M., Mosley, J.D. & Vega-Quinones, A. (1995) Cigarette smoking and bladder cancer in Washington County, Maryland: Ammunition for health educators. *Maryland med. J.*, **44**, 1039–1042

McCredie, M., Ford, J.M., Taylor, J.S. & Stewart, J.H. (1982) Analgesics and cancer of the renal pelvis in New South Wales. *Cancer*, **49**, 2617–2625

McCredie, M., Stewart, J.H. & Ford, J.M. (1983) Analgesics and tobacco as risk factors for cancer of the ureter and renal pelvis. *J. Urol.*, **130**, 28–30

McLaughlin, J.K., Blot, W.J., Mandel, J.S., Schuman, L.M., Mehl, E.S. & Fraumeni, J.F., Jr (1983) Etiology of cancer of the renal pelvis. *J. natl Cancer Inst.*, **71**, 287–291

McLaughlin, J.K., Silverman, D.T., Hsing, A.W., Ross, R.K., Schoenberg, J.B., Yu, M.C., Stemhagen, A., Lynch, C.F., Blot, W.J. & Fraumeni, J.F. (1992) Cigarette smoking and cancer or the renal pelvis and ureter. *Cancer Res.*, **52**, 254–257

McLaughlin, J.K., Hrubec, Z., Blot, W.J. & Fraumeni, J.F., Jr (1995) Smoking and cancer mortality among US veterans: A 26-year follow-up. *Int. J. Cancer.*, **60**, 190–193

Miller, C.T., Neutel, C.I., Nair, R.C., Marrett, L.D., Last, J.M. & Collins, W.E. (1978) Relative importance of risk factors in bladder carcinogenesis. *J. chron. Dis.*, **31**, 51–56

Mills, P.K., Beeson, L., Phillips, R.L. & Fraser, G.E. (1991) Bladder cancer in a low risk population: Results from the Adventist Health Study. *Am. J. Epidemiol.*, **133**, 230–239

Møller-Jensen, O., Knudsen, J.B., Sørensen. B.L. & Clemmesen, J. (1983) Artificial sweeteners and absence of bladder cancer risk in Copenhagen. *Int. J. Cancer*, **32**, 577–582

Møller-Jensen, O., Wahrendorf, J., Blettner, M., Knudsen, J.B. & Sørensen, B.L. (1987) The Copenhagen case–control study of bladder cancer: Role of smoking in invasive and non-invasive bladder tumours. *J. Epidemiol. Community Health*, **41**, 30–36

Momas, I., Daures, J.P., Festy, B., Bontoux, J. & Gremy, F. (1994a) Bladder cancer and black tobacco cigarette smoking. Some results from a French case–control study. *Eur. J. Epidemiol.*, **10**, 599–604

Momas, I., Daurès, J.P., Festy, B., Bontoux, J. & Grémy, G. (1994b) Relative importance of risk factors in bladder carcinogenesis: Some new results about Mediterranean habits. *Cancer Causes Control*, **5**, 326–332

Mommsen, S. & Aagaard, J. (1983) Tobacco as a risk factor in bladder cancer. *Carcinogenesis*, **4**, 335–338

Mommsen, S., Aagaard, J. & Sell, A. (1982) An epidemiological case–control study of bladder cancer in males from a predominantly rural district. *Eur. J. Cancer clin. Oncol.*, **18**, 1205–1210

Mommsen, S., Aagaard, J. & Sell, A. (1983) A case–control study of female bladder cancer. *Eur. J. Cancer clin. Oncol.*, **19**, 725–729

Morgan, R.W. & Jain, M.G. (1974) Bladder cancer: Smoking, beverages and artificial sweeteners. *Can. med. Assoc. J.*, **111**, 1067–1070

Morrison, A.S., Buring, J.E., Verhoek, W.G., Aoki, K., Leck, I., Ohno, Y. & Obata, K. (1984) An international study of smoking and bladder cancer. *J. Urol.*, **131**, 650–654

Murata, M., Takayama, K., Choi, B.C. & Pak, A.W. (1996) A nested case–control study on alcohol drinking, tobacco smoking, and cancer. *Cancer Detect. Prev.*, **20**, 557–565

Najem, R.G., Louria, D.B., Seebode, J.J., Thind, I.S., Prusakowski, J.M., Ambrose, R.B. & Fernicola, A.R. (1982) Life time occupation, smoking, caffeine, saccharine, hair dyes and bladder carcinogenesis. *Int. J. Epidemiol.*, **11**, 212–217

Nordlund, L.A., Carstensen, J.M. & Pershagen, G. (1997) Cancer incidence in female smokers: A 26-year follow-up. *Int. J. Cancer*, **73**, 625–628

Pohlabeln, H., Jöckel, K.-H. & Bolm-Audorff, U. (1999) Non-ocupational risk factors for cancer of the lower urinary tract in Germany. *Eur. J. Epidemiol.*, **15**, 411–419

Pommer, W., Bronder, E., Klimpel, A., Helmert, U., Greiser, E. & Molzahn, M. (1999) Urothelial cancer at different tumour sites: Role of smoking and habitual intake of analgesics and laxatives. Results of the Berlin Urothelial Cancer Study. *Nephrol. Dial. Transplant.*, **14**, 2892–2897

Rebelakos, A., Trichopoulos, D., Tzonou, A., Zavitsanos, X., Velonakis, E. & Trichopoulos, A. (1985) Tobacco smoking, coffee drinking, and occupation as risk factors for bladder cancer in Greece. *J. natl Cancer Inst.*, **75**, 455–461

Rogot, E. & Murray, J.L. (1980) Smoking and causes of death among US veterans: 16 years of observation. *Public Health Rep.*, **95**, 213–222

Sadeghi, A., Behmard, S. & Vesselinovitch, S.D. (1979) Opium: A potential urinary bladder carcinogen in man. *Cancer*, **43**, 2315–2321

Schmauz, R. & Cole, P. (1974) Epidemiology of cancer of the renal pelvis and ureter. *J. natl Cancer Inst.*, **52**, 1431–1434

Schwartz, D., Flamant, R., Lellouch, J. & Denoix, P.F. (1961) Results of a French survey on the role of tobacco, particularly inhalation, in different cancer sites. *J. natl Cancer Inst.*, **26**, 1085–1108

Serra, C., Bonfill, X., Sunyer, J., Urrutia, G., Turuguet, D., Bastús, R., Roqué, M., 't Mannetje, A., Kogevinas, M., Working Group on the Study of Bladder Cancer in the County of Vallès Occidental (2000) Bladder cancer in the textile industry. *Scand. J. Work Environ. Health*, **26**, 476–481

Sorahan, T., Lancashire, R.J. & Sole, G. (1994) Urothelial cancer and cigarette smoking: Findings from a regional case–controlled study. *Br. J. Urol.*, **74**, 753–756

Staszewski, J. (1966) Smoking and cancer of the urinary bladder in males in Poland. *Br. J. Cancer*, **20**, 32–35

Steineck, G., Norell, S.E. & Feychting, M. (1988) Diet, tobacco and urothelial cancer. A 14-year follow-up of 16,477 subjects. *Acta oncol.*, **27**, 323–327

Tola, S., Tenho, M., Korkala, M.-L. & Järvinen, E. (1980) Cancer of the urinary bladder in Finland. Association with occupation. *Int. Arch. occup. environ. Health*, **46**, 43–51

Tulinius, H., Sigfusson, N., Sigvaldson, H., Bjarnadottir, K. & Tryggvadottir, L. (1997) Risk factors for malignant diseases: A cohort study on a populaion of 22,946 Icelanders. *Cancer Epidemiol. Biomarkers Prev.*, **6**, 863–873

Tyrrell, A.B., MacAirt, J.G. & McCaughey, W.T.E. (1971) Occupational and non-occupational factors associated with vesical neoplasms in Ireland. *J. Irish med. Assoc.*, **64**, 213–217

Vena, J.E., Freudenheim, J., Graham, S., Marshall, J., Zielezny, M., Swanson, M. & Sufrin, G. (1993) Coffee, cigarette smoking, and bladder cancer in western New York. *Ann. Epidemiol.*, **3**, 586–591

Vineis, P. & Magnani, C. (1985) Occupation and bladder cancer in males: A case–control study. *Int. J. Cancer*, **35**, 599–606

Vineis, P., Estève, J. & Terracini, B. (1984) Bladder cancer and smoking in males: Types of cigarettes, age at start, effect of stopping and interaction with occupation. *Int. J. Cancer*, **34**, 165–170

Vineis, P., Kogevinas, M., Simonato, L., Brennan, P. & Boffetta, P. (2000) Levelling-off of the risk of lung and bladder cancer in heavy smokers: An analysis based on multicentric case–control studies and a metabolic interpretation. *Mutat. Res.*, **463**, 103–110

Vizcaino, A.P., Parkin, D.M., Boffetta, P. & Skinner, M.E.G. (1994) Bladder cancer: Epidemiology and risk factors in Bulawayo, Zimbabwe. *Cancer Causes Control*, **5**, 517–522

Weir, J.M. & Dunn, J.E., Jr (1970) Smoking and mortality: A prospective study. *Cancer*, **25**, 105–112

Wynder, E.L. & Goldsmith, R. (1977) The epidemiology of bladder cancer. A second look. *Cancer*, **40**, 1246–1268

Wynder, E.L., Onderdonk, J. & Mantel, N. (1963) An epidemiological investigation of cancer of the bladder. *Cancer*, **16**, 1388–1407

Yuan, J.-M., Ross, R.K., Wang, X.-L., Gao, Y.-T., Henderson, B.E. & Yu, M.C. (1996) Morbidity and mortality in relation to cigarette smoking in Shanghai, China. A prospective male cohort. *J. Am. med. Assoc.*, **275**, 1646–1650

2.1.3 *Renal-cell carcinoma*

The evidence available at the time of the *IARC Monograph* on tobacco smoking (IARC, 1986) did not allow the conclusion that there is a causal association between kidney cancer and tobacco smoking.

The designs of the cohort studies are described in the introduction to Section 2 and Table 2.1 and those of the available case–control studies are summarized in Table 2.1.3.1.

Tables 2.1.3.2 and 2.1.3.3 summarize the results of the cohort and case–control studies. Most (12/21) of these studies show a significant increase in risk and a positive association with the number of cigarettes smoked, although tests for trend were rarely reported. The increase in risk associated with smoking 20 cigarettes per day is above 1.3 (e.g. Benhamou *et al.*, 1993; Kreiger *et al.*, 1993; Nordlund *et al.*, 1997). The results are consistent across study designs (cohort studies, hospital- and population-based case–control studies) and in both sexes.

Studies that looked at the effect of duration of smoking and/or age at starting smoking (La Vecchia *et al.*, 1990; McCredie & Stewart, 1992; Benhamou *et al.*, 1993; Kreiger *et al.*, 1993; McLaughlin *et al.*, 1995a; Nordlund *et al.*, 1997; Yuan *et al.*, 1998) found only a weak association. The relative risk for former smokers was investigated in most studies, and all but three studies (Talamini *et al.*, 1990; Schlehofer *et al.*, 1995; Nordlund *et al.*, 1997) showed a lower risk than in current smokers, although it was not always below unity. A significant negative trend was observed with increasing number of years since quitting in five (McLaughlin *et al.*, 1984; La Vecchia *et al.*, 1990; McCredie & Stewart, 1992; McLaughlin *et al.*, 1995a; Yuan *et al.*, 1998) of six studies.

Other known risk factors for kidney cancer include raised body-mass index (obesity) and hypertension. A few studies have adjusted for these potential confounders. La Vecchia *et al.* (1990), Talamini *et al.* (1990), McCredie and Stewart (1992), Kreiger *et al.* (1993), McLaughlin *et al.* (1995a), Yuan *et al.* (1998) and Chow *et al.* (2000) adjusted for body-mass index, whereas Kuller *et al.* (1991) and Chow *et al.* (2000) adjusted for blood pressure. Their results suggest that there is no confounding effect of body-mass index or hypertension. It should be noted that confounding from body-mass index is likely to attenuate the association between kidney cancer and smoking, because smoking tends to induce a decrease in body-mass index. Therefore, an assessment of risk stratified by body-mass index would be more appropriate than adjustment for it. A large cohort study has evaluated the changes in body-mass index and blood pressure on the risk for kidney cancer (Chow *et al.*, 2000). As compared with men in the lowest three-eighths of the cohort for body-mass index, men in the middle three-eighths had a 30–60% greater risk for renal-cell cancer, and men in the highest two-eighths had nearly double the risk. After adjustment for body-mass index and hypertension, current and former smokers still had a greater risk for renal-cell cancer.

Table 2.1.3.1. Case–control studies on tobacco smoking and renal cancer: main characteristics of study design

Reference Country and years of study	Numbers of cases and controls	Criteria for eligibility and comments
Schwartz *et al.* (1961) France started 1954	Men: 69 cases and 69 controls	Hospital-based study; controls had been admitted to hospitals for accidents; matched on age, hospital group, interviewer and date of interview
Bennington & Laubscher (1968) USA 1951–66	Men: 88 cases and 170 controls; women: 12 cases and 20 controls	Hospital-based study; information on smoking habits retrieved from clinical records; information lacking for 22/122 cases and 70/190 controls (the latter were replaced)
Wynder *et al.* (1974) USA 1965–73	Men: 129 cases and 256 controls; women: 73 cases and 138 controls	Hospital-based study; controls were patients admitted for conditions not related to smoking (75% of which were malignant neoplasms) and age-matched to the cases.
Armstrong *et al.* (1976) UK 1972–74	Men: 74 cases and 74 controls; women: 32 cases and 32 controls	Hospital-based study; age- and sex-matched hospital controls (tobacco-related diseases not excluded); 48% of eligible cases in Oxford area and 44% in London could not be interviewed (mostly because of death); 19 lost controls replaced
McLaughlin *et al.* (1984) USA 1974–79	Men: 313 cases and 428 controls; women: 182 cases and 269 controls	Population-based study; all newly diagnosed cases in the Minneapolis-St Paul area; controls: age- and sex-stratified random sample of the population and 495 randomly selected deceased individuals matched (for age, sex and year of death) to deceased cases
La Vecchia *et al.* (1990) Italy 1985–89	Men: 85 cases; women: 46 cases; 394 matched controls	Hospital-based study using interviews. Incident cases confirmed histologically; median age, 60 years. Controls with traumas (30%), non-traumatic orthopaedic conditions (17%), acute medical (13%) and surgical (6%) diseases and others (34%); median age, 60 years. > 97% participation rate for cases and controls
Talamini *et al.* (1990) Italy 1986–89	Men: 150 cases and 445 controls; women: 90 cases and 220 controls	Hospital-based study using interviews. Cases confirmed histologically; aged 20–74 years; 97% response rate. Controls mainly with non-traumatic orthopaedic, traumatic and surgical conditions and eye diseases; matched by age (5-year groups), sex, area of residence and hospital; tobacco-, alcohol- and hormone-related diseases excluded; 96% participation rate

Table 2.1.3.1 (contd)

Reference Country and years of study	Numbers of cases and controls	Criteria for eligibility and comments
McCredie & Stewart (1992) Australia 1989–90	Men: 310 cases and 231 controls; women: 179 cases and 292 controls	Population-based study using interviews. Cases ascertained from Cancer Registry, confirmed by histology (87%), fine needle aspiration cytology (1%) or computerized tomography, ultrasound or contrast radiography (8%); aged 20–79 years; 66% of eligible cases. Controls randomly selected from electoral roll; 65% participation rate
Benhamou et al. (1993) France 1987–91	Men: 138 cases and 235 controls; women: 58 cases and 112 controls	Hospital-based study. Interviews. Cases confirmed histologically; 100% of eligible cases. Controls with malignant diseases (161) and non-malignant diseases (186). Individually matched by age (± 5 years), sex, hospital and interviewer; tobacco-related diseases, liver cirrhosis and diabetes excluded; 99% participation rate
Kreiger et al. (1993) Canada 1986–87	Men: 312 cases and 664 controls; women: 201 cases and 705 controls	Population-based study using a questionnaire. Incident cases confirmed histologically; aged 25–69 years; 81% of eligible cases. Controls randomly selected from general population matched (1:1) for men and (1:2) for women by age, sex and area of residence; 72% participation rate
McLaughlin et al. (1995a) Australia, Denmark, Germany, Sweden and USA 1989–92	Men: 1050 cases and 1429 controls; women: 682 cases and 880 controls	Population-based study using interviews. Cases ascertained from cancer registries, confirmed by histology or cytology; aged 20–79 years; 72% of eligible cases. Controls selected from different population rosters, matched by age (5-year groups) and study area; 75% of eligible controls
Schlehofer et al. (1995) Germany 1989–91	Men: 185 cases; women: 92 cases; 286 matched controls	Population-based study using interviews. Cases confirmed histologically; 70% aged ≥ 55 years; 85% participation rate. Controls randomly selected from population register, matched for age (± 1 year) and sex; 75% participation rate
Yuan et al. (1998) USA 1986–94	Men: 781 cases and 781 controls; women: 423 cases and 423 controls	Population-based study using interviews. Cases ascertained through Cancer Registry, confirmed histologically; non-Asian, aged 25–74 years; 70% of eligible cases. Controls selected from residence area of cases at the time of diagnosis; individually matched on age (± 5 years), sex, race and neighbourhood; 70% were first chosen controls.

Table 2.1.3.2. Cohort studies on tobacco smoking and kidney cancer: intensity of smoking

Reference Country and years of study	No. of subjects (M, F)	No. of events	Smoking categories	Relative risk (95% CI)	Comments
McLaughlin et al. (1990) USA 1954–80	US Veterans' Study 248 046 men	719 deaths	Ever-smoker Former smoker Current smoker *Cigarettes/day* 1–9 10–20 21–39 ≥ 40	1.3 (1.1–1.6) 1.1 (0.9–1.4) 1.5 (1.2–1.8) 1.3 (0.9–1.8) 1.4 (1.1–1.7) 1.6 (1.2–2.1) 2.1 (1.3–3.3)	Adjusted for age at follow-up, calendar time and year of response to questionnaire *p* for trend < 0.001
Kuller et al. (1991) USA 1975–85	MRFIT Study 12 866 men	219 deaths	Nonsmoker Current smoker *Cigarettes/day* 1–15 16–25 26–35 36–45 > 45	Mortality rate 4.8 (113) 1.9† 4.1 (11) 7.0 (30) 12.9 (34) 10.6 (23) 10.1 (8)	Annual mortality rate/10 000 men. Numbers in parentheses represent number of subjects. †RR adjusted for age, blood pressure, cholesterol and ethnicity
Doll et al. (1994) UK 1951–91	British Doctors' Study 34 439 men	113 deaths	Nonsmoker Former smoker Current smoker *Cigarettes/day* 1–14 15–24 ≥ 25	Mortality rate 9 11 13 13 14 12	Annual mortality rate/ 10 000 men χ^2 for trend 0.8 (*p* > 0.05)

Table 2.1.3.2 (contd)

Reference Country and years of study	No. of subjects (M, F)	No. of events	Smoking categories	Relative risk (95% CI)	Comments
McLaughlin et al. (1995b) USA 1954–80	US Veterans' Study 177 903 men	511 deaths	Ever-smoker Former smoker Current smoker *Cigarettes/day* 1–9 10–20 21–39 ≥ 40	1.4 (1.1–1.6) 1.1 (0.9–1.4) 1.5 (1.2–1.9) 1.3 (0.9–2.0) 1.4 (1.1–1.8) 1.6 (1.3–2.2) 2.2 (1.4–3.5)	Adjusted for age attained and calendar year time period (5-year groups) *p* for trend < 0.01
Engeland et al. (1996) Norway 1966–93	Norwegian Cohort Study 11 863 men, 14 269 women	147 cases (87 men, 60 women)	Former smoker Current smoker *Cigarettes/day* 0–4 5–9 ≥ 10	Men 1.3 (0.8–2.4) – 0.9 (0.4–2.1) 1.8 (0.9–3.6) 1.3 (0.7–2.5)	Women 0.2 (0.0–1.7) 1.1 (0.6–2.0) Adjusted for age
Heath et al. (1997) USA 1982–89	Cancer Prevention Study II 434 339 men, 564 565 women	335 deaths (212 men, 123 women)	Current smoker Former smoker	Men 1.7 (1.2–2.6) 1.7 (1.1–2.4)	Women 1.4 (0.9–2.3) 1.2 (0.7–1.9) Adjusted for age

Table 2.1.3.2 (contd)

Reference Country and years of study	No. of subjects (M, F)	No. of events	Smoking categories	Relative risk (95% CI)	Comments
Nordlund et al. (1997) Sweden 1963–89	Swedish Census Study 26 032 women	94 cases	Former smoker	1.9 (0.8–4.7)	Adjusted for age and place of residence
			Current smoker	1.1 (0.6–2.0)	
			Cigarettes/day		
			1–7	0.8 (0.3–1.9)	
			8–15	1.0 (0.4–2.9)	
			≥ 16	3.1 (1.1–8.7)	
			Age at start (years)[†]		[†]Relative risk adjusted for age, place of residence and cigarettes/day *p* for trend = 0.522
			> 24	1.0	
			20–23	2.6 (0.7–9.1)	
			< 19	1.4 (0.3–6.1)	
Chow et al. (2000) Sweden 1971–92	Swedish Construction Worker Cohort 363 992 men	759 cases	Former smoker	1.3 (1.0–1.6)	Adjusted for age, body mass index and blood pressure
			Current smoker	1.6 (1.3–1.9)	

CI, confidence interval

Table 2.1.3.3. Case–control studies on tobacco smoking and kidney cancer: intensity of smoking

Reference Country and years of study	Sex	Smoking categories	Relative risk (95% CI)	Controls	Comments
Schwartz et al. (1961) France started 1954	Men	Smoker	Cases 78[†]	Controls 83[†]	[†]Values represent percentages. Matched analysis; all $p > 0.05$
		Equivalent cigs/day	15.0	15.0	
		Inhaler	44[†]	46[†]	
Bennington & Laubscher (1968) USA 1951–66	Men and women	All tobacco use	5.4		[†]Values represent percentages. No statistical analysis performed on data for women
		> 10 cigs/day	5.1		
		Men	Cases 93[†]	Controls 75[†]	$p < 0.0005$
		Women	66[†]	50[†]	
		Men only			
		> 10 cigs/day	68[†]	54[†]	$p < 0.0005$
		< 10 cigs/day	3.4[†]	4.7[†]	$p < 0.05$
		Former smoker	1.1[†]	6.5[†]	
Wynder et al. (1974) USA 1965–73	Men and women	Cigarettes only	Men 2.0	Women 1.5	$p < 0.005$
		All tobacco	1.7		
		Cigarettes/day			
		1–9	1.5	1.1	
		10–20	1.9	1.5	
		> 20	2.2	1.2	
Armstrong et al. (1976) UK 1972–74	Men and women	Current smoker			
		Men	1.1 (0.5–2.2)		
		Women	1.0 (0.3–3.4)		

Table 2.1.3.3 (contd)

Reference Country and years of study	Sex	Smoking categories	Relative risk (95% CI)	Comments
McLaughlin *et al.* (1984) USA 1974–79	Men and women	**Men**		Odds ratio adjusted for age and type of interview (with subject or next of kin)
		Ever-smoker	1.6 (1.1–2.4)	Relative risk increased with
		Pack–years		intensity (cigarettes/day) and
		0–25.5	1.2 (0.8–2.0)	duration (years smoked) [data not
		> 25.5–50	1.3 (0.8–2.1)	shown]; *p* for trend < 0.01
		> 50	2.3 (1.4–3.8)	
		Women		
		Ever-smoker	1.9 (1.3–3.1)	
		Pack–years		
		0–12	1.8 (1.0–3.9)	
		> 12–33	1.9 (1.0–3.5)	
		> 33	2.1 (1.1–4.6)	*p* for trend < 0.01
		Men		
		Cigarettes only	1.7 (1.1–2.6)	
		Cigarettes and cigars	2.2 (1.1–4.3)	
		Cigarettes and pipes	1.2 (0.7–2.1)	
		Cigarettes, cigars and pipes	1.3 (0.6–3.0)	
		Years since quitting	Men	Women
		> 10	1.1	1.6
		≤ 10	1.7	1.7
		Current	1.8	2.0

Table 2.1.3.3 (contd)

Reference Country and years of study	Sex	Smoking categories	Relative risk (95% CI)		Comments
			Univariate	Multivariate	
La Vecchia *et al.* (1990) Italy 1985–89	Men and women	*Cigarettes/day*			Univariate analysis adjusted for age and sex; multivariate analysis adjusted for area of residence, education and body-mass index
		< 15	1.3 (0.6–2.6)	1.1 (0.5–2.5)	
		15–24	2.0 (1.1–3.8)	1.9 (1.0–3.6)	
		≥ 25	2.1 (1.0–4.6)	2.3 (1.0–5.3)	
		p for trend	0.02	0.02	
		Duration (years)			
		< 30	2.0 (1.1–3.6)	1.7 (0.9–3.0)	
		≥ 30	2.2 (1.2–3.9)	1.8 (1.0–3.2)	
		p for trend	0.01	0.04	
		Age at starting smoking (years)			
		> 20	1.8 (1.0–3.2)	1.7 (1.0–3.0)	
		≤ 20	2.5 (1.3–4.6)	2.0 (1.1–3.7)	
		Years since quitting			
		≥ 10	1.3 (0.6–3.0)	1.3 (0.6–2.7)	
		< 10	2.6 (1.1–5.7)	2.2 (1.1–4.4)	
		Former smoker		1.7 (1.0–3.1)	
Talamini *et al.* (1990) Italy 1986–89	Men and women	Former smoker	1.4 (0.8–2.2)		Adjusted by age, sex, education, body-mass index and residence χ^2 for trend = 0.9
		Current cigarettes/day			
		< 15	1.1 (0.6–1.8)		
		15–24	1.3 (0.8–2.1)		
		≥ 25	1.2 (0.6–2.4)		

Table 2.1.3.3 (contd)

Reference Country and years of study	Sex	Smoking categories	Relative risk (95% CI) Former	Current	Comments
McCredie & Stewart (1992) Australia 1989–90	Men and women	All tobacco	1.4 (1.03–2.0)	2.2 (1.6–3.0)	Adjusted for age, sex, body-mass index and method of interview Model 1 adjusted for duration, cigarettes/day and years since cessation. Model 2 adjusted for age at start, cigarettes/day and years since cessation
		Cigarettes only	1.3 (0.9–1.9)	2.2 (1.5–3.1)	
		Men	1.5 (1.01–2.4)	2.9 (1.8–4.8)	
		Women	1.3 (0.8–2.2)	1.6 (1.00–2.6)	
		Age at diagnosis			
		≤ 58 years	1.3 (0.8–2.4)	2.3 (1.4–3.8)	
		59–67 years	1.7 (0.96–3.0)	2.0 (1.1–3.6)	
		≥ 68 years	1.2 (0.7–2.1)	2.3 (1.1–4.6)	
		Ever-smoker	Model 1	Model 2	
		Duration (years)			
		1–19	1		
		20–34	1.5 (0.9–2.4)		
		≥ 35	1.5 (0.8–3.0)		
		p for trend	0.25		
		Age at starting smoking (years			
		9–17		1	
		≥ 18		1.1 (0.7–1.6)	
		Cigarettes/day			
		1–12	1	1	
		13–20	1.2 (0.7–1.8)	1.2 (0.8–1.9)	
		≥ 21	1.4 (0.9–2.3)	1.5 (0.9–2.4)	
		p for trend	0.14	0.12	
		Years since quitting			
		≥ 25	0.5 (0.2–1.0)	0.4 (0.2–0.7)	
		13–24	0.9 (0.5–1.5)	0.8 (0.5–1.4)	
		1–12	0.9 (0.5–1.4)	0.9 (0.5–1.4)	
		p for trend	0.13	0.003	

Table 2.1.3.3 (contd)

Reference Country and years of study	Sex	Smoking categories	Relative risk (95% CI)		Comments
McCredie & Stewart (1992) (contd)		**Current smoker**			
		Filter status			
		with	2.3 (1.6–3.3)		
		without	2.8 (1.3–6.4)		
		with and without	1.8 (0.95–3.6)		
		Inhalation			
		yes	2.3 (1.6–3.3)		
		no	1.7 (0.8–4.0)		
		Pattern of inhalation			
		deep	1		
		moderate	0.8 (0.4–1.5)		
		light	0.6 (0.3–1.4)		
Benhamou *et al.* (1993) France 1987–91	Men and women		Men	Women	Matched analysis
		Ever-smoker	0.9 (0.6–1.5)	0.7 (0.4–1.5)	
		Current smoker	0.9 (0.4–1.8)	0.8 (0.3–1.8)	3 cases and 12 controls excluded; adjusted for education, Quetelet index and duration of smoking
		Cigarettes/day			
		< 20	0.9 (0.3–3.0)		
		≥ 20	1.2 (0.4–3.7)		Adjusted for education, Quetelet index and cigarettes/day
		Duration (years)			
		< 30	0.7 (0.2–2.0)		
		≥ 30	0.6 (0.2–1.8)		
		Age at starting smoking (years)			Adjusted for education, Quetelet index, cigarettes/day and duration of smoking
		≥ 20	0.7 (0.2–2.9)		
		< 20	0.9 (0.2–3.4)		

Table 2.1.3.3 (contd)

Reference Country and years of study	Sex	Smoking categories	Relative risk (95% CI)		Comments
Kreiger *et al.* (1993) Canada 1986–87	Men and women		Men	Women	Adjusted by age and body-mass index
		Ever-smoker	2.0 (1.4–2.8)	1.9 (1.3–2.6)	
		Current smoker	2.3 (1.5–3.4)	2.2 (1.5–3.2)	
		< 20 years			
		< 20 cigs/day	1.6 (0.9–2.8)	1.5 (0.8–2.9)	
		≥ 20 cigs/day	1.0 (0.5–1.8)	1.8 (0.8–4.2)	
		≥ 20 years			
		< 20 cigs/day	2.2 (1.4–3.5)	1.7 (1.1–2.7)	
		≥ 20 cigs/day	2.2 (1.5–3.3)	2.2 (1.4–3.4)	
		Years since quitting			
		≥ 20	1.3 (0.8–2.1)	1.5 (0.7–3.1)	
		10–19	2.1 (1.3–3.4)	1.9 (0.8–4.2)	
		5–9	1.8 (1.0–3.3)	1.6 (0.7–3.7)	
		1–4	2.1 (1.2–3.8)	1.4 (0.6–2.9)	
McLaughlin *et al.* (1995a) Australia, Denmark, Germany, Sweden and USA 1989–92	Men and women	Ever-smoker	1.3 (1.1–1.5)		Adjusted for age, sex, body-mass index and study centre
		Current smoker	1.4 (1.2–1.7)		
		Former smoker	1.2 (1.0–1.4)		
		Cigarettes/day	Ever-smoker	Current smoker	
		1–10	1.1 (0.9–1.3)	1.1 (0.9–1.5)	
		11–20	1.3 (1.1–1.6)	1.3 (1.1–1.6)	
		> 20	1.5 (1.2–1.9)	2.1 (1.6–2.8)	
		p for trend	< 0.001	< 0.001	
		Pack-years			
		Ever-smoker			
		≤ 9	1.1 (0.9–1.3)		
		9.1–20.1	1.1 (0.9–1.4)		
		20.2–36.9	1.3 (1.0–1.6)		
		≥ 37	1.7 (1.4–2.1)		*p* for trend < 0.001

Table 2.1.3.3 (contd)

Reference Country and years of study	Sex	Smoking categories	Relative risk (95% CI)		Comments
McLaughlin *et al.* (1995a) (contd)		Current smoker			
		< 16	1.1 (0.8–1.5)		
		16–< 28	1.1 (0.8–1.5)		
		28–42.2	1.4 (1.1–1.9)		
		> 42.2	2.0 (1.6–2.7)		*p* for trend < 0.001
		Years since quitting			
		> 25	0.85 (0.6–1.1)		*p* for trend = 0.09
		16–25	0.75 (0.6–1.0)		
		6–15	0.84 (0.7–1.1)		
		≤ 5	0.90 (0.7–1.2)		
		Current	1.0 (reference)		
		Age at starting smoking (years)			
		> 24	0.67 (0.3–1.3)		
		21–24	0.76 (0.4–1.5)		
		17–20	0.77 (0.4–1.4)		
		13–16	0.83 (0.4–1.6)		
		≤ 12	1.0		*p* for trend = 0.20
Schlehofer *et al.* (1995) Germany 1989–91	Men and women	*Pack–years*	Current smoker	Former smoker	Adjusted for age
		Men			
		< 20	1.4 (0.8–2.5)	1.1 (0.6–1.9)	
		20–< 40	1.4 (0.7–3.0)	0.9 (0.5–1.8)	
		≥ 40	1.1 (0.5–2.1)	1.0 (0.4–2.2)	
		Women	2.2 (0.99–4.7)	2.3 (0.9–6.2)	
		< 10	0.8 (0.4–1.8)	1.0 (0.4–1.4)	
		10–< 20	0.5 (0.1–1.9)	0.9 (0.3–2.3)	
		≥ 20	0.3 (0.1–1.2)	0.7 (0.1–4.7)	
			2.2 (0.7–6.8)	3.0 (0.3–30.2)	

Table 2.1.3.3 (contd)

Reference Country and years of study	Sex	Smoking categories	Relative risk (95% CI)	Comments
Yuan *et al.* (1998) USA 1986–94	Men and women		Total	Adjusted for age, sex and education
		Ever-smoker	1.4 (1.1–1.6)	No effect of age at starting
		Former smoker	1.2 (1.02–1.5)	smoking [data not shown]. No
		Current smoker	1.5 (1.2–1.9)	modifying effect of body-mass
		Cigarettes/day		index, history of hypertension,
		1–19	1.5 (1.04–2.1)	regular use of analgesics or use of
		20–39	1.5 (1.1–1.9)	amphetamines in stratified analysis
		≥ 40	1.9 (1.3–2.9)	or in multivariate conditional
		Lifetime exposure (no. of cigs)		analysis
		< 117 000	1.2 (0.97–1.5)	
		117 000–283 000	1.3 (0.99–1.6)	
		≥ 283 000	1.6 (1.3–2.0)	
		Duration (years)		
		< 20	1.1 (0.8–1.4)	
		20–39	1.1 (0.9–1.5)	
		≥ 40	1.2 (0.9–1.7)	
		Years since quitting		
		≥ 20	1.2 (0.9–1.5)	
		10–19	1.3 (0.9–1.6)	
		1–9	1.3 (1.02–1.7)	
		Years since quitting		Compared with current smokers;
		≥ 20	0.7 (0.5–1.0)	adjusted for age, sex, education,
		10–19	0.7 (0.5–1.0)	body-mass index and number of
		< 10	0.8 (0.6–1.1)	cigarettes/day p for trend = 0.01

Table 2.1.3.3 (contd)

Reference Country and years of study	Sex	Smoking categories	Relative risk (95% CI)		Comments
			Men	Women	
Yuan et al. (1998) (contd)		Ever-smoker	1.4 (1.1–1.8)	1.2 (0.9–1.6)	
		Former smoker	1.3 (1.1–1.7)	1.1 (0.8–1.5)	
		Current smoker	1.6 (1.2–2.1)	1.5 (1.0–2.1)	
		Cigarettes/day			
		1–19	1.6 (0.96–2.6)	1.4 (0.8–2.3)	
		20–39	1.5 (1.1–2.0)	1.4 (0.9–2.2)	
		≥ 40	1.9 (1.2–3.2)	1.9 (0.9–4.2)	
		Lifetime exposure (no. of cigs)			
		< 117 000	1.3 (0.96–1.7)	1.1 (0.8–1.6)	
		117 000–283 000	1.3 (0.96–1.7)	1.2 (0.8–1.8)	
		≥ 283 000	1.7 (1.3–2.2)	1.4 (0.9–2.2)	
		Years since quitting			
		≥ 20	1.2 (0.9–1.6)	1.2 (0.7–2.0)	
		10–19	1.3 (0.9–1.8)	1.2 (0.7–2.0)	
		1–9	1.6 (1.2–2.3)	0.9 (0.6–1.4)	

CI, confidence interval

References

Armstrong, B., Garrod, A. & Doll, R. (1976) A retrospective study of renal cancer with special reference to coffee and animal protein consumption. *Br. J. Cancer*, **33**, 127–136

Benhamou, S., Lenfant, M.H., Ory-Paoletti, C. & Flamant, R. (1993) Risk factors for renal-cell carcinoma in a French case–control study. *Int. J. Cancer*, **55**, 32–36

Bennington, J.L. & Laubscher, F.A. (1968) Epidemiologic studies on carcinoma of the kidney. I. Association of renal adenocarcinoma with smoking. *Cancer*, **21**, 1069–1071

Chow, W.H., Gridley, G., Fraumeni, J.F., Jr & Jarvholm, B. (2000) Obesity, hypertension, and the risk of kidney cancer in men. *New Engl. J. Med.*, **343**, 1305–1311

Doll, R., Peto, R., Wheatley, K., Gray, R. & Sutherland, I. (1994) Mortality in relation to smoking: 40 years' observations on male British doctors. *Br. med. J.*, **309**, 901–911

Engeland, A., Andersen, A., Haldorsen, T. & Tretli, S. (1996) Smoking habits and risk of cancers other than lung cancer: 28 years' follow-up of 26,000 Norwegian men and women. *Cancer Causes Control*, **7**, 497–506

Heath, C.W., Jr, Lally, C.A., Calle, E.E., McLaughlin, J.K. & Thun, M.J. (1997) Hypertension, diuretics, and antihypertensive medications as possible risk factor for renal cell cancer. *Am. J. Epidemiol.*, **145**, 607–613

IARC (1986) *IARC Monographs on the Evaluation of the Carcinogenic Risk of Chemicals to Humans*, Vol. 38, *Tobacco Smoking*, Lyon, IARCPress

Kreiger, N., Marrett, L.D., Dodds, L., Hilditch, S. & Darlington, G.A. (1993) Risk factors for renal cell carcinoma: Results of a population-based case–control study. *Cancer Causes Control*, **4**, 101–110

Kuller, L.H., Ockene, J.K., Meilahn, E., Wentworth, D.N., Svendsen, K.H. & Neaton, J.D. for the MRFIT Research Group (1991) Cigarette smoking and mortality. *Prev. Med.*, **20**, 638–654

La Vecchia, C., Negri, E., D'Avanzo, B. & Franceschi, S. (1990) Smoking and renal cell carcinoma. *Cancer Res.*, **50**, 5231–5233

McCredie, M. & Stewart, J.H. (1992) Risk factors for kidney cancer in New South Wales — I. Cigarette smoking. *Eur. J. Cancer*, **28A**, 2050–2054

McLaughlin, J.K., Mandel, J.S., Blot, W.J., Schuman, L.M., Mehl, E.S. & Fraumeni, J.F., Jr (1984) A population-based case–control study of renal cell carcinoma. *J. natl Cancer Inst.*, **72**, 275–284

McLaughlin, J.K., Hrubec, Z., Heineman, E.F., Blot, W.J. & Fraumeni, J.F., Jr (1990) Renal cancer and cigarette smoking in a 26-year followup of US veterans. *Public Health Rep.*, **105**, 535–537

McLaughlin, J.K., Lindblad, P., Mellemgaard, A., McCredie, M., Mandel, J.S., Schlehofer, B., Pommer, W. & Adami, H.O. (1995a) International renal-cell cancer study. I. Tobacco use. *Int. J. Cancer*, **60**, 194–198

McLaughlin, J.K., Hrubec, Z., Blot, W.J. & Frameni, J.F., Jr (1995b) Smoking and cancer mortality among US veterans: A 26-year follow-up. *Int. J. Cancer*, **60**, 190–193

Nordlund, L.A., Carstensen, J.M. & Pershagen, G. (1997) Cancer incidence in female smokers: A 26-year follow-up. *Int. J. Cancer.*, **73**, 625–628

Schlehofer, B., Heuer, C., Blettner, M., Niehoff, D. & Wahrendorf, J. (1995) Occupation, smoking and demographic factors, and renal cell carcinoma in Germany. *Int. J. Epidemiol.*, **24**, 51–57

Schwartz, D., Flamant, R., Lellouch, J. & Denoix, P.F. (1961) Results of a French survey on the role of tobacco, particularly inhalation, in different cancer sites. *J. natl Cancer Inst.*, **26**, 1085–1108

Talamini, R., Barón, A.E., Barra, S., Bidoli, E., La Vecchia, C., Negri, E., Serraino, D. & Franceschi, S. (1990) A case–control study of risk factor for renal cell cancer in northern Italy. *Cancer Causes Control*, **1**, 125–131

Wynder, E.L., Mabuchi, K. & Whitmore, W.F., Jr (1974) Epidemiology of adenocarcinoma of the kidney. *J. natl Cancer Inst.*, **53**, 1619–1634

Yuan, J.M., Castelao, J.E., Gago-Dominguez, M., Yu, M.C. & Ross, R.K. (1998) Tobacco use in relation to renal cell carcinoma. *Cancer Epidemiol. Biomarkers Prev.*, **7**, 429–433

2.1.4   Upper aerodigestive tract

Evidence relating to cancers of the upper aerodigestive tract obtained from relevant cohort and case–control studies on specific sites is described in Sections 2.1.4.a to 2.1.4.f, whereas studies that looked at several subsites combined are described in Section 2.1.4.g.

Most of the cohorts in which these studies were conducted have been described in the introduction to Section 2 and Table 2.1. In addition, in 1975, Tomita *et al.* (1991) established a cohort of 38 621 men, aged 20–55 years, who worked for the East Japan Railway Company. The response rate was 98% and after exclusions and loss to follow-up, 37 645 men were included in the analysis. The health status of the subjects was followed until 1985 using records of medical examinations, mutual-aid pensions and notices of deaths.

The major confounders for the relationship between smoking and several cancers of the upper aerodigestive tract are alcohol consumption and use of any form of smokeless tobacco. In general, the studies examined in the Working Group had adjusted for these two confounders when appropriate.

Some studies also adjusted for dietary intake, especially of fruits and vegetables, although few reported stratified relative risks.

(a)   Oral cancer

Tobacco smoking was shown to be causally related to oral cancer by the previous *IARC Monograph* on tobacco smoking (IARC, 1986) and even earlier by other agencies. Since 1986, many more studies have been reported on the relationship between oral cancer and cigarette smoking. New studies include three cohort studies (Table 2.1.4.1), 16 case–control studies (Tables 2.1.4.2–2.1.4.5), and two case-series reports (Table 2.1.4.6).

(i)   Intensity and duration of smoking

Intensity of smoking was measured in almost all cohort and case–control studies (Tables 2.1.4.1 and 2.1.4.3, respectively). In addition to the number of cigarettes or amount of tobacco smoked daily, cumulative exposure to cigarette smoke was also measured in terms of pack–years, tobacco–years or lifetime tobacco consumption. The link between duration of cigarette consumption and oral cancer was examined in eight case–control studies. Five case–control studies also considered age at starting smoking.

McLaughlin *et al.* (1995) in the US Veterans' Study divided the number of cigarettes smoked per day into four categories and reported a positive, statistically significant trend.

Eleven case–control studies also reported a dose-dependent increase in risk with increasing number of cigarettes smoked daily or increasing daily tobacco consumption (Franceschi *et al.*, 1990; Nandakumar *et al.*, 1990; Zheng *et al.*, 1990; Choi & Kahyo, 1991; Oreggia *et al.*, 1991; Franceschi *et al.*, 1992; Bundgaard *et al.*, 1995; Zheng *et al.*, 1997; De Stefani *et al.*, 1998; Franceschi *et al.*, 1999; Hayes *et al.*, 1999). Whenever analysed, the trend was always statistically significant (Franceschi *et al.*, 1990; Oreggia *et al.*, 1991; Franceschi *et al.*, 1992; Bundgaard *et al.*, 1995; Hayes *et al.*, 1999).

Several case–control studies have reported exposure to tobacco in other ways. Bundgaard *et al.* (1995) used lifetime tobacco consumption divided into four categories and reported a positive, significant trend after adjustment for life-time consumption of alcohol and other risk factors. A positive trend was also found in all studies that have analysed consumption in pack–years or tobacco–years (Zheng *et al.*, 1990; Maier *et al.*, 1992a; Macfarlane *et al.*, 1995; Hung *et al.*, 1997; Zheng *et al.*, 1997; De Stefani *et al.*, 1998).

Eight studies (Franceschi *et al.*, 1990; Nandakumar *et al.*, 1990; Zheng *et al.*, 1990; Choi & Kahyo, 1991; Oreggia *et al.*, 1991; Franceschi *et al.*, 1992; Zheng *et al.*, 1997; De Stefani *et al.*, 1998) classified the duration of smoking in up to four categories, and all but one study (Nandakumar *et al.*, 1990) reported increased relative risks and a positive trend.

Two out of five studies (Choi & Kahyo, 1991; Oreggia *et al.*, 1991; Franceschi *et al.*, 1990, 1992; Zheng *et al.*, 1997) reported a statistically significant trend of increasing risk with decreasing age at starting smoking (Franceschi *et al.*, 1990, 1992).

(ii) *Cessation of smoking*

One cohort study (McLaughlin *et al.*, 1995; Table 2.1.4.1) and eight case–control studies (Zheng *et al.*, 1990; Choi & Kahyo, 1991; Oreggia *et al.*, 1991; Franceschi *et al.*, 1992; Ko *et al.*, 1995; Zheng *et al.*, 1997; De Stefani *et al.*, 1998; Schildt *et al.*, 1998; Table 2.1.4.3) provided point estimates for former smokers. Relative risks among former smokers were always lower than those for current smokers and in half of these studies almost reached unity (Zheng *et al.*, 1990; Choi & Kahyo, 1991; Zheng *et al.*, 1997; Schildt *et al.*, 1998). Seven case–control studies examined the relative risk by years since quitting and all reported a negative trend (Table 2.1.4.4). The risk for oral cancer declines rather rapidly following cessation of smoking, with relative risks compared with those in non-smokers decreasing to near unity after 10 or more years (Franceschi *et al.*, 1990, 1992; De Stefani *et al.*, 1998). When calculated, the trend was always statistically significant (Franceschi *et al.*, 1990; Oreggia *et al.*, 1991; Franceschi *et al.*, 1992).

(iii) *Type of cigarette*

The effect of the type of cigarette smoked was examined in several case–control studies. The characteristics of the cigarettes included the presence of a filter, the type of tobacco, the tar content and whether the product was manufactured or hand-rolled (Table 2.1.4.5). Two studies reported a statistically significantly higher relative risk for black than for blond tobacco (Oreggia *et al.*, 1991; De Stefani *et al.*, 1998). Similarly, a much higher relative risk was found for hand-rolled cigarettes than for manufactured cigarettes, and plain cigarettes had a much higher relative risk than filter-tipped cigarettes (De Stefani *et al.*, 1998). The differences between black and blond tobacco and between hand-rolled and manufactured cigarettes persisted after stratification by duration of smoking (De Stefani *et al.*, 1998). Also smoking cigarettes with a high-tar content led to higher relative risks than smoking cigarettes with a low-tar content (Franceschi *et al.*, 1992).

(iv)   *Sex*

Sex-specific effects were examined in two case–control studies (Zheng *et al.*, 1990; Hayes *et al.*, 1999; Table 2.1.4.3). In both studies, the relative risks for all categories of intensity, duration of smoking and pack–years were higher for women than for men.

(v)   *Case-series reports*

Case-series reports are the only data available from Jordan and Myanmar; the results are given in Table 2.1.4.6. These data are of limited value in assessing causality, but have been included for the sake of completeness.

(*b*)   *Sinonasal cancer*

The Life Span Study in Japan (Akiba, 1994) examined the association of tobacco use with sinonasal cancer (see introduction to Section 2 for cohort description). A total of 26 cases of sinonasal cancer were identified among 61 505 adults during follow-up. Relative risks, adjusted for sex, location, population group, atomic bomb exposure, year of birth and attained age, increased to 2.9 (95% CI, 0.5–) and 4.0 (95% CI, 1.2–) for former and current smokers, respectively, when compared with nonsmokers [upper confidence limits could not be obtained].

A total of nine case–control studies were examined: the study designs and results are presented in Tables 2.1.4.7 and 2.1.4.8, respectively. When histological types were combined, all studies found an increased relative risk associated with cigarette smoking, but only one was statistically significant (Caplan *et al.*, 2000).

Seven studies analysed the dose–response in terms of intensity of smoking (cigarettes/day), duration of smoking or pack–years. A positive significant trend was found in five studies (Brinton *et al.*, 1984; Hayes *et al.*, 1987; Fukuda & Shibata, 1990; Zheng *et al.*, 1993; Caplan *et al.*, 2000) and was suggested in the other two (Strader *et al.*, 1988; Zheng *et al.*, 1992a).

One study (Zheng *et al.*, 1993) examined the residual risk after cessation of smoking and found a significant decrease in risk for sinonasal cancer associated with increasing number of years since cessation. In a previous study, the same authors had found a negative, non-significant association (Zheng *et al.*, 1992a).

Five studies analysed squamous-cell carcinomas and adenocarcinomas separately (Brinton *et al.*, 1984; Hayes *et al.*, 1987; Strader *et al.*, 1988; Zheng *et al.*, 1992b; 't Mannetje *et al.*, 1999). In all studies, there was clearly a significantly increased relative risk for squamous-cell carcinomas, whereas the relative risk was generally not increased for adenocarcinomas.

The evidence of an association between tobacco smoking and sinonasal cancer is based on the results from case–control studies, each of which may be subject to different sources of bias. However, several arguments support the existence of a causal association. These are: presence of a dose–response relationship in most studies; the decrease in relative risk associated with time since quitting; the consistently higher relative risks for squamous-cell carcinoma than for adenocarcinoma; and the lack of potential confounders.

(c)   *Nasopharyngeal carcinoma*

(i)   *Cohort studies*

The risk for nasopharyngeal carcinoma was examined in relation to tobacco use in two cohort studies (Table 2.1.4.9). One study, conducted in a low-risk area (Chow *et al.*, 1993), reported a significant increase in risk among smokers and suggested positive dose–response relationships by duration of smoking and age at starting smoking. The other study, conducted in China, Province of Taiwan, an area in which nasopharyngeal cancer area is endemic, reported a similarly increased risk, but it was not statistically significant (Liaw & Chen, 1998).

(ii)   *Case–control studies*

The study designs and the results of the case–control studies on the association of nasopharyngeal carcinoma with cigarette smoking are given in Tables 2.1.4.10 and 2.1.4.11, respectively.

The results of nine informative case–control studies were available (Lin *et al.*, 1973; Yu *et al.*, 1990; Nam *et al.*, 1992; West *et al.*, 1993; Ye *et al.*, 1995; Zhu *et al.*, 1995; Vaughan *et al.*, 1996; Cao *et al.*, 2000; Yuan *et al.*, 2000). In all these studies, the risk for nasopharyngeal carcinoma was higher in smokers than in nonsmokers.

In the three studies conducted in the USA, where the incidence rate for nasopharyngeal carcinoma is low (Nam *et al.*, 1992; Zhu *et al.*, 1995; Vaughan *et al.*, 1996), the relative risks for current smokers ranged between 2 and 4. In a study conducted in Shanghai, an area of China in which nasopharyngeal carcinoma is not endemic (Yuan *et al.*, 2000), the relative risk was just below 2. One study from the Philippines reported a sevenfold increase in risk after more than 30 years of smoking (West *et al.*, 1993). The four studies (Lin *et al.*, 1973; Yu *et al.*, 1990; Ye *et al.*, 1995; Cao *et al.*, 2000 [small sample size]) conducted in areas of China in which nasopharyngeal carcinoma is endemic (Taiwan, Guangzhou and Sihui) found relative risks for ever smoking ranging between 2 and 5.

A statistically significant dose–response relationship was detected in six studies that reported the effects of daily or cumulative exposure to tobacco smoke (Yu *et al.*, 1990; Nam *et al.*, 1992; Zhu *et al.*, 1995; Vaughan *et al.*, 1996; Cao *et al.*, 2000; Yuan *et al.*, 2000) and suggested in two others (Lin *et al.*, 1973; West *et al.*, 1993). Two studies investigated the effect of quitting smoking and found that the risk of nasopharyngeal carcinoma decreased with increasing time since quitting (Nam *et al.*, 1992; Vaughan *et al.*, 1996).

In the remaining studies, five from areas in which nasopharyngeal carcinoma is endemic (Ng, 1986; Yu *et al.*, 1986; Sriamporn *et al.*, 1992; Zheng *et al.*, 1994 [small sample size]; Cheng *et al.*, 1999) and five from areas in which it was not endemic (Henderson *et al.*, 1976; Lanier *et al.*, 1980; Mabuchi *et al.*, 1985; Ning *et al.*, 1990; Armstrong *et al.*, 2000), the relative risks for nasopharyngeal carcinoma for ever smoking were not significantly increased (Lanier *et al.*, 1980; Mabuchi *et al.*, 1985; Cheng *et al.*, 1999; Armstrong *et al.*, 2000) or were similar to those of nonsmokers (Henderson *et al.*, 1976; Ng, 1986; Yu *et al.*, 1986; Ning *et al.*, 1990; Sriamporn *et al.*, 1992; Zheng *et al.*, 1994).

In the two studies that distinguished between different histological types, relative risks were higher for keratinized (squamous-cell) carcinoma than for unkeratinized carcinoma (Zhu *et al.*, 1995; Vaughan *et al.*, 1996).

In the three studies in which men and women were analysed separately, the relative risks were found to increase similarly in both sexes (Lin *et al.*, 1973; Nam *et al.*, 1992; Yuan *et al.*, 2000).

Although the interpretation of the results is complicated by small sample sizes, the different criteria used for the selection of controls and the problem of control groups with smoking-related diseases, the combined evidence shows an association between tobacco smoking and nasopharyngeal carcinoma in both endemic and non-endemic areas. Infection with Epstein–Barr virus (human herpesvirus 4), a major cause of nasopharyngeal carcinoma worldwide (IARC, 1997), has not been controlled for in any of the available studies. However, it is unlikely that confounding by infection with Epstein–Barr virus would explain the observed association between tobacco smoking and risk for nasopharyngeal carcinoma. On the other hand, most studies have adjusted for other known and suspected causes of nasopharyngeal carcinoma including intake of Chinese-style salted fish, other dietary factors, alcohol drinking and family history of nasopharyngeal carcinoma, suggesting only a limited confounding effect of these factors.

(*d*)   Cancer of the pharynx

Tobacco smoking was considered to be an important cause of oropharyngeal and hypopharyngeal cancers in the previous *IARC Monograph* on tobacco smoking (IARC, 1986). Since then more epidemiological studies have yielded results that lend further support for the association. Many studies, however, combine cancers of the oral cavity and of the pharynx (see Section 2.1.4.g). This section summarizes the evidence from three cohort studies (Table 2.1.4.12) and 12 case–control studies (Tables 2.1.4.13 and 2.1.4.14) that reported results specifically on oropharyngeal and hypopharyngeal cancer, or on pharyngeal cancer in general; the latter may include data on nasopharyngeal cancer.

The risk for pharyngeal cancer was significantly increased in smokers in one cohort study (McLaughlin *et al.*, 1995; Table 2.1.4.12) and all but one of the case–control studies (Rao *et al.*, 1999; Table 2.1.4.14). The trend of increasing risk associated with increasing daily or cumulative consumption of cigarettes was evident from all these studies, particularly those from Europe (Brugere *et al.*, 1986; Tuyns *et al.*, 1988; Franceschi *et al.*, 1990; Maier *et al.*, 1994; Franceschi *et al.*, 1999), Uruguay (De Stefani *et al.*, 1998) and the USA (McLaughlin *et al.*, 1995), and less strongly so in studies from Canada (Elwood *et al.*, 1984) and the Republic of Korea (Choi & Kahyo, 1991).

Two case–control studies showed that the risk increased with decreasing age at starting smoking (Table 2.1.4.14; Franceschi *et al.*, 1990; Choi & Kahyo, 1991), but duration and intensity of smoking were not adjusted for.

The influence of cessation of smoking is also evident in all studies where this aspect has been investigated. Former smokers had consistently lower relative risks than did current smokers in both cohort (McLaughlin *et al.*, 1995) and case–control studies (Choi

& Kahyo, 1991; De Stefani *et al.*, 1998). In comparison with nonsmokers, the relative risks for former smokers who had quit smoking for more than 10 years were between 2 and 4 (Franceschi *et al.*, 1990; De Stefani *et al.*, 1998; La Vecchia *et al.*, 1999a), whereas the relative risks for current smokers in these studies were 10–14. In one study in Brazil (Schlecht *et al.*, 1999), relative risks for former smokers who had stopped smoking for more than 10 years approached 1, whereas that for current smokers was just below 6.

Consumption of black tobacco, hand-rolled cigarettes or plain cigarettes (Table 2.1.4.14) resulted in a higher risk for pharyngeal cancer than consumption of blond tobacco, manufactured cigarettes or filter-tipped cigarettes (De Stefani *et al.*, 1998).

(e)   Cancer of the oesophagus

Early studies on the association of tobacco smoking and oesophageal cancer usually examined the risk for cancer of the oesophagus without further specification; sometimes studies reported on cancer of the oesophagus and gastric cardia combined, or specifically on squamous-cell carcinoma of the oesophagus, which was at that time the predominant histological type of oesophageal cancer. Consequently, the results of the early investigations are mainly applicable to squamous-cell carcinoma of the oesophagus. In the previous *IARC Monograph* on tobacco smoking (IARC, 1986), oesophageal cancer was considered to be causally related to cigarette smoking. Many more epidemiological studies have since been conducted, and results of these studies further support this conclusion.

(i)   *Squamous-cell carcinoma and unspecified cancer of the oesophagus*

The 19 cohort and 35 case–control studies summarized in this section are described in Tables 2.1.4.15 and 2.1.4.16–2.1.4.19, respectively. All but two cohort studies (Doll *et al.*, 1980; Liaw & Chen, 1998), and all case–control studies, conducted in China, Iceland, Japan, Sweden, the United Kingdom and the USA (Table 2.1.4.17), showed that the risk for oesophageal cancer was associated with cigarette smoking. In one study (Li *et al.*, 1989), the elevated risk was observed only in an area with a relatively low incidence rate of oesophageal cancer. However, two later studies in the same area, Lin County, China, found a twofold increase in risk for oesophageal cancer among smokers (Gao *et al.*, 1994; Lu *et al.*, 2000).

In most positive cohort studies and in most case–control studies with relatively large sample sizes, the risk for oesophageal cancer was shown to increase with increasing duration of smoking (one cohort and 12 case–control studies) or number of cigarettes smoked daily (11 cohort and 21 case–control studies), and to decrease with increasing age at starting smoking (six case–control studies; Tables 2.1.4.15 and 2.1.4.17). In comparison with pharyngeal and laryngeal cancers, relative risks for oesophageal cancer estimated by duration and by intensity of smoking were somewhat lower (see Sections 2.1.4.d and 2.1.4.f, respectively).

One cohort (Guo *et al.*, 1994; Table 2.1.4.15) and 10 case–control studies (Table 2.1.4.18) investigated the effect of cessation of smoking on risk for oesophageal cancer. Although not all studies analysed the trend, all found a decreasing risk with increasing number of years since quitting. In some studies, the risk first started to decrease after 10 years of cessation (Brown *et al.*, 1988; Rolón *et al.*, 1995; Gammon *et al.*, 1997; Castellsagué *et al.*, 1999).

Consumption of black tobacco (Table 2.1.4.19) resulted in a higher risk for oeso-phageal cancer than did consumption of blond tobacco (De Stefani *et al.*, 1990; Rolón *et al.*, 1995; Castellsagué *et al.*, 1999). Similarly, smoking untipped cigarettes generally resulted in a higher risk for oesophageal cancer than smoking filter-tipped cigarettes (Vaughan *et al.*, 1995; Gammon *et al.*, 1997; Castellsagué *et al.*, 1999).

One study from the USA reported relative risks separately for blacks and whites (Brown *et al.*, 1994a). Relative risks adjusted for alcohol consumption, age and income were very similar for former and current smokers and for the number of cigarettes smoked per day and duration of smoking (Table 2.1.4.17).

(ii)   *Adenocarcinoma of the oesophagus*

During recent decades incidence rates for adenocarcinoma of the oesophagus and gastric cardia have increased steadily in the USA, whereas the incidence rate for squamous-cell carcinoma of the oesophagus has remained relatively stable (Blot *et al.*, 1991). An increase in the incidence of adenocarcinoma of the distal oesophagus and cardia has also been noted in the United Kingdom (Powell & McConkey, 1990). Since 1990, a number of studies have focused on the risk factors for adenocarcinoma of the oesophagus.

Confounding

The study designs and results of 10 case–control studies on the association of ciga-rette smoking and adenocarcinoma of the oesophagus are presented in Tables 2.1.4.20 and 2.1.4.21, respectively.

With the exception of two studies (Levi *et al.*, 1990; Wu *et al.*, 2001), all studies adjusted for alcohol intake as a potential confounder. Most of these studies were conducted in the USA (Kabat *et al.*, 1993; Brown *et al.*, 1994b; Vaughan *et al.*, 1995; Zhang *et al.*, 1996; Gammon *et al.*, 1997) or in the Netherlands (Menke-Pluymers *et al.*, 1993), where chewing of betel quid with tobacco or use of other forms of smokeless tobacco are probably not strong confounders. One study conducted in Sweden was adjusted for snuff use (Lagergren *et al.*, 2000).

Intensity and duration of smoking

Six studies, three that included only cases of adenocarcinoma of the oesophagus (Menke-Pluymers *et al.*, 1993; Gammon *et al.*, 1997; Wu *et al.*, 2001) and three that included cases of adenocarcinoma of the oesophagus, gastro-oesophageal junction and gastric cardia combined (Kabat *et al.*, 1993; Brown *et al.*, 1994b; Vaughan *et al.*, 1995),

showed a significant positive association of adenocarcinoma of the oesophagus with cigarette smoking; the relative risks were somewhat lower than those for squamous cell carcinoma of the oesophagus. Three studies, one in China (Gao *et al.*, 1994), one in Sweden
(Lagergren *et al.*, 2000) and one in the USA (Zhang *et al.*, 1996), reported similarly
elevated relative risks, but these risks were not statistically significant; in some studies
this was probably because of the relatively small number of cases involved.

Of those studies that reported risks adjusted for alcohol consumption, a positive,
significant dose–response relationship (Table 2.1.4.21) was found with intensity of
smoking (Kabat *et al.*, 1993; Brown *et al.*, 1994b; Gammon *et al.*, 1997), duration of
smoking (Gammon *et al.*, 1997) and/or pack–years (Vaughan *et al.*, 1995; Zhang *et al.*,
1996; Gammon *et al.*, 1997).

Cessation of smoking

Six studies provided point estimates for former smokers (Table 2.1.4.21). In five
studies, relative risks were lower in former smokers than in current smokers, although
they remained elevated (Kabat *et al.*, 1993; Gao *et al.*, 1994; Vaughan *et al.*, 1995;
Gammon *et al.*, 1997; Wu *et al.*, 2001), and were increased in the sixth study (Lagergren
et al., 2000). The decrease in relative risk associated with years since cessation was weak,
but a significant trend was found in two out of four studies (Gammon *et al.*, 1997; Wu
et al., 2001).

Sex

Kabat *et al.* (1993) examined risks for men and women separately and observed
similar patterns in both sexes, although risks among current smokers and heavy smokers
were somewhat higher for women than for men.

Overall, several well-conducted case–control studies, many from the USA, reported a
statistically significantly higher risk for adenocarcinoma of the oesophagus in smokers
than in nonsmokers. Positive dose–response relationships obtained using various
indicators of amount smoked support a causal association, which is further corroborated
by the findings of decreasing risks after smoking cessation. Several of these studies
reported relative risks adjusted for alcohol consumption and other potential confounders.
Further risk factors, such as chewing betel quid with tobacco or use of other forms of
smokeless tobacco, have not been considered, but are not likely to be strong confounders.
Studies from China and Europe also found increased risks for smokers.

(f)   Cancer of the larynx

In the previous *IARC Monograph* on tobacco smoking (IARC, 1986), laryngeal
cancer was one of the cancers strongly associated with cigarette smoking. Since then,
more epidemiological evidence has become available to strengthen the conclusion.

(i)   *Potential confounders*

Other causes of laryngeal cancer include alcohol consumption, some occupational exposures (e.g. sulfuric acid; IARC, 1992) and possibly some dietary habits. In investigating associations between smoking and laryngeal cancer, potential confounding by alcohol consumption is a concern. However, the risks associated with smoking are also modified by alcohol consumption (see Section 2.3). Consequently, the risk should be examined within strata of alcohol consumption and the joint effects of smoking and alcohol should be evaluated.

(ii)   *Intensity and duration of smoking*

In all the cohort studies and case–control studies analysed (Tables 2.1.4.22–2.1.4.24) that were carried out in Asia, Europe and North and South America, the risk for laryngeal cancer was consistently higher in smokers, and a positive significant trend was observed with increasing duration and intensity of smoking.

In most case–control studies, the relative risks for laryngeal cancer were near to or greater than 10 for smokers who had smoked for longer than 40 years (Falk *et al.*, 1989; Zheng *et al.*, 1992c) or had smoked more than 20 cigarettes per day (Tuyns *et al.*, 1988; Falk *et al.*, 1989; Choi & Kahyo, 1991; Zatonski *et al.*, 1991; Muscat & Wynder, 1992; Zheng *et al.*, 1992c; Hedberg *et al.*, 1994; Sokic *et al.*, 1994). Cancer of the larynx in nonsmokers is so rare that several studies used light smokers as the reference category (Herity *et al.*, 1982; Olsen *et al.*, 1985; De Stefani *et al.*, 1987; Zatonski *et al.*, 1991; López-Abente *et al.*, 1992; Maier & Tisch, 1997). Consequently, relative risks were lower in these studies, although the increases were still statistically significant.

Two case–control studies reported odds ratios for cancer of the larynx that increased with decreasing age of starting smoking (Franceschi *et al.*, 1990; Zatonski *et al.*, 1991; Table 2.1.4.24).

(iii)   *Cessation of smoking*

The risk for cancer of the larynx declines rather rapidly after cessation of smoking (Table 2.1.4.25). No detectable elevation compared with never-smokers was seen among subjects who had quit smoking for at least 10 years (Franceschi *et al.*, 1990; Ahrens *et al.*, 1991; Schlecht *et al.*, 1999).

(iv)   *Type of cigarette*

Some investigators considered the role of type of tobacco (Table 2.1.4.26) and reported a 2.5-fold higher risk in smokers of black tobacco than in smokers of blond tobacco (Tuyns *et al.*, 1988; López-Abente *et al.*, 1992; De Stefani *et al.*, 1987). Smoking untipped cigarettes also led to a higher risk than smoking filter-tipped cigarettes (Wynder & Stellman, 1979; Tuyns *et al.*, 1988; Falk *et al.*, 1989).

(v)   *Subsites*

Five studies investigated the risk for glottic and supraglottic cancer separately (Olsen *et al.*, 1985; Tuyns *et al.*, 1988; López-Abente *et al.*, 1992; Maier *et al.*, 1992b; Muscat

& Wynder, 1992). The cancer risk increased with increasing amount smoked per day and with cumulative exposure for both subsites (Table 2.1.4.24). In addition, the observed relative risks were up to 10-fold higher for supraglottic cancer than for glottic cancer (Maier *et al.*, 1992b).

(vi)   *Sex*

Few studies investigated sex-specific effects. One cohort study (Raitiola & Pukander, 1997) reported similar risks for both men and women (Table 2.1.4.22), whereas in two case–control studies (Zheng *et al.*, 1992c; Tavani *et al.*, 1994), the relative risks for women were up to 10-fold higher than for the corresponding categories in men, perhaps because of the small number of cases involved (Table 2.1.4.24).

(g)   *Cancer of the upper aerodigestive tract*

Cancers of the upper aerodigestive tract traditionally comprise cancers of the oral cavity, pharynx, larynx and oesophagus. In epidemiological studies, especially in cohort studies in which there are few cases at some sites, investigators often combine several cancer sites and term these 'cancer of the upper aerodigestive tract'. This section summarizes the data from 16 cohort studies (Table 2.1.4.27), 26 case–control studies (Tables 2.1.4.28–2.1.4.31) and one case-series report (Table 2.1.4.32).

(i)   *Intensity and duration of smoking*

The results from the cohort studies are presented in Table 2.1.4.27. In all but two cohort studies, both from Japan (Kono *et al.*, 1987; Akiba, 1994), the risk for cancer of the upper aerodigestive tract was strongly associated with cigarette smoking. Relative risks increased with increasing daily cigarette consumption (Hammond & Horn, 1958; Doll *et al.*, 1980; Akiba & Hirayama, 1990; Kuller *et al.*, 1991; Doll *et al.*, 1994; Chyou *et al.*, 1995; Engeland *et al.*, 1996; Murata *et al.*, 1996; Yuan *et al.*, 1996; Kjaerheim *et al.*, 1998; Liaw & Chen, 1998), duration of smoking (Chyou *et al.*, 1995) or pack–years (Liaw & Chen, 1998).

Details of the case–control studies are presented in Table 2.1.4.28 and their results in Table 2.1.4.29. Intensity of smoking was measured in most of these studies. In addition to, or instead of, the number of cigarettes or grams of tobacco smoked per day, exposure to tobacco smoke was also measured in terms of pack–years, lifetime consumption or cumulative tar. The link between duration of smoking and cancer of the upper aerodigestive tract was examined in 10 case–control studies (Blot *et al.*, 1988; Merletti *et al.*, 1989; Barra *et al.*, 1991; De Stefani *et al.*, 1992; Franceschi *et al.*, 1992; Day *et al.*, 1993; Mashberg *et al.*, 1993; Kabat *et al.*, 1994; Lewin *et al.*, 1998; Bosetti *et al.*, 2000). Six case–control studies also considered age at starting smoking (Blot *et al.*, 1988; Merletti *et al.*, 1989; Barra *et al.*, 1991; Franceschi *et al.*, 1992; Day *et al.*, 1993; Lewin *et al.*, 1998).

All but one study (Rao *et al.*, 1999) reported an increase in risk for cancer of the upper aerodigestive tract associated with cigarette smoking. A clear dose–response relationship was seen with increasing daily tobacco consumption and duration of smoking as well as with decreasing age at starting smoking in most of the studies examined.

(ii) *Cessation of smoking*

Eight cohort studies (Doll *et al.*, 1980; Tomita *et al.*, 1991; Akiba, 1994; Doll *et al.*, 1994; Chyou *et al.*, 1995; Engeland *et al.*, 1996; Nordlund *et al.*, 1997; Kjaerheim *et al.*, 1998) provided point estimates for former smokers (Table 2.1.4.27). The relative risks for former smokers were always lower than those for current smokers.

Nine case–control studies examined the relative risk by years since quitting and generally reported a negative trend, which was statistically significant whenever analysed (Table 2.1.4.30).

(iii) *Type of cigarette*

The type of cigarette was examined in several case–control studies: characteristics studied included the use of a filter, the type of tobacco, the tar content and whether the product was manufactured or hand-rolled (Table 2.1.4.31). Consumption of black tobacco, untipped cigarettes, hand-rolled cigarettes, or cigarettes with a high-tar yield led to a higher risk than consumption of blond tobacco (Merletti *et al.*, 1989), filter-tipped cigarettes (Merletti *et al.*, 1989; Mashberg *et al.*, 1993; Kabat *et al.*, 1994), manufactured cigarettes (De Stefani *et al.*, 1992) or low-tar cigarettes (Franceschi *et al.*, 1992), respectively, except in one multivariate analysis (Merletti *et al.*, 1989).

(iv) *Sex*

Sex-specific effects were analysed in two cohort studies (Hammond & Seidman, 1980; Akiba & Hirayama, 1990; Table 2.1.4.27) and four case–control studies (Table 2.1.4.29). Both cohort studies reported a higher relative risk for male smokers than for female smokers. One case–control study (Merletti *et al.*, 1989) also reported higher relative risks for men than for women (Table 2.1.4.31), and the trends were generally in the same direction for both men and women in all categories. An exception to the pattern was that for women the relative risk for smoking filter-tipped cigarettes was higher than that for smoking untipped cigarettes.

Three case–control studies (Blot *et al.*, 1988; Kabat *et al.*, 1994; Muscat *et al.*, 1996) found that the relative risks were higher for women than for men in all categories of intensity of smoking (number of cigarettes per day), cumulative exposure (cumulative tar consumption, pack–years, duration of smoking) and age at starting smoking, as well as for former smokers. However, the trends were always in the same direction and of the same order of magnitude.

Overall, the strength of association was generally similar, especially when taking into account the fact that women generally under-report levels of smoking and that most studies included many fewer women than men.

(v)   *Ethnicity*

Relative risks were reported separately for blacks and whites in a large case–control study from the USA (Day *et al.*, 1993; Table 2.1.4.29). Relative risks adjusted for alcohol consumption, sex and other relevant variables were very similar for the number of cigarettes smoked per day, years of cigarette smoking, age at starting smoking and number of years since stopping smoking.

(vi)   *Case-series report*

One case-series report from Saudi Arabia, from where no other information was available, is presented in Table 2.1.4.32. The data are of limited value in assessing causality, but have been included for the sake of completeness.

(vii)   *Second primary tumours*

The occurrence of second primary tumours was investigated in three studies (Day *et al.*, 1994; Barbone *et al.*, 1996; Cianfriglia *et al.*, 1999) and their results are presented in Table 2.1.4.33. All these studies showed an increased risk of second upper aerodigestive tract cancer after a previous cancer in the same organs.

The similarity in the association observed between tobacco smoking and cancers of various upper aerodigestive organs is consistent with the concept of field cancerization, i.e. the concomitant occurrence of carcinogenic alterations in different areas of the mucosa of the upper aerodigestive tract.

Table 2.1.4.1. Cohort studies on tobacco smoking and cancer of the oral cavity

Reference Country and years of study	Subjects	Cancer site ICD code	Smoking categories	Number of cases	Relative risk	95% CI	Comments
Weir & Dunn (1970) 1954–62	Californian Study 68 153 men	Oral cavity ICD: 141 tongue 143 gum 144 floor of mouth	Ever smoker Cigarettes/day 1–14 15–25 > 25	19	2.8 3.7 1.2 5.5		Nonsmokers include cigar and/or pipe only smokers.
McLaughlin et al. (1995) USA 1954–80	US Veterans' Study 248 046 men	Oral cavity ICD-7: 140 lip 141 tongue 142 salivary glands 143 gum 144 floor of mouth	Former smoker Ever-smoker Current smoker Cigarettes/day 1–9 10–20 31–39 ≥ 40	189	1.5 2.6 3.4 0.6 2.5 5.4 8.6	0.9–2.4 1.8–3.9 2.3–5.0 0.2–2.1 1.6–4.0 3.5–8.4 4.7–15.7	Adjusted for attained age and calendar-year time-period at death *p* for trend < 0.01
Nordlund et al. (1997) Sweden 1964–89	Swedish Census Study 26 032 women	Oral cavity ICD-7: 140 lip 141 tongue 142 salivary glands 143 gum 144 floor of mouth	Current smoker	46	1.6	0.7–3.5	Adjusted for age and place of residence

CI, confidence interval

Table 2.1.4.2. Case–control studies on tobacco smoking and oral cancer: main characteristics of study design

Reference Country and years of study	Number of cases and controls	Criteria for eligibility and comments
Franceschi et al. (1990) Italy 1986–89	Men: 157 cases and 1272 controls	Hospital-based study Cases of cancer of the oral cavity, histologically confirmed, aged <75 years; 98% response rate Controls were inpatients with acute conditions unrelated to tobacco or alcohol consumption, without malignant tumours, chosen on the basis of area of residence and age (± 5-year categories); 97% response rate
Nandakumar et al. (1990) India 1982–84	Men: 115 cases and 115 controls; women: 233 cases and 233 controls	Hospital-based study 93% cases histologically confirmed Controls: patients attending the same hospital during the same period, with no diagnosis of cancer, individually matched on sex, age and residence
Zheng et al. (1990) China 1988–89	Men: 248 cases and 248 controls; women: 156 cases and 156 controls	Hospital-based study in seven hospitals from the Beijing area Cases histologically confirmed, mainly squamous-cell carcinoma Controls randomly selected from non-cancer patients diagnosed within 1 year of interview, individually matched on age and sex
Choi & Kahyo (1991) Republic of Korea 1986–89	Men: 113 casess and 339 controls; women: 44 cases and 132 controls	Based on several studies within the Korea Cancer Centre Hospital Some cases histologically confirmed Controls selected from patients excluding individuals with cancers at other sites or tobacco- and alcohol-related diseases, matched 3:1 on age, sex and admission date
Oreggia et al. (1991) Uruguay 1987–89	Men: 57 cases and 353 controls	Hospital-based study in the university hospital at Montevideo Cases histologically confirmed as squamous-cell carcinoma Controls selected from patients with conditions unrelated to tobacco or alcohol consumption

Table 2.1.4.2 (contd)

Reference Country and years of study	Number of cases and controls	Criteria for eligibility and comments
Franceschi et al. (1992) Italy 1986–90	Men: 102 cases and 726 controls	Hospital-based study in the Pordenone province and the greater Milan area (Lombardy region) Cases histologically confirmed Non-cancer controls admitted to the same hospitals for acute illnesses unrelated to tobacco or alcohol consumption
Maier et al. (1992a) Germany 1987–88	Men: 200 cases and 800 controls	Hospital-based study in two university clinics in Giessen and Heidelberg Cases histologically confirmed as squamous-cell carcinoma of the oral cavity, oropharynx, hypopharynx or larynx Non-cancer controls, matched 4:1 on age and residential area
Bundgaard et al. (1995) Denmark 1986–90	Men: 97 cases and 250 controls; women: 64 cases and 150 controls	Population-based study Cases histologically confirmed as primary squamous-cell carcinoma and verrucous carcinoma Controls drawn from the Danish Central Population Register, matched on sex and age
Ko et al. (1995) China, Province of Taiwan 1992–93	Men: 104 cases and 194 controls; women: 3 cases and 6 controls	Hospital-based study in a dentistry department Cases histologically confirmed Controls: non-carcinoma patients treated in the hospital's ophthalmology and physical check-up departments, matched on sex and age
Macfarlane et al. (1995) China, 1988–89 Italy, 1975–83 USA, 1982–84	Men: 549 cases and 834 controls; women, 286 cases and 466 controls	Meta-analysis of three studies in Beijing, Turin and New York Cases histologically confirmed Population and hospital controls

Table 2.1.4.2 (contd)

Reference Country and years of study	Number of cases and controls	Criteria for eligibility and comments
Hung et al. (1997) China, Province of Taiwan 1996	Men: 41 cases and 123 controls	Population-based study Cases histologically confirmed Controls randomly selected from household registration offices in Taipei, matched 3:1 on age and ethnicity
Zheng et al. (1997) China 1988–89	Men: 65 cases and 65 controls; women: 46 cases and 46 controls	Hospital-based study in seven hospitals from the Beijing area Cases histologically confirmed Controls randomly selected from non-cancer patients attending the same hospital for conditions unrelated to smoking or alcohol consumption, matched on age and sex
De Stefani et al. (1998) Uruguay 1992–96	Men: 206 cases and 437 controls	Hospital-based study Cases histologically confirmed as squamous-cell carcinoma of the oral cavity Controls with diseases unrelated to smoking or alcohol consumption, without non-neoplastic lesions of the oral cavity and pharynx, selected from the same hospital, frequency-matched by age (10-year periods), residence and urban/rural status
Schildt et al. (1998) Sweden 1980–89	Men: 237 cases and 237 controls; women: 117 cases and 117 controls	Population-based study Histologically confirmed cases of squamous-cell oral cancer reported to Cancer Registry Living controls drawn from the National Population Registry, deceased controls from the National Registry for Causes of Death; all controls matched on age, sex, residence and year of death (for deceased controls)

Table 2.1.4.2 (contd)

Reference Country and years of study	Number of cases and controls	Criteria for eligibility and comments
Franceschi *et al.* (1999) Italy and Switzerland 1992–97	Men: 274 cases and 1254 controls	Multicentre hospital-based study Cases histologically confirmed Controls admitted for acute non-neoplastic conditions unrelated to alcohol abuse or tobacco smoking, frequency-matched by age and area of residence
Hayes *et al.* (1999) Puerto Rico 1992–95	Men: 298 cases and 417 controls; women: 69 cases and 104 controls	Population-based study Cases histologically confirmed, reported to the Central Cancer Registry Controls younger than 65 years selected from residents of the neighbourhood; controls aged 65 years and over selected from the rosters of the Health Care Financing Administration

Table 2.1.4.3. Case–control studies on tobacco smoking and oral cancer: intensity, duration and age at starting smoking

Reference Country and years of study	Cancer subsite ICD code	No. of cases	No. of controls	Smoking categories	Relative risk	95% CI	Comments
Franceschi et al. (1990) Italy 1986–89	Oral cavity: ICD-9:	147	967	Current smoker	11.1	3.4–34.8	Adjusted for age, area of residence, education, occupation and alcohol intake
	140 lip	26	313	Cigarettes/day ≤ 14	5.3	1.5–17.6	
	141 tongue	79	396	15–24	14.3	4.4–46.7	p for trend < 0.01
	143 gum	42	258	≥ 25	14.3	4.2–48.0	
	144 floor of mouth	34	414	Duration (years) 1–29	5.9	1.8–18.7	
	145 other parts of mouth	49	255	30–39	14.3	4.3–47.7	p for trend < 0.01
		69	300	≥ 40	18.0	5.4–60.4	
		23	224	Age at starting (years) ≥ 25	9.2	2.7–31.7	
		74	498	17–24	10.0	3.1–32.5	p for trend < 0.01
		54	247	< 17	13.6	4.1–44.9	
Nandakumar et al. (1990) India 1982–84	Oral cavity: lip, anterior tongue, alveolus and mouth			Cigarette smoker	3.5	1.5–8.2	
		17	23	Cigarettes/day 1–10	1.2	0.6–2.7	
		37	24	11–20	2.5	1.2–5.4	
		32	25	> 20	2.1	1.0–4.4	
		10	6	Duration (years) 1–5	2.6	0.8–8.6	
		9	14	6–15	0.9	0.3–2.7	
		18	18	16–25	1.5	0.6–3.5	
		49	34	> 25	2.2	1.1–4.3	

Table 2.1.4.3 (contd)

Reference Country and years of study	Cancer subsite ICD code	No. of cases	No. of controls	Smoking categories	Relative risk	95% CI	Comments
Zheng et al. (1990) China 1988–89	Oral cavity: ICD-9: 141 tongue 143 gum 144 floor of mouth 145 other parts of mouth	Men 22 190 168	Men 36 143 107	Former smoker Ever-smoker Current smoker	1.1 2.1 2.4	0.6–2.1 1.3–3.3 1.5–4.0	Adjusted for age, alcohol consumption and education
				Cigarettes/day			
		64	30	< 10	1.2	0.6–2.4	
		61	49	10–19	2.0	1.2–3.6	
		61	46	20	2.2	1.1–4.1	
		44	18	> 20	3.7	1.8–7.9	
				Duration (years)			
		44	48	< 26	1.4	0.8–2.5	
		42	36	26–32	1.9	1.0–3.7	
		49	31	33–41	2.3	1.1–4.6	
		55	28	> 41	4.5	2.1–9.6	
				Pack–years			
		35	49	< 15	1.2	0.7–2.3	
		44	35	15–24	2.0	1.1–3.6	
		49	28	25–34	3.2	1.6–6.7	
		62	31	> 34	3.7	1.8–7.4	

Table 2.1.4.3 (contd)

Reference Country and years of study	Cancer subsite ICD code	No. of cases	No. of controls	Smoking categories	Relative risk	95% CI	Comments
Zheng et al. (1990) (contd)		Women 52	Women 16	Ever-smoker	2.8	1.5–5.4	
				Current smoker			
				Cigarettes/day			
		17	7	< 10	2.1	0.8–5.7	
		22	7	10–19	2.9	1.1–7.4	
		13	2	> 19	5.9	1.1–31.7	
				Duration (years)			
		10	4	< 25	2.0	0.6–0.09 [sic]	
		19	4	25–34	4.7	1.5–15.3	
		23	8	> 34	2.3	0.9–6.2	
				Pack–years			
		15	7	< 13	2.9	0.7–4.7	
		17	6	13–23	3.8	1.1–13.4	
		20	3	> 23	9.0	1.5–27.3	

Table 2.1.4.3 (contd)

Reference Country and years of study	Cancer subsite ICD code	No. of cases	No. of controls	Smoking categories	Relative risk	95% CI	Comments
Choi & Kahyo (1991) Republic of Korea 1986–89	Oral cavity ICD-9:	7	48	Former smoker	0.9	0.4–2.2	Analysis for men only; adjusted for alcohol use
		91	201	Current smoker	2.5	1.3–4.5	Cases in women (44) included
	140 lip			Cigarettes/day			42 nonsmokers and 2 current
	141 tongue	69	196	1–20	1.9	1.02–3.3	smokers. Female controls (131)
	143 gum	27	50	21–40	3.1	1.5–6.5	included 112 nonsmokers, 18
	144 floor of mouth	2	3	≥41	6.1	1.01–37.0	current smokers and 1 former
	145 other parts of			Duration (years)			smoker.
	mouth	16	53	1–19	1.9	0.8–4.3	
		45	128	20–39	2.0	1.01–4.0	
		37	68	≥40	3.0	1.6–5.8	
				Age at starting (years)			
		12	44	≥25	1.8	0.7–4.2	
		75	170	18–24	2.4	1.3–4.4	
		11	35	≤17	1.9	0.8–4.7	
Oreggia et al. (1991) Uruguay 1987–89	Tongue	11	92	Former smoker	11.8	1.4–100.4	Adjusted for age, county, total alcohol consumption, variables analysed and type of tobacco
		45	154	Current smoker	29.4	3.7–234.2	
				Cigarettes/day			
		8	201	≤10	1.0	–	
		9	61	11–20	1.9	0.6–5.4	
		13	42	21–30	3.6	1.3–10.2	
		27	49	≥31	5.2	2.0–13.3	p for trend < 0.001

Table 2.1.4.3 (contd)

Reference Country and years of study	Cancer subsite ICD code	No. of cases	No. of controls	Smoking categories	Relative risk	95% CI	Comments
Oreggia et al. (1991) (contd)				Duration (years)			
		6	144	≤ 29	1.0	–	
		10	67	30–39	1.5	0.5–5.0	
		23	83	40–49	3.1	1.1–9.1	
		18	59	≥ 50	3.6	1.0–12.5	p for trend < 0.01
				Age at starting (years)			
		25	71	≤ 14	1.0	–	
		23	97	15–19	1.1	0.5–2.3	
		8	78	≥ 20	0.5	0.2–1.3	p for trend = 0.25
Franceschi et al. (1992) Italy 1986–90	Tongue ICD-9: 141	15	260	Former smoker	2.1	0.6–7.7	Adjusted for age, area of residence, occupation and alcohol habits
		83	306	Current smoker	10.5	3.2–34.1	
				Cigarettes/day			
		15	206	≤ 14	2.9	0.8–10.2	
		52	229	15–24	9.0	2.7–29.8	
		29	125	≥ 25	9.8	2.8–33.6	p for trend ≤ 0.01
				Duration (years)			
		24	229	≤ 29	3.7	1.1–12.8	
		29	157	30–39	7.7	2.3–26.2	
		43	174	≥ 40	12.4	3.6–43.3	p for trend ≤ 0.01
				Age at starting (years)			
		45	280	≥ 20	6.3	1.9–20.9	
		54	282	≤ 19	7.6	2.3–25.0	p for trend ≤ 0.01

Table 2.1.4.3 (contd)

Reference Country and years of study	Cancer subsite ICD code	No. of cases	No. of controls	Smoking categories	Relative risk	95% CI	Comments
Maier *et al.* (1992a) Germany 1987–88	Oral cavity	47	188	Pack–years			Adjusted for alcohol consumption
				< 5	1.0	–	Study included cigar and pipe smokers (1 pack = 20 cigarettes or 4 cigars or 5 pipes).
				5–50	17.1	3.4–85.3	
				> 50	77.5	11.0–545.6	*p* for trend = 0.0001
Bundgaard *et al.* (1995) Denmark 1986–90	Intra-oral sites: buccal mucosa, upper alveolus and gingiva, lower alveolus and gingiva, hard palate, tongue, retromolar area, floor of mouth	58	128	Daily tobacco consumption (g)			Adjusted for alcohol consumption
		52	41	1–20	2.1	1.3–3.5	1g tobacco equals one cigarette
				≥ 21	5.8	3.1–10.9	*p* for trend < 0.001
				Lifetime tobacco consumption (kg)			
		30	116	1–135	1.7	0.9–3.2	
		32	76	136–235	2.5	1.3–5.0	
		73	68	≥ 236	6.3	3.1–12.9	*p* for trend < 0.001
				Lifetime tobacco consumption (kg)			Adjusted for lifetime consumption of alcohol, marital status, residence and no. of teeth
				1–135	1.7	0.9–3.4	
				136–235	2.2	1.1–4.5	
				≥ 236	6.1	2.8–13.0	*p* for trend < 0.001

Table 2.1.4.3 (contd)

Reference Country and years of study	Cancer subsite ICD code	No. of cases	No. of controls	Smoking categories	Relative risk	95% CI	Comments
Ko et al. (1995) China, Province of Taiwan 1992–93	Oral cavity ICD: 140 lip 141 tongue 143 gum 144 floor of mouth 145 other parts of mouth	11 85	30 98	Former smoker Current smoker	3.6 4.6	0.9–14.6 1.5–14.0	Adjusted for betel quid chewing, alcohol consumption, education and occupation
Macfarlane et al. (1995) China, Italy, USA 1975–89	Oral cavity ICD-9: 141 tongue 143 gum 144 floor of mouth 145 other parts of mouth			Men 1–33 pack-years Tongue Gum Floor of mouth Other/unspec. mouth > 33 pack-years Tongue Gum Floor of mouth Other/unspec. mouth	1.6 1.5 – 1.6 2.9 1.7 – 3.1	0.9–2.8 0.8–2.7 – 0.8–2.9 1.5–5.6 0.8–3.8 – 1.5–6.3	Adjusted for age, study centre, education, alcohol consumption, alcohol–study centre interaction. No cases of floor-of-mouth cancer were found among male nonsmokers.

Table 2.1.4.3 (contd)

Reference Country and years of study	Cancer subsite ICD code	No. of cases	No. of controls	Smoking categories	Relative risk	95% CI	Comments
Macfarlane et al. (1995) (contd)				Women			
				1–33 pack–years			
				Tongue	2.5	1.1–5.3	
				Gum	0.5	0.1–2.3	
				Floor of mouth	8.4	1.6–44.7	
				Other/unspec. mouth	3.6	1.6–8.2	
				> 33 pack–years			
				Tongue	4.9	2.1–11.4	
				Gum	3.8	1.0–14.0	
				Floor of mouth	14.2	2.4–84.3	
				Other/unspec. mouth	7.5	3.2–18.1	
		88 men		Pack–years			Analysis restricted to abstainers from alcohol
				1–33	1.1	0.6–2.2	
				> 33	1.3	0.6–3.1	
		153 women		1–18	2.6	1.2–5.6	
				> 18	4.6	1.9–10.9	
Hung et al. (1997) China, Province of Taiwan 1996	Oral cavity ICD-9: 140 lip 141 tongue 143 gum 144 floor of mouth 145 other parts of mouth	37	81	Ever-smoker	5.0	1.7–15.1	Adjusted for age and ethnicity; 30 cases and 15 controls chewed betel quid, all of whom smoked cigarettes. p for trend = 0.027
				Pack–years			
		14	41	<22.5	4.0	1.2–13.5	
		23	40	≥22.5	5.9	1.9–18.5	

Table 2.1.4.3 (contd)

Reference Country and years of study	Cancer subsite ICD code	No. of cases	No. of controls	Smoking categories	Relative risk	95% CI	Comments
Zheng et al. (1997) China 1988–89	Tongue	3	10	Former smoker	0.5	0.1–2.2	Adjusted for alcohol consumption and education
		63	43	Ever-smoker	2.2	1.1–4.6	
		60	33	Current smoker	2.7	1.3–5.2	
				Cigarette equivalents/day			
		30	22	≤ 15	1.9	0.9–4.2	
		33	21	> 15	2.9	1.2–7.2	
				Duration (years)			
		25	18	< 30	2.1	0.9–4.9	
		38	25	≥ 30	2.4	1.0–5.9	
				Pack–years			
		23	23	≤ 20	1.3	0.6–3.0	
		40	30	> 20	5.1	1.8–14.5	
				Age at starting (years)			
		29	18	≥ 21	2.6	1.1–6.0	
		24	25	< 21	1.9	0.9–4.5	

Table 2.1.4.3 (contd)

Reference Country and years of study	Cancer subsite ICD code	No. of cases	No. of controls	Smoking categories	Relative risk	95% CI	Comments
De Stefani et al. (1998) Uruguay 1992–96	Oral cavity: mucosal surface of the lip, tongue, other parts of mouth	36	105	Former smoker	2.2	1.2–3.9	Adjusted for age, residence, urban/rural status, birthplace, education and total alcohol consumption
		182	287	Ever-moker	4.2	2.6–6.8	
		146	172	Current smoker	5.7	3.4–9.5	
				Cigarettes/day			
		27	91	1–14	1.9	1.0–3.5	
		76	106	15–24	5.1	2.9–8.7	
		79	80	≥ 25	6.1	3.5–10.8	
				Duration (years)			
		51	99	1–39	3.5	1.8–6.5	
		68	98	40–49	4.3	2.5–7.5	
		63	80	≥ 50	4.5	2.5–7.9	
				Pack–years			
		34	100	1–28	2.2	1.2–4.1	
		52	61	29–47	5.5	3.1–9.9	
		47	70	48–76	4.4	2.7–7.9	
		49	46	≥ 77	5.7	3.1–10.6	
Schildt et al. (1998) Sweden 1980–89	Oral cavity ICD-9: 140 lip 141 tongue 143 gum 144 floor of mouth 145 other parts of mouth	80	95	Former smoker	1.0	0.6–1.6	Adjusted for alcohol consumption, oral snuff and chewing tobacco Never snuff-users only
		202	183	Ever-moker	1.3	0.9–1.9	
		122	88	Current smoker	1.8	1.1–2.7	
				Lifetime consumption (kg)			
		48	52	≤ 124.8	1.2	0.7–1.9	
		79	58	> 124.8	1.2	1.1–2.9	

Table 2.1.4.3 (contd)

Reference Country and years of study	Cancer subsite ICD code	No. of cases	No. of controls	Smoking categories	Relative risk	95% CI	Comments
Franceschi et al. (1999) Italy and Switzerland 1992–97	Oral cavity (lip and salivary glands excluded)			Current smoker Cigarettes/day			Adjusted for alcohol consumption
		27		1–14	3.3	1.5–7.2	
		98		15–24	7.7	3.8–15.4	
		72		≥ 25	10.7	5.0–22.8	
Hayes et al. (1999) Puerto Rico 1992–95	Oral cavity ICD-9: 141 tongue 143 gum 144 floor of mouth 145 other parts of mouth	Men 259	Men 270	Ever-smoker	3.9	2.1–7.1	Adjusted for age and alcohol use
				Cigarettes/day			
		9	61	1–9	0.9	0.4–2.4	
		30	53	10–19	2.8	1.3–6.0	
		118	89	20–39	6.0	3.1–11.4	
		101	65	≥ 40	4.9	2.5–9.7	p for trend < 0.0001
		Women 36	Women 30	Ever-smoker	4.9	2.0–11.6	
				Cigarettes/day			
		5	9	1–9	2.2	0.6–8.4	
		6	7	10–19	4.3	1.1–16.1	
		19	12	20–39	6.4	2.1–19.6	
		6	2	≥ 40	28.2	3.7–216.0	p for trend = 0.0001

CI, confidence interval; unspec., unspecified

Table 2.1.4.4. Case–control studies on tobacco smoking and oral cancer: smoking cessation

Reference Country and years of study	Cancer subsite ICD code	No. of cases	No. of controls	Years since quitting	Relative risk	95% CI	Comments
Franceschi et al. (1990) Italy 1986–89	Oral cavity ICD-9: 140 lip 141 tongue 143 gum 144 floor of mouth 145 other parts of mouth	147 20 5	967 203 197	Current smoker < 10 ≥ 10	11.1 5.7 1.1	3.4–34.8 1.6–20.8 0.3–5.1	Adjusted for age, area of residence, education, occupation and alcohol intake p for trend < 0.01
Choi & Kahyo (1991) Republic of Korea 1986–89	Oral cavity ICD-9: 140 lip 141 tongue 143 gum 144 floor of mouth 145 other parts of mouth	91 2 3 2	201 4 15 29	Current smoker 1–4 5–9 ≥ 10	1.0 0.7 0.6 0.2	– 0.1–3.9 0.2–2.2 0.1–0.7	Analysis for men only; adjusted for alcohol use
Oreggia et al. (1991) Uruguay 1987–89	Tongue	45 5 2 4	154 28 23 41	Current smoker 1–4 5–9 ≥ 10	1.0 0.4 0.3 0.2	– 0.1–1.2 0.1–1.4 0.0–0.6	Adjusted for age, county, total alcohol intake, intensity and duration of smoking, age at starting smoking and type of tobacco p for trend < 0.001

Table 2.1.4.4 (contd)

Reference Country and years of study	Cancer subsite ICD code	No. of cases	No. of controls	Years since quitting	Relative risk	95% CI	Comments
Franceschi et al. (1992) Italy 1986–90	Tongue ICD-9: 141	83	306	Current smoker	10.5	3.2–34.1	Adjusted for age, area of residence, occupation and alcohol habits
		12	122	<10	3.8	1.0–14.5	p for trend < 0.01
		3	138	≥10	0.7	0.1–3.8	
Macfarlane et al. (1995) China, Italy, USA 1975–89	Oral cavity ICD-9: 141 tongue 143 gum 144 floor of mouth 145 other parts of mouth			Current smoker	1.0	—	Adjusted for age, sex, study centre, education, alcohol consumption, previous tobacco use and interaction terms for study centre/education and study centre–alcohol use
				<1	1.2	0.7–1.8	
				1–9	0.7	0.5–1.1	
				≥9	0.5	0.3–0.7	
De Stefani et al. (1998) Uruguay 1992–96	Oral cavity: mucosal surface of the lip, tongue, other parts of mouth	146	172	Current smoker	5.8	3.5–9.6	Adjusted for age, residence, urban/rural status, birthplace, education and total alcohol consumption
		20	40	1–4	3.2	1.6–6.5	
		12	28	5–9	2.7	1.2–6.1	
		4	37	≥10	0.7	0.2–2.1	
Hayes et al. (1999) Puerto Rico 1992–95	Oral cavity ICD-9: 141 tongue 143 gum 144 floor of mouth 145 other parts of mouth	Men 259	Men 270	Current smoker	3.9	2.1–7.1	Adjusted for age and alcohol use
		183	103	<2	7.5	3.9–14.4	
		37	38	2–9	4.1	1.8–8.9	
		20	56	10–19	2.0	0.9–4.5	
		18	73	≥20	1.2	0.5–2.7	
		Women 36	Women 30	Current smoker	4.9	2.0–11.6	
		23	10	<2	14.1	4.2–47.2	
		8	5	2–9	8.7	2.2–35.2	
		2	4	10–19	2.1	0.3–13.9	
		2	10	≥20	0.8	0.1–4.2	

CI, confidence interval

Table 2.1.4.5. Case–control studies on tobacco smoking and oral cancer: type of tobacco and/or cigarette

Reference (country and years of study)	Cancer subsite ICD code	No. of cases	No. of controls	Smoking categories	Relative risk	95% CI	Comments
Oreggia et al. (1991) Uruguay 1987–89	Tongue			Type of tobacco			Adjusted for age, county, total alcohol consumption, smoking intensity and duration, age at starting smoking p for trend < 0.25
		10	106	Blond	1.0	–	
		6	23	Mixed	1.8	0.5–6.8	
		40	117	Black	4.0	1.7–9.6	
Franceschi et al. (1992) Italy 1986–90	Tongue ICD-9: 141			Tar yield			Adjusted for age, area of residence, occupation and alcohol habits p for trend < 0.01
		49	364	Low tar (< 22 mg)	5.8	1.8–19.1	
		45	185	High tar (≥ 22 mg)	9.8	2.9–33.1	
De Stefani et al. (1998) Uruguay 1992–96	Oral cavity, mucosal surface of the lip, tongue, other parts of mouth			Type of tobacco			Adjusted for age, residence, urban/rural status, birthplace, education and total alcohol consumption
		91	222	Mainly blond	2.4	1.5–4.1	
		91	55	Mainly black	9.4	5.4–16.3	
				Duration by tobacco type			
		32	85	Blond 1–39 years	2.3	1.2–4.5	
		59	137	Blond ≥ 40 years	2.5	1.4–4.3	
		19	13	Black 1–39 years	8.3	3.5–19.7	
		72	42	Black ≥ 40 years	9.7	5.4–17.3	
				Hand-rolling			
		45	107	Lifelong manufactured	2.9	1.6–5.2	
		31	69	Mixed	2.6	1.4–4.9	
		106	101	Lifelong hand-rolled	6.1	3.6–10.2	
				Duration by hand-rolling			
		17	49	Manufactured 1–39 years	2.6	1.2–5.6	
		28	58	Manufactured ≥ 40 years	3.2	1.7–6.1	
		34	49	Rolled 1–39 years	4.2	2.1–8.2	
		103	121	Rolled ≥ 40 years	4.8	2.9–8.1	

Table 2.1.4.5 (contd)

Reference (country and years of study)	Cancer subsite ICD code	No. of cases	No. of controls	Smoking categories	Relative risk	95% CI	Comments
De Stefani et al. (1998) (contd)				Filter use			Adjusted for age and alcohol use
		6	25	Lifelong filter	1.7	0.6–4.8	
		48	129	Mixed	2.3	1.3–4.1	
		128	123	Lifelong plain	6.0	3.6–10.0	
				Smoking pattern			
		28	96	Blond + manufactured	1.9	0.9–3.5	
		63	126	Blond + hand-rolled	2.8	1.6–4.8	
		17	11	Black + manufactured	10.3	4.2–25.1	
		74	44	Black + hand-rolled	9.2	5.1–16.3	
Hayes et al. (1999) Puerto Rico 1992–95	Oral cavity ICD-9: 141 tongue 143 gum 144 floor of mouth 145 other parts of mouth	Men 259 11 Women 36 6	Men 270 7 Women 30 3	Cigarettes Other tobacco only	3.9 7.6	2.1–7.1 2.1–27.7	
				Cigarettes + other tobacco Other tobacco only	4.9 7.1	2.0–11.6 1.4–34.6	

CI, confidence interval

Table 2.1.4.6. Case-series on smoking and oral cancer

Reference[a] Country and years of study	Cancer subsite	%	No. of cases	Age	Histological types	Exposures			Comments
Sein et al. (1992) Myanmar 1985–88	Alveolar ridge	61	35 men	15–85 years	85.7% squamous-cell carcinoma	*Smoking habit*		%	Incident cases only
	Buccal mucosa	15	35 women			Nonsmoker		32.9	
						Occasional		1.4	
						Regular 65.7			
Ma'aita (2000) Jordan 1989–98	Tongue	23	89 men	35–90 years; mean age, 62.5 years	96% squamous-cell carcinoma	*Smoking habit*		%	
	Buccal mucosa and sulcus	5	29 women			Nonsmoker		24	
	Gingiva	6				Cigarette smoker		55	
	Lower alveolar ridge	19				Pipe/cigar		21	
	Upper alveolar ridge	9							
	Floor of mouth	34							
	Palate	4							

[a] Studies from regions where no other analytical epidemiological data are available

Table 2.1.4.7. Case–control studies on tobacco smoking and sinonasal cancer: main characteristics of study design

Reference Country and years of study	Number of cases and controls	Criteria for eligibility
Brinton et al. (1984) USA 1970–80	Men: 93 cases and 183 controls; women, 67 cases and 1076 controls	Hospital-based study in four hospitals in two states Cases diagnosed as cancer of the nasal cavity (61), maxillary sinus (71) or other sinuses (28), histologically confirmed as squamous-cell carcinomas (54%), adenocarcinomas (15%) or others (31%), aged ≥ 18 years; response rate, 83% Controls (178 hospital controls for living cases and 112 death certificate controls for deceased cases), matched on hospital, admission year, age, sex, race and residence; response rate, 78%; cancers and other conditions of upper aerodigestive tract were excluded.
Ng (1986) Hong Kong SAR 1974–81	Men: 157 cases and 158 controls; women: 68 cases and 68 controls	Hospital-based study at the Institute of Radiology and Oncology Cases of cancers of the nasal fossa (82), maxillary sinus (110) and other sinuses (33), aged ≥ 18 years Controls with all other malignancies except nasopharyngeal cancer, randomly selected and individually matched on admission year, age (± 5 years), sex, race and resident status
Hayes et al. (1987) The Netherlands 1978–81	Men: 92 cases and 195 controls	Population-based study Cases of cancers of the nasal cavity and sinuses, including 28 deceased cases, histologically confirmed as squamous-cell carcinomas (54%) or adenocarcinomas (26%), aged 35–79 years; response rate, 79% Controls included a random sample of residents in the country and of persons deceased during 1980; response rate, 75%
Strader et al. (1988) USA 1979–83	Men: 33 cases and 327 controls; women: 20 cases and 225 controls	Population-based study in Washington Cases identified by the population-based cancer registry, histologically confirmed as squamous-cell carcinomas (51%), adenocarcinomas (11%) or other types (38%), aged 20–74 years; response rate, 72% Controls selected by random-digit dialling and matched by age and sex; 83% of eligible controls participated
Fukuda & Shibata (1990) Japan 1982–86	Men: 125 cases and 250 controls; women: 44 cases and 88 controls	Population-based study in Hokkaido Incident cases of squamous-cell carcinoma of the maxillary sinus, aged 40–79 years; response rate, 96.6% Controls matched by sex, age and area of residence; response rate, 93.4%

Table 2.1.4.7 (contd)

Reference Country and years of study	Number of cases and controls	Criteria for eligibility
Zheng *et al.* (1992b) China 1988–90	Men: 39 cases and 269 controls; women: 21 cases and 145 controls	Population-based study conducted in Shanghai Cases of cancers of the nasal cavity, paranasal sinuses and middle ear, including 40% of squamous-cell carcinomas, aged 20–75 years; response rate, 95.2% Controls frequency matched on sex and age; response rate, 89.6%
Zheng *et al.* (1993) USA 1986	White men: 147 cases and 449 controls	Data from the 1986 US National Mortality Followback Survey Deaths from cancer of the maxillary sinus (76), nasal cavity (11), other sinuses (56) and auditory tube and middle ear (4), aged ≥ 45 years; response rate, 88% Controls aged ≥ 45 years who died from causes unrelated to smoking or alcohol consumption
't Mannetje *et al.* (1999) France, Germany, Italy, Netherlands and Sweden 1979–90	Men: 451 cases and 1464 controls; women: 104 cases and 241 controls	Pooled analysis of eight studies conducted in five European countries Cases of sinonasal cancer, histologically confirmed as squamous-cell carcinomas (43%), adenocarcinomas (29%), other types (26%) and of unknown histology (1%)
Caplan *et al.* (2000) USA 1984–88	Men: 70 cases and 1910 controls	Population-based study (Selected Cancers Study) Cases identified from the registries, histologically confirmed as carcinomas (74%) or non-carcinomas (26%), aged 35–60 years; response rate, 78% of all cases Controls selected by random-digit dialling, frequency-matched to another case group by geographical area and age (5-year groups)

Table 2.1.4.8. Case–control studies on tobacco smoking and cancer of the nasal cavity and sinuses

Reference Country and years of study	Cancer subsite ICD code	Exposure categories	Relative risk	95% CI	Comments
Brinton et al. (1984) USA 1970–80	Nasal cavity, sinuses ICD-8: 160.0; 160.2–5; 160.8–9	Squamous-cell carcinomas (n = 86) Current smoker	1.8		Adjusted for sex
		Duration (years)			
		<30	1.7		
		30–39	1.9		
		40–49	1.9		
		≥50	3.0		
		Adenocarcinomas (n = 24) Current smoker	0.6		
		Duration (years)			
		<30	1.5		
		30–39	0.4		
		40–49	0.8		
		≥50	1.4		
Ng (1986) Hong Kong SAR 1974–81	Nasal cavity, sinuses ICD-8: 160.0, 160.2–5; 160.8–160.9	Current smoker	1.4	0.9–2.3	Referent group included large proportions of smoking-associated malignancies; inconsistent trend with duration or intensity of smoking; relative risk was not reduced after adjusting for confounders.
Hayes et al. (1987) The Netherlands 1978–81	Nasal cavity, accessory sinuses ICD-9: 160.0; 160.2–160.5	Squamous-cell carcinomas (n = 48) Ever-smoker	3.0	0.9–20.8	Adjusted for age; small sample size
		Current smoker	3.1	1.2–9.9	
		Cigarettes/day			
		1–9	1.7		
		10–19	2.6		
		20–34	1.8		
		≥35	5.1		p for trend < 0.005

Table 2.1.4.8 (contd)

Reference Country and years of study	Cancer subsite ICD code	Exposure categories	Relative risk	95% CI	Comments
Hayes *et al.* (1987) (contd)		Adenocarcinomas (*n* = 23)			
		Ever-smoker	3.0	0.5–65.5	
		Current smoker	1.4	0.5–5.5	
		Cigarettes/day			
		1–9	1.8		
		10–19	1.3		
		20–34	1.5		
		≥ 35	0.8		*p* for trend > 0.005
Strader *et al.* (1988) USA 1979–83	Nasal cavity, sinuses ICD-O (1976): 160.0–160.9	≥ 40 pack–years vs ≤ 1 pack–year			Referent group may not be appropriate. Increased relative risk with increasing levels of smoking
		All types (*n* = 53)	1.7	0.8–3.9	
		Squamous-cell (*n* = 27)	6.6	1.7–29.6	
Fukuda & Shibata (1990) Japan 1982–86	Maxillary sinuses ICD-9: 160.2	Cigarettes/day			Analysis for men only; study included only squamous-cell carcinomas.
		< 10	2.7		
		10–19	2.5		
		20–39	2.9		
		> 39	4.6		
		Pack-years			
		< 25	2.1		
		25–50	2.9		
		> 50	4.1		

Table 2.1.4.8 (contd)

Reference Country and years of study	Cancer subsite ICD code	Exposure categories	Relative risk	95% CI	Comments
Zheng et al. (1992b) China 1988–90	Nasal cavity, paranasal sinuses, middle ear ICD-9: 160	All types (n = 60)			Adjusted for age (< 63 vs ≥ 63 years)
		Ever-smoker	0.7	0.4–1.2	
		Cigarettes/day			
		< 20	0.7	0.4–1.2	
		≥ 20	0.7	0.3–1.9	
		Duration (years)			
		< 30	0.6	0.3–1.3	
		≥ 30	0.7	0.4–1.5	
		Squamous-cell carcinomas (n = 24)			
		Ever-smoker	1.7	0.7–3.8	
		Cigarettes/day			
		< 20	1.7	0.7–4.1	
		≥ 20	1.5	0.4–5.6	
		Duration (years)			
		< 30	1.5	0.5–4.1	
		≥ 30	1.8	0.7–4.9	
Zheng et al. (1993) USA 1986	Nasal cavity, paranasal sinuses, middle ear ICD-9: 160	Ever-smoker	1.2	0.7–1.9	
		Cigarettes/day			
		< 15 or occasional	0.6	0.3–1.2	
		15–34	1.1	0.7–1.9	
		> 34	2.0	1.1–3.6	p for trend = 0.01
		Duration (years)			
		≤ 25	0.8	0.4–1.4	
		26–40	1.2	0.7–2.2	
		> 40	1.9	1.1–3.5	p for trend = 0.01
		Years since quitting			
		Current smoker	1.0	–	
		< 5	1.3	0.7–2.2	
		5–9	1.2	0.5–2.8	
		> 10	0.4	0.2–0.7	p for trend < 0.01

Table 2.1.4.8 (contd)

Reference Country and years of study	Cancer subsite ICD code	Exposure categories	Relative risk	95% CI	Comments
't Mannetje *et al.* (1999) France, Germany, Italy, Netherlands and Sweden 1979–90	Nasal cavity and sinuses	All			Adjusted for age (10-year categories), sex, study centre and smoking status
		Former smoker	1.3	1.0–1.8	
		Current smoker	1.2	0.9–1.6	
		Women			
		Former smoker	1.5	0.6–3.4	
		Current smoker	0.8	0.3–1.8	
		Men			
		Former smoker	1.4	1.03–2.0	
		Current smoker	1.3	0.97–1.9	
		Squamous-cell carcinomas (*n* = 241)			
		Former smoker	1.2	0.8–1.8	
		Current smoker	1.7	1.2–2.6	
		Adenocarcinomas (*n* = 160)			
		Former smoker	1.3	0.8–2.2	
		Current smoker	0.7	0.4–1.2	
Caplan *et al.* (2000) USA 1984–88	Nasal cavity	Ever-smoker	2.4	1.1–5.2	Adjusted for age, registry area, living or working on a farm, several other occupations, and household income
		Cigarettes/day			
		1–19	1.5	0.6–3.9	
		20–39	2.1	1.0–4.7	
		≥ 40	3.1	1.3–7.4	
		Pack–years			
		< 15	1.3	0.5–3.3	
		15–29.9	1.6	0.7–3.9	
		30–44.9	2.4	1.0–5.7	
		≥ 45	3.3	1.3–7.4	
		Duration (years)			
		< 15	1.4	0.5–3.6	
		15–24.9	1.9	0.8–4.5	
		25–34.9	3.1	1.3–7.1	
		≥ 35	3.1	1.2–8.2	

CI, confidence interval

Table 2.1.4.9. Cohort studies on tobacco smoking and nasopharyngeal cancer

Reference Country and years of study	Subjects	Smoking categories	Number of cases	Relative risk	95% CI	Comments
Chow et al. (1993) USA 1954–80	US Veterans' Study 248 046 men	Former smoker	48	1.5	0.4–5.1	Adjusted for age and calendar year
		Current smoker		3.9	1.5–10.3	
		Duration (years)				
		< 30		1.5	0.2–10.6	
		30–39		1.8	0.3–10.3	
		≥ 40		1.8	0.3–10.2	
		Age at starting (years)				
		> 24		1.4	0.2–9.2	
		20–24		1.7	0.3–9.8	
		15–19		1.8	0.3–9.7	
		< 15		2.5	0.3–18.0	
Liaw & Chen (1998) China, Province of Taiwan 1982–94	Taiwanese Study 11 096 men, 3301 women	Current smoker	16	3.9	0.9–17.0	Adjusted for age
		Cigarettes/day				
		≤ 10		3.6	0.8–16.3	
		11–20		3.3	0.8–14.0	
		> 20		3.1	0.3–31.5	
		Duration (years)				
		≤ 20		4.4	0.8–23.5	
		21–30		2.6	0.5–14.4	
		> 30		3.5	0.8–15.1	
		Pack–years				
		< 20		3.2	0.7–14.5	
		20–40		3.9	0.9–16.7	
		> 40		2.8	0.4–18.9	
		Age at starting (years)				
		> 24		3.3	0.8–14.1	
		21–24		4.8	1.0–23.5	
		≤ 20		2.8	0.5–14.8	

CI, confidence interval

Table 2.1.4.10. Case–control studies on tobacco smoking and nasopharyngeal cancer: main characteristics of study design

Reference Country and years of study	Number of cases and controls	Criteria for eligibility and comments
Lin *et al.* (1973) China, Province of Taiwan 1969–71	Men and women: 343 cases and 1017 controls	Population-based study in eight cities and counties Cases reported by all the medical facilities in the study areas; 93% histologically confirmed; response rate, 79.4% Controls from neighbourhood individually matched by age (± 5 years) and sex; response rate, 85%
Henderson *et al.* (1976) USA 1960–74	Men: 105 cases and 179 controls; women: 51 cases and 88 controls	Population-based study in California Cases: 88 identified by the Los Angeles Cancer Surveillance Program in 1971–74, 27 by the California Tumor Registry in 1960–70, and 41 incident cases in 1972–74; mean age, 51.4 years Controls were in- and outpatients, individually matched on sex, age, race, area and socioeconomic class; mean age, 52.4 years
Lanier *et al.* (1980) USA 1966–76	Men and women: 13 cases and 13 controls	Population-based study among natives in Alaska Cases identified from pathology files and tumour registries of the Alaska Native Medical Center, aged 32–80 years Controls were apparently healthy, individually matched (1:1) by sex, age (± 2.5 years), race and area of residence
Mabuchi *et al.* (1985) USA 4 years	Men and women: 39 cases and 39 controls	Hospital-based study in five metropolitan areas Cases histologically confirmed; response rate, 64% Controls randomly selected from admissions, matched on age (± 3 years), sex, race, marital status, hospital and admission period
Ng (1986) Hong Kong SAR 1974–81	Men: 159 cases and 158 controls; women: 65 cases and 68 controls	Hospital-based study at the Institute of Radiology and Oncology, among Chinese Cases aged ≥ 18 years; mean age, 57 years Controls with all other malignancies except cancer of the nasal cavity and sinuses, selected in random order from patient's register, matched on admission year, age (± 5 years), sex, race and resident status; mean age, 57 years
Yu *et al.* (1986) Hong Kong SAR 1981	Men: 160 cases and 160 controls; women: 90 cases and 90 controls	Population-based study in 4 hospitals, among Chinese Incident cases histologically confirmed, aged ≤ 35 years; response rate, 94% Controls were friends, individually matched by age and sex
Ning *et al.* (1990) China 1981	Men: 68 cases and 204 controls; women: 32 cases and 96 controls	Population-based study in Tianjin city Cases identified from the population-based cancer registry histologically confirmed, aged ≤ 64 years; response rate, 61.3% Controls individually matched (3:1) on age, sex and race (Han); 97% first chosen controls participated
Yu *et al.* (1990) China 1983–85	Men: 209 cases and 209 controls; women: 97 cases and 97 controls	Population-based study in Guangzhou city Incident cases identified at the Tumor Hospital, histologically confirmed, aged < 50 years; response rate, 93% Controls individually matched by age (± 5 years) and sex

Table 2.1.4.10 (contd)

Reference Country and years of study	Number of cases and controls	Criteria for eligibility and comments
Nam et al. (1992) USA 1986	Men: 141 cases and 282 controls; women: 63 cases and 126 controls	Population-based mortality study among white Americans Cases taken from a random sample of all deaths in 1986, aged ≥ 25 years; response rate, 89% Controls had died from diseases unrelated to smoking or alcohol drinking, aged ≤ 65 years, randomly selected from the sex and age strata, individually matched (2:1)
Sriamporn et al. (1992) Thailand 1987–90	Men: 80 cases and 80 controls: women: 40 cases and 40 controls	Hospital-based study in north-eastern Thailand Cases diagnosed and attending radiation therapy at the hospital Controls admitted for other diseases excluding any cancers and respiratory diseases, matched by sex and age (± 5 years)
West et al. (1993) Philippines	Men: 76 cases; women: 28 cases; 205 controls	Hospital- and population-based study Incident cases recruited from Philippine General Hospital, histologically confirmed, < 10% ethnically Chinese, aged 11–83 years; response rate, 100% Controls: 104 hospital controls matched for sex, age and ward type; response rate, 100%; 101 community controls matched for sex, age and neighbourhood; response rate, 77%
Zheng et al. (1994) China 1986	Men: 64 cases and 128 controls; women: 24 cases and 48 controls	Population-based study in Wuzhou and Zangwu Incident cases, histologically confirmed; mean age, 41.6 years; response rate, 98% Controls from neighbourhood, individually matched (2:1) on sex, age (± 4 years) and place of residence
Ye et al. (1995) China	Men: 114 cases and 114 controls; women: 21 cases and 21 controls	Hospital-based study in teaching hospital Incident cases, histologically confirmed, 82% poorly differentiated Controls from the surgical and orthopaedic departments with non-cancer, non-respiratory diseases, individually matched on sex, age, admission date and residence or ethnicity
Zhu et al. (1995, 1997) USA 1984–88	Men: 113 cases and 1910 controls	Population-based study in eight cancer registries (Selected Cancers Study) Cases histologically confirmed including 73% of squamous-cell carcinomas, aged 15–39 years in 1968; response rate, 86.3% Controls selected by random digit dialling, frequency-matched to another case group; 83.1% of eligible controls
Vaughan et al. (1996) USA 1987–93	Men and women: 231 cases and 244 controls	Population-based study Cases identified by five population-based cancer registries, histologically confirmed as differentiated squamous-cell carcinoma (60%) or undifferentiated and nonkeratinizing carcinomas (28%); aged 18–74 years; response rate, 82% Controls selected by random-digit dialling and frequency-matched on sex and age (± 5 years); response rate, 70%

Table 2.1.4.10 (contd)

Reference Country and years of study	Number of cases and controls	Criteria for eligibility and comments
Cheng et al. (1999) China, Province of Taiwan 1991–94	Men: 114 cases and 104 controls; women: 260 cases and 223 controls	Population-based study in Taipei Incident cases identified in two hospitals, histologically confirmed, aged ≤ 75 years; 99% response rate Controls with no history of nasopharyngeal cancer, randomly selected using the National Household Registration System, individually matched on sex, age (± 5 years) and area of residence; response rate, 88%
Armstrong et al. (2000) Malaysia 1987–92	Men: 195 cases and 195 controls; women: 87 cases and 87 controls	Population-based study among Malaysian Chinese Cases (119 prevalent and 163 incident) diagnosed at four study centres, histologically confirmed, aged 19–74 years; response rate, 53% Controls with no history of cancer of the head, neck or respiratory system, randomly selected and pair-matched by age (± 3 years) and sex; response rate, 90%
Cao et al. (2000) China 1998–99	Men and women: 57 cases and 327 controls	Population-based study in Sihui city Incident cases identified in a highly endemic area Controls were family members of the spouse of case; no matching
Yuan et al. (2000) China 1987–91	Men: 668 cases and 699 controls; women: 267 cases and 333 controls	Population-based study Incident cases identified by the Shanghai cancer registry, aged 15–74 years; response rate, 84% Controls randomly selected from general population and frequency matched by sex and age (5 year groups); response rate, 96.4%

Table 2.1.4.11. Case–control studies on tobacco smoking and nasopharyngeal cancer

Reference Country and years of study	Smoking categories	Relative risk	95% CI	Comments
Lin et al. (1973) China, Province of Taiwan 1969–71	Men Former smoker	0.8		Adjusted for age and area of residence
	Cigarettes/day			
	<10	0.6		
	10–19	1.1		
	20–29	3.2		
	≥30	3.5		
	Women Former smoker	6.6		
	Cigarettes/day			
	<10	1.1		
	10–19	5.0		
	20–29	7.5		
Henderson et al. (1976) USA 1960–74		1.0	p = 0.50	Two-sided p value
Lanier et al. (1980) USA 1966–76	Discrepant pairs: Case/control Case/control		Yes/No 3 No/Yes 1	Very small sample size; no detailed results in the text
Mabuchi et al. (1985) USA 4 years	Ever-smoker	1.9	0.6–5.6	Matched-pair analysis Smokers for > 1 year
	Cigarettes/day			
	1–20	1.4	0.4–4.5	
	21–39	2.8	0.7–12.0	
	≥40	2.8	0.6–13.0	

Table 2.1.4.11 (contd)

Reference Country and years of study	Smoking categories	Relative risk	95% CI	Comments
Ng (1986) Hong Kong SAR 1974–81	Ever-smoker	0.9	0.6–1.4	Adjusted for sex The control group included a large proportion of smoking-related cancers.
Yu et al. (1986) Hong Kong SAR 1981	Similar cigarette smoking habits between cases and controls			Matched-pair analysis
Ning et al. (1990) China 1981	Similar use of cigarettes between cases and controls		p = 0.88	Matched-pair analysis
Yu et al. (1990) China 1983–85	Ever-smoker	1.3		Adjusted for intake of salted fish, mouldy bean curd, preserved plum and tomato intake at age 10 years
	Cigarettes/day			
	1–9	1.3		
	10–19	1.0		
	20–29	1.7	p < 0.05	
	≥ 30	4.3	p < 0.05	
	Pack–years			
	–14	1.2		
	15–29	1.6		
	≥ 30	2.9	p < 0.05	
Nam et al. (1992) USA 1986	Men			Adjusted for sex and alcohol intake
	Pack–years			
	≤ 30	0.9	0.5–1.7	
	31–59	1.8	1.0–3.5	
	≥ 60	3.1	1.6–6.1	p for trend < 0.001

Table 2.1.4.11 (contd)

Reference Country and years of study	Smoking categories	Relative risk	95% CI	Comments
Nam *et al.* (1992) (contd)	Years since quitting			
	Current smoker	1.0	–	
	<5	1.2	0.7–2.2	
	≥5	0.6	0.3–1.1	
	Women			
	Pack–years			
	≤30	1.3	0.6–2.8	
	31–59	3.5	1.3–9.2	
	≥60	4.9	1.2–20.9	*p* for trend < 0.001
	Years since quitting			
	Current smoker	1.0	–	
	<5	1.3	0.5–3.4	
	≥5	0.3	0.1–1.3	
Sriamporn *et al.* (1992) Thailand 1987–90	Manufactured cigarette	0.8	0.3–2.1	Adjusted for education, area of residence, intake of alcohol and salted fish
	Hand-made cigarette	0.9	0.3–2.5	
West *et al.* (1993) Philippines	All controls			Adjusted for education, occupational exposure, intake of fresh fish and processed meats, use of anti-mosquito coils and herbal medicines
	Duration (years)			
	1–20	0.5	0.2–1.5	Hospital controls included patients with smoking-related diseases.
	21–30	0.9	0.3–3.0	
	≥31	2.3	0.7–7.3	
	Community controls			
	Duration (years)			
	1–20	0.8	0.1–4.4	
	21–30	2.9	0.5–18.2	
	≥31	7.2	1.5–34.4	

Table 2.1.4.11 (contd)

Reference Country and years of study	Smoking categories	Relative risk	95% CI	Comments
Zheng et al. (1994) China 1986				No significant association between cigarette smoking and nasopharyngeal cancer
Ye et al. (1995) China	Cigarettes/month			Adjusted for exposure to fumes during cooking, intake of various vegetables and salted fish, family history of cancer and passive smoking during childhood and adulthood
	> 5 vs ≤ 5	1.9	1.1–3.4	
	Duration (years)			
	> 10 vs ≤ 10	1.8	1.01–3.2	
	Smoking index 1			Smoking index 1: duration (years) × intensity (cigarettes/month)/age at starting smoking
	> 25 vs ≤ 25	2.1	1.3–3.5	
	Smoking index 2			Smoking index 2: duration (years)/age at starting smoking
	> 0.5 vs ≤ 0.5	1.9	1.1–3.3	
Zhu et al. (1995, 1997) USA 1984–88	Former smoker	2.3	1.3–4.0	Adjusted for year of birth, cancer registry, existence of home phone, education, ethnic background, growing up in urban/suburban environment, medical history, exposure to asbestos or woodwork, and alcohol consumption. The association was stronger for squamous-cell carcinoma.
	Current smoker	1.4	0.8–2.6	
	Cigarettes/day			
	1–19	1.3	0.7–2.6	
	20–39	1.8	1.0–3.3	
	≥ 40	3.8	2.0–7.3	
	Duration (years)			
	≤ 14	1.7	0.9–3.2	
	15–24	1.5	0.8–2.8	
	25–34	3.0	1.6–5.6	
	≥ 35	2.3	1.0–5.1	
	Pack–years			
	< 15	1.3	0.7–2.5	
	15–29.9	1.8	0.9–3.4	
	30–44.9	2.5	1.3–5.0	
	≥ 45	3.9	2.0–7.8	

Table 2.1.4.11 (contd)

Reference Country and years of study	Smoking categories	Relative risk	95% CI	Comments
Zhu et al. (1995, 1997) (contd)	Age at starting smoking (years)			Further adjusted for pack–years
	≥ 22	1.0	–	
	18–21	0.4	0.2–0.9	
	≤ 17	0.8	0.4–1.5	
Vaughan et al. (1996) USA 1987–93	Former smoker	1.3	0.7–2.2	Adjusted for age, sex, registry, education and alcohol use. The association was much stronger for differentiated squamous-cell carcinoma.
	Current smoker	2.6	1.4–4.6	
	Pack–years			
	1–34	1.9	0.9–4.0	
	35–59	3.0	1.3–6.8	
	≥ 60	4.3	1.5–13.4	p for trend < 0.001
	Years since quitting			The association was much stronger for differentiated squamous-cell carcinoma.
	Current smoker	1.0	–	
	< 5	0.1	0.0–0.6	
	5–14	0.2	0.1–0.7	
	≥ 15	0.2	0.0–0.8	p for trend = 0.003
Cheng et al. (1999) China, Province of Taiwan 1991–94	Former smoker	1.1	0.6–2.1	Adjusted for age, sex, race, education, family history of nasopharyngeal carcinoma and alcohol use
	Current smoker	1.4	0.9–2.1	
	Cigarettes/day			
	< 20	1.4	0.9–2.1	
	≥ 20	1.4	0.9–2.2	p for trend = 0.2
	Duration (years)			
	< 25	1.1	0.7–1.8	
	≥ 25	1.7	1.1–2.9	p for trend = 0.03
	Pack–years			
	< 20	1.3	0.8–2.0	
	≥ 20	1.5	0.9–2.4	p for trend = 0.1

Table 2.1.4.11 (contd)

Reference Country and years of study	Smoking categories	Relative risk	95% CI	Comments
Cheng et al. (1999) (contd)	Age at starting smoking (years)			
	≥ 20	1.4	0.9–2.2	
	< 20	1.3	0.8–2.0	p for trend = 0.1
Armstrong et al. (2000) Malaysia 1987–92	Ever-smoker (> 6 months)	1.8	0.8–4.2	Adjusted for parental smoking and dietary index. Response rate for cases was too low; control group might be biased.
Cao et al. (2000) China 1998–99	Current smoker	5.6	3.3–9.6	No mention of adjustment for age and sex; adjusted for family history of nasopharyngeal carcinoma and separate kitchen
	Cigarettes/day			
	≤ 10	1.0	–	
	> 10	6.4	3.8–10.5	
Yuan et al. (2000) China 1987–91	Men			Adjusted for age, education, intake of preserved foods and oranges/tangerines, exposure to smoke from heated rapeseed oil and burning coal during cooking, occupational exposure to chemical fumes, history of chronic ear and nose condition and family history of nasopharyngeal carcinoma
	Former smoker	1.2	0.8–1.8	
	Ever-smoker	1.3	1.01–1.6	
	Current smoker	1.3	1.01–1.7	
	Cigarettes/day			
	< 10	1.1	0.8–1.7	
	10–19	1.2	0.8–1.6	
	20–29	1.4	1.1–2.0	
	≥ 30	1.8	1.1–3.2	
	Pack–years			
	< 20	1.2	0.9–1.6	
	20–39	1.3	0.96–1.8	
	≥ 40	1.6	1.03–2.6	

Table 2.1.4.11 (contd)

Reference Country and years of study	Smoking categories	Relative risk	95% CI	Comments
Yuan et al. (2000) (contd)	Women			
	Former smoker	1.2	0.4–3.5	
	Ever-smoker	1.3	0.7–2.5	
	Current smoker	1.4	0.6–2.8	
	Cigarettes/day			
	< 10	1.4	0.5–3.8	
	10–19	2.3	0.5–11.7	
	20–29	0.5	0.1–3.0	
	≥ 30	2.9	0.2–47.8	
	Pack–years			
	< 20	1.3	0.7–2.7	
	20–39	0.9	0.2–4.2	
	≥ 40	2.2	0.1–38.2	

CI, confidence interval

Table 2.1.4.12. Cohort studies on tobacco smoking and pharyngeal cancer

Reference Country and years of study	Subjects	Organ subsite ICD code	Smoking categories	Number of cases	Relative risk	95% CI	Comments
Weir & Dunn (1970) USA 1954–62	Californian Study 68 153 men	Pharynx ICD: 145–148	Ever-smoker	13	0.8		Nonsmokers include cigar and/or pipe only smokers.
			Cigarettes/day				
			1–14		–		
			15–25		1.2		
			> 25		0.5		
McLaughlin et al. (1995) USA 1954–80	US Veterans' Study 248 046 men	Pharynx (ICD-1957)	Former smoker	143	2.6	1.1–6.2	Adjusted for attained age and calendar-year time-period at death
			Ever-smoker		9.5	4.6–19.4	
			Current smoker		14.1	6.9–28.9	
			Cigarettes/day				
			1–9		5.2	1.8–15.0	
			10–20		12.6	6.0–26.6	
			31–39 [sic]		18.1	8.5–38.7	
			≥ 40		37.3	15.9–87.5	p for trend < 0.01
Nordlund et al. (1997) Sweden 1963–89	Swedish Census Study 26 032 women	Pharynx ICD-7: 145–148	Current smoker	17	2.9	0.9–9.7	Adjusted for age and place of residence

CI, confidence interval

Table 2.1.4.13. Case–control studies on tobacco smoking and pharyngeal cancer: main characteristics of study design

Reference Country and years of study	Number of cases and controls	Criteria for eligibility and comments
Jussawalla & Deshpande (1971) India 1968	Men and women: 223 cases and 1647 controls	Retrospective study at the Cancer Registry in Mumbai Cases of the oropharynx (185) and hypopharynx (38), histologically confirmed Controls selected among residents from the registered voters' list, matched for age, sex and religion
Elwood et al. (1984) Canada 1977–80	Men: 68 cases and 68 controls; women: 19 cases and 19 controls	Hospital-based study at a cancer referral centre in Vancouver Incident cases of pharyngeal cancer; 95% of identified cases participated. Controls were patients with cancers unrelated to smoking, alcohol use or occupational exposure, individually matched on date of diagnosis, sex and age (± 2 years).
Brugere et al. (1986) France 1975–82	Men: 1000 cases	Population-based study in Paris Cases of oropharyngeal (634) and hypopharyngeal (366) cancer admitted to the head and neck department of the Institut Curie; non- squamous carcinomas and secondary cancers excluded Controls were a random subsample from a large national survey stratified by age.
Tuyns et al. (1988) France, Italy, Spain and Switzerland 1973–80	Men: 281 cases and 3057 controls	Population-based study in six study areas Cases of cancer of the hypopharynx, histologically confirmed; oropharynx excluded; response rate > 80% Controls drawn from the general population within a sample stratified by age and sex; response rate, 56–75%
Franceschi et al. (1990) Italy 1986–89	Men: 134 cases and 1272 controls	Hospital-based study Cases of pharyngeal cancer, including the junction between hypopharynx and larynx, histologically confirmed, aged < 75 years; response rate, 98% Controls were inpatients with acute conditions unrelated to tobacco or alcohol consumption, without malignant tumours, chosen on the basis of area of residence and age (± 5-year categories); response rate, 97%
Choi & Kahyo (1991) Republic of Korea 1986–89	Men: 133 cases and 399 controls; women: 19 cases and 57 controls	Hospital-based study at the Cancer Center Hospital in Seoul Cases of pharyngeal cancer, confirmed histologically or cytologically Controls excluded patients with other cancers or tobacco- and alcohol-related diseases, individually matched (3:1) on year of birth (± 5 years) and admission date (± 3 months).
Maier et al. (1994) Germany 1990–91	Men: 105 cases and 420 controls	Hospital-based study at the Department of Otorhinolaryngology, Head and Neck Surgery of the University of Heidelberg Cases of squamous-cell carcinoma of the oropharynx (40), hypopharynx (44) or both (21), histologically confirmed Controls were outpatients without known cancer, individually matched (4:1) for age and residential area.

Table 2.1.4.13 (contd)

Reference Country and years of study	Number of cases and controls	Criteria for eligibility and comments
De Stefani *et al.* (1998) Uruguay 1992–96	Men: 219 cases and 427 controls	Hospital-based study in four hospitals of Montevideo Cases of squamous-cell carcinoma of the oropharynx (111), hypopharynx (97) or unspecified (11), aged 25–84 years; response rate, 93.8% Controls without diseases related to tobacco and alcohol use or non-neoplastic lesions of the oral cavity and pharynx, aged 25–84 years; frequency-matched on age, area of residence and urban/rural status; response rate, 91.0%
Franceschi *et al.* (1999) Italy & Switzerland 1992–97	Men: 364 cases and 1254 controls	Hospital-based study in major hospitals in three areas Cases of oro- or hypopharyngeal cancer, histologically confirmed, aged 32–74 years Controls were patients with acute non-cancerous illnesses unrelated to tobacco smoking or alcohol abuse, frequency-matched by age and area of residence.
La Vecchia *et al.* (1999a) Italy & Switzerland 1984–97	Men and women: 642 cases; men: 3068 controls; women: 1111 controls	Hospital-based study in a network of hospitals in the study areas Incident cases of pharyngeal cancer, aged < 75 years, histologically confirmed Controls with acute, non-neoplastic conditions unrelated to alcohol or tobacco consumption
Rao *et al.* (1999) India 1980–84	Men: 593 cases and 635 controls	Hospital-based study in Mumbai Cases of cancer of the hypopharynx Controls with infectious diseases and benign tumours, free from cancer, admitted during the same period as controls; no matching
Schlecht *et al.* (1999) Brazil 1986–89	Men and women: 217 cases and 1578 controls	Hospital-based study in three metropolitan areas Incident cases of pharyngeal cancer, histologically confirmed Controls without diagnosis of cancer or mental disorder, individually matched for sex, age and trimester of admission

Table 2.1.4.14. Case–control studies on tobacco smoking and pharyngeal cancer

Reference Country and years of study	Cancer subsite ICD code	Smoking categories	Relative risk	95% CI	Comments
Jussawalla & Deshpande (1971) India 1968	Oro- and hypopharynx	Current smoker Oropharynx Hypopharynx	2.3 0.4	$p < 0.001$ $p > 0.05$	
Elwood et al. (1984) Canada 1977–80	Oro- and hypopharynx ICD-O: 146, 148, 149	Cigarettes/day 1–9 10–19 20–29 ≥ 30	0.5 1.2 1.3 1.5		Adjusted for alcohol, socio-economic group, marital status, dental care and history of tuberculosis p for trend > 0.05
Brugere et al. (1986) France 1975–82	Oro- and hypopharynx ICD-8: 146, 148	Oropharynx Tobacco/day (g) 0–9 10–19 20–29 ≥ 30 Hypopharynx Tobacco/day (g) 0–9 10–19 20–29 ≥ 30	1.0 4.0 7.6 15.2 1.0 7.1 12.6 35.1	– 2.4–6.5 4.8–12.1 9.3–24.9 – 3.1–15.8 5.8–27.4 16.2–75.9	Adjusted for alcohol use Light smokers were included in reference group.
Tuyns et al. (1988) France, Italy, Spain and Switzerland 1973–80	Hypopharynx ICD-9: 148.0, 148.1, 148.3, 149.8	Cigarettes/day 1–7 8–15 16–25 ≥ 26	5.5 13.7 18.0 20.0	2.0–15.1 5.4–34.5 7.2–44.8 7.9–51.0	Adjusted for age, place, age/place interaction and alcohol use

Table 2.1.4.14 (contd)

Reference Country and years of study	Cancer subsite ICD code	Smoking categories	Relative risk	95% CI	Comments
Franceschi et al. (1990) Italy 1986–89	Pharynx, junction between hypopharynx and larynx ICD-9: 146, 148, 161.1	Current smoker	12.9	3.1–52.9	Adjusted for age, area of residence, years of education, occupation and alcohol use
		Cigarettes/day			
		≤ 14	8.0	1.9–34.5	
		15–24	14.2	3.4–59.3	
		≥ 25	17.6	4.1–74.7	p for trend < 0.01
		Duration (years)			
		1–29	6.4	1.5–27.4	
		30–39	15.5	3.6–66.7	
		≥ 40	25.5	6.0–109.9	p for trend < 0.01
		Age at starting smoking (years)			
		≥ 25	7.9	1.7–36.1	
		17–24	12.8	3.1–53.2	
		< 17	16.0	3.8–67.5	p for trend < 0.01
		Years since quitting			
		< 10	11.3	2.6–49.4	
		≥ 10	3.7	0.8–18.0	p for trend < 0.01
Choi & Kahyo (1991) Republic of Korea 1986–89	Pharynx ICD-O: 146–149	Men			
		Former smoker	0.9	0.3–2.1	Adjusted for alcohol use
		Current smoker	1.6	0.9–3.1	
		Cigarettes/day			
		1–20	1.3	0.7–2.5	
		21–40	2.4	1.1–4.9	
		≥ 41	2.9	1.0–9.3	
		Duration (years)			
		1–19	1.2	0.5–2.7	
		20–39	1.2	0.8–2.8	
		≥ 40	2.4	1.2–4.8	

Table 2.1.4.14 (contd)

Reference Country and years of study	Cancer subsite ICD code	Smoking categories	Relative risk	95% CI	Comments
Choi & Kahyo (1991) (contd)		Age at starting smoking (years)			
		≥ 25	1.03	0.5–2.4	
		18–24	1.7	0.9–3.1	
		≤ 17	2.6	1.2–5.9	
		Years since quitting			
		Current smoker	1.0	–	
		1–4	0.1	0.0–0.7	
		5–9	1.1	0.4–2.9	
		≥ 10	0.5	0.1–1.6	
		Women			
		Current smoker	0.98	0.2–4.1	
		Cigarettes/day			
		1–20	1.2	0.3–5.0	
		21–40	0.7	0.1–7.9	
		Duration (years)			
		1–19	0.9	0.2–5.3	
		20–39	0.9	0.1–6.1	
		Age at starting smoking (years)			
		≥ 25	0.98	0.2–4.1	
Maier et al. (1994) Germany 1990–91	Oro- and hypopharynx	Tobacco–years			Adjusted for alcohol use Daily consumption of 20 cigarettes or 4 cigars or 5 pipes for 1 year
		< 5	1.0		
		5–< 20	4.5	1.2–17.3	
		20–< 40	6.1	1.9–18.7	
		40–60	9.5	2.5–35.4	p for trend = 0.0001

Table 2.1.4.14 (contd)

Reference Country and years of study	Cancer subsite ICD code	Smoking categories	Relative risk	95% CI	Comments
De Stefani *et al.* (1998) Uruguay 1992–96	Oro- and hypopharynx, pharynx unspecified	Former smoker	4.3	2.2–8.3	Adjusted for age, residence, urban/rural status, birthplace, education and total alcohol consumption
		Ever-smoker	7.5	4.1–13.6	
		Current smoker	10.2	5.5–18.8	
		Cigarettes/day			
		1–14	3.6	1.8–7.1	
		15–24	7.8	4.1–14.9	
		≥ 25	12.2	6.4–23.3	
		Duration (years)			
		1–39	6.2	2.9–12.8	
		40–49	8.3	4.3–15.9	
		≥ 50	7.5	3.9–14.4	
		Pack–years			
		1–28	3.5	1.7–7.0	
		29–47	8.9	4.5–17.6	
		48–76	6.7	3.4–13.2	
		≥ 77	13.3	6.7–26.2	
		Years since quitting			
		1–4	5.9	2.7–12.8	
		5–9	5.1	2.2–12.0	
		≥ 10	2.1	0.8–5.5	
		Type of tobacco			
		Mainly blond	4.4	2.4–8.1	
		Mainly black	17.8	9.2–34.1	
		Hand-rolling			
		Only manufactured	4.3	2.2–8.5	
		Mixed	2.7	1.3–5.8	
		Only rolled	13.7	7.3–25.5	

Table 2.1.4.14 (contd)

Reference Country and years of study	Cancer subsite ICD code	Smoking categories	Relative risk	95% CI	Comments
De Stefani *et al.* (1998) (contd)		Filter use			Adjusted for area of residence, interviewer, age, education, vegetable and fruit intake, total energy intake and alcohol drinking [†]Smokers of cigars and/or pipes were included.
		Only filter	1.3	0.3–5.2	
		Mixed	4.0	2.1–7.8	
		Only plain	11.3	6.1–20.8	
		Smoking pattern			
		Blond + manufactured	3.4	1.7–6.8	
		Blond + hand-rolled	5.1	2.7–9.6	
		Black + manufactured	9.2	3.4–25.0	
		Black + hand-rolled	20.6	10.5–40.6	
Franceschi *et al.* (1999) Italy & Switzerland 1992–97	Pharynx	Cigarettes/day			
		1–14	7.3	3.3–16.3	
		15–24	14.7	7.0–30.8	
		≥ 25[†]	19.3	8.8–42.4	
La Vecchia *et al.* (1999a) Italy & Switzerland 1984–97	Pharynx	Current smoker	13.5	9.1–19.8	Adjusted for age, sex, study centre, education and alcohol drinking
		Years since quitting			
		1–2	9.9	5.6–17.5	
		3–5	6.3	3.6–11.0	
		6–9	4.8	2.7–8.4	
		10–14	3.2	1.8–5.7	
		≥ 15	2.9	1.7–4.8	

Table 2.1.4.14 (contd)

Reference Country and years of study	Cancer subsite ICD code	Smoking categories	Relative risk	95% CI	Comments
Rao et al. (1999) India 1980–84	Hypopharynx ICD-9: 148.0, 148.1, 148.9	Cigarette smoker	0.8	0.5–1.4	Adjusted for age and residence In the study area, cigarette smoking is not as common as bidi smoking.
Schlecht et al. (1999) Brazil 1986–89	Pharynx ICD-9: 146–149	Current smoker	5.9	2.2–15.3	Adjusted for sex, study location, admission period and alcohol consumption
		Pack–years			
		1–20	5.4	1.9–15.5	
		21–40	5.7	1.9–16.9	
		> 40	7.5	2.4–23.6	
		Years since quitting			
		≤ 5	2.6	0.8–8.5	
		6–10	1.2	0.2–7.0	
		11–15	1.4	0.2–9.8	
		> 15	0.9	0.1–5.5	

CI, confidence interval

Table 2.1.4.15. Cohort studies on tobacco smoking and oesophageal cancer (unspecified)

Reference Country and years of study	Subjects	Smoking categories	Number of cases	Relative risk	95% CI	Comments
Weir & Dunn (1970) USA 1954–62	Californian Study 68153 men	Ever-smoker	32	1.8		Nonsmokers include cigar and/or pipe only smokers.
		Cigarettes/day				
		1–14		1.3		
		15–25		1.7		
		> 25		1.8		
Doll et al. (1980) UK 1951–73 (see also Doll et al., 1994)	British Doctors' Study 6194 women	Nonsmoker	2	Mortality rate 0		Annual mortality rate for 100 000 women
		Former smoker		8		
		Cigarettes/day				
		1–14		4		
		15–24		0		
		≥ 25		0		
Hammond & Seidman (1980) USA 1959–72	Cancer Prevention Study I 1 051 038 adults	Regular smoker		Mortality ratio 4.0		
Kono et al. (1987) Japan 1965–83	Japanese Physicians Study 5477 men	Cigarettes/day				Adjusted for age and alcohol drinking
		1–19		0.5	0.1–3.2	
		≥ 20		2.1	0.5–9.2	

Table 2.1.4.15 (contd)

Reference Country and years of study	Subjects	Smoking categories	Number of cases	Relative risk	95% CI	Comments
Akiba & Hirayama (1990) Japan 1965–81 (see Kinjo et al., 1998)	Six-prefecture Study 265 118 (122 261 men and 142 857 women)	Current smoker	314	2.2	1.6–3.0	Data stratified by prefecture, occupation, attained age and observation period
		Cigarettes/day				
		1–4	3	0.9	0.2–2.5	
		5–14	127	2.0	1.4–2.8	
		15–24	164	2.4	1.7–3.3	
		25–34	13	2.1	1.1–3.8	
		≥ 35	7	2.5	1.0–5.2	
Kuller et al. (1991) USA 1975–85	MRFIT Study 12 866 men			Mortality rate		Annual mortality rate per 10 000 men
		Non- and former smoker	73	3.1		Relative risk adjusted for age, diastolic blood pressure, serum cholesterol level, race (black/non-black)
		Cigarettes/day				
		1–15	15	5.6		
		16–25	29	6.7		
		26–35	17	6.3		
		36–45	18	8.2		
		≥ 46	12	15.9		
		Current smoker		Relative risk		
				2.4	p < 0.0001	
Tomita et al. (1991) Japan 1975–85	37 646 men			Mortality rate		Annual mortality rate per 100 000 men. The authors did not state whether the mortality rates had been adjusted for age.
		Nonsmoker	1	0.2		
		Cigarettes/day				
		1–14	1	0.5		
		15–24	10	1.1		
		25–34	4	1.1		

Table 2.1.4.15 (contd)

Reference Country and years of study	Subjects	Smoking categories	Number of cases	Relative risk	95% CI	Comments
Akiba (1994) Japan 1968–87	Life Span Study 61 505 survivors	Former smoker	103	2.8	1.3–6.3	[Upper limit could not be obtained.]
		Current smoker		3.3	1.7–[†]	
Doll et al. (1994) UK 1951–91 (see also Doll et al., 1980)	British Doctors' Study 30 440 men	Nonsmoker	172	Mortality rate 4		Annual mortality rate for 100 000 men
		Former smoker		19		
		Current smoker		30		
		Cigarettes/day				
		1–14		17		
		15–24		33		
		≥ 25		45		
Guo et al. (1994) China 1985–91	Linxian Intervention Trial Study 29 584 residents	Ever-smoker	150	1.6	1.2–2.2	Adjusted for cancer history in first-degree relatives
		Cigarettes/day[†]				[†]Tobacco smoked in pipe was converted to cigarette equivalent (1 g tobacco = 0.8 cigarette).
		< 10	85	1.8	1.3–2.6	
		10–19	96	1.8	1.3–2.5	
		≥ 20	60	1.9	1.3–2.8	
		Duration (years)				
		< 20	24	1.2	0.7–2.0	
		20–39	145	1.8	1.3–2.5	
		≥ 40	73	2.1	1.4–3.1	
		Pack–years[†]				
		< 10	54	1.5	1.0–2.2	
		10–19	84	2.1	1.5–3.1	p for trend < 0.01
		20–29	43	1.6	1.0–2.4	
		≥ 30	60	2.0	1.4–3.0	

Table 2.1.4.15 (contd)

Reference Country and years of study	Subjects	Smoking categories	Number of cases	Relative risk	95% CI	Comments
Guo et al. (1994) (contd)		Years since quitting				
		Current smoker		1.0	–	
		< 3		1.1	0.6–2.2	
		≥ 3		0.5	0.2–1.2	
McLaughlin et al. (1995) USA 1954–80	US Veterans' Study 248 046 men		318			Adjusted for attained age and calendar-year time-period at death
		Former smoker		1.5	1.0–2.2	
		Ever-smoker		3.0	2.3–4.1	
		Current smoker		4.1	3.0–5.6	
		Cigarettes/day				
		1–9		1.4	0.7–2.7	
		10–20		3.3	2.4–4.7	
		31–39 [sic]		6.7	4.7–9.4	
		≥ 40		6.1	3.5–10.7	p for trend < 0.01
Yuan et al. (1996) China 1986–96	Shanghai Men's Study 18 244 men	Ever-smoker	24	1.4	$p > 0.05$	Adjusted for age and alcohol consumption
		Cigarettes/day				
		< 20		1.0	$p > 0.05$	
		≥ 20		1.7	$p > 0.05$	
Chen et al. (1997) China 1972–93	Shanghai Factory Study 6494 men	Ever-smoker	29	3.6	$p < 0.05$	Adjusted for age, systolic blood pressure, serum cholesterol level and regular alcohol drinking (yes/no)
		Cigarettes/day				
		1–19		2.8	$p > 0.05$	
		≥ 20		4.6	$p < 0.01$	p for trend = 0.009

Table 2.1.4.15 (contd)

Reference Country and years of study	Subjects	Smoking categories	Number of cases	Relative risk	95% CI	Comments
Lam et al. (1997) China 1976–96	Xi'an Factory Study 1124 men	Ever-smoker	12	4.3	0.9–19.9	Adjusted for age, marital status, occupation, education, diastolic blood pressure and triglyceride and total cholesterol levels
Nordlund et al. (1997) Sweden 1963–89	Swedish Census Study 26 032 women	Former smoker	25	3.6	0.8–16.0	Adjusted for age and place of residence
		Current smoker		1.7	0.5–5.3	
Tulinius et al. (1997) Iceland 1968–95	Reykjavik Study 11 366 men	Former smoker		2.0	0.6–6.6	Adjusted for age
		Cigarettes/day				
		1–14		3.6	1.01–12.8	
		15–24		4.1	1.2–14.1	
		≥ 25		1.5	0.2–13.2	
Kinjo et al. (1998) Japan 1966–81 (see also Akiba & Hirayama, 1990)	Six-prefecture Study 220 272 adults (100 840 men and 119 432 women)	Men	328			Adjusted for age, area of residence and occupation
		Former smoker	12	1.9	0.9–3.6	
		Cigarettes/day				
		1–14	117	2.3	1.5–3.3	
		≥ 15	163	2.7	1.8–3.8	p for trend < 0.001
		Women	112			
		1–14 cigarettes/day		1.8	1.1–3.0	
		Men and women	19			Further adjusted for sex, green and yellow vegetable intake, consumption of hot tea and alcohol
		Former smoker		1.5	0.8–2.8	
		Cigarettes/day				
		1–14		1.8	1.3–2.5	
		≥ 15		1.9	1.4–2.7	

Table 2.1.4.15 (contd)

Reference Country and years of study	Subjects	Smoking categories	Number of cases	Relative risk	95% CI	Comments
Liaw & Chen (1998) China, Province of Taiwan 1982–94	Taiwanese Study 11 096 men, 3301 women	Current smoker	26	1.0	0.4–2.6	Adjusted for age and alcohol drinking
		Duration (years)				
		21–30		2.4	0.7–8.9	
		> 30		1.3	0.5–3.4	
		Pack–years				
		< 20		0.4	0.1–2.1	
		20–40		2.1	0.8–5.9	
		> 40		1.2	0.4–4.1	
		Age at starting smoking (years)				
		> 24		1.1	0.3–4.0	
		21–24		1.5	0.4–5.3	
		≤ 20		1.3	0.5–3.6	
Gao et al. (1999) China 1983–94	Shanghai Residential Study 213 800 residents	Ever-smoker				Adjusted for age
		Urban men		2.6[†‡]	$p < 0.05$	Significant linear trend
		Suburban men		3.3[†]	$p < 0.05$	($p < 0.05$) for:
		Rural men		1.8[†‡]	$p < 0.05$	[†], intensity of smoking
		Urban women		1.9	$p > 0.05$	[‡], age at starting smoking

CI, confidence interval

Table 2.1.4.16. Case–control studies on tobacco smoking and oesophageal cancer (unspecified) or squamous-cell carcinoma of the oesophagus: main characteristics of study design

Reference Country and years of study	Number of cases and controls	Criteria for eligibility and comments
Victora *et al.* (1987) Brazil 1985–86	Men: 135 cases and 270 controls; women: 36 cases and 72 controls	Hospital-based study in eight main hospitals in southern Brazil Cases of histologically confirmed squamous-cell carcinoma of the oesophagus aged < 80 years; 90% of eligible cases Controls without disease related to alcohol or tobacco use, or upper gastrointestinal tract diseases, individually matched (2:1) by hospital, age (± 5 years) and sex
Brown *et al.* (1988) USA 1977–84	Men: 74 cases and 157 controls	Hospital-based incidence study combined with mortality study Incident cases of oesophageal cancer (NOS) identified at four hospitals in Charleston (85% squamous-cell carcinoma), aged ≤ 79 years; 85% of eligible cases participated Controls individually matched (2:1) on race, age (± 5 years), hospital and admission period; response rate, 95%; only controls without alcohol- or diet-related conditions or diagnosis of mental disorder were included.
	Men: 133 deaths and 265 controls	Mortality series: deaths from oesophageal cancer (NOS) at age ≤ 79 years Controls randomly selected and individually matched (2:1) by race, age, area of residence and year of death Cases with diagnoses and deaths with causes related to alcohol and/or diet excluded; response rate for deaths and controls combined, 94%
Nakachi *et al.* (1988) Japan 1973–85	Men: 257 cases and 257 controls; women: 86 cases and 86 controls	Population-based study in the Saitama prefecture using interviews Cases were deaths from oesophageal cancer (NOS); participation rate, 54% Controls selected from electoral roll and individually matched on sex, age (± 2 years) and neighbourhood; about 60% of first chosen controls participated.
Yu *et al.* (1988) USA 1975–81	Men: 187 cases and 187 controls; women: 88 cases and 88 controls	Population-based study in Los Angeles County Incident cases of histologically confirmed oesophageal cancer (88% squamous-cell carcinoma), identified through the local Cancer Surveillance Program, aged 20–64 years, mean, 56.5 years; 56% of eligible cases Neighbourhood controls individually matched on sex, age and race; 87% of controls were the first or the second eligible neighbour.
Ferraroni *et al.* (1989) Italy 1983–88	Men: 162 cases and 1334 controls; women: 47 cases and 610 controls	Hospital-based study in four hospitals in Milan Cases of oesophageal cancer (NOS), confirmed histologically, aged ≤ 75 years Controls with traumatic, non-traumatic orthopaedic and acute surgical conditions and ear, nose, throat, skin and dental disorders; malignant tumours, digestive tract disorders or coffee-, alcohol- or tobacco-related conditions were excluded; median age, 56 years
Li *et al.* (1989) China 1984–85	Men: 758 cases and 789 controls; women: 486 cases and 525 controls	Population-based study among residents of Linxian County using interviews Cases of cancer of the oesophageal–gastric junction (mostly squamous-cell carcinoma) or gastric cardia (mostly adenocarcinoma), aged 35–64 years, identified from all hospitals in the county; 98% of eligible cases Controls without cancer, randomly selected from population and roughly matched on age and sex; aged 35–64 years; participation rate, 100%

Table 2.1.4.16 (contd)

Reference Country and years of study	Number of cases and controls	Criteria for eligibility and comments
Rao et al. (1989) India 1980–84	Men: 503 cases and 634 controls	Hospital-based study at the Tata Memorial Hospital Cases with oesophageal cancer (NOS) Controls without cancer or infectious diseases
De Stefani et al. (1990) Uruguay 1985–88	Men: 199 cases and 398 controls; women: 62 cases and 124 controls	Hospital-based study in four main hospitals in Montevideo Cases of squamous-cell carcinoma of the oesophagus; response rate, 92% Controls without diagnosis of tobacco and/or alcohol-related diseases and individually matched (2:1) by age (± 5 years), sex and hospital
Franceschi et al. (1990) Italy 1986–89	Men: 288 cases and 1272 controls	Hospital-based study in two areas of northern Italy Cases of histologically confirmed oesophageal cancer (NOS), aged < 75 years; response rate, 98% Controls with traumatic or non-traumatic orthopaedic conditions, acute conditions, eye disorders and other illnesses unrelated to tobacco and alcohol consumption, matched by area of residence, hospital and age; response rate, 97%
Sankaranaray-anan et al. (1991) India 1983–84	267 cases (207 men and 60 women) and 895 controls (546 men and 349 women)	Hospital-based study at the Regional Cancer Centre of Trivandrum Cases of oesophageal cancer (NOS) confirmed by histology (67%) or radiology (33%); 100% of eligible cases participated. Controls included 271 patients diagnosed with conditions other than cancer or precancerous lesions and 624 patients selected from those attending a teaching hospital with diagnoses of acute respiratory, gastrointestinal and genitourinary infections [no matching]
Cheng et al. (1992) Hong Kong SAR 1989–90	Men: 345 cases and 1378 controls; women: 55 cases and 220 controls	Hospital-based study in four general hospitals in Hong Kong using interviews Cases of histologically confirmed oesophageal cancer (85% squamous-cell carcinoma); 86.8% of all cases participated. Controls individually matched (4:1) by sex and age: 2 controls admitted to the same surgical departments; patients with tobacco- or alcohol-related cancers were excluded; 2 controls selected from private or general practice clinics in the area where case was originally referred to the physician; response rate, 95%
Negri et al. (1992) Italy 1984–90	Men: 244 cases and 901 controls; women: 56 cases and 302 controls	Hospital-based study in several major hospitals in the greater Milan area Cases of histologically confirmed oesophageal cancer (NOS), aged 29–74 years; median, 60 years Controls admitted for traumatic or non-traumatic orthopaedic conditions, acute surgical diseases and various other diseases; patients with cancer or digestive diseases, and diseases related to alcohol or tobacco consumption excluded; aged 25–74 years; median, 55 years
Wang et al. (1992) China 1988–89	Men: 204 cases and 241 controls; women: 122 cases and 155 controls	Population-based study in two major cancer hospitals in two areas Cases of oesophageal cancer (mostly squamous-cell carcinomas), aged 30–87 years (15–20% of all cases); response rate > 90% Controls selected from the population and frequency-matched on gender, age (5-year categories) and residence; response rate > 90%

Table 2.1.4.16 (contd)

Reference Country and years of study	Number of cases and controls	Criteria for eligibility and comments
Kabat et al. (1993) USA 1981–90	Men: 136 cases and 4544 controls; women: 78 cases and 2228 controls	Hospital-based study in 28 hospitals in 8 US cities Cases of histologically confirmed squamous-cell carcinoma of the oesophagus Controls included patients with cancers of breast, endometrium, ovary, prostate and skin, leukaemias, lymphomas and sarcomas and non-cancer diagnosis, individually matched on age ($\pm$ 5 years), sex, race and hospital
Brown et al. (1994a) USA 1986–89	Men: 124 white and 249 black cases, and 750 white and 614 black controls	Population-based study in three areas Cases of histologically confirmed squamous-cell carcinoma of the oesophagus, aged 30–79 years; response rate, 68% Controls selected by random digit dialling and random sampling from Medicare recipients, frequency-matched on race and age; response rates, 78% and 82% for whites and blacks, respectively
Gao et al. (1994) China 1990–93	Men: 624 cases; women: 278 cases; 1552 controls	Population-based study in permanent residents of urban Shanghai Cases of oesophageal cancer (NOS), aged 30–74 years Controls randomly selected from the general population and frequency-matched on sex and age (5-year categories) within a larger case–control study
Hanaoka et al. (1994) Japan 1989–91	Men: 141 cases and 141 controls	Hospital-based study in seven university clinics Cases of histologically confirmed oesophageal cancer (NOS), aged < 85 years Controls selected from patients with diseases supposedly unrelated to alcohol or tobacco use; 54% cancer of the stomach, colon or rectum, and 18% benign gastrointestinal conditions, individually matched (1:1) by age ($\pm$ 3 years), sex, hospital and area of residence
Hu et al. (1994) China 1985–89	Men: 170 cases and 340 controls; women: 26 cases and 52 controls	Hospital-based study at five major hospitals in north-eastern China Cases of histologically confirmed oesophageal cancer (NOS); 100% of eligible cases Controls without cancer or oesophageal diseases, individually matched (2:1) by sex, age ($\pm$ 5 years), hospital and area of residence
Chen et al. (1995) China 1990–92	Men: 117 cases and 234 controls; women: 31 cases and 62 controls	Population-based study in Shichuan Province Incident cases of oesophageal cancer (NOS) registered in Jintang county, aged 26–88 years (mean, 61.5 years) Healthy controls from neighbourhood, individually matched (2:1) by age ($\pm$ 5 years), sex and residence
Cheng et al. (1995) Hong Kong SAR 1989–90	Men: 30 cases and 279 controls; women: 23 cases and 128 controls	Hospital-based study in four general hospitals; cases and controls were abstainers from alcohol. Cases of histologically confirmed oesophageal cancer (NOS) Controls not matched to cases; patients with diabetes mellitus and alcohol- and tobacco-related conditions excluded
Rolón et al. (1995) Paraguay 1988–91	Men: 110 cases and 318 controls; women: 21 cases and 63 controls	Hospital-based study in all medical facilities of Ascunción Cases of oesophageal cancer (NOS) diagnosed by cytology, histology and radiology, aged < 75 years; 100% of eligible cases Controls with cancers thought not to be associated with smoking or alcohol (skin, prostate, leukaemia, lymphomas) and benign conditions, individually matched (3:1) by sex and age ($\pm$ 5 years), hospital and admission period; 97% participation rate

Table 2.1.4.16 (contd)

Reference Country and years of study	Number of cases and controls	Criteria for eligibility and comments
Siemiatycki et al. (1995) Canada 1979–85	Men: 99 cases and 2238 controls	Hospital- and population-based study in Montreal Cases of cancers of the oesophagus (NOS), confirmed histologically, aged 35–70 years Controls: 533 population-based, selected from electoral list stratified by age; participation rate, 72%; 1705 patients with all other cancers
Vaughan et al. (1995) USA 1983–90	Men: 64 cases and 506 controls; women: 42 cases and 218 controls	Population-based study in western Washington State Cases of histologically confirmed squamous-cell carcinoma of the oesophagus, identified by the local Cancer Surveillance System; response rate, 83% Controls identified by random-digit dialling and frequency-matched on age and sex; response rate, 80%
Vizcaino et al. (1995) Zimbabwe 1963–77	Men: 826 cases and 3007 controls; women: 55 cases and 2231 controls	Hospital-based study in Bulawayo using interviews Incident cases of oesophageal cancer registered by the local cancer registry; 86% confirmed histologically, of whom 90% had squamous-cell carcinoma; mean age, 55.7 years; 73% of all cases participated. Controls with all other cancers unrelated to alcohol or tobacco consumption; response rate, 71%
Tavani et al. (1996) Italy 1984–92	Men: 22 cases and 79 controls; women: 18 cases and 72 controls	Hospital-based study in major hospitals in Milan, restricted to abstainers from alcohol Incident cases of oesophageal cancer (NOS), aged 26–74 years; 97% of eligible cases Controls without malignant, digestive or metabolic diseases or diseases known or suspected to be related to alcohol or tobacco consumption; 97% of eligible controls
Gammon et al. (1997) USA 1993–95	Men: 176 cases and 555 controls; women: 45 cases and 140 controls	Population-based study in three areas Cases of histologically confirmed squamous-cell carcinoma of the oesophagus, identified through population-based tumour registries, aged 30–79 years; 74% of eligible cases Controls identified by random-digit dialling or random sampling of Health Care Financing Administration rosters, frequency matched by area, age, sex and/or race, depending on study centre; response rate, 70%
Launoy et al. (1997) France 1991–94	Men: 208 cases and 399 controls	Hospital-based study in three university hospitals Cases of histologically confirmed squamous-cell carcinoma of the oesophagus, aged < 85 years Controls with osteoarthritis, lumbago, sciatica or eye conditions; trauma patients excluded; matched on age and hospital
Castellsagué & Muñoz (1999) Argentina, Brazil, Paraguay & Uruguay 1985–92	Men (76–84%) and women: 179 cases and 776 controls	Pooled analysis of five hospital-based studies in over 30 hospitals and clinics; study restricted to abstainers from alcohol Cases of squamous-cell carcinoma of the oesophagus; response rates, 90–99% Controls with diseases unrelated to alcohol or tobacco use, individually matched (2:1 or 3:1) on age (± 5 years), sex, hospital and residence

Table 2.1.4.16 (contd)

Reference Country and years of study	Number of cases and controls	Criteria for eligibility and comments
Castellsagué et al. (1999) Argentina, Brazil, Paraguay, Uruguay 1985–92	Men (76–84%) and women: 830 cases and 1779 controls	Pooled analysis of five hospital-based studies in over 30 hospitals and clinics Cases of squamous-cell carcinoma of the oesophagus; response rates, 90–99% Controls with diseases unrelated to alcohol or tobacco, individually matched (2:1 or 3:1) by age (± 5 years), sex, hospital, admission period and residence
La Vecchia et al. (1999b) Italy 1984–92	Men: 22 cases and 79 controls; women: 18 cases and 72 controls	Pooled analysis of two hospital-based studies in two regions in northern Italy; study restricted to abstainers from alcohol Incident cases of histologically confirmed oesophageal cancer (NOS) Controls with acute, non-neoplastic conditions; diseases related to tobacco use or alcohol abuse excluded
Shen et al. (1999) China 1994–95	Men: 307 cases and 307 controls; women: 242 cases and 242 controls	Population-based study Incident cases of oesophageal cancer (NOS) confirmed by X-rays or computerized tomography scan (53%) or by histology (47%); 71% of squamous-cell carcinomas; aged 30–74 years; response rate, 90.3% Controls with no history of digestive cancer, individually matched on age (± 3 years), sex and village
Lagergren et al. (2000) Sweden 1995–97	Men: 120 cases; women: 47 cases; 820 controls	Population-based study in the entire population of Sweden using interviews Cases of squamous-cell carcinoma of the oesophagus, born in Sweden on even dates; median age, 67 years; response rate, 73% Controls randomly selected and frequency-matched to total cases of squamous-cell carcinoma and adenocarcinoma of the oesophagus, and adenocarcinoma of the gastric cardia; participation rate, 73%
Lu et al. (2000) China 1995–96	Men: 198 cases and 198 controls; women: 154 cases and 154 controls	Population-based study in Lin County Cases of oesophageal cancer (NOS), confirmed by histology or cytology (87%) or X-rays or surgery (13%) Neighbourhood controls individually matched (1:1) on age (± 3 years) and sex
Zambon et al. (2000) Italy 1992–97	Men: 275 cases and 593 controls	Hospital-based study in three areas of northern Italy using interviews Incident cases of histologically confirmed squamous-cell carcinoma of the oesophagus, aged 39–79 years; 95% of eligible cases Controls admitted for acute illnesses unrelated to tobacco and alcohol use to major hospitals in the same areas, frequency-matched by age (± 5 years) and area of residence; malignant lesions excluded; 95% of eligible controls participated.
Pacella-Norman et al. (2002) South Africa 1995–99	Men: 267 cases and 804 controls; women: 138 cases and 1370 controls	Hospital-based study at 3 major hospitals in greater Johannesburg Incident cases of oesophageal cancer (NOS), 90% confirmed by histology, haematology or cytology, aged 18–74 years Controls with cancers thought to be unrelated to tobacco and alcohol use: breast, prostate, leukaemia, lymphoma, myelomas, ovary, endometrium, vulva, skin, colon, penis and others; aged 18–74 years

Table 2.1.4.17. Case–control studies on tobacco smoking and oesophageal cancer (unspecified) or squamous-cell carcinoma of the oesophagus

Reference Country and years of study	Cancer subsite	Smoking categories	Relative risk	95% CI	Comments
Victora et al. (1987) Brazil 1985–86	Squamous-cell carcinoma	Former smoker Current smoker	1.3 3.9	0.6–2.7 1.9–8.0	Adjusted for cachaça (local beverage) consumption, place of residence, intake of fruit and meat
Brown et al. (1988) USA 1977–84	Oesophagus (unspecified)	Current smoker Cigarettes/day 1–19 20–29 ≥ 30 Duration (years) 1–24 25–44 ≥ 45	1.8 0.8 2.0 2.6 1.4 1.6 1.8	1.0–3.0 0.4–1.5 1.1–3.4 1.4–4.7 0.6–2.9 1.0–2.8 1.0–3.3	Cases and controls from the incidence and mortality series were combined for the analysis. Adjusted for study series (incidence or mortality), use of local beverage and other alcoholic beverages
Nakachi et al. (1988) Japan 1973–85	Oesophagus (unspecified)	Men > 400 000 vs < 400 000 cigarettes smoked Women Ever-smoker vs never	2.4 2.3	0.99–5.7 1.02–5.2	Participation rates for both cases and controls were low. Relevant factors were not fully adjusted for except variables for matching.
Yu et al. (1988) USA 1975–81	Oesophagus (unspecified)	Packs/day ≤ 1 2 ≥ 3	6.6 9.1 5.1	2.3–19.3 2.9–29.0 1.5–16.9	Analysis restricted to directly interviewed pairs (n = 129); relevant factors were not adjusted for except variables for matching (age, sex and race).

Table 2.1.4.17 (contd)

Reference Country and years of study	Cancer subsite	Smoking categories	Relative risk	95% CI	Comments
Ferraroni et al. (1989) Italy 1983–88	Oesophagus (unspecified)	Former smoker	2.9		Adjusted for age, sex, education, social class, marital status, smoking, coffee and alcohol consumption
		Cigarettes/day			$p < 0.01$ for all current smokers combined
		< 15	4.2		
		15–24	4.2		
		≥ 25	7.2		
Li et al. (1989) China 1984–85	Oesophagus (unspecified)	High-risk area			Analysis included only men because of the very small number of women who smoked; cancers of the oesophagus and gastric cardia were combined in the analysis; adjusted for age
		Current smoker	0.9	0.6–1.2	
		Cigarettes/day			
		1–9	1.0	0.6–1.6	
		10–19	0.8	0.5–1.2	
		≥ 20	0.9	0.6–1.4	
		Age at starting smoking (years)			
		≥ 35	1.0	0.6–1.7	
		25–34	1.1	0.7–1.7	
		20–24	0.8	0.5–1.3	
		< 20	0.7	0.4–1.1	
		Low-risk area			
		Current smoker	1.5	1.1–2.0	
		Cigarettes/day			
		1–9	1.4	0.4–2.1	
		10–19	1.3	0.9–2.0	
		≥ 20	1.7	1.2–2.6	

Table 2.1.4.17 (contd)

Reference Country and years of study	Cancer subsite	Smoking categories	Relative risk	95% CI	Comments
Li *et al.* (1989) (contd)		Age at starting smoking (years)			
		≥ 35	1.3	0.7–2.3	
		25–34	2.2	1.5–3.4	
		20–24	2.1	1.3–3.3	
		< 20	0.8	0.5–1.2	
Rao *et al.* (1989) India 1980–84	Oesophagus (unspecified)	Smoker			Adjusted for age and residence. Both bidi and cigarette smokers were included as smokers.
		All	1.7	1.1–2.7	
		Vegetarian	1.2	0.4–3.7	
		Non-vegetarian	2.3	1.3–4.0	
De Stefani *et al.* (1990) Uruguay 1985–88	Squamous-cell carcinoma	Men Cigarettes/day			Adjusted for age, residence and alcohol intake
		1–7	1.9	0.7–5.4	
		8–14	2.7	1.1–6.8	
		15–24	4.3	1.7–10.4	
		≥ 24	4.6	1.9–11.1	
		Women Cigarettes/day			
		1–7	2.3	0.9–6.0	
		≥ 8	3.2	1.1–9.3	
Franceschi *et al.* (1990) Italy 1986–89	Oesophagus (unspecified)	Cigarette smoker Cigarettes/day	3.8	2.2–6.6	Adjusted for age, residence, education, occupation and alcohol intake
		≤ 14	3.0	1.7–5.5	
		15–24	3.8	2.1–6.7	
		≥ 25	4.7	2.6–8.4	*p* for trend < 0.01

Table 2.1.4.17 (contd)

Reference Country and years of study	Cancer subsite	Smoking categories	Relative risk	95% CI	Comments
Franceschi *et al.* (1990) (contd)		Duration (years)			
		1–29	2.4	1.3–4.4	
		30–39	4.0	2.2–7.2	
		≥ 40	5.6	3.1–10.0	*p* for trend < 0.01
		Age at starting smoking (years)			
		≥ 25	3.7	2.0–6.8	
		17–24	4.5	2.5–7.8	
		< 17	2.5	1.4–4.8	*p* for trend < 0.01
Sankaranarayanan *et al.* (1991) India 1983–84	Oesophagus (unspecified)	Cigarette smoker	0.6	0.3–1.2	Only 9 cases were cigarette smokers.
		Duration (years)			
		≤ 20	0.5	0.1–2.1	
		> 21	0.6	0.3–1.4	*p* for trend > 0.05
Cheng *et al.* (1992) Hong Kong SAR 1989–90	Oesophagus (unspecified)	Tobacco/day (g)			Adjusted for age, education, birthplace, alcohol use, consumption of pickled vegetables, green leafy vegetables and citrus fruits, preference for hot drinks or soups, meals taken at home or eaten out
		< 5	1.7	0.8–3.9	
		5–< 10	1.8	1.0–3.2	
		10–< 15	2.2	1.3–3.6	
		15–< 20	1.8	1.1–3.1	
		20–< 25	2.5	1.5–4.1	
		25–< 30	2.3	1.0–5.7	
		30–< 40	3.9	1.9–7.8	
		≥ 40	1.7	0.6–5.1	

Table 2.1.4.17 (contd)

Reference Country and years of study	Cancer subsite	Smoking categories	Relative risk	95% CI	Comments
Negri *et al.* (1992) Italy 1984–90	Oesophagus (unspecified)	Men			Adjusted for age, education, alcohol use and β-carotene intake
		Former smoker and <15 cigarettes/day	3.5	1.9–6.3	
		≥ 15 cigarettes/day	5.1	2.9–9.0	*p* for trend < 0.001
		Women			
		Former smoker and <15 cigarettes/day	1.8	0.8–4.0	
		≥ 15 cigarettes/day	4.8	2.1–10.7	*p* for trend < 0.001
Wang *et al.* (1992) China 1988–89	Oesophagus (unspecified)	High-risk area			Analysis for men only; adjusted for age and occupation; alcohol consumption was a significant risk factor in the high-risk area but was not adjusted for; amount of tobacco consumption too low to show a clear result
		Ever-smoker	0.6	0.3–1.2	
		> 20 cigarettes/month	3.2	0.8–12.6	
		Low-risk area			
		Ever-smoker	1.5	0.7–3.4	
		> 20 cigarettes/month	2.2	0.6–7.6	
Kabat *et al.* (1993) USA 1981–90	Squamous-cell carcinoma	Men			Adjusted for age, education, hospital, time period and alcohol use
		Former smoker	1.3	0.7–2.4	
		Current smoker	4.5	2.5–8.1	
		Cigarettes/day			
		1–20	1.9	1.1–3.5	
		21–30	2.7	1.3–5.4	
		≥ 31	2.7	1.5–5.0	

Table 2.1.4.17 (contd)

Reference Country and years of study	Cancer subsite	Smoking categories	Relative risk	95% CI	Comments
Kabat et al. (1993) (contd)		Women			Adjusted for age, geographical area, alcohol consumption and income
		Former smoker	2.2	1.1–4.3	
		Current smoker	6.8	3.7–12.1	
		Cigarettes/day			
		1–20	3.7	2.0–6.7	
		≥ 21	4.8	2.4–9.5	
Brown et al. (1994a) USA 1986–89	Squamous-cell carcinoma	Whites			
		Former smoker	2.4	0.9–6.5	
		Ever-smoker	3.7	1.4–9.7	
		Current smoker	5.5	2.0–14.9	
		Cigarettes/day			
		1–19	2.9	0.9–8.8	
		20–39	3.8	1.4–10.4	
		≥ 40	3.9	1.4–11.2	p for trend = 0.078
		Duration (years)			
		1–29	2.0	0.7–6.0	
		30–39	3.6	1.3–10.6	
		≥ 40	5.9	2.1–16.3	p for trend < 0.001
		Blacks			
		Former smoker	1.5	0.7–3.6	
		Ever-smoker	3.2	1.5–7.0	
		Current smoker	4.2	1.9–9.2	
		Cigarettes/day			
		1–19	2.2	0.9–4.9	
		20–39	4.0	1.8–8.9	
		≥ 40	3.4	1.3–8.5	p for trend < 0.001

Table 2.1.4.17 (contd)

Reference Country and years of study	Cancer subsite	Smoking categories	Relative risk	95% CI	Comments
Brown et al. (1994a) (contd)		Duration (years)			
		1–29	1.7	0.7–4.1	
		30–39	3.0	1.3–6.9	
		≥40	5.1	2.3–11.6	p for trend < 0.001
Gao et al. (1994) China 1990–93	Oesophagus (unspecified)	Men			Adjusted for age, education, birth place, tea drinking, dietary factors and alcohol intake (for men only)
		Former smoker	1.7	1.1–2.6	
		Current smoker	2.1	1.6–3.0	
		Cigarettes/day			
		1–9	1.4	0.8–2.3	
		10–19	1.7	1.1–2.6	
		20–29	2.5	1.7–3.6	
		≥30	6.0	3.2–11.1	p for trend < 0.001
		Duration (years)			
		0.5–19	1.0	0.5–1.8	
		20–29	1.1	0.7–2.0	
		30–39	2.3	1.5–3.6	
		≥40	2.9	2.0–4.2	p for trend < 0.001
		Pack–years			
		< 15	1.0	0.6–1.7	
		15–34	1.8	1.2–2.7	
		≥35	3.8	2.5–5.6	p for trend < 0.001
		Age at starting smoking (years)			
		≥30	1.3	0.8–2.1	
		20–29	2.6	1.8–3.7	
		<20	2.5	1.6–3.9	p for trend < 0.001

Table 2.1.4.17 (contd)

Reference Country and years of study	Cancer subsite	Smoking categories	Relative risk	95% CI	Comments
Gao et al. (1994) (contd)		Women			
		Former smoker	4.0	1.9–8.3	
		Current smoker	1.6	1.0–2.4	
		Cigarettes/day			
		1–9	1.1	0.5–2.2	
		10–19	2.1	1.1–4.0	
		≥ 20	1.9	0.8–4.6	p for trend < 0.05
		Duration (years)			
		0.5–19	0.5	0.2–1.5	
		20–29	2.4	1.1–5.2	
		30–39	1.2	0.5–3.0	
		≥ 40	2.4	1.2–4.9	p for trend < 0.01
		Pack–years			
		< 10	0.8	0.4–1.7	
		≥ 10	2.4	1.4–4.1	p for trend < 0.01
		Age at starting smoking (years)			
		≥ 25	1.4	0.8–2.3	
		< 25	2.4	1.1–5.2	p for trend < 0.05
Hanaoka et al. (1994) Japan 1989–91	Oesophagus (unspecified)	Cigarettes/day			Adjusted for alcohol intake; controls include patients with tobacco-related diseases. [†]Also includes former smokers
		1–4	1.2[†]	0.6–2.6[†]	
		5–14	1.4	0.6–3.2	
		15–24	1.5	0.8–3.0	
		≥ 25	1.0	0.5–2.2	p for trend = 0.55

Table 2.1.4.17 (contd)

Reference Country and years of study	Cancer subsite	Smoking categories	Relative risk	95% CI	Comments
Hu *et al.* (1994) China 1985–89	Oesophagus (unspecified)	Cigarettes/day[†]			Adjusted for consumption of spirits [†]Former smokers were included in corresponding categories.
		1–10	1.7	1.0–2.9	
		11–20	2.2	1.3–3.7	
		21–30	1.7	0.8–3.7	
		≥ 31	3.3	1.5–7.4	*p* for trend = 0.005
		Duration (years)			
		1–10	1.5	0.5–5.2	
		11–20	2.1	1.1–4.3	
		21–30	2.8	1.6–5.0	
		≥ 31	3.3	2.0–5.3	*p* for trend < 0.0001
		Age at starting smoking (years)			
		≥ 31	2.5	1.3–5.1	
		26–30	2.1	1.1–4.3	
		21–25	2.7	1.5–4.8	
		16–20	3.1	1.8–5.3	
		≤ 15	3.4	1.7–6.6	*p* for trend = 0.03
Chen *et al.* (1995) China 1990–92	Oesophagus (unspecified)	Ever-smoker	1.3	0.8–2.1	Adjusted for age, sex, residence, alcohol use, relevant food items and eating habits. Smoking could not enter into the multivariate analysis. The risk was not significantly associated with daily tobacco consumption, years of smoking, age at starting smoking and type of tobacco smoking.

Table 2.1.4.17 (contd)

Reference Country and years of study	Cancer subsite	Smoking categories	Relative risk	95% CI	Comments
Cheng et al. (1995) Hong Kong SAR 1989–90	Oesophagus (unspecified)	Former smoker	2.4	0.95–6.1	Analysis restricted to abstainers from alcohol; adjusted for sex, age, education, place of birth, preference for hot drinks or soups, consumption of green leafy vegetables, citrus fruits and pickled vegetables
		Current smoker Tobacco/day (g)			
		< 15	3.0	1.1–8.4	
		15–24.99	2.6	0.9–8.1	
		≥ 25	10.3	1.8–57.6	p for trend = 0.019
Rolón et al. (1995) Paraguay 1988–91	Oesophagus (unspecified)	Former smoker	3.6	1.6–7.9	Adjusted for age, sex, hospital group, lifetime alcohol consumption
		Current smoker	4.5	2.2–9.1	
		Cigarettes/day			
		1–14	3.2	1.6–6.5	
		15–39	8.4	3.6–19.3	
		≥ 40	6.1	1.8–20.8	p for trend = 0.01
		Lifetime no. of cigarettes			
		1–49 999	1.8	0.7–4.2	
		50 000–99 999	3.4	1.4–8.5	
		100 000–299 999	9.1	4.0–21.0	
		≥ 300 000	10.0	3.9–25.8	p for trend < 0.00001
		Duration (years)			
		1–29	1.5	0.6–3.7	
		30–39	4.4	1.9–10.0	
		≥ 40	7.3	3.3–16.3	p for trend = 0.00001

Table 2.1.4.17 (contd)

Reference Country and years of study	Cancer subsite	Smoking categories	Relative risk	95% CI	Comments
Siemiatycki et al. (1995) Canada 1979–85	Oesophagus (unspecified)	Ever-smoker	2.4	1.0–5.7	
		Pack-years			
		≤ 25	1.7	0.6–4.7	
		25–49	2.3	0.9–5.8	
		50–74	3.1	1.2–7.9	
		≥ 75	2.8	1.1–7.6	p for trend < 0.01
Vaughan et al. (1995) USA 1983–90	Squamous-cell carcinoma	Pack-years			Adjusted for alcohol intake, body mass index, age, sex, race and education
		1–39	5.2	1.7–16.2	
		40–79	7.9	2.8–22.1	
		≥ 80	16.9	4.1–69.1	p for trend < 0.001
Vizcaino et al. (1995) Zimbabwe 1963–77	Oesophagus (unspecified)	Former smoker	3.1	1.7–5.6	Analysis for men only because of low prevalence of women who smoked; adjusted for age, province, occupation and total alcohol consumption
		Cigarettes/day			
		< 15	3.1	2.4–4.0	
		≥ 15	4.3	2.8–6.7	p for trend < 0.001
Tavani et al. (1996) Italy 1984–92	Oesophagus (unspecified)	Former smoker	0.8	0.2–3.4	Adjusted for age, sex and education
		Current smoker	3.4	1.5–8.1	
		Cigarettes/day			
		< 20	1.3	0.4–4.2	
		≥ 20	7.5	2.7–20.4	p for trend < 0.01
		Duration (years)			
		≤ 30	2.0	0.7–5.3	
		> 30	4.9	1.8–13.6	p for trend < 0.01

Table 2.1.4.17 (contd)

Reference Country and years of study	Cancer subsite	Smoking categories	Relative risk	95% CI	Comments
Tavani *et al.* (1996) (contd)		Age at starting smoking (years)			
		> 25	1.7	0.6–4.7	
		≤ 25	3.9	1.5–10.5	
Gammon *et al.* (1997) USA 1993–95	Squamous-cell carcinoma	Former smoker	2.8	1.5–4.9	Adjusted for age, sex, area, race, body mass index, income and use of alcohol
		Current smoker	5.1	2.8–9.2	
		Cigarettes/day			
		< 16	2.7	1.4–5.1	
		16–20	3.9	2.1–7.2	
		21–30	5.3	2.6–10.7	
		> 30	3.9	2.0–7.6	*p* for trend < 0.05
		Duration (years)			
		< 20	1.8	0.9–3.7	
		20–31	2.0	1.0–4.0	
		32–42	3.3	1.8–6.1	
		> 42	5.9	3.2–10.7	*p* for trend < 0.05
		Pack–years			
		< 14	2.0	1.0–4.0	
		14–31	2.8	1.4–5.5	
		32–54	4.5	2.4–8.5	
		> 54	5.8	3.1–11.0	*p* for trend < 0.05

Table 2.1.4.17 (contd)

Reference Country and years of study	Cancer subsite	Smoking categories	Relative risk	95% CI	Comments
Launoy et al. (1997) France 1991–94	Squamous-cell carcinoma	Duration (years) 1–14 15–29 30–44 ≥ 45	1.0 1.7 3.3 3.2	– 0.7–4.1 1.3–8.3 1.1–10.0	Nonsmokers and abstainers from alcohol were excluded from the analysis, hence the reference group included smokers who had smoked for 1–14 years; adjusted for interviewer, age, place of residence, occupation, education, lifestyle and weekly alcohol consumption p for trend < 0.0001
Castellsagué & Muñoz (1999) Argentina, Brazil, Paraguay & Uruguay 1985–92	Squamous-cell carcinoma	Ever-smoker Cigarettes/day 1–7 8–14 15–24 ≥ 25	2.2 1.5 2.6 3.4 2.5	1.5–3.4 0.8–2.6 1.2–5.4 1.9–6.1 1.2–5.4	Adjusted for hospital, age group, sex and years of schooling p for trend < 0.001
Castellsagué et al. (1999) Argentina, Brazil, Paraguay & Uruguay 1985–92	Squamous-cell carcinoma	Men Former smoker Ever-smoker Current smoker Cigarettes/day 1–7 8–14 15–24 ≥ 25	2.8 4.1 5.1 2.2 4.1 5.3 5.0	1.8–4.3 2.7–6.0 3.4–7.6 1.3–3.5 2.6–6.4 3.4–8.1 3.2–7.7	Adjusted for age, hospital, education and alcohol intake p for trend < 0.00001

Table 2.1.4.17 (contd)

Reference Country and years of study	Cancer subsite	Smoking categories	Relative risk	95% CI	Comments
Castellsagué et al. (1999) (contd)		Duration (years)			
		1–29	2.6	1.7–4.2	
		30–39	3.6	2.3–5.6	
		40–49	4.7	3.0–7.2	
		≥ 50	6.0	3.8–9.5	p for trend < 0.00001
		Age at starting smoking (years)			
		≤ 13	1.0	–	
		14–16	0.7	0.5–0.96	
		17–20	0.8	0.6–1.0	
		≥ 21	0.6	0.4–0.9	p for trend = 0.02
		Women			
		Former smoker	1.6	0.8–3.1	
		Ever-smoker	2.4	1.5–3.7	
		Current smoker	3.1	1.8–5.3	
		Cigarettes/day			
		1–14	2.1	1.2–3.7	
		≥ 15	2.8	1.4–5.4	p for trend = 0.0003
		Duration (years)			
		1–29	1.5	0.8–2.9	
		30–39	2.0	0.9–4.4	
		≥ 40	4.4	2.2–9.0	p for trend < 0.00001

Table 2.1.4.17 (contd)

Reference Country and years of study	Cancer subsite	Smoking categories	Relative risk	95% CI	Comments
Castellsagué et al. (1999) (contd)		Age at starting smoking (years)			
		≤ 13	1.0	–	
		14–16	1.6	0.3–7.5	
		17–20	0.6	0.2–2.4	
		≥ 21	0.2	0.1–0.7	p for trend = 0.003
La Vecchia et al. (1999b) Italy 1984–92	Oesophagus (unspecified)	Cigarettes/day			Analysis restricted to abstainers from alcohol
		< 20	1.3	0.4–4.2	
		≥ 20	7.5	2.7–20.4	p for trend < 0.001
Shen et al. (1999) China 1994–95	Oesophagus (unspecified)	Men			Adjusted for age, education, salted food consumption and fruit intake
		Ever-smoker	1.9	0.9–4.0	
		Current smoker	2.5	1.6–3.8	
		Cigarettes/day			
		1–9	1.5	0.8–3.1	
		10–19	1.9	1.1–3.1	
		20–29	2.5	1.6–4.0	
		≥ 30	7.7	2.8–20.8	p for trend < 0.001
		Duration (years)			
		0.5–19	1.8	0.9–3.4	
		20–29	2.4	1.4–4.3	
		30–39	2.5	1.5–4.2	
		≥ 40	2.7	1.5–4.9	p for trend < 0.001

Table 2.1.4.17 (contd)

Reference Country and years of study	Cancer subsite	Smoking categories	Relative risk	95% CI	Comments
Shen *et al.* (1999) (contd)		Pack–years			
		0.5–13	1.3	0.7–2.4	
		14–29	2.1	1.3–3.5	
		> 29	3.3	2.0–5.5	*p* for trend < 0.001
		Age at starting smoking (years)			
		> 29	2.0	1.2–3.5	
		20–29	2.4	1.5–3.8	
		< 20	2.8	1.6–5.1	*p* for trend < 0.01
		Women			
		Ever-smoker	3.3	0.6–17.6	
		Current smoker	1.2	0.8–1.8	
		Cigarettes/day			
		1–9	1.8	1.0–3.4	
		10–19	0.9	0.6–1.6	
		≥ 20	1.4	0.7–2.8	*p* for trend > 0.05
		Duration (years)			
		0.5–19	0.9	0.5–1.5	
		20–29	1.3	0.7–2.4	
		≥ 30	2.4	1.1–5.1	*p* for trend < 0.05
		Pack–years			
		0.5–13	0.9	0.7–1.6	
		≥ 14	1.9	1.0–3.4	*p* for trend > 0.05

Table 2.1.4.17 (contd)

Reference Country and years of study	Cancer subsite	Smoking categories	Relative risk	95% CI	Comments
Shen et al. (1999) (contd)		Age at starting smoking (years)			
		≥ 30	1.1	0.7–1.7	
		< 30	2.1	1.1–4.1	p for trend > 0.05
Lagergren et al. (2000) Sweden 1995–97	Squamous-cell carcinoma	Former smoker	2.5	1.4–4.7	Adjusted for age, sex, alcohol use, education, body mass index, reflux symptoms, intake of fruit and vegetables, energy intake and physical activity
		Current smoker[†]	9.3	5.1–17.0	
		Cigarettes/day[†]			
		1–9	2.8	1.5–5.2	
		10–19	3.9	2.2–6.9	[†]Also adjusted for pipe smoking and snuff use
		≥ 20	4.9	2.7–9.0	
Lu et al. (2000) China 1995–96	Oesophagus (unspecified)	Ever-smoker	2.0	1.1–3.4	Adjusted for age, sex, occupation, body mass index, dietary factors and habits, depression and hyperplasia
Zambon et al. (2000) Italy 1992–97	Squamous-cell carcinoma	Cigarettes/day			
		1–14	3.2	1.6–6.4	
		15–24	5.4	2.8–10.1	
		≥ 25	7.0	3.2–15.1	p for trend < 0.001
		Duration (years)			
		1–24	1.5	0.4–6.2	
		25–34	2.6	1.2–5.6	
		≥ 35	6.4	3.5–12.0	p for trend < 0.001

Table 2.1.4.17 (contd)

Reference Country and years of study	Cancer subsite	Smoking categories	Relative risk	95% CI	Comments
Zambon et al. (2000) (contd)		Age at starting smoking (years)			
		≥20	4.3	2.2–8.3	
		17–19	3.6	1.8–7.5	
		<17	6.3	3.3–12.3	p for trend = 0.15
Pacella-Norman et al. (2002) South Africa 1995–99	Oesophagus (unspecified)	Men			Adjusted for age, place of birth, education, work category, heating fuel, snuff use and alcohol consumption
		Former smoker	3.8	2.3–6.3	
		Current smoker	3.8	2.3–6.1	
		Tobacco (g/day)			
		1–14	3.3	2.0–5.5	
		≥15	6.0	3.2–11.0	
		Women			
		Former smoker	2.6	1.5–4.5	
		Current smoker	3.1	1.7–5.4	
		Tobacco (g/day)			
		1–14	2.8	1.5–5.2	
		≥15	6.2	1.9–20.2	

CI, confidence interval

Table 2.1.4.18. Case–control studies on tobacco smoking and oesophageal cancer (unspecified) or squamous-cell carcinoma of the oesophagus: smoking cessation

Reference (country and years of study)	Cancer subsite	Years since quitting	Relative risk	95% CI	Comments
Brown et al. (1988) USA 1977–84	Oesophagus (unspecified)	Current smoker	1.8	1.0–3.0	Cases and controls from the incidence and mortality series were combined for the analysis. Adjusted for study series (incidence or mortality), use of local beverage and other alcoholic beverages
		1–9	2.0	1.0–3.7	
		≥ 10	1.0	0.5–2.1	
Yu et al. (1988) USA 1975–81	Oesophagus (unspecified)	< 5	4.1	0.6–28.6	Analysis restricted to directly interviewed pairs (n = 129); relevant factors were not adjusted for, except variables for matching (age, sex and race).
		5–9	3.3	0.8–12.8	
		10–19	2.0	0.6–7.2	
		≥ 20	1.9	0.5–6.6	
		Nonsmoker	1.0	–	
Franceschi et al. (1990) Italy 1986–89	Oesophagus (unspecified)	Current smoker	3.8	2.2–6.6	Adjusted for age, residence, education, occupation and alcohol intake
		< 10	2.5	1.3–4.8	p for trend < 0.01
		≥ 10	2.2	1.1–4.3	
Kabat et al. (1993) USA 1981–90	Squamous-cell carcinoma	Men			Adjusted for age, education, hospital, time period and alcohol use
		Current smoker	1.0	–	
		1–5	0.5	0.3–1.0	
		6–10	0.4	0.2–0.8	
		11–20	0.3	0.2–0.6	
		≥ 21	0.2	0.1–0.3	
		Women			
		Current smoker	1.0	–	
		1–10	0.4	0.2–0.9	
		≥ 11	0.3	0.1–0.5	

Table 2.1.4.18 (contd)

Reference (country and years of study)	Cancer subsite	Years since quitting	Relative risk	95% CI	Comments
Rolón et al. (1995) Paraguay 1988–91	Oesophagus (unspecified)	Current smoker	4.5	2.2–9.1	Adjusted for age, sex, hospital group, lifetime alcohol consumption
		1–7	5.2	2.2–12.4	
		8–19	2.0	0.6–6.7	
		≥ 20	2.0	0.5–7.9	p for trend = 0.06
Gammon et al. (1997) USA 1993–95	Squamous-cell carcinoma	Current smoker	5.1	2.8–9.2	Adjusted for age, sex, area, race, body mass index, income and use of alcohol
		< 11	5.6	2.9–10.8	
		11–20	2.3	1.1–4.8	
		21–30	1.0	0.4–2.7	
		> 30	1.8	0.8–4.2	p for trend < 0.05
Launoy et al. (1997) France 1991–94	Squamous-cell carcinoma	Current smoker	1.0	–	Adjusted for interviewer, age, place of residence, occupation, education, lifestyle and weekly alcohol consumption
		1–5	1.4	0.7–2.6	
		6–10	0.9	0.4–1.9	
		≥ 11	0.5	0.3–1.03	p for trend = 0.06
Castellsagué et al. (1999) Argentina, Brazil, Paraguay & Uruguay 1985–92	Squamous-cell carcinoma	Men Current smoker	1.0	–	Adjusted for age, hospital, education, alcohol intake
		1–4	0.7	0.5–1.0	
		5–9	0.5	0.3–0.8	
		≥ 10	0.5	0.4–0.7	p for trend < 0.00001
		Women Current smoker	1.0	–	
		1–9	1.0	0.3–3.1	
		≥ 10	0.4	0.1–1.2	p for trend = 0.14

Table 2.1.4.18 (contd)

Reference (country and years of study)	Cancer subsite	Years since quitting	Relative risk	95% CI	Comments
Lagergren et al. (2000) Sweden 1995–97	Squamous-cell carcinoma	Current smoker	9.3	5.1–17.0	Adjusted for age, sex, alcohol use, education, body mass index, reflux symptoms, intake of fruit and vegetables, energy intake and physical activity
		< 2	10.3	5.6–19.1	
		3–10	5.2	2.4–11.3	
		11–25	2.1	1.0–4.7	p for trend < 0.0001
		> 25	1.9	0.8–4.0	
Zambon et al. (2000) Italy 1992–97	Squamous-cell carcinoma	< 5	7.7	3.2–18.5	
		5–9	4.1	1.8–9.1	
		≥ 10	1.5	0.8–3.0	
		Nonsmoker	1.0	–	p for trend < 0.001

CI, confidence interval

Table 2.1.4.19. Case–control studies on tobacco smoking and oesophageal cancer (unspecified) or squamous-cell carcinoma of the oesophagus: type of tobacco and/or cigarette

Reference (country and years of study)	Cancer subsite	Cigarette exposure	Relative risk	95% CI	Comments
De Stefani et al. (1990) Uruguay 1985–88	Squamous-cell carcinoma	Type of tobacco Mainly blond Mainly black	1.0 2.6	– 1.7–3.9	Adjusted for age, residence, alcohol intake and duration of smoking
Rolón et al. (1995) Paraguay 1988–91	Oesophagus (unspecified)	Type of tobacco Mainly black Mixed Mainly blond	1.0 1.0 0.5	– 0.3–3.4 0.2–1.1	Adjusted for age, sex, hospital group and lifetime ethanol consumption
Vaughan et al. (1995) USA 1983–90	Squamous-cell carcinoma	Type of cigarettes Filter Mixed Untipped vs filter only vs filter and mixed	1.0 0.6 1.1 1.6	– 0.2–1.9 0.3–3.5 0.8–3.3	Adjusted for alcohol intake, body mass index, age, sex, race and education
Gammon et al. (1997) USA 1993–95	Squamous-cell carcinoma	Filter status Filter only Filter + no filter No filter only	2.9 2.7 3.6	1.7–5.0 1.4–5.6 2.0–6.4	Adjusted for age, sex, area, race, body mass index, income and use of alcohol

Table 2.1.4.19 (contd)

Reference (country and years of study)	Cancer subsite	Cigarette exposure	Relative risk	95% CI	Comments
Castellsagué *et al.* (1999) Argentina, Brazil, Paraguay & Uruguay 1985–92	Squamous-cell carcinoma	Men			Adjusted for age, hospital, education, alcohol intake
		Type of tobacco			
		Only blond	1.0	–	
		Mixed	1.3	0.8–1.9	
		Only black	2.0	1.5–2.7	*p* for trend < 0.00001
		Use of filter			
		Never	1.0	–	
		Ever	0.8	0.6–0.98	
		Women			
		Type of tobacco			
		Blond or mixed	1.0	–	
		Only black	3.4	0.9–13.0	
		Use of filter			
		Never	1.0	–	
		Ever	1.5	0.5–4.4	

CI, confidence interval

Table 2.1.4.20. Case–control studies on tobacco smoking and adenocarcinoma of the oesophagus: main characteristics of study design

Reference Country and years of study	Number of cases and controls	Criteria for eligibility and comments
Levi et al. (1990) Switzerland 1963–85	Men: 21 cases and 85 controls; women: 9 cases and 55 controls	Hospital-based study Cases histologically confirmed as adenocarcinoma in Barrett's oesophagus, aged 37–86 years Controls with Barrett's oesophagus without any malignant features
Kabat et al. (1993) USA 1981–90	Men: 173 cases and 4544 controls; women: 21 cases and 2228 controls	Hospital-based study in 28 hospitals in eight cities Cases histologically confirmed as adenocarcinoma of the distal oesophagus, gastro–oesophageal junction or cardia Controls included cancers of the breast, endometrium, ovary, prostate and skin, leukaemia, lymphomas and sarcomas and non-cancer diagnoses; individually matched on age ($\pm$ 5 years), sex, race and hospital
Menke-Pluymers et al. (1993) Netherlands 1978–85	Men: 47 cases and 53 controls; women: 15 cases and 43 controls	Hospital-based study Cases histologically confirmed as adenocarcinoma in Barrett's oesophagus; mean age, 62 years Controls with cancer-free Barrett's oesophagus; mean age, 61 years
Brown et al. (1994b) USA 1986–89	Men: 174 cases and 750 controls	Population-based study in three areas Cases histologically confirmed as adenocarcinoma of the oesophagus or gastro–oesophageal junction, identified through cancer registries, aged 30–79 years Controls selected from general population by random-digit dialling and random sampling of Medicare recipients, frequency-matched on age and race
Gao et al. (1994) China 1990–93	Men and women: 51 cases and 1552 controls	Population-based study in the urban area of Shanghai Cases histologically confirmed as adenocarcinomas of the oesophagus, identified through Shanghai Cancer Registry, aged 30–74 years Controls randomly selected from Resident Registry, matched on age and sex
Vaughan et al. (1995) USA 1983–90	Men and women: 298 cases and 724 controls	Population-based study in western Washington State Cases histologically confirmed as adenocarcinomas of the oesophagus (133) or gastric cardia/gastro–oesophageal junction (165), identified through the Cancer Surveillance System of the Fred Hutchinson Cancer Research Center Controls identified by random-digit dialling, frequency-matched by age and sex

Table 2.1.4.20 (contd)

Reference Country and years of study	Number of cases and controls	Criteria for eligibility and comments
Zhang *et al.* (1996) USA 1992–94	Men: 79 cases and 62 controls; women: 16 cases and 70 controls	Hospital-based study Cases histologically confirmed as adenocarcinomas of the oesophagus (28) or gastro–oesophageal junction and gastric cardia (67) Controls were patients who had undergone gastrointestinal endoscopy.
Gammon *et al.* (1997) USA 1993–95	Men: 245 cases and 555 controls; women: 48 cases and 140 controls	Population-based study in three areas Cases histologically confirmed as adenocarcinomas of the oesophagus, identified through population-based tumour registries, aged 30–79 years; 81% of eligible cases participated. Controls identified by random-digit dialling or random sampling of Health Care Financing Administration rosters, frequency-matched by geographical area, age, sex and/or race, depending on study centre; response rate, 70%
Lagergren *et al.* (2000) Sweden 1995–97	Men: 164 cases and 681 controls; women: 25 cases and 139 controls	Population-based study Cases histologically confirmed as adenocarcinomas of the oesophagus from the entire population of Sweden; median age, 69 years; 87% of eligible cases participated. Controls randomly selected in general population, from age and sex strata (frequency-matched); participation rate, 73%
Wu *et al.* (2001) USA 1992–97	Men: 202 cases and 999 controls; women: 20 cases and 357 controls	Population-based study in Los Angeles County Cases histologically confirmed as adenocarcinomas of the oesophagus, identified by the Los Angeles County Cancer Surveillance Program; 77% of those approached participated. Controls from neighbourhood, matched on gender, race and age ($\pm$ 5 years); diagnosis of oesophageal or stomach cancer excluded

Table 2.1.4.21. Case–control studies on tobacco smoking and adenocarcinoma of the oesophagus

Reference Country and years of study	Smoking categories	Relative risk	95% CI	Comments
Levi et al. (1990) Switzerland 1963–85	Cigarettes/day			Adjusted for age and sex; the control group used have been inappropriate.
	< 15	1.0	0.3–4.1	
	15–24	0.6	0.2–1.9	
	≥ 25	0.9	0.3–2.9	
Kabat et al. (1993) USA 1981–90	Men			Adjusted for age, education, hospital, time period and alcohol use; adenocarcinomas of the distal oesophagus and gastric cardia were combined.
	Former smoker	1.9	1.2–3.0	
	Current smoker	2.3	1.4–3.9	
	Cigarettes/day			
	1–20	1.8	1.1–2.9	
	21–30	2.1	1.1–3.9	
	≥ 31	2.4	1.5–4.0	
	Years since quitting			
	Current smoker	1.0	–	
	1–5	0.5	0.2–1.1	
	6–10	1.1	0.6–1.9	
	11–20	1.2	0.8–1.9	
	≥ 21	0.5	0.3–0.9	
	Women			
	Former smoker	1.4	0.4–4.4	
	Current smoker	4.8	1.7–14.0	
	Cigarettes/day			
	1–20	1.9	0.7–5.4	
	≥ 21	4.5	1.4–14.2	
	Years since quitting			
	Current smoker	1.0	–	
	1–10	0.3	0.1–1.7	
	≥ 11	0.3	0.1–1.1	

Table 2.1.4.21 (contd)

Reference Country and years of study	Smoking categories	Relative risk	95% CI	Comments
Menke-Pluymers *et al.* (1993) Netherlands 1978–85	Current smoker	2.3	*p* < 0.05	Adjusted for age, sex, alcohol intake and length of Barrett's oesophagus; controls may be inappropriate.
Brown *et al.* (1994b) USA 1986–89	Current smoker	2.1	1.2–3.8	Adjusted for age, area, intake of spirits and income
	Cigarettes/day			
	< 20	1.1	0.5–2.4	
	20–39	2.4	1.3–4.4	
	≥ 40	2.6	1.3–5.0	*p* for trend < 0.01
	Duration (years)			
	< 30	2.5	1.3–4.7	
	30–39	2.5	1.3–4.9	
	≥ 40	1.6	0.8–3.2	*p* for trend > 0.05
	Age at starting smoking (years)			
	≥ 21	2.4	0.5–3.2	
	16–20	1.9	0.9–3.2	
	< 16	2.5	0.9–3.6	*p* for trend > 0.05
	Years since quitting			
	1–9	2.0	1.0–4.1	
	10–19	2.4	1.2–4.9	
	20–29	2.2	1.0–4.7	
	≥ 30	3.1	1.5–6.6	*p* for trend > 0.05

Table 2.1.4.21 (contd)

Reference Country and years of study	Smoking categories	Relative risk	95% CI	Comments
Gao et al. (1994) China 1990–93	Former smoker	1.8		Adjusted for age, sex, education, birthplace, tea drinking, dietary factors and alcohol intake (for men only); for separated histological types, odds ratios were not statistically significant at $p < 0.05$ (numbers too small).
	Current smoker	2.1		
	Cigarettes/day			
	1–9	2.0		
	10–19	1.1		
	20–29	2.0		
	≥ 30	3.5		p for trend > 0.05
	Duration (years)			
	0.5–19	1.8		
	20–29	1.0		
	30–39	2.0		
	≥ 40	2.0		p for trend > 0.05
	Pack–years			
	< 15	1.7		
	15–34	1.4		
	≥ 35	2.4		p for trend > 0.05
	Age at starting smoking (years)			
	≥ 30	2.0		
	20–29	1.6		
	< 20	1.8		p for trend > 0.05
Vaughan et al. (1995) USA 1983–90	Former smoker	1.5	1.0–2.3	Adjusted for age, gender, race, education, alcohol intake and body mass index; cases of adenocarcinoma of the oesophagus, gastro–oesophageal junction and gastric cardia were combined.
	Pack–years			
	1–39	1.4	0.7–2.7	
	40–79	2.4	1.4–4.1	
	≥ 80	3.4	1.4–8.0	p for trend = 0.03

Table 2.1.4.21 (contd)

Reference Country and years of study	Smoking categories	Relative risk	95% CI	Comments
Vaughan *et al.* (1995) (contd)	Type of cigarette			Among ever smokers, further adjusted for pack–years of smoking
	Filter	1.0	–	
	Mixed	0.8	0.4–1.6	
	Untipped			
	vs filter only	1.4	0.7–3.0	
	vs filter and mixed	1.7	1.1–2.7	
Zhang *et al.* (1996) USA 1992–94	Cigarettes/day			Adjusted for age, sex, race, education, alcohol consumption, body-mass index and daily total calories
	1–20	1.1	0.5–2.4	
	21–40	2.8	1.1–7.2	*p* for trend = 0.07
	> 40	1.3	0.1–11.3	
	Duration (years)			
	1–20	0.9	0.3–2.4	
	21–40	2.2	0.99–4.9	
	> 40	1.3	0.4–3.8	*p* for trend = 0.17
	Pack–years			
	1–29	1.5	0.7–3.4	
	30–59	1.6	0.6–3.9	*p* for trend = 0.18
	≥ 60	2.4	0.7–7.9	*p* for trend = 0.034
	continuous variable			
	Age at starting smoking (years)			
	> 20	1.8	0.7–4.7	
	17–20	2.0	0.8–4.9	
	≤ 16	1.0	0.4–2.5	*p* for trend = 0.79

Table 2.1.4.21 (contd)

Reference Country and years of study	Smoking categories	Relative risk	95% CI	Comments
Gammon *et al.* (1997) USA 1993–95	Former smoker	2.0	1.4–2.9	Adjusted for age, sex, area, race, body-mass index, income and use of alcohol
	Current smoker	2.2	1.4–3.3	
	Cigarettes/day			
	< 16	1.5	1.0–2.4	
	16–20	2.2	1.4–3.4	
	21–30	3.1	1.9–5.1	
	> 30	2.1	1.3–3.3	*p* for trend < 0.05
	Duration (years)			
	< 20	1.4	0.9–2.2	
	20–31	1.7	1.0–2.8	
	32–42	2.9	1.8–4.4	
	> 42	2.4	1.5–3.7	*p* for trend < 0.05
	Pack–years			
	< 14	1.4	0.8–2.2	
	14–31	1.6	1.0–2.6	
	32–54	2.9	1.8–4.5	
	> 54	2.8	1.8–4.4	*p* for trend < 0.05
	Years since quitting			
	< 11	2.7	1.6–4.4	
	11–20	2.3	1.4–3.8	
	21–30	1.9	1.1–3.2	
	> 30	1.2	0.7–2.2	*p* for trend < 0.05
	Filter status			
	Filter only	2.0	1.4–2.9	
	Filter + no filter	1.7	1.0–3.0	
	No filter only	1.9	1.2–2.9	

Table 2.1.4.21 (contd)

Reference Country and years of study	Smoking categories	Relative risk	95% CI	Comments
Lagergren et al. (2000) Sweden 1995–97	Former smoker	1.9	1.2–2.9	Adjusted for age, sex, alcohol use, education, body-mass index, reflux symptoms, intake of fruit and vegetables, energy intake, physical activity, pipe smoking and snuff use
	Current smoker	1.6	0.9–2.7	
	Cigarettes/day			
	1–9	1.2	0.7–2.2	
	10–19	1.7	1.0–2.9	
	> 19	1.1	0.6–2.0	
	Duration (years)[†]			[†]Includes cigar and pipe smoking.
	1–20	1.8	1.1–3.1	
	21–35	1.5	0.9–2.6	
	> 35	2.0	1.2–3.3	
	Years since quitting			
	0–2	1.7	1.0–3.0	
	3–10	2.4	1.2–4.8	
	11–25	1.6	0.9–2.5	
	> 25	1.6	0.9–2.8	p for trend = 0.02
Wu et al. (2001) USA 1992–97	Former smoker	1.5	1.0–2.2	Adjusted for age, sex, race, birthplace and education
	Current smoker	2.8	1.8–4.3	
	Cigarettes/day			
	1–19	1.6	0.7–3.3	
	20–39	2.9	1.8–4.8	p for trend < 0.0001
	≥ 40	4.5	2.3–8.7	
	Duration (years)			
	≤ 20	1.4	0.9–2.2	
	21–40	2.1	1.4–3.1	
	≥ 41	2.2	1.3–3.5	p for trend = 0.0001

Table 2.1.4.21 (contd)

Reference Country and years of study	Smoking categories	Relative risk	95% CI	Comments
Wu *et al.* (2001) (contd)	Age at starting smoking (years)			
	≥ 21	1.9	1.2–3.0	
	17–20	1.8	1.2–2.7	
	≤ 16	1.8	1.2–2.8	*p* for trend = 0.003
	Years since quitting			
	1–5	2.2	1.2–3.9	
	6–10	1.1	0.5–2.3	
	11–19	1.7	1.1–2.9	
	≥ 20	1.3	0.8–2.1	*p* for trend = 0.01

CI, confidence interval

Table 2.1.4.22. Cohort studies on tobacco smoking and laryngeal cancer

Reference Country and years of study	Subjects	Smoking categories	Number of cases	Relative risk	95% CI	Comments
Weir & Dunn (1970) USA 1954–62	Californian Study 68 153 men	Cigarettes/day 1–14 15–25 > 25	11	1.0 6.0 5.8		Light smokers were used as the reference group as none of the cases were nonsmokers.
Hirayama (1985); Akiba & Hirayama (1990) Japan 1965–81	Six-prefecture Study 265 118 adults (122 261 men and 142 857 women)	Current smoker Cigarettes/day 1–4 5–14 15–24 25–34 ≥ 35	72 1 23 35 9 4	23.8 13.7 17.0 25.7 76.9 73.4	5.3–420 0.5–346 3.6–304 5.5–458 14–1427 11–1444	Data stratified by prefecture, occupation, attained age and observation period
		Cigarettes/day 1–24 ≥ 25		SMR[†] 31 98.5		[†]Standardized mortality ratio p for trend < 0.0001
Akiba (1994) Japan 1968–87	Life Span Study 61 505 atomic bomb survivors	Former smoker Current smoker	46	> 100 > 100		
McLaughlin et al. (1995) USA 1954–80	US Veterans' Study 293 958 men	Former smoker Ever-smoker Current smoker	167	5.0 10.2 13.7	2.4–10.5 5.2–20.0 7.0–27.1	
Raitiola & Pukander (1997) Finland 1962–91	Data from files of Tampere University Hospital and Finnish Cancer Registry	Current smoker Men Women	244 14	15.9 12.4	10.0–25.4 3.9–39.5	Adjusted for age No description of collection of information on smoking status among reference population; significantly higher proportion of smokers in supra-glottic than in glottic cases ($p = 0.025$)

CI, confidence interval

Table 2.1.4.23. Case–control studies on tobacco smoking and laryngeal cancer: main characteristics of study design

Reference Country and years of study	Number of cases and controls	Criteria for eligibility
Wynder & Stellman (1979) USA 1969–76	Men: 286 cases and 4835 controls; women, 64 cases and 4712 controls	Retrospective study conducted in six cities Cases histologically confirmed Controls with cancers not related to tobacco consumption, benign neoplasms and other non-neoplastic conditions
Burch et al. (1981) Canada 1977–79	Men: 184 cases and 184 controls; women: 20 cases and 20 controls	Population-based study Cases histologically confirmed, ascertained by two Ontario hospitals; response rate, 79% Neighbourhood controls individually matched (1:1) on sex, age (± 5 years) and area of residence; response rate, 78%
Graham et al. (1981) USA 1957–65	White men: 374 cases and 381 controls	Hospital-based study in a major cancer institution Cases histologically confirmed Controls without cancer or respiratory or digestive tract diseases, randomly selected by 5-year age groups
Herity et al. (1982) Ireland	Men only: 68 cases and 68 controls	Hospital-based study Controls with cancers and premalignant skin conditions considered not to be related to tobacco or alcohol consumption
Olsen et al. (1985) Denmark 1980–82	326 cases (276 men and 50 women) and 1134 controls	Population-based study Cases of cancer of the glottis (58%) and supraglottis (34%); aged < 75 years, 91% histologically confirmed; response rate, 96% Controls matched about 4:1 on sex and date of birth; response rate, 78%
Brownson (1987) USA 1984–85	White men: 63 cases and 200 controls	Hospital-based study Cases ascertained through the Missouri Cancer Registry, histologically confirmed Controls with colon cancer, matched about 3:1 by area and admission time period
De Stefani et al. (1987) Uruguay 1985–86	Men: 107 cases and 290 controls	Hospital-based study in the University Hospital in Montevideo Cases histologically confirmed, aged 30–89 years Controls with diseases not related to tobacco or alcohol consumption, admitted to the same hospital in the same time period
Tuyns et al. (1988) France, Italy, Spain and Switzerland 1973–80	Men: 696 cases and 3057 controls	Population-based study in six areas in four countries Cases of cancer of the endolarynx (61% supraglottic, 39% glottic and subglottic); response rate > 80% Controls drawn from the local population as a stratified sample by sex and 10-year age group; response rate, 56–75%

Table 2.1.4.23 (contd)

Reference Country and years of study	Number of cases and controls	Criteria for eligibility
Falk *et al.* (1989) USA 1975–80	Whie men: 151 cases and 235 controls	Population-based study Cases aged 30–79 years, ascertained from 56 hospitals in six counties Controls frequency-matched by area of residence, 5-year age group and ethnicity
Franceschi *et al.* (1990) Italy 1986–89	Men: 162 cases and 1272 controls	Hospital-based study in two hospitals Cases histologically confirmed, aged ≤ 75 years Controls with acute conditions unrelated to tobacco or alcohol consumption from the same hospital, matched by area of residence and age (± 5 years)
Sankaranarayanan *et al.* (1990) India 1983–84	Men: 191 cases and 546 controls	Hospital-based study in two major hospitals Cases histologically confirmed Controls with diagnosis of respiratory, genitourinary and gastrointestinal infections without cancer
Ahrens *et al.* (1991) Germany 1986–87	Men: 85 cases and 100 controls	Hospital-based study in a hospital in Bremen Cases histologically confirmed (55 incident and 30 prevalent) Controls without cancer and with diseases not related to smoking, matched on age
Choi & Kahyo (1991) Republic of Korea 1986–89	Men: 94 cases and 282 controls; women: 6 cases and 18 controls	Hospital-based study in a Cancer Center Hospital in Seoul Cases histologically confirmed Controls without cancer and tobacco- or alcohol-related diseases, matched on sex, year of birth (± 5 years) and admission time period
Zatonski *et al.* (1991) Poland 1986–87	Men: 249 cases and 965 controls	Population-based study Cases identified in Lower Silesia, histologically confirmed, aged < 65 years; response rate, 88% Controls from the same region, aged 25–64 years; response rate, 94%
Freudenheim *et al.* (1992) USA 1975–85	Men: 250 cases and 250 controls	Population-based study in three counties in New York Cases identified from pathology records of the hospitals, Caucasians only; response rate, 30% Neighbourhood controls matched on sex, race and age; response rate, 48%
López-Abente *et al.* (1992) Spain 1982–85	Men: 50 cases and 103 controls	Hospital- and population-based study in Madrid Cases of cancer of the glottis (30%) and supraglottis (54%); aged ≤ 80 years; response rate, 51% Controls matched on sex and age (± 5 years): 45 hospital controls with diseases considered not to be related to tobacco or alcohol consumption, 58 population controls from the general population selected from the electoral roll; response rate, 49%

Table 2.1.4.23 (contd)

Reference Country and years of study	Number of cases and controls	Criteria for eligibility
Maier et al. (1992b) Germany 1988–89	Men: 164 cases and 656 controls	Hospital-based study in Heidelberg Cases of cancer of the glottis and supraglottis, histologically confirmed; mean age, 58.1 years Controls with no known tumorous diseases, selected randomly from outpatient clinics, matched 4:1 by age and residential area
Muscat & Wynder (1992) USA 1985–90	White men: 194 cases and 184 controls	Hospital-based study in eight hospitals in four states Cases of cancer of the glottis (48%) and supraglottis (47%), histologically confirmed Controls with conditions unrelated to tobacco-induced diseases, individually matched on hospital, age (± 5 years) and year of interview
Zheng et al. (1992c) China 1988–90	Men: 177 cases and 269 controls; women: 24 cases and 145 controls	Population-based study among residents of urban Shanghai Cases aged 20–75 years; response rate, 76% Controls randomly selected and frequency-matched by sex and age (5-year groups); response rate, 88%
Hedberg et al. (1994) USA 1983–87	Men: 185 cases and 356 controls; women: 50 cases and 191 controls	Population-based study Cases had response rate of 81%. Controls randomly selected from the population of same area by random-digit dialling and frequency-matched on sex and age (5-year groups); response rate, 75%
Sokic et al. (1994) Yugoslavia 1991–92	Men: 93 cases and 93 controls; women: 7 cases and 7 controls	Hospital-based study in University Clinical Center in Belgrade Cases histologically confirmed Controls with minor injuries, matched on sex, age (5-year groups) and residence
Tavani et al. (1994) Italy 1986–92	Men: 350 cases and 1373 controls; women: 17 cases and 558 controls	Hospital-based study in the greater Milan area Cases histologically confirmed, aged < 80 years Controls without cancer and with diseases or conditions unrelated to smoking, alcohol consumption or long-term dietary modifications, matched by hospital
Dosemeci et al. (1997) Turkey 1979–84	Men: 832 cases and 829 controls	Hospital-based study in an oncology treatment centre in Istanbul Cases histologically confirmed Controls with selected cancers not reported to be related to smoking or alcohol drinking (97%) or without cancer (3%)

Table 2.1.4.23 (contd)

Reference Country and years of study	Number of cases and controls	Criteria for eligibility
Maier & Tisch (1997) Germany 1988–89	Men: 164 cases and 656 controls	Hospital-based study in two clinical departments of the University of Heidelberg Cases histologically confirmed Controls without cancer, randomly selected from outpatients, individually matched (4:1) on age and residential area
Rao *et al.* (1999) India 1980–84	Men: 427 cases and 635 controls	Hospital-based study in Mumbai Cases histologically confirmed Controls free from cancer, infectious diseases or benign tumours, admitted at the same hospital during the same period
Schlecht *et al.* (1999) Brazil 1986–89	Men and women: 194 cases and 1578 controls	Hospital-based study in three metropolitan areas in southern Brazil Cases histologically confirmed Controls without cancer or mental disorders, selected from the same or nearby hospitals, matched on sex, age (± 5 years) and admission period

Table 2.1.4.24. Case–control studies on tobacco smoking and laryngeal cancer

Reference Country and years of study	Smoking categories	Relative risk	95% CI	Comments
Burch et al. (1981) Canada 1977–79	Cigarettes/day 1–14 15–24 ≥25	3.0 3.4 4.5	1.4–6.3 1.7–6.8 2.2–9.2	Adjusted for lifetime alcohol consumption
Graham et al. (1981) USA 1957–65	Cigarettes/day 1–10 11–20 21–39 ≥40	2.1 4.8 8.8 8.5	$p < 0.05$ $p < 0.005$ $p < 0.005$ $p < 0.005$	Adjusted for alcohol consumption. Possible selection bias in controls; p for trend < 0.005
Herity et al. (1982) Ireland	Tobacco consumption None or light Heavy	1.0 4.9	– 2.6–9.0	Analysis restricted to abstainers from alcohol and light drinkers. Consumption of tobacco in pipes and cigars converted into the equivalent of cigarettes/day (1 oz tobacco = 25 cigarettes, 1 cigar = 7 cigarettes, 1 cheroot = 2.5 cigarettes). Smokers whose consumption was at or below the median are referred to as light smokers; those above the median consumption as heavy smokers. Possible selection bias in controls
Olsen et al. (1985) Denmark 1980–82	Tobacco/day (g) 0–10 11–20 ≥21	1.0 1.7 2.3		Adjusted for age, sex and alcohol consumption. One cigarette equals 1 g; one cigar, 3 g, and a pipeful, 2.5 g of tobacco. Effects of smoking cigarettes, cigars and pipe could not be separated. The association was similar for the glottis and supraglottis.
Brownson (1987) USA 1984–85	Cigarettes/day 1–19 20–40 >40	2.6 3.7 7.0	1.1–6.1 1.5–9.2 1.3–37.9	Adjusted for age and alcohol consumption. Former smokers were classified as 1–19 cigarettes/day, cigar and pipe smokers as 20–40 cigarettes/day. Possible selection bias in controls. Effects of cigarette, cigar and pipe smoking could not be separated. p for trend < 0.01

Table 2.1.4.24 (contd)

Reference Country and years of study	Smoking categories	Relative risk	95% CI	Comments
De Stefani et al. (1987) Uruguay 1985–86	Cigarettes/day 0–15 ≥ 16	 1.0 10.9		Adjusted for age and alcohol consumption. Reference group might not have been appropriate. Controls included patients with diseases possibly related to smoking.
Tuyns et al. (1988) France, Italy, Spain and Switzerland 1973–80	Ever-smoker Cigarettes/day 1–7 8–15 16–25 ≥ 26	9.9 2.4 6.7 13.7 16.4	6.4–15.4 1.3–4.3 4.2–10.7 8.7–21.6 10.1–26.6	Adjusted for alcohol intake, age, place and their interaction. The association was stronger (2–3-fold) for the supraglottis than for the glottis.
Falk et al. (1989) USA 1975–80	Cigarettes/day 1–10 11–20 21–30 31–40 > 40	5.4 7.0 6.0 20.8 19.2	1.1–27.1 2.8–18.0 2.0–17.9 6.3–68.1 5.0–73.4	Adjusted for age, residence, fruit and vegetable consumption, high-risk occupations and usual alcohol intake
	Duration (years) For < 20 cigarettes/day < 35 35–44 ≥ 45	 3.4 7.4 9.6	 0.9–13.2 2.4–23.0 3.2–29.1	p for trend < 0.002 p for trend < 0.001
	For > 20 cigarettes/day < 35 35–44 ≥ 45	 11.1 11.3 11.3	 3.1–39.2 3.9–33.3 3.6–35.0	 p for trend < 0.001

Table 2.1.4.24 (contd)

Reference Country and years of study	Smoking categories	Relative risk	95% CI	Comments
Franceschi et al. (1990) Italy 1986–89	Cigarettes/day			Adjusted for age, area of residence, years of education, occupation and alcohol intake
	≤ 14	2.2	1.0–5.2	
	15–24	4.8	2.3–10.4	p for trend < 0.01
	≥ 25	7.1	3.3–15.4	
	Duration (years)			
	1–29	1.9	0.8–4.4	
	30–39	5.2	2.4–11.5	
	≥ 40	7.2	3.3–15.6	p for trend < 0.01
	Age at starting smoking (years)			
	≥ 25	2.4	1.0–5.7	
	17–24	5.1	2.4–10.9	
	< 17	6.5	3.3–14.3	p for trend < 0.01
Sankaranarayanan et al. (1990) India 1983–84	Current smoker	1.4	0.8–2.4	Adjusted for age and religion
	Duration (years)†			†Further adjusted for duration of alcohol and bidi consumption and daily consumption of cigarettes and bidis
	≤ 20	1.6	0.3–7.7	
	> 20	5.2	2.2–12.0	p for trend < 0.005
Ahrens et al. (1991) Germany 1986–87	Current smoker	3.8	0.96–14.7	Adjusted for age; possible selection bias; only 3 cases and 9 controls were nonsmokers, 20 cases and 18 controls smoked both cigarettes and pipe/cigars.
	Pack–years†			†Further adjusted for alcohol intake
	6–29	2.6	1.0–6.6	
	≥ 30	3.0	1.1–7.9	

Table 2.1.4.24 (contd)

Reference Country and years of study	Smoking categories	Relative risk	95% CI	Comments
Choi & Kahyo (1991) Republic of Korea 1986–89	Former smoker	2.2	0.6–8.4	Selection bias could not be excluded.
	Current smoker	5.4	2.1–14.3	
	Cigarettes/day			
	1–20	3.7	1.3–10.0	
	21–40	10.6	3.8–29.9	
	≥ 41	27.3	5.3–141.9	
	Duration (years)			
	1–19	3.8	1.3–23.6	
	20–39	4.8	2.0–15.7	
	≥ 40	5.6	1.8–12.9	
	Age at starting smoking (years)			
	≥ 25	6.6	2.1–21.1	
	18–24	5.2	2.0–13.9	
	≤ 17	3.8	1.2–12.1	
Zatonski et al. (1991) Poland 1986–87	Cigarettes/day			Adjusted for age, residence and education
	0–5	1.0	–	
	6–10	8.4	1.5–46.0	
	11–15	18.1	3.9–83.2	
	16–20	29.9	7.0–128.0	
	21–30	33.7	7.6–150.0	
	> 30	59.7	13.0–274.0	
	Age at starting smoking (years)			
	> 22	0.6	0.3–1.2	
	16–22	1.0	–	
	< 16	1.3	0.7–2.23	

Table 2.1.4.24 (contd)

Reference Country and years of study	Smoking categories	Relative risk	95% CI	Comments
Freudenheim et al. (1992) USA 1975–85	Pack–years			Adjusted for alcohol consumption and education. Response rates too low; possibility of selection bias
	1–12	2.0	0.7–5.9	
	13–29	2.0	0.8–5.3	
	30–45	5.1	1.9–13.6	
	≥ 46	12.6	5.0–31.5	p for trend < 0.001
López-Abente et al. (1992) Spain 1982–85	Cigarettes/day			Adjusted for age, alcohol intake and occupation. Low response rates, small sample size; reference groups may have been inappropriate. The association was stronger for the supraglottis than for the glottis.
	0–9	1.0	–	
	10–19	1.9	0.6–6.0	
	20–29	2.2	0.6–8.0	
	≥30	4.3	1.2–15.4	p for trend = 0.02
	Duration (years)			
	0–20	1.0	–	
	21–40	3.6	0.7–19.6	
	≥41	13.7	2.3–82.6	p for trend = 0.001
	Pack–years			
	≤ 19	1.0	–	
	> 19–41	3.3	0.98–10.8	
	> 41	4.5	1.4–14.9	p for trend = 0.02
Maier et al. (1992b) Germany 1988–89	Pack–years			Adjusted for alcohol consumption. Smokers in case and control groups included 3.5% and 9.5% of cigar or pipe smokers, respectively. The association was much stronger (10-fold) for the supraglottis than for the glottis.
	5–50	5.6	2.9–10.9	
	> 50	9.1	4.5–18.7	
Muscat & Wynder (1992) USA 1985–90	Former smoker	4.8	1.7–13.0	Adjusted for age, education, alcohol and Quetelet index. The association was stronger (3–4-fold) for the supraglottis than for the glottis.
	Current smoker	13.8	2.3–27.1	
	Cigarettes/day			
	1–20	10.3	3.6–29.4	
	21–40	38.5	12.1–122	

Table 2.1.4.24 (contd)

Reference Country and years of study	Smoking categories	Relative risk	95% CI	Comments
Zheng *et al.* (1992c) China 1988–90	**Men**			
	Ever-smoker	8.7	3.8–19.6	Adjusted for age and education
	Cigarettes/day			
	< 10	1.6	0.5–4.9	
	10–19	7.1	3.1–16.6	
	20	12.4	4.6–33.2	
	> 20	25.1	9.9–63.2	*p* for trend < 0.01
	Pack–years			
	< 10	1.4	0.4–4.5	
	10–19	2.9	1.1–7.9	
	20–29	3.1	1.1–8.6	
	30–39	15.4	6.0–39.6	
	≥ 40	25.1	10.3–61.2	*p* for trend < 0.01
	Duration (years)			
	< 20	1.4	0.4–4.6	
	20–29	4.1	1.6–11.1	
	30–39	12.0	4.8–30.1	
	≥ 40	13.2	5.6–31.2	*p* for trend < 0.01
	Women			
	Pack–years			
	1–9	9.4	2.4–37.2	
	≥ 10	20.2	5.3–76.9	

Table 2.1.4.24 (contd)

Reference Country and years of study	Smoking categories	Relative risk	95% CI	Comments
Hedberg et al. (1994) USA 1983–87	Never-smoker + quit	1.0	–	Adjusted for age, sex, alcohol consumption and score in alcoholism screening test
	≥ 15 years			
	Former smoker	2.5	1.4–4.3	
	(< 15 years)			
	Cigarettes/day			
	< 20	6.3	3.1–11.8	
	20–39	10.6	6.5–18.7	
	≥ 40	23.1	9.4–52.6	
Sokic et al. (1994) Yugoslavia 1991–92	≥ 10 years	5.5	0.6–51.6	Multivariate regression model with 25 variables including coffee, alcohol consumption, dietary factors, working conditions, exposure to secondhand smoke and health status; relatively small sample size; referent group not specified
	≥ 10 cigarettes/day	18.2	2.0–169.8	
Tavani et al. (1994) Italy 1986–92	Men			Adjusted for centre, age, education, alcohol intake and β-carotene index. Moderate smokers included former smokers, pipe and/or cigar smokers and current smokers of < 15 cigarettes/day. Estimates in women based on a small number of cases p for trend in men < 0.001
	Moderate smoker	3.3	1.9–5.5	
	Heavy smoker	8.8	5.2–14.8	
	Women			
	Current smoker	23.9	5.2–110.9	

Table 2.1.4.24 (contd)

Reference Country and years of study	Smoking categories	Relative risk	95% CI	Comments
Dosemeci et al. (1997) Turkey 1979–84	Ever-smoker	3.5	2.6–4.4	Adjusted for age and alcohol
	Cigarettes/day			
	1–10	1.6	0.9–2.6	
	11–20	3.5	2.6–4.8	
	≥ 21	6.6	4.2–10.3	p for trend < 0.001
	Pack–years			
	1–10	1.9	1.3–3.0	
	11–20	4.4	2.9–6.7	
	≥ 21	6.0	3.8–9.5	p for trend < 0.001
	Duration (years)			
	1–10	1.1	0.6–1.9	
	11–20	4.8	3.1–7.4	
	≥ 21	4.1	2.8–6.0	p for trend < 0.001
Maier & Tisch (1997) Germany 1988–89	Tobacco–years			Adjusted for alcohol. Tobacco–year defined as 20 cigarettes or 4 cigars or 5 pipes/day for 1 year. Reference group included light smokers; effects of cigarettes, cigars and pipes could not be separated. The categories of tobacco–years are not continuous and appear surprisingly high.
	< 5	1.0		
	5–19	4.0	1.7–9.2	
	50–74 [sic]	6.3	3.0–13.3	
	75–99	7.8	3.6–16.7	
	≥ 100	9.5	4.6–19.6	
Rao et al. (1999) India 1980–84	Current smoker	1.5	0.9–2.4	Adjusted for age and area of residence. Bidi smoking was more common than cigarette smoking in the study area.
Schlecht et al. (1999) Brazil 1986–89	Current smoker	11.7	4.4–31.5	Adjusted for age, sex, study location, admission period, alcohol consumption, race, beverage temperature, religion, wood stove use and consumption of spicy food. One pack = 20 manufactured cigarettes = 4 hand-rolled, black tobacco cigarettes = 4 cigars = 5 pipefuls with regular pipe tobacco. Possible selection bias in controls
	Pack–years			
	1–20	8.2	3.0–22.6	
	21–40	9.4	3.3–26.7	
	> 40	16.3	5.3–49.8	

CI, confidence interval

Table 2.1.4.25. Case–control studies on tobacco smoking and laryngeal cancer: smoking cessation

Reference Country and years of study	Subjects	No. of years since quitting	Relative risk	95% CI	Comments
Tuyns et al. (1988) France, Italy, Spain and Switzerland 1973–80	Men with cancer of the endolarynx	Current smoker	1.0		Adjusted for alcohol intake, daily cigarette consumption, use of filter, type of tobacco and degree of inhalation
		1–4	1.5	1.2–2.0	
		5–9	0.5	0.3–0.8	
		≥ 10	0.3	0.2–0.4	
Falk et al. (1989) USA 1975–80	Men	3–9 years' cessation Cigarettes/day			Adjusted for age, area of residence, fruit and vegetable consumption, high-risk occupations and usual alcohol intake
		1–10	3.0	0.2–40.2	
		11–20	3.6	0.8–15.8	
		21–30	4.0	0.6–29.5	
		31–40	7.2	1.0–54.3	
		> 40	10.9	1.8–68.5	p for trend < 0.002
		≥ 10 years' cessation Cigarettes/day			
		1–10	2.8	0.7–10.7	
		11–20	1.2	0.4–4.0	
		21–30	1.0	0.2–6.4	
		31–40	3.1	0.4–22.4	
		> 40	3.5	0.6–19.1	p for trend = 0.088
Franceschi et al. (1990) Italy 1986–89	Men	< 10	4.6	2.0–10.4	Adjusted for age, area of residence, years of education, occupation and alcohol intake
		≥ 10	1.2	0.4–3.3	
		Nonsmoker	1.0	–	

Table 2.1.4.25 (contd)

Reference Country and years of study	Subjects	No. of years since quitting	Relative risk	95% CI	Comments
Ahrens et al. (1991) Germany 1986–87	Men	Current smoker	3.8	0.96–14.7	Adjusted for age; only 3 cases and 9 controls were nonsmokers.
		1–5	2.4	0.5–12.9	
		6–15	1.4	0.3–7.4	
		≥ 16	0.9	0.2–4.3	p for trend < 0.001
Choi & Kahyo (1991) Republic of Korea 1986–89	Men	Current smoker	1.0	–	Selection bias could not be excluded.
		1–4	0.7	0.2–2.2	
		5–9	0.4	0.1–3.0	
		≥ 10	0.2	0.03–1.02	
Zatonski et al. (1991) Poland 1986–87	Men	Current smoker[†]	1.0	–	Adjusted for age, area of residence and education
		5–10	0.8	0.3–1.8	[†]including former smokers who had quit within the preceding 4 years
		> 10	0.3	0.1–0.6	
		Nonsmoking period of > 6 months			
		No	1.0	–	
		Yes	0.2	0.1–0.5	
López-Abente et al. (1992) Spain 1982–85	Men	Current smoker	1.0	–	Adjusted for age, packs of cigarettes smoked over lifetime, alcohol consumption and occupation; low response rate, small sample size
		1	1.2	0.3–5.5	
		2–5	0.7	0.2–2.9	
		6–15	0.8	0.2–3.0	
		> 15	0.5	0.1–3.2	p for trend = 0.43
Zheng et al. (1992c) China 1988–90	Men	< 2 or current smoker	1.0	–	Adjusted for age and education
		2–4	1.8	0.6–4.9	
		5–9	0.6	0.2–1.5	
		≥ 10	0.6	0.3–1.2	
Schlecht et al. (1999) Brazil 1986–89	Men	Current smoker	10.2	3.7–27.9	Conditional logistic regression (matching variables: age, sex, location and admission period) adjusted for alcohol and tobacco consumption
		≤ 5	11.8	3.7–38.0	
		6–10	5.0	1.3–19.1	
		11–15	6.6	1.0–42.1	
		> 15	1.3	0.3–6.0	

CI, confidence interval

Table 2.1.4.26. Case–control studies on tobacco smoking and laryngeal cancer: type of tobacco and/or cigarette

Reference Country and years of study	Subjects	Type of tobacco	Relative risk	95% CI	Comments
Wynder & Stellman (1979) USA 1969–76	Men	Untipped vs filter	1.5	1.1–2.1	Adjusted for duration, intensity and alcohol consumption
	Women		4.0	2.0–7.7	
De Stefani et al. (1987) Uruguay 1985–86	Men	Dark tobacco			Adjusted for age; controls included patients with diseases possibly related to smoking.
		All smokers	35.4	20.8–60.3	
		Cigarettes/day			
		1–10	1.0	–	
		11–20	24.6	9.0–67.4	
		≥ 21	59.2	25.5–137.3	
		Age at starting smoking (years)			
		> 15	12.3	4.6–32.4	
		≤ 15	100.1	49.6–202.4	
		Light tobacco			
		All smokers	14.7	7.8–27.6	
		Cigarettes/day			
		1–10	1.0	–	
		11–20	14.5	5.3–39.4	
		≥ 21	24.7	7.8–78.4	
		Age at starting smoking (years)			
		> 15	5.0	1.5–16.2	
		≤ 15	51.4	22.4–117.9	

Table 2.1.4.26 (contd)

Reference Country and years of study	Subjects	Type of tobacco	Relative risk	95% CI	Comments
Tuyns *et al.* (1988) France, Italy, Spain and Switzerland 1973–80	Men	Use of filter			Adjusted for alcohol intake, daily cigarette consumption and variables analysed
		Only plain	1.0	–	
		Plain > filter	0.9	0.7–1.2	
		Plain < filter	1.03	0.8–1.4	
		Only filter	0.5	0.3–0.8	
		Type of tobacco			
		Only blond	1.0	–	
		Blond > black	1.6	0.9–2.7	
		Blond < black	1.7	1.0–2.7	
		Inhaler	1.0	–	
		Non-inhaler	0.7	0.5–0.9	
Falk *et al.* (1989) USA 1975–80	Men	Hand-rolled	20.1	5.4–74.6	Adjusted for age, residence, fruit and vegetable consumption, high-risk occupation and usual alcohol intake
		Filter + untipped	13.9	5.1–38.1	
		Untipped only	9.0	3.2–25.1	
		Filter only	5.9	2.4–14.4	
López-Abente *et al.* (1992) Spain 1982–85	Men	Type of tobacco			Adjusted for age, packs of cigarettes smoked over lifetime, alcohol consumption and occupation, low response rate, small sample size
		Blond	1.0	–	
		Mixed	2.4	0.4–14.9	
		Black	2.6	0.4–15.2	
Schlecht *et al.* (1999) Brazil 1986–89	Men	Never-smoker	1.0	–	Conditional logistic regression (matching variables: age, sex, study location and admission period) adjusted for cumulative alcohol and tobacco consumption, race, beverage temperature, religion, wood stove use and consumption of spicy food
		Filter-tipped cigarettes	8.4	3.1–22.8	
		Untipped cigarettes	12.2	4.1–35.9	
		Black tobacco (pack–years)			
		1–20	7.3	2.4–22.4	
		21–40	8.9	2.9–27.2	
		>40	8.5	3.0–23.9	

CI, confidence interval

Table 2.1.4.27. Cohort studies on tobacco smoking and cancers of the upper aerodigestive tract

Reference Country and years of study	Subjects	Cancer site ICD code	Smoking categories	Number of cases	Relative risk	95% CI	Comments
Hammond & Horn (1958) USA 1952–55	American Cancer Society Study 187 783 men	Lip, tongue, oral cavity, pharynx, larynx, oesophagus	Current smoker Cigarettes/day 1–9 10–20 ≥ 21	84 7 21 21	Mortality ratio 7.0 7.8 7.0 10.5		
Doll et al. (1980) UK 1951–73	British Doctors' Study 6194 women	Upper respiratory sites	Nonsmoker Former smoker Cigarettes/day 1–14 15–24 ≥ 25	4	Mortality rate 2 3 0 8 13		Annual mortality rate per 100 000 women p for trend < 0.05
Hammond & Seidman (1980) USA 1967–71	Cancer Prevention Study I 358 422 men and 483 519 women	Oral cavity, pharynx, larynx	Regular smoker Men Women		Mortality ratio 6.5 3.3		
Kono et al. (1987) Japan 1965–83	Japanese Physicians' Study 5477 men	Oral cavity, nasal cavity, pharynx, larynx ICD-8: 140– 150, 161	Cigarettes/day 1–19 ≥ 20	18	1.2 3.0	0.3–4.5 0.9–10.4	Adjusted for age and alcohol drinking

Table 2.1.4.27 (contd)

Reference, Country and years of study	Subjects	Cancer site ICD code	Smoking categories	Number of cases	Relative risk	95% CI	Comments
Akiba & Hirayama (1990) Japan 1966–81	Six-prefecture Study 122 261 men and 142 857 women	Oral cavity ICD-7: 140–149	Men Current smoker Cigarettes/day	64	2.5	1.3–5.7	Adjusted for age, prefecture of residence, occupation and observation period
			1–14	25	2.2	1.0–5.2	
			15–24	32	2.7	1.3–6.3	
			25–34	5	4.2	1.3–12.8	
			≥ 35	2	4.0	0.6–16.2	p for trend = 0.002
			Women Current smoker	5	1.3	0.5–3.2	
Tomita et al. (1991) Japan 1975–85	37 646 men	Lip, oral cavity, pharynx	Nonsmoker	888	Mortality rate 0.19		Annual mortality rates per 10 000 persons Average 6.7 years of follow-up
			Former smoker		0.38		
			Cigarettes/day				
			15–24		0.41		
			25–34		1.34		
			≥ 35		0.59		
Kuller et al. (1991) USA 1972–82	MRFIT Study 361 662 men	Mouth and larynx ICD-9: 140–149; 161	Nonsmoker	35	Mortality rate 1.5		Annual mortality rates per 10 000 persons Reference group includes former smokers at first screen. Relative risk adjusted for age, diastolic blood pressure, serum cholesterol level and race (black/non-black)
			Cigarettes/day				
			1–15	9	3.4		
			16–25	30	7.0		
			26–35	24	9.5		
			36–45	39	17.3		
			≥ 46	16	21.1		
			Current smoker		Relative risk 6.6	$p < 0.0001$	
Akiba (1994) Japan 1968–87	Life Span Study 61 505 survivors	Oral cavity, pharynx ICD-9: 140–49	Former smoker	69	0.4	0.1–1.2	†[Upper limit not obtained]
			Current smoker		1.1	0.6–†	

Table 2.1.4.27 (contd)

Reference Country and years of study	Subjects	Cancer site ICD code	Smoking categories	Number of cases	Relative risk	95% CI	Comments
					Mortality rate		Annual mortality rate per 100 000 men
Doll et al. (1994) UK 1957–91	British Doctors' Study 34 439 men	Upper respiratory sites	Nonsmoker	98	1		
			Former smoker		3		
			Current smoker		24		
			Cigarettes/day				
			1–14		12		
			15–24		18		
			≥ 25		48		*p* for trend < 0.05
Chyou et al. (1995) USA (Hawaii) 1965–68	American Men of Japanese Ancestry Study 7995 men	Upper aero-digestive tract ICD-8: 140–149; 150; 161	Former smoker	21	1.7	0.8–3.5	Adjusted for age and alcohol intake
			Current smoker	59	3.2	1.7–5.9	
			Cigarettes/day				
			1–20	13	2.2	0.99–4.8	
			21–29	31	2.4	1.2–4.7	
			≥ 30	35	3.0	1.5–5.8	*p* for trend = 0.002
			Duration (years)				
			1–24	18	2.1	0.97–4.3	
			25–34	35	2.7	1.4–5.3	
			≥ 35	25	3.0	1.5–5.9	*p* for trend = 0.0006
Murata et al. (1996) Japan 1984–93	Chiba Center Association Study 17 200 male participants	Oral cavity, pharynx, oesophagus, larynx ICD-9: 140–150; 161	Cigarettes/day				
			1–10		1.3		
			11–20		1.8		
			> 21		3.3	*p* < 0.05	*p* for trend < 0.05
Yuan et al. (1996) China 1986–1993	Shanghai Men's Study 18 244 men	Head and neck ICD-9: 140–149; 161	Ever-smoker	43	5.2	*p* < 0.05	Adjusted for age and alcohol consumption
			Current smoker				
			Cigarettes/day				
			< 20	32	3.8	*p* < 0.05	
			≥ 20	53	6.7	*p* < 0.05	

Table 2.1.4.27 (contd)

Reference Country and years of study	Subjects	Cancer site ICD code	Smoking categories	Number of cases	Relative risk	95% CI	Comments
Engeland et al. (1996) Norway 1966–93	Norwegian Cohort Study 26 132 men and women	Upper aero-digestive tract ICD-7: 141; 143–148; 150; 161	Former smoker	15	0.5	0.3–1.1	Analysis for men only because of the small number of cases in women
			Current smoker Cigarettes/day				
			1–4	12	1.2	0.6–2.7	
			5–9	9	1.1	0.5–2.7	
			10–14	16	1.8	0.9–3.8	
			≥ 15	16	5.4	2.5–12.0	
Nordlund et al. (1997) Sweden 1964–89	Swedish Census Study 26 000 women	Upper aero-digestive tract ICD-7: 141; 143-148; 150; 161	Former smoker	94	0.9	0.2–3.8	Adjusted for age and place of residence
			Current smoker Cigarettes/day		2.1	1.3–3.6	
			1–7		1.6	0.8–3.3	
			8–15		3.2	1.6–6.6	
			≥ 16		1.9	0.5–7.9	
			Age at starting smoking (years)				
			> 23		1.0	–	Further adjusted for amount smoked daily
			20–23		0.4	0.1–2.0	
			< 19		1.0	0.3–2.8	p for trend = 0.777

Table 2.1.4.27 (contd)

Reference Country and years of study	Subjects	Cancer site ICD code	Smoking categories	Number of cases	Relative risk	95% CI	Comments
Kjaerheim et al. (1998) Norway 1968–92	10 960 men	Upper aero-digestive tract ICD-7: 141; 143; 144; 145, 147, 148, 150, 161	Never/occasional smoker	5	1.0		Adjusted for age and alcohol consumption All categories include smokers of cigarettes or pipes.
			Former smoker	11	1.7	0.6–4.8	p for trend < 0.002
			Current smoker (g/day)				
			< 15	34	2.6	1.0–6.8	
			≥ 15	15	4.7	1.7–13.2	
			Never/occasional smoker	4	1.0	–	Further adjusted for diet (consumption of oranges and bread)
			Former smoker	11	2.0	0.6–6.4	
			Current smoker (g/day)				
			< 15	30	2.7	1.0–7.7	p for trend = 0.005
			≥ 15	15	4.4	1.4–13.5	Similar results were obtained for cigarettes and pipes analysed separately.
Liaw & Chen (1998) China, Province of Taiwan 1982–94	Taiwanese Study 11 096 men and 3301 women	Lip, oral cavity and pharynx	Current smoker	13 men 0 women	4.2	0.5–32.9	ICD-9 was used, but no codes were reported. Adjusted for age and alcohol consumption
			Cigarettes/day				
			≤ 10		2.3	0.2–25.5	
			11–20		4.7	0.6–38.8	
			> 20		7.5	0.7–86.7	p for trend = 0.05
			Duration (years)				
			21–30		6.0	0.6–55.2	
			> 30		4.5	0.5–38.4	p for trend = 0.08
			Age at starting smoking (years)				
			≤ 20		5.7	0.7–46.1	
			> 24		4.5	0.5–43.5	p for trend = 0.11
			Pack–years				
			≤ 20		1.9	0.2–21.2	
			20–40		3.9	0.4–34.4	
			> 41		11.6	1.2–109.1	p for trend = 0.01

CI, confidence interval

Table 2.1.4.28. Case–control studies on tobacco smoking and cancers of the upper aerodigestive tract: main characteristics of study design

Reference Country and years of study	Number of cases and controls	Criteria for eligibility and comments
Blot et al. (1988) USA 1984–85	Men: 762 cases and 837 controls; women: 352 cases and 431 controls	Population-based study in four regions Incident cases of pathologically confirmed oral and pharyngeal cancer identified through local cancer registries; aged 18–79 years; 75% of all incident cases Controls selected by random-digit dialling (aged 18–64 years) and from Health Care Financing Administration rosters (aged 65–79 years), frequency-matched by age, sex and race
Ferraroni et al. (1989) Italy 1983–88	Men: 43 cases and 1334 controls; women: 7 cases and 710 controls	Hospital-based study in four hospitals in Milan Cases confirmed histologically, aged ≤ 75 years Controls with traumatic, non-traumatic orthopaedic and acute surgical conditions and ear, nose, throat, skin and dental disorders included; malignant tumours, digestive tract disorders and coffee-, alcohol- or tobacco-related conditions excluded; median age, 56 years
Merletti et al. (1989) Italy 1982–84	Men: 86 cases and 385 controls; women: 36 cases and 221 controls	Population-based study Cases histologically confirmed as squamous invasive carcinoma Controls selected from random samples of files of residents of Turin stratified by sex and age
Talamini et al. (1990) Italy 1986–89	Men: 291 cases and 1272 controls; women: 45 cases and 380 controls	Hospital-based study in two areas of northern Italy; study restricted to abstainers from alcohol Cases histologically confirmed as cancer of oral cavity (183) or pharynx (153) Controls: patients from the same hospitals admitted for acute illnesses, without malignant tumours or conditions related to tobacco or alcohol consumption
Barra et al. (1991) Italy 1985–90	Men: 236 cases, 577 cancer controls and 1122 non-cancer controls; women: 36 cases, 446 cancer controls and 762 non-cancer controls	Hospital-based study in the Pordenone province Cases histologically confirmed Cancer controls with cancers not related to tobacco or alcohol consumption: colorectal, renal cell, prostate, thyroid, and haematological. Non-cancer controls admitted for acute illnesses, without malignant tumours or conditions related to tobacco or alcohol consumption

Table 2.1.4.28 (contd)

Reference Country and years of study	Number of cases and controls	Criteria for eligibility and comments
La Vecchia *et al.* (1991) Italy 1987–89	Men: 89 cases and 875 controls; women: 16 cases and 294 controls	Hospital-based study in five hospitals in Milan Incident cases of histologically confirmed oral (35) or oropharyngeal (70) cancer, aged <75 years Controls admitted for acute, non-neoplastic or digestive diseases unrelated to alcohol or tobacco consumption; aged 21–74 years
De Stefani *et al.* (1992) Uruguay 1988–90	Men: 109 cases and 273 controls	Hospital-based study in a cancer institute Cases of cancer of the mouth and pharynx Controls with diseases unrelated to tobacco or alcohol use, admitted to the same hospital during the same time period
Franceschi *et al.* (1992) Italy 1986–90	Men: 104 cases and 726 controls	Hospital-based study in the Pordenone province and the greater Milan area (Lombardy region) Cases histologically confirmed Non-cancer controls admitted to the same hospitals for acute illnesses unrelated to tobacco or alcohol consumption
Marshall *et al.* (1992) USA 1975–83	Men: 201 cases and 201 controls; women: 89 cases and 89 controls	Population-based study Cases from 20 major hospitals in three New York counties, histologically confirmed (90% squamous-cell carcinoma) Controls selected by sampling dwellings, individually matched on neighbourhood, age and sex
Zheng *et al.* (1992a) China 1988–90	Men: 115 cases and 269 controls; women: 89 cases and 145 controls	Population-based study in the urban Shanghai area, linked to the Shanghai Cancer Registry Controls randomly selected from the Shanghai Resident Registry
Day *et al.* (1993) USA 1984–85	Men: 729 cases and 785 controls; women: 336 cases and 397 controls	Population-based study in four regions Incident cases of histologically confirmed oral and pharyngeal cancer identified through local cancer registries Controls selected by random-digit dialling (aged 18–64 years) and Health Care Administration rosters (aged 65–79 years), frequency-matched by age, sex and race

Table 2.1.4.28 (contd)

Reference Country and years of study	Number of cases and controls	Criteria for eligibility and comments
Kune *et al.* (1993) Germany 1982	Men: 41 cases and 398 controls	Population-based study Incident cases of histologically confirmed squamous-cell oral and pharyngeal cancer at a general hospital in Heidelberg; mean age, 64 years Community controls from Melbourne Colorectal Cancer Study; mean age, 65 years
Mashberg *et al.* (1993) USA 1972–83	Men: 359 cases and 2280 controls	Hospital-based study in a veterans' medical centre in New Jersey Cases histologically confirmed as invasive squamous-cell carcinoma or carcinoma *in situ* Controls without evidence of cancer or dysplasia of the pharynx, larynx, lung or oesophagus
Negri *et al.* (1993) Italy 1984–92	Men: 372 cases and 1575 controls; women: 67 cases and 531 controls	Hospital-based study Cases histologically confirmed Controls: patients admitted to the same network of hospitals for acute, non-neoplastic, non-digestive conditions
Spitz *et al.* (1993) USA 1987–91	Men: 70 cases and 70 controls; women: 38 cases and 38 controls	Population-based study in Texas Cases histologically confirmed as squamous-cell carcinoma Controls selected from blood and platelet donors, matched on age, sex and ethnicity
De Stefani *et al.* (1994) Uruguay 1988–92	Men: 246 cases and 253 controls	Hospital-based study in a cancer institute Incident cases of histologically confirmed squamous-cell carcinoma of the oral cavity and pharynx, aged 40–89 years; participation rate, 100% Controls free of benign oral tumours, non-neoplastic conditions of the mouth and pharynx, digestive diseases, or diseases related to tobacco and alcohol consumption; frequency-matched by age; participation rate, 100%
Kabat *et al.* (1994) USA 1977–90	Men: 1097 cases and 2075 controls; women: 463 cases and 873 controls	Hospital-based study in 28 hospitals in eight cities Cases histologically confirmed Controls: patients with diseases unrelated to tobacco or alcohol consumption, and without history of tobacco-related cancer, matched on age, sex, race, hospital and date of interview

Table 2.1.4.28 (contd)

Reference Country and years of study	Number of cases and controls	Criteria for eligibility and comments
Muscat et al. (1996) USA 1981–90	Men: 687 cases and 619 controls; women: 322 cases and 304 controls	Hospital-based study Cases histologically confirmed Controls with conditions unrelated to tobacco use, identified from daily hospital admission logs, matched on sex, age, race and date of admission
Sanderson et al. (1997) Netherlands 1980–90	Women: 303 cases	Population-based study Cases of squamous-cell carcinoma of the oral cavity and oropharynx Controls: data from a large national survey on public health conducted by the National Central Bureau of Statistics; matched on sex and age
Lewin et al. (1998) Sweden 1988–91	Men: 545 cases and 641 controls	Population-based study in two areas Cases identified at weekly conferences at all ear, nose and throat departments in the study area (90%) and from regional cancer registers (10%); aged 40–79 years; 90% eligible cases Controls selected by random sampling from a population register stratified by region and age; response rate, 85%
Talamini et al. (1998) Italy and Switzerland 1992–97	Men: 10 cases and 79 controls; women: 22 cases and 145 controls	Multicentre hospital-based study; analysis restricted to abstainers from alcohol Cases histologically confirmed Controls admitted for acute non-neoplastic conditions unrelated to alcohol consumption or tobacco use
Rao et al. (1999) India 1980–84	678 cases and 635 controls (men only)	Hospital-based study in Mumbai Cases of cancer of the oral cavity and pharynx Controls with infectious diseases and benign tumours, free from cancer, admitted during the same period as controls [no matching]
Bosetti et al. (2000) Italy and Switzerland 1984–97	Women: 195 cases and 1113 controls	Two multicentre hospital-based studies Cases histologically confirmed Controls admitted for acute non-neoplastic conditions, frequency-matched by age and residence

Table 2.1.4.28 (contd)

Reference Country and years of study	Number of cases and controls	Criteria for eligibility and comments
Dikshit & Kanhere (2000) India 1986–92	Men: 247 cases and 260 controls	Population-based study in Bhopal Cases of oropharyngeal cancer collected by a population-based cancer registry Controls randomly selected from a group of 2500 men surveyed for tobacco habits in the general population, stratified by age
Moreno-Lopez et al. (2000) Spain	Men: 63 cases; women: 12 cases; 150 controls	Hospital-based study in three hospitals in the Madrid community Cases histologically confirmed Controls selected from healthy subjects with no history of cancer or oral disease, in health care centres corresponding to the hospitals
Zavras et al. (2001) Greece 1995–98	Men: 68 cases and 69 controls; women: 42 cases and 46 controls	Hospital-based study in three university hospitals in Athens Cases histologically confirmed Controls hospitalized for conditions unrelated to cancer, matched on age and sex

Table 2.1.4.29. Case–control studies on tobacco smoking and cancers of the upper aerodigestive tract

Reference Country and years of study	Cancer subsite ICD code	No. of cases	No. of controls	Smoking categories	Relative risk	95% CI	Comments
Blot et al. (1988) USA 1984–85	Oral cavity and pharynx ICD-9: 141 tongue 143 gum 144 floor of mouth 145 other 146 oropharynx 148 hypopharynx 149 other sites within lip, oral cavity and pharynx			**Men**			Adjusted for age, race, study location, alcohol consumption and respondent status
		659	593	Ever-smoker	1.9	1.3–2.9	
		485	239	Current smoker	3.4	2.3–5.1	
				Cigarettes/day			
		80	173	1–19	1.2	0.7–1.8	
		312	288	20–39	2.1	1.4–3.1	
		262	130	≥ 40	2.8	2.8–4.4	
				Duration (years)			
		45	138	1–19	0.8	0.5–1.3	
		286	281	20–39	1.9	1.2–2.8	
		313	171	≥ 40	3.6	2.3–5.6	
				Age at starting smoking (years)			
		38	47	≥ 25	1.8	0.9–3.3	
		279	285	17–24	1.8	1.2–2.7	
		325	258	< 17	2.1	1.4–3.2	
				Women			
		298	229	Ever-smoker	3.0	2.0–4.5	
		258	129	Current smoker	4.7	3.0–7.3	
				Cigarettes/day			
		60	104	1–19	1.8	1.1–2.9	
		145	94	20–39	3.6	2.3–5.8	
		93	31	≥ 40	6.2	3.6–11.3	
				Duration (years)			
		15	59	1–19	1.0	0.5–1.9	
		127	105	20–39	2.9	1.8–4.6	
		153	64	≥ 40	5.0	3.0–8.3	
				Age at starting smoking (years)			
		54	54	≥ 25	2.8	1.6–4.8	
		153	116	17–24	3.1	2.0–4.9	
		89	59	< 17	2.9	1.7–4.9	

Table 2.1.4.29 (contd)

Reference Country and years of study	Cancer subsite ICD code	No. of cases	No. of controls	Smoking categories	Relative risk	95% CI	Comments
Ferraroni et al. (1989) Italy 1983–88	Mouth and pharynx	2	380	Former smoker	0.9	0.2–3.9	Adjusted for age, sex, education, marital status, social class, coffee and alcohol consumption
				Cigarettes/day			p < 0.01 for all current cigarette smokers combined
		5	267	< 15	3.6		
		25	332	15–24	11.1		
		12	159	≥ 25	11.0		
Merletti et al. (1989) Italy 1982–84	Oral cavity and oropharynx	Men	Men	Tobacco/day (g)			Adjusted for age
	ICD-9:	3	58	1–7	0.9	0.2–3.9	
	140.3 upper lip	27	91	8–15	4.6	1.8–11.9	
	140.4 lower lip	37	106	16–25	5.2	2.1–13.3	
	141 tongue	14	45	> 25	5.2	1.9–14.6	
	143 gum			Duration (years)			
	144 floor of mouth	4	54	1–20	1.0	0.2–5.1	
	145 other parts of mouth	5	52	21–30	1.7	0.4–6.9	
	146 oropharynx	29	79	31–40	5.0	1.6–16.2	
		26	77	41–50	5.0	1.8–13.8	
		17	38	> 50	7.1	1.9–26.0	
				Age at starting smoking (years)			
		9	42	> 20	3.4	1.1–10.6	
		24	119	18–20	3.1	1.2–8.4	
		27	91	15–17	4.6	1.8–12.2	
		21	48	< 15	7.0	2.6–18.4	

Table 2.1.4.29 (contd)

Reference Country and years of study	Cancer subsite ICD code	No. of cases	No. of controls	Smoking categories	Relative risk	95% CI	Comments
Merletti et al. (1989) (contd)		Women	Women	Tobacco/day (g)			Adjusted for age
		10	32	1–7	5.6	2.0–15.3	
		13	52	≥8	5.9	2.3–15.0	
				Duration (years)			
		9	60	1–30	5.5	1.8–16.8	
		8	15	31–40	6.1	2.1–18.1	
		6	9	>40	5.7	1.9–16.9	
				Age at starting smoking (years)			
		10	31	>20	4.7	1.8–12.4	
		13	53	≤20	6.7	2.4–18.4	
		Men	Men	Tobacco (g/day)			Multivariate logistic regression model; adjusted for age, educational level, area of birth, alcohol consumption and type of alcoholic beverage
				1–7	1.0	–	Trends not seen for women for any variable
				8–15	4.4	1.0–18.3	
				16–25	5.1	1.2–21.0	
				>25	6.2	1.4–28.3	
				Duration (years)			
				1–20	1.0	–	
				21–30	0.7	0.1–4.4	
				31–40	2.5	0.3–18.4	
				41–50	3.9	0.4–34.6	
				>50	34.0	2.6–436.4	
				Age at starting smoking (years)			
				<15	1.0	–	
				15–17	0.6	0.3–1.5	
				18–20	0.4	0.2–0.9	
				>20	0.4	0.1–1.1	

Table 2.1.4.29 (contd)

Reference Country and years of study	Cancer subsite ICD code	No. of cases	No. of controls	Smoking categories	Relative risk	95% CI	Comments
Talamini et al. (1990) Italy 1986–89	Oral cavity and pharynx (nasopharynx and salivary glands excluded)	3	34	Former smoker	4.1	0.5–93.6	Non-drinkers only; adjusted for age and sex
				Current smoker Cigarettes/day			
		2	12	< 15	3.8	0.2–58.2	
		10	22	≥ 15	12.9	2.3–106.3	p for trend < 0.001
Barra et al. (1991) Italy 1985–90	Oral cavity and pharynx			Cigarettes/day Cancer controls			Adjusted for age, sex, education, occupation and alcohol consumption
		58	134	≤ 14	5.2	2.9–9.2	
		73	119	15–24	5.8	3.2–10.5	
		49	48	≥ 25	9.6	4.9–18.9	p for trend < 0.01
				Non-cancer controls			
		58	254	≤ 14	5.8	3.3–10.1	
		73	268	15–24	6.1	3.5–10.9	
		49	87	≥ 25	12.2	6.4–23.2	p for trend < 0.01
				Duration (years) Cancer controls			
		57	237	< 30	2.7	1.5–4.9	
		78	123	30–39	7.0	3.9–12.6	
		107	186	≥ 40	7.4	4.0–13.6	p for trend < 0.01
				Non-cancer controls			
		57	537	< 30	2.7	1.5–4.7	
		78	258	30–39	6.9	3.9–12.1	
		107	288	≥ 40	8.8	4.9–15.6	p for trend < 0.01

Table 2.1.4.29 (contd)

Reference Country and years of study	Cancer subsite ICD code	No. of cases	No. of controls	Smoking categories	Relative risk	95% CI	Comments
Barra *et al.* (1991) (contd)				Age at starting smoking (years)			
				Cancer controls			
		26	121	≥ 25	2.8	1.4–5.4	
		122	298	17–24	4.7	2.7–8.1	
		101	155	≤ 16	6.8	3.8–12.2	*p* for trend < 0.01
				Non-cancer controls			
		26	192	≥ 25	3.3	1.7–6.2	
		122	583	17–24	4.9	2.9–8.4	
		101	331	≤ 16	6.6	3.8–11.5	*p* for trend < 0.01
La Vecchia *et al.* (1991) Italy 1987–89	Oral cavity and oropharynx (nasopharynx and salivary glands excluded)	11	244	Former smoker	4.3		Data stratified by sex and decade of age
				Cigarettes/day			
		61	372	≤ 25	11.0		
		23	123	> 25	17.9		
De Stefani *et al.* (1992) Uruguay 1988–90	Mouth and pharynx	87	122	Current smoker	1.0	–	Adjusted for age, county, area of residence, education, income and alcohol consumption; light smokers used as reference group
		19	112	Former smoker	0.3	0.1–0.6	
				Cigarettes/day			
		16	74	1–10	1.0	–	
		41	74	11–20	2.0	0.9–4.4	
		26	34	21–30	3.1	1.3–7.6	
		23	52	≥ 31	1.9	0.8–4.5	
				Duration (years)			
		7	58	1–29	1.0	–	
		20	58	30–39	2.3	0.8–6.4	
		40	47	40–49	4.8	1.7–13.4	
		39	71	≥ 50	4.3	1.5–12.3	

Table 2.1.4.29 (contd)

Reference Country and years of study	Cancer subsite ICD code	No. of cases	No. of controls	Smoking categories	Relative risk	95% CI	Comments
Franceschi et al. (1992) Italy 1986–90	Mouth ICD-9:	18 78	260 306	Former smoker Current smoker	3.6 11.8	1.0–12.6 3.6–38.4	Adjusted for age, area of residence, occupation and alcohol use
	143 gum 144 floor of mouth 145 other parts of mouth	18 51 26	206 229 125	Cigarettes/day ≤ 14 15–24 ≥ 25	4.5 11.0 9.6	1.3–15.8 3.3–36.4 2.8–33.1	p for trend ≤ 0.01
	149 other parts within lip, oral cavity and pharynx	17 36 41	229 157 174	Duration (years) ≤ 29 30–39 ≥ 40	3.5 11.0 14.3	1.0–12.3 3.2–36.3 4.1–49.6	p for trend ≤ 0.01
		40 59	280 282	Age at starting smoking (years) ≥ 20 ≤ 19	6.5 11.0	2.0–21.8 3.3–36.4	p for trend ≤ 0.01
Marshall et al. (1992) USA 1975–83	Oral cavity: tongue, oropharynx, floor of mouth, pharynx, hypopharynx	290	290	Pack–years 1–20 21–30 31–40 41–50 51–70 ≥ 71	1.3 2.7 2.9 7.0 7.7 5.7	0.7–2.4 1.2–6.0 1.5–5.9 3.3–15.1 3.7–15.9 2.7–12.1	Matched pairs analysis p for trend < 0.0001

Table 2.1.4.29 (contd)

Reference Country and years of study	Cancer subsite ICD code	No. of cases	No. of controls	Smoking categories	Relative risk	95% CI	Comments
Zheng et al. (1992a) China 1988–90	Oral cavity and pharynx ICD-9: 141 tongue 143 gum 144 floor of mouth 145 other parts of mouth 146 oropharynx 148 hypopharynx 149 other parts within lip, oral cavity and pharynx	115	269	Pack–years < 25 ≥ 25	0.8 2.2	0.4–1.4 1.2–4.1	Analysis for men only p for trend ≤ 0.05
Day et al. (1993) USA 1984–85	Oral cavity and pharynx ICD-9: 141 tongue 143 gum 144 floor of mouth 145 other parts of mouth 146 oropharynx 148 hypopharynx 149 other sites within lip, oral cavity and pharynx	Whites 568 90 349 306 38 313 386 71 356 308	Whites 256 186 308 144 152 293 191 74 322 241	Current smoker Cigarettes/day 1–19 20–39 ≥ 40 Duration (years) 1–19 20–39 ≥ 40 Age at starting smoking (years) ≥ 25 17–24 < 17	3.6 1.2 2.2 2.8 0.6 1.9 3.3 2.2 1.9 2.0	2.6–4.8 0.8–1.7 1.6–2.9 2.0–4.0 0.4–1.0 1.3–2.5 2.3–4.6 1.4–3.5 1.4–2.6 1.4–2.7	Adjusted for age, sex, study location, alcohol consumption and respondent status

Table 2.1.4.29 (contd)

Reference Country and years of study	Cancer subsite ICD code	No. of cases	No. of controls	Smoking categories	Relative risk	95% CI	Comments
Day et al. (1993) (contd)		Blacks 147	Blacks 81	Current smoker	2.3	1.1–4.7	
				Cigarettes/day			
		39	62 *	1–19	1.2	0.5–2.6	
		93	57	20–39	2.1	1.0–4.4	
		36	14	≥40	2.8	1.0–7.7	
				Duration (years)			
		14	28	1–19	0.9	0.3–2.4	
		84	72	20–39	1.6	0.7–3.3	
		66	33	≥40	2.9	1.2–7.2	
				Age at starting smoking (years)			
		14	18	≥25	1.2	0.4–3.6	
		67	56	17–24	1.7	0.8–3.8	
		84	59	<17	1.8	0.8–3.9	
Kune et al. (1993) Germany 1982	Oral cavity and pharynx			Former smoker	3.9	0.5–34.0	Adjusted for age, alcohol consumption, vitamin C and fibre intake
				Current smoker	13.8	1.1–112.5	

Table 2.1.4.29 (contd)

Reference Country and years of study	Cancer subsite ICD code	No. of cases	No. of controls	Smoking categories	Relative risk	95% CI	Comments
Mashberg et al. (1993) USA 1972–83	Oral cavity and oropharynx	9	309	Minimal smoking	1.0	–	Adjusted for age, race and alcohol drinking; reference groups may have been inappropriate.
		9	307	Former smoker	0.8	0.3–2.2	
				Current smoker Cigarettes/day			Trends seen and commented upon, but not analysed
		41	269	6–15	4.0	1.9–8.5	
		109	538	16–25	4.4	2.2–8.9	
		61	216	26–35	5.6	2.7–11.7	
		94	381	≥36	4.0	1.9–8.2	Further adjusted for average cigarette consumption
				Duration (years)			
		23	438	Nonsmoker and 1–15	1.0	–	
		55	440	16–30	0.7	0.3–3.6	
		203	1017	31–45	1.5	0.4–5.3	
		78	385	≥46	1.9	0.5–7.1	
				Pack–years			
		25	419	Nonsmoker and 1–5	1.0	–	
		37	395	5–25	3.1	1.3–7.3	
		143	708	25–50	5.5	2.5–12.1	
		78	378	50–75	4.5	2.0–10.2	
		76	380	>75	4.0	1.8–9.0	
Negri et al. (1993) Italy 1984–92	Oral cavity and pharynx ICD-9: 141–149			Moderate/former smoker	3.6		Adjusted for alcohol consumption
				Heavy and/or pipe/cigar smoker	9.4		
Spitz et al. (1993) USA 1987–91	Upper aero-digestive tract			Cigarettes/day			Univariate analysis
				1–14	4.2	1.4–12.8	
				15–24	7.9	3.2–19.1	
				≥25	11.0	4.4–27.4	p for trend < 0.001
				≥25	4.8	2.3–10.0	Adjusted for alcohol, mutagen sensitivity and educational level

Table 2.1.4.29 (contd)

Reference Country and years of study	Cancer subsite ICD code	No. of cases	No. of controls	Smoking categories	Relative risk	95% CI	Comments
De Stefani et al. (1994) Uruguay 1988–92	Oral cavity and pharynx (lip, salivary glands and nasopharynx excluded)			Pack–years			Adjusted for age, area of residence and education
		36	82	1–26	1.5	0.6–3.9	
		62	55	27–45	3.3	1.3–8.3	
		70	44	46–70	4.2	1.6–10.9	
		71	38	≥71	4.5	1.7–11.6	
Kabat et al. (1994) USA 1977–90	Oral cavity and pharynx: tongue, floor of mouth, gums, gingiva, buccal mucosa, palate, retromolar area, tonsil, other pharynx (nasopharynx excluded)	Men	Men				Adjusted for age, years of schooling, alcohol consumption, race, time period and type of hospital
		246	811	Former smoker	1.1	0.8–1.5	
		676	667	Current smoker	3.3	2.4–4.3	
				Cigarettes/day			
		284	376	1–20	1.0	–	
		128	116	21–30	1.5	1.1–2.1	
		264	175	≥31	1.8	1.4–2.4	
				Duration (years)			Also adjusted for amount smoked and smoking status
		97	355	1–20	1.0	–	
		469	776	21–40	1.3	0.96–1.7	
		355	347	≥41	1.8	1.3–2.7	
		Women	Women				Adjusted for age, years of schooling, alcohol consumption, race, time period and type of hospital
		79	210	Former smoker	1.4	1.0–2.0	
		271	192	Current smoker	4.3	3.2–5.9	
				Cigarettes/day			
		143	132	1–20	1.0	–	
		54	28	21–30	1.7	0.9–2.9	
		74	32	≥31	1.9	1.1–3.2	
				Duration (years)			Also adjusted for amount smoked and smoking status
		35	108	1–20	1.0	–	
		201	216	21–40	1.5	0.9–2.4	
		114	79	≥41	1.8	0.97–3.4	

Table 2.1.4.29 (contd)

Reference Country and years of study	Cancer subsite ICD code	No. of cases	No. of controls	Smoking categories	Relative risk	95% CI	Comments
Muscat et al. (1996) USA 1981–90	Oral cavity and pharynx ICD-9: 141 tongue 143 gum 144 floor of mouth 145 other parts of mouth 146 oropharynx 148 hypopharynx 149 other sites within lip, oral cavity and pharynx	Men	Men	Cumulative tar (kg)			Adjusted for age, residence, urban/rural status, birthplace, education and total alcohol consumption
		61	99	< 1.4	1.0	0.6–1.6	
		99	119	1.4–3.5	0.9	0.6–1.6	
		174	122	3.5–6.8	1.6	1.0–2.5	
		283	141	> 6.8	2.1	1.4–3.2	p for trend < 0.01
				Pack–years			
		69	131	1–19	0.7	0.5–1.1	
		142	132	20–39	1.4	0.9–2.1	
		186	108	40–59	2.0	1.3–3.1	
		219	110	> 60	2.2	1.4–3.3	p for trend < 0.01
		Women	Women	Cumulative tar (kg)			
		47	55	< 1.4	1.8	1.1–3.0	
		60	34	1.4–3.5	2.8	1.6–4.9	
		85	33	3.5–6.8	3.2	1.9–5.6	
		53	15	> 6.8	4.6	2.5–8.7	p for trend < 0.01
				Pack–years			
		49	66	1–19	1.6	1.0–2.6	
		72	37	20–39	3.3	2.0–5.9	
		76	21	40–59	5.5	2.9–10.1	
		48	13	> 60	5.3	2.5–11.3	p for trend < 0.01
Sanderson et al. (1997) Netherlands 1980–90	Oral cavity and oropharynx			Cigarettes/day			Adjusted for age and alcohol
		57	350	1–19	1.3	0.9–2.0	
		79	241	> 19	2.2	1.5–3.3	

Table 2.1.4.29 (contd)

Reference Country and years of study	Cancer subsite ICD code	No. of cases	No. of controls	Smoking categories	Relative risk	95% CI	Comments
Lewin et al. (1998) Sweden 1988–91	Head and neck	116	234	Former smoker	1.9	1.3–2.8	Adjusted for age, region and alcohol
		501	448	Ever-smoker	4.0	2.8–5.7	
		385	214	Current smoker	6.5	4.4–9.5	
				Tobacco/day (g)			
		202	211	<15	3.4	2.3–5.1	
		230	189	15–24	4.4	2.9–6.5	
		69	48	≥25	4.8	2.9–8.1	
				Duration (years)			
		50	156	<30	1.2	0.7–1.9	
		168	148	30–44	3.9	2.6–5.9	
		283	144	≥45	7.2	4.8–10.8	
				Age at starting smoking (years)			
		33	49	≥25	2.6	1.5–4.6	
		101	102	20–24	3.8	2.4–5.9	
		257	220	15–19	4.0	2.7–5.9	
		110	77	<15	5.0	3.2–7.9	
				Total consumption (kg tobacco)			
		53	145	<125	1.5	1.0–2.4	
		181	146	126–250	4.3	2.9–6.5	
		267	157	>250	5.9	4.0–8.8	
Talamini et al. (1998) Italy and Switzerland 1992–97	Oral cavity and pharynx; naso-pharynx and salivary gland excluded	7	33	Former smoker	2.2	0.8–6.2	Analysis restricted to abstainers from alcohol; Adjusted for study centre, age, sex and education; p for trend = 0.07
				Current smoker Cigarettes/day			
		6	44	<25	1.5	0.5–4.6	
		3	5	≥25	7.2	1.1–46.6	
Rao et al. (1999) India 1980–84	Oropharynx ICD-9: 141.0, 145.3, 146.9	45	98	Cigarette smoker	1.3	0.8–2.2	Adjusted for age and area of residence; in the study area, cigarette smoking was not as common as bidi smoking.

Table 2.1.4.29 (contd)

Reference Country and years of study	Cancer subsite ICD code	No. of cases	No. of controls	Smoking categories	Relative risk	95% CI	Comments
Bosetti *et al.* (2000) Italy and Switzerland 1984–97	Oral cavity and pharynx	19	111	Former smoker Current smoker Cigarettes/day	1.6	0.9–2.9	Adjusted for education, body-mass index and alcohol consumption
		57	139	1–14	3.6	2.3–5.6	
		47	93	≥ 15	4.6	2.7–7.6	*p* for trend < 0.0001
				Duration (years)			
		29	138	< 28	1.6	1.0–2.7	
		75	88	≥ 28	5.1	3.3–7.7	*p* for trend < 0.0001
Dikshit & Kanhere (2000) India 1986–92	Oropharynx ICD-9: 141.0, 141.6, 145.3, 145.4, 146.0– 146.9, 147.0–147.9, 148.0–149.0			Cigarettes/day			Adjusted for age and bidi smoking
		15		1–10	1.5	0.5–4.4	
		18		11–20	5.7	2.2–15.0	
		9		> 20	11.4	2.7–48.8	
Moreno-Lopez *et al.* (2000) Spain	Oral cavity ICD-9: 140 lip 141 tongue 143 gum 144 floor of mouth 145 other parts of mouth 146 oropharynx			Cigarettes/day			Adjusted for alcohol consumption and daily tooth brushing
		22	38	1–20	3.1	1.4–6.7	
		23	13	≥ 20	8.3	3.4–20.4	*p* for trend < 0.05

Table 2.1.4.29 (contd)

Reference Country and years of study	Cancer subsite ICD code	No. of cases	No. of controls	Smoking categories	Relative risk	95% CI	Comments
Zavras et al. (2001) Greece 1995–98	Oral cavity ICD-9:	Men	Men	Former smoker	0.4	0.1–1.3	Adjusted for age, hospital and alcohol consumption; very few cases in women
	141 tongue	8	22	Current smoker	3.0	1.2–7.9	
	143 gum	56	46	Pack–years			
	144 floor of mouth	10	17	1–25	1.0	0.3–3.0	
	145 other parts of	14	14	> 25–50	1.4	0.5–4.3	
	mouth	32	15	> 50	2.8	1.0–8.0	p for trend = 0.03
	148 hypopharynx	Women	Women				
	149 other parts	8	3	Former smoker	6.2	1.2–31.4	
	within lip, oral	5	5	Current smoker	0.7	0.1–3.7	
	cavity and pharynx			Pack–years			
		7	5	1–25	1.9	0.5–7.8	
		5	2	26–50	4.1	0.6–26.9	
		1	1	> 50	0.9	0.0–24.6	p for trend = 0.30
				Men and women combined			Also adjusted for sex
		16	25	Former smoker	0.9	0.4–2.1	
		61	51	Current smoker	3.0	1.4–6.6	p for trend = 0.01
				Pack–years			
		17	22	1–25	1.3	0.6–3.0	
		19	16	26–50	1.7	0.7–4.3	
		33	16	> 50	3.3	1.3–8.5	

CI, confidence interval

Table 2.1.4.30. Case–control studies on tobacco smoking and cancers of the upper aerodigestive tract cancer: smoking cessation

Reference (country and years of study)	Cancer subsite ICD code	No. of cases	No. of controls	Years since quitting	Relative risk	95% CI	Comments
Blot et al. (1988) USA 1984–85	Oral cavity and pharynx ICD-9:	Men	Men				Adjusted for age, race, study location, alcohol consumption and respondent status
		485	239	Current smoker	3.4	2.3–5.1	
	141 tongue	64	98	1–9	1.1	0.7–1.9	
	143 gum	56	114	10–19	1.1	0.7–1.9	
	144 floor of mouth	43	141	≥ 20	0.7	0.4–1.2	
	145 other	Women	Women				
	146 oropharynx	258	129	Current smoker	4.7	3.0–7.3	
	148 hypopharynx	24	39	1–9	1.8	0.9–3.6	
	149 other sites within lip, oral cavity and pharynx	10	35	10–19	0.8	0.4–1.9	
		4	26	≥ 20	0.4	0.1–1.4	
Merletti et al. (1989) Italy 1982–84	Oral cavity and oropharynx ICD-9:	Men	Men	0–1	5.4	2.3–16.8	Adjusted for age
	140.3 upper lip	68	195	2–5	4.4	1.6–12.4	
	140.4 lower lip	11	42	> 5	0.4	0.1–2.7	
	141 tongue	2	63	Nonsmoker	1.0	–	
	143 gum	5	85				Adjusted for age
	144 floor of mouth	Women	Women	0–1	7.4	3.0–18.3	
	145 other parts of mouth	18	68	> 1	3.7	1.3–10.8	
	146 oropharynx	5	16	Nonsmoker	1.0	–	
		13	137	0–1	0.7	0.3–1.8	Multivariate logistic regression model adjusted for age, educational level, area of birth, alcohol consumption and type of alcoholic beverage
		Men		2–5	0.3	0.1–1.8	
				> 5	1.0	–	
		Women		0–1	1.0	–	
				> 1	1.5	0.3–8.9	

Table 2.1.4.30 (contd)

Reference (country and years of study)	Cancer subsite ICD code	No. of cases	No. of controls	Years since quitting	Relative risk	95% CI	Comments
Barra *et al.* (1991) Italy 1985–90	Oral cavity and pharynx			Cancer controls			Adjusted for age, sex, education, occupation and alcohol consumption
		43	120	< 10	3.9	2.0–7.8	*p* for trend < 0.01 with both groups of
		22	151	≥ 10	1.4	0.6–3.1	controls
		21	445	Nonsmoker	1.0	–	
				Non-cancer controls			
		43	239	< 10	3.9	2.0–7.8	
		22	261	≥ 10	1.6	0.8–3.5	
		21	769	Nonsmoker	1.0	–	
De Stefani *et al.* (1992) Uruguay 1988–90	Mouth and pharynx	84	121	Current smoker	1.0	–	Adjusted for age, county, residence, education, income and alcohol consumption
		10	25	1–4	0.6	0.2–1.4	
		7	11	5–9	1.1	0.4–3.3	
		5	77	≥ 10	0.1	0.0–0.3	
Franceschi *et al.* (1992) Italy 1986–90	Mouth ICD-9: 143 gum 144 floor of mouth 145 other parts of mouth 149 other parts within lip, oral cavity and pharynx	78	306	Current smoker	11.8	3.6–38.4	Adjusted for age, area of residence, occupation and alcohol use
		13	122	< 10	3.8	1.0–14.4	*p* for trend ≤ 0.01
		3	138	≥ 10	0.7	0.1–3.9	

Table 2.1.4.30 (contd)

Reference (country and years of study)	Cancer subsite ICD code	No. of cases	No. of controls	Years since quitting	Relative risk	95% CI	Comments
Day et al. (1993) USA 1984–85	Oral cavity and pharynx ICD-9: 141 tongue 143 gum 144 floor of mouth 145 other 146 oropharynx 148 hypopharynx 149 other sites within lip, oral cavity and pharynx	Whites 568 70 63 41 Blacks 147 13 1 3	Whites 256 107 128 147 Blacks 81 24 13 15	Current smoker 1–9 10–19 ≥ 20 Current smoker 1–9 10–19 ≥ 20	3.6 1.1 1.1 0.6 2.3 1.1 0.1 0.3	2.6–4.8 0.7–1.6 0.7–1.6 0.3–0.9 1.1–4.7 0.4–3.1 0.0–1.3 0.1–1.7	Adjusted for age, sex, study location, alcohol consumption and respondent status
Mashberg et al. (1993) USA 1972–83	Oral cavity and oropharynx	9 6 3	309 147 160	3–10 ≥ 11 Minimal smoking	1.3 0.5 1.0	0.3–6.5 0.1–2.6 –	
Kabat et al. (1994) USA 1977–90	Oral cavity and pharynx	Men 676 113 59 70 Women 271 40 24 15	Men 668 225 276 306 Women 193 69 82 59	Current smoker 1–9 10–19 ≥ 20 Current smoker 1–9 10–19 ≥ 20	1.0 0.6 0.3 0.5 1.0 0.5 0.3 0.3	– 0.4–0.8 0.2–0.5 0.3–0.9 – 0.3–0.8 0.2–0.5 0.1–0.8	Adjusted for age, years of schooling, alcohol consumption, race, time period, type of hospital, and intensity and duration of smoking
Lewin et al. (1998) Sweden 1988–90	Head and neck	385 61 32 23	214 75 76 83	Current smoker 1–10 11–20 ≥ 21	6.5 3.2 1.7 0.9	4.4–9.5 2.0–5.2 1.0–2.9 0.5–1.7	Adjusted for age, region and alcohol

CI, confidence interval

Table 2.1.4.31. Case–control studies on tobacco smoking and cancers of the upper aerodigestive tract: type of tobacco and/or cigarette

Reference (country and years of study)	Cancer subsite ICD code	No. of cases	No. of controls	Smoking categories	Relative risk	95% CI	Comments
Merletti et al. (1989) Italy 1982–84	Oral cavity and oropharynx ICD-9: 140.3 upper lip 140.4 lower lip 141 tongue 143 gum 144 floor of mouth 145 other parts of mouth 146 oropharynx	Men 13 7 48 20 13 35 Women 12 4 7 15 3 5 Men	Men 84 37 142 97 42 124 Women 63 9 12 69 6 9 Men	Type of tobacco > 66% blond Mixed > 66% black Use of filter > 66% with filter Mixed > 66% without filter Type of tobacco > 66% blond Mixed > 66% black Use of filter > 66% with filter Mixed > 66% without filter Type of tobacco > 66% blond Mixed > 66% black Use of filter > 66% with filter Mixed > 66% without filter	2.4 2.9 4.8 3.2 4.7 4.2 6.0 4.7 6.9 6.3 5.4 5.2 1.0 0.7 1.0 1.0 1.2 1.2	0.8–7.2 0.9–10.1 1.9–12.1 1.2–9.0 1.5–14.9 1.6–11.0 2.2–16.1 1.3–16.3 2.5–19.1 2.4–16.6 1.3–22.2 1.8–15.1 – 0.2–2.7 0.4–2.6 – 0.4–3.5 0.5–2.8	Adjusted for age Multivariate analysis adjusted for age, education, area of birth, alcohol consumption and type of alcoholic beverage

Table 2.1.4.31 (contd)

Reference (country and years of study)	Cancer subsite ICD code	No. of cases	No. of controls	Smoking categories	Relative risk	95% CI	Comments
De Stefani et al. (1992) Uruguay 1988–90	Mouth and pharynx			Type of cigarette			Adjusted for age, county, residence, education, income and alcohol consumption
		16	72	Manufactured	1.0	–	
		90	162	Hand-rolled	2.5	1.2–5.2	
Franceschi et al. (1992) Italy 1986–90	Mouth ICD-9: 143 gum 144 floor of mouth 145 other parts of mouth 149 other parts within lip, oral cavity and pharynx			Tar yield			Adjusted for age, area of residence, occupation and alcohol use p for trend ≤ 0.01
		53	364	Low tar (< 22 mg)	7.1	2.2–23.3	
		42	185	High tar (≥ 22 mg)	14.4	4.2–49.5	
Mashberg et al. (1993) USA 1972–83	Oral cavity and oropharynx			Untipped cigarettes (cigarettes/day)			Adjusted for age, race and alcohol drinking
				6–15	7.8	2.4–19.0	
				16–25	7.7	3.6–16.5	
				26–35	12.3	5.3–28.6	
				≥ 36	7.6	3.5–16.8	
				Filter-tipped cigarettes (cigarettes/day)			
				6–15	1.5	0.5–4.2	
				16–25	3.6	1.6–7.7	
				26–35	1.9	0.7–5.0	
				≥ 36	2.3	1.0–5.2	

Table 2.1.4.31 (contd)

Reference (country and years of study)	Cancer subsite ICD code	No. of cases	No. of controls	Smoking categories	Relative risk	95% CI	Comments
Kabat et al. (1994) USA 1977–90	Oral cavity and pharynx	Men	Men				Adjusted for age, years of schooling, alcohol consumption, race, time period and hospital
		221	126	Non-filter only	1.0	–	
		96	105	Filter for 1–9 years	0.5	0.4–0.8	
		280	334	Filter for ≥ 10 years	0.5	0.4–0.7	
		57	80	Filter only	0.6	0.4–0.9	
		Women	Women				
		46	17	Non-filter only	1.0	–	
		38	20	Filter for 1–9 years	0.8	0.3–1.8	
		125	89	Filter for ≥ 10 years	0.5	0.2–1.0	
		57	63	Filter only	0.6	0.3–1.2	

CI, confidence interval

Table 2.1.4.32. Case-series on tobacco smoking and cancers of the upper aerodigestive tract

Reference Country and years of study	Cancer subsites	%	No. of cases	Age	Histological types	Exposures		Comments
al-Idrissi (1990) Saudi Arabia 1982–89	Nasopharynx	43	42 men	Mean age, 48.6 ± 14.9 years	100% squamous-cell carcinoma; all others excluded	No tobacco habit	% 32.3	Cases histologically confirmed
	Tongue	17	23 women			Tobacco smoking	41.5	Al-Shamma (mixture
	Oral cavity	15				Al-Shamma	26.2	of tobacco, pepper
	Larynx	14						and oil) is frequently
	Pharynx	6						chewed instead of
	Oropharynx	5						smoking tobacco.

Table 2.1.4.33. Case–control studies on tobacco smoking and second primary tumours in patients with a primary cancer of the upper aerodigestive tract

Reference Country, cohort collection period and follow-up period	Initial population study	Cases (second primary tumours)	Controls (no second primary tumours)	Exposure categories	Relative risk	95% CI	Factors adjusted for; comments

Day et al. (1994) USA 1984–85 follow-up until 1989	1090 patients with cancer of the oral cavity or pharynx (ICD-9: 141, 143–146, 148–149); follow-up of at least 6 months	80 meta-chronous cases in the oral cavity, pharynx, larynx, oesophagus and lung (56 men and 24 women)	189 controls (132 men and 57 women) matched by sex and study area	Ever-smoker
				Current smoker
				Cigarettes/day†
				  0–20
				  20–39
				  ≥40
				Duration (years)†
				  0–20
				  20–39
				  ≥40
					3.8
					4.3
					
					1.0
					1.8
					3.6
					
					1.0
					3.2
					4.7
						0.6–5.2
						1.6–12
						
						–
						0.5–6.2
						0.9–14.0
						
						–
						0.9–12
						1.3–17
							Matched analysis; model adjusted for age at index cancer diagnosis and index tumour stage; odds ratios adjusted for age, stage of disease and alcohol intake; adjustment for race, education, marital status, occupation, location or radiation therapy had no effect. †ever-smokers

Barbone et al. (1996) Italy 1984–91 follow-up until 1994	380 patients with incident first cancer of the oral cavity, larynx or pharynx; median follow-up, 40 months	62 multiple second primary tumours, of which 39 were meta-chronous cases in the oral cavity, pharynx, larynx, oesophagus and nasal cavities (34 men and 5 women)	Not available	Never or very light smoker Light Intermediate Heavy	1.0 2.3 2.7 4.3	– 0.4–12.2 0.5–13.4 0.7–26.9	Hazard ratios adjusted for age, sex, area of residence, occupation, smoking habits, alcohol intake, β-carotene intake, index tumour grade and stage p for trend = 0.08
Cianfriglia et al. (1999) Italy 1989–92 follow-up until 1997	200 patients with first incident cancer of the oral cavity and oro-pharynx (ICD-10: C01–C06; C09) and curative-intended treatment; median follow-up, 3.2 years	28 cases: 24 second, 3 third and 1 fourth primary tumour (22 men and 6 women)	Population covered by southern and central Italian cancer registries	Site of second tumour: Oropharynx Oral cavity Lip Larynx Lung	SIR† 250.0 137.5 22.2 8.0 2.5	 208.7–291.2 103.7–171.3 17.7–29.8 6.9–9.4 2.2–2.8	†Standardized incidence ratios Heavy smokers accounted for higher incidence rates of second primary tumours, but the results were not adjusted for alcohol consumption. Information on multiple synchronous tumours available

CI, confidence interval

References

Ahrens, W., Jockel, K.-H., Patzak, W. & Elsner, G. (1991) Alcohol, smoking, and occupational factors in cancer of the larynx: A case–control study. *Am. J. ind. Med.*, **20**, 477–493

Akiba, S. (1994) Analysis of cancer risk related to longitudinal information on smoking habits. *Environ. Health Perspect.*, **102** (Suppl 8), 15–20

Akiba, S. & Hirayama, T. (1990) Cigarette smoking and cancer mortality risk in Japanese men and women — Results from reanalysis of the six-prefecture cohort study data. *Environ. Health Perspect.*, **87**, 19–26

al-Idrissi, H.Y. (1990) Head and neck cancer in Saudi Arabia: Retrospective analysis of 65 patients. *J. int. med. Res.*, **18**, 515–519

Amstrong, R.W., Imrey, P.B., Lye, M.S., Armstrong, M.J., Yu, M.C. & Sani, S. (2000) Nasopharyngeal carcinoma in Malaysian Chinese: Occupational exposures to particles, formaldehyde and heat. *Int. J. Epidemiol.*, **29**, 991–998

Barbone, F., Franceschi, S., Talamini, R., Barzan, L., Franchin, G., Favero, A. & Carbone, A. (1996) A follow-up study of determinants of second tumor and metastasis among subjects with cancer of the oral cavity, pharynx and larynx. *J. clin. Epidemiol.*, **59**, 367–372

Barra, S., Baron, A.E., Franceschi, S., Talamini, R. & La Vecchia, C. (1991) Cancer and non-cancer controls in studies on the effect of tobacco and alcohol consumption. *Int. J. Epidemiol.*, **20**, 845–851

Blot, W.J., McLaughlin, J.K., Winn, D.M., Austin, D.F., Greenberg, R.S., Preston-Martin, S., Bernstein, L., Schoenberg, J.B., Stemhagen, A. & Fraumeni, J.F., Jr (1988) Smoking and drinking in relation to oral and pharyngeal cancer. *Cancer Res.*, **48**, 3282–3287

Blot, W.J., Devesa, S.S., Kneller, R.W. & Fraumeni, J.F., Jr (1991) Rising incidence of adenocarcinoma of the esophagus and gastric cardia. *J. Am. med. Assoc.*, 265, 1287–1289

Bosetti, C., Negri, E., Franceschi, S., Conti, E., Levi, F., Tomei, F. & La Vecchia, C. (2000) Risk factors for oral and pharyngeal cancer in women: A study from Italy and Switzerland. *Br. J. Cancer*, **82**, 204–207

Brinton, L.A., Blot, W.J., Becker, J.A., Winn, D.M., Browder, J.P., Farmer, J.C., Jr & Fraumeni, J.F., Jr (1984) A case–control study of cancers of the nasal cavity and paranasal sinuses. *Am. J. Epidemiol.*, **119**, 896–906

Brown, L.M., Blot, W.J., Schuman, S.H., Smith, V.M., Ershow, A.G., Marks, R.D. & Fraumeni, J.F., Jr (1988) Environmental factors and high risk of esophageal cancer among men in coastal South Carolina. *J. natl Cancer Inst.*, **80**, 1620–1625

Brown, L.M., Hoover, R.N., Greenberg, R.S., Schoenberg, J.B., Schwartz, A.G., Swanson, G.M., Liff, J.M., Silverman, D.T., Hayes, R.B. & Pottern, L.M. (1994a) Are racial differences in squamous cell esophageal cancer explained by alcohol and tobacco use? *J. natl Cancer Inst.*, **86**, 1340–1345

Brown, L.M., Silverman, D.T., Pottern, L.M., Schoenberg, J.B., Greenberg, R.S., Swanson, G.M., Liff, J.M., Schwartz, A.G., Hayes, R.B., Blot, W.J. & Hoover, R.N. (1994b) Adenocarcinoma of the esophagus and esophagogastric junction in white men in the United States: Alcohol, tobacco, and socioeconomic factors. *Cancer Causes Control*, **5**, 333–340

Brownson, R.C. (1987) Exposure to alcohol and tobacco and the risk of laryngeal cancer. *Arch. environ. Health*, **42**, 192–196

Brugere, J., Guenel, P., Leclerc, A. & Rodriguez, J. (1986) Differential effects of tobacco and alcohol in cancer of the larynx, pharynx, and mouth. *Cancer*, **57**, 391–395

Bundgaard, T., Wildt, J., Frydenberg, M., Elbrond, O. & Nielsen, J.E. (1995) Case–control study of squamous cell cancer of the oral cavity in Denmark. *Cancer Causes Control*, **6**, 57–67

Burch, J.D., Howe, G.R., Miller, A.B. & Semenciw, R. (1981) Tobacco, alcohol, asbestos, and nickel in the etiology of cancer of the larynx: A case-control study. *J. natl Cancer Inst.*, **67**, 1219–1224

Cao, S.M., Liu, Q., Huang, Q.H., Yang, C.W. & Huang, T.B. (2000) [Analysis for risk factors of nasopharyngeal carcinoma in Sihui city.] *Cancer*, **19**, 987–989 (in Chinese)

Caplan, L.S., Hall, H.I., Levine, R.S. & Zhu, K. (2000) Preventable risk factors for nasal cancer. *Ann. Epidemiol.*, **10**, 186–191

Castellsagué, X. & Muñoz, N. (1999) Re: Cancer of the oral cavity and pharynx in nonsmokers who drink alcohol and in nondrinkers who smoke tobacco. *J. natl Cancer Inst.*, **91**, 1336–1337

Castellsagué, X., Muñoz, N, de Stefani, E., Victora, C.G., Castelletto, R., Rolón, P.A. & Quintana, M.J. (1999) Independent and joint effects of tobacco smoking and alcohol drinking on the risk of esophageal cancer in men and women. *Int. J. Cancer*, **82**, 657–664

Chen, K.L., Yin, H.Y., Yi, D.D., Lan, Y.J., Wu, B.Z., Wang, Z.S., Ju, X.G., Fan, Z.J. & Wu, D.X. (1995) [Association of esophageal cancer risk in non-endemic area with smoking, alcohol drinking and dietary habit.] *China Cancer*, **4**, 7–9 (in Chinese)

Chen, Z.M., Xu, Z., Collins, R., Li, W.X. & Peto, R. (1997) Early health effects of the emerging tobacco epidemic in China. A 16-year prospective study. *J. Am. med. Assoc.*, **278**, 1500–1504

Cheng, K.K., Day, N.E., Duffy, S.W., Lam, T.H., Fok, M. & Wong J. (1992) Pickled vegetables in the aetiology of oesophageal cancer in Hong Kong Chinese. *Lancet*, **339**, 1314–1318

Cheng, K.K., Duffy, S.W., Day, N.E. & Lam, T.H. (1995) Oesophageal cancer in never-smokers and never-drinkers. *Int. J. Cancer*, **60**, 820–822

Cheng, Y.J., Hildesheim, A., Hsu, M.M., Chen, I.H., Brinton, L.A., Levine, P.H., Chen, C.J. & Yang, C.S. (1999) Cigarette smoking, alcohol consumption and risk of nasopharyngeal carcinoma in Taiwan. *Cancer Causes Control*, **10**, 201–207

Choi, S.Y. & Kahyo, H. (1991) Effect of cigarette smoking and alcohol consumption in the aetiology of cancer of the oral cavity, pharynx and larynx. *Int. J. Epidemiol.*, **20**, 878-885.

Chow, W.H., McLaughlin, J.K., Hrubec, Z., Nam, J.-M. & Blot, W.J. (1993) Tobacco use and nasopharyngeal carcinoma in a cohort of US veterans. *Int. J. Cancer*, **55**, 538–540

Chyou, P.H., Nomura, A.M. & Stemmermann, G.N. (1995) Diet, alcohol, smoking and cancer of the upper aerodigestive tract: A prospective study among Hawaii Japanese men. *Int. J. Cancer*, **60**, 616–621

Cianfriglia, F., Di Gregorio, D.A. & Manieri, A. (1999) Multiple primary tumours in patients with oral squamous cell carcinoma. *Oral Oncol.*, **35**, 157–163

Day, G.L., Blot, W.J., Austin, D.F., Bernstein, L., Greenberg, R.S., Preston-Martin, S., Schoenberg, J.B., Winn, D.M., McLaughlin, J.K. & Fraumeni, J.F., Jr (1993) Racial differences in risk of oral and pharyngeal cancer: Alcohol, tobacco, and other determinants. *J. natl Cancer Inst.*, **85**, 465–473

Day, G.L., Blot, W.J., Shore, R.E., McLaughlin, J.K., Austin, D.F., Greenberg, R.S., Liff, J.M., Preston-Martin, S., Sarkar, S. & Schoenberg, J.B. (1994) Second cancers following oral and pharyngeal cancers: Role of tobacco and alcohol. *J. natl Cancer Inst.*, **86**, 131–137

De Stefani, E., Correa, P., Oreggia, F., Leiva, J., Rivero, S., Fernandez, G., Deneo-Pellegrini, H., Zavala, D. & Fontham, E. (1987) Risk factors for laryngeal cancer. *Cancer*, **60**, 3087–3091

De Stefani, E., Muñoz, N., Estève, J., Vasallo, A. & Victora, C.G. & Teuchmann, S. (1990) Mate drinking, alcohol, tobacco, diet, and esophageal cancer in Uruguay. *Cancer Res.*, **50**, 426–431

De Stefani, E., Oreggia, F., Rivero, S. & Fierro, L. (1992) Hand-rolled cigarette smoking and risk of cancer of the mouth, pharynx, and larynx. *Cancer*, **70**, 679–682

De Stefani, E., Oreggia, F., Ronco, A., Fierro, L. & Rivero, S. (1994) Salted meat consumption as a risk factor for cancer of the oral cavity and pharynx: A case–control study from Uruguay. *Cancer Epidemiol. Biomark. Prev.*, **3**, 381–385

De Stefani, E., Boffetta, P., Oreggia, F., Mendilaharsu, M. & Deneo-Pellegrini, H. (1998) Smoking patterns and cancer of the oral cavity and pharynx: A case–control study in Uruguay. *Oral Oncol.*, **34**, 340–346

Dikshit, R.P. & Kanhere, S. (2000) Tobacco habits and risk of lung, oropharyngeal and oral cavity cancer: A population-based case–control study in Bhopal, India. *Int. J. Epidemiol.*, **29**, 609–614

Doll, R., Gray, R., Hafner, B. & Peto, R. (1980) Mortality in relation to smoking: 22 years' observations on female British doctors. *Br. med. J.*, **280**, 967–971

Doll, R., Peto, R., Wheatley, K., Gray, R. & Sutherland, I. (1994) Mortality in relation to smoking: 40 years' observations on male British doctors. *Br. med. J.*, **309**, 901–911

Dosemeci, M., Gokmen, I., Unsal, M., Hayes, R.B. & Blair, A. (1997) Tobacco, alcohol use, and risks of laryngeal and lung cancer by subsite and histologic type in Turkey. *Cancer Causes Control*, **8**, 729–737

Elwood, J.M., Pearson, J.C.G., Skippen, D.H. & Jackson, S.M. (1984) Alcohol, smoking, social and occupational factors in the aetiology of cancer of the oral cavity, pharynx and larynx. *Int. J. Cancer*, **34**, 603–612

Engeland, A., Andersen, A., Haldorsen, T. & Tretli, S. (1996) Smoking habits and risk of cancers other than lung cancer: 28 years' follow-up of 26,000 Norwegian men and women. *Cancer Causes Control*, **7**, 497–506

Falk, R.T., Pickle, L.W., Brown, L.M., Mason, T.J., Buffler, P.A. & Fraumeni, J.F., Jr (1989) Effect of smoking and alcohol consumption on laryngeal cancer risk in coastal Texas. *Cancer Res.*, **49**, 4024–4029

Ferraroni, M., Negri, E., La Vecchia, C., D'Avanzo, B. & Franceschi, S. (1989) Socioeconomic indicators, tobacco and alcohol in the aetiology of digestive tract neoplasms. *Int. J. Epidemiol.*, **18**, 556–562

Franceschi, S., Talamini, R., Barra, S., Barón, A.E., Negri, E., Bidoli, E., Serraino, D. & La Vecchia, C. (1990) Smoking and drinking in relation to cancers of the oral cavity, pharynx, larynx, and esophagus in northern Italy. *Cancer Res.*, **50**, 6502–6507

Franceschi, S., Barra, S., La Vecchia, C., Bidoli, E., Negri, E. & Talamini, R. (1992) Risk factors for cancer of the tongue and the mouth. A case–control study from northern Italy. *Cancer*, **70**, 2227–2233

Franceschi, S., Levi, F., La Vecchia, C., Conti, E., Dal Maso, L., Barzan, L. & Talamini, R. (1999) Comparison of the effect of smoking and alcohol drinking between oral and pharyngeal cancer. *Int. J. Cancer*, **83**, 1–4

Freudenheim, J.L., Graham, S., Byers, T.E., Marshall, J.R., Haughey, B.P., Swanson, M.K. & Wilkinson, G. (1992) Diet, smoking, and alcohol in cancer of the larynx: A case–control study. *Nutr. Cancer*, **17**, 33–45

Fukuda, K. & Shibata, A. (1990) Exposure–response relationships between woodworking, smoking or passive smoking, and squamous cell neoplasms of the maxillary sinus. *Cancer Causes Control*, **1**, 165–168

Gammon, M.D., Schoenberg, J.B., Ahsan, H., Risch, H.A., Vaughan, T.L., Chow, W.H., Rotterdam, H., West, A.B., Dubrow, R., Stanford, J.L., Mayne, S.T., Farrow, D.C., Niwa, S., Blot, W.J. & Fraumeni, J.F., Jr (1997) Tobacco, alcohol, and socioeconomic status and adenocarcinomas of the esophagus and gastric cardia. *J. natl Cancer Inst.*, **89**, 1277–1284

Gao, Y.T., McLaughlin, J.K., Blot, W.J., Ji, B.T., Benichou, J., Dai, Q. & Fraumeni, J.F., Jr (1994) Risk factors for esophageal cancer in Shanghai, China. I. Role of cigarette smoking and alcohol drinking. *Int. J. Cancer*, **58**, 192–196

Graham, S., Mettlin, C., Marshall, J., Priore, R., Rzepka, T. & Shedd, D. (1981) Dietary factors in the epidemiology of cancer of the larynx. *Am. J. Epidemiol.*, **113**, 675–680

Guo, W., Blot, W.J., Li, J.-Y., Taylor, P.R., Liu, B.Q., Wang, W., Wu, Y.P., Zheng, W., Dawsey, S.M., Li, B. & Fraumeni, J.F., Jr (1994) A nested cse–control study of oesophageal and stomach cancers in the Linxian nutrition intervention study. *Int. J. Epidemiol.*, **23**, 444–450

Hammond, E.C. & Horn, D. (1958) Smoking and death rates — Report on forty-four months of follow-up of 187 783 men. II. Death rates by cause. *J. Am. med. Assoc.*, **166**, 1294–1308

Hammond, E.C. & Seidman, H. (1980) Smoking and cancer in the United States. *Prev. Med.*, **9**, 169–173

Hanaoka, T., Tsugane, S., Ando, N., Ishida, K., Kakegawa, T., Isono, K., Takiyama, W., Takagi, I., Ide, H., Watanabe, H. & Iizuka, T. (1994) Alcohol consumption and risk of esophageal cancer in Japan: A case–control study in seven hospitals. *Jpn. J. clin. Oncol.*, **24**, 241–246

Hayes, R.B., Kardaun, J.W.P.F. & de Bruyn, A. (1987) Tobacco use and sinonasal cancer: A case–control study. *Br. J. Cancer*, **56**, 843–846

Hayes, R.B., Bravo-Otero, E., Kleinman, D.V., Brown, L.M., Fraumeni, J.F., Harty, L.C. & Winn, D.M. (1999) Tobacco and alcohol use and oral cancer in Puerto Rico. *Cancer Causes Control*, **10**, 27–33

Hedberg, K., Vaughan, T.L., White, E., Davis, S. & Thomas, D.B. (1994) Alcoholism and cancer of the larynx: A case–control study in western Washington (United States). *Cancer Causes Control*, **5**, 3–8

Henderson, B.E., Louie, E., Jing, J.S.H., Buell, P. & Gardner, M.B. (1976) Risk factors associated with nasopharyngeal carcinoma. *New Engl. J. Med.*, **295**, 1101–1106

Herity, B., Moriarty, M., Daly, L., Dunn, J. & Bourke, G.J. (1982) The role of tobacco and alcohol in the aetiology of lung and larynx cancer. *Br. J. Cancer*, **46**, 961–964

Hirayama, T. (1985) A cohort study on cancer in Japan. In: Blot, W.J., Hirayama, T. & Hoel, D.G., eds, *Statistical Methods in Cancer Epidemiology*, Hiroshima, Radiation Effects Research Foundation, pp. 73–91

Hu, J., Nyrén, O., Wolk, A., Bergström, R., Yuen, J., Adami, H.O., Guo, L., Li, H., Huang, G., Xu, X., Zhao, F., Chen, Y., Wang, C., Qin, H., Hu, C. & Li, Y. (1994) Risk factors for oesophageal cancer in northeast China. *Int. J. Cancer*, **57**, 38–46

Hung, H.C., Chuang, J., Chien, Y.C., Chern, H.D., Chiang, C.P., Kuo, Y.S., Hildesheim, A. & Chen, C.J. (1997) Genetic polymorphisms of CYP2E1, GSTM1 and GSTT1; environmental factors and risk of oral cancer. *Cancer Epidemiol. Biomarkers Prev.*, **6**, 901–905

IARC (1986) *IARC Monographs on the Evaluation of the Carcinogenic Risk of Chemicals to Humans*, Vol. 38, *Tobacco Smoking*, Lyon, IARCPress

IARC (1992) *IARC Monographs on the Evaluation of Carcinogenic Risks to Humans*, Vol. 54, *Occupational Exposures to Mists and Vapours from Strong Inorganic Acids; and Other Industrial Chemicals*, Lyon, IARCPress

IARC (1997) *IARC Monographs on the Evaluation of Carcinogenic Risks to Humans*, Vol. 70, *Epstein-Barr Virus and Kaposi's Sarcoma Herpesvirus/Human Herpesvirus 8*, Lyon, IARC Press, pp. 47–373

Jussawalla, D.J. & Deshpande, V.A. (1971) Evaluation of cancer risk in tobacco chewers and smokers: An epidemiologic assessment. *Cancer*, **28**, 244–252

Kabat, G.C., Ng, S.K.C. & Wynder, E.L. (1993) Tobacco, alcohol intake, and diet in relation to adenocarcinoma of the esophagus and gastric cardia. *Cancer Causes Prev.*, **4**, 123–132

Kabat, G.C., Chang, C.J. & Wynder, E.L. (1994) The role of tobacco, alcohol use, and body mass index in oral and pharyngeal cancer. *Int. J. Epidemiol.*, **23**, 1137–1144

Kinjo, Y., Cui, Y., Akiba, S., Watanabe, S., Yamaguchi, N., Sobue, T., Mizuno, S. & Beral, V. (1998) Mortality risks of oesophageal cancer associated with hot tea, alcohol, tobacco and diet in Japan. *J. Epidemiol.*, **8**, 235–243

Kjaerheim, K., Gaard, M. & Andersen, A. (1998) The role of alcohol, tobacco, and dietary factors in upper aerogastric tract cancers: A prospective study of 10 900 Norwegian men. *Cancer Causes Control*, **9**, 99–108

Ko, Y.C., Huang, Y.L., Lee, C.H., Chen, M.J., Lin, L.M. & Tsai, C.C. (1995) Betel quid chewing, cigarette smoking and alcohol consumption related to oral cancer in Taiwan. *J. oral Pathol. Med.*, **24**, 450–453

Kono, S., Ikeda, M., Tokudome, S., Nishizumi, M. & Kuratsune, M. (1987) Cigarette smoking, alcohol and cancer mortality: A cohort study of male Japanese physicians. *Jpn. J. Cancer Res.*, **78**, 1323–1328

Kuller, L.H., Ockene, J.K., Meilahn, E., Wentworth, D.N., Svendsen, K.H. & Neaton, J.D. (1991) Cigarette smoking and mortality. MRFIT Research Group. *Prev. Med.*, **20**, 638–654

Kune, G.A., Kune, S., Field, B., Watson, L.F., Cleland, H., Merenstein, D. & Vitetta, L. (1993) Oral and pharyngeal cancer, diet, smoking, alcohol, and serum vitamin A and β carotene levels: A case–control study in men. *Nutr. Cancer*, **20**, 61–70

Lagergren, J., Bergström, R., Lindgren, A. & Nyrén, O. (2000) The role of tobacco, snuff and alcohol use in the aetiology of cancer of the oesophagus and gastric cardia. *Int. J. Cancer*, **85**, 340–346

Lam, T.H., He, Y., Li, L.S., Li, L.S., He, S.F. & Liang, B.Q. (1997) Mortality attributable to cigarette smoking in China. *J. Am. med. Assoc.*, **278**, 1505–1508

Lanier, A., Bender, T., Talbot, M., Wilmeth, S., Tschopp, C., Henle, W., Henle, G., Ritter, D. & Terasaki, P. (1980) Nasopharyngeal carcinoma in Alaskan Eskimos, Indians, and Aleuts: A review of cases and study of Epstein-Barr virus, HLA, and environmental risk factors. *Cancer*, **46**, 2100–2106

Launoy, G., Milan, C.H., Faivre, J., Pienkowski, P., Milan, C.I. & Gignoux, M. (1997) Alcohol, tobacco and oesophageal cancer: Effects of the duration of consumption, mean intake and current and former consumption. *Br. J. Cancer*, **75**, 1389–1396

La Vecchia, C., Negri, E., D'Avanzo, B., Boyle, P. & Franceschi, S. (1991) Dietary indicators of oral and pharyngeal cancer. *Int. J. Epidemiol.*, **20**, 39–44

La Vecchia, C., Franceschi, S., Bosetti, C., Levi, F., Talamini, R. & Negri, E. (1999a) Time since stopping smoking and the risk of oral and pharyngeal cancers (Correspondence). *J. nat. Cancer Inst.*, **91**, 726–728

La Vecchia, C., Talamini, R., Bosetti, C., Negri, E. & Franceschi, S. (1999b) Response. *J. natl Cancer Inst.*, **91**, 1337–1338

Levi, F., Ollyo, J.B., La Vecchia, C., Boyle, P., Monnier, P. & Savary, M. (1990) The consumption of tobacco, alcohol and the risk of adenocarcinoma in Barrett's oesophagus. *Int. J. Cancer*, **45**, 852–854

Lewin, F., Norell, S.E., Johansson, H., Gustavsson, P., Wennerberg, J., Biörklund, A. & Rutqvist, L.E. (1998) Smoking tobacco, oral snuff, and alcohol in the etiology of squamous cell carcinoma of the head and neck. A population-based case–referent study in Sweden. *Cancer*, **82**, 1367–1375

Li, J.Y., Ershow, A.G., Chen, Z.J., Wacholder, S., Li, G.Y., Guo, W., Li, B. & Blot, W.J. (1989) A case–control study of cancer of the esophagus and gastric cardia in Linxian. *Int. J. Cancer*, **43**, 755–761

Liaw, K.M. & Chen, C.J. (1998) Mortality attributable to cigarette smoking in Taiwan: A 12-year follow-up study. *Tob. Control*, **7**, 141–148

Lin, T.M., Chen, K.P., Lin, C.C., Hsu, M.M., Tu, S.M., Chiang, T.C., Jung, P.F. & Hirayama, T. (1973) Retrospective study on nasopharyngeal carcinoma. *J. natl Cancer Inst.*, **51**, 1403–1408

López-Abente, G., Pollan, M., Monge, V. & Martinez-Vidal, A. (1992) Tobacco smoking, alcohol consumption, and laryngeal cancer in Madrid. *Cancer Detect. Prev.*, **16**, 265–271

Lu, J.B., Lian, S.Y., Sun, X.B., Zhang, Z.X., Dai, D.X., Li, B.X., Chen, L.P., Wei, J.R. & Duan, W.J. (2000) [A case–control study on the risk factors of esophageal cancer in Linzhou.] *Chin. J. Epidemiol.*, **21**, 434–436 (in Chinese)

Ma'aita, J.K. (2000) Oral cancer in Jordan: A retrospective study of 118 patients. *Croat. med. J.*, **41**, 64–69

Mabuchi, K., Bross, D.S. & Kessler, I.I. (1985) Cigarette smoking and nasopharyngeal carcinoma. *Cancer*, **55**, 2874–2876

Macfarlane, G.J., Zheng, T., Marshall, J.R., Boffetta, P., Niu, S., Brasure, J., Merletti, F. & Boyle, P. (1995) Alcohol, tobacco, diet and the risk of oral cancer: A pooled analysis of three case-control studies. *Eur. J. Cancer*, **31B**, 181–187

Maier, H. & Tisch, M. (1997) Epidemiology of laryngeal cancer: Results of the Heidelberg case–control study. *Acta otolaryngol.*, **Suppl. 527**, 160–164

Maier, H., Dietz, A., Gewelke, U., Heller, W.D. & Weidauer, H. (1992a) Tobacco and alcohol and the risk of head and neck cancer. *Clin. Invest.*, **70**, 320–327

Maier, H., Gewelke, U., Dietz, A. & Heller, W.-D. (1992b) Risk factors of cancer of the larynx: Results of the Heidelberg case–control study. *Otolaryngol. Head Neck Surg.*, **107**, 577–582

Maier, H., Sennewald, E., Fischer, G., Heller, W.D. & Weidauer, H. (1994) Chronic alcohol consumption — The key risk factor for pharyngeal cancer. *Otolaryngol. Head Neck Surg.*, **110**, 168–173 't Mannetje, A., Kogevinas, M., Luce, D., Demers, P.A., Begin, D., Bolm-Audorff, U., Comba, P., Gerin, M., Hardell, L., Hayes, R.B., Leclerc, A., Magnani, C., Merler, E., Tobias, A. & Boffetta, P. (1999) Sinonasal cancer, occupation, and tobacco smoking in European women and men. *Am. J. ind. Med.*, **36**, 101–107

Marshall, J.R., Graham, S., Haughey, B.P., Shedd, D., O'Shea, R., Brasure, J., Wilkinson, G.S. & West, D. (1992) Smoking, alcohol, dentition and diet in the epidemiology of oral cancer. *Eur. J. Cancer*, **28B**, 9–15

Mashberg, A., Boffetta, P., Winkelman, R. & Garfinkel, L. (1993) Tobacco smoking, alcohol drinking, and cancer of the oral cavity and oropharynx among US veterans. *Cancer*, **72**, 1369–1375

McLaughlin, J.K., Hrubec, Z., Blot, W.J. & Fraumeni, J.F. (1995) Smoking and cancer mortality among US veterans: A 26-year follow-up. *Int. J. Cancer*, **60**, 190–193

Menke-Pluymers, M.B.E., Hop, W.C.J., Dees, J., van Blankenstein, M., Tilanus, H.W. & The Rotterdam Esophageal Tumor Study Group (1993) Risk factors for the development of an adenocarcinoma in columnar-lined (Barrett) esophagus. *Cancer*, **72**, 1155–1158

Merletti, F., Boffetta, P., Ciccone, G., Mashberg, A. & Terracini, B. (1989) Role of tobacco and alcoholic beverages in the etiology of cancer of the oral cavity/oropharynx in Torino, Italy. *Cancer Res.*, **49**, 4919–4924

Moreno-Lopez, L.A., Esparza-Gomez, G.C., Gonzalez-Navarro, A., Cerero-Lapiedra, R., Gonzalez-Hernandez, M.J. & Dominguez-Rojas,V. (2000) Risk of oral cancer associated with tobacco smoking, alcohol consumption and oral hygiene: A case–control study in Madrid, Spain. *Oral Oncol.*, **36**, 170–174

Murata, M., Takayama, K., Choi, B.C.K. & Pak, A.W.P. (1996) A nested case–control study on alcohol drinking, tobacco smoking, and cancer. *Cancer Detect. Prev.*, **20**, 557–565

Muscat, J.E. & Wynder, E.L. (1992) Tobacco, alcohol, asbestos, and occupational risk factors for laryngeal cancer. *Cancer*, **69**, 2244–2251

Muscat, J.E., Richie, J.P., Thompson, S. & Wynder, E.L. (1996) Gender differences in smoking and risk for oral cancer. *Cancer Res.*, **56**, 5192–5197

Nakachi, K., Imai, K., Hoshiyama, Y. & Sasaba, T. (1988) The joint effects of two factors in the etiology of oesophageal cancer in Japan. *J. Epidemiol. Community Health*, **42**, 355–364

Nam, J.-M., McLaughlin, J.K. & Blot, W.J. (1992) Cigarette smoking, alcohol, and nasopharyngeal carcinoma: A case–control study among US whites. *J. natl Cancer Inst.*, **84**, 619–622

Nandakumar, A., Thimmasetty, K.T., Sreeramareddy, N.M., Venugopal, T.C., Rajanna, Vinutha, A.T., Srinivas & Bhargava, M.K. (1990) A population-based case–control investigation on cancers of the oral cavity in Bangalore, India. *Br. J. Cancer*, **62**, 847–851

Negri, E., La Vecchia, C., Franceschi, S., Decarli, A. & Bruzzi, P. (1992) Attributable risks for oesophageal cancer in northern Italy. *Eur. J. Cancer*, **28A**, 1167–1171

Negri, E., La Vecchia, C., Franceschi, S. & Tavani, A. (1993) Attributable risk for oral cancer in northern Italy. *Cancer Epidemiol. Biomark. Prev.*, **2**, 189–193

Ng, T.P. (1986) A case–referent study of cancer of the nasal cavity and sinuses in Hong Kong. *Int. J. Epidemiol.*, **15**, 171–175

Ning, J.P., Yu, M.C., Wang, Q.S. & Henderson, B.E. (1990) Consumption of salted fish and other risk factors for nasopharyngeal carcinoma (NPC) in Tianjin, a low-risk region for NPC in the People's Republic of China. *J. natl Cancer Inst.*, **82**, 291–296

Nordlund, L.A., Carstensen, J.M. & Pershagen, G. (1997) Cancer incidence in female smokers: A 26-year follow-up. *Int. J. Cancer*, **73**, 625–628

Olsen, J., Sabreo, S. & Fasting, U. (1985) Interaction of alcohol and tobacco as risk factors in cancer of the laryngeal region. *J. Epidemiol. Community Health*, **39**, 165–168

Oreggia, F., De Stefani, E., Correa, P. & Fierro, L. (1991) Risk factors for cancer of the tongue in Uruguay. *Cancer*, **67**, 180–183

Pacella-Norman, R., Urban, M.I., Sitas, F., Carrara, H., Sur, R., Hale, M., Ruff, P., Patel, M., Newton, R., Bull, D. & Beral, V. (2002) Risk factors for oesophageal, lung, oral and laryngeal cancers in black south Africans. *Br. J. Cancer*, **86**, 1751–1756

Powell, J. & McConkey, C.C. (1990) Increasing incidence of adenocarcinoma of the gastric cardia and adjacent sites. *Br. J. Cancer*, **59**, 440–443

Raitiola, H.S. & Pukander, J.S. (1997) Etiological factors of laryngeal cancer. *Acta otolaryngol.*, **Suppl. 529**, 215–217

Rao, D.N., Sanghvi, L.D. & Desai, P.B. (1989) Epidemiology of esophageal cancer. *Sem. surg. Oncol.*, **5**, 351–354

Rao, D.N., Desai, P.B. & Ganesh, B. (1999) Alcohol as an additional risk factor in laryngo-pharyngeal cancer in Mumbai — A case–control study. *Cancer Detect. Prev.*, **23**, 37–44

Rolón, P.A., Castellsagué, X., Benz, M. & Muñoz, N. (1995) Hot and cold mate drinking and eso-phageal cancer in Paraguay. *Cancer Epidemiol. Biomarkers Prev.*, **4**, 595–605

Sanderson, R.J., de Boer, M.F., Damhuis, R.A., Meeuwis, C.A. & Knegt, P.P. (1997) The influence of alcohol and smoking on the incidence of oral and oropharyngeal cancer in women. *Clin. Otolaryngol.*, **22**, 444–448

Sankaranarayanan, R., Duffy, S.W., Nair, M.K., Padmakumary, G. & Day, N.E. (1990) Tobacco and alcohol as risk factors in cancer of the larynx in Kerala, India. *Int. J. Cancer*, **45**, 879–882

Sankaranarayanan, R., Duffy, S.W., Padmakumary, G., Nair, S.M., Day, N.E. & Padmanabhan, T.K. (1991) Risk factors for cancer of the oesophagus in Kerala, India. *Int. J. Cancer*, **49**, 485–489

Schildt, E.B., Eriksson, M., Hardell, L. & Magnuson, A. (1998) Oral snuff, smoking habits and alcohol consumption in relation to oral cancer in a Swedish case–control study. *Int. J. Cancer*, **77**, 341–346

Schlecht, N., Franco, E.L., Pintos, J. & Kowalski, L.P. (1999) Effect of smoking cessation and tobacco type on the risk of cancers of the upper areo-digestive tract in Brazil. *Epidemiology*, **10**, 412–418

Sein, K., Maung, K.K. & Aung, T.H. (1992) An epidemiologic study of 70 oral cancer cases at the Institute of Dental Medicine, Yangon, Myanmar, 1985–88. *Odontostomatol. trop. Mar.*, **15**, 5–8

Shen, Y.P., Gao, Y.T., Dai, Q., Wu, X., Xu, T.L., Xiang, Y.B., Tang, Z.L. & Li. W.L. (1999) A case–control study on esophageal cancer in Huaian city, Jiangsu province. I. Role of cigarette smoking and alcohol drinking. *Tumor*, **19**, 363–367 (in Chinese)

Siemiatycki, J., Krewski, D., Franco, E. & Kaiserman, M. (1995) Associations between cigarette smoking and each of 21 types of cancer: A multi-site case–control study. *Int. J. Epidemiol.*, **24**, 504–514

Sokic, S.I., Adanja, B.J., Marinkovic, J.P. & Vlajinac, H.D. (1994) Case–control study of risk factors in laryngeal cancer. *Neoplasma*, **41**, 43–47

Spitz, M.R., Fueger, J.J., Halabi, S., Schantz, S.P., Sample, D. & Hsu, T.C. (1993) Mutagen sensitivity in upper aerodigestive tract cancer: A case–control analysis. *Cancer Epidemiol. Biomarkers Prev.*, **2**, 329–333

Sriamporn, S., Vatanasapt, V., Pisani, P., Yongchaiyudha, S. & Rungpitarangsri, V. (1992) Environmental risk factors for nasopharyngeal carcinoma: A case–control study in northeastern Thailand. *Cancer Epidemiol. Biomarkers Prev.*, **1**, 345–348

Strader, C.H., Vaughan, T.L. & Stergachis, A.A. (1988) Use of nasal preparations and the incidence of sinonasal cancer. *J. Epidemiol. Community Health*, **42**, 243–248

Talamini, R., Franceschi, S., Barra, S. & La Vecchia, C. (1990) The role of alcohol in oral and pharyngeal cancer in non-smokers, and of tobacco in non-drinkers. *Int. J. Cancer*, **46**, 391–393

Talamini, R., La Vecchia, C., Levi, F., Conti, E., Favero, A. & Franceschi, S. (1998) Cancer of the oral cavity and pharynx in nonsmokers who drink alcohol and in nondrinkers who smoke tobacco. *J. natl Cancer Inst.*, **90**, 1901–1903

Tavani, A., Negri, E., Franceschi, S., Barbone, F. & La Vecchia, C. (1994) Attributable risk for laryngeal cancer in northern Italy. *Cancer Epidemiol. Biomarkers Prev.*, **3**, 121–125

Tavani, A., Negri, E., Franceschi, S. & La Vecchia, C. (1996) Tobacco and other risk factors for oesophageal cancer in alcohol non-drinkers. *Eur. J. Cancer Prev.*, **5**, 313–318

Tomita, M., Odaka, M., Matsumoto, M., Yamaguchi, M., Hosoda, Y. & Mizuno, S. (1991) [Cigarette smoking and mortality among Japanese males in a prospective cohort study.] *Nippon Koshu Eisei Zasshi*, **38**, 492–497 (in Japanese)

Tulinius, H., Sigfússon, N., Sigvaldason, H., Bjarnadóttir, K. & Tryggvadóttir, L. (1997) Risk factors for malignant diseases: A cohort study on a population of 22,946 Icelanders. *Cancer Epidemiol. Biomarkers Prev.*, **6**, 863–873

Tuyns, A.J., Esteve, J., Raymond, L., Berrino, F., Benhamou, E., Blanchet, F., Boffetta, P., Crosignani, P., del Moral, A., Lehmann, W., Merletti, F., Pequignot, G., Riboli, E., Bancho-Garnier, H., Terracini, B., Zubiri, A. & Zubiri, L. (1988) Cancer of the larynx/hypopharynx, tobacco and alcohol: IARC International case-control study in Turin and Varese (Italy), Zaragoza and Navarra (Spain), Geneva (Switzerland) and Calvados (France). *Int. J. Cancer*, **41**, 483–491

Vaughan, T.L., Davis, S., Kristal, A. & Thomas, D.B. (1995) Obesity, alcohol, and tobacco as risk factors for cancers of the esophagus and gastric cardia: Adenocarcinoma *versus* squamous cell carcinoma. *Cancer Epidemiol. Biomarkers Prev.*, **4**, 85–92

Vaughan, T.L., Shapiro, J.A., Burt, R.D., Swanson, G.M., Berwick, M., Lynch, C.F. & Lyon, J.L. (1996) Nasopharyngeal cancer in a low-risk population: Defining risk factors by histological type. *Cancer Epidemiol. Biomarkers Prev.*, **5**, 587–593

Victora, C.G., Muñoz, N., Day, N.E., Barcelos, L.B., Peccin, D.A., Braga, N.M. (1987) Hot beverages and oesophageal cancer in southern Brazil: A case–control study. *Int. J. Cancer*, **39**, 710–716

Vizcaino, A.P., Parkin, D.M., Skinner, M.E.G. (1995) Risk factors associated with oesophageal cancer in Bulawayo, Zimbabwe. *Br. J. Cancer*, **72**, 769–773

Wang, Y.P., Han, X.Y., Su, W., Wang, Y.L., Zhu, Y.W., Sasaba, T., Nakachi, K., Hoshiyama, Y. & Tagashira, Y. (1992) Esophageal cancer in Shanxi Province, People's Republic of China: A case–control study in high and moderate risk areas. *Cancer Causes Control*, **3**, 107–113

Weir, J.M. & Dunn, J.E., Jr (1970) Smoking and mortality: A prospective study. *Cancer*, **25**, 105–112

West, S., Hildesheim, A. & Dosemeci M. (1993) Non-viral risk factors for nasopharyngeal carcinoma in the Philippines: Results from a case–control study. *Int. J. Cancer*, **55**, 722–727

Wu, A.H., Wan, P. & Bernstein, L. (2001) A multiethnic population-based study of smoking, alcohol and body size and risk of adenocarcinomas of the stomach and esophagus (United States). *Cancer Causes Control*, **12**, 721–732

Wynder, E.L. & Stellman, S.D. (1979) Impact of long-term filter cigarette usage on lung and larynx cancer risk: A case–control study. *J. natl Cancer Inst.*, **62**, 471–477

Ye, W.M., Ye, Y.N., Lin, R.D., Zhou, T.S. & Lu, Y.B. (1995) [Case–control study on naso-pharyngeal cancer in southern region of Fujian Province.] *Chin. J. prev. Control chron. Dis.*, **3**, 158–161 (in Chinese)

Yu, M.C., Ho, J.H.C., Lai, S.-H. & Henderson, B.E. (1986) Cantonese-style salted fish as a cause of nasopharyngeal carcinoma: Report of a case–control study in Hong Kong. *Cancer Res.*, **46**, 956–961

Yu, M.C., Garabrant, D.H., Peters, J.M. & Mack, T.M. (1988) Tobacco, alcohol, diet, occupation, and carcinoma of the esophagus. *Cancer Res.*, **48**, 3843–3848

Yu, M.C., Garabrant, D.H., Huang, T.B. & Henderson, B.E. (1990) Occupational and other non-dietary risk factors for nasopharyngeal carcinoma in Guangzhou, China. *Int. J. Cancer*, **45**, 1033–1039

Yuan, J.M., Ross, R.K., Wang, X.L., Gao, Y.T., Henderson, B.E. & Yu, M.C. (1996) Morbidity and mortality in relation to cigarette smoking in Shanghai, China. A prospective male cohort study. *J. Am. med. Assoc.*, **275**, 1646–1650

Yuan, J.M., Wang, X.L., Xiang, Y.B., Gao, Y.T., Ross, R.K. & Yu, M.C. (2000) Non-dietary risk factors for nasopharyngeal carcinoma in Shanghai, China. *Int. J. Cancer*, **85**, 364–369

Zambon, P., Talamini, R., La Vecchia, C., Dal Maso, L., Negri, E., Tognazzo, S., Simonato, L. & Franceschi, S. (2000) Smoking, type of alcoholic beverage and squamous-cell oesophageal cancer in northern Italy. *Int. J. Cancer*, **86**, 144–149

Zatonski, W., Becher, H., Lissowska, J. & Wahrendorf, J. (1991) Tobacco, alcohol, and diet in the etiology of laryngeal cancer: A population-based case–control study. *Cancer Causes Prev.*, **2**, 3–10

Zavras, A.I., Douglass, C.W., Joshipura, K., Wu, T., Laskaris, G., Petridou, E., Dokianakis, G., Segas, J., Lefantzis, D., Nomikos, P., Wang, Y.F. & Diehl, S.R. (2001) Smoking and alcohol in the etiology of oral cancer: Gender specific risk profiles in the south of Greece. *Oral Oncol.*, **37**, 28–35

Zhang, Z.F., Kurtz, R.C., Sun, M., Karpeh, M., Jr, Yu, G.P., Gargon, N., Fein, J.S., Georgopoulos, S.K. & Harlap, S. (1996) Adenocarcinomas of the esophagus and gastric cardia: Medical conditions, tobacco, alcohol, and socio-economic factors. *Cancer Epidemiol. Biomarkers Prev.*, **5**, 761–768

Zheng, T.Z., Boyle, P., Hu, H.F., Duan, J., Jiang, P.J., Ma, D.Q., Shui, L.P., Niu, S.R. & MacMahon, B. (1990) Tobacco smoking, alcohol consumption, and risk of oral cancer: A case-control study in Beijing, People's Republic of China. *Cancer Causes Control*, **1**, 173–179

Zheng, W., Blot, W.J., Shu, X.O., Diamond, E.L., Gao, Y.T., Ji, B.T. & Fraumeni, J.F. (1992a) Risk factors for oral and pharyngeal cancer in Shanghai, with emphasis on diet. *Cancer Epidemiol. Biomarkers Prev.*, **1**, 441–448

Zheng, W., Blot, W.J., Shu, X.O., Diamond, E.L., Gao, Y.T., Ji, B.T. & Fraumeni, J.F., Jr (1992b) A population-based case–control study of cancers of the nasal cavity and paranasal sinuses in Shanghai. *Int. J. Cancer*, **52**, 557–561

Zheng, W., Blot, W.J., Shu, X.O., Gao, Y.T., Ji, B.T., Zieler, R.G. & Fraumeni, J.F., Jr (1992c) Diet and other risk factors for laryngeal cancer in Shanghai, China. *Am. J. Epidemiol.*, **136**, 178–191

Zheng, W., McLaughlin, J.K., Chow, W.H., Chien, H.T.C. & Blot, W.J. (1993) Risk factors for cancers of the nasal cavity and paranasal sinuses among white men in the United States. *Am. J. Epidemiol.*, **138**, 965–972

Zheng, Y.M., Tuppin, P., Hubert, A., Jeannel, D., Pan, Y.J., Zeng, Y., & de Thé, G. (1994) Environmental and dietary risk factors for nasopharyngeal carcinoma: A case–control study in Zangwu County, Guangxi, China. *Br. J. Cancer*, **69**, 508–514

Zheng, T., Holford, T., Chen, Y., Jiang, P., Zhang, B. & Boyle, P. (1997) Risk of tongue cancer associated with tobacco smoking and alcohol consumption: A case–control study. *Oral Oncol.*, **33**, 82–85

Zhu, K., Levine, R.S., Brann, E.A., Gnepp, D.R. & Baum, M.K. (1995) A population-based case-control study of the relationship between cigarette smoking and nasopharyngeal cancer (United States). *Cancer Causes Control*, **6**, 507–512

Zhu, K., Levine, R.S., Brann, E.A., Gnepp, D.R. & Baum, M.K. (1997) Cigarette smoking and nasopharyngeal cancer: An analysis of the relationship according to age at starting smoking and age at diagnosis. *J. Epidemiol.*, **7**, 107–111

2.1.5   *Cancer of the pancreas*

(*a*)   *Cohort and case–control studies*

The designs of the case–control and cohort studies are summarized in Table 2.1.5.1 and 2.1, respectively. Additional data have come from the Alpha-Tocopherol Beta-Carotene Cancer Prevention Study (Stolzenberg-Solomon *et al.*, 2001), which followed a cohort of more than 27 000 male smokers between 1985 and 1997. Pancreatic cancer cases were ascertained from the Finnish Cancer Registry, which hold records of almost 100% of all cases in Finland.

All but two of the published cohort and case–control studies (Murata *et al.*, 1996; Liaw & Chen, 1998) showed an increased risk for pancreatic cancer in ever-smokers (Tables 2.1.5.2 and 2.1.5.3). The conclusion that smoking is a cause of this cancer reached in the *IARC Monograph* on tobacco smoking (IARC, 1986) remains unchanged; smokers have about twice as high a risk for this cancer as never-smokers.

A number of cohort studies have reported associations between smoking and the subsequent development of pancreatic cancer. Pancreatic cancer was ascertained mainly by linkage to population-based cancer registries, death notification systems or pathology laboratories. Some studies only recorded smoking habits at time of enrolment; thus data on prolonged tobacco consumption were not readily available.

Several case–control studies on the relationship between smoking and pancreatic cancer have also been published since 1986. These studies were designed to measure the effect of smoking, alcohol consumption and coffee drinking. Some studies also measured the effect of certain dietary items. Two types of control group were used: hospital-based controls, mainly with conditions not thought to be associated with smoking or tobacco, or neighbourhood-matched controls selected using electoral rolls or random-digit telephone dialling. Verification of pancreatic cancers ranged from 100% (i.e. only those with histological verification were included in a study) to about 30%. However, whether or not subanalyses were carried out on cases diagnosed with histology, this made little difference to the results. Because pancreatic cancer is rapidly fatal, most studies questioned proxies for the case about the smoking characteristics of the patients. Some studies also interviewed proxies of the control patients, but again, restricting the analyses to direct interviews rather than proxy interviews made little difference to the direction of the association.

(*b*)   *Factors affecting risk*

(i)   *Duration and intensity*

Table 2.1.5.3 shows the results of studies that considered dose–response relationships. Most studies found clear evidence demonstrating that the risk for cancer of the pancreas increases with daily cigarette consumption and the number of years of smoking.

(ii)   Cessation

Eight studies (Mack *et al.*, 1986; Cuzick & Babiker, 1989; Bueno de Mesquita *et al.*, 1991; Howe *et al.*, 1991; Silverman *et al.*, 1994; Ji *et al.*, 1995; Muscat *et al.*, 1997; Partanen *et al.*, 1997) reported on the risk of pancreatic cancer according to the number of years since quitting. Five of these studies found a decreasing monotonic trend in risk associated with the number of years for which the subjects had stopped smoking (Mack *et al.*, 1986; Howe *et al*, 1991; Silverman *et al.*, 1994; Ji *et al.*, 1995; Partanen *et al.*, 1997). A further study reported that the excess risk in former smokers disappeared after less than 10 years since quitting, but did not provide quantitative estimates (Fuchs *et al.*, 1996) (Table 2.5.1.4).

(iii)   *Type of cigarette*

Friedman *et al.* (1998) compared rates of pancreatic cancer development between those who reported smoking mentholated cigarettes and those who smoked non-mentholated cigarettes. The rate ratio was 0.6 for men (95% CI, 0.3–1.4) and 0.8 for women (95% CI, 0.3–1.8); the difference in risk between mentholated and non-mentholated cigarettes was not statistically significant and the confidence intervals were wide, so that no firm conclusion can be made.

Three case–control studies (Table 2.1.5.5; Bueno de Mesquita *et al.*, 1991; Ghadirian *et al.*, 1991; Howe *et al.*, 1991) compared filter-tipped with untipped cigarettes. Ghadirian *et al.* (1991) observed an approximately twofold higher risk for pancreatic cancer in heavy smokers of untipped cigarettes than in smokers of filter-tipped cigarettes. Overall, however, there was no difference in effect.

(c)   *Population characteristics*

(i)   *Sex*

The effect of sex on risk was investigated in two case–control studies (Mack *et al.*, 1986; Clavel *et al.*, 1989) and four cohort studies (Akiba & Hirayama, 1990; Engeland *et al.*, 1996; Fuchs *et al.*, 1996; Tulinius *et al.*, 1997). Relative risks were similar for men and women and no consistent evidence of an effect of sex on risk was observed.

(ii)   *Ethnic group*

The role of ethnic group in the association between tobacco smoking and pancreatic cancer was investigated among African Americans and Caucasians in the USA (Silverman *et al.*, 1994). No evidence of heterogeneity by ethnic group was obtained.

(d)   *Confounding factors*

In addition to age and sex, other potential confounding factors considered in several studies included consumption of alcohol and coffee. The excess risk due to smoking remained after adjustment for some or all of these factors (Hiatt *et al.*, 1988; Lyon *et al.*, 1992; Zheng *et al.*, 1993; Silverman *et al.*, 1994; Engeland *et al.*, 1996).

Five studies were carried out simultaneously in Utrecht, The Netherlands (Bueno de Mesquita *et al.*, 1991), Toronto, Canada (Howe *et al.*, 1991), Montreal, Canada (Ghadirian *et al.*, 1991), Opole, Poland (Zatonski *et al.*, 1993) and Adelaide, Australia (Baghurst *et al.*, 1991), as part of the Surveillance of Environmental Aspects Related to Cancer in Humans (SEARCH) programme of the IARC, to elucidate the roles of alcohol and tobacco in the development of pancreatic cancer. These were reviewed by Boyle *et al.* (1996).

Table 2.1.5.1. Case–control studies on tobacco smoking and cancer of the pancreas: main characteristics of study design

Reference Country and years of study	Number of cases and controls	Criteria for eligibility and comments
Wynder *et al.* (1973) USA 1950–64	Men: 100 cases and 200 controls; women: 42 cases and 107 controls	Hospital-based study. Cases from nine hospitals. Controls: hospitalized patients without tobacco-related disease, matched for age, sex and ethnicity
MacMahon *et al.* (1981) USA 1974–79	Men: 218 cases and 306 controls; women: 149 cases and 337 controls	Hospital-based study. Cases from 11 hospitals. Controls: hospitalized patients without tobacco or alcohol-related disease
Durbec *et al.* (1983) France 1979–80	Men: 37 cases and 100 controls; women: 32 cases and 99 controls	Cases selected in three hospitals; neighbourhood controls
Whittemore *et al.* (1983) USA 1962–66	Men: 122 cases and 781 controls	Population-based study. Cases from the University of Harvard and University of Pennsylvania. Data obtained by postal survey. Controls: randomly selected classmates
Wynder *et al.* (1983) USA 1981	Men: 153 cases; women: 122 cases; 7994 controls	Hospital-based study. Cases from 15 hospitals. Controls: hospitalized patients without tobacco-related disease
Kinlen & McPherson (1984) UK 1952–54	Men: 109 cases and 218 controls; women: 107 cases and 214 controls	Cases not specified. Controls: patients with cancers unrelated to smoking
Gold *et al.* (1985) USA 1978–80	Men and women: 201 cases, 201 hospital controls and 201 community controls	Hospital-based study in 16 hospitals; 62% cases histologically confirmed. Hospital controls: patients with heart, other circulatory and digestive diseases excluding any type of cancer; matched to cases on age, ethnicity, sex, hospital and date of admission. Community controls: selected by random-digit dialling, matched to cases on age, ethnicity, sex and telephone exchange
Hsieh *et al.* (1986) USA 1981–84	Men and women: 176 cases and 273 controls	Hospital-based study in 11 large hospitals 100% cases histologically confirmed Controls: patients with cancers of the breast, colon, stomach, uterus, benign tumours, hernia, colitis enteritis or other minor conditions

Table 2.1.5.1 (contd)

Reference Country and years of study	Number of cases and controls	Criteria for eligibility and comments
Mack et al. (1986) USA 1976–81	Men and women: 490 cases and 490 controls	Population-based study. Histologically confirmed cases identified by cancer registry; neighbourhood controls matched on age, sex, ethnicity and place
Wynder et al. (1986) USA 1981–84	Men: 127 cases and 371 controls; women: 111 cases and 325 controls	Hospital-based study in 18 hospitals in six cities. Cases: identified by histology or discharge summary. About three controls/case, matched for sex, age, ethnicity, hospital, year of admission, without tobacco-related disease
La Vecchia et al. (1987) Italy 1983–86	Men: 99 cases and 471 controls; women: 51 cases and 134 controls	Hospital-based study. Cases histologically confirmed. Controls admitted to hospitals for traumatic or surgical conditions, orthopaedic disorders, disorders of ear, nose and throat, skin or teeth
Clavel et al. (1989) France 1982–85	Men: 98 cases and 161 controls; women: 63 cases and 107 controls	Hospital-based study; 63% of cases histologically confirmed; controls had cancers and benign conditions unrelated to smoking or alcohol; two controls matched to each case by age, sex, hospital and interviewer
Cuzick & Babiker (1989) UK 1983–86	Men: 123 cases and 150 controls; women: 93 casess and 129 controls	Hospital-based study in 3 major city hospitals; 30.1% of cases histologically confirmed. Hospital controls and general practitioner controls had diseases unrelated to smoking
Ferraroni et al. (1989) Italy 1983–88	Men: 136 cases and 1334 controls; women: 78 cases and 610 controls	Hospital-based study. All cases histologically confirmed
Falk et al. (1990) USA 1979–83	Men and women: 198 cases and 209 controls	Hospital-based study in 29 hospitals; 83% cases histologically confirmed. Hospital controls matched for ethnicity, age, sex and hospital
Baghurst et al. (1991) Australia 1984–87	Men and women: 104 cases and 253 controls	Population-based study within the IARC SEARCH[a] programme. Controls obtained from a random sample of the electoral roll. Analysis matched by age and sex
Bueno de Mesquita et al. (1991) Netherlands 1984–88	Men and women: 176 cases and 487 controls	Population-based study within the IARC SEARCH[a] programme; 68% of cases histologically confirmed. Controls selected from municipal population registries
Ghadirian et al. (1991) Canada 1984–88	Men: 97 cases and 239 controls; women: 82 cases and 116 controls	Population-based study within the IARC SEARCH[a] Programme; 83% of cases histologically confirmed. Controls selected by random-digit dialling and from telephone directories, and matched to cases on age, sex and residence

Table 2.1.5.1 (contd)

Reference Country and years of study	Number of cases and controls	Criteria for eligibility and comments
Howe et al. (1991) Canada 1983–86	Men: 141 cases and 270 controls; women: 108 cases and 235 controls	Population-based study within the IARC SEARCH[a] Programme; 69% of cases histologically confirmed. Controls selected randomly from population lists in the same study area
Vioque & Walker (1991) Multinational; early 1960s to beginning of 1980s	Men and women: 108 cases and 374 controls	Hospital-based study. Data collected by the Boston Collaborative Drug Surveillance Programme in six countries: Canada, Israel, New Zealand, Scotland, USA and former West Germany; age-sex- and hospital-matched controls
Lyon et al. (1992) USA 1984–87	Men and women: 149 cases and 363 controls	Population-based study. Cases from the Utah Cancer Registry. Controls selected by random-digit dialling
Mizuno et al. (1992) Japan 1989–90	Men: 68 cases and 68 controls; women: 56 cases and 56 controls	Hospital-based study in seven hospitals. Cases and hospital controls matched on age, sex and institute. Controls: patients with benign digestive, circulatory and other disorders
Kalapothaki et al. (1993) Greece 1991–92	Men: 115 cases, 115 hospital controls and 115 visitor controls; women: 66 cases, 66 hospital controls and 66 visitor controls	Hospital-based study in eight major teaching hospitals. Cases (all histologically confirmed) and controls matched by hospital, gender and age. Controls: patients with fractures, appendicitis, ear, nose and throat conditions, goitre, varicose veins and sciatica
Zatonski et al. (1993) Poland 1985–88	Men: 68 cases and 89 controls; women: 42 cases and 106 controls	Population-based study within the IARC SEARCH[a] programme; 43.6% cases histologically confirmed
Silverman et al. (1994) USA 1986–89	Men: 244 cases and 1328 controls; women: 235 cases and 774 controls	Population-based study; 85% cases histologically confirmed. Controls aged 30–64 years selected by random-digit dialling, those aged 65–79 years selected by stratified random sampling from the Health Care Financing Administration's rosters. Cases and controls matched by area, age, sex and ethnicity
Gullo et al. (1995) Italy 1987–89	Men: 319 cases; women: 251 cases; 570 matched controls	Hospital-based study in 14 university and community hospitals. Cases and controls matched for age, sex, socioeconomic status and area; 70% cases histologically confirmed. Controls: patients with minor trauma or disorders unrelated to alcohol, coffee or tobacco consumption
Ji et al. (1995) China 1990–93	Men: 264 cases and 852 controls; women: 187 cases and 701 controls	Population-based study among permanent residents of 10 urban districts; cases identified by the Shanghai Cancer Registry; 37% of cases histologically confirmed. Controls randomly selected from Shanghai residents' registry

Table 2.1.5.1 (contd)

Reference Country and years of study	Number of cases and controls	Criteria for eligibility and comments
Siemiatycki *et al.* (1995) Canada 1979–86	Men: 116 cases, 1705 hospital controls with cancer and 533 population controls	All cases histologically confirmed. Control group had cancer at sites not previously demonstrated as affected by cigarette smoking
Fernandez *et al.* (1996) Italy 1983–92	Men: 229 cases and 1031 controls; women: 133 cases and 377 controls	All cases histologically confirmed. Controls: hospital patients with acute, non-neoplastic, non-digestive, non-smoking- and non-alcohol-related disorders
Lee *et al.* (1996) China, Province of Taiwan 1989–94	Men and women: 282 cases and 282 controls	Hospital-based study; 45.7% of cases histologically confirmed. Controls matched on age and sex had no history of pancreatic cancer.
Nishi *et al.* (1996) Japan 1987–92	Men and women: 141 cases and 282 controls	Population-based study. Controls matched for sex, age and place of residence selected using random-digit dialling
Ohba *et al.* (1996) Japan 1987–92	Men: 85 cases; women: 56 cases; and 282 controls	Cases: data obtained by direct interview; 41.8% of cases histologically confirmed. Controls matched on age, sex and residence randomly selected from telephone directories, data collected from self-administered questionnaires and telephone back-up
Fryzek *et al.* (1997) USA 1994–95	Men and women: 66 cases and 131 controls	Hospital-based study in five large hospitals and two teaching hospitals. Cases diagnosed by cytology. Controls selected by random-digit dialling. Cases and controls matched by age, sex, ethnicity and county of residence
Muscat *et al.* (1997) USA 1985–93	Men: 290 cases and 572 controls; women: 194 cases and 382 controls	Hospital-based study; all cases histologically confirmed. Controls without pancreatic cancer hospitalized for conditions unrelated to tobacco use. Cases and controls matched by hospital, sex, age, ethnicity and year of diagnosis
Partanen *et al.* (1997) Finland 1984–87	Men and women: 662 cases and 1770 controls	Population-based study. Cases from the Finnish Cancer Registry diagnosed 1984–87 and decedent in 1990. Cancer controls include 1014 patients with stomach, 441 with colon and 315 with rectum cancers
Mori *et al.* (1999) India 1994–96	Men and women: 79 cases and 146 controls	Hospital-based study; 100% of cases of histologically confirmed pancreatic ductal adenocarcinoma. Controls selected from healthy hospital visitors, matched to cases on sex and age
Villeneuve *et al.* (2000) Canada 1994–97	Men: 322 cases and 2452 controls; women: 261 cases and 2361 controls	Population-based study in 8 provinces, within the Canadian National Enhanced Cancer Surveillance System (NECSS); all cases histologically confirmed. Strategies for selection of controls varied by province.

[a] SEARCH, Surveillance of Environmental Aspects Related to Cancer in Humans

Table 2.1.5.2. Additional cohort studies on tobacco smoking and cancer of the pancreas

Reference Country and years of study	Subjects	No. of cases and/or deaths	Covariates adjusted for	Smoking category and/or amount smoked	Relative risk (95% CI)	Comments
Hammond & Horn (1958a,b) USA 1952–55	American Cancer Society Study 187 783 men	117 deaths		Regular smoker	1.5	
Hammond (1966) USA 1959–63	Cancer Prevention Study (CPS) I 440 558 men and 562 671 women	274 men, 108 women		Men Ever-smoker aged 45–64 years aged 65–79 years Women Ever-smoker Heavy smoker	Mortality ratio 2.7 2.7 1.8 2.6	
Kahn (1966) USA 1954–62	US Veterans' Study 293 958 men	415 deaths		Former smoker Occasional smoker Cigarettes/day 1–9 10–20 21–39 ≥ 40	1.3 1.1 1.4 1.8 2.2 2.7	
Lossing et al. (1966) Canada 1956–62	Canadian War Veterans Study 78 000 men	28 deaths in cigarette smokers		Cigarettes/day 1–9 10–20 ≥ 21	1.4 2.0 2.4	Number of nonsmoking men not given
Weir & Dunn (1970) USA 1954–62	Californian Study 68 153 men	71 deaths		Ever-smoker Cigarettes/day 1–10 20 ≥ 30	2.4 2.9 2.5 1.4	Decreasing relative risk with increasing consumption unexplained

Table 2.1.5.2 (contd)

Reference Country and years of study	Subjects	No. of cases and/or deaths	Covariates adjusted for	Smoking category and/or amount smoked	Relative risk (95% CI)	Comments
Cederlöf et al. (1975) Sweden 1963–72	Swedish Census Study 25 444 men, 26 467 women	46 deaths in men		Former smoker Cigarettes/day 1–7 8–15 ≥16	4.8 ($p < 0.05$) 1.6 3.4 5.9	
		37 deaths in women		Former smoker Cigarettes/day 1–7 8–15 ≥16	5.5 2.4 2.5 3.0	
Doll & Peto (1976) UK 1951–71	British Doctors' Study 34 440 men	78 deaths		Tobacco (g)/day 0 1–14 15–24 ≥25 Former smoker	Mortality rate 14 14 18 27 12	Annual mortality rate per 100 000 men p for trend < 0.1
Doll et al. (1980) UK 1951–73	British Doctors' Study 6194 women	14 deaths		Tobacco (g)/day 0 1–14 15–24 ≥25 Former smoker	Mortality rate 9 4 24 16 11	Annual mortality rate per 100 000 women
Hirayama (1981) Japan 1965–78	Six-prefecture Study 122 261 men, 142 857 women	251 deaths in men		Never-smoker Former smoker Occasional smoker Cigarettes/day 1–9 10–19 ≥20	Mortality rate 13.3 15.4 12.8 14.7 19.8 20.3	Annual mortality rate per 100 000 men

Table 2.1.5.2 (contd)

Reference Country and years of study	Subjects	No. of cases and/or deaths	Covariates adjusted for	Smoking category and/or amount smoked	Relative risk (95% CI)	Comments
Hirayama (1981) (contd)		417 deaths (251 men, 166 women)		Current smoker	Relative risk 1.6	Relative risk for men and women combined. Effect persisted after adjustment for social class and meat and green/leafy vegetable consumption
Heuch et al. (1983) Norway 1967–78	[About 11 000] Norwegian men (some overlap with Norwegian Cohort Study)	22 cases		≥ 10 cigarettes/day	2.0 (p = 0.087)	Analysis confined to histologically confirmed cases
Hiatt et al. (1988) USA 1978–85	Kaiser Permanente Medical Care Program Study II 122 894 persons	49 cases	Age, sex, ethnic origin, blood glucose, alcohol, coffee and tea	Former smoker Current smoker < ½ pack/day ½–1 pack/day 1–2 packs/day > 2 packs/day	0.8 (0.4–2.0) 1.8 (0.4–8.1) 1.9 (0.6–6.2) 2.1 (0.6–8.2) 6.6 (1.4–31.8)	Nested case–control study
Mills et al. (1988) USA 1976–82	Adventists' Health Study 34 198 persons	40 cases	Age and sex	Former smoker Current smoker	1.5 (0.7–3.4) 5.4 (1.8–16.5)	

Table 2.1.5.2 (contd)

Reference Country and years of study	Subjects	No. of cases and/or deaths	Covariates adjusted for	Smoking category and/or amount smoked	Relative risk (95% CI)	Comments
Hirayama (1989) Japan 1965–81	Six-prefecture Study 122 261 men, 142 857 women	679 deaths (399 men, 280 women)	Age	Daily smoker Men Women	1.6 (1.2–2.0) 1.5 (1.0–1.9) Mortality rate	
				1–14 cigarettes/day 15–29 cigarettes/day 30–39 cigarettes/day 40–49 cigarettes/day ≥ 50 cigarettes/day	24.6 26.5 28.4 30.7 43.9	p for trend = 0.002
Akiba & Hirayama (1990) Japan 1965–81	Six-prefecture Study 122 261 men, 142 857 women	554 deaths (322 men, 232 women)	Age, prefecture of residence, occupation and observation period	Ever-smokers (men) 1–4 cigarettes/day 5–14 cigarettes/day 15–24 cigarettes/day 25–34 cigarettes/day ≥ 35 cigarettes/day	1.5 (1.1–2.1) 1.1 (0.3–2.7) 1.5 (1.1–2.1) 1.6 (1.2–2.2) 1.2 (0.6–2.2) 1.3 (0.4–2.9)	p for trend = 0.04 p for heterogeneity = 0.07
				Ever-smokers (women) 1–4 cigarettes/day 5–14 cigarettes/day ≥ 15 cigarettes/day	1.6 (1.1–2.3) 0.6 (0.1–1.9) 1.9 (1.2–2.8) 1.4 (0.4–3.4)	p for trend = 0.02 p for heterogeneity = 0.03
Kuller et al. (1991) USA 1975–85	MRFIT Study		Age, diastolic blood pressure, serum cholesterol levels and race	Current smoker	2.0 (p < 0.0001)	

Table 2.1.5.2 (contd)

Reference Country and years of study	Subjects	No. of cases and/or deaths	Covariates adjusted for	Smoking category and/or amount smoked	Relative risk (95% CI)	Comments
Friedman & van den Eeden (1993) USA 1964–88	Kaiser Permanente Medical Care Program Study I 175 000 persons	450 cases, 2687 controls	Ethnicity and age	Former smoker Current smoker > 20 years < 1 pack/day 1–2 packs/day > 2 packs/day	1.3 1.6 (1.1–2.2) 1.8 ($p < 0.01$) 1.6 ($p < 0.01$) 3.0 ($p < 0.01$)	Nested case–control study; controls matched for sex, age, examination site, date of check-up
Tverdal et al. (1993) Norway 1972–88	Norwegian Screening Study 44 290 men, 24 535 women	57 deaths	Age and area	Never-smoker Former smoker Current smoker 1–9 cigarettes/day 10–19 cigarettes/day ≥ 20 cigarettes/day Relative risk per 10 cigarettes/day	Mortality rate 4.4 (127 325 person–years) 6.3 (144 776 person–years) 13.5 (248 159 person–years) 5.5 (56 350 person–years) 17.2 (135 167 person–years) 14.9 (56 441 person–years) 1.5 (0.9–2.3)	Annual mortality rate per 100 000 persons
Zheng et al. (1993) USA 1966–86	Lutheran Brotherhood Insurance Study 17 633 men 286 731 person–years	57 deaths	Age and alcohol	Former smoker Current smoker < 25 cigarettes/day ≥ 25 cigarettes/day	1.0 (0.4–2.2) 1.4 (0.6–3.2) 3.9 (1.5–10.3)	p for trend ≤ 0.01
Doll et al. (1994) UK 1951–91	British Doctors' Study 34 439 men	205 deaths		Nonsmoker Former cigarette smoker Current cigarette smoker 1–14 cigarettes/day 15–24 cigarettes/day ≥ 25 cigarettes/day	Mortality rate 16 23 35 30 29 49	Annual mortality rate per 100 000 men p for trend = 0.001 p for trend = 0.001

Table 2.1.5.2 (contd)

Reference Country and years of study	Subjects	No. of cases and/or deaths	Covariates adjusted for	Smoking category and/or amount smoked	Relative risk (95% CI)	Comments
Shibata et al. (1994) USA 1981–90	Leisure World Study 13 979 persons 100 921 person–years	65 cases (28 men, 37 women)	Sex and age	Former smoker (quit ≥ 20 years) Recent quitter (< 20 years) and current smoker	1.4 (0.7–2.6) 1.2 (0.7–2.2)	
McLaughlin et al. (1995) USA 1954–80	US Veterans' Study 248 046 men 3 252 983 person–years	1264 deaths	Attained age and calendar-year time-period	Former smoker Current smoker 1–9 cigarettes/day 10–20 cigarettes/day 31–39 cigarettes/day ≥ 40 cigarettes/day	1.1 (0.9–1.3) 1.7 (1.5–1.9) 1.4 (1.1–1.8) 1.7 (1.4–1.9) 1.8 (1.5–2.2) 1.6 (1.1–2.3)	p for trend < 0.01
Engeland et al. (1996) Norway 1966–93	Norwegian Cohort Study 11 857 men and 14 269 women Person–years: about 230 000 men and 310 000 women	224 cases (109 men, 115 women, 55% histo-logically verified)		Men Former smoker Current smoker 1–4 cigarettes/day 5–9 cigarettes/day 10–14 cigarettes/day ≥ 15 cigarettes/day Unknown consumption Women Former smoker Current smoker 1–4 cigarettes/day ≥ 5 cigarettes/day	0.9 (0.6–1.5) 0.9 (0.5–1.8) 1.0 (0.5–2.1) 1.3 (0.7–2.4) 1.6 (0.8–3.2) 7.9 (1.1–58) 0.6 (0.2–1.5) 0.9 (0.4–1.8) 1.8 (1.1–3.0)	

Table 2.1.5.2 (contd)

Reference Country and years of study	Subjects	No. of cases and/or deaths	Covariates adjusted for	Smoking category and/or amount smoked	Relative risk (95% CI)	Comments
Fuchs *et al.* (1996) USA 1980–92	Nurses' Health Study (1976–92) and Health Professionals Follow Up Study (1986–94) 49 428 men 2 116 229 person–years	186 cases	Sex, body-mass index, history of diabetes mellitus and age	**Men**		
				Former smoker	1.3 (0.7–2.3)	
				Current smoker	3.0 (1.6–6.3)	
				1–10 pack–years	0.9 (0.3–2.6)	
				11–25 pack–years	1.3 (0.7–2.7)	
				26–50 pack–years	1.5 (0.7–3.1)	
				> 50 pack–years	2.8 (1.3–5.7)	*p* for trend = 0.004
				Women		
				Former smoker	1.1 (0.7–1.7)	
				Current smoker	2.4 (1.6–3.6)	
				1–10 pack–years	1.1 (0.6–1.9)	
				11–25 pack–years	1.6 (1.0–2.7)	
				26–50 pack–years	2.1 (1.4–3.3)	
				> 50 pack–years	1.3 (0.7–2.7)	*p* for trend = 0.01
				All		
				Former smoker	1.2 (0.8–1.7)	
				Current smoker	2.5 (1.7–3.6)	
				1–10 pack–years	1.0 (0.6–1.6)	
				11–25 pack–years	1.5 (1.0–2.3)	
				26–50 pack–years	1.9 (1.3–2.8)	
				> 50 pack–years	1.8 (1.1–3.0)	*p* for trend = 0.04
				Current consumption		
				Men		
				1–10 pack–years	1.3 (0.3–5.4)	
				11–25 pack–years	2.7 (1.4–5.1)	
				26–50 pack–years	2.8 (1.8–4.4)	
				> 50 pack–years	2.1 (1.2–3.8)	*p* for trend < 0.001

Table 2.1.5.2 (contd)

Reference Country and years of study	Subjects	No. of cases and/or deaths	Covariates adjusted for	Smoking category and/or amount smoked	Relative risk (95% CI)	Comments
Fuchs et al. (1996) (contd)				Women		
				1–10 pack–years	1.0 (0.6–1.7)	
				11–25 pack–years	1.2 (0.7–2.0)	
				26–50 pack–years	1.2 (0.7–2.1)	
				> 50 pack–years	1.3 (0.6–2.9)	p for trend = 0.03
				Past consumption		
				< 15 years		
				1–5 pack–years	0.6 (0.5–6.5)	
				6–15 pack–years	3.9 (0.9–16)	
				16–25 pack–years	4.8 (1.1–22)	
				> 25 pack–years	5.5 (1.1–27)	p for trend = 0.01
				≥ 15 years		
				1–5 pack–years	1.6 (0.3–8.1)	
				6–15 pack–years	0.5 (0.2–2.3)	
				16–25 pack–years	0.8 (0.2–3.3)	
				> 25 pack–years	0.5 (0.1–2.2)	p for trend = 0.69
Murata et al. (1996) Japan 1984–93	Chiba Center Association Study			Cigarettes/day		Small study; small number of cases
		2		1–10	0.3	
		12		11–20	0.7	
		5		≥ 21	0.8	
Yuan et al. (1996) China 1986–93	Shanghai Men's Study 18 244 98 267 person– years	21 cases	Age and alcohol consumption	Ever-smoker	1.8	No significant dose–response relationship
				< 20 cigarettes/day	1.5	
				≥ 20 cigarettes/day	2.1	
Harnack et al. (1997) USA 1986–94	Iowa Women's Health Study 33 976 women 291 598 person– years	66 cases	Age	Former smoker	1.1 (0.6–2.1)	
				Ever-smoker	2.4 (1.3–4.2)	
				Current smoker		
				< 20 pack–years	1.1 (0.5–2.5)	
				≥ 20 pack–years	1.9 (1.1–3.3)	p for trend = 0.02

Table 2.1.5.2 (contd)

Reference Country and years of study	Subjects	No. of cases and/or deaths	Covariates adjusted for	Smoking category and/or amount smoked	Relative risk (95% CI)	Comments
Liaw & Chen (1997) China, Province of Taiwan 1982–94	Taiwanese Study	15 cases		Current smoker	0.3 (0.1–0.9)	Analysis for men only because of small number of deaths in women; small number of cases
Nordlund et al. (1997) Sweden 1963–89	Swedish Census Study 26 032 women 600 000 person–years	144 cases	Age and place of residence	Former smoker Current smoker 1–7 cigarettes/day 8–15 cigarettes/day ≥ 16 cigarettes/day	2.5 (1.1–5.3) 1.8 (1.1–2.9) 2.0 (1.2–3.5) 1.4 (0.6–3.4) 1.6 (0.4–6.7)	
			Age, place of residence and amount of tobacco smoked daily	Age at starting smoking (years) 20–23 < 19	1.1 (0.3–3.2) 0.6 (0.1–2.8)	p for trend = 0.6
Tulinius et al. (1997) Iceland 1968–95	Reykjavik Study 11 366 men, 11 580 women	101 cases (65 men, 36 women)	Age	Men Former smoker 1–14 cigarettes/day 15–24 cigarettes/day ≥ 25 cigarettes/day Women Former smoker 1–14 cigarettes/day 15–24 cigarettes/day ≥ 25 cigarettes/day	2.4 (0.7–7.6) 7.2 (2.3–22.3) 10.2 (3.4–30.6) 12.5 (3.7–41.7) 0.9 (0.3–2.8) 1.5 (0.7–3.5) 1.7 (0.6–4.4) 4.5 (1.0–20.1)	

Table 2.1.5.2 (contd)

Reference Country and years of study	Subjects	No. of cases and/or deaths	Covariates adjusted for	Smoking category and/or amount smoked	Relative risk (95% CI)	Comments
Stolzenberg-Solomon et al. (2001) Finland 1985–88	Alpha-Tocopherol Beta-Carotene Cancer Prevention Study 27101 men	157 cases	Age (continuous) and intervention (α-tocopheral and β-carotene supplements)	Cigarettes/day		All reference groups comprise light smokers.
				< 14	1.0	
				14–19	1.4 (0.9–2.4)	
				20	1.1 (0.7–1.9)	
				21–25	1.3 (0.8–2.3)	
				> 25	1.8 (1.1–3.0)	p for trend = 0.05
				Duration (years)		
				< 30	1.0	
				30–34	1.1 (0.6–2.1)	
				35–39	1.2 (0.7–2.0)	
				40–42	1.5 (0.9–2.5)	
				> 42	1.4 (0.8–2.6)	p for trend = 0.22
				Pack–years		
				< 22	1.0	
				22–31	1.2 (0.7–2.0)	
				32–39	1.3 (0.7–2.1)	
				40–49	1.3 (0.7–2.1)	
				> 49	1.7 (1.0–2.7)	p for trend = 0.04
				Age at starting smoking (years)		
				< 17	1.0	
				17–18	0.9 (0.6–1.4)	
				19	1.0 (0.5–1.9)	
				20–21	0.9 (0.5–1.4)	
				> 21	1.0 (0.6–1.6)	p for trend = 0.85
				Smoke inhalation		
				Never/seldom	1.0	
				Often	0.9 (0.5–1.7)	
				Always	1.3 (0.7–2.2)	p for trend = 0.14

CI, confidence interval

Table 2.1.5.3. Case–control studies on tobacco smoking and cancer of the pancreas

Reference Country and years of study	Subjects	Smoking categories	Odds ratio (95% CI)	Comments
Wynder et al. (1973) USA 1950–64	Men	*Cigarettes/day* 1–10 11–20 21–40 ≥ 41	2.0 2.2 3.6 5.0	$p < 0.25$ $p < 0.5$ Calculated by the Working Group
	Women	1–10 11–20 21–40 ≥ 41	0.7 5.3 1.6 0	Adjusted for age and sex
MacMahon et al. (1981) USA 1974–79	Men	*Cigarettes/day* 1–19 ≥ 20 Former smoker	1.1 1.4 1.4	
	Women	1–19 ≥ 20 Former smoker	1.5 1.6 1.3	
Durbec et al. (1983) France 1979–80	Men and women		1.3 per 10 g/day current intake	Adjusted for age, sex, neighbourhood and alcohol consumption
Whittemore et al. (1983) USA 1962–66		*Packs/year* 1–19 10–19 20–29 ≥ 30	1.0 2.1 2.4 2.5	Adjusted for age and years of schooling Overall $p < 0.05$
Wynder et al. (1983) USA 1981	Men	*Cigarettes/day* 1–10 11–20 21–30 > 31 Former smoker	0.9 2.1 ($p < 0.05$) 2.3 ($p < 0.05$) 3.0 ($p < 0.05$) 1.7 ($p < 0.05$)	Adjusted for age

Table 2.1.5.3 (contd)

Reference Country and years of study	Subjects	Smoking categories	Odds ratio (95% CI)	Comments
Wynder et al. (1983) (contd)	Women	*Cigarettes/day* 1–10 11–20 21–30 Former smoker	1.8 1.5 2.0 ($p < 0.05$) 1.4	Adjusted for age and sex
Kinlen & McPherson (1984) UK 1952–54	Men	*Cigarettes/week* 10–49 50–149 ≥ 150 Pipe	1.3 (0.5–3.2) 1.6 (0.8–3.1) 1.05 (0.4–3.0) 1.2 (0.6–2.6)	
	Women	10–49 50–149	1.1 (0.4–2.9) 1.6 (0.6–4.1)	
Gold et al. (1985) USA 1978–80	Men and women	Ever-smoker Smoker > 5 years Smoker ≥ 1 pack/day Never quitter	1.4 (0.8–2.3) 1.1 (0.1–1.9) 0.9 (0.6–1.5) 1.7 (0.9–3.4) ($p = 0.092$)	Hospital controls
	Men and women	Ever-smoker Smoker > 5 years Smoker ≥ 1 pack/day Never quitter	1.2 (0.7–2.0) 1.2 (0.7–2.0) 1.3 (0.8–2.2) 2.7 (1.3–5.7) ($p = 0.0064$)	Community controls
Hsieh et al. (1986) USA 1981–84	Men and women	Former smoker Current smoker <1 pack/day Current smoker ≥ 1 pack/day χ^2 for trend	1.0 (0.6–1.7) 1.8 (0.8–3.9) 1.9 (1.1–3.3) 5.0 ($p = 0.03$)	Adjusted for age and sex

Table 2.1.5.3 (contd)

Reference Country and years of study	Subjects	Smoking categories	Odds ratio (95% CI)	Comments
Mack et al. (1986) USA 1976–81	Men and women	*Pack/day* ≤ 1 > 1	2.4 (1.7–3.6) 2.1 (1.4–3.2)	
	Men Women	≤ 1 ≤ 1	1.8 (1.3–20.8) 2.9 (1.5–5.8)	
Wynder et al. (1986) USA 1981–84	Men	Former smoker *Cigarettes/day* 1–20 ≥ 21	1.3 (0.7–2.4) 3.5 (1.8–6.5) 2.9 (1.5–5.7)	
	Women	Former smoker *Cigarettes/day* 1–20 ≥ 21	1.2 (0.7–2.1) 1.5 (0.8–2.7) 4.8 (2.4–9.5)	
La Vecchia et al. (1987) Italy 1983–86	Men and women	≥ 15 cigarettes/day	1.4 (0.9–2.1)	Adjusted for sex and age
Clavel et al. (1989) France 1982–85	Men	Former smoker *Cigarettes/day* 1–20 ≥ 21	1.0 (0.5–2.14) 1.7 (0.8–3.7) 1.4 (0.6–3.5)	Adjusted for foreign origin, educational level, coffee and alcohol consumption
		Years of cigarette smoking 1–29 30–39 ≥ 40	0.8 (0.4–1.9) 1.0 (0.5–2.3) 1.9 (0.8–4.3)	
		Years at first cigarette ≤ 17 18–19 ≥ 20	1.8 (0.7–4.3) 0.9 (0.4–2.2) 1.5 (0.7–3.0)	

Table 2.1.5.3 (contd)

Reference Country and years of study	Subjects	Smoking categories	Odds ratio (95% CI)	Comments
Clavel *et al.* (1989) (contd)	Women	Former smoker	0.8 (0.3–2.5)	
		Cigarettes/day		
		1–20	1.0 (0.3–3.3)	
		≥ 21	2.7 (0.5–14.1)	
		Years of cigarette smoking		
		1–29	1.0 (0.4–2.6)	
		30–39	0.9 (0.2–3.7)	
		≥ 40	1.7 (0.4–6.7)	
		Years at first cigarette		
		≤ 17	3.4 (0.7–15.9)	
		18–19	0.4 (0.0–6.0)	
		≥ 20	0.9 (0.4–2.2)	
Cuzick & Babiker (1989) UK 1983–86	Men	*Cigarettes/day*		Adjusted for age, sex and social class
		< 10	1.3	
		10–20	1.7	
		> 20	4.1 ($p < 0.01$)	
		χ^2 for trend	5.74 ($p < 0.05$)	
	Women	< 10	0.8	
		10–20	1.1	
		> 20	5.5 ($p < 0.1$)	
		χ^2 for trend	1.11 ($p > 0.05$)	
	Men and women	< 10	1.1	
		10–20	1.3	
		> 20	4.4 ($p < 0.01$)	
		χ^2 for trend	5.80 ($p < 0.01$)	

Table 2.1.5.3 (contd)

Reference Country and years of study	Subjects	Smoking categories	Odds ratio (95% CI)	Comments
Ferraroni et al. (1989) Italy 1983–88	Men and women	Former smoker	1.2	Adjusted for age, sex, alcohol, education, marital status, coffee consumption; p for trend: 1.25. No difference when adjusted for age and sex only
		Current cigarette smoker		
		Cigarettes/day		
		< 15	0.8	
		15–24	1.2	
		≥ 25	1.4	
Falk et al. (1990) USA 1979–1983	Men	*Cigarettes/day*		Adjusted for age, type of respondent, ethnicity, area of residence, income, and pork and fruit intake
		1–19	1.7	
		20–29	2.3 ($p = 0.05$)	
		≥ 30	1.8	
Baghurst et al. (1991) Australia 1984–87	Men and women	Former smoker	1.1 (0.6–2.2)	χ^2 for trend with increasing alcohol consumption: 8.26 ($p = 0.004$)
		Current smoker	1.8 (0.9–3.3)	
Bueno de Mesquita et al. (1991) The Netherlands 1984–88	Men and women	All smokers		Adjusted for age, sex, response type, energy intake and vegetable consumption
		Cigarettes in lifetime		
		Low ≤ 111 200	1.4 (0.8–2.5)	
		High > 111 200	1.7 (1.0–3.1)	
		χ^2 for trend	3.26	
		Current smoker		
		Low	1.6 (0.7–3.8)	
		High	2.0 (1.0–4.0) ($p < 0.05$)	
		χ^2 for trend	4.02 ($p < 0.05$)	
		Current smoker ≤ 43 years		
		Low	2.1 (0.8–5.5)	
		High	2.3 (0.9–6.1)	
		χ^2 for trend	3.52	
		Current smoker ≥ 44 years		
		Low	0.7 (0.1–6.7)	
		High	1.8 (0.8–4.4)	
		χ^2 for trend	1.69	

Table 2.1.5.3 (contd)

Reference Country and years of study	Subjects	Smoking categories	Odds ratio (95% CI)	Comments
Bueno de Mesquita *et al.* (1991) (contd)		Former smoker		
		Cigarettes in lifetime		
		Low ≤ 111 200	1.4 (0.7–2.6)	
		High > 111 200	1.1 (0.4–2.7)	
		χ^2 for trend	0.24	
Ghadirian *et al.* (1991) Canada 1984–88	Men and women	Former smoker		Adjusted for age, sex, schooling and response type
		Cigarettes (lifetime)		
		< 104 025	1.0 (0.3–2.8)	
		104 025–219 000	3.4 (1.2–9.4)	
		219 000–405 150	5.4 (1.8–16.7)	
		> 405 150	4.0 (1.3–12.2)	
		χ^2 for trend	11.70	
		Years of smoking		
		1–20	1.2 (0.4–3.4)	
		21–32	2.9 (1.0–8.1)	
		33–39	3.0 (1.1–8.7)	
		> 39	6.2 (2.0–19.5)	
		χ^2 for trend	11.97	
		Current smoker		
		Cigarettes (lifetime)		
		<146 000	3.6 (1.3–10.0)	
		146 000–301 125	1.9 (0.7–5.4)	
		301 125–459 900	2.4 (0.9–6.2)	
		> 459 900	5.2 (1.7–16.1)	
		χ^2 for trend	8.30	
		Years of smoking		
		1–28	2.1 (0.6–7.2)	
		29–40	2.9 (1.0–8.3)	
		41–48	3.0 (1.1–8.7)	
		> 48	3.2 (1.1–9.2)	
		χ^2 for trend	9.03	

Table 2.1.5.3 (contd)

Reference Country and years of study	Subjects	Smoking categories	Odds ratio (95% CI)	Comments
Howe et al. (1991) Canada 1983–86	Men	*Packs/year* 0–17.9 17.9–37.5 > 37.5	0.9 (0.4–1.9) 1.6 (0.8–3.1) 1.6 (0.8–3.2)	Adjusted for calorie and fibre intakes
	Women	0–17.9 17.9–37.5 > 37.5	1.4 (0.7–2.8) 3.4 (1.5–7.5) 4.7 (2.0–11.4)	
	Men and women	Former smoker *Packs/year* 0–17.9 17.9–37.5 > 37.5	0.7 (0.4–1.3) 1.6 (0.8–3.2) 1.2 (0.6–2.6)	
		Current smoker *Packs/year* 0–17.9 17.9–37.5 > 37.5	2.1 (1.0–4.5) 2.9 (1.6–5.4) 3.4 (1.9–6.1)	
Vioque & Walker (1991) Multinational; early 1960s to beginning of 1980s	Men and women	Former smoker Current smoker *Packs/day* 0.5 1 ≥ 2	0.9 (0.4–1.7) 2.3 (0.7–7.3) 1.2 (0.5–3.0) 1.6 (0.8–3.3) 1.8 (0.7–4.7)	Adjusted for blood type, age, sex and hospital
Lyon et al. (1992) USA 1984–87	Men and women	*Packs/year* 1–25 ≥ 25	1.0 (0.5–2.1) 2.7 (1.4–5.2)	Adjusted for age, coffee consumption and religion

Table 2.1.5.3 (contd)

Reference Country and years of study	Subjects	Smoking categories	Odds ratio (95% CI)	Comments
Mizuno et al. (1992) Japan 1989–90	Men, at onset of study	Ever-smoker Current smoker *Cigarettes/day* Light smoker (1–12) Medium smoker (13–22) Heavy smoker (≥ 23)	2.4 (1.1–5.3) 2.8 (1.2–6.4) 6.2 (1.7–22.8) 1.8 (0.7–4.9) 2.5 (0.8–7.6)	Adjusted for age, sex and place of enrolment
	Men, 10 years prior study	Former smoker *Cigarettes/day* Light smoker (1–12) Medium smoker (13–22) Heavy smoker (≥ 23)	1.2 (0.4–3.4) 4.5 (1.5–13.2) 2.6 (1.0–6.5) 2.6 (0.9–7.0)	
Kalapothaki et al. (1993) Greece 1991–92	Men and women versus hospital controls	*Cigarettes/day* 1–10 11–20 ≥ 21	1.3 (0.5–2.9) 1.5 (0.9–2.7) 1.4 (0.8–2.4)	Adjusted for age, sex and hospital
	Men and women versus visitor controls	1–10 11–20 ≥ 21	1.0 (0.5–2.3) 1.9 (1.0–3.5) 1.8 (0.9–3.6)	
Zatonski et al. (1993) Poland 1985–88	Men and women	Ever-smoker Quartile 2 Quartile 3 Quartile 4 χ^2 for trend	1.5 (0.8–2.8) 0.8 (0.4–1.8) 2.9 (1.3–6.6) 1.5 (0.7–3.5) 3.52 (p = 0.06)	Quartiles lifetime cigarette consumption. Adjusted for schooling, age and sex
Silverman et al. (1994) USA 1986–89	Men	Years of smoking < 20 20–39 ≥ 40 p for trend	1.4 (0.8–2.3) 1.6 (1.1–2.4) 1.7 (1.1–2.7) 0.009	Adjusted for age, ethnicity, sex, area, income, alcohol consumption and gallbladder disease
	Women	< 20 20–39 ≥ 40 p for trend	0.7 (0.3–1.3) 2.0 (1.3–3.0) 2.8 (1.8–4.3) < 0.0001	

Table 2.1.5.3 (contd)

Reference Country and years of study	Subjects	Smoking categories	Odds ratio (95% CI)	Comments
Silverman *et al.* (1994) (contd)	Men and women	Ever-smoker	1.7 (1.3–2.2)	
		Former smoker	1.4 (1.1–1.9)	
		Current smoker	2.0 (1.5–2.6)	
		Cigarettes/day		
		<20	1.3 (0.9–1.7)	
		20–39	2.2 (1.7–3.0)	
		≥40	1.8 (1.2–2.8)	
		p for trend	< 0.0001	
		Years of smoking		
		<20	1.1 (0.7–1.6)	
		20–39	1.8 (1.3–2.4)	
		≥40	2.1 (1.6–2.9)	
		p for trend	< 0.0001	
		Packs/year		
		<20	1.3 (0.9–1.7)	
		20–44	1.9 (1.4–2.6)	
		≥45	2.2 (1.6–3.1)	
		p for trend	< 0.0001	
Gullo *et al.* (1995) Italy 1987–89	Men	Former smoker	0.6 (0.4–0.9)	Adjusted for age
		Current cigarette smoker		
		Cigarettes/day		
		≤ 20	0.9 (0.6–1.5)	
		> 20	1.6 (0.9–2.8)	
	Women	Former smoker	1.0 (0.5–1.9)	
		Current cigarette smoker		
		Cigarettes/day		
		≤ 20	2.2 (1.3–3.7)	
		> 20	0.6 (0.1–2.7)	

Table 2.1.5.3 (contd)

Reference Country and years of study	Subjects	Smoking categories	Odds ratio (95% CI)	Comments
Gullo et al. (1995) (contd)	Men and women	Former smoker	0.7 (0.5–1.0)	Adjusted for age and sex
		Current cigarette smoker		
		Cigarettes/day		
		≤ 20	1.3 (1.0–1.9)	
		> 20	1.4 (0.8–2.4)	
Ji et al. (1995) China 1990–93	Men	Former smoker	1.2 (0.8–2.0)	Adjusted for income and age (men), income, age, education and green tea drinking (women). Results not affected when analysis restricted to cases with histological confirmation; or whether or not interviews were conducted with next of kin or directly with the subject. Attributable risk: 24.3% (men, 95% CI, 7.1–41.3); 5.9% (women, 95% CI, 1.6–13.4)
		Current smoker	1.6 (1.1–2.2)	
		Cigarettes/day		
		1–9	0.9 (0.5–1.6)	
		10–19	1.3 (0.8–2.0)	
		20–29	1.7 (1.1–2.4)	
		≥ 30	5.0 (2.7–9.3)	
		p for trend	< 0.0001	
		Years of smoking		
		0.5–19	0.8 (0.4–1.5)	
		20–29	1.4 (0.8–2.3)	
		30–39	1.7 (1.0–2.7)	
		≥ 40	2.3 (1.5–3.5)	
		p for trend	< 0.001	
		Packs/year		
		< 15	0.8 (0.5–1.4)	
		15–34	1.5 (1.0–2.2)	
		≥ 35	2.4 (1.6–3.6)	
		p for trend	< 0.0001	
		Age at starting smoking (years)		
		≥ 30	1.5 (1.0–2.3)	
		20–29	1.6 (1.1–2.3)	
		< 20	1.7 (1.0–2.6)	
		p for trend	0.01	

Table 2.1.5.3 (contd)

Reference Country and years of study	Subjects	Smoking categories	Odds ratio (95% CI)	Comments
Ji *et al.* (1995) (contd)	Women	Former smoker	1.6 (0.6–4.0)	
		Current smoker	1.4 (0.9–2.4)	
		Cigarettes/day		
		1–9	1.1 (0.5–2.3)	
		10–19	1.3 (0.5–3.2)	
		≥ 20	2.8 (1.1–7.0)	
		p for trend	0.05	
		Years of smoking		
		0.5–19	0.6 (0.2–2.2)	
		20–29	1.4 (0.5–4.0)	
		30–39	1.7 (0.7–4.4)	
		≥ 40	2.0 (0.9–4.4)	
		p for trend	0.06	
		Packs/year		
		< 10	1.0 (0.5–2.0)	
		≥ 10	2.0 (1.0–3.8)	
		p for trend	0.07	
		Age at starting smoking (years)		
		≥ 25	1.2 (0.6–2.1)	
		< 25	2.4 (1.0–5.6)	
		p for trend	0.07	
Siemiatycki *et al.* (1995) Canada 1979–86	Men	Ever-smoker	1.6 (0.9–3.0)	Adjusted for age
		Packs/year		*p* for trend < 0.05
		≤ 25	1.2 (0.5–2.6)	
		25–49	1.7 (0.9–3.5)	
		50–74	1.8 (0.8–3.7)	
		≥ 75	1.9 (0.9–4.1)	

Table 2.1.5.3 (contd)

Reference Country and years of study	Subjects	Smoking categories	Odds ratio (95% CI)	Comments
Fernandez et al. (1996) Italy 1983–92	Men	Former smoker	1.4 (0.9–1.2)	Adjusted for sex, age, area, education and risk factors for pancreatic cancer identified in this population
		Current smoker	1.3 (0.9–1.9)	
	Women	Former smoker	0.9 (0.4–2.0)	
		Current smoker	1.3 (0.8–2.2)	
	Men and women	Former smoker	1.3 (0.9–1.9)	
		Current smoker	1.3 (0.9–1.7)	
Lee et al. (1996) China, Province of Taiwan 1989–94	Men and women (all cases)	Ever-smoker	2.3 (1.6–3.3) $(p < 0.01)$	Multivariate model unspecified. Odds ratios for histologically confirmed cases were similar
		Cigarettes/day		
		< 10	2.0 (1.0–4.0)	
		10–20	2.2 (1.4–3.4)	
		> 20	2.7 (1.6–4.7)	
		χ^2 for trend	22.02 $(p < 0.001)$	
		Years of smoking		
		≤ 10	1.4 (0.3–6.8)	
		11–20	1.3 (0.5–3.3)	
		21–30	2.7 (1.1–6.4)	
		> 30	2.5 (1.7–3.7)	
		χ^2 for trend	24.37 $(p < 0.001)$	
		Smoking index (consumption × duration)		
		< 500	1.7 (1.0–3.2)	
		500–999	2.4 (1.5–4.1)	
		≥ 1000	2.6 (1.6–4.4)	
		χ^2 for trend	22.45 $(p < 0.001)$	
Nishi et al. (1996) Japan 1987–92	Men and women	Current smoker	1.5 (0.8–3.1)	Among never-drinkers of coffee Among drinkers of ≥ 3 cups of coffee/day Adjusted for age and sex
			2.0 (0.9–4.2)	
Ohba et al. (1996) Japan 1987–92	Men and women	Former smoker	1.3 (0.7–2.1)	Univariate model. Smoking rates of the study place (Hokkaido) higher than national average
		Current smoker	1.3 (0.8–2.0)	

Table 2.1.5.3 (contd)

Reference Country and years of study	Subjects	Smoking categories	Odds ratio (95% CI)	Comments
Fryzek et al. (1997) USA 1994–95		Former smoker	1.8 (0.9–3.6)	Included cases who quit within 1 year prior to interview
		Ever-smoker	2.0 (1.1–3.8)	
		Current smoker	2.5 (1.1–5.4) ($p < 0.05$)	
		p for trend	0.02	
Muscat et al. (1997) USA 1985–93	Men	Former smoker	1.0 (0.7–1.5)	Adjusted for age and education
		Current smoker	1.6 (1.1–2.4)	
		Cigarettes/day		
		1–19	1.5 (0.9–2.4)	
		20–39	1.4 (0.7–2.8)	
		≥ 40	1.8 (0.9–3.6)	
		Years of smoking		
		1–9	0.8 (0.4–1.5)	
		10–19	1.0 (0.6–1.8)	
		20–29	1.3 (0.8–2.0)	
		30–39	1.4 (0.9–2.2)	
		≥ 40	1.3 (0.8–2.1)	
		p for trend	< 0.14	
	Women	Former smoker	1.9 (1.3–2.9)	
		Current smoker	2.3 (1.4–3.5)	
		Cigarettes/day		
		1–19	2.1 (1.3–3.6)	
		20–39	2.3 (0.8–6.3)	
		≥ 40	5.6 (2.0—5.8)	
		Years of smoking		
		1–9	1.3 (0.5–3.6)	
		10–19	1.7 (0.8–3.7)	
		20–29	2.4 (1.3–4.4)	
		30–39	2.2 (1.4–3.7)	
		≥ 40	2.1 (1.3–3.4)	
		p for trend	< 0.01	

Table 2.1.5.3 (contd)

Reference Country and years of study	Subjects	Smoking categories	Odds ratio (95% CI)	Comments
Partanen *et al.* (1997) Finland 1984–87	Men and women	Occasional smoker	1.7 (1.0–2.9)	Adjusted for age and sex
		Cigarettes/day		
		1–9	1.6 (1.2–2.2)	
		10–20	1.9 (1.5–2.5)	
		≥ 20	2.3 (1.7–3.2)	
		All smokers (includes smokers of cigarettes, pipes and cigars)	2.0 (1.6–2.4)	Adjusted for age and sex
		Age at starting smoking (years)		
		≤ 14	1.2 (0.8–2.0)	
		15–19	1.03 (1.0–1.7)	
		20–29	1.5 (1.1–1.9)	
		30–39	2.1 (1.2–3.7)	
		≥ 40	2.4 (1.0–5.4)	Adjusted for age, sex and duration of smoking
		≤ 14	0.6 (0.3–1.1)	
		15–19	0.6 (0.4–1.1)	
		20–29	0.8 (0.5–1.3)	
		30–39	1.3 (0.7–2.4)	
		≥ 40	1.6 (0.6–3.8)	
Mori *et al.* (1999) India 1994–96	Men and women	Current smoker	1.0 (0.6–1.6)	
		Cigarettes/day		
		0–9	1.0 (reference)	
		10–19	1.6 (0.6–4.2)	
		≥ 20	5.8 (2.2–15.4)	

Table 2.1.5.3 (contd)

Reference Country and years of study	Subjects	Smoking categories	Odds ratio (95% CI)	Comments
Villeneuve *et al.* (2000) Canada 1994–97	Men	*Duration of smoking (years)*		Adjusted for age, province, number of live births, alcohol, coffee, energy intake and dietary fat
		< 20	0.8 (0.5–1.2)	
		20–39	1.3 (0.9–1.9)	
		≥ 40	1.1 (0.8–1.7)	
		Cigarettes/day		
		1–9	0.8 (0.5–1.4)	
		10–24	1.1 (0.8–1.5)	
		≥ 25	1.2 (0.8–1.8)	
		Packs/year		
		0–14	0.7 (0.5–1.1)	
		15–34	1.2 (0.8–1.7)	
		≥ 35	1.5 (1.0–2.1)	
	Women	*Duration of smoking (years)*		
		< 20	1.1 (0.7–1.7)	
		20–39	1.4 (1.0–2.1)	
		≥ 40	1.8 (1.1–2.8)	
		Cigarettes/day		
		1–9	1.1 (0.7–1.7)	
		10–24	1.5 (1.1–2.1)	
		≥ 25	1.5 (0.9–2.6)	
		Packs/year		
		0–7	0.9 (0.5–1.4)	
		8–22	1.4 (1.0–2.2)	
		≥ 23	1.8 (1.3–2.7)	

CI, confidence interval

Table 2.1.5.4. Case–control studies on tobacco smoking and cancer of the pancreas: smoking cessation

Reference Country and years of study	No. of years since quitting	Odds ratio (relative to never-smokers) (95% CI)		
Mack *et al.* (1986) USA 1976–81	0–4 5–9 ≥ 10 (smoked ≤ 1 pack/day) (smoked > 1 pack/day)	3.3 (1.6–6.9) 2.3 (1.2–4.3) 1.1 (0.7–1.4) 0.9 (0.5–1.7)		
Cuzick & Babiker (1989) UK 1983–86	 < 10 10–20 > 20 χ^2 for trend	*Men* 3.6 (*p* < 0.01) 3.6 (*p* < 0.05) 1.3 8.64 (*p* < 0.01)	*Women* 0.8 1.0 1.1 0.23	*Men and women* 1.7 1.8 1.0 3.14 (*p* < 0.1)
Bueno de Mesquita *et al.* (1991) Netherlands 1984–88	 2–14 ≥ 15	*Low consumption* *(≤ 111 200 ciga-* *rettes in lifetime)* 2.0 (0.8–5.0) 1.0 (0.5–2.2)	*High consumption* *(> 111 200 cigarettes* *in lifetime)* 1.7 (0.6–4.6)	
Howe *et al.* (1991) Canada 1983–86	2–9 10–19 ≥ 20	1.8 1.4 0.7		
Silverman *et al.* (1994) USA 1986–89	1–2 3–5 6–10 11–20 > 20	3.1 (2.0–5.0) 2.0 (1.1–3.5) 1.8 (1.1–2.9) 1.2 (0.8–1.9) 1.3 (0.8–1.9)		
Ji *et al.* (1995) China 1990–93	≤ 1 2–9 ≥ 10 *p* for trend	3.8 (1.4–10.2) 1.6 (0.8–3.0) 0.7 (0.3–1.5) 0.02		
Muscat *et al.* (1997) USA 1985–93	 1–2 3–5 6–10 > 10 *p* for trend	*Men* 1.7 (0.8–3.7) 0.5 (0.2–1.1) 1.2 (0.6–2.3) 1.1 (0.7–1.6) NS	*Women* 10.6 (2.9–39.2) 1.5 (0.6–3.7) 2.1 (0.9–4.5) 1.6 (1.0–2.7) < 0.05	
Partanen *et al.* (1997) Finland 1984–87	*Any tobacco* Early quitters (before 1975) Late quitters (quit 1975–83) Continued smoking	 1.2 (0.9–1.6) 1.8 (1.3–2.6) 2.5 (1.9–3.2)		
	Cigarettes Early quitters (before < 1975) Late quitters (quit 1975–83) Continued smoking	 1.2 (0.9–1.5) 1.8 (1.3–2.5) 2.5 (1.9–3.3)		

Table 2.1.5.5. Case–control studies on tobacco smoking and cancer of the pancreas: type of tobacco and/or cigarettes

Reference Country and years of study	Type of tobacco	Odds ratio (relative to never smokers) (95% CI)				
Bueno de Mesquita *et al.* (1991) Netherlands 1984–88	Filter-tipped cigarettes	1.4 (0.9–2.1)				
	Untipped cigarettes	1.9 (1.2–3.2)				
	Low-tar cigarettes	1.8 (0.7–4.5)				
Ghadirian *et al.* (1991) Canada 1984–88		Quintiles (total cigarettes in lifetime)				
		Q2 (83 850)	Q3 (193 450)	Q4 (319 875)	Q5 (1 814 963)	χ2 for trend
	Filter-tipped cigarettes	0.9	2.5	1.6	2.9 (1.5–5.9)	9.73
	Untipped cigarettes	1.3	1.4	1.4	5.1 (2.0–13.1)	8.88
	Low-tar cigarettes	0.5	2.5	3.0	2.4 (1.1–5.5)	7.07
Howe *et al.* (1991) Canada 1983–86	Packs/year of untipped cigarettes					
	0–17.9	0.9 (0.6–1.4)				
	17.9–37.5	2.1 (1.1–4.2)				
	> 37.5	0.9 (0.4–2.0)				
	Packs/year of filter-tipped cigarettes					
	0–17.9	1.3 (0.8–2.1)				
	17.9–37.5	2.3 (1.4–3.7)				
	> 37.5	2.4 (1.3–4.2)				

References

Akiba, S. & Hirayama, T. (1990) Cigarette smoking and cancer mortality risk in Japanese men and women — Results from reanalysis of the six-prefecture cohort study data. *Environ. Health Perspect.*, **87**,19–26

Baghurst, P.A., McMichael, A.J., Slavotinek, A.H., Baghurst, K.I., Boyle, P. & Walker, A.M. (1991) A case–control study of diet and cancer of the pancreas. *Am. J. Epidemiol.*, **134**, 167–179

Boyle, P., Maisonneuve, P., Bueno de Mesquita, B., Ghadirian, P., Howe, G.R., Zatonski, W., Baghurst, P., Moerman, C.J., Simard, A., Miller, A.B., Przewoniak, K., McMichael, A.J., Hsieh, C.-C. & Walker, A.M. (1996) Cigarette smoking and pancreas cancer: A case–control study of the SEARCH programme of the IARC. *Int. J. Cancer*, **67**, 63–71

Bueno de Mesquita, H.B., Masonneuve, P., Moerman, C.J., Runia, S. & Boyle, P. (1991) Life-time history of smoking and exocrine carcinoma of the pancreas: A population-based case–control study in the Netherlands. *Int. J. Cancer*, **49**, 816–822

Cederlöf, R., Friberg, L., Hrubec, Z. & Lorich, U. (1975) *The Relationship of Smoking and Some Social Covariables to Mortality and Cancer Morbidity. A Ten Year Follow-up in a Probability Sample of 55 000 Swedish Subjects, Age 18-69, Part 1 and Part 2*, Stockholm, Department of Environmental Hygiene, The Karolinska Institute

Clavel, F., Benhamou, E., Auquier, A., Tarayre, M. & Flamant, R. (1989) Coffee, alcohol, smoking and cancer of the pancreas: A case–control study. *Int. J. Cancer*, **43**, 17–21

Cuzick, J. & Babiker, A.G. (1989) Pancreatic cancer, alcohol, diabetes mellitus and gall-bladder disease. *Int. J. Cancer*, **43**, 415–421

Doll, R. & Peto, R. (1976) Mortality in relation to smoking: 20 years' observations on male British doctors. *Br. med. J.*, **ii**, 1525–1536

Doll, R., Gray, R., Hafner, B. & Peto, R. (1980) Mortality in relation to smoking: 22 years' observations on female British doctors. *Br. med. J.*, **i**, 967–971

Doll, R., Peto, R., Wheatley, K., Gray, R. & Sutherland, I. (1994) Mortality in relation to smoking: 40 years' observations in male British doctors. *Br. med. J.*, **309**, 901–911

Durbec, J.P., Chevillotte, G., Bidart, J.M., Berhezene, P. & Sarles, H. (1983) Diet, alcohol, tobacco and risk of cancer of the pancreas: A case–control study. *Br. J. Cancer*, **47**, 463–470

Engeland, A., Andersen, A., Haldorsen, T. & Tretli, S. (1996) Smoking habits and risk of cancers other than lung cancer: 28 years' follow-up of 26,000 Norwegian men and women. *Cancer Causes Control*, **7**, 497–506

Falk, R.T., Pickle, L.W., Fontham, E.T., Correa, P., Morse, A., Chen, V. & Fraumeni, J.F., Jr (1990) Occupation and pancreatic risk in Louisiana. *Am. J. ind. Med.*, **18**, 565–576

Fernandez, E., La Vecchia, C. & Decarli, A. (1996) Attributable risks for pancreatic cancer in northern Italy. *Cancer Epidemiol. Biomarkers Prev.*, **5**, 23–27

Ferraroni, M., Negri, E., La Vecchia, C., D'Avanzo, B. & Franceschi, S. (1989) Socioeconomic indicators, tobacco and alcohol in the aetiology of digestive tract neoplasms. *Int. J. Epidemiol.*, **18**, 556–562

Friedman, G.D. & van den Eeden, S.K. (1993) Risk factors for pancreatic cancer: An exploratory study. *Int. J. Epidemiol.*, **22**, 30–37

Friedman, G.D., Sadler, M., Tekawa, I.S. & Sidney, S. (1998) Mentholated cigarettes and non-lung smoking related cancers in California, USA. *J. Epidemiol. Community Health*, **52**, 202

Fryzek, J.P., Garabrant, D.H., Harlow, S.D., Severson, R.K., Gillespie, B.W., Schenk, M. & Schottenfeld, D. (1997) A case–control study of self-reported exposures to pesticides and pancreas cancer in southeastern Michigan. *Int. J. Cancer*, **72**, 62–67

Fuchs, C.S., Colditz, G.A., Stampfer, M.J., Giovannucci, E.L., Hunter, D.J., Rimm, E.G., Willett, W.C. & Speizer, F.E. (1996) A prospective study of cigarette smoking and the risk of pan-creatic cancer. *Arch. intern. Med.*, **156**, 2255–2260

Ghadirian, P., Simard, A. & Baillargeon, J. (1991) Tobacco, alcohol, and coffee and cancer of the pancreas. A population-based, case–control study in Quebec, Canada. *Cancer*, **67**, 2664–2670

Gold, E.B., Gordis, L., Diener, M.D., Seltser, R., Boitnott, J.K., Bynum, T.E. & Hutcheon, D.F. (1985) Diet and other risk factors for cancer of the pancreas. *Cancer*, **55**, 460–467

Gullo, L., Pezzilli R., Morselli-Labate, A.M. & the Italian Pancreatic Cancer Study Group (1995) Coffee and cancer of the pancreas: An Italian multicencer study. *Pancreas*, **11**, 223–229

Hammond, E.C. (1966) Smoking in relation to the death rates of one million men and women. *Natl. Cancer Inst. Monogr.*, **19**, 127–204

Hammond, E.C. & Horn, D. (1958a) Smoking and death rates — Report on forty-four months of follow-up of 187 783 men. I. Total mortality. *J. Am. med. Assoc.*, **166**, 1159–1172

Hammond, E.C. & Horn, D. (1958b) Smoking and death rates — Report on forty-four months of follow-up of 187 783 men. II. Death rates by cause. *J. Am. med. Assoc.*, **166**, 1294–1308

Harnack, L.J., Anderson, K.E., Zheng, W., Folsom, A.R., Sellers, T.A. & Kushi, L.H. (1997) Smoking, alcohol, coffee, and tea intake and incidence of cancer of the exocrine pancreas: The Iowa Women's Health Study. *Cancer Epidemiol. Biomarkers Prev.*, **6**, 1081–1086

Heuch, I., Kvåle, G., Jacobsen, B.K. & Bjelke, E. (1983) Use of alcohol, tobacco and coffee, and risk of pancreatic cancer. *Br. J. Cancer*, **48**, 637–643

Hiatt, R.A., Klatsky, A.L. & Armstrong, M.A. (1988) Pancreatic cancer, blood glucose and beverage consumption. *Int. J. Cancer*, **41**, 794–797

Hirayama, T. (1981) A large-scale cohort study on the relationship between diet and selected cancers of digestive organs. In: Bruce, W.R., Correa, P., Lipkin, M., Tannenbaum, S.R. & Wilkins, T.D., eds, *Gastrointestinal Cancer: Endogenous Factors* (Banbury Report 7), Cold Spring Harbor, NY, Cold Spring Harbor Laboratory, pp. 409–426

Hirayama, T. (1989) Epidemiology of pancreatic cancer in Japan. *Jpn. J. clin. Oncol.*, **19**, 208–215

Howe, G.R., Jain, M., Burch, J.D. & Miller, A.B. (1991) Cigarette smoking and cancer of the pancreas: Evidence from a population-based case–control study in Toronto, Canada. *Int. J. Cancer*, **47**, 323–328

Hsieh, C.C., MacMahon, B., Yen, S., Trichopoulos, D., Warren, K. & Nardi, G. (1986) Coffee and pancreatic cancer. *New Engl. J. Med.*, **315**, 587–589

IARC (1986) *IARC Monographs on the Evaluation of the Carcinogenic Risk of Chemicals to Humans*, Vol. 38, *Tobacco Smoking*, Lyon, IARCPress

Ji, B.T., Chow, W.H., Dai, Q., McLaughlin, J.K., Benichou, J., Hatch, M.C., Gao, Y.T. & Fraumeni, J.F., Jr (1995) Cigarette smoking and alcohol consumption and the risk of pancreatic cancer: A case–control study in Shanghai, China. *Cancer Causes Control*, **6**, 369–376

Kahn, H.A. (1966) The Dorn study of smoking and mortality among US veterans: Report on eight and one-half years of observation. *Natl Cancer Inst. Monogr.*, **19**, 1–125

Kalapothaki, V., Tzonou, A., Hsieh, C.C., Toupadaki, N., Karakatsani, A. & Trichopoulos, D. (1993) Tobacco, ethanol, coffee, pancreatitis, diabetes mellitus, and cholelithiasis as risk factors for pancreatic carcinoma. *Cancer Causes Control*, **4**, 375–382

Kinlen, L.J. & McPherson, K. (1984) Pancreas cancer and coffee and tea consumption: A case–control study. *Br. J. Cancer*, **49**, 93–96

Kuller, L.H., Ockene, J.K., Meilahn, E., Wentworth, D.N., Svendsen, K.H. & Neaton, J.D. for the MRFIT Research Group (1991) Cigarette smoking and mortality. *Prev. Med.*, **20**, 638–654

La Vecchia, C., Liati, P., Decarli, A., Negri, E. & Franceschi, S. (1987) Coffee consumption and risk of pancreatic cancer. *Int. J. Cancer*, **40**, 309–313

Lee, C.T., Chang, F.Y. & Lee, S.D. (1996) Risk factors for pancretic cancer in orientals. *J. Gastroenterol. Hepatol.*, **11**, 491–495

Liaw, K.M. & Chen, C.J. (1998) Mortality attributable to cigarette smoking in Taiwan: A 12-year follow-up study. *Tob. Control,* **7**, 141–148

Lossing, E.H., Best, E.W.R., McGregor, J.T., Josie, G.H., Walker, C.B., Delaquis, F.M., Baker, P.M. & McKenzie, A.C. (1966) *A Canadian Study of Smoking and Health*, Ottawa, Department of National Health and Welfare

Lyon, J.L., Mahoney, A.W., French, T.K. & Moser, R. (1992) Coffee consumption and the risk of cancer of the exocrine pancreas: A case–control study in a low-risk population. *Epidemiology*, **3**, 164–170

Mack, R.M., Yu, M.C., Hanisch, R. & Henderson, B.E. (1986) Pancreas cancer and smoking, beverage consumption, and past medical history. *J. natl Cancer Inst.*, **76**, 49–60

MacMahon, B., Yen, S., Trichopoulos, D., Warren, K. & nardi, G. (1981) Coffee and cancer of the pancreas. *New Engl. J. Med.*, **304**, 630–633

McLaughlin, J.K., Hrubec, Z., Blot, W.J. & Fraumeni, J.F. (1995) Smoking and cancer mortality among US veterans: A 26-year follow-up. *Int. J. Cancer*, **60**, 190–193

Mills, P.K., Beeson, W.L., Abbey, D.E., Fraser, G.E. & Phillips, R.L. (1988) Dietary habits and past medical history as related to fatal pancreas cancer risk among Adventists. *Cancer*, **61**, 2578–2585

Mizuno, S., Watanabe, S., Nakamura, K., Omata, M., Oguchi, H., Ohashi, K. Ohyanagi, H., Fujiki, T. & Motojima, K. (1992) A multi-institute case–control study on the risk factors of developing pancreatic cancer. *Jpn. J. clin. Oncol.*, **22**, 286–291

Mori, M., Hariharan, M., Anandakumar, M., Tsutsumi, M., Ishikawa, O., Konishi, Y., Chellam, V.G., John, M., Praseeda, I., Priya, R. & Narendranathan, M. (1999) A case–control study on risk factors for pancreatic diseases in Kerala, India. *Hepatogastroenterology*, **46**, 25–30

Murata, M., Takayama, K., Choi, B.C.K. & Pak, A.W.P. (1996) A nested case–control study on alcohol drinking, tobacco smoking, and cancer. *Cancer Detect. Prev.*, **20**, 557–565

Muscat, J.E., Stellman, S.D., Hoffmann, D. & Wynder, E.L. (1997) Smoking and pancreatic cancer in men and women. *Cancer Epidemiol. Biomarkers Prev.*, **6**, 15–19

Nishi, M., Ohba, S., Hirata, K. & Miyake, H. (1996) Dose–response relationship between coffee and the risk of pancreas cancer. *Jpn. J. clin. Oncol.*, **26**, 42–48

Nordlund, L.A., Carstensen, J.M. & Pershagen, G. (1997) Cancer incidence in female smokers: A 26-year follow-up. *Int. J. Cancer*, **73**, 625–628

Ohba, S., Nishi, M. & Miyake, H. (1996) Eating habits and pancreas cancer. *Int. J. Pancreatol.*, **20**, 37–42

Partanen, T.J., Vainio, H.U., Ojajarvi, I.A. & Kauppinen, T.P. (1997) Pancras cancer, tobaco smoking and consumption of alcoholic beverages: A case–control study. *Cancer Lett.*, **116**, 27–32

Siemiatycki, J., Krewski, D., Franco, E. & Kaiserman, M. (1995) Associations between cigarette smoking and each of 21 types of cancer: A multi-site case–control study. *Int. J. Epidemiol.*, **24**, 504–514

Shibata, A., Mack, T.M., Paganini-Hill, A., Ross, R.K. & Henderson, B.E. (1994) A prospective study of pancreatic cancer in the elderly. *Int. J. Cancer*, **58**, 46–49

Silverman, D.T., Dunn, J.A., Hoover, R.N., Schiffman, M., Lillemoe, K.D., Schoenberg, J.B., Brown, L.M., Greenberg, R.S., Hayes, R.B. & Swanson, G.M. (1994) Cigarette smoking and pancreas cancer: A case–control study based on direct interviews. *J. natl Cancer Inst.*, **86**, 1510–1516

Stolzenberg-Solomon, R.Z., Pietinen, P., Barrett, M.J., Taylor, P.R., Virtamo, J. & Albanes, D. (2001) Dietary and other methyl-group availability factors and pancreatic cancer risk in a cohort of male smokers. *Am. J. Epidemiol.*, **153**, 680–687

Tulinius, H., Sigfusson, N., Sigvaldason, H., Bjarnadottir, K. & Tryggvadottir, L. (1997) Risk factors for malignant diseases: A cohort study on a population of 22,946 Icelanders. *Cancer Epidemiol. Biomarkers Prev.*, **6**, 863–973

Tverdal, A., Thelle, D., Stensvold, I., Leren, P. & Bjartveit, K. (1993) Mortality in relation to smoking history: 13 years' follow-up of 68,000 Norwegian men and women 35–49 years. *J. clin. Epidemiol.*, **46**, 475–487

Villeneuve, P.J., Johnson, K.C., Hanley, A.J., Mao, Y. & the Canadian Cancer Registries Epidemiology Research Group (2000) Alcohol, tobacco and coffee consumption and the risk of pancreatic cancer: Results from the Canadian Enahnced Surveillance System case–control project. *Eur. J. Cancer Prev.*, **9**, 49–58

Vioque, J. & Walker, A.M. (1991) [Pancreatic cancer and ABO blood types: a case–control study.] *Med. clin.*, **96**, 761–764 (in Spanish)

Weir, J.M. & Dunn, J.E., Jr (1970) Smoking and mortality: A prospective study. *Cancer*, **25**, 105–112

Whittemore, A.S., Paffenbarger, R.S., Jr, Anderson, K. & Halpern, J. (1983) Early precursors of pancreatic cancer in college men. *J. chron. Dis.*, **36**, 251–256

Wynder, E.L., Mabuchi, K., Maruchi, N. & Fortner, J.G. (1973) A case control study of cancer of the pancreas. *Cancer*, **31**, 641–648

Wynder, E.L., Hall, N.E. & Polansky, M. (1983) Epidemiology of coffee and pancreatic cancer. *Cancer Res.*, **43**, 3900–3906

Wynder, E.L., Dieck, G.S. & Hall, N.E.L. (1986) Case–control study of decaffeinated coffee consumption and pancreatic cancer. *Cancer Res.*, **46**, 5360–5363

Yuan, J.M., Ross, R.K., Wang, X.L., Gao, Y.T., Henderson, B.E. & Yu, M.C. (1996) Morbidity and mortality in relation to cigarette smoking in Shanghai, China. A prospective male cohort study. *J. Am. med. Assoc.*, **275**, 1646–1650

Zatonski, W.A., Boyle, P., Przewozniak, K., Maisonneuve, P., Drosik, K. & Walker, A.M. (1993) Cigarette smoking, alcohol, tea and coffee consumption and pancreas cancer risk: A case–control study from Opole, Poland. *Int. J. Cancer*, **53**, 601–607

Zheng, W., McLaughlin, J.K., Gridley, G., Bjelke, E., Schuman, L.M., Silverman, D.T., Wacholder, S., Co-Chien, H.T., Blot, W.J. & Fraumeni, J.F. (1993) A cohort study of smoking, alcohol consumption, and dietary factors for pancreatic cancer (United States). *Cancer Causes Control*, **4**, 477–482

2.1.6   Cancer of the stomach

(a)   Cohort studies

A total of 29 prospective cohort studies have examined the association between smoking and stomach cancer. The details of the design of these studies are described in Table 2.1 and Table 2.1.6.1. Summary findings are presented in Table 2.1.6.2.

(i)   Intensity and duration of smoking

Intensity (cigarettes/day), age at starting smoking and/or duration of smoking were studied in almost all of the cohorts. Sixteen cohort studies reported a statistically significant association between smoking and the risk for stomach cancer, with odds ratios ranging from 1.4 to 2.6 in current smokers (Kahn, 1966; Hirayama, 1982, 1985; Kono et al., 1987; Akiba & Hirayama, 1990; McLaughlin et al., 1990; Nomura et al., 1990a,b; Kneller et al., 1991; Kato et al., 1992a; Doll et al., 1994; McLaughlin et al., 1995; Nomura et al., 1995; Liaw & Chen, 1998; Gao et al., 1999; You et al., 2000; Chao et al., 2002). In eight of these studies, significant dose–response relationships were observed between intensity of smoking and the risk for stomach cancer (Kahn, 1966; Hirayama, 1985; Akiba & Hirayama, 1990; McLaughlin et al., 1990; Kneller et al., 1991; Doll et al., 1994; McLaughlin et al., 1995; Gao et al., 1999) and in five studies between duration of smoking and risk for stomach cancer (McLaughlin et al., 1990; Nomura et al., 1995; Liaw & Chen, 1998; You et al., 2000; Chao et al., 2002). In eight cohort studies, the increase in risk associated with smoking was statistically non-significant (Hammond, 1966; Doll & Peto, 1976; Kato et al., 1992b; Tverdal et al., 1993; Engeland et al., 1996; Yuan et al., 1996; Nordlund et al., 1997; Mizoue et al., 2000). Five studies did not find any association between smoking and stomach cancer (Guo et al., 1994; Murata et al., 1996; Chen et al., 1997; Tulinius et al., 1997; Terry et al., 1998).

Many studies that have tested the statistical significance of trend in risk with duration of smoking or number of cigarettes/day have included nonsmokers in the analysis. [The Working Group noted that the preferred approach is to limit testing for trend to exposed persons across gradients of exposure.]

(ii)   Smoking cessation

Relative risks in former smokers have been examined in 16 studies and two studies have assessed the effect of number of years since quitting (Guo et al., 1994; Chao et al., 2002). The risk in former smokers ranged from 1.2 to 2.6 in men and women combined, from 0.9 to 2.2 in men and from 0.2 to 1.4 in women. Increasing number of years since cessation and younger age at cessation were associated with a significant trend in decreasing risk (Chao et al., 2002).

(iii)   Effect of sex

Data for men and women were combined in five studies, seven studies presented data separated by sex, 16 studies presented results for men only and one study for women only.

Generally, the numbers of incident cases and of deaths from stomach cancer in women were small. The risks for stomach cancer associated with smoking were assessed separately for women in only seven cohort studies and, of these, only three reported significant increases in risk (Akiba & Hirayama, 1990; Gao *et al.*, 1999; Chao *et al.*, 2002). In three studies, increases in risk were statistically non-significant (Hirayama, 1982; Kato *et al.*, 1992a; Nordlund *et al.*, 1997) and, in one study, smoking was not associated with risk for stomach cancer (Engeland *et al.*, 1996).

(iv)   *Bias and misclassification*

Several limitations of cohort studies should be considered. First, some studies reported a low response rate in the initial survey and a high proportion of individuals who were lost to follow-up, leading to selection bias. Second, most cohorts were followed passively and the information on smoking habits was based only on the initial survey, although many cohort members could have subsequently changed their smoking habits. Therefore, misclassification of former smokers as current smokers is possible. Thus, the risk for stomach cancer is most probably underestimated in most, if not all, cohort studies. The results of cohort studies could also be confounded by the effects of alcohol consumption. Only seven studies adjusted relative risks for alcohol consumption (Kono *et al.*, 1987; Kato *et al.*, 1992a; Nomura *et al.*, 1995; Chen *et al.*, 1997; Liaw & Chen, 1998; Mizoue *et al.*, 2000; You *et al.*, 2000). In most of these studies, the risk for stomach cancer in smokers was significantly different from unity.

(b)   *Case–control studies*

Forty-five case–control studies detailed in Tables 2.1.6.3 and 2.1.6.4 have reported results regarding the influence of smoking on the risk for stomach cancer. Some very weak, early studies, although reported in Tables 2.1.6.3 and 2.1.6.4 for completeness, will not be considered further here (Wynder *et al.*, 1963; Staszewski, 1969; Ames & Gamble, 1983). Twenty-three studies were hospital-based, one was a retrospective mortality study and 18 studies were population-based. In most studies, odds ratios were adjusted for variables such as sex, age, residence, socioeconomic status, income, diet and consumption of fresh fruits and vegetables. Odds ratios were adjusted for alcohol consumption in 18 studies (Hoey *et al.*, 1981; Correa *et al.*, 1985; Hu *et al.*, 1988; You *et al.*, 1988; Ferraroni *et al.*, 1989; De Stefani *et al.*, 1990; Lee *et al.*, 1990; Jedrychowski *et al.*, 1993; Kabat *et al.*, 1993; Siemiatycki *et al.*, 1995; Ji *et al.*, 1996; Zhang *et al.*, 1996; Gammon *et al.*, 1997; De Stefani *et al.*, 1998; Inoue *et al.*, 1999; Ye *et al.*, 1999; Lagergren *et al.*, 2000; Zaridze *et al.*, 2000).

(i)   *Intensity and duration*

Thirty-one case–control studies (Haenszel *et al.*, 1972; Hoey *et al.*, 1981; Correa *et al.*, 1985; Risch *et al.*, 1985; Hu *et al.*, 1988; You *et al.*, 1988; De Stefani *et al.*, 1990; Kato *et al.*, 1990; Lee *et al.*, 1990; Wu-Williams *et al.*, 1990; Dockerty *et al.*, 1991; Saha, 1991; Yu & Hsieh, 1991; Kabat *et al.*, 1993; Hansson *et al.*, 1994; Inoue *et al.*, 1994;

Siemiatycki *et al.*, 1995; Yu *et al.*, 1995; Gajalakashmi & Shanta, 1996; Ji *et al.*, 1996; Zhang *et al.*, 1996; Gammon *et al.*, 1997; De Stefani *et al.*, 1998; Liu *et al.*, 1998; Chow *et al.*, 1999; Inoue *et al.*, 1999; Ye *et al.*, 1999; Lagergren *et al.*, 2000; Mathew *et al.*, 2000; Zaridze *et al.*, 2000; Wu *et al.*, 2001) reported a statistically significant association between smoking and the risk for stomach cancer. Most studies published after 1990 examined the effect of intensity and duration of smoking on the risk for stomach cancer. In most of them, there was a statistically significant dose–response trend between the number of cigarettes smoked daily, duration of smoking and/or age at start and the risk for stomach cancer (Hu *et al.*, 1988; You *et al.*, 1988; De Stefani *et al.*, 1990; Kato *et al.*, 1990; Lee *et al.*, 1990; Wu-Williams *et al.*, 1990; Yu & Hsieh, 1991; Kabat *et al.*, 1993; Hansson *et al.*, 1994; Gajalakashmi & Shanta, 1996; Ji *et al.*, 1996; Zhang *et al.*, 1996; Gammon *et al.*, 1997; De Stefani *et al.*, 1998; Ye *et al.*, 1999; Lagergren *et al.*, 2000; Mathew *et al.*, 2000; Zaridze *et al.*, 2000; Wu *et al.*, 2001). In nine studies, no association was found between smoking and the risk for stomach cancer (Jedrychowski *et al.*, 1986; Buiatti *et al.*, 1989; Ferraroni *et al.*, 1989; Boeing *et al.*, 1991; Buiatti *et al.*, 1991; Agudo *et al.*, 1992; Palli *et al.*, 1992; Jedrychowski *et al.*, 1993; Gao *et al.*, 1999).

(ii) *Smoking cessation*

Twenty-five studies examined relative risks in former smokers and several also examined the effect of cessation of smoking (De Stefani *et al.*, 1990; Kabat *et al.*, 1993; Hansson *et al.*, 1994; Inoue *et al.*, 1994; Ji *et al.*, 1996; Gammon *et al.*, 1997; De Stefani *et al.*, 1998; Chow *et al.*, 1999; Ye *et al.*, 1999; Lagergren *et al.*, 2000; Wu *et al.*, 2001). Quitting smoking was found to decrease the risk for cancer. A significant negative trend for increasing number of years since cessation was reported in six studies (De Stefani *et al.*, 1990; Hansson *et al.*, 1994; Inoue *et al.*, 1994; Gammon *et al.*, 1997; De Stefani *et al.*, 1998; Lagergren *et al.*,. 2000), whereas two studies found no effect (Kabat *et al.*, 1993; Ji *et al.*, 1996). However, in examining temporal trends in risk with time since cessation, some studies did not exclude persons who had quit recently, among whom increased risk may reflect cessation due to smoking-attributable disease.

(iii) Subsites of stomach cancer

Several case–control studies presented studies by subsites (De Stefani *et al.*, 1990; Wu-Williams *et al.*, 1990; Saha, 1991; Palli *et al.*, 1992; Kabat *et al.*, 1993; Inoue *et al.*, 1994; Zhang *et al.*, 1996; Gammon *et al.*, 1997; De Stefani *et al.*, 1998; Ye *et al.*, 1999; Zardize *et al.*, 2000; Wu *et al.*, 2001). In all the studies that distinguished between cancer of the gastric cardia and distal stomach, an effect of smoking was seen on the risk for cancers at both sites. Dose–response relationships were observed between number of cigarettes smoked per day, duration of smoking and time since quitting for cancers of both sites. The significant association between smoking and cancer risk persisted when relative risks were examined separately for intestinal and diffuse histological types (Kato *et al.*, 1990; Ye *et al.*, 1999).

(iv)   *Effect of sex*

Most studies included both men and women; seven studies reported results for men only and only eight reported results for men and women separately (Haenszel *et al.*, 1972; Kato *et al.*, 1990; Kabat *et al.*, 1993; Inoue *et al.*, 1994; Ji *et al.*, 1996; Liu *et al.*, 1998; Chow *et al.*, 1999; Inoue *et al.*, 1999). The number of cases of stomach cancer in women was generally small and the increase in risk estimates was generally lower than that for men and was not statistically significant (Kato *et al.*, 1990; Inoue *et al.*, 1994; Ji *et al.*, 1996; Liu *et al.*, 1998). However, in the studies in which a sufficient number of cases of stomach cancer in women were included, the relative risks were significant and comparable with those in men (Kabat *et al.*, 1993; Chow *et al.*, 1999; Inoue *et al.*, 1999).

(v)   *Effect of ethnicity*

The only study that investigated ethnicity reported a significantly higher risk for African Americans than for Caucasians (Correa *et al.*, 1985).

(vi)   *Type of tobacco and type of cigarette*

The effects of black and blond tobacco were distinguished only by De Stefani *et al.* (1990, 1998). Five studies evaluated the effect of filter tips (De Stefani *et al.*, 1990; Jedrychowski *et al.*, 1993; Gammon *et al.*, 1997; De Stefani *et al.*, 1998; Chow *et al.*, 1999) and one study looked at the effect of swallowing tobacco smoke (Saha, 1991). The risk associated with smoking black tobacco was higher than that for smoking blond tobacco (De Stefani *et al.*, 1990, 1998). There was no clear difference in risk between smokers of filter-tipped or untipped cigarettes or whether or not smoke is swallowed.

(vii)   *Bias and misclassification*

The relative risk for stomach cancer associated with smoking is most probably underestimated, particularly in hospital-based case–control studies, because of a substantial proportion of controls with smoking-related diseases. Of special concern are the studies in which prevalence of smoking was higher in controls than in cases and in which controls with smoking-associated diseases were included (Haenszel *et al.*, 1976; Correa *et al.*, 1985; Jedrychowski *et al.*, 1986; Lee *et al.*, 1990; Boeing *et al.*, 1991; Agudo *et al.*, 1992; Zaridze *et al.*, 2000) or in which the diagnoses of hospital controls were not reported (Haenszel *et al.*, 1972).

(c)   Helicobacter pylori *infection*

A positive association between smoking and the risk for stomach cancer could be confounded by the effect of *Helicobacter pylori* infection status. A large body of evidence supports a causative role for *H. pylori* in stomach cancer. In 1994, IARC recognized *H. pylori* as a class 1 human carcinogen (IARC, 1994).

None of the available cohort studies have assessed *H. pylori* infection status. Two case–control studies investigated the interaction between *H. pylori* seropositivity and smoking in relation to the risk for stomach cancer (Zaridze *et al.*, 2000; Siman *et al.*,

2001). The relative risk for stomach cancer was higher in *H. pylori*-infected men (Zaridze *et al.*, 2000). These results suggest that smoking may potentiate the carcinogenic effect of *H. pylori*.

Several studies have shown that *H. pylori* infection status is not associated with smoking habit. Limburg *et al.* (2001) examined the association between seropositivity for *H. pylori* and different risk factors. The proportion of seropositive individuals was similar in nonsmokers (58%) and in smokers (61%). Moreover, the prevalence of CagA-sero-positive individuals was higher in nonsmokers (32%) than in smokers (24%). Another study in China looked at the association between the prevalence of *H. pylori* infection and smoking, alcohol consumption and diet. The prevalence of *H. pylori* positivity was lower among ever-smokers than never-smokers, with an odds ratio for ever-smokers of 0.9 (95% CI, 0.7–1.0). In the highest category of smokers, who had a lifetime exposure of more than 14 235 packs, the odds ratio was 0.8 (95% CI, 0.6–1.1) (Brown *et al.*, 2002).

Similar evidence has been obtained in Europe. The prevalence of seropositive subjects is similar among never- (50.9%), former (48.7%) and current smokers (45.1%). In fact, the percentage of *H. pylori* seropositivity is somewhat lower among current smokers than among never-smokers (crude odds ratio, 0.8; 95% CI, 0.7–0.9) (EUROGAST Study Group, 1993). In only one study conducted in northern England was smoking more than 35 cigarettes/day found to be associated with higher risk for *H. pylori* positivity (Moayyedi *et al.*, 2002). However, it should be noted that the proportion of subjects infected was identical in all categories of low smoking intensity. Overall, there is no association between *H. pylori* infection status and smoking. Therefore, *H. pylori* is of little or no relevance with regard to potential confounding of the association between smoking and stomach cancer.

(*d*)   *Precursor lesions*

According to one widely accepted model of gastric carcinogenesis, development of stomach cancer is preceded by several precursor stages, including chronic atrophic gastritis, intestinal metaplasia and dysplasia. An increase in the relative risk for developing these lesions has been shown to be associated with smoking, with a significant positive trend associated with intensity and duration of smoking. The magnitude of the association was stronger for dysplasia than for metaplasia (Kneller *et al.*, 1991). You *et al.* (2000) found an increased risk for the progression of precursor lesions to dysplasia and cancer for subjects who had smoked for more than 25 years and a significant trend with increasing duration of smoking.

Overall, the results from both cohort and case–control studies are consistent with a causal role of tobacco smoking in the development of stomach cancer.

Table 2.1.6.1. Additional cohort studies on tobacco smoking and stomach cancer: main characteristics of study design

Reference Country and years of follow-up	Cohort sample	Cases/deaths identification	Comments
Kato et al. (1992a) Japan 1985–91	9753 male (≥ 40 years) and female (≥ 30 years) inhabitants of a mountainous area of Aichi prefecture	Death certificates	Questionnaires linked to data from another questionnaire survey conducted in 1983–84 that included information on smoking habits
Kato et al. (1992b) Japan 1985–89	5395 patients receiving gastroscopic examination at Aichi Centre Hospital	Linkage with gastro-endoscopic records at Aichi Cancer Centre Hospital, Aichi Cancer Registry and death certificates	Diagnoses at baseline included: atrophic gastritis (mild, moderate/severe), 'extension on the greater curvature', 'extension on the lesser curvature', gastric ulcer and gastric polyp (none with normal gastric mucosa)
You et al. (2000) China 1989–94	3433 subjects participating in a gastric cancer-screening study, residents in 14 villages randomly selected within Linqu County, aged 35–64 years	Cases identified by pathological examination of biopsies and endoscopic examination	Diagnosis of cohort members divided into superficial gastritis or chronic atrophic gastritis, intestinal metaplasia and dysplasia (none with normal gastric mucosa)

Table 2.1.6.2. Cohort studies on tobacco smoking and stomach cancer

Reference Country and years of study	No. of subjects	No. of cases	Exposure estimates	Relative risk (95% CI)	Comments
Hammond (1966) USA 1959–62	Cancer Prevention Study I 440 558 men, 562 671 women 1 639 211 person–years	562 deaths (343 men, 219 women); 283 deaths in men aged ≥ 45 years	Aged 45–64 (n = 131) Aged 65–79 (n = 79)	Mortality ratio 1.4 1.3	Data presented for men only
Kahn (1966) USA 1954–62	US Veterans' Study 293 658 men 2 265 674 person–years	420 deaths	Non- or occasional smoker	Mortality ratio 1.0	Crude mortality ratio
			Current cigarette smoker[†]		[†]'Current and former 'cigarette
			Total	1.5 (p < 0.01)	smoker' refer to combined use
			Occasional	0.7	of cigarettes and other forms
			Cigarettes/day		of tobacco
			1–9	1.7	
			10–20	1.4 (p < 0.01)	
			21–39	1.6 (p < 0.01)	
			≥ 40	1.8 (p < 0.01)	p for trend < 0.01
			Current cigarette-only smoker		
			Total	1.6	
			Occasional	0.6	
			Cigarettes/day		
			1–9	2.2	
			10–20	1.6	
			21–39	1.4	
			≥ 40	1.9	
			Former cigarette smoker[†]		
			Total	1.03	
			Cigarettes/day		
			1–9	0.98	
			10–20	0.8	
			21–39	1.1	
			≥ 40	2.0	

Table 2.1.6.2 (contd)

Reference Country and years of study	No. of subjects	No. of cases	Exposure estimates	Relative risk (95% CI)	Comments
Kahn (1966) (contd)			*Former cigarette only-smoker* *Cigarettes/day* 1–9 10–20 21–39 ≥40	0.9 0.96 0.7 0.8 2.1	Annual mortality rate/100 000 men standardized for age p for trend > 0.1
Doll & Peto (1976) United Kingdom 1951–71	British Doctors' Study 34 439 men	163 deaths	Nonsmoker Former smoker Current smoker *Cigarettes/day* 1–14 15–24 ≥25	Mortality rate 23 21 32 28 38 32	Inconsistency between table and text for values in women
Hirayama (1982) Japan 1965–78	Six-prefecture Study 122 261 men, 142 857 women 3 060 499 person–years	Not given	Men Women *Age at starting smoking (years)* ≥20 <19	SMR 1.5 (p < 0.001) 1.3 (p < 0.01) **Men** **Women** 1.4 1.2 1.7 1.6	
Hirayama (1985) Japan 1965–81	Six-prefecture Study 122 261 men, 142 847 women 3 659 588 person–years	Not given	Current smoker *Cigarettes/day* 1–24 ≥25	1.5 (p < 0.001) 1.48 1.5	p for trend = 4×10^{-8}
Kono et al. (1987) Japan 1965–83	Japanese Physicians' Study 5130 men	116 deaths	*Cigarettes/day* 1–19 ≥20	1.7 (1.1–2.6) 1.8 (1.1–3.0)	Never- and former smokers combined used as referents. Low response rate. Relative risks adjusted for age and alcohol drinking

Table 2.1.6.2 (contd)

Reference Country and years of study	No. of subjects	No. of cases	Exposure estimates	Relative risk (95% CI)	Comments
Akiba & Hirayama (1990) Japan 1965–81	Six-prefecture Study 122 261 men, 142 857 women	4426 deaths (2839 men, 1587 women)	**Men** *Cigarettes/day* 1–4	1.4 (1.0–1.8)	Relative risks stratified by prefecture of residence, occupation, attained age and observation period.
			5–14	1.4 (1.3–1.6)	
			15–24	1.5 (1.4–1.7)	
			25–34	1.4 (1.1–1.7)	
			≥ 35	1.7 (1.3–2.2)	*p* for trend < 0.001
			Total	1.5 (1.3–1.6)	*p* for heterogeneity < 0.001
			Women *Cigarettes/day* 1–4	1.2 (0.8–1.7)	
			5–14	1.3 (1.1–1.5)	
			≥ 15	0.8 (0.5–1.3)	*p* for trend > 0.1
			Total	1.2 (1.0–1.4)	*p* for heterogeneity = 0.04
McLaughlin *et al.* (1990) USA 1954–80	US Veterans' Study 293 916 men 4 531 000 person–years	1520 deaths	Former smoker	1.0 (0.9–1.2)	Relative risks for age at start and duration adjusted for number of cigarettes smoked.
			Current smoker	1.4 (1.2–1.6)	
			Cigarettes/day 1–9	1.3 (1.1–1.7)	
			10–19	1.4 (1.2–1.6)	
			20–39	1.5 (1.2–1.8)	
			≥ 40	1.8 (1.3–2.6)	
				p for trend < 0.001	
			Age at starting smoking (years) ≥ 20	1.3 (1.0–1.6)	
			15–19	1.5 (1.1–1.9)	
			< 15	1.9 (1.4–2.7)	
				p for trend < 0.01	

Table 2.1.6.2 (contd)

Reference Country and years of study	No. of subjects	No. of cases	Exposure estimates	Relative risk (95% CI)	Comments
McLaughlin et al. (1990) (contd)			*Duration (years)* < 25 ≥ 25	1.1 (0.7–1.6) 1.4 (1.1–1.8) *p* for trend < 0.01	
Nomura et al. (1990a,b) USA 1965–84	American Men of Japanese Ancestry Study 7990 men 140 190 person–years	150 cases	Former smoker Former smoker[†] Current smoker *Cigarettes/day* 1–10 11–20 > 20 *Duration (years)* ≤ 25 26–35 > 35	1.0 (0.6–1.7) 0.9 (0.4–2.0) 2.7 (1.8–4.1) 2.7 (1.5–5.1) 2.9 (1.9–4.6) 2.4 (1.4–4.1) 3.5 (1.9–6.6) 1.5 (0.9–2.7) 3.5 (2.2–5.6)	Relative risks adjusted for age. [†]Subjects who had quit ≤ 5 years before interview
Kneller et al. (1991) USA 1966–86	Lutheran Brotherhood Insurance Study 17 633 men 287 000 person–years	75 deaths	Ever-smoker Occasional smoker Former smoker *Cigarettes/day* Total 1–19 20–29 ≥ 30	2.1 (0.98–4.4) 0.7 (0.2–2.8) 2.2 (0.99–4.9) 2.6 (1.1–5.8) 2.2 (0.8–6.0) 2.0 (0.7–5.6) 5.8 (2.1–16.2) *p* for trend < 0.01	Response rate, 68%; 23% of cohort lost to follow-up. Diagnosis not confirmed histologically. Data stratified by year of birth (5-year intervals). Stratification by education, immigrant status, occupation or residential region did not alter results.

Table 2.1.6.2 (contd)

Reference Country and years of study	No. of subjects	No. of cases	Exposure estimates	Relative risk (95% CI)		Comments
Kneller et al. (1991) (contd)			*Pack–years*			
			< 0.01	1.0		
			0.01–17.99	1.3 (0.6–2.7)		
			18.00–32.99	1.4 (0.7–3.1)		
			≥ 33	2.3 (1.2–4.3)		
				p for trend < 0.01		
			Current smoker	≤ 67 years	> 67 years	
			All	4.8 (1.1–21.4)	1.6 (0.5–4.6)	
			≥ 30 cigarettes/day	9.4 (1.8–48.7)	3.8 (0.8–18.9)	
Kato et al. (1992a) Japan 1985–91	9753 men and women 55 284 person–years	57 deaths (35 men, 22 women)	Former smoker	2.6 (0.97–7.0)		Information on smoking habits taken from another survey unrelated to study. Small number of observations. Relative risks adjusted for age and sex. Multivariate analysis adjusted for alcohol intake, diet, cooking methods and family history of stomach cancer
			Current smoker	2.3 (1.2–4.6)		
			Cigarettes/day			
			1–19	2.6		
			≥ 20	1.9		
				Men	**Women**	
			Former smoker	2.6 (0.8–8.1)	4.9 (0.6–36.8)	
			Current smoker	2.6 (1.1–6.1)	1.7 (0.4–7.3)	
				Multivariate analysis		
			Current smoker	2.2 (1.1–4.4)		
			Former smoker	2.6 (0.97–7.1)		
Kato et al. (1992b) Japan 1985–89	3194 patients (1851 men, 2063 women) 17 289 person–years	45 cases (35 men, 10 women)	Former smoker	1.2 (0.5–2.9)		Relative risk adjusted for age, sex and residence
			≤ 19 cigarettes/day	1.1 (0.4–3.3)		
			≥ 20 cigarettes/day	2.2 (0.9–5.4)		

Table 2.1.6.2 (contd)

Reference Country and years of study	No. of subjects	No. of cases	Exposure estimates	Relative risk (95% CI)		Comments
				Mortality rate		
				Men	**Women**	
Tverdal *et al.* (1993) Norway 1972–88	Norwegian Screening Study 44 290 men, 24 535 women	98 deaths (78 men, 20 women)				Mortality rate/100 000 person-years adjusted for age and area. No statistical analysis performed. Relative risks per 10 cigarettes/day adjusted for age, cholesterol, systolic blood pressure, physical activity during leisure, body-mass index, height and number of cigarettes smoked
			Never-smoker	6.9	7.3	
			Former smoker	7.5	10.5	
			Current smoker	18.8	4.1	
			Pipe and cigarettes	22.9		
			Cigarettes/day			
			1–9	20.7		
			10–19	17.2		
			≥ 20	21.3		
			RR per 10 cig./day	1.2 (0.7–1.8)		
				Mortality rate		
Doll *et al.* (1994) UK 1951–91	British Doctors' study 34 439 men	277 deaths				Annual mortality rate/100 000 men standardized for age and calendar period
			Never-smoker	26		
			Former smoker	25		
			Current smoker	43		
				p for trend ≤ 0.01		
			Cigarettes/day			
			1–14	40		
			15–24	46		
			≥ 25	44		
				p for trend < 0.05		

Table 2.1.6.2 (contd)

Reference Country and years of study	No. of subjects	No. of cases	Exposure estimates	Relative risk (95% CI)	Comments
Guo et al. (1994) China 1985–91	Linxian Intervention Trial Study 29 584 men and women	539 cases in men	Ever-smoker Cigarettes only Cigarettes and pipe *Cigarettes/day* < 10 10–19 ≥ 20 *Duration (years)* < 20 20–39 ≥ 40 *Pack–years* < 10 1–19 20–29 ≥ 30 *Years since quitting* ≥ 3 < 3	1.1 (0.8–1.4) 1.0 (0.7–1.3) 1.3 (1.0–1.8) 1.2 (0.9–1.6) 1.0 (0.8–1.4) 1.1 (0.8–1.5) 0.9 (0.5–1.4) 1.0 (0.8–1.4) 1.3 (0.9–1.9) *p* for trend = 0.19 1.0 (0.7–1.5) 1.0 (0.7–1.4) 1.1 (0.8–1.7) 1.2 (0.9–1.8) 0.8 (0.4–1.7) 1.0 (0.4–2.3)	Nested case–control study. Analysis for men only. Odds ratios adjusted for participation in intervention group and cancer history in first-degree relatives
McLaughlin et al. (1995) USA 1954–80	US Veterans' Study 177 903 men 3 252 983 person–years	1058 deaths	Ever-smoker Former smoker Current smoker *Cigarettes/day* 1–9 10–20 21–39 ≥ 40	1.3 (1.1–1.4) 1.0 (0.9–1.2) 1.4 (1.2–1.6) 1.3 (1.0–1.7) 1.4 (1.2–1.6) 1.4 (1.2–1.8) 1.9 (1.3–2.7) *p* for trend < 0.01	Relative risks adjusted for attained age and calendar-year time-period.

Table 2.1.6.2 (contd)

Reference Country and years of study	No. of subjects	No. of cases	Exposure estimates	Relative risk (95% CI)	Comments
Nomura *et al.* (1995) USA 1965–94	American Men of Japanese Ancestry Study 7972 men 177 080 person–years	250 cases	Former smoker Current smoker *Age at starting smoking (years)* ≥ 21 18–20 ≤ 17	1.1 (0.7–1.6) 2.3 (1.7–3.2) 1.9 (1.3–2.9) 2.5 (1.7–3.7) 2.6 (1.7–3.9) *p* for trend < 0.0001	Adjusted for age and alcohol intake. No trend observed for pack–years [data not shown]
Engeland *et al.* (1996) Norway 1966–93	Norwegian Cohort Study 11 863 men, 14 269 women About 540 000 person–years	417 cases (258 men, 159 women)	Former smoker Current smoker	**Men** **Women** 1.3 (0.9–2.0) 0.8 (0.4–1.6) 1.3 (0.9–1.9) 1.0 (0.6–1.4)	Response rate, 76%. Relative risks adjusted for age.
Murata *et al.* (1996) Japan 1984–93	Chiba Center Association Study	23 65 32	Cigarettes/day 1–10 11–20 ≥ 21	1.0 1.1 1.1	
Yuan *et al.* (1996) China 1986–93	Shanghai Men's Study 18 244 men 98 267 person–years	113 cases	Ever-smoker < 20 cigarettes/day ≥ 20 cigarettes/day	1.4 (0.9–2.1) 1.4 1.3	Relative risks adjusted for age.
Nordlund *et al.* (1997) Sweden 1963–89	Swedish Census Study 26 032 women Almost 600 000 person–years	226 cases	Former smoker Current smoker *Cigarettes/day* 1–7 8–15 ≥ 16	0.2 (0.0–1.3) 1.3 (0.8–1.9) 1.2 (0.7–2.0) 1.2 (0.6–2.3) 1.9 (0.8–4.7)	Relative risks adjusted for age and place of residence.

Table 2.1.6.2 (contd)

Reference Country and years of study	No. of subjects	No. of cases	Exposure estimates	Relative risk (95% CI)	Comments
Nordlund *et al.* (1997) (contd)			*Age at starting smoking (years)*		Relative risks for age at starting smoking adjusted for amount of tobacco smoked daily
			20–23	0.5 (0.1–1.5)	
			< 19	0.9 (0.4–2.3)	
				p for trend = 0.559	
Chen *et al.* (1997) China 1972–93	Shanghai Factory Study 6494 men, 2857 women 101 949 person–years	86 deaths in men	*Ever-smoker*	1.0	Analysis for men only because of few of the women smoked. Relative risks adjusted for factories, age, systolic blood pressure, serum cholesterol and regular alcohol drinking
			Cigarettes/day		
			1–19	1.1	
			≥ 20	0.9	
				p for trend = 0.81	
Tulinius *et al.* (1997) Iceland 1968–95	Reykjavik Study 11 366 men, 11 580 women	246 cases (171 men, 75 women)	Former smoker	1.2 (0.8–1.8)	Analysis for men only because of small no. of deaths in women. Relative risks adjusted for age
			Cigarettes/day		
			1–14	1.5 (0.8–2.5)	
			15–24	1.9 (1.1–3.1)	
			≥ 25	1.0 (0.4–2.4)	
Liaw & Chen (1998) China, Province of Taiwan 1982–94	Taiwanese Study 11 096 men, 3301 women 140 493 person–years	69 deaths (57 men, 12 women)	*Ever-smoker*	1.9 (1.0–3.5)	Analysis for men only because of small no. of deaths in women. Relative risks adjusted for age and alcohol drinking.
			Cigarettes/day		
			≤ 10	1.7 (0.9–3.4)	
			11–20	1.6 (0.8–3.1)	
			> 20	3.0 (1.1–8.3)	
				p for trend = 0.06	
			Duration (years)		
			≤ 20	1.7 (0.7–4.4)	
			21–30	0.7 (0.2–2.4)	
			> 30	2.0 (1.1–3.7)	
				p for trend = 0.04	

Table 2.1.6.2 (contd)

Reference Country and years of study	No. of subjects	No. of cases	Exposure estimates	Relative risk (95% CI)	Comments
Liaw & Chen (1998) (contd)			*Age at starting smoking (years)*		
			> 24	1.5 (0.7–3.3)	
			21–24	0.6 (0.2–2.2)	
			≤ 20	2.2 (1.2–4.2)	
				p for trend = 0.02	
			Pack–years		
			< 20	1.3 (0.6–2.8)	
			20–40	1.5 (0.7–3.1)	
			≥ 41	2.8 (1.4–5.8)	
				p for trend < 0.01	
Terry *et al.* (1998) Sweden 1967–92	Swedish Twin Registry Study 11 546 individuals	116 cases	Current smoker	0.8 (0.4–2.3)	
Gao *et al.* (1999) China 1983–94	Shanghai Residential Study		Men		*p* for trend < 0.05 for intensity of smoking and age at starting smoking for men
			urban	1.9[†]	[†]CI does not include 1.0
			suburban	1.3	
			rural	1.3	
			Women (urban)	1.2	
Mizoue *et al.* (2000) Japan 1986–96	Fukuoka Study 4050 men 35 785 person–years	53 cases		**SMR**	Standardized mortality ratio (SMR) adjusted for study area, age and alcohol consumption.
			Former smoker	2.2 (0.8–6.0)	
			Current smoker	2.2 (0.8–5.7)	
			Cigarettes/day		
			1–24	2.2 (0.8–6.0)	
			≥ 25	1.9 (0.6–6.4)	

Table 2.1.6.2 (contd)

Reference Country and years of study	No. of subjects	No. of cases	Exposure estimates	Relative risk (95% CI)		Comments
You et al. (2000) China 1989–94	2628 participants with: 1240 superficial or chronic atrophic gastritis 842 intestinal metaplasia 546 gastric displasia 805 normal	34 cases 1 18 15 0	*Cigarettes/day* 1–19 ≥ 20 *p* for trend = 0.12 *Duration (years)* 1–24 ≥ 25 *p* for trend = 0.04	1.2 (0.7–1.9) 1.4 (0.9–2.3) 1.1 (0.7–1.7) 1.6 (1.0–2.7)		Information about smoking habit available for only 2436 subjects. Relative risks for progression to dysplasia or stomach cancer, adjusted for sex, age, alcohol consumption and baseline histopathology.
Chao et al. (2002) USA 1982–96	Cancer Prevention Study II 467 788 men, 588 053 women	1505 deaths (996 men, 509 women)	**Current smoker** *Cigarettes/day* < 20 20 21–39 ≥ 40 *p* for trend *Duration (years)* < 20 20–29 30–39 ≥ 40 *p* for trend *Age at starting smoking (years)* ≥ 20 16–19 ≤ 15 *p* for trend	**Men** 2.2 (1.8–2.7) 1.7 (1.2–2.3) 2.5 (1.9–3.3) 2.7 (2.0–3.8) 1.8 (1.3–2.7) 0.539 1.2 (0.4–3.4) 1.0 (0.5–2.0) 2.1 (1.5–2.9) 2.4 (1.8–3.0) 0.059 1.9 (1.4–2.5) 2.4 (1.9–3.1) 2.2 (1.6–3.0) 0.075	**Women** 1.5 (1.2–1.9) 1.3 (0.9–1.8) 1.3 (0.8–1.9) 2.2 (1.3–3.5) 2.2 (1.2–3.9) 0.038 1.4 (0.7–3.0) 1.2 (0.7–2.2) 1.8 (1.3–2.6) 1.5 (1.02–2.1) 0.074 1.5 (1.1–2.0) 1.6 (1.2–2.3) 1.6 (0.8–3.0) 0.672	Multivariate models include age, race, education, family history of stomach cancer, consumption of high-fibre cereal products, vegetables, citrus fruits and juices, and use of vitamin C, multivitamins and aspirin. Estimates of *p* for trend excluded non-users of tobacco.

Table 2.1.6.2 (contd)

Reference Country and years of study	No. of subjects	No. of cases	Exposure estimates	Relative risk (95% CI)	Comments
Chao et al. (2002) (contd)			*Pack–years*		
			≤ 19	1.4 (0.9–2.3)	1.6 (1.0–2.4)
			20–39	2.0 (1.4–2.7)	1.3 (0.8–1.9)
			40–59	2.7 (2.0–3.6)	1.2 (0.7–2.0)
			≥ 60	2.1 (1.5–2.8)	2.8 (1.8–4.5)
			p for trend	0.401	0.053
			Former smoker	1.6 (1.3–1.9)	1.4 (1.1–1.7)
			Cigarettes/day			
			< 20	1.3 (0.96–1.7)	1.2 (0.9–1.6)	†Two highest categories (21–39 and ≥ 40 cigarettes/ day) grouped together because of small numbers
			20	1.6 (1.2–2.1)	1.5 (1.02–2.3)
			21–39	1.6 (1.1–2.3)	1.6 (0.95–2.6)†
			≥ 40	1.8 (1.4–2.4)	
			p for trend	0.064	0.165
			Duration (years)		
			< 20	1.1 (0.8–1.5)	1.4 (0.96–2.0)
			20–29	1.5 (1.2–2.0)	1.7 (1.2–2.6)
			30–39	1.7 (1.3–2.3)	1.2 (0.8–1.8)†
			≥ 40	2.0 (1.5–2.7)	
			p for trend	0.0017	0.3208
			Age at starting smoking (years)		
			≥ 20	1.7 (1.3–2.2)	1.5 (1.1–2.0)
			16–19	1.6 (1.2–2.0)	1.3 (0.9–1.8)
			≤ 15	1.3 (0.9–1.8)	0.9 (0.4–2.1)
			p for trend	0.608	0.605

Table 2.1.6.2 (contd)

Reference Country and years of study	No. of subjects	No. of cases	Exposure estimates	Relative risk (95% CI)	Comments
Chao et al. (2002) (contd)			*Pack–years*		
			≤ 19	1.1 (0.9–1.5)	1.4 (1.0–1.9)
			20–39	1.6 (1.3–2.1)	1.4 (0.9–2.2)
			40–59	1.9 (1.4–2.6)	1.2 (0.7–2.2)[†]
			≥ 60	1.9 (1.4–2.6)	
			p for trend	0.0037	0.828
			Age at quitting smoking (years)		
			≤ 30	1.2 (0.8–1.7)	1.1 (0.7–1.9)
			31–40	1.3 (0.9–1.7)	1.8 (1.2–2.7)
			41–50	1.6 (1.2–2.1)	1.3 (0.8–2.0)
			≥ 51	1.9 (1.5–2.4)	1.3 (0.9–1.8)
			p for trend	0.0015	0.683
			Years since cessation		
			≥ 20	1.2 (0.95–1.6)	1.3 (0.95–1.9)
			11–19	1.6 (1.3–2.1)	1.5 (1.00–2.1)
			≤ 10	1.9 (1.5–2.5)	1.3 (0.9–1.9)
			p for trend	0.0015	0.683

CI, confidence interval

Table 2.1.6.3. Case–control studies on tobacco smoking and stomach cancer: main characteristics of study design

Reference Country and years of study	Number of cases and controls	Criteria for eligibility and comments
Wynder et al. (1963) Slovenia, Iceland, Japan and USA Years of study not specified	Men: 367 cases and 401 controls; women: 154 cases and 252 controls	Hospital-based study Cases from Japan (51%), New York (30%), Slovenia (10%) and Iceland (9%) Controls with malignant and non-malignant diseases, individually matched by age and hospital; cancers of the respiratory and upper alimentary tract excluded
Staszewski (1969) Poland 1957–68	Men: 450 cases and 771 controls; women: 178 cases and 383 controls	Hospital-based study Cases confirmed by histopathology (72%) or surgery and/or radiology (28%) as cancer of the cardia (17%), middle part (27%), pylorus (33%) or all stomach (23%) Controls hospitalized for diseases not connected with smoking; cancers of the colon and rectum excluded
Haenszel et al. (1972) USA 1963–69	Men: 135 cases and 270 controls; women: 85 cases and 170 controls	Hospital-based study among Japanese Hawaiian migrants (120) and their offspring (100) Cases: 96% confirmed histologically as cancer of the cardia (6%), fundus (8%), prepylorus (10%), antrum (33%), lesser or greater curvatures (25%) or other/unknown site (18%) Controls individually matched by age, sex, hospital and time of visit; gastric ulcer, other stomach diseases and cancer of digestive system excluded
Haenszel et al. (1976) Japan 1962–65	Men: 526 cases and 1052 controls; women: 257 cases and 514 controls	Hospital-based study from eight hospitals in Hiroshima (247) and Miyagi (416) Cases: 98% confirmed microscopically as cancer of the cardia (9%), fundus (4%), antrum (40%), prepylorus (31%), or lesser or greater curvatures (14%); aged ≥ 35 years Controls with neoplasms, gastrointestinal, infectious and circulatory diseases and conditions affecting nervous system and sense organs; individually matched for age, sex, hospital and time of visit; gastric ulcer, other stomach diseases and cancer of digestive system excluded
Hoey et al. (1981) France 1978–80	Men: 40 cases and 168 controls	Hospital-based study in endoscopy department among French residents of Lyon Cases confirmed histologically; mean age, 65.4 years; 91% of eligible cases Controls with other gastrointestinal diagnoses (hiatal hernia (29%), colorectal polyps (33%), gallstones (17%) and colorectal cancer (21%); mean age, 59.9 years

Table 2.1.6.3 (contd)

Reference Country and years of study	Number of cases and controls	Criteria for eligibility and comments
Ames & Gamble (1983) USA Years of study not specified	Men: 46 cases and 92 controls	Prospective mortality study on white coal miners Controls: deaths from other cancers (1:1) and from non-cancer/non-accidents (1:1), individually matched by age at death and year of birth (± 3 years)
Correa et al. (1985) USA 1979–83	Men: 264 cases and 264 controls; women: 127 cases and 127 controls	Hospital-based study in 26 counties of South Louisiana Cases: 98% confirmed histologically as cancer of the antrum/corpus (87%), cardia (6.5%) or other/unknown site (6.5%) Controls mainly with cardiovascular (20%), gastrointestinal (12%), infectious (11%) or respiratory (10%) diseases; individually matched on age (± 5 years), sex, race and hospital
Risch et al. (1985) Canada 1979–82	Men: 163 cases and 163 controls; women: 83 cases and 83 controls	Population-based study Cases confirmed histologically; aged 35–79 years Controls randomly selected from electoral lists, individually matched by age (± 4 years), sex, province of residence and neighbourhood; participation rate, 58%
Jedrychowski et al. (1986) Poland 1980–81	Men: 70 cases and 140 controls; women: 40 cases and 80 controls	Hospital- and population-based study using interviews Cases confirmed histologically Controls individually matched by age (± 5 years) and sex: hospital-based (1:1), with orthopaedic problems, heart or endocrinological disorders; obvious gastrointestinal diseases and recent dietary abnormality excluded; population-based (1:1), randomly selected from healthy participants of a medical survey on chronic chest diseases
You et al. (1988) China 1984–86	Men: 443 cases and 888 controls; women: 121 cases and 243 controls	Population-based study among residents of Linqu for ≥ 10 years Cases confirmed by histology (50%), endoscopy or surgery (32%) or radiological and clinical examination (17%); aged 35–64 years; 82% of eligible cases Controls randomly selected using rosters, frequency-matched by age and sex; participation rate, 100%

Table 2.1.6.3 (contd)

Reference Country and years of study	Number of cases and controls	Criteria for eligibility and comments
Hu et al. (1988) China 1985–86	Men: 170 cases and 170 controls; women: 71 cases and 71 controls	Hospital-based study from two hospitals in Harbin and Heilongjiang province using interviews. Cases confirmed histologically; aged 25–80 years. Controls with non-neoplastic diseases (chest diseases, general surgery, urological and orthopaedic diseases, trauma); individually matched by sex, age and area of residence
Buiatti et al. (1989, 1991) Italy 1985–87	1989 study: men: 640 cases; women: 376 cases; 1991 study: men: 597 cases; women: 326; 1159 controls (705 men and 454 women)	Population-based study among residents of four areas with varying incidence of stomach cancer using interviews. Cases confirmed histologically as intestinal (55%), diffuse (23%) or mixed/unclassified (22%); mean age, 65 years; 83% of eligible cases. Controls randomly selected from general population, frequency-matched on 5-year age-groups and sex; participation rate, 81%
Ferraroni et al. (1989) Italy 1983–88	Men: 243 cases and 1334 controls; women: 154 cases and 610 controls	Hospital-based study from four major hospitals in Milan. Cases confirmed histologically; aged ≤ 75 years. Controls with traumatic (38%), non-traumatic orthopaedic (15%) and acute surgical conditions (34%) and ear, nose, throat, skin and dental disorders (13%); malignant tumours, digestive tract disorders or any coffee-, alcohol- or tobacco-related conditions excluded; median age, 56 years
De Stefani et al. (1990) Uruguay 1985–88	Men: 138 cases and 414 controls; women: 72 cases and 216 controls	Hospital-based study from the University Hospital in Montevideo using interviews. Cases confirmed histologically as cancer of the cardia (13%), corpus (9%), antrum (15%) and unclassified (63%); aged 30–89 years; 100% of eligible cases participated. Controls individually matched (1:3) by age (± 5 years) and sex; tobacco- or alcohol-related diseases or gastric conditions excluded
Kato et al. (1990) Japan 1985–89	Men: 289 cases and 2013 controls; women: 138 cases and 2415 controls	Hospital-based study at gastroscopy department in Aichi prefecture; self-administered questionnaire. Cases confirmed histologically, mainly of diffuse (48%) or intestinal (50%) type. Controls with normal gastric mucosa (3014) or atrophic gastritis (1414); other cancers, resected stomach and gastroduodenal diseases excluded; 89% participation rate for cases and controls
Lee et al. (1990) China, Province of Taiwan 1954–88	Men: 123 cases and 478 controls; women: 87 cases and 332 controls	Hospital-based study in four major hospitals in Taipei using interviews. Cases confirmed histologically; 90% of eligible cases participated. Controls from ophthalmic service, group matched by sex and age; participation rate, 96%

Table 2.1.6.3 (contd)

Reference Country and years of study	Number of cases and controls	Criteria for eligibility and comments
Wu-Williams et al. (1990) USA 1975–82	Men: 137 cases and 137 controls	Population-based study among white men from Los Angeles County using interviews Cases confirmed histologically as cancer of the cardia (58), fundus/body (10), antrum/pylorus (22) or other site (47); aged < 55 years; 52 % of eligible cases participated. Controls individually matched by age (± 5 years), sex and race (Hispanic white and other white)
Boeing et al. (1991) Germany 1985–87	Men and women: 143 cases (almost equal number of men and women) and 579 controls (slightly more women)	Hospital-based study from five hospitals in Bavaria and Hesse using interviews Cases confirmed histologically as cancer of the cardia (17%), corpus (32%), antrum/pylorus (40%) or multiple sites (11%); aged 32–80 years; 85% of eligible cases Controls: 251 visitors and 328 patients with other cancers (12%), metabolic (13%), cardiovascular (30%) and respiratory (5%) diseases, and diseases of digestive organs other than stomach (23%); matched by sex and age (± 3 years); patients with history of atrophic gastritis or intestinal metaplasia excluded; participation rate, 90%
Dockerty et al. (1991) New Zealand 1980–84	Men: 797 cases and 8398 controls	Cases and controls from New Zealand Cancer Registry Cases aged ≥ 20 years; 78% of all cases registered at the Registry. Controls with other types of cancer; smoking-related cancers excluded
Saha (1991) UK 8 years	Men: 81 cases and 162 controls; women: 36 cases and 72 controls	Hospital-based study at four hospitals using interviews Cases confirmed histologically as cancer of the cardia (46), body (24) or antrum (47); aged 35–89 years Controls with benign surgical conditions, individually matched by age (± 5 years), sex and social class; respiratory, upper gastrointestinal and vascular diseases excluded
Yu & Hsieh (1991) China 1976–80	Men: 52 cases and 2676 controls; women: 32 cases and 1843 controls	Population-based study among primary and middle-school staff in Shanghai using interviews for cases and self-administered questionnaire for controls Cases confirmed histologically as cancer of the lesser curvature (73%), pylorus (17%), antrum (6%) or other site (4%); 89% of eligible cases participated. Controls from 55 randomly selected schools stratified by districts; participation rate, 91%

Table 2.1.6.3 (contd)

Reference Country and years of study	Number of cases and controls	Criteria for eligibility and comments
Agudo et al. (1992) Spain 1987–89	Men: 235 cases and 235 controls; women: 119 cases and 119 controls	Hospital-based study in 4 regions with varying incidences of stomach cancer using a questionnaire Cases confirmed histologically mainly as intestinal (56%) or diffuse (26%) type; mean age, 65.2 years Controls with a wide variety of diagnoses; individually matched by hospital, sex, age (± 3 years) and area of residence; cancers of digestive and respiratory tracts, and chronic respiratory illnesses excluded; aged 31–88 years (mean, 65.5 years)
Hoshiyama & Sasaba (1992a,b) Japan 1984–90	Men: 251 cases and 483 controls	Population-based study among people living in Saitama Prefecture for ≥ 10 years using interviews Cases confirmed histologically as single (216) or multiple (35) cancer; 73% of eligible cases participated. Controls randomly selected from electoral roll with stratification by sex and age; participation rate, 28%
Palli et al. (1992) Italy 1985–87	Men: 597 cases and 705 controls; women: 326 cases and 454 controls	Population-based study using interviews Cases from study by Buiatti et al. (1991); histologically confirmed as cancer of the cardia (68) or other site (819); cancer of the stump (36) excluded from the analysis Controls randomly selected from 5-year age and sex strata; history of gastric surgery excluded
Jedrychowski et al. (1993) Poland 1986–90	Men: 520 cases and 520 controls	Hospital-based study from nine university hospitals in Poland using interviews Cases confirmed histologically as cancer of the cardia (137, of which 58% of intestinal and 20% of diffuse type) or of non-cardia (383, of which 51% of intestinal and 36% of diffuse type); aged < 75 years; 100% of eligible cases participated. Controls admitted mostly for accidents, orthopaedic problems or general surgery; individually matched by age (± 5 years); diseases of the gastrointestinal tract and other cancers excluded; participation rate, 100%
Kabat et al. (1993) USA 1981–90	Men: 295 cases and 4544 controls; women: 52 cases and 2228 controls	Hospital-based study in 28 hospitals of seven states using interviews Cases confirmed histologically as cancer of distal oesophagus/gastric cardia (194) or of distal stomach (153) Controls with non-tobacco-related cancers (43%) and non-cancer diagnoses (57%), including fractures, disc problems, eye problems, acute infections and trauma; matched by age (± 5 years), sex, race and hospital; cancers and other diseases of the gastrointestinal tract excluded

Table 2.1.6.3 (contd)

Reference Country and years of study	Number of cases and controls	Criteria for eligibility and comments
Hansson et al. (1994) Sweden 1989–92	Men: 218 cases; women: 120 cases; and 679 controls [no information on sex distribution]	Population-based study among residents of five counties in central and northern Sweden using interviews Cases confirmed histologically; aged 40–70 years (mean, 67.7 years); 74% of eligible cases Controls randomly selected from population registers, frequency-matched by sex and age strata; mean age, 67.0 years; participation rate, 77%
Inoue et al. (1994) Japan 1988–91	Men: 420 cases and 420 controls; women: 248 cases and 248 controls	Hospital-based study at Aichi Cancer Centre Hospital using self-administered questionnaire Cases identified through Cancer Registry database; confirmed histologically as cancer of the cardia, middle part or antrum; aged ≥ 18 years (mean, 58.0 years) Controls randomly selected from first-visit outpatients, individually matched by sex, age (± 2 years) and date of first visit (± 2 months); history of cancer or any other specific disease excluded; mean age, 57.8 years; participation rate, 98%
Siemiatycki et al. (1995) Canada 1979–85	Men: 251 cases and 2238 controls	Hospital- and population-based study among residents of Montreal area using interviews Cases confirmed histologically; aged 35–70 years Controls: 533 population-based, selected from electoral lists stratified by age; participation rate, 72%; 1705 hospital-based; cancers of the lung, bladder, oesophagus, pancreas, liver and kidney excluded
Yu et al. (1995) China 1991–93	Men: 453 cases and 453 controls; women: 258 cases and 258 controls	Population-based study among residents of Hongkou district and Nanhui county (Shanghai) using interviews Cases confirmed; aged < 80 years; 91% of eligible cases participated. Controls individually matched for age (± 3 years), sex and residence (street); participation rate, 99%
Gajalakshmi & Shanta (1996) India 1998–90	Men: 287 cases and 287 controls; women: 101 cases and 101 controls	Hospital-based study from Cancer Institute in Chennai (Madras) using interviews Cases confirmed histologically (75%) or by barium meal evidence, exploratory surgery or endoscopy (25%) Controls with cancer mainly of the penis, bone and connective tissue, skin and cervix; individually matched for age (± 5 years), sex, religion and mother tongue; cancers of the gastrointestinal tract, bladder and pancreas and smoking-related cancers excluded

Table 2.1.6.3 (contd)

Reference Country and years of study	Number of cases and controls	Criteria for eligibility and comments
Ji *et al.* (1996) China 1988–89	Men: 770 cases and 819 controls; women: 354 cases and 632 controls	Population-based study among permanent residents in Shanghai using interviews Cases identified through Shanghai cancer registry; confirmed histologically (52%) or by surgery, endoscopy, X-rays or ultrasound (48%) as cancer of the cardia (16%), distal stomach (70%) or unspecified site (14%); aged 20–69 years; 66% of eligible cases participated. Controls randomly selected, frequency-matched for age (5-year categories) and sex; participation rate, 86%
Zhang *et al.* (1996) USA 1992–94	Men: 122 cases and 62 controls; women: 40 cases and 70 controls	Hospital-based study at endoscopy department in New York using self-administered questionnaire Cases confirmed histologically as cancer of oesophagus/cardia (95) or distal stomach (67) Controls were cancer-free, with atrophic/chronic or other types of gastritis (71%) or disease-free (29%)
Gammon *et al.* (1997) USA 1993–95	Men: 477 cases and 555 controls; women: 152 cases and 140 controls	Population-based study using interviews Cases confirmed histologically as cancer of the cardia (261) or other sites (368); aged 30–79 years; 81% of eligible cases participated. Controls aged 30–65 years identified by random-digit dialling and those aged 65–79 years by random sampling of rosters; frequency-matched by age (5-year group) and sex; participation rate, 70%
De Stefani *et al.* (1998) Uruguay 1992–96	Men: 311 cases and 622 controls	Hospital-based study from four major hospitals in Montevideo using interviews Cases confirmed microscopically as cancer of the cardia (24), antrum (240), fundus (25) or of diffuse type (22); aged 25–84 years Controls mainly with eye disorders (33%), hernia (17%), osteoarticular diseases (11%) and skin (9%) and ear (7%) disorders; frequency-matched for age (10-year group), hospital, time of visit and residence; tobacco- and alcohol-related diseases and digestive tract conditions excluded; aged 25–84 years; participation rate for cases and controls, 93%
Liu *et al.* (1998) China 1986–88	Men: 20 195 cases and 52 775 controls; women: 9009 cases and 34 560 controls	Retrospective mortality study Cases aged 35–69 years Controls: death from neoplastic, respiratory and cardiovascular diseases excluded

Table 2.1.6.3 (contd)

Reference Country and years of study	Number of cases and controls	Criteria for eligibility and comments
Chow et al. (1999) Poland 1994–97	Men: 302 cases and 314 controls; women: 162 cases and 166 controls	Population-based study among Warsaw residents using interviews Cases from 22 hospitals in Warsaw, confirmed histologically mainly as intestinal (67%) or diffuse (14%); aged 21–79 years; 90% of eligible cases participated. Controls randomly selected from registry, frequency-matched by age (5-year categories) and sex; participation rate, 82%
Gao et al. (1999) China 1995	Men: 110 cases and 154 controls; women: 43 cases and 80 controls	Population-based study among Yangzhong residents using interviews Cases from Regional Cancer Registry, confirmed histologically; aged 30–79 years Controls from household registration office, individually matched for sex, age (± 2 years) and town or area of residence; participation rate for cases and controls, 100%
Inoue et al. (1999) Japan 1988–95	Men: 651 cases and 12 041 controls; women: 344 cases and 31 805 controls	Hospital-based study at Aichi Cancer Centre Hospital Cases from cancer registry and surgical records, confirmed histologically mainly as differentiated (46%) or non-differentiated (53%) Controls with benign tumours or non-neoplastic polyps (13%), benign and non-specific diseases (43%), or no abnormal findings (44%); cancers or past history of cancer excluded; aged ≥ 18 years
Ye et al. (1999) Sweden 1989–95	Men: 348 cases and 779 controls; women: 166 cases and 385 controls	Population-based study using interviews Cases confirmed histologically as cancer of the cardia (90), and distal cancer of intestinal (260) or diffuse (164) type; aged 40–79 years; 62% of eligible cases participated. Controls randomly selected from registers, frequency-matched by age and sex; participation rate, 76%
Lagergren et al. (2000) Sweden 1995–97	Men: 223 cases and 681 controls; women: 39 cases and 139 controls	Population-based study among people born in Sweden using interviews Cases of cardia; aged ≤ 80 years, mean 66 years; 83% of eligible cases participated. Controls randomly selected from whole population of Sweden, frequency-matched for age and sex; mean age, 68 years; participation rate, 73%
Mathew et al. (2000) India 1988–91	Men: 151 cases and 228 controls; women: 43 cases and 77 controls	Hospital-based study at the Regional Cancer Centre in Trivandrum using interviews Cases confirmed by histology and/or endoscopy or barium meal evidence, aged ≥ 20 years Controls selected from visitors, individually matched for age (± 5 years), sex, religion and residential area; controls with gastric complaints excluded

Table 2.1.6.3 (contd)

Reference Country and years of study	Number of cases and controls	Criteria for eligibility and comments
Zaridze et al. (2000) Russia 1996–97	Men: 248 cases and 292 controls; women: 200 cases and 318 controls	Hospital-based study in two cancer hospitals (cases) and two general hospitals (controls) among Moscow residents using self-administered questionnaire Cases confirmed histologically as cancer of the cardia (92) or non-cardia (356); aged < 75 years; 98% of eligible cases participated. Controls with a variety of conditions including respiratory (10%) and heart (10%) diseases, diseases of the nervous system (10%) and hypertension and stroke (9%); cancer and/or gastrointestinal diseases excluded; participation rate, 97%
Wu et al. (2001) USA 1992–97	Men: 492 cases and 999 controls; women: 228 cases and 357 controls	Population-based study among whites, Latino-, African and Asian Americans from Los Angeles county using interviews Cases confirmed histologically as cancer of the cardia (277) or distal stomach (443); aged 30–74 years; 56% of eligible cases participated. Controls individually matched by neighbourhood, sex, age (± 5 years) and ethnicity; diagnosis of stomach or oesophageal cancer excluded

Table 2.1.6.4. Case–control studies on tobacco smoking and stomach cancer

Reference Country and years of study	Subjects	Exposure estimates	Relative risk (95% CI)	Comments, variables adjusted for, significance, limitations of the study
Wynder et al. (1963) Slovenia, Iceland, Japan, USA	Men and women			No definition of smoking habit. No participation rate for cases or controls. No relative risk calculated. No consistent difference between cases and controls in terms of type or quantity of tobacco smoked
Staszewski (1969) Poland 1957–68	Men and women	Ever-smoker % of smokers % of heavy smokers† Index of smoking‡	1.6 Cases Controls 90.0 84.8 $p \leq 0.01$ 71.9 63.0 $p \leq 0.01$ 472 428 $p < 0.05$	No definition of smoking habit. No participation rate for cases or controls. The majority of cases among men were cancer of the cardia and pylorus, and among women cancer of the cardia. †Index of smoking ≥ 300 ‡Index of smoking = daily amount of tobacco × years of smoking
Haenszel et al. (1972) USA, Hawaii 1963–69	Men and women	Any tobacco use Hawaiian Japanese Migrant Offspring ≥ 20 vs < 20 cigarettes/day	Men and women Men Women 1.5* 1.4 1.7 1.9* 1.9* 1.7 1.1 0.9 1.8 0.9	* $p < 0.05$ No definition of tobacco use. No response rate for cases or controls. Odds ratios adjusted for sex and age, and for birthplace for Hawaiian Japanese
Haenszel et al. (1976) Japan 1962–65	Men and women	Any tobacco use Hiroshima Miyagi Hawaii†	1.1 1.3 1.4 All $p > 0.05$	Odds ratio reported for men only, probably because of low prevalence of smoking among women in Japanese populations. Same questionnaire used as in previous study. No response rate for cases or controls. Odds ratios adjusted for prefecture, occupation (farm, non-farm), age and sex. Relative risks probably underestimated because of high proportion of controls with smoking-related diseases. †Data from previous study

Table 2.1.6.4 (contd)

Reference Country and years of study	Subjects	Exposure estimates	Relative risk (95% CI)	Comments, variables adjusted for, significance, limitations of the study
Hoey et al. (1981) France 1978–80	Men	≥ 7 cigarettes/week	4.8 (1.6–14.8)	Very small study. No participation rate for controls. Significant difference between cases and controls in mean age and weekly alcohol consumption. Little information about potential confounding. Relative risk reduced to 3.8 after adjustment for wine intake, but still statistically significant [95% CI not given].
Ames & Gamble (1983) USA	Men	Current smoker	0.7 (0.2–2.0)	Very small study. Deaths from other cancers used as controls, leading to underestimation of risk

Correa et al. (1985) USA 1979–83	Men and women	*Cigarette smoker*
		Ever-smoker
		Former smoker
		Current smoker
			Whites
			1.3 (0.8–2.2)
			1.0 (0.5–2.0)
			1.4 (0.8–2.4) **Blacks**
			  2.6 (1.4–5.0)
			  1.9 (0.8–4.2)
			  2.7 (1.3–5.3)
				No response rate for cases or controls. No definition of smoking habit. High proportion of interviews with proxies. Odds ratios adjusted for age, sex, current alcohol consumption, respondent type, education and income. About 30% of controls had cardiac or respiratory diseases. No significant linear trend for no. of cigarettes/day, pack–years or age at starting smoking. Increasing risk with increasing duration of smoking for blacks only ($p < 0.05$). Relative risk for deep inhalers of 1.8 compared with nonsmokers and non-inhalers. Adjustment for vitamin C intake had no effect on relative risk [data not shown].

Risch et al. (1985) Canada 1979–82	Men and women	20 pack–years	1.3 (1.01–1.6)	No definition of smoking habit or smoking history. Low response rate for controls. Odds ratios adjusted for ethnicity, various foods and type of water supply.
Jedrychowski et al. (1986) Poland 1980–81	Men and women	Former smoker Current smoker	0.8 (0.3–2.1) 0.7 (0.4–1.2)	No definition of smoking habit. No response rate for cases or controls. Analysis performed with hospital controls only. Odds ratio adjusted for residence only. Relative risk could be underestimated because hospital controls included patients with smoking-related diseases

Table 2.1.6.4 (contd)

Reference Country and years of study	Subjects	Exposure estimates	Relative risk (95% CI)		Comments, variables adjusted for, significance, limitations of the study
You et al. (1988) China 1984–86	Men and women	*Cigarettes /day* < 20 ≥ 20 *p* for trend	1.3 (0.9–1.9) 1.5 (1.0–2.1) 0.01		Analysis for men only because there were few women who smoked. Odds ratios adjusted for age, family income and alcohol drinking. Association stronger when analysis restricted to histologically confirmed cases [data not shown].
Hu et al. (1988) China 1985–86	Men and women	*Cigarettes/day* < 6 ≥ 6 *Duration (years)* < 14 14–25 > 25 *p* for trend *Age at starting smoking (years)* > 21 6–21 < 6 *p* for trend *Index of smoking*[a] < 7 ≥ 7	**Univariate** 1.0 1.8 (1.2–2.6) 1.0 1.6 (0.7–3.6) 2.3 (1.6–3.5) *p* for trend < 0.001 2.2 (1.1–4.4) 1.6 (0.8–3.2) 1.0 < 0.001 1.0 2.0 (1.4–2.9)	**Multivariate** 1.0 2.0 (1.4–2.7)	No definition of smoking status. No participation rate for cases or controls. Multivariate analysis adjusted for Chinese cabbage and alcohol consumption. Inconsistency between table and text in direction of trend for age at starting analysis, and limit of category surprisingly low.
Buiatti et al. (1989, 1991) Italy 1985–87	Men and women	Former smoker Current smoker Low High	0.9 (0.7–1.1) 1.0 (0.8–1.4) 1.2 (0.9–1.7)		No definition of smoking history or smoking habit. Odds ratios adjusted for age, sex, study area and place of residence, migration from the south, socioeconomic status, family history of stomach cancer and Quetelet index. Results not presented in tables. No association found for specific histological types separately.

Table 2.1.6.4 (contd)

Reference Country and years of study	Subjects	Exposure estimates	Relative risk (95% CI)		Comments, variables adjusted for, significance, limitations of the study
			Univariate	Multivariate	
Ferraroni et al. (1989) Italy 1983–88	Men and women	Former smoker	0.9	0.9	No participation rate for cases or controls. Univariate analysis adjusted for age and sex. Multivariate analysis adjusted for age, sex, social class, education, marital status, alcohol and coffee consumption.
		Cigarettes/day			
		<15	0.9	1.0	
		15–20	1.0	1.0	
		> 25	1.1	1.1	
		χ^2 for trend	0.18	1.19	
			All subsites	**Cardia and corpus**	
De Stefani et al. (1990) Uruguay 1985–88	Men and women			($n = 46$)	Analysis for men only because there were few women who smoked. No participation rate for controls. Odds ratios adjusted for age, area of residence, wine intake and vegetable consumption.
		Former smoker	1.9 (0.9–3.8)	1.8 (0.4–8.8)	
		Current smoker	2.7 (1.3–5.5)	5.3 (1.2–24.1)	
		p for trend	0.004	0.002	
		Age at starting smoking (years)			
		≥ 20	0.7 (0.4–1.3)		
		15–19	0.8 (0.5–1.3)		
		≤ 14	1.0		
		p for trend	0.01		
		Cigarettes/day			
		1–9	1.3 (0.5–3.4)	2.9 (0.6–14.8)	
		10–19	1.7 (0.7–4.3)	3.0 (0.6–15.0)	
		≥ 20	1.6 (0.6–3.8)	3.8 (0.8–17.1)	
		p for trend	0.92		
		Duration (years)			
		1–29	1.7 (0.7–4.2)	2.0 (0.3–12.0)	
		30–39	2.3 (0.9–5.4)	2.3 (0.4–12.6)	
		40–49	2.3 (1.0–5.2)	4.1 (0.9–19.4)	
		≥ 50	3.4 (1.5–7.5)	4.0 (0.8–19.4)	
		p for trend	0.002		

Table 2.1.6.4 (contd)

Reference Country and years of study	Subjects	Exposure estimates	Relative risk (95% CI)		Comments, variables adjusted for, significance, limitations of the study
De Stefani et al. (1990)		*Years since quitting*			
		≥ 10	0.6 (0.3–1.0)		
		5–9	0.5 (0.2–1.1)		
		1–4	1.2 (0.6–2.3)		
		p for trend	0.028		
		Filter-tipped			
		Non-user	1.0		
		User	1.2 (0.7–2.1)		
		Type of tobacco			
		Blond	1.0		
		Black	1.4 (0.9–2.3)		
Kato et al. (1990) Japan 1985–89	Men and women	**All types**	Men	Women	Many more cases than controls were aged ≥ 55 years. Odds ratios adjusted for age and residence. [†]Group 1, healthy controls; group 2, patients with atrophic gastritis. In a multivariate analysis, odds ratios additionally adjusted for type of breakfast, consumption of salted fish gut and cod roe and past history of gastric ulcer were significantly different from unity for all categories of smokers [data not shown].
		Compared with group 1[†]			
		Former smoker	1.8 (1.2–2.8)	1.3 (0.5–3.1)	
		Cigarettes/day			
		1–19	1.9 (1.1–3.3)	0.6 (0.2–1.8)	
		≥ 20	2.8 (1.8–4.3)	1.5 (0.6–3.7)	
		Compared with group 2			
		Former smoker	2.1 (1.4–3.3)	1.1 (0.4–2.9)	
		Cigarettes/day			
		1–19	2.5 (1.5–4.4)	0.6 (0.2–1.8)	
		≥ 20	3.5 (2.3–5.5)	2.5 (0.9–6.9)	
			(*n* = 117)	(*n* = 86)	
		Diffuse type			
		Compared with group 1			
		Former smoker	2.7 (1.4–5.5)	1.0 (0.3–3.4)	
		Cigarettes/day			
		1–19	1.8 (0.7–4.2)	0.5 (0.1–2.1)	
		≥ 20	3.3 (1.7–6.4)	1.1 (0.3–3.6)	

Table 2.1.6.4 (contd)

Reference Country and years of study	Subjects	Exposure estimates	Relative risk (95% CI)		Comments, variables adjusted for, significance, limitations of the study
Kato et al. (1990) (contd)		**Intestinal type**	(n = 166)	(n = 49)	
		Compared with group 1			
		Former smoker	1.6 (0.9–2.8)	1.2 (0.3–5.3)	
		Cigarettes/day			
		1–19	2.3 (1.2–4.3)	0.8 (0.2–3.6)	
		≥ 20	3.0 (1.7–5.1)	2.7 (0.8–9.9)	
		Compared with group 2			
		Former smoker	2.0 (1.2–3.4)	0.9 (0.2–4.3)	
		Cigarettes/day			
		1–19	3.1 (1.6–6.0)	0.7 (0.2–3.2)	
		≥ 20	3.8 (2.2–6.6)	6.4 (1.5–27.4)	
Lee et al. (1990) China, Province of Taiwan 1954–88	Men and women	Current smoker	1.6 ($p < 0.05$)		No definition of smoking habit. Multivariate analysis adjusted for alcohol drinking, green tea habit and salted meat, fried food, fermented beans and milk, as well as other variables not listed. Relative risks probably underestimated by use of controls with eye diseases possibly causally associated with smoking
		Duration (years)			
		1–30	1.4		
		31–40	1.4		
		≥ 41	1.9 ($p < 0.05$)		
		Cigarettes/day			
		1–10	1.4		
		11–20	1.5		
		≥ 21	1.8 ($p < 0.05$)		
Wu–Williams et al. (1990) USA 1975–82	Men		**All pairs**	**Excl. proxies**	Very small study. Very low response rate for cases; no participation rate for controls. High proportion of interviews with proxies (42% of cases, 12% of controls). Numbers in analyses by subsites too small for meaningful conclusion. Matched analysis made without adjustment.
		Former smoker	1.3 (0.6–2.5)	1.8	†Values for which the 95% CI does not include 1.0
		Current smoker (packs/day)			
		1	2.2 (1.1–4.7)	5.4†	
		2	2.1 (1.0–4.5)	4.0†	
		≥ 3	5.2 (1.4–8.6)	17.7†	
		Any tobacco			
		Former smoker	1.1 (0.5–2.2)	1.9	
		Current smoker (g/day)			
		1–20	2.3 (1.1–4.8)	6.2†	
		> 20–40	2.0 (1.0–4.3)	3.3†	
		> 40	5.0 (1.4–17.5)	17.1†	

Table 2.1.6.4 (contd)

Reference Country and years of study	Subjects	Exposure estimates	Relative risk (95% CI) Cardia	Fundus/body	Comments, variables adjusted for, significance, limitations of the study
Wu-Williams et al. (1990) (contd)		Former smoker	1.0	3.4	
		Current smoker (packs/day)			
		1	2.3	2.0	
		2	2.2	4.4	
		≥3	7.0†	9.3	
		Any tobacco			
		Former smoker	0.9	3.5	
		Current smoker (g/day)			
		1–20	2.3	2.1	
		> 20–40	2.6	4.2	
		> 40	7.0†	9.3	

			Antrum/pylorus	**All others**	
		Former smoker	0.8	1.4	
		Current smoker (packs/day)			
		1	4.0	1.7	
		2	4.1	1.8	
		≥3	7.2	1.8	
		Any tobacco			
		Former smoker	0.4	1.2	
		Current smoker (g/day)			
		1–20	4.8	1.8	
		> 20–40	2.9	1.8	
		> 40	12.1†	1.9	
Boeing et al. (1991) Germany 1985–87	Men and women	Former smoker	0.6 (0.3–1.2)		Higher proportion of nonsmokers in cases from two study centres; higher proportion of smokers in hospital controls than in visitor controls; 47% of hospital controls had tobacco-related diseases. Odds ratios adjusted for age, sex and hospital. Significant positive trend observed for pack–years [data not shown]
		Current smoker	0.5 (0.3–0.9)		

Table 2.1.6.4 (contd)

Reference Country and years of study	Subjects	Exposure estimates	Relative risk (95% CI)	Comments, variables adjusted for, significance, limitations of the study
Dockerty et al. (1991) New Zealand 1980–84	Men	Ever-smoker	1.4 (1.2–1.6)[b] 1.4 (1.2–1.7)[c]	Information on smoking habit abstracted from Cancer Registry records. No definition of smoking habit. No information on histological confirmation of diagnoses
Saha (1991) UK 8 years	Men and women	Former smoker Current smoker Non-swallower Swallower Cigarettes/day 10–19 20–30 *Age at starting smoking (years)* 16–20 21–30 10–15 *Swallowers* Compared with non-swallower Compared with nonsmoker	1.4 (1.7–3.6) 2.6 (1.2–5.5) 1.3 (1.5–2.4) 6.4 (3.3–12.5) **Body**[†] **Antrum**[†] 0.6 (0.9–3.9) 2.1 (0.6–7.5) 1.9 (0.5–7.5) 2.9 (0.9–9.3) 0.5 (0.1–3.3) 1.3 (0.3–4.7) 2.0 (0.6–6.9) 1.2 (0.4–3.9) 1.3 (0.3–5.2) 2.5 (0.3–7.8) 7.2 (1.3–41.0) 2.4 (0.6–9.0)	Small no. of cases for the period of study. No participation rate for cases or controls. Statistical analysis limited. Odds ratios not adjusted. Small study †Cancer of cardia used as reference (odds ratio, 1.0)
Yu & Hsieh (1991) China 1976–80	Men and women	*Cigarettes/day* 1–20 > 20	**Crude** **Adjusted** 3.7 2.1 (0.9–4.6) 20.7 6.2 (2.2–17.0) *p* for trend = 0.003	57% of interviews for cases with proxies. Odds ratios adjusted for age, sex, family income, family history of cancer or tuberculosis, blood type and consumption of alcohol, strong tea, fruit and milk
Agudo et al. (1992) Spain 1987–89	Men and women	Former smoker Current smoker Ever-smoker	0.9 (0.5–1.7) 0.9 (0.6–1.5) 0.9 (0.6–1.7)	Analysis for men only because few women smoked. No participation rate for cases or controls. Odds ratios adjusted for total caloric intake (including alcohol) and consumption of fruit, vegetables, cold cuts and preserved fish.

Table 2.1.6.4 (contd)

Reference Country and years of study	Subjects	Exposure estimates	Relative risk (95% CI)	Comments, variables adjusted for, significance, limitations of the study
Hoshiyama & Sasaba (1992a,b) Japan 1984–90	Men		**Single** **Multiple**	No definition of smoking status. Very low response rate for controls. No comparison of demographic variables such as education or socioeconomic status between cases and controls. Odds ratios adjusted for sex, age and administrative division.
		Former smoker	1.1 (0.6–1.8) 0.9 (0.3–3.0)	
		Current smoker	1.5 (0.9–2.6) 1.4 (0.5–4.3)	
		Pack–years		
		≤ 40	1.4 (0.8–2.3) 1.1 (0.3–3.3)	
		> 40	1.3 (0.8–2.4) 1.3 (0.4–4.2)	
Palli *et al.* (1992) Italy 1985–87	Men and women		**Gastric cardia** **Other subsites**	Study population from Buatti *et al.* (1989, 1991). Odds ratios adjusted for age, sex, area and place of residence, migration from the south, socioeconomic status, family history of stomach cancer and Quetelet index. Similar results with pack–years variable [data not shown]
		Current smoker	1.1 (0.6–2.3) 0.9 (0.7–1.1)	
		Former smoker	1.1 (0.5–2.2) 1.1 (0.8–1.4)	
Jedrychowski *et al.* (1993) Poland 1986–90	Men	*Filter status*		Current and former smokers combined because of insufficient distinction in questionnaire. Odds ratios adjusted for hospital, age, sex, occupation, education, sausage consumption, fruit and vegetable consumption and vodka drinking. No relative risks for ever-smokers. No increased relative risk for cigarettes/day, age at starting smoking or smoking before breakfast [data not shown]. Odds ratios seem overadjusted
		With filter/unknown	1.0 (0.7–1.5)	
		With and without filter	1.1 (0.8–1.6)	
		Without filter	1.4 (0.9–2.1)	
		p for trend	0.14	
		Pack–years		
		< 20	1.2 (0.8–1.7)	
		≥ 20	1.1 (0.8–1.6)	
		p for trend	0.58	

Table 2.1.6.4 (contd)

Reference Country and years of study	Subjects	Exposure estimates	Relative risk (95% CI)	Comments, variables adjusted for, significance, limitations of the study
Kabat *et al.* (1993) USA 1981–90	Men and women	**Men**	**Distal stomach**	Analysis limited to Caucasians. No participation rate for controls. Odds ratios adjusted for age, education, alcohol consumption, hospital and time of interview.
		Current smoker	1.7 (1.0–3.0)	
		Former smoker	1.4 (0.9–2.4)	
		Cigarettes/day		
		1–20	1.7 (1.0–2.8)	
		21–30	0.8 (0.3–1.8)	
		≥ 31	1.6 (0.9–2.9)	
		Years since quitting[†]		[†]Relative to current smokers
		≥ 21	0.6 (0.3–1.2)	
		11–20	1.1 (0.6–1.9)	
		6–10	1.1 (0.6–2.4)	
		1–5	1.0 (0.5–2.0)	
		Women		
		Current smoker	3.2 (1.3–7.7)	
		Former smoker	2.0 (0.8–4.9)	
		Cigarettes/day		
		1–20	1.6 (0.6–3.8)	
		≥ 21	4.8 (1.9–11.9)	
		Years since quitting[†]		[†]Relative to current smokers
		1–10	0.7 (0.2–2.2)	
		≥ 11	0.7 (0.2–2.1)	
Hansson *et al.* (1994) Sweden 1989–92	Men and women	Former smoker	1.1 (0.8–1.6)	Odds ratios adjusted for age, sex, socioeconomic status and use of other tobacco
		Current smoker	1.7 (1.2–2.5)	
		Age at starting smoking (years)		
		≥ 21	1.2 (0.7–1.9)	
		16–20	1.4 (0.9–2.0)	
		≤ 15	1.5 (0.9–2.5)	
		p for trend	0.38	

Table 2.1.6.4 (contd)

Reference Country and years of study	Subjects	Exposure estimates	Relative risk (95% CI)	Comments, variables adjusted for, significance, limitations of the study
Hansson et al. (1994) (contd)		*Duration (years)*		
		1–10	1.1 (0.6–2.1)	
		11–20	1.1 (0.6–2.0)	
		21–30	0.8 (0.5–1.4)	
		31–40	1.8 (1.2–3.0)	
		≥ 41	1.6 (1.1–2.5)	
		p for trend	0.01	
		Cigarettes/day		
		1–5	1.1 (0.7–1.7)	
		6–10	1.4 (0.9–2.1)	
		11–15	2.1 (1.2–3.5)	
		≥ 16	1.2 (0.8–1.8)	
		p for trend	0.10	
		Years since quitting		
		> 31	0.9 (0.5–1.7)	
		21–31	0.9 (0.5–1.7)	
		11–20	1.2 (0.7–2.1)	
		≤ 10	1.3 (0.7–2.2)	
		Current smoker	1.7 (1.2–2.5)	
		p for trend	0.02	
Inoue et al. (1994) Japan 1988–91	Men and women	**Men**	**All**	No definition of smoking habit. Odds ratios adjusted for age (continuous) and intake of fresh vegetables. According to the authors, prevalence of smoking in general population in Japan is slightly higher than in hospital controls used (81.6% vs 77% in men), possibly leading to a slight overestimation of risks
		Ever-smoker	2.6 (1.7–3.8)	**Cardia** (*n* = 79)
		Current smoker	2.7 (1.8–4.1)	4.4 (1.8–11.3)
		Former smoker	2.4 (1.6–3.6)	4.7 (1.8–12.3)
		Cigarettes/day		4.1 (1.6–11.0)
		< 20	2.7 (1.6–4.5)	5.9 (2.0–17.3)
		≥ 20	2.7 (1.8–4.1)	4.3 (1.6–11.5)
		Years since quitting		
		≥ 10	2.3 (1.4–3.7)	2.8 (0.9–8.6)
		1–9	2.5 (1.5–4.1)	4.7 (1.6–13.7)
		< 1	2.6 (1.2–5.2)	6.9 (1.9–25.0)

Table 2.1.6.4 (contd)

Reference Country and years of study	Subjects	Exposure estimates	Relative risk (95% CI)		Comments, variables adjusted for, significance, limitations of the study
Inoue et al. (1994) (contd)			**Middle** (n = 133)	**Antrum** (n = 170)	
		Ever-smoker	1.8 (1.0–3.1)	2.9 (1.7–5.1)	
		Current smoker	1.9 (1.1–3.4)	3.0 (1.7–5.4)	
		Former smoker	1.6 (0.9–2.9)	2.7 (1.5–5.0)	
		Cigarettes/day			
		< 20	1.4 (0.6–3.0)	3.0 (1.5–6.1)	
		≥ 20	2.2 (1.2–3.9)	3.0 (1.6–5.5)	
		Years since quitting			
		≥ 10	1.7 (0.9–3.4)	2.7 (1.4–5.4)	
		1–9	1.4 (0.7–3.0)	3.0 (1.5–6.1)	
		< 1	3.6 (0.8–5.8)	2.1 (0.7–6.1)	
		Women	**All**	**Cardia** (n = 44)	Because of the small number of women who smoked, no detailed analyses were performed
		Ever-smoker	1.2 (0.7–2.0)	1.3 (0.5–3.1)	
			Middle (n = 85)	**Antrum** (n = 86)	
			1.0 (0.5–2.1)	1.3 (0.7–2.6)	
Siemiatycki et al. (1995) Canada 1979–85	Men	Ever-smoker	1.7 (1.1–2.6)		Odds ratios adjusted for age, ethnic group, socioeconomic status, consumption of β-carotene, coffee and alcohol. Odds ratios shown are with population controls only. Difference in odds ratios between population and hospital controls was negligible.
		Pack-years			
		≤ 25	1.6 (0.9–2.8)		
		26–49	1.6 (1.0–2.7)		
		50–74	1.7 (1.0–2.9)		
		≥ 75	1.9 (1.0–3.3)		
Yu et al. (1995) China 1991–93	Men and women	*Cigarettes/day*			No definition of smoking habit. Odds ratios adjusted for age and sex
		1–9	1.2 (0.8–1.9)		
		10–19	1.1 (0.8–1.5)		
		≥ 20	1.9 (1.4–2.5)		

Table 2.1.6.4 (contd)

Reference Country and years of study	Subjects	Exposure estimates	Relative risk (95% CI)		Comments, variables adjusted for, significance, limitations of the study
Gajalakshmi & Shanta (1996) India 1988–90	Men and women	*Any tobacco* Former smoker Current smoker Ever-smoker Current cigarette smoker	**Model 1** 1.8 (1.1–3.1) 2.7 (1.8–4.1) 2.5 (1.7–3.6) 2.0 (1.1–3.6)	**Model 2** 1.5 (0.7–3.5) 2.5 (1.4–4.4) 2.2 (1.3–3.8)	Any tobacco included bidi, cigarette and/or chutta. Conditional logistic regression models: Model 1, adjusted for income, education and area of residence; Model 2, additionally adjusted for betel-quid chewing habit and significant dietary factors. Absence of trend with age at starting smoking probably caused by reference age of 20 years or less being too high
		Age at starting smoking (years) > 30 21–30 ≤ 20 *p* for trend	1.5 (0.4–5.6) 2.1 (0.9–5.1) 2.4 (0.9–5.9) < 0.1		
		Lifetime exposure (no. of cigarettes) < 50 000 (mild) 50 000–100 000 (moderate) > 100 000 (heavy) *p* for trend	1.6 (0.7–3.6) 2.0 (0.7–5.4) 3.1 (0.9–10.5) < 0.01		
Ji *et al.* (1996) China 1988–89	Men and women	Former smoker Current smoker	**Men** 1.3 (0.9–1.8) 1.4 (1.1–1.7)	**Women** 2.0 (0.7–5.6) 0.9 (0.5–1.4)	Odds ratios adjusted for age, education and income (and alcohol drinking for men only)
		Cigarettes/day 1–9 10–19 20–29 ≥ 30 *p* for trend	1.0 (0.7–1.4) 1.1 (0.8–1.4) 1.8 (1.4–2.3) 1.4 (0.9–2.1) 0.0002	1.1 (0.6–2.0) 0.5 (0.2–1.2) 2.1 (0.7–6.3)[†] 0.80	[†] ≥ 20 cigarettes/day
		Duration (years) 0.5–19 20–29 30–39 ≥ 40 *p* for trend	1.0 (0.7–1.5) 1.4 (1.02–2.0) 1.3 (0.9–1.7) 1.6 (1.2–2.2) 0.002	1.0 (0.4–2.6) 1.0 (0.4–2.1) 1.1 (0.5–2.4) 0.9 (0.4–2.2) 0.91	

Table 2.1.6.4 (contd)

Reference Country and years of study	Subjects	Exposure estimates	Relative risk (95% CI)		Comments, variables adjusted for, significance, limitations of the study
Ji *et al.* (1996) (contd)		*Pack–years*			
		< 10	1.0 (0.7–1.4)	< 10	0.9 (0.4–1.6)
		10–19	1.1 (0.8–1.5)	10–19	1.0 (0.5–2.1)
		20–39	1.5 (1.2–2.1)	≥ 20	1.3 (0.5–3.1)
		≥ 40	1.7 (1.2–2.3)		
		p for trend	0.0002	0.62	
		Age at starting smoking (years)			
		≥ 30	1.0 (0.7–1.4)	≥ 25	0.7 (0.4–1.3)
		25–29	1.4 (0.9–1.9)	< 25	1.8 (0.9–3.6)
		20–24	1.6 (1.2–2.2)		
		< 20	1.3 (0.95–1.7)		
		p for trend	0.005	0.37	
		Years since quitting			
		≥ 20	0.7 (0.3–1.6)	≥ 10	3.7 (0.9–14.7)
		10–19	1.5 (0.8–2.7)	< 10	0.7 (0.1–4.1)
		5–9	0.9 (0.5–1.9)		
		< 5	2.7 (1.4–5.4)		
		p for trend	0.10	0.48	
		Men	**Cardia** (*n* = 145)	**Distal** (*n* = 530)	
		Former smoker	1.8 (0.97–3.4)	1.1 (0.7–1.7)	
		Current smoker	1.2 (0.8–1.9)	1.4 (1.1–1.9)	
		Cigarettes/day			
		1–9	1.0 (0.5–2.1)	1.0 (0.7–1.6)	
		10–19	1.1 (0.7–1.9)	1.0 (0.8–1.5)	
		20–29	1.4 (0.9–2.3)	1.9 (1.4–2.6)	
		≥ 30	1.9 (0.96–3.7)	1.3 (0.8–2.1)	
		p for trend	0.06	0.0004	

Table 2.1.6.4 (contd)

Reference Country and years of study	Subjects	Exposure estimates	Relative risk (95% CI)	Comments, variables adjusted for, significance, limitations of the study
		Duration (years)		
		0.5–19	1.4 (0.7–2.7)	
		20–29	1.2 (0.6–2.3)	
		30–39	1.1 (0.6–1.9)	
		≥ 40	1.4 (0.9–2.4)	
		p for trend	0.28	
		Pack–years		
		< 10	1.4 (0.8–2.6)	
		10–19	0.8 (0.4–1.6)	
		20–24	1.3 (0.8–2.2)	
		≥ 25	1.6 (0.9–2.7)	
		p for trend	0.14	
		Age at starting smoking (years)		
		≥ 30	1.0 (0.5–1.8)	
		25–29	2.0 (1.1–3.6)	
		20–24	1.5 (0.9–2.5)	
		< 20	1.0 (0.5–1.7)	
		p for trend	0.52	
		Years since quitting		
		≥ 20	1.5 (0.5–5.2)	
		10–19	1.3 (0.5–4.0)	
		5–9	1.3 (0.4–4.3)	
		< 5	5.5 (1.9–15.9)	
		p for trend	0.01	
			1.0 (0.6–1.4)	
			1.5 (1.02–2.2)	
			1.4 (1.2–2.5)	
			1.8 (1.2–2.5)	
			0.001	
			1.0 (0.7–1.5)	
			1.1 (0.7–1.6)	
			1.7 (1.2–2.3)	
			1.7 (1.2–2.4)	
			0.0002	
			1.0 (0.7–1.5)	
			1.2 (0.8–1.9)	
			1.8 (1.3–2.4)	
			1.4 (0.99–1.9)	
			0.002	
			0.5 (0.2–1.5)	
			1.4 (0.7–2.8)	
			0.7 (0.3–1.8)	
			2.5 (1.1–5.4)	
			0.10	
Zhang *et al.* (1996) USA 1992–94	Men and women	Ever-smoker	**Distal stomach** 1.8 (0.9–3.8)	Odds ratios adjusted for age, sex, race, education, alcohol intake, body-mass index and total calorie intake
		Cigarettes/day		
		1–20	1.6 (0.7–3.5)	
		21–40	3.3 (1.2–9.2)	
		> 40	4.0 (0.6–25.2)	
		p for trend	0.0220	

Table 2.1.6.4 (contd)

Reference Country and years of study	Subjects	Exposure estimates	Relative risk (95% CI)		Comments, variables adjusted for, significance, limitations of the study
Zhang et al. (1996) (contd)		Continuous variable cigarettes/day			
		Years of smoking			
		1–20	1.2 (0.5–3.2)		
		21–40	1.7 (0.7–4.0)		
		> 40	2.6 (0.9–7.8)		
		p for trend	0.0485		
		Pack–years			
		1–29	1.1 (0.5–2.5)		
		30–59	2.7 (1.1–6.9)		
		> 60	4.6 (1.3–16.6)		
		p for trend	0.0074		
		Continuous variable; pack–years			
		Age at starting smoking (years)			
		> 20	1.4 (0.5–3.9)		
		17–20	2.6 (1.03–6.7)		
		≤ 16	1.8 (0.7–4.5)		
		p for trend	0.1332		
Gammon et al. (1997) USA 1993–95	Men and women		**Cardia**	**Other**	Odds ratios adjusted for age, sex, geographical area, race, body-mass index, income and alcohol intake
		Current smoker	2.6 (1.7–4.0)	1.8 (1.2–2.7)	
		Former smoker	1.9 (1.3–2.9)	1.5 (1.1–2.1)	
		Years since quitting			
		> 30	1.1 (0.6–2.0)	1.0 (0.6–1.8)	
		21–30	2.2 (1.3–3.7)	1.5 (0.9–2.4)	
		11–30	1.6 (0.9–2.8)	1.7 (1.0–2.7)	
		< 10	2.9 (1.8–4.8)	1.8 (1.2–2.9)	
		p for trend	< 0.05	< 0.05	

Table 2.1.6.4 (contd)

Reference Country and years of study	Subjects	Exposure estimates	Relative risk (95% CI)	Comments, variables adjusted for, significance, limitations of the study
Gammon *et al.* (1997) (contd)		*Cigarettes/day*		
		< 16	1.4 (0.9–2.2)	1.5 (1.0–2.2)
		16–20	2.2 (1.4–3.4)	1.7 (1.2–2.6)
		21–30	3.1 (1.9–5.2)	1.4 (0.9–2.5)
		> 30	2.0 (1.2–3.3)	1.5 (1.0–2.4)
		p for trend	< 0.05	
		Duration (years)		
		< 20	1.6 (1.0–2.6)	1.0 (0.7–1.6)
		20–31	1.8 (1.1–2.9)	1.6 (1.0–2.4)
		32–42	2.7 (1.7–4.2)	1.8 (1.2–2.7)
		> 42	2.9 (1.8–4.7)	2.1 (1.4–3.1)
		p for trend	< 0.05	< 0.05
		Pack–years		
		< 14	0.9 (0.5–1.6)	1.2 (0.8–1.8)
		14–31	2.3 (1.4–3.6)	1.5 (1.0–2.4)
		32–54	2.8 (1.8–4.4)	1.7 (1.2–2.6)
		> 54	2.5 (1.5–4.1)	2.1 (1.3–3.2)
		p for trend	< 0.05	< 0.05
		Filter status		
		With filter	2.1 (1.4–3.1)	1.6 (1.1–2.2)
		With and without filter	1.5 (0.8–2.7)	1.1 (0.6–1.9)
		Without filter	2.1 (1.3–3.2)	1.5 (1.0–2.3)

Table 2.1.6.4 (contd)

Reference Country and years of study	Subjects	Exposure estimates	Relative risk (95% CI)	Comments, variables adjusted for, significance, limitations of the study
De Stefani et al. (1998) Uruguay 1992–96	Men	Former smoker	1.3 (0.8–2.2)	Odds ratios adjusted for age, residence, urban/rural status, total alcohol consumption and vegetable intake
		Current smoker	2.6 (1.6–3.1)	
		Ever-smoker	1.8 (1.2–2.8)	
		Cigarettes/day		
		1–10	1.6 (0.9–2.8)	
		11–20	1.8 (1.2–3.1)	
		21–30	2.5 (1.5–4.5)	
		≥ 31	1.2 (0.7–2.2)	
		p for trend	0.23	
		Duration (years)		
		1–29	1.2 (0.7–2.2)	
		30–39	1.7 (0.9–3.0)	
		40–49	1.9 (1.1–3.0)	
		≥ 50	2.2 (1.3–3.6)	
		p for trend	< 0.001	
		Pack–years		
		1–13	1.6 (0.9–2.6)	
		14–25	1.7 (1.0–2.8)	
		26–50	2.1 (1.3–3.6)	
		≥ 51	2.3 (1.4–3.8)	
		p for trend	< 0.001	
		Years since quitting		
		≥ 15	1.1 (0.7–1.9)	
		10–14	1.0 (0.5–2.1)	
		5–9	1.5 (0.8–2.9)	
		1–4	2.4 (1.3–4.3)	
		Current smoker	2.6 (1.6–4.1)	
		p for trend	< 0.001	

Table 2.1.6.4 (contd)

Reference Country and years of study	Subjects	Exposure estimates	Relative risk (95% CI)	Comments, variables adjusted for, significance, limitations of the study
De Stefani et al. (1998) (contd)		*Age at starting smoking (years)*		
		≥ 20	1.8 (1.1–3.0)	
		15–19	1.9 (1.2–3.1)	
		10–14	1.9 (1.2–3.1)	
		< 10	2.3 (1.2–4.3)	
		p for trend	0.01	
		Type of cigarette		
		Blond	1.6 (1.0–2.6)	
		Black	2.0 (1.3–3.3)	
		Manufactured	1.2 (0.6–2.1)	
		Hand-rolled	1.9 (1.2–3.1)	
		Filter-tipped	1.4 (0.9–2.5)	
		Untipped	1.9 (1.3–3.1)	
		Duration (years)	**Cardia** / **Antrum/pylorus**	
		0–31	1.0 / 1.0	
		32–47	2.9 (0.8–11.6) / 1.6 (1.1–2.4)	
		≥ 48	5.3 (1.4–20.2) / 2.1 (1.4–3.2)	
		p for trend	0.006 / < 0.001	
			Fundus / **Diffuse**	
		0–31	1.0 / 1.0	
		32–47	0.4 (0.1–1.3) / 2.6 (0.9–7.7)	
		≥ 48	1.4 (0.5–3.7) / 1.4 (0.4–5.5)	
		p for trend	0.64 / 0.50	
Liu et al. (1998) China 1986–88	Men and women		**Men†** / **Women†**	†Values in parentheses represent standard errors. Odds ratios stratified by 5-year age groups of age at death and study area (county or city district)
		Current Smoker	1.4 (0.03) / 1.2 (0.06)	
		Urban	1.4 (0.03) / 1.3 (0.05)	
		Rural	1.4 (0.04) / 1.1 (0.07)	
		Cigarettes/day	**Urban** / **Rural**	
		1–19	1.3 (0.04) / 1.3 (0.05)	
		20	1.4 (0.04) / 1.6 (0.06)	
		> 20	1.5 (0.08) / 1.7 (0.13)	

Table 2.1.6.4 (contd)

Reference Country and years of study	Subjects	Exposure estimates	Relative risk (95% CI)		Comments, variables adjusted for, significance, limitations of the study
Liu et al. (1998) (contd)		*Duration (years)*			
		<20	1.5 (0.05)		
		20–24	1.3 (0.04)		
		≥25	1.3 (0.05)		
Chow et al. (1999) Poland 1994–97	Men and women		**Men**	**Women**	Odds ratios adjusted for age, education, years lived on a farm, family history of cancer; p values for trend not calculated
		Ever-smoker	1.2 (0.8–1.8)	1.8 (1.1–3.0)	
		Former smoker	0.9 (0.6–1.4)	1.8 (0.9–3.7)	
		Current smoker	1.7 (1.1–2.7)	1.8 (1.0–3.3)	
		Cigarettes/day			
		≤10	0.7 (0.4–1.2)	1.3 (0.7–2.5)	
		11–20	1.5 (1.0–2.3)	2.5 (0.9–3.7)	
		≥21	1.5 (0.9–2.6)	1.8 (1.0–3.3)	
		Duration (years)			
		<20	0.6 (0.3–1.1)	2.3 (1.0–5.4)	
		20–29	1.0 (0.6–1.8)	1.8 (0.8–3.8)	
		30–39	1.1 (0.7–1.9)	1.6 (0.7–3.7)	
		40–49	2.0 (1.2–3.4)	1.8 (0.7–4.4)[†]	[†] ≥ 40 years
		≥50	2.0 (1.0–3.9)		
		Age at starting smoking (years)			
		≥25	0.6 (0.3–1.3)	1.7 (0.8–3.4)	
		20–24	1.1 (0.7–1.9)	1.1 (0.5–2.4)	
		18–19	1.7 (1.0–2.8)	3.5 (1.5–8.0)	
		<18	1.3 (0.8–2.1)	2.1 (0.7–6.3)	
		Years since quitting			
		≥30	0.7 (0.4–1.5)	3.0 (1.0–9.2)[‡]	[‡] ≥ 20 years
		20–29	0.8 (0.4–1.6)	1.5 (0.5–4.3)	
		10–19	0.9 (0.5–1.7)	1.3 (0.4–4.0)	
		<10	1.0 (0.5–1.8)		

Table 2.1.6.4 (contd)

Reference Country and years of study	Subjects	Exposure estimates	Relative risk (95% CI)		Comments, variables adjusted for, significance, limitations of the study
Chow et al. (1999) (contd)		*Pack–years*			
		< 10	0.8 (0.4–1.5)		
		10–< 20	0.9 (0.5–1.9)		
		20–< 30	1.0 (0.6–1.8)		§≥ 30 pack–years
		30–< 40	1.0 (0.6–1.8)		
		40–< 50	2.1 (1.2–3.8)		
		≥ 50	1.9 (1.1–3.3)		
		Filter status			
		With filter	1.2 (0.8–1.9)		
		Without filter	0.8 (0.5–1.3)		
		With and without filter	1.9 (1.1–3.2)		
Gao et al. (1999) China 1995	Men and women	Ever-smoker	0.9 (0.5–1.7)		Odds ratios adjusted for age and sex
Inoue et al. (1999) Japan 1988–95	Men and women		**Men**	**Women**	Odds ratios adjusted for age, year and season at first hospital visit, family history of gastric cancer, alcohol drinking, preference for salty food and fruit intake
		Former smoker	1.7 (1.3–2.3)	1.4 (0.8–2.3)	
		Current smoker	2.5 (1.9–3.3)	1.7 (1.3–2.4)	
		< 60 years old	(n = 314)	(n = 182)	
		Former smoker	2.2 (1.4–3.4)	2.1 (1.1–4.1)	
		Current smoker	3.3 (2.2–4.9)	1.7 (1.1–2.5)	
		≥ 60 years old	(n = 337)	(n = 162)	
		Former smoker	1.4 (0.9–2.0)	0.8 (0.3–2.0)	
		Current smoker	1.9 (1.3–2.7)	2.0 (1.2–3.2)	

Table 2.1.6.4 (contd)

Reference Country and years of study	Subjects	Exposure estimates	Relative risk (95% CI)			Comments, variables adjusted for, significance, limitations of the study
Ye et al. (1999) Sweden 1989–95	Men and women		**Cardia**	**Distal (intestinal)**	**Distal (diffuse)**	Odds ratios adjusted for age, sex, residence area, body-mass index 20 years before interview, socioeconomic status, use of smokeless tobacco and use of beer, wine and spirits. About 30% of eligible cases died or became too ill to be interviewed; if smoking affects the prognosis of stomach cancer, relative risks could be underestimated
		Former smoker	0.8 (0.4–1.5)	1.4 (0.9–2.0)	1.2 (0.8–2.0)	
		Cigarettes/day				
		1–10	1.7 (0.7–3.8)	1.6 (0.9–2.8)	1.9 (1.0–3.4)	
		11–15	1.2 (0.4–3.8)	1.8 (0.9–3.7)	2.5 (1.2–5.5)	
		≥ 16	2.2 (1.0–4.8)	2.0 (1.1–3.9)	2.7 (1.4–5.1)	
		p for trend	0.04	0.005	0.0004	
		Duration (years)				
		1–30	1.3 (0.5–3.6)	1.2 (0.5–2.9)	1.9 (0.9–3.8)	
		≥ 31	2.2 (1.1–4.3)	2.1 (1.3–3.4)	2.6 (1.5–4.5)	
		p for trend	0.03	0.002	0.0003	
Lagergren et al. (2000) Sweden 1995–97	Men and women		**Univariate**	**Multivariate**		Smokers include cigarette, cigar and pipe smokers. Univariate analysis adjusted for age and sex; multivariate analysis further adjusted for alcohol use, educational level, body-mass index, reflux symptoms, intake of fruit and vegetables, energy intake and physical activity. Multivariate analysis for no. of cigarettes/day included adjustments for cigarette smoking, pipe smoking, and snuff use. *p* values for trend not always shown. Odds ratios in multivariate analysis not significantly different from univariate analysis [data not shown]
		Former smoker	3.1 (2.1–4.5)	3.4 (2.2–5.2)		
		Current smoker	3.9 (2.6–5.8)	4.5 (2.9–7.1)		
		Duration (years)				
		1–20	1.8 (1.1–2.9)	2.1 (1.2–3.4)		
		21–35	3.6 (2.3–5.5)	3.9 (2.4–6.2)		
		> 35	4.6 (3.0–6.9)	5.7 (3.6–9.1)		
		Cigarettes/day				
		1–9	2.2 (1.4–3.4)	2.3 (1.4–3.7)		
		10–19	3.0 (2.0–4.5)	3.1 (2.0–4.9)		
		> 19	3.5 (2.3–5.2)	3.6 (2.3–5.7)		
		Years since quitting				
		> 25	1.9 (1.1–3.1)	2.1 (1.2–3.6)		
		11–25	3.7 (2.3–5.8)	4.2 (2.6–7.0)		
		3–10	4.1 (2.4–7.0)	4.9 (2.8–8.7)		
		0–2	4.2 (2.8–6.4)	5.0 (3.2–8.0)		
		p for trend	< 0.0001			

Table 2.1.6.4 (contd)

Reference Country and years of study	Subjects	Exposure estimates	Relative risk (95% CI)	Comments, variables adjusted for, significance, limitations of the study
Mathew et al. (2000) India 1988–91	Men and women	*Smoking index*[†] 1–199 200–399 400–599 ≥ 600 *p* for trend	0.8 (0.4–1.8) 2.3 (1.2–4.6) 1.8 (0.9–3.7) 2.6 (1.4–4.7) 0.0008	No response rate for cases or controls. No definition of smoking status. Odds ratios adjusted for age, sex, religion, education and income [†]No. of cigarettes and bidis/week × years of smoking
Zaridze et al. (2000) Russia 1996–97	Men and women	Former smoker Current smoker *Cigarettes/day* 1–11 12–19 ≥ 20 *p* for trend *Pack–years* 1–18 19–32 ≥ 33 *p* for trend *Duration (years)* 1–26 27–39 ≥ 40 *p* for trend *Age at starting smoking (years)* ≥ 20 16–19 < 16 *p* for trend	**All types** 1.1 (0.6–1.9) 1.4 (0.9–2.2) 1.0 (0.6–1.7) 1.6 (0.9–2.8) 1.2 (0.8–2.0) 0.24 0.9 (0.5–1.5) 1.5 (0.9–2.5) 1.5 (0.9–2.5) 0.06 1.0 (0.6–1.8) 1.7 (1.0–2.8) 1.1 (0.7–1.9) 0.30 1.2 (0.7–2.1) 1.1 (0.7–1.9) 1.4 (0.8–2.3) 0.57 **Cardia** 1.2 (0.5–3.1) 2.0 (0.9–4.5) 1.2 (0.5–3.0) 1.5 (0.6–4.0) 2.4 (1.0–5.3) 0.03 1.1 (0.4–2.8) 1.2 (0.4–3.1) 3.1 (1.3–7.2) 0.01 1.0 (0.4–2.7) 2.6 (1.1–6.1) 1.7 (0.7–4.1) 0.08 2.1 (0.9–5.0) 1.2 (0.5–3.2) 1.9 (0.8–4.4) 0.21	Controls significantly younger and better educated than cases (*p* < 0.01). Odds ratios adjusted for age, education and vodka consumption. Relative risk may be underestimated because of substantial proportion of controls had smoking-associated diseases (> 20%). Relative risks for sites other than cardia show similar trend but no statistically significant increases [data not shown]. Relative risk for women around 1.0

Table 2.1.6.4 (contd)

Reference Country and years of study	Subjects	Exposure estimates	Relative risk (95% CI)		Comments, variables adjusted for, significance, limitations of the study
			Cardia	**Distal stomach**	
Wu et al. (2001) USA 1992–97	Men and women	Former smoker	1.2 (0.9–1.6)	1.1 (0.8–1.5)	Very low participation rate for cases; no response rate for controls. Odds ratios adjusted for age, sex, race, birthplace and education
		Cigarettes/day			
		1–19	1.1 (0.7–1.6)	1.1 (0.8–1.6)	
		≥ 20	1.3 (0.9–1.8)	1.0 (0.7–1.5)	
		Current smoker	2.1 (1.5–3.1)	1.5 (1.1–2.1)	
		Cigarettes/day			
		1–19	2.2 (1.3–3.8)	1.3 (0.8–2.1)	
		20–39	1.6 (1.0–2.6)	1.4 (0.9–2.3)	
		≥ 40	3.8 (2.1–7.0)	2.4 (1.1–4.9)	
		p for trend	< 0.0001	< 0.02	
		Duration (years)			
		≤ 20	1.1 (0.8–1.6)	0.8 (0.6–1.2)	
		21–40	1.4 (1.0–1.9)	1.5 (1.1–2.1)	
		≥ 41	2.3 (1.5–3.4)	1.6 (1.1–2.4)	
		p for trend	< 0.0002	0.002	
		Age at starting smoking (years)			
		≥ 21	1.4 (0.9–2.1)	1.1 (0.8–1.6)	
		17–20	1.2 (0.9–1.8)	1.3 (0.9–1.7)	
		≤ 16	1.7 (1.2–2.4)	1.3 (0.9–1.8)	
		p for trend	0.008	0.09	
		Years since quitting			
		≥ 20	1.1 (0.7–1.7)	1.1 (0.8–1.6)	
		11–19	1.2 (0.8–1.9)	0.9 (0.6–1.4)	
		6–10	1.6 (0.9–2.7)	1.4 (0.9–2.2)	
		1–5	1.4 (0.8–2.4)	1.2 (0.7–2.0)	
		p for trend	0.08	0.31	

CI, confidence interval
[a] Index of smoking = no. of cigarettes × years of smoking/age at starting smoking
[b] Logistic regression adjusted for age, ethnic group and socioeconomic level
[c] Stratified analysis adjusted for age

References

Agudo, A., González, C.A., Marcos, G., Sanz, M., Saigi, E., Verge, J., Boleda, M. & Ortega, J. (1992) Consumption of alcohol, coffee, and tobacco, and gastric cancer in Spain. *Cancer Causes Control*, **3**, 137–143

Akiba, S. & Hirayama, T. (1990) Cigarette smoking and cancer mortality risk in Japanese men and women — Results from reanalysis of the six-prefecture cohort study data. *Environ. Health Perspect.*, **87**, 19–26

Ames, R.G. & Gamble, J.F. (1983) Lung cancer, stomach cancer, and smoking status among coal miners. *Scand. J. Work Environ. Health*, **9**, 443–448

Armijo, R., Orellana, M., Medina, E., Coulson, A.H., Sayre, J.W. & Detels, R. (1981) Epidemiology of gastric cancer in Chile: I. Case–control study. *Int. J. Epidemiol.*, **10**, 53–56

Boeing, H., Frentzel-Beyme, R., Berger, M., Berndt, V., Göres, W., Körner, M., Lohmeier, R., Menarcher, A., Männl, H.F.K., Meinhardt, M., Müller, R., Ostermeier, H., Paul, F., Schwemmle, K., Wagner, K.H. & Wahrendorf, J. (1991) Case–control study on stomach cancer in Germany. *Int. J. Cancer*, **47**, 858–864

Brown, L.M., Thomas, T.L., Ma, J., Chang, Y., Yopu, W., Liu, W., Zhang, L., Pee, D. & Gail, M.H. (2002) *Helicobacter pylori* infection in rural China: Demographic, lifestyle and environmental fators. *Int. J. Epidemiol.*, **31**, 638–646

Buiatti, E., Palli, D., Decarli, A., Amadori, D., Avellini, C., Bianchi, S., Biserni, R., Cipriani , F., Cocco, P., Giacosa, A., Marubini, E., Puntoni, R., Vindigni, C., Fraumeni, J., Jr & Blot, W. (1989) A case–control study of gastric cancer and diet in Italy. *Int. J. Cancer*, **44**, 611–616

Buiatti, E., Palli, D., Bianchi, S., Decarli, A., Amadori, D., Avellini, C., Cipriani, F., Cocco, P., Giacosa, A., Lorenzini, L., Marubini, E., Puntoni, R., Saragoni, A., Fraumeni, J.F., Jr & Blot, W.J. (1991) A case–control study of gastric cancer and diet in Italy. III. Risk patterns by histologic type. *Int. J. Cancer*, **48**, 369–374

Chao, A., Thun, M.J., Henley, S.J., Jacobs, E.J., McCullough, M.L. & Calle, E.E. (2002) Cigarette smoking, use of other tobacco products and stomach cancer mortality in US adults: The Cancer Prevention Study II. *Int. J. Cancer*, **101**, 380–389

Chen, Z.-M., Xu, Z., Collins, R., Li, W.-X. & Peto, R. (1997) Early health effects of the emerging tobacco epidemic in China. A 16-year prospective study. *J. Am. med. Assoc.*, **278**, 1500–1504

Chow, W.-H., Swanson, C.A., Lissowska, J., Groves, F.D., Sobin, L.H., Nasierowska-Guttmejer, A., Radziszewski, J., Regula, J., Hsing, A.W., Jagannatha, S., Zatonski, W. & Blot, W.J. (1999) Risk of stomach cancer in relation to consumption of cigarettes, alcohol, tea and coffee in Warsaw, Poland. *Int. J. Cancer*, **81**, 871–876

Correa, P., Fontham, E., Pickle, L.W., Chen, V., Lin, Y. & Haenszel, W. (1985) Dietary determinants of gastric cancer in South Louisiana inhabitants. *J. natl Cancer Inst.*, **75**, 645–654

De Stefani, E., Correa, P., Fierro, L., Carzoglio, J., Deneo-Pellegrini, H. & Zavala, D. (1990) Alcohol drinking and tobacco smoking in gastric cancer. A case–control study. *Rev. Epidemiol. Santé publique*, **38**, 297–307

De Stefani, E., Boffetta, P., Carzoglio, J., Mendilaharsu, S. & Deneo-Pellegrini, H. (1998) Tobacco smoking and alcohol drinking as risk factors for stomach cancer: A case–control study in Uruguay. *Cancer Causes Control*, **9**, 321–329

Dockerty, J.D., Marshall, S., Fraser, J. & Pearce, N. (1991) Stomach cancer in New Zealand: Time trends, ethnic group differences and a cancer registry-based case–control study. *Int. J. Epidemiol.*, **20**, 45–53

Doll, R. & Peto, R. (1976) Mortality in relation to smoking: 20 years' observations on male British doctors. *Br. med. J.*, **ii**, 1525–1536

Doll, R., Peto, R., Wheatey, K., Gray, R. & Sutherland, E. (1994) Mortality in relation to smoking: 40 years' observation on male British doctors. *Br. med. J.*, **309**, 901–912

Engeland, A., Andersen, A., Haldorsen, T. & Tretli, S. (1996) Smoking habits and risk of cancers other than lung cancer: 28 years' follow-up of 26,000 Norwegian men and women. *Cancer Causes Control*, **7**, 497–506

EUROGAST Study Group (1993) The epidemiology of, and risk factors for, *Helicobacter pylori* infection among 3194 asymptomatic subjects in 17 populations. *Gut*, **34**, 1672–1676

Ferraroni, M., Negri, E., La Vecchia, C., D'Avanzo, B. & Franceschi, S. (1989) Socioeconomic indicators, tobacco and alcohol in the aetiology of digestive tract neoplasms. *Int. J. Epidemiol.*, **18**, 556–562

Gajalakshmi, C.K. & Shanta, V. (1996) Lifestyle and risk of stomach cancer: A hospital-based case–control study. *Int. J. Epidemiol.*, **25**, 1146–1153

Gammon, M.D., Schoenberg, J.B., Ahsan, H., Risch, H.A., Vaughan, T.L., Chow, W.-H., Rotterdam, H., West, A.B., Dubrow, R., Stanford, J.L., Mayne, S.T., Farrow, D.C., Niwa, S., Blot, W.J. & Fraumeni, J.F., Jr (1997) Tobacco, alcohol, and socioeconomic status and adenocarcinomas of the esophagus and gastric cardia. *J. natl Cancer Inst.*, **89**, 1277–1284

Gao, C.M., Takezaki, T., Ding, J.H., Li, M.S. &Tajima, K. (1999) Protective effect of allium vegetables against both esophageal and stomach cancer: A simultaneous case–referent study of a high-epidemic area in Jiangsu province, China. *Jpn. J. Cancer Res.*, **90**, 614–621

Guo, W., Blot, W.J., Li, J.-Y., Taylor, P.R., Liu, B.Q., Wang, W., Wu, Y.P., Zheng, W., Dawsey, S.M., Li, B. & Fraumeni, J.F., Jr (1994) A nested case–control study of oesophageal and stomach cancers in the Linxian Nutrition Intervention Trial. *Int. J. Epidemiol.*, **23**, 444–450

Haenszel, W., Kurihara, M., Segi, M. & Lee, R.K.C. (1972) Stomach cancer among Japanese in Hawaii. *J. natl Cancer Inst.*, **49**, 969–988

Haenszel, W., Kurihara, M., Locke, F.B., Shimuzu, K. & Segi, M. (1976) Stomach cancer in Japan. *J. natl Cancer Inst.*, **56**, 265–278

Hammond, E.C. (1966) Smoking in relation to the death rates of one million men and women. *Natl Cancer Inst. Monogr.*, **19**, 127–204

Hansson, L.E., Baron, J., Nyrén, O., Bergström, R., Wolk, A. & Adami, H.O. (1994) Tobacco, alcohol and the risk of gastric cancer. A population-based case–control study in Sweden. *Int. J. Cancer*, **57**, 26–31

Hirayama, T. (1982) Smoking and cancer in Japan. A prospective study on cancer epidemiology based on census population in Japan. Results of 13 years follow up. In: Tominaga, S. & Aoki, K., eds, *The UICC Smoking Control Workshop, Nagoya, Japan, August 24–25, 1981*, Nagoya, University of Nagoya Press, pp. 2–8

Hirayama, T. (1985) A cohort study on cancer in Japan. In: Blot, W.J., Hirayama, T. & Hoel, D.G., eds, *Statistical Methods in Cancer Epidemiology*, Hiroshima, Radiation Effects Research Foundation, pp. 73–91

Hoey, J., Montvernay, C. & Lambert, R. (1981) Wine and tobacco: Risk factors for gastric cancer in France. *Am. J. Epidemiol.*, **113**, 668–674

Hoshiyama, Y. & Sasaba, T. (1992a) A case–control study of stomach cancer and its relation to diet, cigarettes, and alcohol consumption in Saitama Prefecture, Japan. *Cancer Causes Control*, **3**, 441–448

Hoshiyama, Y. & Sasaba, T. (1992b) A case–control study of single and multiple stomach cancers in Saitama Prefecture, Japan. *Jpn. J. Cancer Res.*, **83**, 937–943

Hu, J., Zhang, S., Jia, E., Wang, Q., Liu, S., Liu, Y., Wu, Y. & Cheng, Y. (1988) Diet and cancer of the stomach: A case–control study in China. *Int. J. Cancer*, **41**, 331–335

IARC (1994) *IARC Monographs on the Evaluation of Carcinogenic Risks to Humans*, Vol. 61, *Schistosomes, Liver Flukes and* Helicobacter pylori, Lyon, *IARC*Press

Inoue, M., Tajima, K., Hirose, K., Kuroishi, T., Gao, C.M. & Kitoh, T. (1994) Life-style and subsite of gastric cancer — Joint effect of smoking and drinking habits. *Int. J. Cancer*, **56**, 494–499

Inoue, M., Tajima, K., Yamamura, Y., Hamajima, N., Hirose, K., Nakamura, S., Kodera, Y., Kito, T. & Tominaga, S. (1999) Influence of habitual smoking on gastric cancer by histologic sub-type. *Int. J. Cancer*, **81**, 39–43

Jedrychowski, W., Wahrendorf, J., Popiela, T. & Rachtan, J. (1986) A case–control study of dietary factors and stomach cancer risk in Poland. *Int. J. Cancer*, **37**, 837–842

Jedrychowski, W., Boeing, H., Wahrendorf, J., Popiela, T., Tobiasz-Adamczyk, B. & Kulig, J. (1993) Vodka consumption, tobacco smoking and risk of gastric cancer in Poland. *Int. J. Epi-demiol.*, **22**, 606–613

Ji, B.T., Chow, W.H., Yang, G., McLaughlin, J.K., Gao, R.N., Zheng, W., Shu, X.O., Jin, F., Fraumeni, J.F., Jr & Gao, Y.T. (1996) The influence of cigarette smoking, alcohol, and green tea consumption on the risk of carcinoma of the cardia and distal stomach in Shanghai, China. *Cancer*, **77**, 2449–2457

Kabat, G.C., Ng, S.K.C. & Wynder, E.L. (1993) Tobacco, alcohol intake, and diet in relation to adenocarcinoma of the esophagus and gastric cardia. *Cancer Causes Control*, **4**, 123–132

Kahn, H.A. (1966) The Dorn study of smoking and mortality among US veterans: Report of eight and one-half years of observation. *Natl Cancer Inst. Monogr.*, **19**, 1–125

Kato, I., Tominaga, S., Ito, Y., Kobayashi, S., Yoshii, Y., Matsuura, A., Kameya, A. & Kano, T. (1990) A comparative case–control analysis of stomach cancer and atrophic gastritis. *Cancer Res.*, **50**, 6559–6564

Kato, I., Tominaga, S. & Matsumoto, K. (1992a) A prospective study of stomach cancer among a rural Japanese population: A 6-year survey. *Jpn. J. Cancer Res.*, **83**, 568–575

Kato, I., Tominaga, S., Ito, Y., Kobayashi, S., Yoshii, Y., Matsuura, A., Kameya, A., Kano, T. & Ikari, A. (1992b) A prospective study of atrophic gastritis and stomach cancer risk. *Jpn. J. Cancer Res.*, **83**, 1137–1142

Kneller, R.W., McLaughlin, J.K., Bjelke, E., Schuman, L.M., Blot, W.J., Wacholder, S., Gridley, G., Co Chien, H.T. & Fraumeni, J.F. (1991) A cohort study of stomach cancer in a high-risk American population. *Cancer*, **68**, 672–678

Kono, S., Ikeda, M., Tokudome, M. & Keratsune, M. (1987) Cigarette smoking, alcohol consumption and mortality: A cohort study of male Japanese physicians. *Jpn. J. Cancer Res.*, **78**, 1323–1328

Lagergren, J., Bergström, R., Lindgren, A. & Nyrén, O. (2000) The role of tobacco, snuff and alcohol use in the aetiology of cancer of the oesophagus and gastric cardia. *Int. J. Cancer*, **85**, 340–346

Lee, H.H., Wu, H.Y., Chuang, Y.C., Chang, A.S., Chao, H.H., Chen, K.Y., Chen, H.K., Lai, G.M., Huang, H.H. & Chen, C.J. (1990) Epidemiologic characteristics and multiple risk factors of stomach cancer in Taiwan. *Anticancer Res.*, **10**, 875–881

Liaw, K.-M. & Chen, C.-J. (1998) Mortality attributable to cigarette smoking in Taiwan: A 12-year follow-up study. *Tob. Control*, **7**, 141–148

Limburg, P.J., Qiao, Y.L., Mark, S.D., Wang, G.Q., Perez-Perez, G.I., Blaser, M.J., Wu, Y.P., Zou, X.N., Dong, Z.W., Taylor, P.R. & Dawsey, S.M. (2001) *Helicobacter pylori* seropositivity and subsite-specific gastric cancer risks in Linxian, China. *J. natl Cancer Inst.*, **93**, 226–233

Liu, B.-Q., Peto, R., Chen, Z.-M., Boreham, J., Wu, Y.-P., Li, J.-Y., Campbell, T.C. & Chen, J.-S. (1998) Emerging tobacco hazards in China: 1. Retrospective proportional mortality study of one million deaths. *Br. med. J.*, **317**, 1411–1422

Mathew, A., Gangadharan, P., Varghese, C. & Nair, M.K. (2000) Diet and stomach cancer: A case–control study in South India. *Eur. J. Cancer Prev.*, **9**, 89–97

McLaughlin, J.K., Hrubec, Z., Blot, W.J. & Fraumeni, J.F. (1990) Stomach cancer and cigarette smoking among US veterans, 1954–1980. *Cancer Res.*, **50**, 3804

McLaughlin, J.K., Hrubec, Z., Blot, W.J. & Fraumeni, J.F. (1995) Smoking and cancer mortality among US veterans: A 26-year follow-up. *Int. J. Cancer*, **60**, 190–193

Mizoue, T., Tokui, N., Nishisaka, K., Nishisaka, S.I., Ogimoto, I., Ikeda, M. & Yoshimura, T. (2000) Prospective study on the relation of cigarette smoking with cancer of the liver and stomach in an endemic region. *Int. J. Epidemiol.*, **29**, 232–237

Moayyedi, P., Axon, A.T.R., Feltbower, R., Duffett, S., Crocombe, W., Braunholtz, D., Richards, I.D.G., Dowell, A.C. & Forman, D. for the Leeds HELP Study Group (2002) Relation of adult lifestyle and socioeconomic factors to the prevalence of *Helicobacter pylori* infection. *Int. J. Epidemiol.*, **31**, 624–631

Murata, M., Takayama, K., Choi, B.C.K. & Pak, A.W.P. (1996) A nested case–control study on alcohol drinking, tobacco smoking, and cancer. *Cancer Detect. Prev.*, **20**, 557–565

Nomura, A., Grove, J.S., Stemmermann, G.N. & Severson, R.K. (1990a) A prospective study of stomach cancer and its relation to diet, cigarettes, and alcohol consumption. *Cancer Res.*, **50**, 627–631

Nomura, A., Grove, J.S., Stemmermann, G.N. & Severson, R.K. (1990b) Cigarette smoking and stomach cancer. *Cancer Res.*, **50**, 7084

Nomura, A.M., Stemmermann, G.N. & Chyou, P.H. (1995) Gastric cancer among the Japanese in Hawaii. *Jpn. J. Cancer Res.*, **86**, 916–923

Nordlund, L.A., Carstensen, J.M. & Pershagen, G. (1997) Cancer incidence in female smokers: A 26-year follow-up. *Int. J. Cancer*, **73**, 625–628

Palli, D., Bianchi, S., Decarli, A., Cipriani, F., Avellini, C., Cocco, P., Falcini, F., Puntoni, R., Russo, A., Vindigni, C., Fraumeni, J.F., Jr, Blot, W.J. & Buiatti, E. (1992) A case–control study of cancers of the gastric cardia in Italy. *Br. J. Cancer*, **65**, 263–266

Risch, H.A., Jain, M., Choi, N.W., Fodor, J.G., Pfeiffer, C.J., Howe, G.R., Harrison, L.W., Craib, K.J.P. & Miller, A.B. (1985) Dietary factors and the incidence of cancer of the stomach. *Am. J. Epidemiol.*, **122**, 947–959

Saha, S.K. (1991) Smoking habits and carcinoma of the stomach: a case–control study. *Jpn. J. Cancer Res.*, **82**, 497–502

Siemiatycki, J, Krewski, D., Franco, E. & Kaiserman, M. (1995) Associations between cigarette smoking and each of 21 types of cancer: A multi-site case–control study. *Int. J. Epidemiol.*, **24**, 504–514

Siman, J.H., Forsgren, A., Berglund, G. & Floren, C.H. (2001) Tobacco smoking increases the risk for gastric adenocarcinoma among *Helicobacter pylori*-infected individuals. *Scand. J. Gastroenterol.*, **36**, 208–213

Staszewski, J. (1969) Smoking and cancer of the alimentary tract in Poland. *Br. J. Cancer*, **23**, 247–253

Terry, P., Nyrén, O. & Yuen, J. (1998) Protective effect of fruits and vegetables on stomach cancer in a cohort of Swedish twins. *Int. J. Cancer*, **76**, 35–37

Tulinius, H., Sigfússon, N., Sigvaldason, H., Bjarnadóttir, K. & Tryggvadóttir, L. (1997) Risk factors for malignant diseases: A cohort study on a population of 22,946 Icelanders. *Cancer Epidemiol. Biomarkers Prev.*, **6**, 863–873

Tverdal, A., Thelle, D., Stensvold, I., Leren, P. & Bjartveit, K. (1993) Mortality in relation to smoking history: 13 years' follow-up of 68,000 Norwegian men and women 35–49 years. *J. clin. Epidemiol.*, **46**, 475–487

Wu, A.H., Wan, P. & Berstein, L. (2001) A multiethnic population-based study of smoking, alcohol and body size and risk of adenocarcinomas of the stomach and esophagus (United States). *Cancer Causes Control*, **12**, 721–732

Wu-Williams, A.H., Yu, M.C. & Mack, T.M. (1990) Life-style, workplace, and stomach cancer by subsite in young men of Los Angeles County. *Cancer Res.*, **50**, 2569–2576

Wynder, E.L., Kmet, J., Dungal, N. & Segi, M. (1963) An epidemiological investigation of gastric cancer. *Cancer*, **16**, 1461–1496

Ye, W., Ekström, A.M., Hansson, L.-E., Bergström, R. & Nyrén, O. (1999) Tobacco, alcohol and the risk of gastric cancer by sub-site and histologic type. *Int. J. Cancer*, **83**, 223–229

You, W.C., Blot, W.J., Chang, Y.S., Ershow, A.G., Yang, Z.T., An, Q., Henderson, B., Xu, G.W., Fraumeni, J.F., Jr & Wang, T.G. (1988) Diet and high risk of stomach cancer in Shandong, China. *Cancer Res.*, **48**, 3518–3523

You, W., Zhang, L., Gail, M.H., Chang, Y.-S., Liu, W.-D., Ma, J.-L., Li, J.-Y., Jin, M.-L., Hu, Y.-R., Yang, C.-S., Blaser M.J., Correa, P., Blot, W.J., Fraumeni, J.F., Jr & Xu, G.-W. (2000) Gastric dysplasia and gastric cancer: *Helicobacter pyrlori*, serum vitamin C, and other risk factors. *J. natl Cancer Inst.*, **92**, 1607–1612

Yu, G.P. & Hsieh, C.C. (1991) Risk factors for stomach cancer: A population-based case–control study in Shanghai. *Cancer Causes Control*, **2**, 169–174

Yu, G.P., Hsieh, C.C., Wang, L.Y., Yu, S.Z., Li, X.L. & Jin, T.H. (1995) Green-tea consumption and risk of stomach cancer: A population-based case–control study in Shanghai, China. *Cancer Causes Control*, **6**, 532–538

Yuan, J.M., Ross, R.K., Wang, X.L., Gao, Y.T., Henderson, B.E. & Yu, M.C. (1996) Morbidity and mortality in relation to cigarette smoking in Shanghai, China. A prospective male cohort study. *J. Am. med. Assoc.*, **275**, 1646–1650

Zaridze, D., Borisova, E., Maximovitch, D. & Chkhikvadze, V. (2000) Alcohol consumption, smoking and risk of gastric cancer: Case–control study from Moscow, Russia. *Cancer Causes Control*, **11**, 363–371

Zhang, Z.F., Kurtz, R.C., Sun, M., Karpeh, M., Yu, G.P., Gargon, N., Fein, J.S., Georgopoulos, S.K. & Harlap, S. (1996) Adenocarcinomas of the esophagus and gastric cardia: Medical conditions, tobacco, alcohol, and socioeconomic factors. *Cancer Epidemiol. Biomarkers Prev.*, **5**, 761–768

2.1.7   Colorectal cancer

(a)   Overview

In the last three decades, a total of 60 epidemological studies have investigated the relationship between tobacco smoke and colorectal cancer, but few were specifically designed to study the effects of tobacco smoking. Although most of the earlier studies did not show any consistent association between tobacco use and risk, several prospective cohort and case–control studies published since the late 1980s have found a significantly increased risk for colorectal cancer among smokers. Also, since the late 1980s, smoking has emerged as a risk factor for colorectal adenomas, a well-established precursor for colorectal cancer. On the basis of these new findings on smoking and colorectal cancer and adenomas, Giovannucci et al. (1994a,b) hypothesized that smoking may act as an initiator of colorectal cancer and that an induction period of 35–40 years may be needed to increase incidence. Giovannucci explained that if a long induction is needed for tobacco to play a role in colorectal carcinogenesis, this may explain the lack of association between smoking and colorectal cancer found in earlier cohort studies that had a short follow-up time and in case–control studies that did not obtain complete lifetime smoking histories.

The epidemiological evidence on tobacco smoke and colorectal cancer from prospective cohort and case–control studies is summarized below. Relevant information on each of the cohort studies (source of the cohort, years of follow-up, number of cases) is summarized in Tables 2.1 and 2.1.7.1 and the data obtained are reported in Table 2.1.7.2. Relevant information on case–control study design and results is summarized in Tables 2.1.7.3 and 2.1.7.4, respectively. Site-specific relative risks were presented in the majority of studies. Results for colorectal cancers combined were reported in 12 prospective cohort studies (Hammond, 1966; Garland et al., 1985; Wu et al., 1987; Giovannucci et al., 1994a,b; Chen et al., 1997; Kato et al., 1997; Liaw & Chen, 1998; Nordlund et al., 1997; Tulinius et al., 1997; Chao et al., 2000; Stürmer et al., 2000) and six case–control studies (Dales et al., 1979; Olsen & Kronborg, 1993; Boutron et al., 1995; Yamada et al., 1997; Nusko et al., 2000; Lam et al., 2001).

(b)   Factors affecting risk

Virtually all the cohort and case–control studies reported risks for colorectal cancer in former and current smokers relative to never-smokers (Tables 2.1.7.2 and 2.1.7.4). Sixteen of the prospective cohort studies were conducted in the USA, 10 in Europe and three in Japan. In most studies, a small elevated risk for colon, rectal or colorectal cancer was found for smokers, but results were statistically significant in only a few studies. In these latter studies, former and/or current smokers experienced a significantly increased risk of 1.2–1.4 for colon cancer (Heineman et al., 1994; Chyou et al., 1996), rectal cancer (Akiba & Hirayama, 1990; Doll et al., 1994; Heineman et al., 1994; Chyou et al., 1996; Engeland et al., 1996) or colorectal cancer (Wu et al., 1987; Chao et al., 2000; Stürmer et al., 2000), relative to never-smokers (Table 2.1.7.4). Of all cohort studies, four showed a lower risk for colorectal cancer among smokers (Hammond & Horn, 1958a,b; Williams *et al.*, 1981; Garland *et al.*, 1985; Kono *et al.*, 1987); the result was statistically significant in one (Williams *et al.*, 1981).

A total of 31 case–control studies have examined the association between active smoking and cancer of the colon and rectum (Tables 2.1.7.3 and 2.1.7.4). [The Working Group excluded from their review studies that did not present point risk estimates in association with smoking.]

Nine European case–control studies on tobacco use and colorectal cancer were identified. They were conducted in Yugoslavia (Jarebinski *et al.*, 1988; 1989), Denmark (Olsen & Kronborg, 1993), Sweden (Baron *et al.*, 1994), France (Tuyns *et al.*, 1982; Boutron *et al.*, 1995), Italy (Ferraroni *et al.*, 1989; D'Avanzo *et al.*, 1995; Tavani *et al.*, 1998) and Germany (Nusko *et al.*, 2000). Ten case–control studies were conducted in Asia, eight in Japan (Tajima & Tominaga, 1985; Kato *et al.*, 1990a,b; Hoshiyama *et al.*, 1993; Inoue *et al.*, 1995; Kotake *et al.*, 1995; Murata *et al.*, 1996; Yamada *et al.*, 1997) and one each in the Republic of Korea (Choi & Kahyo, 1991) and Hong Kong SAR (Lam *et al.*, 2001). Eight case–control studies on tobacco use and colorectal cancer have been carried out in the USA; two of these were hospital-based (Williams & Horm, 1977; Dales *et al.*, 1979). The population-based studies were conducted among whites in Los Angeles County (Peters *et al.*, 1989), Utah (Slattery *et al.*, 1990), Wisconsin (Newcomb *et al.*, 1995), northern California, Utah and Minnesota (Slattery *et al.*, 1997) and Iowa (Chiu *et al.*, 2001) and among the multiethnic population in Hawaii (Le Marchand *et al.*, 1997).

Of the case–control studies, statistically significant increased risks among former or current smokers or ever-smokers were reported in two studies each on colon cancer (Slattery *et al.*, 1990, 1997; Chiu *et al.*, 2001), rectal cancer (Inoue *et al.*, 1995; Chiu *et al.*, 2001) and colorectal cancer (Newcomb *et al.*, 1995; Nusko *et al.*, 2000). However, one investigator reported a statistically significant reduction in risk for cancer of the colon (Hoshiyama *et al.*, 1993) and rectum among smokers (Vobecky *et al.*, 1983). Because smokers may stop or reduce smoking because of disease-related symptoms, case–control studies that presented data on smoking status only without data on duration/intensity (i.e. ever-smoked only or former/current smoking only) (Dales *et al.*, 1979; Tuyns *et al.*, 1983; Vobecky *et al.*, 1983; Kato *et al.*, 1990a,b; Inoue *et al.*, 1995; Ghadirian *et al.*, 1998; Nusko *et al.*, 2000) are of limited value.

(i)   *Intensity of smoking*

The evidence for an association between cigarette smoking and colorectal cancer would be strengthened if dose–response relationships could be demonstrated. In only one cohort study, were parameters including number of cigarettes smoked, pack–years of smoking, duration of smoking and age at which smoking started investigated separately in current and former smokers (Chao *et al.*, 2000). In most of the other cohort studies, one or two parameters of intensity of exposure were assessed. Number of cigarettes smoked per day was most frequently assessed (Hammond, 1966; Doll *et al.*, 1980; Williams *et al.*, 1981; Carstensen *et al.*, 1987; Klatsky *et al.*, 1988; Akiba & Hirayama, 1990; Doll *et al.*,

1994; Heineman *et al.*, 1994; Chyou *et al.*, 1996; Nyrén *et al.*, 1996; Tulinius *et al.*, 1997; Knekt *et al.*, 1998; Chao *et al.*, 2000; Terry *et al.*, 2001). Statistically significant dose–response trends with amount smoked daily were reported for colon cancer (Heineman *et al.*, 1994; Chyou *et al.*, 1996), rectal cancer (Doll *et al.*, 1994; Heineman *et al.*, 1994; Chyou *et al.*, 1996) and colorectal cancer (Chao *et al.*, 2000; Stürmer *et al.*, 2000).

Number of cigarettes smoked daily was evaluated in over half of the case–control studies (Williams & Horm, 1977; Jarebinski *et al.*, 1989; Peters *et al.*, 1989; Slattery *et al.*, 1990; Choi & Kahyo, 1991; Kune *et al.*, 1992; Hoshiyama *et al.*, 1993; Baron *et al.*, 1994; D'Avanzo *et al.*, 1995; Kotake *et al.*, 1995; Newcomb *et al.*, 1995; Murata *et al.*, 1996; Slattery *et al.*, 1997; Yamada *et al.*, 1997; Tavani *et al.*, 1998; Chiu *et al.*, 2001; Lam *et al.*, 2001). Statistically significant positive trends of increasing risk with increasing number of cigarettes smoked daily were reported for colon cancer (Newcomb *et al.*, 1995; Slattery *et al.*, 1997), rectal cancer (Newcomb *et al.*, 1995) and colorectal cancer (Yamada *et al.*, 1997). In two studies, this pattern of increasing risks was apparent only in men (Slattery *et al.*, 1990) or older men (aged $\geq$ 70 years) (Lam *et al.*, 2001) but not among women in the same study.

(ii)   *Duration of smoking*

Studies on colorectal cancer have been varied in their assessment of duration of smoking. Only a few studies actually evaluated years of smoking whereas others considered age at starting smoking, years since initiation of smoking or pack–years, combining duration and intensity of smoking. Five of the cohort studies have looked at years of smoking (Hsing *et al.*, 1998; Chao *et al.*, 2000), age at starting smoking (Heineman *et al.*, 1994; Chao *et al.*, 2000), years since initiation of smoking (Giovannucci *et al.*, 1994a,b) and pack–years of smoking (Giovannucci *et al.*, 1994a ; Heineman *et al.*, 1994; Chao *et al.*, 2000; Stürmer *et al.*, 2000). Some evidence exists to suggest that risk for colorectal cancer increased with earlier age at initiation (Heineman *et al.*, 1994; Chao *et al.*, 2000) and with increasing number of years of smoking (Chao *et al.*, 2000). In one study, risk increased with years since smoking initiation but this was observed among heavier smokers (i.e. subjects who smoked at least 10 cigarettes per day at starting smoking) only (Giovannucci *et al.*, 1994a). Three studies showed a statistically significant trend of increasing risk with increasing pack–years of smoking (Heineman *et al.*, 1994; Chao *et al.*, 2000; Stürmer *et al.*, 2000) but, in a fourth study, this association was limited to those who started smoking before the age of 30 years (Giovannucci *et al.*, 1994b).

Some case–control studies have examined risk patterns in relation to years of smoking (Jarebinski *et al.*, 1989; Choi & Kahyo, 1991; Olsen & Kronborg, 1993; Baron *et al.*, 1994; D'Avanzo *et al.*, 1995; Newcomb *et al.*, 1995; Slattery *et al.*, 1997; Tavani *et al.*, 1998; Chiu *et al.*, 2001), age at starting smoking (Tajima & Tominaga, 1985; Choi & Kahyo, 1991; D'Avanzo *et al.*, 1995; Newcomb *et al.*, 1995; Slattery *et al.*, 1997; Tavani *et al.*, 1998) and pack–years of smoking (Tajima & Tominaga, 1985; Kune *et al.*, 1992; Hoshiyama *et al.*, 1993; Baron *et al.*, 1994; Boutron *et al.*, 1995; D'Avanzo *et al.*, 1995; Siemiatycki *et al.*, 1995; Le Marchand *et al.*, 1997; Slattery *et al.*, 1997; Yamada *et al.*, 1997; Chiu *et al.*, 2001). The risk for colon and rectal cancer increased significantly with increasing number of years of smoking in one study; this relationship was observed even after adjustment for other smoking variables including number of cigarettes smoked per day (Newcomb *et al.*, 1995). In two studies, risk for colon cancer (Newcomb *et al.*, 1995; Slattery *et al.*, 1997) and rectal cancer (Newcomb *et al.*, 1995) increased significantly with earlier age at initiation. In one study that included both sexes, this association was found in men only (Slattery *et al.*, 1997) whereas in the study of women only (Newcomb *et al.*, 1995), any effect of age at initiation was eliminated after adjusting for years of smoking for both colon and rectal cancer. In three studies, the risk for colon cancer (Slattery *et al.*, 1997) and rectal cancer (Le Marchand *et al.*, 1997; Yamada *et al.*, 1997) increased significantly with increasing pack–years of smoking.

(iii)   *Smoking cessation*

Modest differences in risk exist between former and current smokers (Tables 2.1.7.2 and 2.1.7.4). The benefit of smoking cessation by years since stopping was evaluated in two cohort studies (Wu *et al.*, 1987; Chao *et al.*, 2000). The risks in both men and women remained substantially elevated (relative risk, 1.6–1.7) even after 20 years of smoking cessation in one study (Wu *et al.*, 1987) but the risk was substantially reduced (to near unity) in another (Chao *et al.*, 2000).

Results from case–control studies are also somewhat inconsistent. Risk patterns by years of cessation (D'Avanzo *et al.*, 1995; Newcomb *et al.*, 1995; Slattery *et al.*, 1997; Tavani *et al.*, 1998) or age at stopping (Choi & Kahyo, 1991) have been investigated. Cessation was not associated with risk in two studies (Choi & Kahyo, 1991; Tavani *et al.*, 1998), but was significantly associated with reduced risk in one (D'Avanzo *et al.*, 1995). In one study, women who stopped smoking for 20 or more years still showed an elevation in risk of 10–30% compared with never-smokers (Newcomb *et al.*, 1995). In another study, relative to never-smokers, former smokers who had stopped smoking within the first 15 years of starting smoking actually showed a higher risk than current smokers (Slattery *et al.*, 1997).

(iv)   *Length of follow-up*

Giovannuci *et al.* (1994a,b) proposed that smoking may act as an initiator of colorectal cancer and that a long induction period (i.e. 35–40 years) is needed before an effect on risk can be observed. However, the available results are not entirely compatible with their hypothesis. Of the cohort studies in which smoking was a significant risk factor for colon cancer (Heineman *et al.*, 1994; Chyou *et al.*, 1996), rectal cancer (Doll *et al.*, 1994; Heineman *et al.*, 1995; Chyou *et al.*, 1996) or colorectal cancer (Wu *et al.*, 1987 (men only); Giovannuci *et al.*, 1994a; Chao *et al.*, 2000; Stürmer *et al.*, 2000), the length of follow-up was 6 years or less in two studies (Wu *et al.*, 1987; Giovannuci *et al.*, 1994a), between 13 and 14 years in two studies (Chao *et al.*, 2000; Stürmer *et al.*, 2000) and greater than 20 years in three studies (Doll *et al.*, 1994; Heineman *et al.*, 1994; Chyou *et al.*, 1996). In the British Doctors' study, an elevated but non-significant risk for rectal cancer in smokers had already been observed after the first 20 years of follow-up ($p = 0.09$). The magnitude of risk for rectal cancer in smokers was essentially the same after 20 years as after 40 years of follow-up (Doll & Peto, 1976; Doll *et al.*, 1994) although the result became statistically significant with longer follow-up (Doll *et al.*, 1994).

(c)   Population characteristics

(i)   Sex

There is some suggestion that the association between smoking and colorectal cancer may be stronger in men than in women although the evidence for this is far from consistent. Nine cohort studies showed sex-specific results (Hammond, 1966; Wu *et al.*, 1987; Sandler *et al.*, 1988; Akiba & Hirayama, 1990, Tverdal *et al.*, 1993; Doll *et al.*, 1994; Engeland *et al.*, 1996; Tulinius *et al.*, 1997; Chao *et al.*, 2000). In one study, a significantly increased risk associated with smoking was observed only in women and not in men (Tulinius *et al.*, 1997). In three other studies, an increased risk was more apparent in men than in women (Wu *et al.*, 1987; Akiba & Hirayama, 1990; Tverdal *et al.*, 1993). In another study, the association between smoking and colorectal cancer was equally strong in both sexes (Chao *et al.*, 2000). Ten case–control studies also presented sex-specific results (Williams *et al.*, 1977; Slattery *et al.*, 1990; Kune *et al.*, 1992; Boutron *et al.*, 1995; D'Avanzo *et al.*, 1995; Inoue *et al.*, 1995; Le Marchand *et al.*, 1997; Slattery *et al.*, 1997; Chiu *et al.*, 2001; Lam *et al.*, 2001). Of the studies in which smoking was implicated as a risk factor, three showed no clear gender differences (Le Marchand *et al.*, 1997; Slattery *et al.*, 1997; Chiu *et al.*, 2001) but in two studies, smoking was a risk factor only in men (Slattery *et al.*, 1990) or older men (Lam *et al.*, 2001).

(ii)   Ethnicity

Almost all the cohort and case–control studies were conducted in Australia, Canada, Europe, the United Kingdom and the USA and included only Caucasian study subjects. One case–control study in the USA was conducted in African Americans (Dales *et al.*, 1979) and another included Caucasians and various Asian groups (Le Marchand *et al.*, 1997). Approximately one-fourth of the cohort studies (Kono *et al.*, 1987; Akiba & Hirayama, 1990; Akiba, 1994) and of the case–control studies (Tajima & Tominaga, 1985; Kato *et al.*, 1990a,b; Choi *et al.*, 1991; Hoshiyama *et al.*, 1993; Inoue *et al.*, 1995; Kotake *et al.*, 1995; Murata *et al.*, 1996; Yamada *et al.*, 1997; Lam *et al.*, 2001) were conducted in Asia, mostly in native Japanese. There are no apparent differences in the association between smoking and colorectal cancer in members of different racial or ethnic groups.

(d)   Subsites of colorectal cancer

Smoking and risk for cancer of the colon and for rectal cancer were investigated separately in the majority of cohort and case–control studies. Risk patterns are generally consistent between rectal and colon cancer in most of the cohort studies (Hammond & Horn, 1958a,b; Carstersen *et al.*, 1987; Tverdal *et al.*, 1993; Akiba, 1994; Heineman *et al.*, 1994; Chyou *et al.*, 1996; Nyren *et al.*, 1996; Chao *et al.*, 2000; Terry *et al.*, 2001) and case–control studies (Tuyns *et al.*, 1982; Vobecky *et al.*, 1983; Tajima & Tominaga, 1985; Peters *et al.*, 1989, Kato *et al.*, 1990a; Choi & Kahyo, 1991; Kune *et al.*, 1992; Baron *et al.*, 1994; D'Avanzo *et al.*, 1995; Le Marchand *et al.*, 1997; Tavani *et al.*, 1998). However, in four cohort studies (Klatsky *et al.*, 1988; Akiba & Hirayama, 1990; Doll *et al.*, 1994; Engeland *et al.*, 1996) and eight case–control studies (Williams *et al.*, 1977; Kato *et al.*, 1990b; Hoshiyama *et al.*, 1993; Inoue *et al.*, 1995; Kotake *et al.*, 1995; Newcomb *et al.*, 1995; Siemiatycki *et al.*, 1995; Murata *et al.*, 1996), any effect of smoking was more apparent for rectal cancer than for colon cancer. A stronger smoking association for colon cancer was found in two cohort studies (Hsing *et al.*, 1998; Knekt *et al.*, 1998) but in none of the case–control studies.

In three large population-based case–control studies and one cohort study (Heineman *et al.*, 1994) in which smoking was also implicated as a cause of colon cancer, the effect of smoking by colon subsite was investigated. In two studies, there were no clear differences in the effects of smoking by colon subsite (Heineman *et al.*, 1994; Slattery *et al.*, 1997). In one case–control study, any effect of smoking was limited to the left colon (Newcomb *et al.*, 1995). In another case–control study, the effects of smoking varied by colon subsite and were not consistent in men and women (Le Marchand *et al.*, 1997).

(e)   Confounding

It is of note that even among the 'positive' cohort and case–control studies, the magnitude of risk between the highest and lowest exposure (i.e. in people who have never used tobacco) was modest (20–60% increase in risk). The treatment of potential confounders is particularly important when evaluating the overall evidence on the association of smoking with colorectal cancer. Inadequate adjustment for various potential confounders (e.g. alcohol, physical activity, body size, dietary factors) or unidentified confounders could account for the small increase in risk found with smoking in some studies. For example, smokers are more likely than nonsmokers to be physically inactive (IARC, 2002), to use alcohol, to have poorer dietary habits (e.g. low consumption of fruits and vegetables and high consumption of fat and meat) and they are less likely to be screened for colorectal cancer (Margetts & Jackson, 1993). Each of these factors, in turn, is positively associated with colorectal cancer risk (Potter *et al.*, 1993). Thus, smoking may appear to increase the risk for colorectal cancer even if it has no direct effect on risk, if these potential confounders are inadequately controlled for or not controlled for in the analysis.

Few potential confounders were adjusted in most of the cohort studies. In some one-third of the published studies, only age or other relevant demographic factors were considered (Hammond & Horn, 1958a,b; Hammond, 1966; Doll *et al.*, 1980; Williams *et al.*, 1981; Garland *et al.*, 1985; Carstensen *et al.*, 1987; Sandler *et al.*, 1988; Akiba & Hirayama, 1990; Tverdal *et al.*, 1993; Akiba, 1994; Doll *et al.*, 1994; Engeland *et al.*, 1996). Some studies adjusted only for demographic factors and alcohol use (Kono *et al.*, 1987; Chyou *et al.*, 1996; Hsing *et al.*, 1998). Less than half of the studies considered two or more of the potential confounders mentioned above (Wu *et al.*, 1987; Klatsky *et al.*, 1988; Bostick *et al.*, 1994; Giovannucci *et al.*, 1994a,b; Heineman *et al.*, 1994; Nyrén *et al.*, 1996; Knekt *et al.*, 1998; Singh & Fraser, 1998; van Wayenburg *et al.*, 2000; Chao *et al.*, 2000; Stürmer *et al.*, 2000; Terry *et al.*, 2001). The extent to which residual effects of potential confounders can explain the small increase in risk associated with smoking cannot be determined for certain. In some studies, adjustment for alcohol (Hirayama, 1989) and other risk factors (Giovannucci *et al.*, 1994a) substantially reduced the magnitude and the significance of the effect of smoking. In other studies, the risk estimate associated with smoking was reduced by up to 10% although the association remained statistically significant (Chao *et al.*, 2000; Stürmer *et al.*, 2000). None of the prospective studies has evaluated whether the association between smoking and colorectal cancer was modified by other characteristics such as alcohol intake, body size, and others.

In about half of the case–control studies, demographic factors and at least two of the potential confounders discussed above were adjusted for the analyses (Slattery *et al.*, 1990; Choi & Kahyo, 1991; Kune *et al.*, 1992; Olsen & Kronborg, 1993; Baron *et al.*, 1994; D'Advanzo *et al.*, 1995; Newcomb *et al.*, 1995; Siemiatycki *et al.*, 1995; Le Marchand *et al.*, 1997; Slattery *et al.*, 1997; Yamada *et al.*, 1997; Ghadirian *et al.*, 1998; Tavani *et al.*, 1998; Chiu *et al.*, 2001). In addition, two studies investigated whether the association between smoking and colorectal cancer was modified by other characteristics (Newcomb *et al.*, 1995; Slattery *et al.*, 1997). Newcomb and coworkers reported a significant interaction between body-mass index and risk for rectal cancer (but not colon cancer) such that the risk for cancer at this site was significantly greater among heavier women. In the study of colon cancer by Slattery *et al* (1997), smokers with a high body-mass index displayed higher risk than those with a low body-mass index. However, the influence of β-carotene and other antioxidants on risk appeared to vary by smoking levels, but the nature of the effect differed according to whether the sources of antioxidants were dietary or from supplements. Although no systematic confounding factor has been identified, limited results (Newcomb *et al.*, 1995; Slattery *et al.*, 1997) show that body size, dietary factors and other potential confounders need to be adequately controlled for in the analysis before any association between smoking and colorectal cancer can be accepted.

(f)   Colorectal polyps

Twenty-seven informative studies have investigated the association between tobacco smoking and risk of colorectal polyps, mostly of the adenomatous type, a well-established precursor for colorectal cancer. These studies are presented in Table 2.1.7.5. Prevalent cases were investigated in most of the studies, although the risk of reccurrence was the end-point in two studies (Jacobson *et al.*, 1994; Baron *et al.*, 1998). In contrast to the weak and inconsistent findings on tobacco use and risk of colon and rectal cancer, the epidemiological evidence on the relationship between smoking and colorectal polyps is generally consistent and more compelling. A significant positive association between smoking and risk of polyps has been found in all but five studies (Kato *et al.*, 1990b; Kono *et al.*, 1990; Sandler *et al.*, 1993; Baron *et al.*, 1998; Breuer-Katschinski *et al.*, 2000). In five studies that presented results separately for men and women (Lee *et al.*, 1993; Jacobson *et al.*, 1994; Boutron *et al.*, 1995; Kahn *et al.*, 1998; Nagata *et al.*, 1999), the association appeared equally strong in men and women. Significant positive dose–response trends with number of cigarettes smoked daily (Kikendall *et al.*, 1989; Monnet *et al.*, 1991; Zahm *et al.*, 1991; Kearney *et al.*, 1995; Kahn *et al.*, 1998), years of smoking (Monnet *et al.*, 1991; Zahm *et al.*, 1991; Olsen & Kronborg, 1993; Nagata *et al.*, 1999) and pack–years of smoking (Kikendall *et al.*, 1989; Monnet *et al.*, 1991; Zahm *et al.*, 1991; Honjo *et al.*, 1992; Lee *et al.*, 1993; Giovannucci *et al.*, 1994a,b; Jacobson *et al.*, 1994; Boutron *et al.*, 1995; Honjo *et al.*, 1995; Martínez *et al.*, 1995; Longnecker *et al.*, 1996; Nagata *et al.*, 1999; Almendingen *et al.*, 2000) have been found.

The benefit of smoking cessation has been evaluated. Point estimates for former smokers were calculated in 14 studies. Some studies found a decrease relative to current smokers to a non-significantly elevated risk (Zahm *et al.*, 1991; Kearney *et al.*, 1995; Longnecker *et al.*, 1996; Martínez *et al.*, 1997; Almendingen *et al.*, 2000), while the risk remained significantly elevated in others (Monnet *et al.*, 1991; Honjo *et al.*, 1992; Olsen & Kronborg, 1993; Martínez *et al.*, 1995; Kahn *et al.*, 1998).

A few studies also investigated trends, and the results are inconclusive. In one study, the risk for colorectal adenomas was higher than for current smokers after 10 years of smoking cessation (Monnet *et al.*, 1991), whereas in another study, the risk was close to unity after only 2 years of smoking cessation (Kikendall *et al.*, 1989).

Studies also varied in the potential confounders that were considered. In about half of the studies, demographic factors and several of the potential confounders discussed for colorectal cancer (physical activity, alcohol consumption, body size, dietary factors and screening history) were controlled for in the analysis (Olsen & Kronborg, 1993; Giovannucci *et al.*, 1994a,b; Jacobson *et al.*, 1994; Honjo *et al.*, 1995; Kearney *et al.*, 1995; Martínez *et al.*, 1995; Nelson *et al.*, 1995; Longnecker *et al.*, 1996; Martínez *et al.*, 1997; Kahn *et al.*, 1998; Almendingen *et al.*, 2000; Breuer-Katschinski *et al.*, 2000). Several studies adjusted for demographic factors and alcohol use only (Kikendall *et al.*, 1989; Kono *et al.*, 1990; Cope *et al.*, 1991; Zahm *et al.*, 1991; Honjo *et al.*, 1992; Sandler *et al.*, 1993; Boutron *et al.*, 1995), whereas only age was adjusted for in other studies (Hoff *et al.*, 1987; Demers *et al.*, 1988; Stemmermann *et al.*, 1988; Kato *et al.*, 1990b; Monnet *et al.*, 1991; Lee *et al.*, 1993; Manus *et al.*, 1997; Nagata *et al.*, 1999). In a study that examined the joint effect of smoking and alcohol, a statistically significant increase in risk was found only among subjects who were both smokers and drinkers (Cope *et al.*, 1991) although a non-significant twofold increase in risk was also found among smokers who were non-drinkers.

Most relative risk estimates for smoking and colorectal polyps range between 2 and 3, whereas the risk estimates for colorectal cancer range between 1.2 and 1.4. The reasons for the apparent paradox have stimulated considerable discussion (Boutron *et al.*, 1995; Terry & Neugut, 1998; Potter, 1998; Boutron-Ruault, 1999; Poole, 1999; Boutron-Ruault & Rabkin, 2000; Stürmer *et al.*, 2000; Terry *et al.*, 2000). The probable high prevalence of adenomas in most unscreened control groups selected for colorectal cancer studies may have diluted the association between colorectal cancer and smoking (Terry & Neugut, 1998). The strength of an association between a risk factor and a causal intermediate (e.g.

colorectal polyp) may be stronger than the association with the end-point of interest (e.g. colorectal cancer) if other pathways to that end-point exist (Poole, 1999; Terry *et al.*, 2000). Finally, because prevalences of colorectal polyps of at least 20% have been estimated for subjects aged 50 years or older in the USA, the rare disease assumption may not apply and the odds ratios reported would be inflated estimates of the relative risk (Terry *et al.*, 2000).

Table 2.1.7.1. Additional cohort studies on tobacco smoking and colorectal cancer: main characteristics of study design

Reference Country and years of study	Name of study (if available)	Cohort sample	Cases/deaths identification	Comments
Garland *et al.* (1985) USA 1957–77	Western Electric Health Study	1954 male employees at the Western Electric Company in Chicago, aged 40–55 years	Death certificates and medical and hospital records	Study primarily investigating dietary vitamin D and calcium intake and risk of colorectal cancer
Sandler *et al.* (1988) USA 1963–75		91 909 residents in Washington County, aged ≥ 25 years	County-wide cancer register or death certificates	
Kato *et al.* (1997) USA 1985–94	New York University Women's Health Study	15 785 women recruited from New York City and Florida, aged 34–65 years	Active follow-up and linkage to state cancer registries and National Death Index	Study mainly investigating diet and colorectal cancer
Stürmer *et al.* (2000) USA 1982–95	Physicians' Health Study	22 071 male physicians, aged 40–84 years	Yearly questionnaires	
Baron *et al.* (1998) USA 4 years		751 participants in a multi-centre clinical trial of β-carotene and vitamins C and E, with at least one recent large bowel adenoma	Cases ascertained by colonoscopy	Randomized intervention trial
Nagata *et al.* (1999) Japan 1992–95		31 552 (14 427 men, 17 125 women) residents of Takayama, aged ≥ 35 years	Cases ascertained by colonoscopy at two major hospitals	
Olsen & Kronborg (1993) Denmark 1986–90		17 284 residents of Funen Island, participating in a randomized control trial for colorectal cancer screening, aged 45–74 years	Cases ascertained by Haemoccult-II test	Nested case–control study; controls matched by age, sex and date of testing

Table 2.1.7.2. Cohort studies on smoking and risk of colorectal cancer

Reference Country and years of study	Cohort No. of subjects	No. of deaths from cancer of colon or rectum/incident cancers	Smoking categories	Relative risks (95% CI or p value)			Adjustment factors/ comments
				Colon cancer	Rectal cancer	Colorectal cancer	
Hammond & Horn (1958a,b) USA 1952–55	American Cancer Society Study 187 783 men	84 colon, 55 rectal deaths	Ever-smoker	0.8	0.9		Age
Hammond (1966) USA 1959–63	Cancer Prevention Study 1 440 558 men, 562 671 women	Colorectal deaths 572 men, 349 women	*Men* Regular smoker			1.0 (age: 45–64 years) 1.2 (age: 65–79 years)	Stratified by age and sex. Baseline group included those who never smoked regularly
			Heavy smoker				
			Women Regular smoker			0.8 (age: 45–64 years) 0.7 (age: 45–64 years)	
			Heavy smoker				
Kahn (1966) USA 1954–62	US Veterans' Study 248 195 men	513 colon, 216 rectal deaths	Former smoker	1.3	1.0		A few cancers of the small intestines were included with colon cancers
			Current smoker	1.2	0.9		
			Cigarettes/day				
			10–20	1.1	0.7		
			21–39	1.3	1.0		
Doll & Peto (1976) UK 1951–71	British Doctors' Study 34 440 men	195 colon, 78 rectal deaths	Former smoker	1.0	1.0		Age, calendar year
			Ever-smoker	1.3	2.3		
			Current, any tobacco smoking	1.3	2.3		
			g tobacco/day				
			1–14	1.3	1.7		
			15–24	1.2	2.3		
			≥ 25	1.2	4.5		
			p for trend	> 0.05	0.09		

Table 2.1.7.2 (contd)

Reference Country and years of study	Cohort No. of subjects	No. of deaths from cancer of colon or rectum/incident cancers	Smoking categories	Relative risks (95% CI or p value)			Adjustment factors/ comments
				Colon cancer	Rectal cancer	Colorectal cancer	
Doll et al. (1980) UK 1951–73	British Doctors' Study 6194 women	7 rectal deaths	Current smoker *Cigarettes/day* 1–14 15–24 ≥25 p for trend	Not available	0.8 3.0 9.6 > 0.05		Age, calendar year
Rogot & Murray (1980) USA 1954–69	US Veterans' Study 248 195 men	1093 colon, 370 rectal deaths in smokers	Former smoker Current smoker	1.3 1.1	1.1 1.1		A few cases of cancers of the small intestine were included with colon cancers; no. of deaths in never smokers not given
Williams et al. (1981) USA 1948–82 24 years	Framingham Heart Study 5209 men and women	58 colon (28 men, 30 women)	Packs/day <1 1 >1	0.5 0.3 0.3	Not available		Age, not sure about sex. Not all colon (n = 88) and none of rectal (n = 26) were included in analysis
Garland et al. (1985) USA 1957–77	Western Electric Company Study 1954 men	49 colorectal deaths	Non-cancer comparison group, Colorectal cancer group Cigarettes/day			9.5† 7.4†	†No relative risk calculated Numbers indicate average number of cigarettes smoked per day.
Carstensen et al. (1987) Sweden 1963–79	Swedish Census Study 25 129 men	117 colon, 69 rectal deaths	Former smoker *Current, any tobacco, g/day* 1–7 8–15 ≥15 p for trend	1.1 1.4 1.5 1.5 0.07	1.0 2.0 1.1 1.3 0.65		Age, residence Former smokers were excluded in test for trends.

Table 2.1.7.2 (contd)

Reference Country and years of study	Cohort No. of subjects	No. of deaths from cancer of colon or rectum/incident cancers	Smoking categories	Relative risks (95% CI or p value)			Adjustment factors/ comments
				Colon cancer	Rectal cancer	Colorectal cancer	
Kono et al. (1987) Japan 1965–83	Japanese Physicians' Study 5130 men	39 colorectal deaths	Never/past/ occasional Current smoker 1–19 cigs/day ≥ 20 cigs/day			1.0 0.9 (0.4–1.9) 0.9 (0.4–2.2)	Age, alcohol use
Wu et al. (1987) USA 1981–85	Leisure World Study 11 644 men and women	126 colorectal cancers (58 men, 68 women)	Men Former >20 years Former ≤ 20 years Current Women Former >20 years Former ≤ 20 years Current			1.7 (0.8–3.6) 2.6 (1.3–5.3) 1.8 (0.6–5.2) 1.6 (0.8–3.0) 0.7 (0.3–1.5) 1.4 (0.7–1.0)	Age; odds ratio for smoking in men was significant (1.49) after adjustment for sex, alcohol consumption, physical activity and body mass index
Klatsky et al. (1988) USA 1978–84	Kaiser Permanente Medical Care Program Study 106 203 men and women	203 colon cancers (92 men, 111 women), 66 rectal cancers (33 men, 33 women)	Former smoker Current smoker < 1 pack/day ≥ 1 pack/day	1.0 (0.7–1.4) 0.8 (0.5–1.3) 1.4 (0.8–2.3)	1.3 (0.7–2.3) 1.1 (0.5–2.3) 1.0 (0.4–2.8)		Age, race, alcohol and coffee intake, body size, education, serum cholesterol; 10% random sample of controls used in analyses
Sandler et al. (1988) USA 1963–75	22 773 men, 25 369 women	Colorectal deaths (194 men, 286 women)	Current smoker Men Women			1.4 (0.9–2.2) 0.8 (0.5–1.1)	Age Nonsmokers were never smokers who did not live with smokers.
Hirayama (1989) Japan 1965–81	Six-prefecture Study 122 261 men, 142 847 women	574 colon deaths (256 men, 318 women) (91 sigmoid cancers)	Daily smoker	Proximal colon, 1.2 (0.9–1.6); Sigmoid colon, 1.4 (0.7–2.8)			Age Smoking was not significant after adjusting for alcohol and dietary factors (1.2; 95% CI, 0.6–2.3).

Table 2.1.7.2 (contd)

Reference Country and years of study	Cohort No. of subjects	No. of deaths from cancer of colon or rectum/incident cancers	Smoking categories	Relative risks (95% CI or p value)			Adjustment factors/ comments
				Colon cancer	Rectal cancer	Colorectal cancer	
Akiba & Hirayama (1990) Japan 1965–81	Six-prefecture Study 122 261 men, 142 847 women	Colon (190 men, 257 women) and rectal (254 men, 211 women) cancer deaths	*Men* Any cigarettes *Cigarettes/day* 1–4 5–14 15–24 25–34 ≥ 35 p for trend	1.1 (0.8–1.5) 0.9 (0.2–2.6) 1.0 (0.7–1.6) 1.1 (0.7–1.6) 1.2 (0.5–2.4) 1.8 (0.6–4.2) > 0.1	1.4 (1.0–1.9) 1.4 (0.5–3.2) 1.3 (0.9–1.9) 1.4 (1.0–2.0) 1.5 (0.7–2.9) 1.1 (0.3–2.9) 0.09		Prefecture of residence, occupation, attained age (5-year interval), observation period (see Hirayama, 1989)
			Women Any cigarettes *Cigarettes/day* 1–4 5–14 ≥ 15 p for trend	0.9 (0.6–1.3) 1.1 (0.4–2.4) 0.9 (0.5–1.4) 0.5 (0.1–1.6) > 0.1	0.9 (0.6–1.5) 0.5 (0.1–1.7) 0.9 (0.5–1.5) 2.1 (0.8–4.3) > 0.1		
Chute et al. (1991) USA 1976–84	Nurses' Health Study 118 404 women	191 colon, 49 rectal cancers	Former smoker Current smoker *Cigarettes/day* 1–14 15–24 > 24 p for trend	1.2 (0.9–1.7) 1.0 (0.7–1.4) 1.0 (0.6–1.7) 1.0 (0.0–1.6) 1.0 (0.6–1.7) 0.88	1.9 (1.0–3.6) 1.1 (0.5–1.3) 1.2 (0.4–3.7) 1.1 (0.5–2.5)† 0.65		Age †for ≥ 15 cigarettes/day

Table 2.1.7.2 (contd)

Reference Country and years of study	Cohort No. of subjects	No. of deaths from cancer of colon or rectum/incident cancers	Smoking categories	Relative risks (95% CI or p value)			Adjustment factors/ comments
				Colon cancer	Rectal cancer	Colorectal cancer	
Tverdal et al. (1993) Norway 1972–88	Norwegian Screening Study 44 290 men, 24 535 women	Colon (53 men, 30 women), rectal (50 men, 16 women) cancer deaths	*Men* Former smoker Current smoker **Cigarettes/day** 1–9 10–19 ≥ 20 *Women* Former smoker Current smoker	1.2 1.5 0.7[†] 1.7 1.3 0.9 1.1	1.4 1.8 1.7[†] 1.7 1.7 NA 0.6		Age, area [†]Among male current smokers of cigarettes only, the relative risk per 10 cigarettes was 1.2 (95% CI, 0.7–2.2) for colon and 0.8 (95% CI, 0.4–1.6) for rectal cancers [assuming this was calculated using 1–9 cigarettes per day as the baseline group]
Akiba (1994) Japan 1963–87	Life Span Study 61 505 men and women	324 colon (172 men, 152 women), 218 rectal (122 men, 96 women) cancers	Former smoker Current smoker	0.9 (0.6–1.4) 1.2 (0.9–1.6)	1.3 (0.8–2.0) 1.0 (0.7–1.4)		City, sex, population group, atomic bomb exposure, birth year (10-year interval), attained age (5-year interval)
Bostick et al. (1994) USA 1986–92	Iowa Women's Health Study 35 215 women	212 colon cancers	Former smoker Current smoker	0.9 (0.6–1.3) 1.1 (0.7–1.6)			Age, total energy, height, parity, total vitamin E intake; total vitamin E by age interaction term; vitamin A supplement

Table 2.1.7.2 (contd)

Reference, Country and years of study	Cohort No. of subjects	No. of deaths from cancer of colon or rectum/incident cancers	Smoking categories	Relative risks (95% CI or p value) Colon cancer	Rectal cancer	Colorectal cancer	Adjustment factors/comments
Doll et al. (1994) UK 1951–91	British Doctors' Study 34 439 men	437 colon and 168 rectal deaths	Former smoker	1.4	1.5		Age, calendar period
			Current smoker	1.3	2.3		
			p for trend	0.37	0.06		
			Current smoker **Cigarettes/day**				
			1–14	1.4	1.3		
			15–24	1.1	1.9		
			≥ 25	1.4	4.5		
			p for trend	0.06	0.03		
Giovannucci et al. (1994a) USA 1976–90	Nurses' Health Study 118 334 women	586 colorectum deaths	Current smoker			0.9 (0.7–1.2)	
			Years since starting smoking				
			≤ 10 cigarettes/ day				
			1–19 years			0.8 (0.4–1.4)	
			20–29 years			1.0 (0.7–1.4)	
			30–34 years			0.8 (0.5–1.1)	
			35–39 years			0.8 (0.6–1.2)	
			40–44 years			1.0 (0.7–1.5)	
			≥ 45 years			1.1 (0.6–2.0)	
			≥ 10 cigarettes/ day				
			1–19 years			0.4 (0.1–1.3)	
			20–29 years			1.1 (0.7–1.6)	
			30–34 years			0.8 (0.5–1.2)	
			35–39 years			1.5 (1.1–2.0)	
			40–44 years			1.6 (1.1–2.3)	
			≥ 45 years			2.0 (1.1–3.5)	
			Smoking > *10 pack–years*				
			Before age 30	1.2 (0.9–1.5)	2.1 (1.2–3.4)	1.3 (1.0–1.8)	
			After age 30			1.0 (0.8–1.3)	

Table 2.1.7.2 (contd)

Reference Country and years of study	Cohort No. of subjects	No. of deaths from cancer of colon or rectum/incident cancers	Smoking categories	Relative risks (95% CI or p value)			Adjustment factors/ comments
				Colon cancer	Rectal cancer	Colorectal cancer	
Giovannucci et al. (1994b) USA 1986–92	Health Professionals' Follow-up Study 47 935 men	239 colorectum deaths (44 rectal)	Current smoker			1.4 (0.8–2.2)	Age, family history of colorectal cancer, body-mass index, intake of saturated fat, fibre, folate, and alcohol
			Pack–years				
			1–9			1.3 (0.8–2.1)	
			10–19			1.5 (1.0–2.3)	
			20–29			1.7 (1.1–2.5)	
			30–39			1.4 (0.8–2.2)	
			≥ 40			1.5 (1.0–2.1)	
			p for trend			0.12	
			Before age 30				All the risk estimates for pack–years smoked after age 30 years were < 1.0 when also adjusted for smoking before age 30 years.
			1–4			1.6 (1.0–2.6)	
			5–10			1.6 (1.0–2.6)	
			11–15			2.1 (1.2–3.4)	
			≥ 16			2.0 (1.3–3.2)	
			p for trend			0.001	
			After age 30				
			1–4			0.8 (0.5–1.5)	
			5–10			0.9 (0.6–1.5)	
			11–15			0.8 (0.5–1.3)	
			≥ 16			0.7 (0.4–1.1)	
			p for trend			0.18	
			Years since starting smoking				Age, body-mass index, family history of colorectal cancer, intake of saturated fat, folate, dietary fibre and alcohol
			≤ 10 cigarettes/day				
			1–19 years			–	
			20–29 years			1.3 (0.6–2.6)	
			30–34 years			1.3 (0.6–2.7)	
			35–39 years			1.2 (0.7–2.1)	
			40–44 years			1.8 (1.2–2.9)	
			≥ 45			1.6 (1.1–2.0)	

Table 2.1.7.2 (contd)

Reference Country and years of study	Cohort No. of subjects	No. of deaths from cancer of colon or rectum/incident cancers	Smoking categories	Relative risks (95% CI or *p* value)			Adjustment factors/ comments
				Colon cancer	Rectal cancer	Colorectal cancer	
Giovannucci *et al.* (1994b) (contd)			**≥ 10 cigarettes/day**				
			1–19 years			1.9 (0.6–6.3)	
			20–29 years			0.8 (0.3–2.2)	
			30–34 years			0.8 (0.2–2.6)	
			35–39 years			1.2 (0.6–2.3)	
			40–44 years			1.7 (0.9–3.3)	
			≥ 45 years			2.6 (1.5–4.4)	
Heineman *et al.* (1994) USA 1954–80	US Veterans' Study 248 046 men	3812 colon and 1100 rectal deaths	Current smoker	1.2 (1.1–1.4)	1.4 (1.2–1.7)		Age, social class, physical activity. [Note that 'unknown' cigarette use was also associated with an increased risk.]
			Former smoker	1.3 (1.2–1.5)	1.4 (1.1–1.7)		
			Unknown	1.2 (1.1–1.4)	1.4 (1.1–1.8)		
			Cigarettes/day				
			1–9	1.1 (1.0–1.3)	1.3 (1.0–1.7)		
			10–20	1.2 (1.1–1.4)	1.4 (1.1–1.7)		
			21–39	1.3 (1.1–1.4)	1.6 (1.3–2.1)		
			≥ 40	1.6 (1.2–2.0)	1.7 (1.1–2.6)		
			p for trend	< 0.001	< 0.001		
			Pack-years				
			0–8	1.0 (0.8–1.3)	0.8 (0.5–1.3)		
			> 8–18	1.2 (1.1–1.4)	1.6 (1.2–2.1)		
			> 18–98	1.4 (1.2–1.6)	1.7 (1.4–2.2)		
			p for trend	< 0.001	< 0.001		
			Age at starting smoking				
			≥ 25 years	1.1 (1.0–1.3)	1.2 (0.9–1.6)		
			20–24 years	1.3 (1.1–1.5)	1.4 (1.1–1.7)		
			15–19 years	1.2 (1.1–1.4)	1.6 (1.3–1.9)		
			< 15	1.4 (1.2–1.8)	1.5 (1.0–2.2)		
			p for trend	< 0.001	0.006		

Table 2.1.7.2 (contd)

Reference Country and years of study	Cohort No. of subjects	No. of deaths from cancer of colon or rectum/incident cancers	Smoking categories	Relative risks (95% CI or p value)			Adjustment factors/comments
				Colon cancer	Rectal cancer	Colorectal cancer	
McLaughlin et al. (1995) USA 1954–80	US Veterans' Study 177 903 men (excluded 34 219 pipe/cigar smokers and 35924 with unknown smoking habits)	2596 colon and 735 rectal deaths	Former smoker	1.4 (1.2–1.5)	1.3 (1.0–1.5)		Age, calendar-year time-period. Relative risks were lower for 1954–69 than for 1970–80: colon cancer, 1.1 (95% CI, 1.0–1.3) and 1.4 (95% CI, 1.2–1.6), respectively; rectal cancer, 1.2 (95% CI, 1.0–1.5) and 2.0 (95% CI, 1.5–2.8), respectively.
			Current smoker	1.2 (1.1–1.4)	1.4 (1.2–1.7)		
			Ever-smoker	1.3 (1.2–1.4)	1.4 (1.2–1.6)		
			Cigarettes/day				
			1–9	1.1 (0.9–1.3)	1.3 (1.1–1.9)		
			10–20	1.2 (1.1–1.4)	1.3 (1.1–1.6)		
			31–39	1.3 (1.1–1.5)	1.6 (1.2–2.0)		
			≥40	1.7 (1.3–2.1)	1.5 (0.9–2.4)		
			p for trend	< 0.01	< 0.01		
Chyou et al. (1996) USA 1965–95	American Men of Japanese Ancestry Study 7945 men	330 colon and 123 rectal cancers	Former smoker	1.3 (1.0–1.7)	1.3 (0.8–2.2)		Age
			Current smoker	1.4 (1.1–1.9)	2.0 (1.3–3.0)		
			Pack-years				
			1–15	1.3 (0.9–1.9)	1.1 (0.4–2.1)		
			16–30	1.1 (0.8–1.5)	1.6 (0.9–2.7)		
			≥31	1.5 (1.1–1.9)	1.9 (1.2–3.0)		
			p for trend	0.0008	0.0034		Age, alcohol consumption, body-mass index, serum cholesterol, heart rate, intake of mono unsaturated fatty acid
			Per 10 pack-years	1.1 (1.0–1.1)	1.1 (1.0–1.2)		
Engeland et al. (1996) Norway 1966–93	Norwegian Cohort Study 11 863 men, 14 269 women	Colon (230 men, 300 women) and rectum (139 men, 141 women) cancers	*Men*				Age
			Former smoker	1.0 (0.6–1.5)	0.8 (0.4–1.6)		
			Current smoker	1.2 (0.8–1.6)	1.6 (1.0–2.6)		
			Women				
			Former smoker	1.3 (0.9–2.0)	1.3 (0.8–2.4)		
			Current smoker	1.1 (0.8–1.4)	0.8 (0.5–1.3)		

Table 2.1.7.2 (contd)

Reference Country and years of study	Cohort No. of subjects	No. of deaths from cancer of colon or rectum/incident cancers	Smoking categories	Relative risks (95% CI or p value)			Adjustment factors/ comments
				Colon cancer	Rectal cancer	Colorectal cancer	
Murata et al. (1996) Japan 1984–93	Chiba Center Association Study 17 200 men	61 colon, 43 rectum	*Cigarettes/day* 1–10 11–20 ≥ 21 *p* for trend	0.8 (0.3–2.2) 1.1 (0.5–2.4) 1.0 (0.3–2.8) 0.98	1.3 (0.3–6.0) 1.1 (0.5–2.7) 3.0 (0.7–13.4) 0.37		Crude 95% CI calculated by Working Group based on the data presented. No effect of smoking by levels of alcohol intake
Nyrén et al. (1996) Sweden 1971–91	Swedish Construction Workers Cohort 134 985 men for colon, 135 009 men for rectum	713 colon, 505 incident rectal cancers	Former smoker Current smoker *Cigarettes/day* 1–4 5–14 15–24 ≥ 25 **Duration (years)** *Former smoker* 1–10 11–20 ≥ 21 *Current smoker* 1–10 11–20 21–30 31–40 ≥ 41	1.0 (0.8–1.2) 1.0 (0.8–1.2) 0.9 (0.7–1.2) 0.8 (0.7–1.0) 1.1 (0.9–1.4) 1.1 (0.6–1.8) 0.8 (0.4–1.1) 1.1 (0.9–1.5) 1.1 (0.8–1.4) 0.8 (0.4–1.3) 0.7 (0.5–1.1) 1.0 (0.8–1.3) 1.1 (0.8–1.3) 1.0 (0.7–1.4)	1.2 (1.0–1.5) 1.1 (0.9–1.4) 1.1 (0.81–1.4) 0.8 (0.6–1.0) 1.2 (0.9–1.5) 1.1 (0.6–2.0) 1.3 (0.9–1.9) 1.4 (1.0–1.9) 1.1 (0.8–1.5) 0.8 (0.4–1.7) 1.0 (0.7–1.6) 1.2 (0.8–1.6) 1.3 (1.0–1.7) 1.1 (0.7–1.6)		Body-mass index, height, normal and maximum pulse rate, marital status and asbestos exposure
Yuan et al. (1996) China 1986–93	Shanghai Men's Study 18 244 men	26 colon, 31 rectal cancers	Ever-smoker *Cigarettes/day* < 20 ≥ 20	1.1 1.5 0.7	0.6 0.5 0.7		Adjusted for age and alcohol consumption
Chen et al. (1997) China 1972–93	Shanghai Factory Study 1696 men and women	22 colorectal cancers	*Cigarettes/day* 1–19 ≥ 20			1.5 *p* > 0.05 2.6 *p* > 0.05	Adjusted for age, systolic blood pressure, serum cholesterol and regular alcohol drinking (yes/no)

Table 2.1.7.2 (contd)

Reference Country and years of study	Cohort No. of subjects	No. of deaths from cancer of colon or rectum/incident cancers	Smoking categories	Relative risks (95% CI or *p* value)			Adjustment factors/ comments
				Colon cancer	Rectal cancer	Colorectal cancer	
Kato *et al.* (1997) USA 1985–94	New York University Women's Health Study 14 727 women	73 colon and 27 rectum	Former smoker Current smoker			1.0 (0.6–1.6) 1.0 (0.5–1.9)	Age, place of enrolment
Liaw & Chen (1998) China, Province of Taiwan 1982–94	Taiwanese Study 17 538 men and women	42 colorectal cancers	Current smoker			0.8 (0.4–1.5)	Analysis for men only because of the small number of cases in women
Norlund *et al.* (1997) Sweden 1963–89	Swedish Census Study 26 032 women	559 incident colorectal cancers	Former smoker Current smoker *Cigarettes/day* 1–7 8–15 > 15 *Age at starting smoking (years)* 20–23 < 19 *p* for trend			1.2 (0.7–1.9) 0.9 (0.7–1.2) 0.9 (0.6–1.3) 0.7 (0.4–1.1) 1.4 (0.8–2.6) 1.2 (0.6–2.3) 1.0 (0.5–1.9) 0.95	Age, place of residence
Tulinius *et al.* (1997) Iceland 1968–95	Reykjavík Study 11 366 men, 11 580 women	Colorectal cancers (193 men, 145 women)	*Women* Former smoker *Cigarettes/day* 1–14 15–24 ≥ 25	1.1 (0.7–1.9) 1.4 (0.9–2.1) 1.5 (1.0–2.5) 2.5 (1.0–6.2)			Age, glucose levels. Results for men were not presented: presumably not statistically significant

Table 2.1.7.2 (contd)

Reference Country and years of study	Cohort No. of subjects	No. of deaths from cancer of colon or rectum/incident cancers	Smoking categories	Relative risks (95% CI or p value) Colon cancer	Rectal cancer	Colorectal cancer	Adjustment factors/ comments
Hsing et al. (1998) USA 1966–86	Lutheran Brotherhood Insurance Study 17 633 men	120 colon, 25 rectal deaths	Former smoker	1.5 (0.8–2.7)		1.1 (0.7–1.8)	Age, urban/rural residence, alcohol intake Occasional users smoked less than 1 cigarette, pipe or cigar per day
			Occasional smoker	1.4 (0.7–2.9)		1.1 (0.6–2.0)	
			Current smoker	1.4 (0.7–2.7)		1.0 (0.6–1.7)	
			Cigarettes/day				
			1–19	1.1 (0.5–2.5)		0.8 (0.4–1.6)	
			20–29	1.6 (0.7–3.4)		1.1 (0.5–2.1)	
			≥30	2.3 (0.9–5.7)		1.7 (0.7–3.8)	
			p for trend	0.3		0.5	
			Duration (years)				
			1–19	1.3 (0.2–9.7)		0.8 (0.1–6.0)	
			20–29	2.4 (1.0–5.3)		1.0 (0.7–3.2)	
			≥30	1.2 (0.6–2.4)		0.9 (0.5–1.6)	
			p for trend	0.8		0.8	
Knekt et al. (1998) Finland 1966–94	Mobile Health Clinic Study 56 973 men and women	241 colon and 216 incident rectal cancers	Former smoker	1.2 (0.8–1.9)	0.9 (0.6–1.4)	1.0 (0.7–1.4)	Sex, age, body-mass index, occupation, area, type of population, marital status 17 291 subjects in second health examination between 1973 and 1976
			Cigarettes/day				
			<15	1.1 (0.7–1.7)	1.1 (0.7–1.7)	1.1 (0.8–1.5)	
			≥15	1.4 (0.8–2.1)	0.9 (0.5–1.4)	1.0 (0.7–1.5)	
			Smoker in 1966 and 1973	1.9 (1.1–3.5)	1.5 (0.8–2.9)	1.7 (1.1–2.7)	
			Follow-up (years)			Smokers	
			<10			1.0 (0.6–1.6)	
			11–20			1.6 (1.1–2.2)	
			>20			0.8 (0.5–1.1)	
Singh & Fraser (1998) USA 1976–82	Adventists' Health Study 32 051 men and women	157 colon (135 colon, 22 recto-sigmoid)	Former smoker	1.1 (0.8–1.7)			Age, sex, parental history of colon cancer
			Current smoker	1.4 (0.5–3.8)			

Table 2.1.7.2 (contd)

Reference Country and years of study	Cohort No. of subjects	No. of deaths from cancer of colon or rectum/incident cancers	Smoking categories	Relative risks (95% CI or p value)			Adjustment factors/ comments
				Colon cancer	Rectal cancer	Colorectal cancer	
Chao et al. (2000) USA 1982–96	Cancer Prevention Study (CPS) II 312 332 men and 469 019 women	Colorectal deaths (2156 men, 2276 women)	*Men*				Age, race, body-mass index, education, family history of colorectal cancers, exercise, aspirin and multivitamin use, intake of alcohol, vegetables, high-fibre cereal products, and fatty meats; hormone replacement therapy in women; no. of colon and rectal cancers not specified
			Former smoker	1.3 (1.2–1.5)		1.2 (1.0–1.3)	
			Current smoker		1.2 (0.9–1.7)	1.3 (1.2–1.5)	
			Women				
			Former smoker			1.2 (1.1–1.4)	
			Current smoker	1.4 (1.3–1.6)	1.3 (1.0–1.8)	1.4 (1.3–1.6)	
			Men and women				
			Cigarettes/day				
			< 20			1.3 (1.2–1.5)	
			20			1.4 (1.2–1.6)	
			21–39			1.3 (1.1–1.6)	
			≥ 40			1.5 (1.3–1.8)	
			p for trend			0.03	
			Pack–years				
			< 20			1.3 (1.1–1.5)	
			20–39			1.3 (1.1–1.5)	
			40–59			1.4 (1.2–1.6)	
			≥ 60			1.5 (1.3–1.7)	
			p for trend			0.05	
			Duration (years)				
			< 20			1.1 (0.8–1.5)	
			20–29			1.3 (1.1–1.6)	
			30–39			1.4 (1.2–1.6)	
			≥ 40			1.4 (1.3–1.6)	
			p for trend			0.24	
			Age at starting smoking (years)				
			≥ 20			1.3 (1.2–1.5)	
			16–19			1.4 (1.3–1.6)	
			≤ 15			1.5 (1.3–1.7)	
			p for trend			0.02	

Table 2.1.7.2 (contd)

Reference Country and years of study	Cohort No. of subjects	No. of deaths from cancer of colon or rectum/incident cancers	Smoking categories	Relative risks (95% CI or *p* value)			Adjustment factors/ comments
				Colon cancer	Rectal cancer	Colorectal cancer	
Chao *et al.* (2000) (contd)			*Former smokers* **Years since quitting**				Similar patterns of increased risk with years smoked and pack–years smoked among former smokers.
			≤ 10			1.3 (1.2–1.5)	
			11–19			1.2 (1.1–1.4)	
			≥ 20			1.0 (0.9–1.2)	
			p for trend			0.0001	
			Age at quitting smoking				
			≤ 30			0.9 (0.8–1.1)	
			31–40			1.1 (1.0–2.3)	
			41–50			1.2 (1.0–1.3)	
			51–60			1.4 (1.2–1.6)	
			≥ 61			1.3 (1.1–1.6)	
			p for trend			0.0001	
Stürmer *et al.* (2000) USA 1982–95	Physicians' Health Study 22 071 men	351 colorectal cancers	Former smoker			1.5 (1.2–1.9)	Body-mass index, alcohol intake, exercise, use of vitamins and aspirin, and selected dietary factors
			Current smoker			1.8 (1.3–2.6)	
			p for trend			< 0.001	
			Former smoker				
			< 20 cigarettes/day			1.5 (1.1–2.1)	
			> 20 cigarettes/day			1.3 (1.0–1.7)	
			Current smoker				
			< 20 cigarettes/day			1.3 (0.7–2.4)	
			> 20 cigarettes/day			2.1 (1.5–3.1)	
			p for trend			0.002	
			Pack–years				
			0–≤ 10			1.5 (1.1–2.2)	
			10–≤ 20			1.6 (1.1–2.2)	
			20–≤ 40			1.2 (0.9–1.7)	
			> 40			1.7 (1.2–2.4)	
			p for trend			0.009	

Table 2.1.7.2 (contd)

Reference Country and years of study	Cohort No. of subjects	No. of deaths from cancer of colon or rectum/incident cancers	Smoking categories	Relative risks (95% CI or p value)			Adjustment factors/ comments
				Colon cancer	Rectal cancer	Colorectal cancer	
van Wayenburg et al. (2000) Netherlands 1974–96	Dutch Study 20 555 women	95 colorectal deaths	Ever-smoker			1.4 (0.9–2.2)	Age, age at first birth, use of oral contraceptives, natural or artificial menopause, social class, body-mass index
Terry et al. (2001) Sweden 1961–97	Swedish Twin Registry Study 10 945 pairs	318 colon, 180 rectal cancers	Former smoker *Cigarette smoker* Light smoker Moderate smoker Heavy smoker	1.1 (0.8–1.5) 1.0 (0.7–1.5) 1.0 (0.6–1.8) 1.7 (0.4–7.0)	1.0 (0.6–1.6) 0.9 (0.6–1.7) 1.2 (0.6–2.4) 5.3 (1.9–15.0)	1.0 (0.8–1.4) 1.0 (0.7–1.3) 1.1 (0.7–1.7) 3.1 (1.4–7.1)	Age (5-year age groups), sex, body-mass index, physical activity

CI, confidence interval

Table 2.1.7.3. Case–control studies on tobacco smoking and colorectal cancer: main characteristics of study design

Reference Country and years of study	No. of cases and controls	Comments
Williams & Horm (1977) USA Early 1960s	Men: 333 colon, 185 rectum; women: 389 colon, 154 rectum; and about 4700 controls	Data from the Third National Cancer Survey personal interviews Controls included patients with all other cancers, excluding 'tobacco-related cancers' (lung, larynx, oesophagus, bladder and oral cavity).
Dales et al. (1979) USA 1973–76	Men and women: 99 colorectum cases and 280 controls	Hospital-based study among African Americans in the San Francisco Bay Area Cases with colon cancer (72), rectosigmoid cancer (5) and rectal cancer (22); response rate, 40% Controls were hospital patients matched 2:1 (189) and from multiphasic health check-ups matched 1:1 (91), all matched on age, sex and ethnicity; response rate, 50%
Tuyns et al. (1982) France 1973–80	Men: 80 colon, 104 rectum and 923 controls; women: 62 colon, 94 rectum and 1053 controls	Population-based study in Calvados Controls represented a random sample of 2% of the total adult population, aged ≥ 20 years,; response rate, 75%
Vobecky et al. (1983) Canada 1965–76	Men: 103 colorectum and 103 controls; women: 104 colorectum and 104 controls	Population-based study in St Laurent River Area Cases had 93% response rate. Controls randomly selected in area, individually matched 1:1 by age and sex
Tajima & Tominaga (1985) Japan 1981–83	Men: 27 colon, 25 rectume and 111 controls; women: 15 colon, 26 rectum and 75 controls	Hospital-based study in Aichi Cancer Centre Cases aged 40–70 years Controls were non-cancer patients
Jarebinski et al. (1988, 1989) Yugoslavia 1984–86	1988: men: 97 colorectum and 97 controls; women: 87 colorectum and 87 controls; 1989: men: 56 rectum and 112 controls; women: 42 rectum and 84 controls	Population- and hospital-based study in Belgrade Controls from case's neighbourhood (98) and hospital (98), individually matched by sex and age
Ferraroni et al. (1989) Italy 1985–88	Men: 221 colon, 170 rectum and 1334 controls; women: 234 colon, 125 rectum and 610 controls	Hospital-based study in northern Italy Cases aged < 75 years Controls were cancer-free (all subjects included in D'Avanzo et al., 1995)
Peters et al. (1989) USA 1974–82	Men: 106 colon, 41 rectum and 106 controls	Population-based study among young white men in Los Angeles County Cases aged 25–44 years; response rate, 63% Controls individually matched for neighbourhood, race, sex, date of birth; response rate, 63%

Table 2.1.7.3 (contd)

Reference Country and years of study	No. of cases and controls	Comments
Kato *et al.* (1990a) Japan 1986–90	Men: 79 colon, 60 rectum and 377 controls; women: 53 colon, 31 rectum and 201 controls	Population-based study in Aichi Cancer Centre among 1776 patients receiving colonoscopy; response rate for cases, 86% Controls from telephone directories matched by sex, age (5-year groups) and municipality; response rate, 91%
Kato *et al.* (1990b) Japan 1979–87	Men: 1716 colon, 1611 rectum and 16 600 controls	Hospital-based study in Aichi Cancer Centre among patients receiving colonoscopy Cases with cancer of the colon (445 proximal, 765 distal, 506 not specified), or rectum aged ≥ 20 years; response rate, 89% Controls with other cancers, excluding sites related to smoking (larynx, lung, pancreas, bladder) and alcohol consumption
Slattery *et al.* (1990) USA 1979–83	Men: 112 colon and 185 controls; women: 119 colon and 206 controls	Population-based study in Utah Cases of primary cancer, histologically confirmed, aged 40–79 years; response rate, 71% Controls selected by random-digit dialling; response rate, 74%
Choi & Kahyo (1991) Republic of Korea 1986–90	Men: 63 colon, 67 rectum, 189 controls for colon cases, 201 controls for rectal cases	Hospital-based study in Korea Cancer Centre Controls were cancer-free, matched 3:1 on birth years (± 5 years), sex and admission date.
Kune *et al.* (1992) Australia 1980–81	Men: 202 colon, 186 rectum; women: 190 colon, 137 rectum; and 727 controls	Population-based study in Melbourne Incident, histologically confirmed cases; response rate, 62% Controls from community, matched by age and sex; response rate, 71%
Hoshiyama *et al.* (1993) Japan 1984–90	Men: 37 colon, 61 rectum and 343 controls; women: 42 colon, 41 rectum and 310 controls	Population-based study in Saitama Prefecture Incident cases aged 40–69 years Controls from general population; response rate, 28%
Olsen & Kronborg (1993) Denmark 1986, 1988, 1990	Men: 21 colorectum and 156 controls; women 28 colorectum and 206 controls	Randomized control trial using Hemaoccult II as screening test for colorectal cancer 30 970 to screening and 30 968 to control group Cases tested positive for Hemaoccult II test and colonoscopy, aged 45–74 years (mean, 66.7 years) Controls tested negative for Hemaoccult II test, matched to cases on age and sex; mean age, 63.8 years

Table 2.1.7.3 (contd)

Reference Country and years of study	No. of cases and controls	Comments
Baron *et al.* (1994) Sweden 1986–88	Men and women: 352 colon, 217 rectum (262 men, 307 women) and 512 controls (236 men, 276 women)	Population-based study in Stockholm County All cases diagnosed in the area during that period identified through the regional cancer registry; age, 40–79 years; response rate, 79% Controls from population register; response rate, 82%
Boutron *et al.* (1995) France 1985	Men: 109 colorectum and 159 controls; women: 62 colorectum and 150 controls	Population-based study in a clinic in Côte d'Or Cases aged 30–79 years; response rate, 80% Controls selected from the 1975 census list; response rate, 54%
D'Avanzo *et al.* (1995) Italy 1985–91 (see also Ferraroni *et al.*, 1989)	Men: 498 colon, 337 rectum and 1863 controls; women: 457 colon, 252 rectum and 1016 controls	Hospital-based study in northern Italy (Greater Milan and Pordenone Province) Cases aged 20–74 years; response rate, 95% Controls with a wide spectrum of acute non-malignant conditions, excluding diseases of the gastrointestinal tract or diseases related to coffee, alcohol or tobacco consumption; response rate, 95%
Inoue *et al.* (1995) Japan 1988–92	Men and women: 94 proximal and 137 distal colon, 201 rectum (257 men, 175 women) and 31 782 controls (8621 men, 23 161 women)	Hospital-based study in Aichi Cancer Centre; response rate for cases, 94% Controls were non-cancer outpatients on first hospital visit; response rate, 94%
Kotake *et al.* (1995) Japan 1992–94	Men and women: 187 colon, 176 rectum (214 men, 149 women) and 363 controls	Hospital-based study in 10 hospitals Controls included cancer (94), non-cancer (56) and screening controls (213) individually matched by age and sex
Newcomb *et al.* (1995) USA 1990–91	Women: 536 colon, 243 rectum and 2315 controls	Population-based study in Wisconsin Incident cases aged 30–74 years; response rate, 74% Controls randomly selected from driver's licences and Health Care Financing Administration listings; response rate, 90%
Siemiatycki *et al.* (1995) Canada 1979–85	Men: 505 colon, 256 rectum and 1492 controls	Study based in major hospitals in Montreal Cases aged 35–70 years; response rate, 82% (including next of kin) Controls selected among cancer patients (959) and from electoral lists (533); response rate, 72%
Le Marchand *et al.* (1997) USA 1987–92	Men: 698 colorectum and 698 controls; women: 494 colorectum and 494 controls	Population-based study among residents of Oahu, Hawaii Cases histologically confirmed, aged < 85 years; response rate, 66% Controls individually matched on sex, ethnicity and age; response rate, 71%

Table 2.1.7.3 (contd)

Reference Country and years of study	No. of cases and controls	Comments
Slattery et al. (1997) USA 1991–94	Men: 1097 colon and 1290 controls; women: 892 colon and 1220 controls	Population-based study in northern California, Utah and Minnesota Cases with first primary cancer, excluding rectosigmoid junction or rectum, aged 30–79 years; response rate, 76% Controls selected by random-digit dialling, Health Care Financing Administration and drivers' licence listings; response rate, 64%
Yamada et al. (1997) Japan 1991–93	Men: 108 cancers in situ, 55 colorectum; women: 21 cancers in situ, 11 colorectum; and 390 controls	Study based on a multiphasic health check-up in Tokyo Cases and controls selected among 79 082 persons receiving a faecal occult blood test Controls with no history of colorectal cancer or inflammatory bowel disease, matched 2:1 on sex, age and history of prior health check-up
Ghadirian et al. (1998) Canada 1989–93	Men: 200 colon and 239 controls; women: 202 colon and 429 controls	Population-based study in Greater Montreal Cases selected from five teaching hospitals, aged 35–79; response rate, 60% Controls selected by random-digit dialling, matched by age, sex, place of residence and language; response rate, 50%
Tavani et al. (1998) Italy 1991–96	Men: 688 colon, 437 rectum and 2073 controls; women: 537 colon, 219 rectum and 2081 controls	Hospital-based study in six centres in northern Italy Cases aged < 75 years Controls were non–cancer patients Response rate for cases and controls, > 95%
Nusko et al. (2000) Germany 1993–96	Men: 126 colorectum and 100 controls; women: 76 colorectum and 134 controls	Hospital-based study among patients undergoing colonoscopy Cases aged ≥ 40 years Controls were polyp-free patients
Chiu et al. (2001) USA 1986–89	Men: 317 colon, 362 rectum and 1503 controls; women: 338 colon, 267 rectum and 833 controls	Population-based study in Iowa Incident cases, histologically confirmed; aged 40–85 years; response rate, 86% Controls selected from driver's licence and Health Care Financing Administration listings, frequency-matched by sex and age; response rate, 80%
Lam et al. (2001) Hong Kong SAR 1997–99	Men: 636 colorectum; women: 563 colorectum; and 13 054 controls	Mortality study among 27 507 cancer deaths Cases aged ≥ 35 years; information retrieved from next of kin; response rate, 81% Controls were relatives of cases or other informants.

Table 2.1.7.4. Case–control studies on tobacco smoking and colorectal cancer

Reference Country and years of study	Smoking variables	Odds ratio (95% CI or p value)			Variables adjusted for and other comments
		Colon	Rectum	Colorectum	
Williams & Horm (1977) USA Early 1960s	Pack–years *Men* <20 20–40 >40 *Women* <20 20–40 >40	0.7 ($p < 0.05$) 0.7 0.8 1.2 0.9 0.7	1.6 ($p < 0.05$) 1.5 0.8 0.8 0.7 0.9		Age, race
Dales et al. (1979) USA 1973–76	Ever–smoker			58% cases versus 58% controls	Crude percentages
Tuyns et al. (1982) France 1973–80	Current smoker	1.0 (0.4–2.7)	1.1 (0.4–2.6)		Age, sex. Risks were non-significantly increased with alcohol intake; 44% of controls were younger than cases.
Vobecky et al. (1983) Canada 1965–76	*Men* Former smoker Current smoker *Women* Former smoker Current smoker	0.5 ($p >0.05$) 2.0 ($p > 0.05$) Not available 1.3 ($p > 0.05$)	0.2 ($p = 0.03$) 1.4 ($p > 0.05$) Not available 1.0 ($p > 0.05$)		Age, sex, city. Alcohol was not a risk factor for colon cancer but was for rectal cancer in men (not significant); information and selection bias

Table 2.1.7.4 (contd)

Reference Country and years of study	Smoking variables	Odds ratio (95% CI or p value) Colon	Rectum	Colorectum	Variables adjusted for and other comments
Tajima & Tominaga (1985) Japan 1981–83	Ever-smoker *Pack-years* < 30 30 *Age at starting smoking (years)* < 20 > 20	0.6 0.3 0.8 0.2 0.7	1.0 1.1 0.9 0.8 1.2		Age, education. All odds ratios were non-significant
Jarebinski et al. (1988, 1989) Yugoslavia 1984–86	*Cigarettes/day (current smokers only)* 1–14 15–24 ≥ 25 *Duration (years) (former + current smokers)* 1–30 ≥ 31		N† H† 0.7 1.0 1.3 1.0 1.3 1.8 1.0 1.0 2.7 2.3 All p > 0.05	N H 0.6 0.7 1.1 1.2 1.5 1.3 1.0 1.0 2.0 1.5 All p > 0.05	Age, sex. Adjusted for cigarettes/day and duration, respectively. Extent of overlap of subjects unknown †N, neighbourhood controls; H, hospital controls
Ferraroni et al. (1989) (see also D'Avanzo et al. 1995) Italy 1985–88	Former smoker *Cigarettes/day* < 15 15–24 ≥ 25 p for trend	0.7 0.7 0.8 0.8 > 0.05	0.9 0.7 0.8 1.1 > 0.05		Age, sex, education, marital status, coffee and alcohol consumption
Peters et al. (1989) USA 1974–82	Former smoker *Pack/day* ≤ 1 ≥ 2	0.6 (0.3–1.3) 0.4 (0.2–1.0) 1.1 (0.5–2.1)	0.7 (0.3–1.8) 0.9 (0.3–2.5) 0.5 (0.2–1.5)	0.7 (0.4–1.4) 0.7 (0.3–1.4) 0.9 (0.4–1.8)	Age and education. Effect for alcohol consumption only with ≥ 70 g/day

Table 2.1.7.4 (contd)

Reference, Country and years of study	Smoking variables	Odds ratio (95% CI or p value) Colon	Rectum	Colorectum	Variables adjusted for and other comments
Kato et al. (1990a) Japan 1986–90	Former smoker	1.1 (0.6–2.1)	1.5 (0.7–3.4)		Sex, age, residence; not adjusted for alcohol. Increased risk for colon and rectal cancer with former, but not current drinking
	Current smoker	0.6 (0.3–1.1)	1.4 (0.7–3.0)		
Kato et al. (1990b) Japan 1979–87	Current smoker	*Proximal* 0.7 (0.6–0.9)	0.9 (0.8–1.1)		Age Approximately 50% of control subjects had stomach cancer.
		Distal 0.8 (0.7–1.0)			
		All 0.8 (0.7–0.9)			
Slattery et al. (1990) USA 1979–83	*Men* Any tobacco	1.7 (1.0–2.8)			No adjustments No effect of alcohol, but an effect of coffee intake
	Cigarettes/day				
	1–16	1.2 (0.6–2.4)			
	17–20	1.4 (0.8–2.6)			
	>20	2.0 (1.0–3.9)			
	p for trend	0.04			
	Women Current smoker	1.2 (0.7–2.2)			
	Cigarettes/day				
	1–16	0.8 (0.3–1.8)			
	17–20	2.0 (0.8–4.7)			
	>20	1.5 (0.5–4.8)			
	p for trend	0.24			
	Men Cigarette smoker	1.3 (0.8–2.3)			Age, body-mass index, calories, crude fibre intake

Table 2.1.7.4 (contd)

Reference Country and years of study	Smoking variables	Odds ratio (95% CI or *p* value)			Variables adjusted for and other comments
		Colon	Rectum	Colorectum	
Choi & Kahyo (1991) Republic of Korea 1986–90	Former smoker	0.6 (0.2–1.7)	1.4 (0.5–3.3)		Age, marital status, education, diet, alcohol intake
	Current smoker	0.8 (0.4–1.6)	0.7 (0.4–1.5)		
	Cigarettes/day				
	1–20	0.7 (0.3–1.3)	0.7 (0.3–1.4)		
	21–40	1.4 (0.5–4.0)	1.3 (0.5–3.1)		
	> 40	–	0.4 (0.1–3.8)		
	Duration (years)				
	1–19	1.1 (0.4–3.3)	1.2 (0.5–2.9)		
	20–39	0.7 (0.3–1.6)	0.7 (0.3–1.4)		
	≥ 40	0.6 (0.3–1.6)	1.0 (0.4–2.8)		
	Age at starting smoking (years)				
	≥ 25	1.0 (0.4–2.5)	1.6 (0.7–3.9)		
	18–24	0.8 (0.4–1.6)	0.6 (0.2–1.3)		
	<18	0.6 (0.2–1.7)	1.2 (0.4–3.5)		
	Years of cessation				
	1–4	1.1 (0.2–5.9)	2.8 (0.9–9.1)		
	5–9	–	1.3 (0.3–5.3)		
	≥ 10	1.6 (0.5–4.9)	1.6 (0.5–5.7)		
Kune *et al.* (1992) Australia 1980–81	*Men*				Age, alcohol, dietary factors. Only significant increased risk with combination of hand-rolled and ready-made cigarettes. No significant association with pack–years or cigarettes/day
	Former smoker	1.0	1.2	1.1	
	Ever-smoker	0.9	1.1	1.0	
	Current smoker	0.7	1.0	0.9	
	Women				
	Former smoker	0.7	0.6	0.7	
	Ever-smoker	0.7	0.7	0.8	
	Current smoker	0.8	0.9	0.8	

Table 2.1.7.4 (contd)

Reference Country and years of study	Smoking variables	Odds ratio (95% CI or p value)			Variables adjusted for and other comments
		Colon	Rectum	Colorectum	
Hoshiyama et al. (1993) Japan 1984–90	Current smoker	0.3 (0.1–0.8)	1.4 (0.6–3.1)		Sex and age
	Cigarettes/day				
	1–29	0.3 (0.1–0.7)	1.7 (0.9–3.4)		
	≥ 30	0.3 (0.1–1.0)	(0.3–2.6)		
	Pack–years				
	≤ 40	0.3 (0.1–0.7)	1.6 (0.8–3.0)		
	> 40	0.2 (0.0–0.7)	1.5 (0.6–3.6)		
	p for trend	< 0.01	0.31		
Olsen & Kronborg (1993) Denmark 1986, 1988, 1990	Former smoker			1.2 (0.5–3.1)	Age, sex, dietary fibre and coffee intake. Controls were younger (mean age, 63.8 versus 66.7 for colorectal cases)
	Current smoker			0.9 (0.4–2.1)	
	Duration (years)				
	1–19			2.8 (0.9–8.7)	
	20–39			0.7 (0.3–1.9)	
	≥ 40			0.7 (0.3–1.7)	
Baron et al. (1994) Sweden 1986–88	Former smoker	0.9 (0.7–1.3)	0.9 (0.6–1.3)	0.9 (0.7–1.3)	Age, gender, fat and fibre consumption, body-mass index, exercise [†]Questions on smoking starting from 1950
	Current smoker	0.9 (0.6–1.3)	0.8 (0.6–1.3)	0.9 (0.7–1.2)	
	Cigarettes/day				
	1–10	1.1 (0.7–1.7)	1.0 (0.6–1.7)	1.1 (0.7–1.6)	
	≥ 11	0.8 (0.5–1.2)	0.7 (0.4–1.2)	0.8 (0.5–1.1)	
	Duration (years)[†]				
	< 20	1.0 (0.7–1.5)	1.0 (0.6–1.6)	1.0 (0.7–1.4)	
	25–35	0.9 (0.6–1.3)	0.8 (0.5–1.4)	0.9 (0.6–1.3)	
	≥ 40	0.9 (0.6–1.3)	0.8 (0.5–1.3)	0.9 (0.6–1.2)	
	Pack–years[†]				
	< 11.05	0.8 (0.5–1.2)	0.9 (0.6–1.5)	0.9 (0.6–1.2)	
	11.05–< 22.74	1.0 (0.7–1.6)	0.9 (0.5–1.3)	1.0 (0.7–1.4)	
	≥ 22.74	0.9 (0.6–1.4)	0.8 (0.5–1.3)	0.9 (0.6–1.3)	

Table 2.1.7.4 (contd)

Reference Country and years of study	Smoking variables	Odds ratio (95% CI or p value)			Variables adjusted for and other comments
		Colon	Rectum	Colorectum	
Boutron et al. (1995) France 1985	Pack–years *Men* 1–20 > 20 *Women* 1–20 > 20			1.4 (0.7–2.8) 1.5 (0.8–2.9) 0.2 (0.03–2.0) 0.6 (0.2–1.9)	Age; not clear if alcohol was adjusted for. Smoking was a risk factor for polyps
D'Avanzo et al. (1995) (see also Ferraroni et al., 1989) Italy 1985–91	Former smoker Current smoker *Cigarettes/day* < 15 15–24 ≥ 25 *Duration (years)* < 10 10–19 20–29 ≥ 30 *Time since starting (years)* < 30 > 30 *Time since quitting (years)* < 10 > 10 *Pack–years* 1–9 10–19 20–29 30–39 ≥ 40	1.1 (0.8–1.3) 0.7 (0.5– 0.8) 0.6 (0.5–0.8) 0.7 (0.5–0.9) 0.6 (0.4–0.9) 0.9 (0.6–1.2) 0.7 (0.6–1.0) 0.9 (0.7–1.1) 0.7 (0.5–0.9) 0.7 (0.6–0.9) 0.8 (0.7–1.0) 0.9 (0.7–1.2) 1.2 (0.9–1.6) 0.9 (0.7–1.3) 0.9 (0.7–1.4) 0.7 (0.5–1.0) 0.7 (0.5–1.0) 0.8 (0.6–1.0)	0.8 (0.6–1.0) 0.7 (0.6–0.9) 0.7 (0.6–0.9) 0.7 (0.5–0.9) 0.9 (0.6–1.2) 0.7 (0.5–1.1) 0.8 (0.6–1.1) 0.7 (0.5–0.9) 0.7 (0.5–0.9) 0.7 (0.5–1.0) 0.7 (0.6–0.9) 0.9 (0.6–1.2) 0.7 (0.6–0.9) 0.9 (0.6–1.2) 0.7 (0.5–1.0) 0.5 (0.3–0.7) 0.6 (0.4–0.9) 0.8 (0.6–1.1)	0.9 (0.8–1.1) 0.7 (0.6–0.8) 0.7 (0.5–0.8) 0.7 (0.6–0.9) 0.8 (0.6–1.0) 0.8 (0.7–1.1) 0.7 (0.6–0.9) 0.8 (0.6–1.0) 0.7 (0.6–0.9) 0.7 (0.6–0.9) 0.8 (0.7–0.9) 1.1 (0.8–1.4) 0.7 (0.6–0.8) 0.9 (0.7–1.2) 0.8 (0.6–1.0) 0.6 (0.5–0.8) 0.7 (0.5–0.9) 0.8 (0.6–1.0)	Age, sex, education, area of residence, food score, fat intake, calorie intake, meat and alcohol, family history of cancer. Results similar in men and women

Table 2.1.7.4 (contd)

Reference Country and years of study	Smoking variables	Odds ratio (95% CI or *p* value)				Variables adjusted for and other comments
		Colon	Rectum	Colorectum		
Inoue *et al.* (1995) Japan 1988–92	Nonsmoker versus ever-smoker					Age. No association with alcohol consumption
	Men	*Proximal* 0.7 (0.4–1.4)	1.9 (1.1–3.2)			
	Women	0.9 (0.4–2.4)	1.7 (1.0–3.1)			
	Men	*Distal* 1.0 (0.6–1.7)				
	Women	1.1 (0.6–2.3)				
Kotake *et al.* (1995) Japan 1992–94	Current smoker	1.3 (0.3–5.2)	1.4 (0.3–6.8)			Age, sex. Potential for selection bias of control groups
	> 20 pack–years	0.8 (0.2–2.8)	2.7 (0.9–8.3)			
Newcomb *et al.* (1995) USA 1990–91	Former smoker	1.2 (1.0–1.6)	1.3 (0.9–1.8)			Age, body-mass index, consumption of beer, wine and spirits, family history of cancer, sigmoidoscopy biopsy. Trends for amount smoked, age at start or time since cessation not significant after adjusting for duration. Increased risk mainly for cancer of left colon and not right colon
	Ever-smoker	1.3 (1.0–1.6)	1.4 (1.1–1.9)			
	Current smoker	1.3 (1.0–1.8)	1.7 (1.2–2.4)			
	Cigarettes/day					
	≤ 10	1.2 (0.9–1.5)	1.3 (0.9–1.9)			
	11–20	1.4 (1.0–1.8)	1.6 (1.1–2.3)			
	21–30	1.2 (0.7–2.1)	1.3 (0.6–2.7)			
	> 30	1.7 (1.0–2.8)	1.6 (0.8–3.2)			
	p for trend	0.01	0.02			
	Duration (years)					
	1–20	1.1 (0.8–1.5)	1.1 (0.7–1.7)			
	21–30	1.1 (0.7–1.6)	1.0 (0.6–1.8)			
	31–40	1.7 (1.2–2.3)	1.5 (0.9–2.3)			
	> 40	1.4 (0.9–1.9)	2.2 (1.4–3.5)			
	p for trend	0.005	< 0.001			

Table 2.1.7.4 (contd)

Reference, Country and years of study	Smoking variables	Odds ratio (95% CI or p value)			Variables adjusted for and other comments
		Colon	Rectum	Colorectum	
Newcomb et al. (1995) (contd)	*Age at starting smoking (years)*				
	>30	1.4 (0.9–2.2)	0.6 (0.4–1.5)		
	26–30	0.8 (0.5–1.5)	1.1 (0.6–2.0)		
	21–25	1.3 (1.0–1.9)	1.9 (1.3–2.9)		
	≤20	1.4 (1.0–1.8)	1.5 (1.1–2.2)		
	p for trend	0.02	0.002		
	Years of cessation				
	>20	1.1 (0.8–1.7)	1.3 (0.8–2.2)		
	11–20	1.3 (0.9–1.9)	1.0 (0.5–1.8)		
	1–10	1.3 (0.9–1.9)	1.4 (0.9–2.3)		
	Current smoker	1.3 (1.0–1.8)	1.7 (1.2–2.4)		
	p for trend	0.02	0.004		
Siemiatycki et al. (1995) Canada 1979–85	Ever-smoker	1.0 (0.8–1.4)	1.1 (0.7–1.6)		Age, ethnic group, social class, blue collar/white collar dirtiness score, consumption of coffee, alcohol and β-carotene
	Cigarette-years				
	1–500	1.2 (0.8–1.8)	1.1 (0.7–1.8)		
	501–1000	1.1 (0.8–1.6)	1.1 (0.7–1.8)		
	1001–1500	0.9 (0.6–1.3)	0.9 (0.5–1.4)		
	≥1501	0.9 (0.6–1.5)	1.1 (0.6–1.9)		
Le Marchand et al. (1997) USA 1987–92	*Men*	Right colon (*n* = 197)	Left colon (*n* = 270)	Rectum (*n* = 221)	Age, family history of colorectal cancer, alcohol, physical activity, body-mass index, intake of eggs, dietary fibre, calcium, calories. Tertile cuts differed for men and women. Interquartile range was 0–39 pack–years in men and 0–28 in women.
	Former smoker	1.0 (0.5–1.9)	1.4 (0.9–2.4)	1.4 (0.8–2.3)	
	Current smoker	0.7 (0.3–1.6)	0.9 (0.4–1.9)	0.8 (0.4–1.8)	
	Pack-years				
	Tertile 1	1.0	1.0	1.0	
	Tertile 2	1.1 (0.6–2.2)	0.9 (0.5–1.6)	1.2 (0.7–2.1)	
	Tertile 3	0.8 (0.4–1.6)	2.0 (1.1–3.5)	1.3 (0.7–2.5)	
			p = 0.006	*p* = 0.41	
	Women	(*n* = 164)	(*n* = 194)	(*n* = 129)	
	Former smoker	2.4 (1.0–5.6)	1.1 (0.6–2.0)	1.6 (0.7–3.4)	
	Current smoker	1.1 (0.4–2.6)	0.7 (0.3–1.5)	1.4 (0.5– 3.7)	

Table 2.1.7.4 (contd)

Reference / Country and years of study	Smoking variables	Odds ratio (95% CI or p value)			Variables adjusted for and other comments
		Colon	Rectum	Colorectum	
Le Marchand et al. (1997) (contd)	*Pack–years*				
	Tertile 1	1.0	1.0	1.0	
	Tertile 2	2.1 (0.9–5.1)	0.5 (0.3–1.2)	1.5 (0.5–4.4)	
	Tertile 3	1.6 (0.7–3.6)	1.3 (0.7–2.5)	1.5 (0.7–3.0)	
		$p = 0.47$	$p = 0.41$	$p = 0.35$	
Slattery et al. (1997) USA 1991–94	**Men**				Age, body-mass index, activity, intake of energy, fibre and calcium, family history of cancer, non-steroidal anti-inflammatory drugs. Cigarettes/day and years smoked were mutually adjusted. No consistent differences between colon subsites. [Identical values of relative risk and confidence intervals for pack–years in men and women]
	Ever-smoker	1.3 (1.1–1.5)			
	Cigarettes/day				
	≤ 10	1.0 (0.8–1.4)			
	11–20	1.2 (0.9–1.7)			
	> 20	1.5 (1.1–1.8)			
	Duration (years)				
	< 15	0.8 (0.6–1.1)			
	15–34	1.1 (0.9–1.5)			
	≥ 35	0.9 (0.7–1.2)			
	Pack–years				
	≤ 20	1.1 (0.9–1.4)			
	21–35	1.3 (1.0–1.7)			
	> 35	1.4 (1.1–1.7)			
	Age at starting smoking (years)				
	≤ 16	1.3 (1.0–1.6)			
	17–20	1.4 (1.1–1.7)			
	> 20	1.1 (0.8–1.5)			
	Years of cessation				
	≥ 15	1.3 (1.0–1.6)			
	11–14	1.4 (1.0–2.1)			
	5–10	1.3 (1.0–1.8)			
	Current smoker	1.2 (0.9–1.5)			
	Women				
	Ever-smoker	1.1 (0.9–1.3)			

Table 2.1.7.4 (contd)

Reference Country and years of study	Smoking variables	Odds ratio (95% CI or *p* value)			Variables adjusted for and other comments
		Colon	Rectum	Colorectum	
Slattery *et al.* (1997) (contd)	*Cigarettes/day*				
	≤ 10	1.1 (0.7–1.5)			
	11–20	1.0 (0.7–1.6)			
	> 20	1.5 (0.9–2.4)			
	Duration (years)				
	< 15	0.9 (0.6–1.2)			
	15–34	0.9 (0.7–1.3)			
	≥ 35	0.9 (0.6–1.3)			
	Pack–years				
	≤ 20	1.1 (0.9–1.4)			
	21–35	1.3 (1.0–1.7)			
	> 35	1.4 (1.1–1.7)			
	Age at starting smoking (years)				
	≤ 16	1.2 (0.9–1.7)			
	17–20	1.1 (0.8–1.3)			
	> 20	1.1 (0.8–1.5)			
	Years of cessation				
	≥ 15	1.0 (0.7–1.2)			
	11–14	1.4 (0.8–2.3)			
	5–10	1.5 (1.0–2.1)			
	Current smoker	1.1 (0.8–1.4)			

Table 2.1.7.4 (contd)

Reference Country and years of study	Smoking variables	Odds ratio (95% CI or p value)			Variables adjusted for and other comments
		Colon	Rectum	Colorectum	
Yamada et al. (1997) Japan 1991–93	*Pack–years*		**Cancer *in situ***	**Cancer**	Gender, age, body mass index, cumulative alcohol consumption. Current alcohol intake associated with small increased risk for colorectal cancer (*p* for trend = 0.09), but not for cancer *in situ*
	1–20		1.4 (0.7–2.7)	0.8 (0.3–2.2)	
	21–40		2.8 (1.4–5.4)	1.2 (0.5–3.0)	
	> 41		2.5 (1.3–5.1)	2.6 (0.9–7.1)	
	p for trend		0.006	0.02	
	Cigarettes/day				
	Past				
	Current: 1–15		1.0 (0.5–1.9)	1.8 (0.7–4.4)	
	16–30		2.2 (1.0–4.6)	1.2 (0.4–3.8)	
	≥ 31		2.6 (1.3–5.1)	0.8 (0.3–2.1)	
			3.1 (1.3–7.5)	2.4 (0.7–8.6)	
	p for trend		0.006	0.8	
	Pack–years				
	Within past 20 years				
	1–15		1.3 (0.7–2.4)	1.1 (0.5–2.7)	
	16–30		2.2 (1.2–4.1)	1.2 (0.5–2.9)	
	≥ 31		3.7 (1.6–8.5)	2.9 (0.9–9.4)	
	p for trend		0.0003	0.1	
	Until 20 years ago				
	1–15		1.2 (0.7–2.0)	1.0 (0.4–2.4)	
	16–30		2.1 (1.0–4.0)	3.4 (1.2–9.2)	
	≥ 31		0.7 (0.3–2.0)	5.0 (1.3–18.3)	
	p for trend		0.9	0.005	
Ghadirian et al. (1998) Canada 1989–93	*Ever-smoker*				Age, sex, marital status, family history of colon cancer. Matching not clearly reported
	Any tobacco	1.0 (0.7–1.3)			
	Cigarettes	1.0 (0.7–1.3)			

Table 2.1.7.4 (contd)

Reference Country and years of study	Smoking variables	Odds ratio (95% CI or p value)			Variables adjusted for and other comments
		Colon	Rectum	Colorectum	
Tavani et al. (1998) Italy 1991–96	Former smoker	1.0 (0.9–1.2)	1.1 (0.9–1.4)		Centre, age, sex, education, body-mass index, alcohol and energy intake, consumption of vegetables and coffee, meals/day, physical activity, family history of cancer. No association in analysis by colon subsites
	Current smoker	0.8 (0.7–1.0)	0.7 (0.6–0.9)		
	Cigarettes/day				
	< 15	0.8 (0.6–1.0)	0.6 (0.5–0.9)		
	15–24	0.8 (0.6–1.0)	0.8 (0.6–1.1)		
	≥ 25	0.9 (0.6–1.3)	0.9 (0.6–1.4)		
	Duration (years)				
	< 20	1.1 (0.8–1.3)	1.1 (0.8–1.4)		
	20–29	0.9 (0.8–1.2)	0.8 (0.6–1.0)		
	30–39	0.9 (0.7–1.1)	0.9 (0.7–1.1)		
	≥ 40	0.8 (0.6–1.0)	0.9 (0.7–1.1)		
	p for trend	< 0.05	> 0.05		
	Pack–years				
	< 20	0.9 (0.8–1.1)	0.9 (0.7–1.1)		
	20–39	0.9 (0.7–1.1)	1.0 (0.8–1.2)		
	≥ 40	0.9 (0.7–1.2)	0.9 (0.7–1.2)		
	Age at starting smoking (years)				
	< 18	1.0 (0.8–1.3)	1.0 (0.8–1.3)		
	18–20	0.9 (0.7–1.1)	0.9 (0.7–1.1)		
	≥ 21	0.8 (0.6–1.0)	0.8 (0.6–1.1)		
	Years since starting				
	< 30	0.9 (0.7–1.1)	0.7 (0.5–1.0)		
	30–39	0.9 (0.7–1.1)	0.8 (0.6–1.1)		
	≥ 40	0.9 (0.8–1.1)	1.1 (0.8–1.3)		
	Years since cessation				
	< 10	1.0 (0.8–1.3)	1.1 (0.8–1.5)		
	> 10	1.0 (0.8–1.3)	1.1 (0.9–1.4)		

Table 2.1.7.4 (contd)

Reference Country and years of study	Smoking variables	Odds ratio (95% CI or p value)			Variables adjusted for and other comments
		Colon	Rectum	Colorectum	
Nusko et al. (2000) Germany 1993–96	Smoker			1.5 (1.0–2.1)	Crude Definition of smoker not given. Cases were older, higher percentage of men; no adjustment for age, sex or other relevant covariates
Chiu et al. (2001) USA 1986–89	Men				Age, total energy, farming, fibre intake, colitis, no. of first degree relatives with colorectal cancer, body-mass index at age 20 years
	Former smoker	1.5 (1.1–2.0)	1.4 (1.1–1.8)		
	Ever-smoker	1.3 (1.0–1.8)	1.3 (1.0–1.8)		
	Current smoker	1.0 (0.7–1.5)	1.3 (0.9–1.9)		
	Cigarettes/day				
	≤ 10	1.5 (1.0–2.4)	1.5 (1.0–2.2)		
	11–20	1.3 (0.9–1.8)	1.3 (1.0–1.8)		
	21–40	1.3 (0.9–1.9)	1.2 (0.9–1.8)		
	> 40	1.3 (0.7–2.3)	1.2 (0.7–2.0)		
	Duration (years)				
	≤ 20	1.5 (1.0–2.3)	1.2 (0.8–1.8)		
	21–40	1.1 (1.0–1.4)	1.1 (1.0–1.4)		
	> 40	1.1 (1.0–1.2)	1.1 (1.0–1.2)		
	Pack–years				
	≤ 20	1.5 (1.0–2.2)	1.4 (1.0–2.0)		
	21–40	1.6 (1.1–2.3)	1.5 (1.1–2.1)		
	> 40	1.1 (0.8–1.6)	1.2 (0.9–1.7)		
	Women				
	Former smoker	1.6 (1.1–2.2)	1.2 (0.8–1.8)		
	Ever-smoker	1.3 (0.9–1.7)	1.0 (0.7–1.3)		
	Current smoker	1.0 (0.7–1.4)	0.7 (0.5–1.1)		
	Cigarettes/day				
	≤ 10	1.1 (0.7–1.6)	1.0 (0.6–1.6)		
	11–20	1.3 (0.9–1.9)	1.2 (0.8–1.8)		
	21–40	1.2 (0.7–2.0)	0.5 (0.2–0.9)		
	> 40	1.5 (0.7–9.9)	1.2 (0.2–9.7)		

Table 2.1.7.4 (contd)

Reference Country and years of study	Smoking variables	Odds ratio (95% CI or *p* value)			Variables adjusted for and other comments
		Colon	Rectum	Colorectum	
Chiu *et al.* (2001) (contd)	*Duration (years)*				
	≤ 20	1.3 (0.7–2.4)	1.4 (0.8–2.6)		
	21–40	1.1 (0.9–1.4)	0.9 (0.8–1.2)		
	> 40	1.1 (0.9–1.2)	0.9 (0.8–1.1)		
	Pack–years				
	≤ 20	1.4 (0.9–2.1)	1.3 (0.8–2.0)		
	21–40	1.1 (0.7–1.8)	0.9 (0.6–1.5)		
	> 40	1.2 (0.8–1.9)	0.7 (0.4–1.1)		
Lam *et al.* (2001) Hong Kong SAR 1997–99	*Ever-smoker*				Age, education
	Men aged 35–69 years			0.8 (0.6–1.1)	
	Men aged ≥ 70 years			1.2 (0.9–1.5)	
	Women aged 35–69 years			1.0 (0.6–1.7)	
	Women aged ≥ 70 years			1.1 (0.8–1.4)	
				Men *Women*	
	Cigarettes/day			Aged ≥ 70 years	
	1–14			1.1 1.1	
	15–24			1.2 0.9	
	≥ 25			1.7 1.3	
	p for trend			< 0.05 0.63	
				Aged 35–69 years	
	1–14			0.9 1.1	
	15–24			0.7 0.5	
	≥ 25			1.2 2.5	
	p for trend			0.29 0.98	

CI, confidence interval

Table 2.1.7.5. Tobacco smoking and risk of colorectal polyps

Reference Country and years of study	Initial study population	Case patients (M, F)	Polyp-free patients (M, F)	Smoking categories	Relative risk (95% CI)	Adjustment factors, comments
Hoff et al. (1987) Norway	400 individuals randomly selected from population registry, aged 50–59 years; 324 (81%) underwent sigmoidoscopy.	90 (55 M, 35 F) adenomas and/or hyperplastic polyps 71 (50 M, 21 F) adenomas and/or hyperplastic polyps	69 (32 M, 37 F) 38 (23 M, 15 F)	*Duration (years)* Men Women *Age at start (years)* Men Women	Cases vs non-cases 31.3 ± 1.7 vs 17.3 ± 2.8; $p < 0.01$ 17.6 ± 2.8 vs 8.9 ± 2.2; $p < 0.05$ 17.9 ± 0.6 vs 19.0 ± 1.2; $p > 0.05$ 23.1 ± 1.9 vs 27.7 ± 2.3; $p > 0.05$	Crude analysis. No significant differences in risk according to amount smoked daily
Demers et al. (1988) USA 1981–85	1380 male aerospace workers screened for colorectal cancer by sigmoidoscopy	246 polyps, including 94 adenomatous polyps	1134	Ever-smoker Adenomatous polyps Any polyp	1.7 (1.3–2.3) 1.5 (1.2–1.8)	Adjusted for age
Stemmermann et al. (1988) USA 1966–83	American Men of Japanese Ancestry Study 163 deaths with detailed autopsy of the colon	79 adenomatous polyps	84	Ever-smoker Current smoker	Cases vs non-cases 32.1 vs 30.7; $p = 0.74$ 13.2 vs 12.3; $p = 0.70$	
Kikendall et al. (1989) USA 1984–87	204 patients referred for colonoscopy; 185 with complete colonoscopy, adequate biopsy and smoking history	98 adenomas or adenocarcinomas	87	*Cigarettes/day* 1–19 ≥ 20 *Pack–years* 1–19 20–39 ≥ 40 *Years since quitting* > 2 < 2	2.0 (1.3–3.2) 4.2 (1.7–10.3) 1.5 (1.1–2.0) 2.2 (1.3–3.9) 3.3 (1.4–7.8) 1.2 2.8	Adjusted for age, sex and beer consumption [number of cases and non-cases not clear; sex distribution not reported]

Table 2.1.7.5 (contd)

Reference Country and years of study	Initial study population	Case patients (M, F)	Polyp-free patients (M, F)	Smoking categories	Relative risk (95% CI)	Adjustment factors, comments
Kato *et al.* (1990b) Japan 1986–90	2052 patients undergoing colonoscopy; 1776 (87%) responded to postal questionnaire.	525 adenomas[†] 163 proximal (124 M, 39 F) 351 distal (219 M, 132 F) 118 rectum (80 M, 38 F)	578 (377 M, 201 F) selected through telephone directories; 91% responded to postal questionnaire	Former smoker Current smoker Former smoker Current smoker Former smoker Current smoker	Proximal colon 1.03 (0.6–1.9) 0.8 (0.4–1.3) Distal colon 0.9 (0.6–1.5) 0.8 (0.6–1.3) Rectum 0.95 (0.5–1.9) 1.1 (0.6–2.0)	Adjusted for age, sex and residence [†]Inconsistency between total number of adenomas and numbers at specific sites
Kono *et al.* (1990) Japan 1986–88	1348 male self-defence officials aged 49–56 years, undergoing colonoscopy for health check-up	86 adenomatous polyps of sigmoid colon	1184	*Pack-years* < 20 ≥ 20–< 40 ≥ 40	0.8 (0.4–1.6) 0.9 (0.5–1.6) 0.8 (0.4–1.7)	Adjusted for rank, alcohol and rice consumption
Cope *et al.* (1991) UK	152 patients undergoing routine colonoscopy	66 (36 M, 30 F) adenomatous polyps	86 (38 M, 48 F)	Nonsmoker/non-drinker Smoker/non-drinker Nonsmoker/drinker Smoker/drinker	1.0 2.1 (0.5–8.3) 3.0 (1.1–8.2) 12.7 (3.0–53.4)	Adjusted for age and sex; categories refer to current alcohol drinkers and/or smokers.

Table 2.1.7.5 (contd)

Reference Country and years of study	Initial study population	Case patients (M, F)	Polyp-free patients (M, F)	Smoking categories	Relative risk (95% CI)	Adjustment factors, comments
Monnet et al. (1991) France 1983–87	302 male inpatients or outpatients referred for colonoscopy; 211 (70%) responded to survey by phone or post.	103 adenomas	108	Former smoker	2.7 (1.3–5.7)	Adjusted for age; diagnosis of adenoma confirmed by biopsy
				Ever-smoker	2.2 (1.1–4.4)	
				Current smoker	1.9 (0.9–4.0)	
				Cigarettes/day		
				1–9	1.5 (0.6–3.9)	
				10–19	2.0 (1.0–4.3)	
				> 19	3.4 (1.5–7.9)	
				p for trend	< 0.02	
				Duration (years)		
				1–19	1.3 (0.5–3.6)	
				> 19	2.5 (1.3–4.9)	
				p for trend	< 0.02	
				Pack–years		
				1–19	1.4 (0.6–3.0)	
				> 19	3.0 (1.5–6.1)	
				p for trend	< 0.004	
				Years of cessation		
				> 10	2.2 (0.9–5.3)	
				< 10	3.2 (1.3–7.7)	

Table 2.1.7.5 (contd)

Reference Country and years of study	Initial study population	Case patients (M, F)	Polyp-free patients (M, F)	Smoking categories	Relative risk (95% CI)	Adjustment factors, comments
Zahm et al. (1991) USA 1981–83	1465 white male pattern makers examined by flexible sigmoidoscopy; 48% completed questionnaire; 549 with smoking history	76 polyps (adenomatous, hyperplastic or other not specified)	470	Former smoker Ever-smoker Current smoker *Cigarettes/day* ≤19 20–39 ≥40 *p* for trend *Duration (years)* ≤10 11–25 ≥26 *p* for trend *Pack-years* ≤20 21–40 ≥41 *p* for trend	1.4 (0.8–2.5) 1.7 (1.0–2.9) 2.2 (1.2–4.1) 5.5 (2.5–12.1) 1.5 (0.7–3.3) 5.7 (2.6–12.9) 0.0035 Not available 3.3 (1.3–8.3) 2.8 (1.4–5.5) 0.0006 2.4 (0.9–6.4) 4.5 (2.2–9.4) 2.1 (1.0–4.5) 0.0014	Adjusted for age and alcohol consumption; relative risks available for former smokers by number of cigarettes per day, years of smoking and pack–years, and for former and current smokers according to duration of employment
Honjo et al. (1992) Japan 1989–90	1296 male self-defence officials aged 48–54 years; 1203 received routine colonoscopy.	116 adenomatous polyps in sigmoid colon	930	Former smoker Current smoker *Cigarettes/day* <25 ≥25 *Pack-years* <20 20–<40 ≥40	2.2 (1.1–4.3) 3.3 (1.8–6.3) 2.8 (1.3–5.9) 2.3 (1.1–4.6) 2.9 (1.5–5.4) 3.2 (1.6–6.5)	Adjusted for alcohol drinking, official rank and body-mass index
Kono et al. (1990); Honjo et al. (1992) Japan	Combined data from both studies 202 polyps with information on size	Adenomas 86 small (< 5mm) 72 large (≥ 5 mm)	2114	*Pack-years* <20 20–<40 ≥40	Small Large 1.5 (0.7–3.3) 1.7 (0.8–3.8) 2.1 (1.1–4.1) 1.7 (0.8–3.4) 2.5 (1.2–5.3) 1.4 (0.6–3.3)	Adjusted for alcohol intake, official rank and body-mass index

Table 2.1.7.5 (contd)

Reference Country and years of study	Initial study population	Case patients (M, F)	Polyp-free patients (M, F)	Smoking categories	Relative risk (95% CI)	Adjustment factors, comments
Lee et al. (1993) USA 1986–88	2879 patients referred for colonoscopy beyond splenic flexure, aged 35–84 years; 1892 (81%) interviewed	303 polyps 271 (153 M, 118 F) with smoking data	509 457 (202 M, 255 F) with smoking data	*Pack–years* ≤ 10 > 10–≤ 40 > 40 *p* for trend *Pack–years* ≤ 7.5 > 7.5–≤ 30 > 30 *p* for trend	Men 1.0 (0.5–1.9) 1.8 (0.3–3.3) 2.2 (1.2–3.8) 0.002 Women 0.9 (0.5–1.8) 1.2 (0.6–2.1) 1.4 (0.8–2.5) > 0.05	Adjusted for age. Significant trend by intensity of smoking for right side colon, severe atypia, multiplicity and polyps ≥ 10 mm
Olsen & Kronborg (1993) Denmark 1986	20 672 individuals randomly selected for Haemoccult II screening test; 397 (85%) with positive test had complete colonoscopy.	171 polyps (57 M, 114 F)	362 (157 M, 205 F)	Former smoker Current smoker *Duration (years)* 1–19 20–39 ≥ 40	2.1 (1.1–3.9) 2.0 (1.1–3.5) 2.1 (0.8–5.6) 2.0 (1.1–3.6) 2.7 (1.6–4.7)	Adjusted for age, sex and consumption of dietary fibre, coffee, tea and alcohol. Controls were participants with negative screening test result.
Sandler et al. (1993) USA 1988–91	2094 patients undergoing colonoscopy, aged ≥ 30 years; 645 eligible with reliable interviews	236 (105 M, 131 F) adenomatous polyps, including 39 adenomatous and hyperplastic polyps	409 (165 M, 244 F), including 46 with hyper-plastic polyps	Ever-smoker Ever-smoker[†] *Cigarettes/day* 1–10 11–20 ≥ 21 *Pack–years* 1–20 21–40 ≥ 41	1.1 (0.8–1.6) 1.2 (0.9–1.7) 1.3 (0.8–2.1) 1.00 (0.6–1.6) 0.96 (0.6–1.7) 1.2 (0.8–1.9) 0.9 (0.5–1.4) 1.4 (0.8–2.4)	Adjusted for age and sex. [†]Excluding controls with hyperplastic polyps. Similar results in men and women. Little change in results after adjusting for alcohol consumption. No difference between cases and controls for age at start, mean number of cigarettes per day, mean years of smoking and mean pack–years by sex. No difference between ever-smoker, former smoker and current smoker

Table 2.1.7.5 (contd)

Reference Country and years of study	Initial study population	Case patients (M, F)	Polyp-free patients (M, F)	Smoking categories	Relative risk (95% CI)	Adjustment factors, comments
Giovannucci et al. (1994a) USA 1980–90 (see also Kearney et al., 1995)	Nurses' Health Study 12 143 women undergoing endoscopy (primarily sigmoido-scopy)	564 prevalent and incident adenomatous polyps of distal colon and rectum		Current smoker *Pack–years* 1–9 10–19 20–29 30–39 ≥ 40 p for trend	2.1 (1.7–2.6) 1.2 (0.9–1.7) 1.5 (1.1–2.0) 1.3 (0.9–1.8) 2.2 (1.6–3.1) 2.4 (1.8–3.1) < 0.0001	Adjusted for age, intake of dietary fat, fibre, folate and alcohol, body-mass index and family history of colorectal cancer. Diagnosis confirmed with histopathological reports. Significant trend for large (≥ 1 cm) adenomas with total pack–years ($p < 0.0001$), pack–years smoked before age 30 years ($p = 0.05$) and pack–years smoked after age 30 years ($p < 0.0001$) Significant trend for small (< 1 cm) adenomas with total pack–years ($p < 0.0001$) and pack–years smoked after age 30 years ($p < 0.0001$)
Giovannucci et al. (1994b) USA 1986–92 (see also Kearney et al., 1995)	Health Professionals Follow-up Study 12 854 men undergoing endoscopy (primarily sigmoidoscopy)	499 prevalent adenomatous polyps of distal colon and rectum		Current smoker *Pack–years* 1–9 10–19 20–29 30–39 ≥ 40 p for trend *Pack–years ≥ 20 years* *ago* 1–4 5–9 10–15 ≥ 16 p for trend	1.6 (1.2–2.1) 1.5 (1.1–2.0) 1.3 (0.9–1.7) 1.4 (0.99–1.9) 1.9 (1.4–2.7) 1.7 (1.3–2.2) < 0.0001 Large Small 1.9 (0.9–3.8) 1.7 (1.03–2.9) 1.3 (0.8–2.4) 1.2 (0.8–1.9) 1.4 (0.7–2.7) 0.8 (0.5–1.5) 2.4 (1.6–3.6) 0.96 (0.7–1.4) 0.004 0.95	Adjusted for age, family history of colorectal cancer, body-mass index and intake of fat, fibre, folate and alcohol. Diagnosis confirmed by histopathological reports Significant trend for small ($p = 0.05$) and large ($p = 0.0002$) polyps by total pack–years

Table 2.1.7.5 (contd)

Reference Country and years of study	Initial study population	Case patients (M, F)	Polyp-free patients (M, F)	Smoking categories	Relative risk (95% CI)		Adjustment factors, comments
					Large	Small	
Giovannucci et al. (1994b) (contd)				*Pack-years < 20 years ago*			
				1–9	0.9 (0.5–1.6)	1.2 (0.8–1.9)	
				10–19	0.9 (0.5–1.6)	1.2 (0.7–2.0)	
				20–34	1.3 (0.8–2.2)	1.3 (0.8–2.2)	
				≥ 35	0.5 (0.1–1.9)	3.0 (1.5–6.0)	
				p for trend	0.56	0.04	
				Pack-years before 30 years			
				1–4	1.9 (0.9–3.9)	1.4 (0.8–2.5)	
				5–10	1.6 (0.9–2.9)	1.2 (0.8–2.0)	
				11–15	1.8 (1.1–3.1)	1.0 (0.7–1.6)	
				≥ 16	2.3 (1.2–4.2)	0.97 (0.6–1.7)	
				p for trend	0.02	0.56	
				Pack-years after 30 years			
				1–9	0.8 (0.4–1.6)	0.99 (0.6–1.7)	
				10–19	1.1 (0.6–1.9)	0.9 (0.6–1.5)	
				20–34	1.2 (0.7–2.1)	1.1 (0.7–1.9)	
				≥ 35	1.1 (0.6–2.1)	1.6 (0.96–2.7)	
				p for trend	0.23	0.03	
Jacobson et al. (1994) USA 1986–88	3008 patients with self-reported history of polypectomy, undergoing colonoscopy for adenoma recurrence, aged 35–84 years	186 (130 M, 56 F) recurrent adenomas	330 (187 M, 143 F)		Men		Adjusted for age, time since previous polypectomy, body-mass index, alcohol intake and percentage of fat/calories consumed
				Pack-years			
				1–12	1.3 (0.7–2.6)		
				13–40	2.4 (1.3–4.4)		
				> 40	1.9 (1.0–3.7)		
				p for trend	0.03		
					Women		
				Pack-years			
				1–7	0.5 (0.1–1.7)		
				8–30	1.7 (0.6–4.5)		
				> 30	2.8 (1.2–6.5)		
				p for trend	0.005		

Table 2.1.7.5 (contd)

Reference Country and years of study	Initial study population	Case patients (M, F)	Polyp-free patients (M, F)	Smoking categories	Relative risk (95% CI)	Adjustment factors, comments
Boutron et al. (1995) France	1232 patients undergoing colonoscopy, aged 30–79 years	208 (129 M, 79 F) large adenomas (≥ 10 mm) 154 (85 M, 69 F) small adenomas (< 10 mm)	427 (182 M, 245 F)	**Small adenomas** *Pack–years* 1–20 > 20 *p* for trend *Pack–years* 1–5 > 5 *p* for trend **Large adenomas** *Pack–years* 1–20 > 20 *p* for trend	Men 1.9 (0.9–4.1) 3.6 (1.8–7.3) < 0.0001 Women 1.3 (0.5–3.1) 1.4 (0.6–3.2) > 0.1 Men 2.3 (1.2–4.5) 2.1 (1.1–4.2) < 0.01	Small adenomas: adjusted for age; large adenomas: adjusted for age and alcohol intake; data available for men only
Honjo et al. (1995) Japan 1986–92	4981 male self-defence officials undergoing sigmoidoscopy or colonoscopy, aged 48–56 years	429 sigmoid adenomas, 75 rectal adenomas	3101	*Pack–years* ≤ 22.5 > 22.5–≤ 33 > 33 *p* for trend *Pack–years* ≤ 22.5 > 22.5–≤ 33 > 33 *p* for trend	Sigmoid adenoma 1.7 (1.2–2.3) 2.3 (1.7–3.2) 2.3 (1.6–3.2) < 0.01 Rectal adenoma 0.6 (0.3–1.2) 1.7 (0.9–3.2) 1.0 (0.5–2.0) 0.28	Adjusted for body-mass index, official rank, hospital, study period and alcohol consumption. Seventeen patients had both sigmoid and rectal adenomas and were included in both groups.

Table 2.1.7.5 (contd)

Reference Country and years of study	Initial study population	Case patients (M, F)	Polyp-free patients (M, F)	Smoking categories	Relative risk (95% CI)	Adjustment factors, comments
Kearney et al. (1995) USA 1986–92 (see also Giovannucci et al., 1994a,b) 1980–90	Health Professionals Follow-up Study 12 922 men undergoing endoscopy Nurses' Health Study 15 984 women undergoing endoscopy	219 hyperplastic polyps of the distal colon and rectum 175 hyperplastic polyps of the distal colon and rectum		Former smoker Current smoker *Cigarettes/day* 1–14 ≥ 15 Former smoker Current smoker *Cigarettes/day* 1–14 ≥ 15 *p* for trend	Men 1.1 (0.9–1.5) 2.5 (1.6–3.8) 2.3 (1.2–4.4) 2.1 (1.3–3.6) Women 1.3 (0.9–2.0) 2.0 (1.2–2.9) 2.2 (1.3–3.7) 2.4 (1.6–3.7) < 0.0001	Adjusted for age, energy intake, family history of colorectal cancer, previous endoscopy; [discrepancies in relative risks between text and table]
Martinez et al. (1995) USA 1991–93	4698 patients undergoing colonoscopy or sigmoidoscopy, identified by medical records; 200 eligible cases, 673 eligible controls (aged > 35 years)	157 (98 M, 59 F) adenomatous polyps	480 (229 M, 251 F)	Former smoker Current smoker *Pack–years* 1–10 11–20 > 20 *p* for trend	1.6 (1.03–2.5) 2.3 (1.3–4.1) 1.7 (0.5–5.7) 2.1 (0.6–6.5) 2.6 (1.3–5.1) = 0.008	Adjusted for age, sex, race, intake of dietary fibre, vitamin C and alcohol, body-mass index, family history of colorectal cancer, physical activity and non-steroidal anti-inflammatory drugs. Relative risks available for interaction with alcohol
Nelson et al. (1995) USA 1984–87 (see also Kikendall et al., 1989)	Patients undergoing colonoscopy, aged 26–87 years [number not specified]	137 (109 M, 28 F) adenomas	136 (86 M, 50 F)	Smoker	2.0 (1.1–3.8)	Adjusted for age, sex, family history of cancer, race, alcohol consumption, serum ferritin, β-carotene, α-tocopheral and selenium. Controls included patients with hyperplastic polyps.

Table 2.1.7.5 (contd)

Reference Country and years of study	Initial study population	Case patients (M, F)	Polyp-free patients (M, F)	Smoking categories	Relative risk (95% CI)	Adjustment factors, comments
Longnecker et al. (1996) USA 1991–93	1317 patients undergoing sigmoidoscopy, aged 50–74 years; 488 matched pairs with complete smoking and diet data	488 (325 M, 163 F) (response rate, 84%)	488 matched by age, sex, date of sigmoidoscopy and medical centre (response rate, 82%)	Former smoker Current smoker *Ever-smoker (pack-years)* Total 1–9 10–29 ≥30 *p* for trend ≤ 20 years ago 1–9 10–30 > 30 *p* for trend > 20 years ago 1–9 10–30 > 30 *p* for trend	1.2 (0.9–1.7) 2.4 (1.6–3.8) 1.2 (0.8–1.8) 1.3 (0.9–1.9) 1.8 (1.2–2.5) 0.002 1.5 (1.00–2.3) 2.3 (1.4–3.7) 2.4 (1.02–5.6) 0.0007 1.2 (0.7–1.8) 0.7 (0.5–1.2) 1.1 (0.6–1.9) 0.65	Adjusted for race, alcohol intake, body-mass index, vigorous leisure-time activity, intake of energy, saturated fat and fruits and vegetables. Results by period of tobacco consumption similar for small (< 1 cm) and large (≥ 1 cm) polyps 55% of cases and 54% of controls were whites.
Manus et al. (1997) Germany 1990–91	1166 patients in clinical rehabilitation centre, aged 50–60 years; 665 (57%) underwent sigmoidoscopy.	146 (97 M, 49 F) adenomatous polyps	519 (308 M, 211 F)	Ever-smoker	Cases vs non-cases 33.6% vs 24.1% (*p* = 0.03)	Large number of subjects with diabetes or hypertension
Martinez et al. (1997) USA 1991–93 (see also Martinez et al., 1995)	4698 patients undergoing colonoscopy or sigmoidoscopy, identified by medical records; 113 eligible cases, 719 eligible controls (aged > 35 years)	81 (44 M, 37 F) hyperplastic polyps	480 (229 M, 251 F)	Former smoker Current smoker *Pack-years* ≤ 10 11–20 > 20	1.3 (0.8–2.3) 2.5 (1.2–5.0) 1.2 (0.6–2.3) 1.7 (0.8–3.7) 2.0 (1.02–3.8)	Adjusted for age, sex, race, intake of dietary fibre, energy and alcohol, body-mass index, physical activity and non-steroidal anti-inflammatory drugs

Table 2.1.7.5 (contd)

Reference Country and years of study	Initial study population	Case patients (M, F)	Polyp-free patients (M, F)	Smoking categories	Relative risk (95% CI)	Adjustment factors, comments
Baron et al. (1998) USA 4 years	864 participants in an ongoing clinical trial with prior history of colorectal polypectomy; 751 subjects had colonoscopy 1 and 4 years after the excision	260 (212 M, 48 F) recurrent adenomas	449 (344 M, 105 F)	Former smoker Current smoker *Cigarettes/day* ≤ 20 21–40 > 40 *Duration (years)* ≤ 20 > 20–≤ 30 > 30–≤ 40 > 40	1.1 (0.8–1.6) 0.95 (0.6–1.5) 1.2 (0.8–1.8) 0.8 (0.5–1.2) 1.6 (0.9–2.7) 1.5 (0.9–2.5) 0.7 (0.4–1.2) 1.1 (0.7–1.7) 0.97 (0.6–1.6)	Adjusted for age, sex, clinical centre, intake of fat, total dietary fibre, energy intake and colonoscopy interval. Similar results for polyp recurrence in right and left colon
Kahn et al. (1998) USA 1982–92	Cancer Prevention Study II 72 868 men and 81 356 women without polyps at baseline, aged 40–64 years	12 615 (7504 M, 5111 F) polyps		Former smoker Current smoker *(cigarettes/day)* 1–20 ≥ 21 Former smoker Current smoker *(cigarettes/day)* 1–20 ≥ 21	Men 1.25 (1.17–1.34) 1.30 (1.18–1.43) 1.34 (1.21–1.47) Women 1.21 (1.13–1.30) 1.37 (1.25–1.50) 1.50 (1.32–1.70)	Adjusted for age, education, race, gallbladder status, body-mass index, exercise, alcohol and coffee consumption, aspirin use, multivitamin use, family history of colorectal cancer, diet change, diet (intake of eggs, vegetables, meat, fibre, chicken, fish), and for women, parity, estrogen replacement therapy and menopausal status
Terry & Neugut (1998) USA 1986–88	3008 subjects undergoing complete colonoscopy beyond splenic flexure, aged 35–84 years; 2443 (81%) eligible; 2001 interviewed	269 (155 M, 114 F) polyps	508 (225 M, 283 F)	Ever-smoker *Pack–years* 1–19 20–39 ≥ 40	1.3 (0.97–1.8) 1.2 (0.8–1.8) 1.2 (0.7–1.9) 1.6 (1.1–2.4)	Adjusted for gender, age and Quetelet index. Study investigated the hypothesis that control groups in many studies on tobacco smoking and colorectal cancer included a high proportion of individuals with adenomatous polyps.

Table 2.1.7.5 (contd)

Reference Country and years of study	Initial study population	Case patients (M, F)	Polyp-free patients (M, F)	Smoking categories	Relative risk (95% CI)	Adjustment factors, comments
Nagata et al. (1999) Japan 1993–95	14 427 M, 17 125 F residents of Takayama, aged ≥ 35 years; 593 under-went colonoscopy	259 (181 M, 78 F) histologically proven adenomas		Former smoker	Men 1.2 (0.8–2.0)	Adjusted for age
				Current smoker	1.4 (0.9–2.3)	
				Cigarettes/day		
				1–19	1.4 (0.9–2.2)	
				≥ 20	1.3 (0.8–2.2)	
				Duration (years)		
				1–29	1.1 (0.7–1.8)	
				≥ 30	1.6 (1.02–2.6)	
					p = 0.02	
				Pack–years		
				1–19	1.1 (0.7–1.9)	
				≥ 20	1.5 (0.97–2.5)	
				p for trend	0.04	
				Ever-smoker	Women 2.2 (1.2–3.7)	
				Cigarettes/day		
				1–4	2.4 (1.2–4.5)	
				≥ 5	2.1 (0.9–4.5)	
				Duration (years)		
				1–29	1.5 (0.7–2.9)	
				≥ 30	4.5 (2.0–9.1)	
				p for trend	0.0002	
				Pack–years		
				1–14	2.1 (1.00–3.8)	
				≥ 15	2.9 (1.2–6.0)	
				p for trend	0.002	

Table 2.1.7.5 (contd)

Reference Country and years of study	Initial study population	Case patients (M, F)	Polyp-free patients (M, F)	Smoking categories	Relative risk (95% CI)	Adjustment factors, comments
Almendingen *et al.* (2000) Norway 3 years	116 subjects with polyps at baseline participating in a 3-year follow-up intervention study, aged 50–76 years	87 histologically confirmed adenomas	35 hospital outpatients with abdominal pain; 35 healthy controls; both groups matched by age and sex		*Healthy controls*	Adjusted for body-mass index, familial colonic cancer, energy, fat, fibre, dietary vitamin C, cruciferous vegetables, coffee and alcohol
				Former smoker	1.4 (0.4–4.4)	
				Current smoker	3.8 (0.9–14.4)	
				Duration (years)		
				0.1–15	1.7 (0.4–7.3)	
				16–25	1.4 (0.3–6.6)	
				≥ 26	2.7 (0.8–9.0)	
				p for trend	0.1	
				Pack–years[†]		[†]Referent category included former smokers.
				0.1–15	1.1 (0.2–5.9)	
				> 15	5.5 (1.3–24.3)	
				p for trend	0.03	
					Hospital controls	
				Former smoker	1.4 (0.5–3.9)	
				Current smoker	3.6 (1.1–12.6)	
				Duration (years)		
				0.1–15	0.9 (0.3–3.4)	
				16–25	2.1 (0.5–9.4)	
				≥ 26	2.8 (0.9–8.4)	
				p for trend	0.05	
				Pack–years[†]		
				0.1–15	1.6 (0.3–9.0)	
				> 15	4.1 (1.1–15.9)	
				p for trend	0.04	

Table 2.1.7.5 (contd)

Reference Country and years of study	Initial study population	Case patients (M, F)	Polyp-free patients (M, F)	Smoking categories	Relative risk (95% CI)	Adjustment factors, comments
Breuer-Katschinski *et al.* (2000) Germany 1993–95	Patients undergoing colonoscopy at 5 major hospitals in Essen	182 (94 M, 88 F) polyps; response rate, 69%	178 (88 M, 90 F) hospital controls; response rate, 50% 182 (92 M, 90 F) population controls; response rate, 66%	Former smoker Current smoker *Cigarettes/day* 1–10 11–20 > 20 Former smoker Current smoker Ever-smoker *Cigarettes/day* 1–10 11–20 > 20	*Population controls* 0.9 (0.5–1.4) 0.97 (0.5–1.8) 0.8 (0.4–1.4) 1.2 (0.6–2.1) 0.7 (0.4–1.4) *Hospital controls* 1.0 (0.6–1.7) 2.3 (1.1–4.6) 1.3 (0.9–2.1) 1.2 (0.7–2.3) 1.5 (0.8–2.8) 1.1 (0.6–2.2)	Adjusted for age, sex, social class, intake of fat, fibre and energy, relative weight, consumption of red meat, vitamin A, carotene and folate Data available for men and women separately, and for large and small polyps separately with each control group

M, men; F, women; CI, confidence interval

References

Akiba, S. (1994) Analysis of cancer risk related to longitudinal information on smoking habits. *Environ. Health Perspect.*, **102** (Suppl. 8), 15–20

Akiba, S. & Hirayama, T. (1990) Cigarette smoking and cancer mortality risk in Japanese men and women — Results from reanalysis of the six-prefecture cohort study data. *Environ. Health Perspect.*, **87**, 19–26

Almendingen, K., Hofstad, B., Trygg, K., Hoff, G., Hussain, A. & Vatn, M.H. (2000) Smoking and colorectal adenomas: A case–control study. *Eur. J. Cancer Prev.*, **9**, 193–203

Baron, J.A., Gerhardsson de Verdier, M. & Ekbom, A. (1994) Coffee, tea, tobacco, and cancer of the large bowel. *Cancer Epidemiol. Biomarkers Prev.*, **3**, 565–570

Baron, J.A., Sandler, R.S., Haile, R.W., Mandel, J.S., Mott, L.A. & Greenberg, E.R. (1998) Folate intake, alcohol consumption, cigarette smoking, and risk of colorectal adenomas. *J. natl Cancer Inst.*, **90**, 57–62

Bostick, R.M., Potter, J.D., Kushi, L.H., Sellers, T.A., Steinmetz, K.A., McKenzie, D.R., Gapstur, S.M. & Folsom, A.R. (1994) Sugar, meat, and fat intake, and non-dietary risk factors for colon cancer incidence in Iowa women (United States). *Cancer Causes Control*, **5**, 38–52

Boutron, M.C., Faivre, J., Dop, M.C., Quipourt, V. & Senesse, P. (1995) Tobacco, alcohol, and colorectal tumors: A multistep process. *Am. J. Epidemiol.*, **141**, 1038–1046

Boutron-Ruault, M.C. (1999) Re: 'Cigarette smoking and the colorectal adenoma–carcinoma sequence: A hypothesis to explain the paradox'. *Am. J. Epidemiol.*, **149**, 787–788

Boutron-Ruault, M.C. & Rabkin, C.S. (2000) Re: 'Controls who experienced hypothetical causal intermediates should not be excluded from case–control studies'. *Am. J. Epidemiol.*, **151**, 436

Breuer-Katschinski, B., Nemes, K., Marr, A., Rump, B., Leiendecker, B., Breuer, N. & Goebell, H. (2000) Alcohol and cigarette smoking and the risk of colorectal adenomas. *Dig. Dis. Sci.*, **45**, 487–493

Carstensen, J.M., Pershagen, G. & Eklund, G. (1987) Mortality in relation to cigarette and pipe smoking: 16 years' observation of 25,000 Swedish men. *J. Epidemiol. Community Health*, **41**, 166–172

Chao, A., Thun, M.J,. Jacobs, E.J., Henley, S.J., Rodriguez, C. & Calle, E.E. (2000) Cigarette smoking and colorectal cancer mortality in the cancer prevention study II. *J. natl Cancer Inst.*, **92**, 1888–1896

Chen, Z.M., Xu, Z., Collins, R., Li, W.X. & Peto, R. (1997) Early health effects of the emerging tobacco epidemic in China. A 16-year prospective study. *J. Am. med. Assoc.*, **278**, 1500–1504

Chiu, B.C., Lynch, C.F., Cerhan, J.R. & Cantor, K.P. (2001) Cigarette smoking and risk of bladder, pancreas, kidney, and colorectal cancers in Iowa. *Ann. Epidemiol.*, **11**, 28–37

Choi, S.Y. & Kahyo, H. (1991) Effect of cigarette smoking and alcohol consumption in the etiology of cancers of the digestive tract. *Int. J. Cancer*, **49**, 381–386

Chute, C.G., Willett, W.C., Colditz, G.A., Stampfer, M.J., Baron, J.A., Rosner, B. & Speizer, F.E. (1991) A prospective study of body mass, height, and smoking on the risk of colorectal cancer in women. *Cancer Causes Control*, **2**, 117–124

Chyou, P.H., Nomura, A.M. & Stemmermann, G.N. (1996) A prospective study of colon and rectal cancer among Hawaii Japanese men. *Ann. Epidemiol.*, **6**, 276–282

Cope, G.F., Wyatt, J.I., Pinder, I.F., Lee, P.N., Heatley, R.V. & Kelleher, J. (1991) Alcohol consumption in patients with colorectal adenomatous polyps. *Gut*, **32**, 70–72

Dales, L.G., Friedman, G.D., Ury, H.K., Grossman, S. & Williams, S.R. (1979) A case–control study of relationships of diet and other traits to colorectal cancer in American blacks. *Am. J. Epidemiol.*, **109**, 132–144

D'Avanzo, B., La Vecchia, C., Franceschi, S., Gallotti, L. & Talamini, R. (1995) Cigarette smoking and colorectal cancer: A study of 1,584 cases and 2,879 controls. *Prev. Med.*, **24**, 571–579

Demers, R.Y., Neale, A.V., Demers, P., Deighton, K., Scott, R.O., Dupuis, M.H. & Herman, S. (1988) Serum cholesterol and colorectal polyps. *J. clin. Epidemiol.*, **41**, 9–13

Doll, R. & Peto, R. (1976) Mortality in relation to smoking: 20 years' observations on male British doctors. *Br. med. J.*, **ii**, 1525–1536

Doll, R., Gray, R., Hafner, B. & Peto, R. (1980) Mortality in relation to smoking: 22 years' observation on female British doctors. *Br. med. J.*, **280**, 967–971

Doll, R., Peto, R., Wheatley, K., Gray, R. & Sutherland, I. (1994) Mortality in relation to smoking: 40 years' observations on male British doctors. *Br. med. J.*, **309**, 901–911

Engeland, A., Andersen, A., Haldorsen, T. & Tretli, S. (1996) Smoking habits and risk of cancers other than lung cancer: 28 years' follow-up of 26,000 Norwegian men and women. *Cancer Causes Control*, **7**, 497–506

Ferraroni, M., Negri, E., La Vecchia, C., D'Avanzo, B. & Franceschi, S. (1989) Socio-economic indicators, tobacco and alcohol in the aetiology of digestive trace neoplasm. *Int. J. Epidemiol.*, **18**, 556–562

Garland, C., Barrett-Connor, E., Rossof, A.H., Shekelle, R.B., Criqui, M.H. & Oglesby, P. (1985) Dietary vitamin D and calcium and risk of colorectal cancer: A 19-year prospective study in men. *Lancet*, **i**, 307–309

Ghadirian, P., Maisonneuve, P., Perret, C., Lacroix, A. & Boyle, P. (1998) Epidemiology of socio-demographic characteristics, lifestyle, medical history, and colon cancer: A case–control study among French Canadians in Montreal. *Cancer Detect. Prev.*, **22**, 396–404

Giovannucci, E., Colditz, G.A., Stampfer, M.J., Hunter, D., Rosner, B.A., Willett, W.C. & Speizer, F.E. (1994a) A prospective study of cigarette smoking and risk of colorectal adenoma and colorectal cancer in US women. *J. natl Cancer Inst.*, **86**, 192–199

Giovannucci, E., Rimm, E.B., Stampfer, M.J., Colditz, G.A., Ascherio, A., Kearney, J. & Willett, W.C. (1994b) A prospective study of cigarette smoking and risk of colorectal adenoma and colorectal cancer in US men. *J. natl Cancer Inst.*, **86**, 183–191

Hammond, E.C. (1966) Smoking in relation to the death rates of one million men and women. *Natl Cancer Inst. Monogr.*, **19**, 127–204

Hammond, E.C. & Horn, D. (1958a) Smoking and death rates — Report on forty-four months of follow-up of 187,783 men. I. Total mortality. *J. Am. med. Assoc.*, **166**, 1159–1172

Hammond, E.C. & Horn, D. (1958b) Smoking and death rates — Report on forty-four months of follow-up of 187,783 men. II. Death rates by causes. *J. Am. med. Assoc.*, **166**, 1294–1308

Heineman, E.F., Zahm, S.H., McLaughlin, J.K. & Vaught, J.B. (1994) Increased risk of colorectal cancer among smokers: Results of a 26-year follow-up of US veterans and a review. *Int. J. Cancer*, **59**, 728–738

Hirayama, T. (1989) Association between alcohol consumption and cancer of the sigmoid colon: Observations from a Japanese cohort study. *Lancet*, **2**, 725–727

Hoff, G., Vatn, M.H. & Larsen, S. (1987) Relationship between tobacco smoking and colorectal polyps. *Scand. J. Gastroenterol.*, **22**, 13–16

Honjo, S., Kono, S., Shinchi, K., Imanishi, K. & Hirohata, T. (1992) Cigarette smoking, alcohol use and adenomatous polyps of the sigmoid colon. *Jpn J. Cancer Res.*, **83**, 806–811

Honjo, S., Kono, S., Shinchi, K., Wakabayashi, K., Todoroki, I., Sakurai, Y., Imanishi, K., Nishikawa, H., Ogawa, S. & Katsurada, M. (1995) The relation of smoking, alcohol use and obesity to risk of sigmoid colon and rectal adenomas. *Jpn. J. Cancer Res.*, **86**, 1019–1026

Hoshiyama, Y., Sekine, T. & Sasaba, T. (1993) A case–control study of colorectal cancer and its relation to diet, cigarettes, and alcohol consumption in Saitama Prefecture, Japan. *Tohoku J. exp. Med.*, **171**, 153–165

Hsing, A.W., McLaughlin, J.K., Chow, W.H., Schuman, L.M., Co Chien, H.T., Gridley, G., Bjelke, E., Wacholder, S. & Blot, W.J. (1998) Risk factors for colorectal cancer in a prospective study among US white men. *Int. J. Cancer*, **77**, 549–553

IARC (2002) *IARC Handbooks of Cancer Prevention*, Vol. 6, *Weight Control and Physical Activity*, Lyon, *IARC*Press

Inoue, M., Tajima, K., Hirose, K., Hamajima, N., Takezaki, T., Hirai, T., Kato, T. & Ohno, Y. (1995) Subsite-specific risk factors for colorectal cancer: A hospital-based case–control study in Japan. *Cancer Causes Control*, **6**, 14–22

Jacobson, J.S., Neugut, A.I., Murray, T., Garbowski, G.C., Forde, K.A., Treat, M.R., Waye, J.D., Santos, J. & Ahsan, H. (1994) Cigarette smoking and other behavioral risk factors for recurrence of colorectal adenomatous polyps (New York City, NY, USA). *Cancer Causes Control*, **5**, 215–220

Jarebinski, M., Klajinac, H. & Adanja, B. (1988) Biosocial and other characteristics of the large bowel cancer patients in Belgrade (Yugoslavia). *Arch. Geschwulstforsch.*, **58**, 411–417

Jarebinski, M., Adanja, B. & Vlajinac, H. (1989) Case–control study of relationship of some bio-social correlates to rectal cancer patients in Belgrade, Yugoslavia. *Neoplasma*, **36**, 369–374

Kahn, H.A. (1966) The Dorn study of smoking and mortality among US veterans: Report of eight and one-half years of observation. *Natl Cancer Inst. Monogr.*, **19**, 1–126

Kahn, H.S., Tatham, L.M., Thun, M.J. & Health, C.W., Jr (1998) Risk factors for self-reported colon polyps. *J. gen. intern. Med.*, **13**, 303–310

Kato, I., Tominaga, S. & Ikari, A. (1990a) A case–control study of male colorectal cancer in Aichi Prefecture, Japan: With special reference to occupational activity level, drinking habits and family history. *Jpn. J. Cancer Res.*, **81**, 115–121

Kato, I., Tominaga, S., Matsuura, A., Yoshii, Y., Shirai, M. & Kobayashi, S. (1990b) A comparative case–control study of colorectal cancer and adenoma. *Jpn. J. Cancer Res.*, **81**, 1101–1108

Kato, I., Akhmedkhanov, A., Koenig, K., Toniolo, P.G., Shore, R.E. & Riboli, E. (1997) Prospective study of diet and female colorectal cancer: The New York University Women's Health Study. *Nutr. Cancer*, **28**, 276–281

Kearney, J., Giovannucci, E., Rimm, E.B., Stampfer, M.J., Colditz, G.A., Ascherio, A., Bleday, R. & Willett, W.C. (1995) Diet, alcohol, and smoking and the occurrence of hyperplastic polyps of the colon and rectum (United States). *Cancer Causes Control*, **6**, 45–56

Kikendall, J.W., Bowen, P.E., Burgess, M.B., Magnetti, C., Woodward, J. & Langenberg, P. (1989) Cigarettes and alcohol as independent risk factors for colonic adenomas. *Gastroenterology*, **97**, 660–664

Klatsky, A.L., Armstrong, M.A., Friedman, G.D. & Hiatt, R.A. (1988) The relations of alcoholic beverage use to colon and rectal cancer. *Am. J. Epidemiol.*, **128**, 1007–1015

Knekt, P., Hakama, M., Jarvinen, R., Pukkala, E. & Heliovaara, M. (1998) Smoking and risk of colorectal cancer. *Br. J. Cancer*, **78**, 136–139

Kono, S., Ikeda, M., Tokudome, S., Nishizumi, M. & Kuratsune, M. (1987) Cigarette smoking, alcohol and cancer mortality: A cohort study of male Japanese physicians. *Jpn. J. Cancer Res.*, **78**, 1323–1328

Kono, S., Ikeda, N., Yanai, F., Shinchi, K. & Imanishi, K. (1990) Alcoholic beverages and adenomatous polyps of the sigmoid colon: A study of male self-defence officials in Japan. *Int. J. Epidemiol.*, **19**, 848–852

Kotake, K., Koyama, Y., Nasu, J., Fukutomi, T. & Yamaguchi, N. (1995) Relation of family history of cancer and environmental factors to the risk of colorectal cancer: A case–control study. *Jpn. J. clin. Oncol.*, **25**, 195–202

Kune, G.A., Kune, S., Vitetta, L. & Watson, L.F. (1992) Smoking and colorectal cancer risk: Data from the Melbourne Colorectal Cancer Study and brief review of literature. *Int. J. Cancer*, **50**, 369–372

Lam, T.H., Ho, S.Y. & Hedley, A.J. (2001) Mortality and moking in Hong Kong: Case–control study of all adult deaths in 1998. *Br. med. J.*, **326**, 1–6

Le Marchand, L., Wilkens, L.R., Kolonel, L.N., Hankin, J.H. & Lyu, L.C. (1997) Associations of sedentary lifestyle, obesity, smoking, alcohol use, and diabetes with the risk of colorectal cancer. *Cancer Res.*, **57**, 4787–4794

Lee, W.C., Neugut, A.I., Garbowski, G.C., Forde, K.A., Treat, M.R., Waye, J.D. & Fenoglio-Preiser, C. (1993) Cigarettes, alcohol, coffee, and caffeine as risk factors for colorectal adenomatous polyps. *Ann. Epidemiol.*, **3**, 239–244

Liaw, K.M. & Chen, C.J. (1998) Mortality attributable to cigarette smoking in Taiwan: A 12-year follow-up study. *Tob. Control*, **7**, 141–148

Longnecker, M.P., Chen, M.J., Probst-Hensch, N.M., Harper, J.M., Lee, E.R., Frankl, H.D. & Haile, R.W. (1996) Alcohol and smoking in relation to the prevalence of adenomatous colorectal polyps detected at sigmoidoscopy. *Epidemiology*, **7**, 275–280

Manus, B., Adang, R.P., Ambergen, A.W., Brägelmann, R., Armbrecht, U. & Stockbrügger, R.W. (1997) The risk factor profile of recto-sigmoid adenomas: A prospective screening study of 665 patients in a clinical rehabilitation centre. *Eur. J. Cancer Prev.*, **6**, 38–43

Margetts, B.M. & Jackson, A.A. (1993) Interactions between people's diet and their smoking habits: The dietary and nutritional survey and British adults. *Br. med. J.*, **307**, 1381–1384

Martínez, M.E., McPherson, R.S., Annegers, J.F. & Levin, B. (1995) Cigarette smoking and alcohol consumption as risk factors for colorectal adenomatous polyps. *J. natl Cancer Inst.*, **87**, 274–279

Martínez, M.E., McPherson, R.S., Levin, B. & Glober, G.A. (1997) A case–control study of dietary intake and other lifestyle risk factors for hyperplastic polyps. *Gastroenterology*, **113**, 423–429

McLaughlin, J.K., Hrubec, Z., Blot, W.J. & Fraumeni, J.F. (1995) Smoking and cancer mortality among US veterans: A 26-year follow-up. *Int. J. Cancer*, **60**, 190–193

Monnet, E., Allemand, H., Farina, H. & Carayon, P. (1991) Cigarette smoking and the risk of colorectal adenoma in men. *Scand. J. Gastroenterol.*, **26**, 758–762

Murata, M., Takayama, K., Choi, B.C. & Pak, A.W. (1996) A nested case–control study on alcohol drinking, tobacco smoking, and cancer. *Cancer Detect. Prev.*, **20**, 557–565

Nagata, C., Shimizu, H., Kametani, M., Takeyama, N., Ohnuma, T. & Matsushita, S. (1999) Cigarette smoking, alcohol use, and colorectal adenoma in Japanese men and women. *Dis. Colon Rectum*, **42**, 337–342

Nelson, R.L., Davis, F.G., Sutter, E., Kikendall, J.W., Sobin, L.H., Milner, J.A. & Bowen, P.E. (1995) Serum selenium and colonic neoplastic risk. *Dis. Colon Rectum*, **38**, 1306–1310

Newcomb, P.A., Storer, B.E. & Marcus, P.M. (1995) Cigarette smoking in relation to risk of large bowel cancer in women. *Cancer Res.*, **55**, 4906–4909

Nordlund, L.A., Carstensen, J.M. & Pershagen, G. (1997) Cancer incidence in female smokers: A 26-year follow-up. *Int. J. Cancer*, **73**, 625–628

Nusko, G., Schneider, B., Schneider, I., Wittekind, C. & Hahn, E.G. (2000) Anthranoid laxative use is not a risk factor for colorectal neoplasia: Results of a prospective case–control study. *Gut*, **46**, 651–655

Nyrén, O., Bergstrom, R., Nystrom, L., Engholm, G., Ekbom, A., Adami, H.O., Knutsson, A. & Stjernberg, N. (1996) Smoking and colorectal cancer: A 20-year follow-up study of Swedish construction workers. *J. natl Cancer Inst.*, **88**, 1302–1307

Olsen, J. & Kronborg, O. (1993) Coffee, tobacco and alcohol as risk factors for cancer and adenoma of the large intestine. *Int. J. Epidemiol.*, **22**, 398–402

Peters, R.K., Garabrant, D.H., Yu, M.C. & Mack, T.M. (1989) A case–control study of occupational and dietary factors in colorectal cancer in young men by subsite. *Cancer Res.*, **49**, 5459–5468

Poole, C. (1999) Controls who experienced hypothetical causal intermediates should not be excluded from case–control studies. *Am. J. Epidemiol.*, **150**, 547–551

Potter, J.D. (1998) Invited commentary: Old problem, new wrinkles. *Am. J. Epidemiol.*, **147**, 911–913

Potter, J.D., Slattery, M.L., Bostick, R.M. & Gapstur, S.M. (1993) Colon cancer: A review of the epidemiology. *Epidemiol. Rev.*, **15**, 499–545

Rogot, E. & Murray, J.L. (1980) Smoking and cause of death among US veterans: 16 years of observation. *Public Health Rep.*, **95**, 213–222

Sandler, R.S., Sandler, D.P., Comstock, G.W., Helsing, K.J. & Shore, D.L. (1988) Cigarette smoking and the risk of colorectal cancer in women. *J. natl Cancer Inst.*, **80**, 1329–1333

Sandler, R.S., Lyles, C.M., McAuliffe, C., Woosley, J.T. & Kupper, L.L. (1993) Cigarette smoking, alcohol, and the risk of colorectal adenomas. *Gastroenterology*, **104**, 1445–1451

Siemiatycki, J., Kreski, D., Franco, E. & Kaiserman, M. (1995) Associations between cigarette smoking and each of 21 types of cancer: A multi-site case–control study. *Int. J. Epidemiol.*, **24**, 504–514

Singh, P.N. & Fraser, G.E. (1998) Dietary risk factors for colon cancer in a low-risk population. *Am. J. Epidemiol.*, **148**, 761–774

Slattery, M.L., West, D.W., Robison, L.M., French, T.K., Ford, M.H., Schuman, K.L. & Sorenson, A.W. (1990) Tobacco, alcohol, coffee, and caffeine as risk factors for colon cancer in a low-risk population. *Epidemiology*, **1**, 141–145

Slattery, M.L., Potter, J.D., Friedman, G.D., Ma, K.N. & Edwards, S. (1997) Tobacco use and colon cancer. *Int. J. Cancer*, **70**, 259–264

Stemmermann, G.N., Heilbrun, L.K. & Nomura, A.M.Y. (1988) Association of diet and other factors with adenomatous polyps of the large bowel: A prospective autopsy study. *Am. J. clin. Nutr.*, **47**, 312–317

Stürmer, T., Glynn, R.J., Lee, I.M., Christen, W.G. & Hennekens, C.H. (2000) Lifetime cigarette smoking and colorectal cancer incidence in the Physicians' Health Study I. *J. natl Cancer Inst.*, **92**, 1178–1181

Tajima, K. & Tominaga, S. (1985) Dietary habits and gastro-intestinal cancers: A comparative case–control study of stomach and large intestinal cancers in Nagoya, Japan. *Jpn. J. Cancer Res.*, **76**, 705–716

Tavani, A., Gallus, S., Negri, E., Franceschi, S., Talamini, R. & La Vecchia, C. (1998) Cigarette smoking and risk of cancers of the colon and rectum: A case–control study from Italy. *Eur. J. Epidemiol.*, **14**, 675–681

Terry, M.B. & Neugut, A.I. (1998) Cigarette smoking and the colorectal adenoma–carcinoma sequence: A hypothesis to explain the paradox. *Am. J. Epidemiol.*, **147**, 903–910

Terry, M.B., Neugut, A.I., Schwartz, S. & Susser, E. (2000) Risk factors for a causal intermediate and an endpoint: Reconciling differences. *Am. J. Epidemiol.*, **151**, 339–345

Terry, P., Ekbom, A., Lichtenstein, P., Feychting, M. & Wolk, A. (2001) Long-term tobacco smoking and colorectal cancer in a prospective cohort study. *Int. J. Cancer*, **91**, 585–587

Tulinius, H., Sigfusson, N., Sigvaldason, H., Bjarnadottir, K. & Tryggvadottir, L. (1997) Risk factors for malignant diseases: A cohort study on a population of 22,946 Icelanders. *Cancer Epidemiol. Biomarkers Prev.*, **6**, 863–873

Tuyns, A.J., Péquignot, G., Gignoux, M. & Valla, A. (1982) Cancers of the digestive tract, alcohol and tobacco. *Int. J. Cancer*, **30**, 9–11

Tverdal, A., Thelle, D., Stensvold, I., Leren, P. & Bjartveit, K. (1993) Mortality in relation to smoking history: 13 years' follow-up of 68 000 Norwegian men and women 35–49 years. *J. clin. Epidemiol.*, **46**, 475–487

Vobecky, J., Caro, J. & Devroede, G. (1983) A case–control study of risk factors for large bowel carcinoma. *Cancer*, **51**, 1958–1963

van Wayenburg, C.A., van der Schouw, Y.T., van Noord, P.A. & Peeters, P.H. (2000) Age at menopause, body mass index, and the risk of colorectal cancer mortality in the Dutch Diagnostich Onderzoek Mammacarcinoom (DOM) cohort. *Epidemiology*, **11**, 304–308

Williams, R.R. & Horm, J.W. (1977) Association of cancer sites with tobacco and alcohol consumption and socioeconomic status of patients: Interview study from the Third National Cancer Survey. *J. natl Cancer Inst.*, **58**, 525–547

Williams, R.R., Sorlic, P.D., Feinlieb, M., McNamara, P.M., Kannel, W.D. & Dawber, T.R. (1981) Cancer incidence by levels of cholesterol. *J. Am. med. Assoc.*, **245**, 247–252

Wu, A.H., Paganini-Hill, A., Ross, R.K. & Henderson, B.E. (1987) Alcohol, physical activity and other risk factors for colorectal cancer: A prospective study. *Br. J. Cancer*, **55**, 687–694

Yamada, K., Araki, S., Tamura, M., Sakai, I., Takahashi, Y., Kashihara, H. & Kono, S. (1997) Case–control study of colorectal carcinoma in situ and cancer in relation to cigarette smoking and alcohol use (Japan). *Cancer Causes Control*, **8**, 780–785

Yuan, J.M., Ross, R.K., Wang, X.L., Gao, Y.T., Henderson, B.E. & Yu, M.C. (1996) Morbidity and mortality in relation to cigarette smoking in Shanghai, China. A prospective male cohort study. *J. Am. med. Assoc.*, **275**, 1646–1650

Zahm, S.H., Cocco, P. & Blair, A. (1991) Tobacco smoking as a risk factor for colon polyps. *Am. J. public Health*, **81**, 846–849

2.1.8   Cancer of the liver

(a)   Overall risk

An association between cigarette smoking and liver cancer was reported in two cohort studies, one in Japan and one in the USA, and in four case–control studies on the topic (IARC, 1986). In one of the cohort studies (Hirayama, 1981), the relative risks associated with smoking were statistically significant in each alcohol-specific stratum; in another (Trichopoulos et al., 1980), a relative risk of 5.5 remained among hepatitis B surface antigen (HBsAg)-positive individuals who smoked > 20 cigarettes/day after adjustment for alcohol consumption. At the time, however, it was thought that the available data did not convincingly exclude residual confounding.

Twenty-eight additional cohort studies have been published since or after 1985, including 10 from Japan (Kono et al., 1987; Akiba & Hirayama, 1990; Hiyama et al., 1990; Shibata et al., 1990; Kato et al., 1992; Goodman et al., 1995; Chiba et al., 1996; Murata et al., 1996; Mizoue et al., 2000; Mori et al., 2000), nine from China (Tu et al., 1985; Ross et al., 1992; London et al., 1995; Yuan et al., 1996; Chen et al., 1997; Lam et al., 1997; Gao et al., 1999; Sun et al., 1999; Evans et al., 2002), four from China, Province of Taiwan (Yu & Chen, 1993; Chang et al., 1994; Liaw & Chen, 1998; Yang et al., 2002), two each from the USA (Hsing et al., 1990; McLaughlin et al., 1995) and Sweden (Carstensen et al., 1987; Nordlund et al., 1997) and one from the United Kingdom (Doll et al., 1994). In some studies, the cohort included patients with decompensated cirrhosis or post-transfusional hepatitis (Kato et al., 1992), persons with chronic hepatitis or cirrhosis (Chiba et al., 1996) or HBsAg-positive healthy patients (Hiyama et al., 1990). The design of these cohort studies is described in Tables 2.1 and 2.1.8.1, and the results are summarized in Table 2.1.8.2.

Most of the new cohort studies show an increased relative risk among current smokers.

Twenty-six additional case–control studies (Tables 2.1.8.3 and 2.1.8.4) published after 1985 provide information on smoking and liver cancer: six were conducted in Japan (Hiyama et al., 1990; Tsukuma et al., 1990; Tanaka et al., 1992; Pyong et al., 1994; Tanaka et al., 1995; Mukaiya et al., 1998), three each in Africa (Kew et al., 1990; Olubuyide & Bamgboye, 1990; Mohamed et al., 1992), China or Hong Kong SAR (Lin et al., 1991; Liu et al., 1998; Lam et al., 2001) and the USA (Austin et al., 1986; Yu, M.C. et al., 1991; Chen et al., 2003), two each in Greece (Tzonou et al., 1991; Kuper et al., 2000), Italy (La Vecchia et al., 1988; Ferraroni et al., 1989), the Republic of Korea (Choi & Kahyo, 1991; Shin et al., 1996) and China, Province of Taiwan (Chen et al., 1991; Yu, M.W. et al., 1991) and one each in Canada (Siemiatycki et al., 1995), Germany (Peters et al., 1994) and Spain (Vall Mayans et al., 1990). The majority of these studies used hospital controls. Five studies included community controls; two large Chinese studies (Liu et al., 1998; Lam et al., 2001) include controls who had died of causes other than neoplastic respiratory or vascular diseases. Risks in current smokers that were higher than those in never-smokers were found in 17 studies and attained statistical significance in 10 studies. An association between smoking and increased risk of liver cancer is thus consistently demonstrated in nearly all cohort studies and in a number of case–control studies, particularly the largest ones from Asia, Greece and the USA. These studies used different approaches to consider other established risk factors for liver cancer such as infection with hepatitis B virus (HBV) and with hepatitis C virus (HCV) infection and alcohol consumption.

(i)   Confounding and effect modification

Covariates that may potentially confound and/or modify the relationship between smoking and liver cancer include chronic infection with HBV and HCV (IARC, 1994) and heavy alcohol consumption (IARC, 1988). Consideration of each of these factors presents a challenge, however, because analyses that adjust for alcohol consumption may over-control for cigarette smoking, and stratification on hepatitis infection status rather than adjustment may be the preferred approach for differentiating confounding from effect modification by HBV or HCV infection.

Heavy, although not moderate, intake of alcoholic beverages is associated with an increased risk for liver cancer (IARC, 1988). The excess of liver cancer in populations where drinking alcohol is common could thus reflect an insufficient adjustment for drinking habits (Doll et al., 1994; McLaughlin et al., 1995). However, several recent case–control and cohort studies have found an association between smoking and liver cancer after controlling for alcohol consumption (Yu, M.C. et al., 1991; Yuan et al., 1996; Chen et al., 1997; Liaw & Chen, 1998; Mizoue et al., 2000) and among persons who reported no alcohol consumption. Chen et al. (1991) showed that subjects who consumed no alcohol, but smoked 20 cigarettes or more daily had a relative risk of 2.7 of developing liver cancer relative to nonsmokers who drank no alcohol. Those who both drank and smoked heavily had a relative risk of 11.7. Further supportive evidence is provided by the association between smoking and liver cancer observed among Chinese women (Liu et al., 1998) and Japanese women (Tanaka et al., 1995), in whom heavy alcohol drinking is extremely rare.

Infection with HBV is the main cause of liver cancer worldwide, whereas HCV infection causes a large fraction of liver cancer in Japan, northern Africa and southern Europe (IARC, 1994). Infection with HCV is increasing in many countries. To distinguish the strong effect of infection with HBV and HCV (relative risks of the order of 20; IARC, 1994) from the association with smoking, stratification and/or adjustment for HBsAg and anti-HCV have been made in some studies (Yu, M.C. et al., 1991; Yu, M.W. et al., 1991; Liaw & Chen, 1998; Kuper et al., 2000). The association between smoking and liver cancer was not generally weakened by adjustment for HBV and HCV. Infection with HBV was less frequent among smokers than nonsmokers in a large population survey in China (Evans et al., 2002). The possibility that tobacco smoking may potentiate the progression of chronic HBV and HCV infections to liver cirrhosis (Yu et al., 1997) and/or liver cancer (Tsukuma et al., 1993) has been examined in relatively few studies. The increase in risk for liver cancer associated with cigarette smoking appears to be greater among HBV carriers than among uninfected persons in some studies (Tu et al., 1985), but not in others (Kuper et al., 2000).

No information on confounding from exposure to aflatoxin was available.

(ii) *Bias*

The most frequent bias that can arise in studies of associations between smoking and cancer are described in the General Remarks. Many of the case–control studies that have not found an association between smoking and liver cancer are hospital-based, so that the control series may include tobacco-related diseases. Morbidity and symptoms resulting from prevalent liver cirrhosis or undiagnosed liver cancer can lead to lifestyle changes, including a reduction in number of cigarettes smoked per day or cessation of smoking. This phenomenon would lead to underestimation of the relative risk for current smokers and to overestimation of the relative risk for former smokers. It can also distort the association of liver cancer with the number of cigarettes smoked per day. The detection of liver cancer in a cirrhotic liver presents substantial difficulties of under- or over-diagnosis in cohort studies. Differential ascertainment of liver cancer according to smoking status, however, is unlikely.

A varying, but often substantial, proportion of liver cancer cases in the studies considered in this section was not pathologically confirmed. Liver cancer is a common site for metastases. If a high proportion of liver cancer for which pathological confirmation was not acquired were in reality metastases from smoking-related cancers (e.g. of the lung, oesophagus or stomach), the association between smoking and liver cancer in some studies would be overestimated. In the vast majority of the examined studies, however, diagnosis of liver cancer was confirmed by cytological findings or by the combined presence of elevated concentrations of α-fetoprotein (> 400 ng/mL) and at least one positive image obtained by angiography, sonography, liver scan or computerize tomography scan.

(b) *Factors affecting risk*

(i) *Duration and intensity*

The US Veterans Study (Hsing *et al.*, 1990) found a substantial increase in the association with increased smoking duration. A clear trend of increasing risk of liver cancer with the increase in pack–years was reported by Chiba *et al.* (1996). Many more studies reported relative risk by number of cigarettes smoked per day. An increased risk in heavy smokers relative to light smokers was shown in several studies (Hiyama *et al.*, 1990; Hsing *et al.*, 1990; Chen *et al.*, 1991; Tzonou *et al.*, 1991; Yu, M.W. *et al.*, 1991; Tanaka *et al.*, 1992; Chiba *et al.*, 1996; Liu *et al.*, 1998; Kuper *et al.*, 2000). In other studies, especially those from Asia, however, the relative risk among smokers did not vary by category of cigarettes smoked per day. The reasons for this are unknown but they may include the relatively low power of most studies to detect small relative risks, and the inclusion of persons who smoke up to 25 cigarettes per day in the referent group. Hsing *et al.* (1990) showed higher relative risk among smokers who started smoking earlier (generally before age 20 years) than in those who started at age 25 years or older.

(ii)   *Smoking cessation*

Nine cohort and 10 case–control studies provided information on the relative risk for former smokers. Most studies showed a lower risk for liver cancer among former smokers than in current smokers. In four studies, however, the relative risk for former smokers was of similar magnitude or even higher than the relative risk for current smokers (Ferraroni *et al.*, 1989; Tanaka *et al.*, 1992, 1995; Kuper *et al.*, 2000). The only study that examined relative risks by number of years since quitting showed a decrease in risk with time since cessation (Goodman *et al.*, 1995).

(iii)   *Type of cigarettes*

No data were available to the Working Group.

(c)   *Population characteristics*

(i)   *Sex*

The absolute risk of liver disease (hepatitis, cirrhosis, and cancer) is substantially greater in men than women in all populations. The data available suggest, however, that the association between smoking and liver cancer is similar in men and women (Liu *et al.*, 1998; Kuper *et al.*, 2000), after taking into account different levels of smoking in the two sexes.

(ii)   *Ethnicity*

Some disparities have been described in the relative risks observed in different racial and ethnic populations. [Such variations may reflect factors other than race such as different smoking and alcohol drinking patterns, variations in prevalence of HBV and HCV infection, and the greater probability of residual confounding from alcohol drinking in populations from Europe and North America.]

Table 2.1.8.1. Additional cohort studies on tobacco smoking and liver cancer

Reference Country and years of study	Hepatitis B virus (HBV) status	Cohort sample	Cases/deaths identification	Comments
Basa et al. (1977) Philippines 1968–73	HBV/HCV status unknown	16 492 cancer cases registered at the Central Tumour Registry of the Philippines	Registry	Retrospective study
Tu et al. (1985) China 1980–82	16% HBV-positive Stratified data	Male residents of Chongming Island, aged ≥ 40 years	Deaths ascertained by local Anti-Epidemic Station	
Hiyama et al. (1990) Japan 1969–85 1972–92	Unknown status All HBsAg-positive	Male patients admitted to mental hospitals for alcoholism [age range not reported] 8646 men who donated blood in 1972–75	Deaths	Nested case–control study
Shibata et al. (1990) Japan 1958–86 1960–86	Status unknown	Men aged 40–69 years from: Farming areas (cohort I) Fishing areas (cohort II)	Deaths ascertained with resident's cards and other materials at municipal offices	
Kato et al. (1992) Japan 1987–90	Status known No adjustment No stratification	Patients with decompensated liver cirrhosis, 343 with post-transfusion hepatitis, aged ≥ 16 years	Cases	
Ross et al. (1992) China 1986–90	HBsAg-positive: 55% cases, 11% controls	All men aged 45–64 years living in 4 defined areas of metropolitan Shanghai	Cases of primary liver cancer identified through Shanghai municipality and Shanghai Cancer Registry	Nested case–control study; adjustment for HBsAg status in a multivariate regression model
Yu & Chen (1993) China, Province of Taiwan 1984–90	HBsAg-positive: 57% cases, 55% controls Anti-HCV: 20% cases, 3% controls No stratification	Men aged 30–85 years	Cases	Nested case–control study, adjustment for HBsAg and anti-HCV status in multivariate regression model

Table 2.1.8.1. (contd)

Reference Country and years of study	Hepatitis B virus (HBV) status	Cohort sample	Cases/deaths identification	Comments
Chang et al. (1994) China, Province of Taiwan 1984–92	HBsAg-positive: 63% cases, 7% controls Anti-HCV: 13% cases, 3% controls	Men aged 30–85 years	Cases	Same cohort as Yu & Chen (1993). Nested case–control study without adjustment for HBsAg or anti-HCV status
London et al. (1995); Evans et al. (2002) China 1992–2000	81% HBsAg-positive 11–15% HBsAg-positive, 1.5% HCV-positive No adjustment, no stratification	Residents of Haimen City, the world highest incidence area for hepatocellular carcinoma; aged 30–64 years	Deaths certificates confirmed by hospital records	London et al. (1995) conducted a nested case–control study with matching for HBV status.
Chiba et al. (1996) Japan 1977–93	HBsAg-negative, anti-HCV-positive	412 patients with chronic liver disease, including 232 chronic hepatitis and 180 cirrhosis	Cases ascertained by medical follow-up	
Sun et al. (1999) China 1987–98	16% HBsAg-positive, 7% HCV-positive	Men with chronic hepatitis B (72% of all men with hepatitis B in two townships)	Cases identified by twice-yearly examinations	
Mori et al. (2000) Japan 1992–97	1.8% HBsAg-positive 22% HCVAb-positive	Baseline survey during liver disorder screening	Cases	
Yang et al. (2002) China, Province of Taiwan 1991–2000	Known HBV and HCV status	Men aged 30–65 years	Cases ascertained by yearly mass screening	Nested case–control study

HCV, hepatitis C virus; HBsAg, hepatitis B surface antigen

Table 2.1.8.2. Cohort studies on tobacco smoking and liver cancer

Reference Country and years of study	Cohort No. of subjects	No. deaths/ incident cancers	Smoking categories and other variables	Relative risk (95% CI)		Adjustment factors/ comments
Hammond (1966) USA 1959–63	Cancer Prevention Study (CPS) I 440 558 men, 562 671 women		Ever-smoker Aged 45–64 years Aged 65–79 years	**Mortality ratio** 2.8 1.3		Mortality ratio of age-standardized death rates. Study based on examination of death certificates on which secondary liver cancers may have been included in the category 'liver cancer' (many smoking-related cancers metastasize to the liver).
Basa et al. (1977) Philippines 1968–73	16 492 cancer cases (6771 men, 9721 women)	541 men, 213 women	Ever-smoker Current smoker	**Men** 1.5 (p = 0.01) 1.3	**Women** 2.6 (p = 0.001) 1.9 (p = 0.01)	Adjusted for age
Hirayama (1981) Japan 1965–78	Six-prefecture Study 265 118 men and women	865 deaths	*Lifelong no. of cigarettes smoked* None 1–190 000 200 000–390 000 400 000	**Alcohol use** *Occasional, rare, none* 26.5 38.8 39.9 45.2	*Daily* 24.0 49.4 45.8 66.9	Standardized mortality ratios
Tu et al. (1985) China 1980–82	12 222 men	70 deaths	*HBV carrier* Nonsmoker Current smoker ≤ 19 cigs/day ≥ 20 cigs/day *HBV non-carrier* Nonsmoker Current smoker ≤ 19 cigs/day ≥ 20 cigs/day	**Mortality rate** 332.8 737.9 660.1 1519 (p < 0.05) 115.1 99.9 96.3 145.2		Adjusted for age and alcohol consumption

Table 2.1.8.2 (contd)

Reference Country and years of study	Cohort No. of subjects	No. deaths/ incident cancers	Smoking categories and other variables	Relative risk (95% CI)		Adjustment factors/ comments
Carstensen et al. (1987) Sweden 1963–79	Swedish Census Study 25 129 men	54 deaths	Former smoker Current smoker *Cigarettes/day* 1–7 8–15 > 15	1.7 3.0 1.6 3.3 4.1		Relative death rates Categories in grams of any tobacco/day combined: 1 cigarette = 1 g; 1 small cigar = 3 g; 1 large cigar = 5 g
Kono et al. (1987) Japan 1965–83	Japanese Physicians' Study 5130 men	51 deaths	1–19 cigarettes/day ≥ 20 cigarettes/day	1.1 (0.6–2.2) 1.0 (0.5–2.2)		Adjusted for age and alcohol
Akiba & Hirayama (1990) Japan 1965–81	Six-prefecture Study 122 261 men, 142 857 women ~3 975 000 person–years	1060 deaths (662 men, 398 women)	Current smoker *Cigarettes/day* **Men** 1–4 5–14 15–24 25–34 ≥ 35 **Women** 1–4 5–14 ≥ 15	1.5 (1.2–1.9) 1.1 (0.5–2.0) 1.6 (1.3–2.0) 1.4 (1.2–1.8) 1.6 (1.1–2.4) 1.9 (1.1–3.2) [*p* for trend = 0.002] 1.4 (0.7–2.5) 1.4 (1.0–2.0) 2.5 (1.3–4.1) [*p* for trend = 0.001]		Adjusted for prefecture, occupation, age and observation period. No trend observed in the relative risk in relation to calendar period. Unclear whether former smokers were included in analysis or not
Hiyama et al. (1990) Japan 1969–85	13 171 men	93 cases		*Ratio observed/expected* 1.4 (1.1–1.7)		
1972–92	8646 men	22 cases, 44 controls	*Cigarettes/day* 10–29 ≥ 30	*Crude odds ratio* 1.7 (0.4–6.4) 5.8 (1–34.2)	*Adjusted for alcohol* 1.2 6.3	Nested case–control study; controls matched by age

Table 2.1.8.2 (contd)

Reference Country and years of study	Cohort No. of subjects	No. deaths/ incident cancers	Smoking categories and other variables	Relative risk (95% CI)	Adjustment factors/ comments
Hsing et al. (1990) USA 1954–80	US Veterans' Study 293 916 men	289 deaths	Former smoker	1.9 (1.2–2.9)	Adjusted for age and calendar period
			Current smoker	2.4 (1.6–3.5)	
			Cigarettes/day		
			< 10	2.2 (1.2–3.8)	
			10–20	2.0 (1.3–3.0)	
			21–39	2.9 (1.8–4.5)	
			> 39	3.8 (1.9–8.0)	
			Duration (years)		
			< 35	0.9 (0.4–2.1)	
			35–39	2.6 (1.4–4.9)	
			> 39	2.7 (1.5–4.9)	
			Age at starting smoking (years)		
			< 20	2.9 (1.6–5.3)	
			20–24	2.3 (1.2–4.3)	
			> 24	1.0 (0.4–2.3)	
Shibata et al. (1990) Japan 1958–86 (I)	Cohort I 639 men 17 480 person– years	11 deaths	Current smoker	1.1 (0.2–4.7)	Adjusted for age. Calculations based on small number of liver cancer cases. No information on HBV/HCV
			Cigarettes/day		
			1–9	0.6 (0.1–3.7)	
			≥ 10	1.2 (0.2–5.7) [*p* for trend ~0.6]	
1960–86 (II)	Cohort II 677 men 17 172 person– years	22 deaths	Former smoker	2.9 (0.3–29.0)	
			Current smoker	3.6 (0.6–22.3)	
			Cigarettes/day		
			1–9	11.9 (1.5–96.8)	
			10–19	1.1 (0.1–10.6)	
			20–29	2.7 (0.4–19.2)	
			≥ 30	3.2 (0.4–23.7) [*p* for trend ~0.5]	
			1–19	2.1 (0.4–10.0)	Adjusted for age and alcohol
			≥ 20	1.9 (0.4–9.4)	

Table 2.1.8.2 (contd)

Reference Country and years of study	Cohort No. of subjects	No. deaths/ incident cancers	Smoking categories and other variables	Relative risk (95% CI)	Adjustment factors/ comments
Kato et al. (1992) Japan 1987–90	1441 patients with decompensated liver cirrhosis, 343 with post-transfusion hepatitis 4386 person–years	122 cases	Former smoker Current smoker *Pack–years* < 30 ≥ 30	0.9 (0.4–2.0) 1.0 (0.5–1.8) 0.8 (0.4–1.7) 0.9 (0.5–1.9) *p* for trend = 0.824	Adjusted for sex and age. Record linkage study. Patients at high risk for development of hepatocellular carcinoma
Ross et al. (1992) China 1986–89	18 244 men 35 299 person–years	22 cases, 140 controls	Ever-smoker *Cigarettes/day* 1–19 ≥ 20 *Duration (years)* 1–29 ≥ 30 Ever-smoker	2.6 (0.9–7.2) 3.1 (1.0–10.3) 2.1 (0.6–6.9) 2.6 (0.7–9.4) 2.5 (0.9–7.6) 1.8 (0.6–5.6)	No adjustment; nested case–control study. Population-based controls matched on age, sample collection and residence Adjusted for HBV, alcohol consumption, aflatoxin exposure and education
Yu & Chen (1993) China, Province of Taiwan 1987–90	9691 men	35 cases, 140 controls	Current smoker	1.2 (0.4–3.1)	Nested case–control study; controls matched by age, date of interview and residence. Adjusted for testosterone, alcohol consumption, HCV status, HBsAg status, vegetable consumption and history of liver disease
Chang et al. (1994) China, Province of Taiwan 1984–92	9775 men	38 cases, 152 controls	Ever-smoker	1.2 (0.6–2.7)	Nested case–control study; controls matched for age, residence and date of recruitment. Cases confirmed pathologically or α-fetoprotein ≥ 400 mg/mL and ultrasound

Table 2.1.8.2 (contd)

Reference Country and years of study	Cohort No. of subjects	No. deaths/ incident cancers	Smoking categories and other variables	Relative risk (95% CI)	Adjustment factors/ comments
Doll et al. (1994) UK 1951–91	British Doctors' Study 34 439 men	76 deaths		**Mortality rate**	Annual mortality rate per 100 000 men
			Never-smoker	7	
			Former smoker	9	
			Current smoker	11	
			Cigarettes/day		
			1–14	17	
			15–24	3	
			≥25	15 [*p* for trend = 0.7]	
Goodman et al. (1995) Japan 1980–89	Life Span Study 36 133 men and women 311 086 person–years	252 cases (156 men, 86 women)	**Men**		Adjusted for city, age at time of bombing and radiation dose to liver. Relative risk among non-drinkers of alcohol for ever smoking, 1.9 (95% CI, 1.2–2.9); among men, 7.2 (95% CI, 1.0–53.3); among women, 1.3 (95% CI, 1.0–1.7). [CIs calculated by the Working Group]
			Former smoker	4.2 (2.0–10.7)	
			Current smoker	4.3 (1.9–9.7)	
			Ever-smoker	4.4 (1.9–9.9)	
			Pack–years		
			<23	6.5 (2.7–15.3)	
			23–40	4.4 (1.9–10.5)	
			>40	3.1 (1.3–7.3)	
			Years since quitting		
			≥24	4.0 (1.5–10.6)	
			14–23	4.1 (1.6–10.7)	
			<14	5.6 (2.2–14.6)	
			Women		
			Former smoker	1.7 (0.8–3.6)	
			Current smoker	1.6 (0.9–2.9)	
			Ever-smoker	1.6 (1.0–2.7)	
			Pack–years		
			<16	1.8 (0.9–3.8)	
			≥16	1.5 (0.7–3.2)	
			Years since quitting		
			≥25	2.3 (0.7–7.4)	
			10–24	1.0 (0.3–4.2)	
			<10	10.4 (2.5–43.5)	

Table 2.1.8.2 (contd)

Reference Country and years of study	Cohort No. of subjects	No. deaths/ incident cancers	Smoking categories and other variables	Relative risk (95% CI)	Adjustment factors/ comments
London et al. (1995) China 1992–95	60 984 men	183 cases (2% histologically verified), 868 controls	Current smoker	0.7 (0.5–1.0)	Nested case–control study; controls matched 5:1 by age, area of residence and HBV status; strong inverse association between recent hepatitis and current smoking
McLaughlin et al. (1995) USA 1954–80	US Veterans' Study 248 046 men 3 252 983 person–years	363 deaths	Former smoker Current smoker *Cigarettes/day* 1–9 10–20 21–30 ≥40	1.5 (1.4–2.3) 1.8 (1.4–2.3) 1.8 (1.1–2.8) 1.4 (1.1–2.0) 2.3 (1.6–3.1) 2.6 (1.4–4.6) p for trend < 0.01	Adjusted for age and calendar-year time-period
Chiba et al. (1996) Japan 1977–93	249 men, 163 women ~2000 person-years	63 cases (54 men, 9 women)	*Pack–years* < 20 ≥ 20	1.7 (0.8–3.7) 2.5 (1.1–5.5)	Adjusted for age, sex, alcohol consumption, clinical stage of liver disease, serum α-fetoprotein value, antibodies against HBV, history of blood transfusion, history of surgical procedures and family history of liver cancer
Murata et al. (1996) Japan 1983–94	Chiba Cancer Association Study 17 200 men	Cases 8 26 3	*Cigarettes/day* 1–10 11–20 ≥21	1.4 2.0 $p < 0.05$ 0.4	
Yuan et al. (1996) China 1986–93	Shanghai Men's Study 18 244 men 98 267 person–years	79 cases	Ever-smoker *Cigarettes/day* < 20 ≥ 20	1.8 $p < 0.05$ 1.8 1.8	Adjusted for age and alcohol consumption

Table 2.1.8.2 (contd)

Reference Country and years of study	Cohort No. of subjects	No. deaths/ incident cancers	Smoking categories and other variables	Relative risk (95% CI)	Adjustment factors/ comments
Chen et al. (1997) China 1972–93	Shanghai Factory Study 6494 men, 2857 women 149 616 person–years	66 deaths	Current smoker *Cigarettes/day* 1–19 ≥ 20 *p* for trend	2.0 *p* < 0.05 2.1 2.1 0.07	Adjusted for age, blood pressure, cholesterol and alcohol at baseline
Lam et al. (1997) China 1976–96	Xi'an Factory Study 1124 men, 572 women 32 428 person–years	17 deaths	Ever-smoker	1.1 (0.4–2.9)	Adjusted for age, marital status, occupation, blood pressure, triglycerides and total cholesterol
Nordlund et al. (1997) Sweden 1963–89	Swedish Census Study 26 000 women 600 000 person–years	41 cases	Current smoker	0.7 (0.2–2.0)	Adjusted for age and place of residence
Liaw & Chen (1998) China, Province of Taiwan 1982–94	Taiwanese Study 11 096 men, 3301 women 140 493 person–years	128 deaths (110 men, 18 women)	Current smoker **Men** *Cigarettes/day* ≤ 10 11–20 > 20 *Duration (years)* ≤ 20 21–30 > 30	2.2 (1.4–3.6) 2.1 (1.2–3.5) 1.9 (1.2–3.2) 1.8 (1.2–3.5) *p* for trend = 0.02 1.6 (0.8–3.2) 1.0 (0.5–2.1) 2.5 (1.6–4.1)	Adjusted for age, HBV status and alcohol

Table 2.1.8.2 (contd)

Reference Country and years of study	Cohort No. of subjects	No. deaths/ incident cancers	Smoking categories and other variables	Relative risk (95% CI)	Adjustment factors/ comments
Liaw & Chen (1998) (contd)			*Age at starting smoking (years)*		
			> 24	1.4 (0.8–2.6)	
			21–24	2.3 (1.2–4.2)	
			≤ 20	2.2 (1.4–3.7) *p* for trend < 0.01	
			Pack–years		
			< 20	1.7 (1.0–2.9)	
			20–40	2.1 (1.2–3.5)	
			≥ 41	2.5 (1.3–4.6)	
Gao *et al.* (1999) China 1983–94	Shanghai Residential Study 213 800 men and women		**Men**		†CI does not include 1.0. *p* for trend < 0.05 for intensity of smoking for men and women and for age at starting smoking for men only
			Urban	1.5†	
			Suburban	1.4	
			Rural	1.5†	
			Women (urban)	2.4†	
Sun *et al.* (1999) China 1987–98	145 men	22 cases, 45% histolo- gically confirmed	Never-smoker	**Incidence rate** 2.3	Rate per 100 person–years
			Current smoker	1.6 *p* = 0.5	
Mizoue *et al.* (2000) Japan 1986–96	Fukuoka Study 4050 men 35 785 person– years	59 deaths	Former smoker	2.9 (1.0–8.4)	Adjusted for age, alcohol consumption and area of residence
			Current smoker	3.3 (1.2–9.5)	
			Cigarettes/day		
			1–24	3.5 (1.2–10.2)	
			≥ 25	2.8 (0.8–9.6)	
Mori *et al.* (2000) Japan 1992–97	974 men, 2078 women 13 984 person– years	22 (14 men, 8 women)	Former smoker	2.1 (0.6–7.2)	Adjusted for age and sex
			Pack–years		
			< 10	3.3 (0.4–28.2)	
			≥ 10	2.0 (0.6–6.9) *p* for trend = 0.3	

Table 2.1.8.2 (contd)

Reference Country and years of study	Cohort No. of subjects	No. deaths/ incident cancers	Smoking categories and other variables	Relative risk (95% CI)	Adjustment factors/ comments
Evans et al. (2002) China 1992–2000	48 454 men, 25 430 women	977 deaths (900 men, 77 women)	*Current smoker* Men Women	0.9 (0.8–1.1) 2.0 (0.9–4.2)	Smoking was not significantly associated with liver cancer as assessed by present consumption, duration of smoking or pack–years
Yang et al. (2002) China, Province of Taiwan 1991–2000	11 83 men 92 359 person– years	111 cases, 222 controls	Current smoker	1.5 (1.0–2.2)	Nested case–control study; population-based controls matched on age, date of enrolment and township. Adjusted for HBV and HCV status, age and alcohol consumption

HBV, hepatitis B virus; HCV, hepatitis C virus

Table 2.1.8.3. Case–control studies on tobacco smoking and liver cancer: main characteristics of study design

Reference Country and years of study	No. of cases and controls	Source of cases and controls
Williams & Horm (1977) USA 1969–71	Men: 31 cases and 1739 controls; women: 14 cases and 3164 controls	Study with the Third National Survey Cases and controls aged ≥ 35 years; response rate, 57% Controls were patients with other cancers, excluding lung, larynx, oral cavity, oesophagus and bladder
Trichopoulos et al. (1980) Greece 1976–77	Men: 35 cases and 169 controls; women: 5 cases and 35 controls	Hospital-based study among HBsAg-negative Cases histologically confirmed (58%); mean age, 62 years Controls matched on age and sex
Lam et al. (1982) Hong Kong SAR 1977–80	Men: 17 cases and 94 controls; women: 2 cases and 13 controls	Hospital-based study among HBsAg-negative patients Cases histologically confirmed (99%); mean age, 50 years Controls matched on age and sex
Stemhagen et al. (1983) USA 1975–80	Men: 178 cases and 356 controls; women: 87 cases and 174 controls	Hospital-based study Cases histologically confirmed; mean age, 64 years Controls matched on age, race, sex and area of residence
Yu et al. (1983) USA 1975–79	Men and women: 78 cases and controls	Population-based study among black and white non-Asians Incident cases histologically confirmed (70.6%); aged ≥ 70 years Controls matched on age, sex, race and neighbourhood
Hardell et al. (1984) Sweden 1974–81	Men: 98 cases and 200 controls	Population-based study Deceased cases of hepatocellular carcinoma (83) or cholangiocarcinoma (15), 100% histologically confirmed; aged 25–80 years Controls randomly selected from population
Austin et al. (1986) Cuba, USA (years of study not specified)	Men: 60 cases; women: 26 cases; 172 controls	Hospital-based study Cases confirmed histologically (93%); aged 19–84 years Controls matched by age, sex and race
La Vecchia et al. (1988) Italy 1984–87	Men: 115 cases and 776 controls; women: 36 cases and 275 controls	Hospital-based study Cases aged 24–74 years Controls with acute conditions excluding malignant disorders, digestive tract diseases and conditions related to tobacco or alcohol; aged 22–74 years
Ferraroni et al. (1989) Italy 1983–88	Men: 115 cases and 1334 controls; women: 36 cases and 610 controls	Hospital-based study Cases histologically confirmed (100%); aged < 75 years Controls with no cancer, digestive tract disorders or conditions related to coffee, alcohol and tobacco consumption; comparable catchment areas

Table 2.1.8.3 (contd)

Reference Country and years of study	No. of cases and controls	Source of cases and controls
Hiyama *et al.* (1990) Japan 1984–87	Men: 192 cases and 192 controls; women: 37 cases and 74 controls	Population-based study (in Japanese)
Kew *et al.* (1990) South Africa (years of study not specified)	Women: 46 cases and 92 controls	Hospital-based study Cases aged 19–54 years Controls with various medical disorders, excluding diseases related to contraceptive steroids, matched on sex, race, exact tribe, place of birth (rural/urban), migration, hospital and ward
Vall Mayans *et al.* (1990) Spain 1986–88	Men: 67 cases and 133 controls; women: 29 cases and 57 controls	Hospital-based study Cases histologically confirmed (77%) Controls were diagnosed with 76 different conditions (including other cancers, AIDS, liver disease, stomach ulcer, pancreatitis), all unrelated to study exposure, matched on age and sex
Olubuyide & Bamgboye (1990) Nigeria 1987–88	Men: 85 cases and 85 controls; women: 15 cases and 15 controls	Hospital-based study Cases of primary hepatocellular carcinoma, 100% histologically confirmed; aged 42–55 years Controls were patients admitted to orthopaedic clinic, matched for sex and age
Tsukuma *et al.* (1990) Japan 1983–87	Men: 192 cases and 192 controls; women: 37 cases and 74 controls	Hospital-based study Cases histologically confirmed (38%); aged < 74 years Controls from gastroenterology department, excluding liver disease and smoking- or alcohol-related diseases
Chen *et al.* (1991) China, Province of Taiwan 1985–87	Men: 200 cases and 200 controls	Population-based study Cases recruited at teaching hospitals Controls selected from household registration offices, with no history of hepatocellular carcinoma, matched on age, sex, ethnic group and area of residence
Choi & Kahyo (1991) Republic of Korea 1986–90	Men: 216 cases and 648 controls	Hospital-based study Cases; average age, 49 years Controls matched on age and date of admission to hospital
Lin *et al.* (1991) China 1984–86	Men: 200 cases and 200 controls	Hospital-based study in a polyclinic Cases with primary hepatoma; aged ≥ 20 years Controls were patients with conditions unrelated to smoking

Table 2.1.8.3 (contd)

Reference Country and years of study	No. of cases and controls	Source of cases and controls
Tzonou et al. (1991) Greece 1976–84	Men: 166 cases and 381 controls; women: 19 cases and 51 controls	Hospital-based study in nine major hospitals Cases histologically confirmed (58%) Controls were patients without cancer or liver disease
Yu, M.C. et al. (1991b) USA 1984–90	Men: 49 cases and 104 controls; women: 25 cases and 58 controls	Population-based study Cases histologically confirmed (100%); aged 18–74 years Controls from neighbourhood, matched by age, sex and race
Yu, M.W. et al. (1991) China, Province of Taiwan 1986–87	Men: 121 cases and 121 controls; women: 6 cases and 6 controls	Population-based study Cases histologically confirmed (80%); aged 38–62 years Health community controls from household registration offices, individually matched for sex, age, ethnicity and area of residence
Mohamed et al. (1992) South Africa (years of study not specified)	Men: 77 cases and 77 controls; women: 24 cases and 24 controls	Hospital-based study in a major teaching hospital Cases histologically confirmed (95%); aged 20–87 years Controls with conditions unrelated to alcohol consumption, matched for age, sex and ethnicity
Tanaka et al. (1992) Japan 1985–89	Men: 168 cases and 291 controls; women: 36 cases and 119 controls	Hospital-based study Cases histologically confirmed (40%); aged 40–69 years
Peters et al. (1994) Germany 1986–93	Men: 72 cases and 72 controls; women: 14 ccases, and 14 controls	Hospital-based study Cases histologically confirmed (74%) Controls with cirrhosis, matched on age and sex (mean age: men, 62.8 years; women 65.0 years)
Pyong et al. (1994) Japan 1989–92	Men: 68 cases and 109 controls; women: 22 cases and 140 controls	Study among Koreans Cases aged 40–89 years Controls matched by age
Siemiatycki et al. (1995) Canada 1979–86	Men: 48 cases and 2238 controls	Hospital-based study Cases histologically confirmed (100%); aged 35–70 years Controls were hospital controls with other cancers (1705) and population controls (533)
Tanaka et al. (1995) Japan 1983–89	Women: 120 cases and 257 controls	Hospital-based study Cases aged 35–74 years

Table 2.1.8.3 (contd)

Reference Country and years of study	No. of cases and controls	Source of cases and controls
Shin *et al.* (1996) Republic of Korea 1990–93	Men: 159 cases and 318 controls; women: 44 cases and 88 controls	Hospital-based study Cases histologically confirmed (53%) Controls were healthy patients from check-up at hospital (159 men, 44 women) and in-patients (159 men, 44 women), individually matched for sex and age
Liu *et al.* (1998) China 1989–91	Men and women: 28 187 cases and 87 315 controls	Population-based study in rural and urban areas of China Cases: 17 523 (13 478 men, 4045 women) from urban and 10 664 (7979 men, 2685 women) from rural areas Controls: 51 880 (30 709 men, 21 171 women) from urban and 35 435 (22 046 men, 13 389 women) from rural areas
Mukaiya *et al.* (1998) Japan 1991–93	Men: 104 cases and 104 controls	Hospital-based study Cases with chronic liver disease; aged 51–69 years Controls with chronic disease but no hepatocellular carcinoma, matched for age
Kuper *et al.* (2000) Greece 1995–98	Men: 283 cases and 298 controls; women: 50 cases and 62 controls	Hospital-based study Cases histologically confirmed (47%) Non-cancer controls with injuries, eye/ear/nose/throat conditions, unrelated to smoking, alcohol or coffee consumption
Lam *et al.* (2001) Hong Kong SAR 1998	Men: 15 296 cases and 3918 controls; women: 12 211 cases and 9136 controls	Population-based study among ethnic Chinese Cases from death registries; aged ≥ 35 years Controls were spouses or relatives; aged ≥ 60 years
Chen *et al.* (2003) China 1986–88	Men: 26 294 cases and 11 321 controls; women: 9642 cases and 5619 controls	Retrospective population-based study in 24 cities and 74 rural counties Cases aged ≥ 35 years Controls with cirrhosis

Table 2.1.8.4. Case–control studies on tobacco smoking and liver cancer

Reference Country and years of study	No. of cases and controls	Smoking categories	Relative risk (95% CI)	Adjustment/comments
Williams & Horn (1977) USA 1969–71	40/204	*Pack–years* < 20 20–39 ≥ 40	Men Women 0.6 0.3 2.3 – 3.1 1.6	Adjusted for age and sex. Non-significant odds ratios
Trichopoulos *et al.* (1980) Greece 1976–77	19/107	*Cigarettes/day* 1–10 11–20 21–30 ≥ 31	1.3 2.5[†] 3.7[†] 8.4[†]	Persistence of effect after adjusting for alcohol consumption [†]significantly higher than 1
Lam *et al.* (1982) Hong Kong 1977–80	265/530	≥ 20 cigarettes/day	3.3 (1.0–13.4)	Overall, no significant association between alcohol consumption and liver cancer. Peanuts not considered as important source of aflatoxin
Stemhagen *et al.* (1983) USA 1975–80	78/78	Ever-smoker	Men Women 0.7 (0.5–1.1) 1.0 (0.6–1.7)	No difference when adjusted for alcohol consumption. No dose–response
Yu *et al.* (1983) USA 1975–79		Former smoker ≤ 20 cigarettes/day > 20 cigarettes/day	1.1 (0.3–4.0) 1.2 (0.6–2.5) 2.6 (1.0–6.7)	Adjusted for alcohol. Nonsmokers and former smokers combined. [The Working Group considered that because only 4 controls drank ≥ 80 g/day ethanol, there were insufficient data to study the effect of smoking among heavy drinkers. Among lighter drinkers, the effect does not reach significance, is lower in magnitude that the unstratified effect and may be influenced by residual confounding.]
Hardell *et al.* (1984) Sweden 1974–81	98/200			The small positive association between HCC and smoking disappeared after controlling for alcohol consumption. Strong association between smoking and cholangiocarcinoma

Table 2.1.8.4 (contd)

Reference, Country and years of study	No. of cases and controls	Smoking categories	Relative risk (95% CI)	Adjustment/comments
Austin et al. (1986) USA	86/172	Ever-smoker	1.3 (NS)	Unadjusted
		Current smoker	1.5 (0.7–3.7)	
		Former smoker	0.9 (NS)	Adjusted for alcohol consumption
		Ever-smoker	1.0 (0.5–1.8)	
		Current smoker	1.1 (0.5–2.4)	Adjusted for HBsAg status and alcohol consumption
		Pack–years		
		1–24	0.9 (NS)	
		25–49	2.6 (NS)	
		≥ 50	0.8 (NS)	
La Vecchia et al. (1988) Italy 1984–87	151/1051	Former smoker	0.7 (0.4–1.0)	Adjusted for age, sex, geographical area, hepatitis, cirrhosis and alcohol consumption
		Current smoker	0.9 (0.6–1.5)	
Ferraroni et al. (1989) Italy 1983–88	151/1944	Former smoker	0.9	Adjusted for age, sex, alcohol, education, marital status and coffee consumption. No difference when adjusted for age and sex only
		Cigarettes/day		
		< 15	0.9 (NS)	
		15–24	0.7 (NS)	
		≥ 25	0.8 (NS)	
Hiyama et al. (1990) Japan 1984–87	229/266	*Pack–years*		Adjusted for HBsAg status, age, sex, alcohol consumption and family history of liver cancer
		< 20	1.0 (baseline)	
		20–39	1.9 (1.1–3.3)	
		40–59	2.0 (1.1–3.6)	
		≥ 60	1.0 (0.5–1.9)	
Kew et al. (1990) South Africa	46/92	Current smoker	2.2 (0.8–6.1)	
		Cigarettes/day		
		< 10	2.1 (0.8–7.1)	
		≥ 10	2.1 (0.4–10.7)	
Vall Mayans et al. (1990) Spain 1986–88	96/190	*Cigarettes/day*		χ² for trend = 0.01. No difference after adjustment for HBV or alcohol consumption
		1–20	1.4	
		> 20	1.1	

Table 2.1.8.4 (contd)

Reference Country and years of study	No. of cases and controls	Smoking categories	Relative risk (95% CI)			Adjustment/comments
Olubuyide & Bamgboye (1990) Nigeria 1987–88	100/100	*Current smoker*				Adjusted for age and sex
		All	1.7 (0.9–3.1) $p < 0.1$			
		Men	1.5 (0.8–2.8)			
		Women	7.1 (0.7–26.5)			
Tsukuma *et al.* (1990) Japan 1983–87	229/266	**Men and women**				
		Former smoker	0.7			
		Current smoker	2.5 (1.4–4.5)			
		Cigarettes/day				
		1–19	4.2			
		20–39	2.2			
		≥ 40	1.1			
		Pack–years	*All*	*Men*	*Women*	
		0–19	1.0	1.0	1.0	
		20–39	1.7 (1.0–2.8)	1.6 (0.9–2.8)	[2.4]	
		40–50	1.8 (1.0–3.1)	1.9 (1.1–3.4)		
		≥ 50	1.0 (0.5–1.8)	0.9 (0.5–1.7)	[1.6]	
		Men				Adjusted for age
		Former smoker	0.8			
		Current smoker	2.3 (1.1–4.8)			
		Cigarettes/day				
		1–19	3.4			
		20–39	2.5			
		≥ 40	1.0			
		Women				Crude risk estimates
		Current smoker	2.9 (1.1–7.9)			
		Cigarettes/day				
		1–19	[6.1]			
		≥ 20	[1.1]			

Table 2.1.8.4 (contd)

Reference Country and years of study	No. of cases and controls	Smoking categories	Relative risk (95% CI)	Adjustment/comments
Chen et al. (1991) China, Province of Taiwan 1985–87	200/200	*Cigarettes/day* 1–10 11–20 ≥ 21	1.1 (0.6–2.0) 1.9 (1.2–3.1) 3.0 (1.5–5.8)	Matched univariate analysis
Choi & Kahyo (1991) Republic of Korea 1986–90	216/648	Former smoker Current smoker *Cigarettes/day* 1–20 21–40 ≥ 41 *Duration (years)* 1–19 20–39 ≥ 40	0.7 (0.4–1.2) 1.0 (0.7–1.6) 1.2 (0.8–1.8) 0.6 (0.3–1.2) 0.5 (0.1–2.6) 0.7 (0.4–1.3) 1.0 (0.6–1.6) 1.9 (0.4–1.8)	Adjusted for HBV status, age, alcohol consumption, education and marital status
Lin et al. (1991) China 1984–86	200/200	Current smoker	2.1 (1.3–3.2)	Adjusted for age; study in an aflatoxin-endemic region of China
Tzonou et al. (1991) Greece 1976–84	185/432	HCC cases with cirrhosis HCC cases without cirrhosis HBsAg-positive cases and controls HBsAg-negative cases and controls	2.3 (0.9–5.9) 2.1 (1.1–4.0) 1.7 (0.5–5.6) 2.4 (1.2–4.7)	Adjusted for age and sex Adjusted for HBsAg and HCV status Adjusted for age and sex Adjusted for HCV status [Crude odds ratio, 1.7 (95% CI, 1.1–2.6)]

Table 2.1.8.4 (contd)

Reference Country and years of study	No. of cases and controls	Smoking categories	Relative risk (95% CI)		Adjustment/comments
Yu, M.W. et al. (1991) China, Province of Taiwan 1986–87	127 pairs of cases and controls	*Cigarettes/day* 1–10 11–20 > 20	1.1 (0.5–2.2) 1.8 (1.0–3.4) 1.7 (0.7–4.5)		Matched odds ratio
		1–10 11–20 > 20	0.4 (0.1–1.9) 1.3 (0.4–4.2) 2.1 (0.3–13.5)		Adjusted for HBV and HCV status, alcohol and peanut consumption
Yu, M.C. et al. (1991) USA 1984–90	74/162	Former smoker Current smoker	*All* 1.6 (0.7–3.5) 2.5 (1.2–5.0)	*Men* 1.8 (0.7–4.8) 2.8 (1.0–7.9)	*Women* 1.4 (0.3–6.5) 2.4 (0.8–6.9)	Unadjusted
		Cigarettes/day ≤ 19 ≥ 20 Former smoker Current smoker *Current smoker* HBV/HCV-positive HBV/HCV-negative	2.8 (1.2–6.9) 2.2 (1.0–5.0) 1.1 (0.4–2.6) 2.1 (1.1–4.3) 1.8 (0.5–6.2) 3.4 (0.9–12.5)	3.7 (1.0–13.3) 2.4 (0.8–7.4) 1.1 (0.4–3.3) 2.2 (0.8–6.0)	2.1 (0.6–7.7) 2.9 (0.7–11.7) 0.8 (0.1–8.9) 2.4 (0.9–6.7)	Adjusted for alcohol consumption Adjusted for age, sex and ethnicity
Mohamed et al. (1992) South Africa	101/101	*Cigarettes/day* 0–19 ≥ 20	*Men* 1.3 (0.5–3.4) 0.7 (0.2–2.5)	*Women* 2.2 (0.3–6.3) –		Adjusted for alcohol, age and HBV status
Tanaka et al. (1992) Japan 1985–89	204/410	Former smoker Current smoker *Pack–years* < 10.9 11–26.2 26.3–35.9 ≥ 36	*All* 1.6 (0.9–2.8) 1.5 (0.5–2.5) 1 1.4 (0.8–2.3) 1.2 (0.7–2.1) 1.4 (0.8–2.4)	*Men* 1.8 (0.9–3.5) 1.7 (0.9–3.2)	*Women* 1.7 (0.4–7.1) 1.0 (0.3–3.2)	Adjusted for age and sex. Subjects with chronic hepatitis and cirrhosis exluded from control group. Histologically confirmed cases (82) did not differ from the remaining cases of liver cancer in their smoking habits.

Table 2.1.8.4 (contd)

Reference Country and years of study	No. of cases and controls	Smoking categories	Relative risk (95% CI)	Adjustment/comments
Peters et al. (1994) Germany 1986–93	86/86	Current smoker of > 40 pack–years	1.2 (0.5–2.9)	Adjusted for alcohol and HBV and HCV status
Pyong et al. (1994) Japan 1989–92	90/249	*Cigarettes/day* 1–20 > 20	 0.7 (0.2–2.4) 0.4 (0.1–1.6)	Adjusted for age, sex, HBV and HCV status, transfusion and alcohol consumption
Siemiatycki et al. (1995) Canada 1979–86	48/2238	Ever-smoker *Pack–years* <25 25–49 50–74 ≥ 75	0.9 (0.4–2.1) 1.4 (0.5–3.8) 0.7 (0.3–1.9) 0.7 (0.2–2.2) 0.8 (0.3–2.7)	Adjusted for age; cancer control group had cancer at sites not previously associated with cigarette smoking
Tanaka et al. (1995) Japan 1983–89	120/257	Former smoker Current smoker Male ever-smoker *Pack–years* 0.1–12.9 ≥ 13.0	2.2 (1.2–4.1) 2.8 (1.1–6.9) 1.9 (1.2–2.8) 2.4 (1.1–4.9) 1.8 (0.8–3.7)	Adjusted for age, study category (except for ever-smokers), HBV, history of transfusion, family history of liver cancer and alcohol consumption. Combined analysis of 3 studies; partial overlap with Tanaka et al. (1992)
Shin et al. (1996) Republic of Korea 1990–93	203/406	*Current smoker* Moderate High (> 20 cigs/day for > 10 years)	 2.3 (0.4–11.7) 1.1 (0.3–2.5)	Adjusted for HBV/HCV status, *Clonorchis sinensis*, history of hepatitis, liver, alcohol consumption and socioeconomic status

Table 2.1.8.4 (contd)

Reference, Country and years of study	No. of cases and controls	Smoking categories	Relative risk (95% CI)		Adjustment/comments
Liu et al. (1998) China 1989–91	29 187/ 87 215	*Ever-smoker*[†]	*Men*	*Women*	Adjusted for age and study area (county or city). Retrospective proportional mortality study. Latency, 6–8 years. [†]Values in parentheses are standard errors.
		Urban	1.4 (0.03)	1.5 (0.06)	
		Rural	1.4 (0.04)	1.1 (0.08)	
		All China weighted	1.4 (0.03)	1.2 (0.06)	
		Current smoker	*Urban men*	*Rural men*	
		Cigarettes/day			
		1–19	1.4 (0.03)	1.5 (0.05)	
		20	1.5 (0.04)	1.6 (0.06)	
		> 20	1.6 (0.07)	1.8 (0.12)	
		Age at starting smoking (years)			
		< 20	1.4 (0.04)	1.4 (0.06)	
		20–24	1.4 (0.03)	1.4 (0.04)	
		≥ 25	1.4 (0.04)	1.4 (0.05)	
Mukaiya et al. (1998) Japan 1991–93	104/104	≥ 5 years vs < 5 years	3.3 (1.3–8.3)		Adjusted for age and sex
		≥ 10 pack/years vs < 10 pack–years	3.3 (1.3–8.3)		
Kuper et al. (2000) Greece 1995–98	333/360		*< 40 cigarettes/day*	*≥ 40 cigarettes/day*	
		Former smoker	1.2 (0.7–1.9)	1.5 (0.7–3.0)	
		Current smoker	1.2 (0.8–1.9)	1.6 (0.9–2.9)	
		Ever-smoker	1.6 (0.8–2.9)	2.5 (1.1–5.5)	Adjusted for age, sex and HBV and HCV status
		Current smoker			Adjusted for age, sex, education and HBV and HCV status
		HBV- and HCV-negative	1.8 (0.9–3.6)	2.8 (1.1–6.9)	
		HBV- and/or HCV-positive	1.3 (0.3–5.6)	2.1 (0.3–17.1)	
		All, adjusted for HBV/HCV	1.6 (0.8–2.9)	2.5 (1.1–5.5)	

Table 2.1.8.4 (contd)

Reference Country and years of study	No. of cases and controls	Smoking categories	Relative risk (95% CI)		Adjustment/comments
Lam et al. (2001) Hong Kong SAR 1998	27 507/ 13 054	*Ever-smoker* Aged 35–59 Aged ≥ 70	*Men* 1.6 (1.3–1.9) 1.2 (0.9–1.5)	*Women* 1.4 (0.8–2.4) 1.4 (0.9–2.0)	Adjusted for age and education
Chen et al. (2003) USA 1986–88	36 000 cases/ 17 000 controls with cirrhosis	Ever-smoker *Cigarettes/day (approx.)* 10 20 30 *p* for trend	*Men* 1.4 (1.3–1.4) 1.3 1.5 1.6 < 0.001	*Women* 1.2 (1.1–1.3) 1.1 (0.9–1.3) 1.5 (1.2–1.8) –	Adjusted for age and locality. Relative risk independent of age, urban/rural status or age at start of smoking

CI, confidence interval; NS, not significant; HBsAg, hepatitis B surface antigen; HBV, hepatitis B virus; HCC, hepatocellular carcinoma; HCV, hepatitis C virus

References

Akiba, S. & Hirayama, T. (1990) Cigarette smoking and cancer mortality risk in Japanese men and women — Results from reanalysis of the six-prefecture cohort study data. *Environ. Health Perspect.*, **87**, 19–26

Austin, H., Delzell, E., Grufferman, S., Levine, R., Morrison, A.S., Stolley, P.D. & Cole, P. (1986) A case–control study of hepatocellular carcinoma and the hepatitis B virus, cigarette smoking, and alcohol consumption. *Cancer Res.*, **46**, 962–966

Basa, G.F., Hirayama, T. & Cruz-Basa, A.G. (1977) Cancer epidemiology in the Philippines. *Natl Cancer Inst. Monogr.*, **47**, 45–56

Carstensen, J.M., Pershagen, G. & Eklund, G. (1987) Mortality in relation to cigarette and pipe smoking: 16 years' observation of 25 000 Swedish men. *J. Epidemiol. Community Health*, **41**, 166–172

Chang, C.C., Yu, M.W., Lu, C.F., Yang, C.S. & Chen, C.J. (1994) A nested case–control study on association between hepatitis C virus antibodies and primary liver cancer in a cohort of 9775 men in Taiwan. *J. med. Virol.*, **43**, 276–280

Chen, C.J., Liang, K.Y., Chang, A.S., Chang, Y.C., Lu, S.N., Liaw, Y.F., Chang, W.Y., Sheen, M.C. & Lin, T.M. (1991) Effects of hepatitis B virus, alcohol drinking, cigarette smoking and familial tendency on hepatocellular carcinoma. *Hepatology*, **13**, 398–406

Chen, Z.M., Xu, Z., Collins, R., Li, W.X. & Peto, R. (1997) Early health effects of the emerging tobacco epidemic in China. A 16-year prospective study. *J. Am. med. Assoc.*, **278**, 1500–1504

Chen, Z.M., Liu, B.Q., Boreham, J., Wu, Y.P., Chen, J.S. & Peto, R. (2003) Smoking and liver cancer in China: Case–control comparison of 36 000 liver cancer deaths vs. 17 000 cirrhosis deaths. *Int. J. Cancer*, **107**, 106–112

Chiba, T., Matsuzaki, Y., Abei, M., Shoda, J., Tanaka, N., Osuga, T. & Aikawa, T. (1996) The role of previous hepatitis B virus infection and heavy smoking in hepatitis C virus-related hepatocellular carcinoma. *Am. J. Gastroenterol.*, **91**, 1195–1203

Choi, S.Y. & Kahyo, H. (1991) Effect of cigarette smoking and alcohol consumption in the etiology of cancers of the digestive tract. *Int. J. Cancer*, **49**, 381–386

Doll, R., Peto, R., Wheatley, K., Gray, R. & Sutherland, I. (1994) Mortality in relation to smoking: 40 years' observations on male British doctors. *Br. med. J.*, **309**, 901–911

Evans, A.A., Chen, G., Ross, E.A., Shen, F.M., Lin, W.Y. & London, W.T. (2002) Eight-year follow-up of the 90 000-person Haimen City cohort: I. Hepatocellular carcinoma mortality, risk factors, and gender differences. *Cancer Epidemiol. Biomarkers Prev.*, **11**, 369–76

Ferraroni, M., Negri, E., La Vecchia, C., D'Avanzo, B. & Franceschi, S. (1989) Socioeconomic indicators, tobacco and alcohol in the aetiology of digestive tract neoplasms. *Int. J. Epidemiol.*, **18**, 556–562

Gao, Y.T., Den, J., Xiang, Y., Ruan, Z., Wang, Z., Hu, B., Guo, M., Teng, W., Han, J. & Zhang, Y. (1999) [Smoking, related cancers, and other diseases in Shanghai: A 10-year prospective study.] *Chin. J. Prev. Med.*, **33**, 5–8 (in Chinese)

Goodman, M.T., Moriwaki, H., Vaeth, M., Akiba, S., Hayabuchi, H. & Mabuchi, K. (1995) Prospective cohort study of risk factors for primary liver cancer in Hiroshima and Nagasaki, Japan. *Epidemiology*, **6**, 36–41

Hammond, E.C. (1966) Smoking in relation to the death rates of one million men and women. *Natl Cancer Inst. Monogr.*, **19**, 127–204

Hardell, L., Bengtsson, N.O., Jonsson, U., Eriksson, S. & Larsson, L.G. (1984) Aetiological aspects on primary liver cancer with special regard to alcohol, organic solvents and acute intermittent porphyria — An epidemiological investigation. *Br. J. Cancer*, **50**, 389–397

Hiyama, T., Tsukuma, H., Oshima, A. & Fujimoto, I. (1990) Liver cancer and life style — Drinking habits and smoking habits. *Gan No Rinsho*, **Spec. No.**, 249–256

Hirayama, T. (1981) A large scale cohort study on the relationship between diet and selected cancers of digestive organs. In: Bruce, W. R., Correa, P., Lipkin, M., Tannenbaum, S.R. & Wilkins, T.D., eds, *Gastrointestinal Cancer: Endogenous Factors* (Banbury Report 7), Cold Spring Harbor, NY, Cold Spring Harbor Laboratory, pp. 409–426

Hsing, W., McLaughlin, J.K., Hrubec, Z., Blot, W.J. & Fraumeni, J.F. (1990) Cigarette smoking and liver cancer among US veterans. *Cancer Causes Control*, **1**, 217–221

IARC (1986) *IARC Monographs on the Evaluation of the Carcinogenic Risk of Chemicals to Humans*, Vol. 38, *Tobacco Smoking*, Lyon, IARCPress

IARC (1988) *IARC Monographs on the Evaluation of Carcinogenic Risks Humans*, Vol. 44, *Alcohol Drinking*, Lyon, IARCPress

IARC (1994) *IARC Monographs on the Evaluation of Carcinogenic Risks Humans*, Vol. 59, *Hepatitis Viruses*, Lyon, IARCPress

Kato, I., Tominaga, S. & Ikari, A. (1992) The risk and predictive factors for developing liver cancer among patients with decompensated liver cirrhosis. *Jpn. J. clin. Oncol.*, **22**, 278–285

Kew, M.C., Song, E., Mohammed, A. & Hodkinson, J. (1990) Contraceptive steroids as a risk factor for hepatocellular carcinoma: A case–control study in South African black women. *Hepatology*, **11**, 298–302

Kono, S., Ikeda, M., Tokudome, S., Nishizumi, M. & Kuratsune, M. (1987) Cigarette smoking, alcohol and cancer mortality: A cohort study of male Japanese physicians. *Jpn. J. Cancer Res.*, **78**, 1323–1328

Kuper, H., Tzonou, A., Kaklamani, E., Hsieh, C.C., Lagiou, P., Adami, H.O., Trichopoulos, D. & Stuver, S.O. (2000) Tobacco smoking, alcohol consumption and their interaction in the causation of hepatocellular carcinoma. *Int. J. Cancer*, **85**, 498–502

Lam, K.C., Yu, M.C., Leung, J.W. & Henderson, B.E. (1982) Hepatitis B virus and cigarette smoking: Risk factors for hepatocellular carcinoma in Hong Kong. *Cancer Res.*, **42**, 5246–5248

Lam, T.H., He, Y., Li, L.S., Li, L.S., He, S.F. & Liang, B.Q. (1997) Mortality attributable to cigarette smoking in China. *J. Am. med. Assoc.*, **278**, 1505–1508

Lam, T.H., Ho, S.Y. & Hedley, A.J. (2001) Mortality and smoking in Hong Kong: Case control study of all adult deaths in 1998. *Br. med. J.*, **326**, 1–6

La Vecchia, C., Negri, E., Decarli, A., D'Avanzo, B. & Franceschi, S. (1988) Risk factors for hepatocellular carcinoma in northern Italy. *Int. J. Cancer*, **42**, 872–876

Liaw, K.M. & Chen, C.J. (1998) Mortality attributable to cigarette smoking in Taiwan: A 12-year follow-up study. *Tob. Control*, **7**, 141–148

Lin, L., Yang, F., Ye, Z., Xu, E., Yang, C., Zhang, C., Wu, D. & Nebert, D.W. (1991) Case–control study of cigarette smoking and primary hepatoma in an aflatoxin-endemic region of China: A protective effect. *Pharmacogenetics*, **1**, 79–85

Liu, Q., Peto, R., Chen, Z.M., Boreham, J., Wu, Y.P., Li, J.Y., Campbell, T.C. & Chen, J.S. (1998) Emerging tobacco hazards in China: 1. Retrospective proportional mortality study of one million deaths. *Br. med. J.*, **317**, 1411–1422

London, W.T., Evans, A.A., McGlynn, K., Buetow, K., An, P., Gao, L., Lustbader, E., Ross, E., Chen, G. & Shen, F. (1995) Viral, host and environmental risk factors for hepatocellular carcinoma: a prospective study in Haimen City, China. *Intervirology*, **38**, 155–161

McLaughlin, J.K., Hrubec, Z., Blot, W.J. & Fraumeni, J.F. (1995) Smoking and cancer mortality among US veterans: A 26-year follow-up. *Int. J. Cancer*, **60**, 190–193

Mizoue, T., Tokui, N., Nishisaka, K., Nishisaka, S., Ogimoto, I., Ikeda, M. & Yoshimura, T. (2000) Prospective study on the relation of cigarette smoking with cancer of the liver and stomach in an endemic region. *Int. J. Epidemiol.*, **29**, 232–237

Mohamed, E., Kew, M.C. & Groeneveld, H.T. (1992) Alcohol consumption as a risk factor for hepatocellular carcinoma in urban southern African blacks. *Int. J. Cancer*, **51**, 537–541

Mori, M., Hara, M., Wada, I., Hara, T., Yamamoto, K., Honda, M. & Naramoto, J. (2000) Prospective study of hepatitis B and C viral infections, cigarette smoking, alcohol consumption, and other factors associated with hepatocellular carcinoma risk in Japan. *Am. J. Epidemiol.*, **151**, 131–139

Mukaiya, M., Nishi, M., Miyake, H. & Hirata, K. (1998) Chronic liver diseases for the risk of hepatocellular carcinoma: A case–control study in Japan. Etiologic association of alcohol consumption, cigarette smoking and the development of chronic liver diseases. *Hepatogastroenterology*, **45**, 2328–2332

Murata, M., Takayama, K., Choi, B.C.K. & Pak, A.W.P. (1996) A nested case–control study on alcohol drinking, tobacco smoking, and cancer. *Cancer Detect. Prev.*, **20**, 557–565

Nordlund, L.A., Carstensen, J.M. & Pershagen, G. (1997) Cancer incidence in female smokers: A 26-year follow-up. *Int. J. Cancer*, **73**, 625–628

Olubuyide, O. & Bamgboye, E.A. (1990) A case–controlled study of the current role of cigarette smoking and alcohol consumption in primary liver cell carcinoma in Nigerians. *Afr. J. Med. med. Sci.*, **19**, 191–194

Peters, M., Wellek, S., Dienes, H.P., Junginger, T., Meyer, J., Meyer-Zum-Buschendfelde, K.H. & Gerken, G. (1994) Epidemiology of hepatocellular carcinoma. Evaluation of viral and other risk factors in a low-endemic area for hepatitis B and C. *Z. Gastroenterol.*, **32**, 146–151

Pyong, S.J., Tsukuma, H. & Hyama, T. (1994) Case–control study of hepatocellular carcinoma among Koreans living in Osaka, Japan. *Jpn. J. Cancer Res.*, **85**, 674–679

Ross, R.K., Yuan, J.M., Yu, M.C., Wogan, G.N., Qian, G.S., Tu, J.T., Groopman, J.D., Gao, Y.T. & Henderson, B.E. (1992) Urinary aflatoxin biomarkers and risk of hepatocellular carcinoma. *Lancet*, **339**, 943–946

Shibata, A., Fukuda, K., Toshima, H., Tashiro, H. & Hirohata, T. (1990) The role of cigarette smoking and drinking in the development of liver cancer: 28 years of observations on male cohort members in a farming and fishing area. *Cancer Detect. Prev.*, **14**, 617–623

Shin, H.R., Lee, C.U., Park, H.J., Seol, S.Y., Chung, J.M., Choi, H.C., Ahn, Y.O. & Shigemastu, T. (1996) Hepatitis B and C virus, Clonorchis sinensis for the risk of liver cancer: A case–control study in Pusan, Korea. *Int. J. Epidemiol.*, **25**, 933–940

Siemiatycki, J., Krewski, D., Franco, E. & Kaiserman, M. (1995) Associations between cigarette smoking and each of 21 types of cancer: A multi-site case–control study. *Int. J. Epidemiol.*, **24**, 504–514

Stemhagen, A., Slade, J., Altman, R. & Bill, J. (1983) Occupational risk factors and liver cancer. A retrospective case–control study of primary liver cancer in New Jersey. *Am. J. Epidemiol.*, **117**, 443–454

Sun, Z., Lu, P., Gail, M.H., Pee, D., Zhang, Q., Ming, L., Wang, J., Wu, Y., Liu, G., Wu, Y. & Zhu, Y. (1999) Increased risk of hepatocellular carcinoma in male hepatitis B surface antigen carriers with chronic hepatitis who have detectable urinary aflatoxin metabolite M1. *Hepatology*, **30**, 379–383

Tanaka, K., Hirohata, T., Takeshita, S., Hirohata, I., Koga, S., Sugimachi, K., Kanematsu, T., Ohryohji, F. & Ishibashi, H. (1992) Hepatitis B virus, cigarette smoking and alcohol consumption in the development of hepatocellular carcinoma: A case–control study in Fukuoka, Japan. *Int. J. Cancer*, **51**, 509–514

Tanaka, K., Hirohata, T., Fukuda, K., Shibata, A., Tsukuma, H. & Hiyama, T. (1995) Risk factors for hepatocellular carcinoma among Japanese women. *Cancer Causes Control*, **6**, 91–98

Trichopoulos, D., MacMahon, B., Sparros, L. & Merikas, G. (1980) Smoking and hepatitis B-negative primary hepatocellular carcinoma. *J. natl Cancer Inst.*, **65**, 111–114

Tsukuma, H., Hiyama, T., Oshima, A., Sobue, T., Fujimoto, I., Kasugai, H., Kojima, J., Sasaki, Y., Imaoka, S., Horiuchi, N. & Okuda, S. (1990) A case–control study of hepatocellular carcinoma in Osaka, Japan. *Int. J. Cancer*, **45**, 231–236

Tsukuma, H., Hiyama, T., Tanaka, S., Nakao, M., Tabuuchi, T., Kitamura, T., Nakahishi, K., Fujimoto, I., Inoue, A., Yamazaki, H. & Kawashima, T. (1993) Risk factors for hepatocellular carcinoma among patients with chronic liver disease. *New Engl. J. Med.*, **328**, 1797–1801

Tu, J.T., Gao, R.N. & Zhang, D.H. (1985) Hepatitis B virus and primary liver cancer. *Natl Cancer Inst. Monogr.*, **69**, 213–215

Tzonou, A., Trichopoulos, D., Kaklamani, E., Zavitsanos, X., Koumantaki, Y. & Hsieh, C.C. (1991) Epidemiologic assessment of interactions of hepatitis-C virus with seromarkers of hepatitis-B and -D viruses, cirrhosis and tobacco smoking in hepatocellular carcinoma. *Int. J. Cancer*, **49**, 377–380

Vall Mayans, M., Calvet, X., Bruxi, J., Bruguera, M., Costa, J., Estève, J., Bosch, F.X., Bru, C. & Rodés, J. (1990) Risk factors for hepatocellular carcinoma in Catalonia, Spain. *Int. J. Cancer*, **46**, 378–381

Williams, R.R. & Horm, J.W. (1977) Association of cancer sites with tobacco and alcohol consumption and socioeconomic status of patients: Interview study from the Third National Cancer Survey. *J. natl Cancer Inst.*, 58, 525–547

Yang, H.-I., Lu, S.-N., Liaw, Y.-F., You, S.-L., Sun, C.-A., Wang, L.-Y., Hsiao, C. K., Chen, P.-J., Chen, D.-S., Chen, C.-J. & the Taiwan Community-Based Cancer Screening Project Group (2002) Hepatitis B e antigen and the risk of hepatocellular carcinoma. *New Engl. J. Med.*, **347**, 168–174

Yu, M.W. & Chen, C.J. (1993) Elevated serum testosterone levels and risk of hepatocellular carcinoma. *Cancer Res.*, **53**, 790–794

Yu, M.C., Mack, T., Hanisch, R., Peters, R.L., Henderson, B.E. & Pike, M.C. (1983) Hepatitis, alcohol consumption, cigarette smoking, and hepatocellular carcinoma in Los Angeles. *Cancer Res.*, **43**, 6077–6079

Yu, M.C., Tong, M.J., Govindarajan, S. & Henderson, B.E. (1991) Nonviral risk factors for hepatocellular carcinoma in a low-risk population, the non-Asians of Los Angeles County, California. *J. natl Cancer Inst.*, **83**, 1820–1826

Yu, M.W., You, S.L., Chang, A.S., Lu, S.N., Liaw, Y.F. & Chen, C.J. (1991) Association between hepatitis C virus antibodies and hepatocellular carcinoma in Taiwan. *Cancer Res.*, **51**, 5621–5625

Yu, M.W., Hsu, F.C., Sheen, I.S., Chu, C.M., Lin, D.Y., Chen, C.J. & Liaw, Y.F. (1997) Prospective study of hepatocellular carcinoma and liver cirrhosis in asymptomatic chronic hepatitis B virus carriers. *Am. J. Epidemiol.*, **145**, 1039–47

Yuan, J.M., Ross, R.K., Wang, X.L., Gao, Y.T., Henderson, B.E. & Yu, M.C. (1996) Morbidity and mortality in relation to cigarette smoking in Shanghai, China. A prospective male cohort study. *J. Am. med. Assoc.*, **275**, 1646–1650

2.1.9   Breast cancer

Indirect evidence suggests that smoking could conceivably reduce the risk for breast cancer. It is recognized that high levels of estrogens, particularly of estrone and estradiol, contribute to an increased risk for breast cancer and smoking is thought to have an anti-estrogenic effect. The occurrence of menopause at an earlier age among smokers than among nonsmokers is also well established, and late age at menopause has been consistently related to an increased risk for breast cancer. Conversely, cigarette smoke contains carcinogens that could plausibly affect the breast (US Department of Health and Human Services, 2001). Research is in progress to determine whether some population groups are placed genetically at a higher risk for breast cancer associated with smoking (see Section 4).

A total of 18 case–control and cohort studies that addressed the association of tobacco smoke with breast cancer were reviewed by the IARC Working Group on Tobacco Smoke in 1986 (IARC, 1986). A suggestion of a decreased risk was noted, but the reported relative risks were distributed on both sides of unity, ranging from 0.7 to 1.4. While the epidemiological evidence was consistent with a decrease in risk, it could not be concluded that this had been demonstrated.

Thirty-six case–control studies and eight cohort studies as well as one large pooled analysis of data from 10 cohort and 29 case–control studies from the Collaborative Group on Hormonal Factors in Breast Cancer Study (2002) were examined to assess the relationship between smoking and breast cancer risk. The characteristics of the case–control studies and the principal findings relative to the association with smoking are shown in Tables 2.1.9.1 and 2.1.9.2, respectively. Descriptions of all cohort studies are presented at the beginning of Section 2 and in Tables 2.1 and 2.1.9.3, and the results for breast cancer are given in Table 2.1.9.4. The studies included in the analysis by the Oxford Collaboration and the results of the pooled analysis are shown in Table 2.1.9.5 and Figure 2.1.9.1 (Collaborative Group on Hormonal Factors in Breast Cancer, 2002).

The Oxford Collaborative Study included over 80% of the worldwide epidemiological data on breast cancer and on alcohol and tobacco consumption. Overall, the analyses for tobacco exposure included 58 515 women with invasive breast cancer and 95 067 controls from 53 studies, in which individual data on both alcohol and tobacco consumption had been recorded. Case–control and cohort studies were eligible for the collaborative analysis if they included at least 100 women with incident invasive breast cancer and had information on reproductive factors and on use of hormonal therapies. Cohort studies were included using a nested case–control design, in which four controls were selected at random, matched on follow-up to the age of the case at diagnosis and, where appropriate, matched on broad geographical region. Only active smoking was considered and no attention was given to the reported associations with passive exposures, nor was information obtained on the age when women started or stopped smoking, or the amount smoked. Relative risks of breast cancer were estimated, after stratifying by study, age, parity and, when indicated, women's age at time of first birth and their consumption of alcohol and tobacco.

Figure 2.1.9.1. Relative risk of breast cancer in relation to tobacco consumption in various subgroups of women

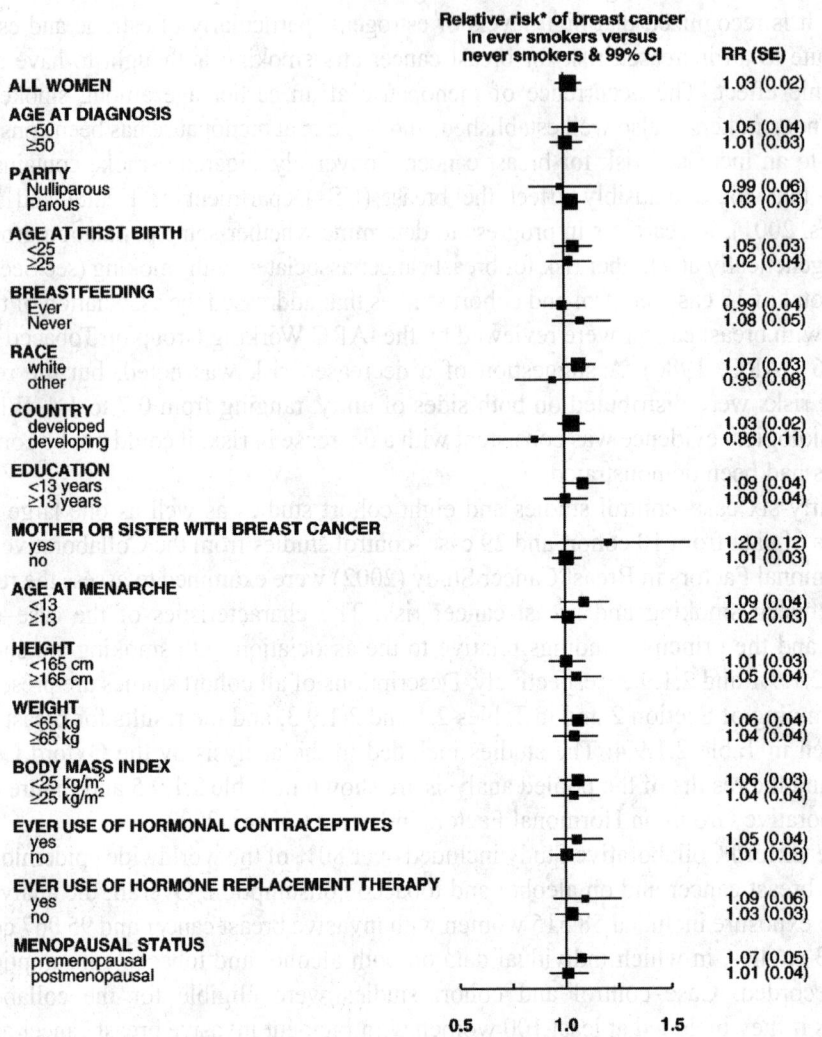

Relative risk* of breast cancer
in ever smokers versus
never smokers & 99% CI

	RR (SE)
ALL WOMEN	1.03 (0.02)
AGE AT DIAGNOSIS	
<50	1.05 (0.04)
≥50	1.01 (0.03)
PARITY	
Nulliparous	0.99 (0.06)
Parous	1.03 (0.03)
AGE AT FIRST BIRTH	
<25	1.05 (0.03)
≥25	1.02 (0.04)
BREASTFEEDING	
Ever	0.99 (0.04)
Never	1.08 (0.05)
RACE	
white	1.07 (0.03)
other	0.95 (0.08)
COUNTRY	
developed	1.03 (0.02)
developing	0.86 (0.11)
EDUCATION	
<13 years	1.09 (0.04)
≥13 years	1.00 (0.04)
MOTHER OR SISTER WITH BREAST CANCER	
yes	1.20 (0.12)
no	1.01 (0.03)
AGE AT MENARCHE	
<13	1.09 (0.04)
≥13	1.02 (0.03)
HEIGHT	
<165 cm	1.01 (0.03)
≥165 cm	1.05 (0.04)
WEIGHT	
<65 kg	1.06 (0.04)
≥65 kg	1.04 (0.04)
BODY MASS INDEX	
<25 kg/m²	1.06 (0.03)
≥25 kg/m²	1.04 (0.04)
EVER USE OF HORMONAL CONTRACEPTIVES	
yes	1.05 (0.04)
no	1.01 (0.03)
EVER USE OF HORMONE REPLACEMENT THERAPY	
yes	1.09 (0.06)
no	1.03 (0.03)
MENOPAUSAL STATUS	
premenopausal	1.07 (0.05)
postmenopausal	1.01 (0.01)

0.5   1.0   1.5

*Stratified by study, age, parity and age at first birth; analyses restricted to women who reported drinking no alcohol

RR, relative risk; SE, standard error

The collaborative analysis examined the relationship between smoking and breast cancer and found it to be substantially confounded by the effect of alcohol consumption. When the analyses were restricted to 22 255 cases and 40 832 controls reported to drink no alcohol, smoking was not associated with breast cancer (compared with never-smokers, the relative risk for ever-smokers was 1.03 (95% CI, 0.98–1.07) and the relative risk for current smokers was 0.99 (95% CI, 0.92–1.05)). The findings for tobacco were not substantially confounded by any other factors, including family history of breast cancer, race, height, weight, age at menarche, menopause or use of hormonal preparations. Furthermore, the results for tobacco exposure and breast cancer did not vary substantially between studies, study designs or by the 15 personal characteristics of the women that were examined (Figure 2.1.9.1).

Among women who reported drinking alcohol, it was difficult to distinguish the independent effects of smoking (Collaborative Group on Hormonal Factors in Breast Cancer Study, 2002). For example, when ever-smokers were compared with never-smokers, the relative risk for breast cancer was 1.09 before stratification by alcohol consumption and was reduced to 1.05 after stratification. Moreover, the corresponding χ^2 (Chi squared) value declined by 75% from 23.4 to 6.4. Among ever-smokers in the 48 studies that gave information on current and past smoking, 54% were current smokers and 46% were past smokers. Compared with never-smokers, the relative risk for breast cancer was 0.99 for current smokers and 1.07 for past smokers.

Eleven studies, comprising a total of 4781 cases and 12 713 controls, contributed data on tobacco consumption for each woman, but no data on alcohol consumption, and were not included in the pooled analysis. The relative risk for breast cancer in ever-smokers compared with never-smokers in this subset of 11 studies was 1.05.

The results of some individual studies, particularly hospital-based case–control studies, must be interpreted cautiously (see General Remarks). Furthermore, questions have been raised about the results of some studies of women who participated in breast cancer screening programmes because the extent to which early detection methods are used may be correlated with smoking behaviour. Population-based case–control studies are generally believed to provide the most valid results.

Confounding

The most serious constraint in the interpretation of results from most studies that have attempted to evaluate the association of exposure to tobacco smoking with breast cancer risk results from the strong correlation of alcohol consumption, an established risk factor for breast cancer, with smoking behaviour, and the imprecision in estimates of the amount of alcohol consumed, especially those based on self-reports. The Oxford Collaborative analysis addressed this constraint by limiting the analysis of the association of breast cancer with tobacco consumption to study subjects who reported never drinking alcohol.

Table 2.1.9.1. Case–control studies on tobacco smoking and breast cancer: main characteristics of study design

Reference Country and years of study	Number of cases and controls	Criteria for eligibility and comments
Rosenberg et al. (1984) USA and Canada 1976–82	2160 cases diagnosed in the last 6 months, and 717 controls, aged 30–69 years	Case–control surveillance programme in medical centers Controls admitted for cancers unrelated to smoking and to age at menopause (e.g. endometrium)
Smith et al. (1984) USA 1980–82	429 cases and 612 controls, aged 20–54 years, matched by age	National population-based study conducted by the CDC Cases histologically confirmed Controls with no previous cancer of the breast, endometrium and ovary 95% response rate for both cases and controls
Schechter et al. (1985) Canada Up to 1982	123 cases and 369 controls, aged 40–59 years, matched by age group and screening center	Multicenter randomized controlled trial (National Breast Screening Study) Criteria for eligibility: no history of breast cancer, not pregnant, no mammogram in the last 12 months Cases histologically confirmed Controls selected among women allocated to mammography
Brinton et al. (1986) USA 1973–1980	1547 cases and 1930 controls, matched by center, ethnicity, age group, time of entry and length of participation in the programme	Multicenter screening programme (Breast Cancer Detection Demonstration Project) Controls selected among women not having received a biopsy 74% response rate for cases and 90% for controls
McTiernan et al. (1986) USA 1981–82	329 cases and 332 controls, aged 25–54 years, matched by age	Population-based study (CDC Cancer and Steroid Hormone Study) Controls selected among women of the county by Waxberg's random-digit dialling method 79% response rate for cases and 87% for controls
O'Connell et al. (1987) USA 1977–78	276 cases and 1519 controls, aged 30 years or older	Population-based study Cases (patients admitted to North Carolina hospitals) histologically confirmed Controls selected from a stratified sample of households within the catchment area of the hospitals where the cases were identified 93% response rate for cases and 88% for controls
Stockwell & Lyman (1987) USA 1981	5246 cases and 3921 controls	Population-based study Controls were residents of the state of Florida diagnosed with colon or rectal cancers, or melanoma, or endocrine neoplasms

Table 2.1.9.1 (contd)

Reference Country and years of study	Number of cases and controls	Criteria for eligibility and comments
Stanford et al. (1987) USA 1980–82	458 cases and 568 controls, aged 20–54 years, matched by age group	Population-based study (Cancer and Steroid Hormone Study) Cases histologically confirmed Controls selected by random-digit dialling in the same geographical area as cases 85% response rate for cases and 90% for controls
Adami et al. (1988) Sweden & Norway 1984–85	422 cases and 527 controls, aged less than 45 years (Sweden) and less than 40 years (Norway), matched by age (Sweden) and day and year of birth (Norway)	Population-based study Cases histologically confirmed Controls with no history of cancer selected from population registers 89% response rate for cases and 81% for controls
Brownson et al. (1988) USA 1979–86	456 cases (88% prevalent) and 1693 controls, matched by age group and county of residence	Screening programme (Columbia Women's Cancer Control Programme) Cases histologically confirmed Controls randomly selected from participants to the programme Near 100% response rates for cases [controls not specified]
Cooper et al. (1989); Rohan & Baron (1989) Australia 1982–84	451 case–control pairs, aged 20–74 years, matched by age	Population-based study Cases histologically confirmed Controls randomly selected from the electoral roll of the Adelaide area 81% response rate for cases; 648 controls approached to achieve a final number of 451
Kato et al. (1989) Japan 1980–86	1740 cases and 8920 controls, aged 20 years and older	No detailed information on study design Cases selected from cancer registry Controls with cancers of known primary site, unrelated to alcohol
Meara et al. (1989) UK 1980–84	998 cases (hospital study) and 118 cases (screening), aged 25–59 years (hospital study) and 45–69 years (screening), and 998 controls matched by age group	Hospital-based study and mammographic screening Controls selected among patients from the same hospital with conditions unrelated to breast cancer or contraceptive practice, and among normal screenees Near 100% response rates in both studies for cases and controls
Schechter et al. (1989) Canada 1982–85 (prevalence study) 1981–87 (incidence study)	254 prevalent cases and 762 controls; 317 incident cases and 951 controls; age 40–59 years	Multicentre randomized controlled trial (National Breast Screening Study) Criteria for eligibility: no history of breast cancer, not pregnant, no mammogram in the last 12 months Cases histologically confirmed Controls selected among women allocated to mammography

Table 2.1.9.1 (contd)

Reference Country and years of study	Number of cases and controls	Criteria for eligibility and comments
Chu *et al.* (1990) USA 1980–82	4720 cases and 4682 controls, aged 20–54 years, matched by age group and geographic location	Population-based study (CDC Cancer and Steroid Hormone Study) Controls selected among women of the county by Waxberg's random-digit dialling method 80% response rate for cases and 88% for controls
Ewertz (1990) Denmark 1983–84	1480 cases and 1332 controls, aged less than 70 years, matched by age	Population-based study Controls with no history of breast cancer identified from the Central Population Register 87% response rate for cases and 78% for controls
Palmer *et al.* (1991) Canada and USA 1982–86	**Canada** 607 cases and 1214 controls under age 70, matched by age and neighbourhood **USA** 1955 cases and 805 controls, aged 30–69 years	**Population-based study in Canada** English-speaking women with no history of cancer were eligible Controls identified from tax assessment rolls 76% response rate for cases and 65% for controls **Hospital-based study in the USA** Controls admitted to hospital for cancers unrelated to smoking (colon, rectum, melanoma, lymphoma, bone or connective tissues) diagnosed in the last 6 months and having no previous history of cancer
Field *et al.* (1992) USA 1982–84	1617 case–control pairs aged 20–79 years, matched by year of birth and county of residence	Population-based study Cases histologically confirmed Controls selected using state driver's licence files 79% response for cases and 72% for controls
Smith *et al.* (1994) UK 1984–88	755 case–control pairs (cases under age 36 at date of diagnosis), matched by date of birth (within 6 months)	Population-based study Cases diagnosed in 1982–85 Controls randomly chosen from each case's general practioner list of patients 72% response rate for cases and 89% for controls
Ranstam & Olsson (1995) Sweden 1981–84	177 premenopausal and 216 postmenopausal cases; 195 premenopausal and 254 postmenopausal controls	Population-based study Controls randomly selected from the national population register 90% response rate for cases and 80% for controls
Baron *et al.* (1996) USA 1988–91	6888 cases and 9529 controls, aged less than 75 years	Population-based study Controls randomly selected from state driver's licence lists (aged < 65 years) and among women enrolled in Medicare in the participating state (aged 65–74 years) 81% response rate for cases and 84% for controls

Table 2.1.9.1 (contd)

Reference Country and years of study	Number of cases and controls	Criteria for eligibility and comments
Braga *et al.* (1996) Italy 1991–94	2569 cases and 2588 controls, aged 23–74 years (cases) and 20–74 years (controls)	Multicentre hospital-based study in six Italian areas Cases histologically confirmed Controls with no history of cancer admitted to hospitals for acute, non-neoplastic, non-hormonal, non-gynaecological diseases, smoking-related conditions excluded > 96% response rate for both cases and controls
Haile *et al.* (1996) Canada and USA 1970–89 (Los Angeles) 1975–89 (Quebec) 1935–89 (Connecticut)	144 cases and 232 controls, aged less than 50 years	Population-based study Cases histologically confirmed Controls were cases' sister(s) who were alive in 1989 (≥ 1 sister by case) and unaffected by breast cancer ~70% response rate for cases and controls combined
Morabia *et al.* (1996) Switzerland 1992–93	244 cases and 1032 controls, aged less than 75 years	Population-based study Cases histologically confirmed Controls were residents of Geneva, aged 30–74 years 71% response rate for cases and 70% for controls
Yoo *et al.* (1997) Japan 1988–92	1154 cases and 21714 controls, aged 25 years or older	Hospital-based study Cases histologically confirmed Controls were cancer-free hospital patients with no history of cancer
Brunet *et al.* (1998) Canada and USA [years of study not specified]	186 case–control pairs, mean age 49.7 years, matched by age and mutation in the same BRCA gene	Study involving genetic counselling centers Cases with past diagnosis of invasive breast cancer and no previous diagnosis of ovarian cancer Controls: women with no history of breast cancer, carriers of BRCA1 or BRCA2 mutations
Ghadirian *et al.* (1998) Canada 1989–93	414 cases and 429 controls, aged 35–79 years, matched by age and residence	Population-based study in the Francophone Community of greater Montreal Cases histologically confirmed Controls selected by random-digit dialling 77% response rate for cases
Gammon *et al.* (1998) USA 1990–92	2199 cases and 2009 controls, under 45 years, matched by age group and geographic area	Population-based study (Women's Interview Study of Health) Controls identified by random-digit dialling 86% response rate for cases and 71% for controls

Table 2.1.9.1 (contd)

Reference Country and years of study	Number of cases and controls	Criteria for eligibility and comments
Millikan *et al.* (1998) USA 1993–96	498 cases and 473 controls	Population-based study (Carolina Breast Cancer Study) Cases histologically confirmed Controls selected from lists from the North Carolina Division of Motor Vehicles (aged 20–64 years) and the Health Care Financing Administration (aged 65–74 years) Randomized recruitment among cases and controls to have equivalent numbers of white and African Americans as well as < 50 and ≥ 50 years of age 77% response rate for cases and 68% for controls
Gammon *et al.* (1999) USA 1990–92	378 cases (168 TP53-positive and 210 TP53-negative) and 462 controls, under the age of 45 years, matched by age group	Multicentre population-based study Cases histologically confirmed Controls identified by random-digit dialling 83% response rate for cases and 77% for controls
Lash & Aschengrau (1999) USA 1983–86	265 cases and 763 controls	Population-based study Controls identified by random-digit dialling (aged < 65 years); from the Health Care Financing Administration lists (aged ≥ 65 years); and from the Massachusets Department of Vital Statistics lists (deceased subjects 1983–89) 79% response rate for cases and 77% for controls
Johnson *et al.* (2000) Canada 1994–97	2617 cases (805 premenopausal and 1512 postmenopausal) and 2438 controls, aged 25–74 years	Population-based study Cases histologically confirmed Controls randomly selected from provincial health insurance plans; or random-digit dialling; or population research laboratory 77% response rate for cases and 71% for controls
Marcus *et al.* (2000) USA 1993–96	864 cases and 790 controls, aged 20–74 years	Population-based study (Carolina Breast Cancer Study) see Millikan *et al.* (1998) 77% response rate for cases and 68% for controls
Innes & Byers (2001) USA 1989–95	319 cases and 768 controls, aged 26–45 years	Record-linkage study Cases had completed a first pregnancy after 1987 Primiparous controls who resided and delivered in the same county as the case and were not subsequently diagnosed with breast or endometrial cancer were identified from infants' birth records
Kropp & Chang-Claude (2002) Germany 1992–95 and 1999–2000	468 mostly premenopausal cases and 1093 controls, matched by age and region	Population-based study Cases histologically confirmed Controls selected from regional population registries 70% response rate for cases and 61% for controls

Table 2.1.9.2. Case–control studies on tobacco smoking and breast cancer

Reference Country and years of study	Smoking categories	Relative risk (95% CI)	Comments
Rosenberg *et al.* (1984) USA Canada 1976–82	Former smoker *Cigarettes/day* 1–14 15–24 ≥ 25	1.1 (0.8–1.3) 1.3 (0.9–1.8) 1.0 (0.8–1.4) 1.1 (0.8–1.7)	Adjusted for all identified potential confounders
Smith *et al.* (1984) USA 1980–82	Occasional smoker Current smoker	0.9 (0.7–1.3) 1.2 (0.9–1.6)	Continuous smokers
Schechter *et al.* (1985) Canada Up to 1982	*All* Former smoker Ever-smoker Current smoker *Premenopausal* Former smoker Ever-smoker Current smoker *Postmenopausal* Former smoker Ever-smoker Current smoker	1.0 (0.6–1.7) 1.4 (0.9–2.1) 1.9 (1.2–3.1) 1.0 (0.5–2.7) 2.1 (1.1–4.0) 3.6 (1.7–7.7) 1.0 (0.5–2.0) 1.1 (0.6–1.9) 1.3 (0.7–2.4)	
Brinton *et al.* (1986) USA 1973–80	Former smoker Ever-smoker Current smoker *Cigarettes/day* < 10 10–19 20–29 30–39 ≥ 40 *Duration (years)* < 10 10–19 20–29 30–39 ≥ 40 Age at starting smoking (years) ≥ 23 20–22 17–19 < 17	1.2 (1.0–1.5) 1.2 (1.0–1.4) 1.2 (0.9–1.4) 1.2 (0.9–1.4) 1.4 (1.1–1.8) 1.2 (0.9–1.4) 1.2 (0.9–1.8) 1.2 (0.8–1.6) 1.4 (1.0–1.9) 1.2 (0.9–1.5) 1.2 (0.9–1.4) 1.1 (0.9–1.4) 1.3 (0.9–1.7) 1.1 (0.9–1.4) 1.1 (0.9–1.5) 1.3 (1.0–1.6) 1.3 (1.0–1.6)	Adjusted for age *p* for trend = 0.2 *p* for trend = 0.02

Table 2.1.9.2 (contd)

Reference Country and years of study	Smoking categories	Relative risk (95% CI)	Comments
McTiernan *et al.* (1986) USA 1981–82	*Estrogen receptor-positive cases (n = 143)*		Cases identified via population-based cancer registry, aged 25–54 years at diagnosis. Part of CASH study. Adjusted for age and use of alcohol
	Former smoker	0.96 (0.6–1.6)	
	Current smoker	1.1 (0.7–1.8)	
	Estrogen receptor-negative cases (n = 97)		
	Former smoker	0.8 (0.5–1.6)	
	Current smoker	0.8 (0.4–1.3)	
	Estrogen receptor status unknown (n = 89)		
	Former smoker	0.8 (0.5–1.5)	
	Current smoker	0.8 (0.5–1.5)	
O'Connell *et al.* (1987) USA 1977–78	Former smoker	1.2 (0.8–1.7)	Adjusted for age, race, estrogen use, oral contraceptive use and alcohol consumption
	Cigarettes/day		
	1–20	0.8 (0.5–1.1)	
	> 20	0.6 (0.3–1.1)	
Stockwell & Lyman (1987) USA 1981	Former smoker	1.0 (0.8–1.1)	Adjusted for age, race and marital status
	Cigarettes/day		
	> 20	1.3 (1.1–1.5)	
	20–40	1.2 (1.0–1.5)	
	> 40	1.3 (1.0–1.8)	
Stanford *et al.* (1987) USA 1980–82	Estrogen receptor-positive ever-smoker (*n* = 204)	1.03 (0.7–1.4)	Women aged 20–54 years. Part of CASH study. Ever-smoker defined as having smoked ≥ 100 cigarettes/lifetime Adjusted for age
	Estrogen receptor-negative ever-smoker (*n* = 254)	1.00 (0.7–1.4)	
Adami *et al.* (1988) Sweden, Norway 1984–85	*Cigarettes/day*		Adjusted for age, education, alcohol consumption and reproductive factors
	1–4	1.1 (0.5–2.1)	
	5–9	1.3 (0.8–2.0)	
	10–14	1.0 (0.6–1.5)	
	15–19	0.7 (0.4–1.2)	
	≥ 20	1.1 (0.7–1.8)	
	Duration (years)		
	0–4	1.2 (0.6–2.3)	
	5–9	0.7 (0.3–1.3)	
	10–14	1.0 (0.6–1.8)	
	15–19	1.1 (0.7–1.7)	
	≥ 20	1.2 (0.8–1.7)	
	Age at starting smoking (years)		
	≥ 25	1.6 (0.8–3.3)	
	20–24	0.8 (0.5–1.3)	
	15–19	1.0 (0.7–1.5)	
	< 15	1.3 (0.7–2.5)	

Table 2.1.9.2 (contd)

Reference Country and years of study	Smoking categories	Relative risk (95% CI)	Comments
Brownson *et al.* (1988) USA 1979–86	Former smoker Ever-smoker Current smoker	0.9 (0.6–1.2) 1.1 (0.9–1.4) 1.4 (1.01–1.9)	Adjusted for age, age at first pregnancy, parity, age at menarche, ever being married, family history of breast cancer and oral contraceptive use

Cooper *et al.* (1989); Rohan & Baron (1989) Australia 1982–84	*Estrogen receptor-positive* (*n* = 238)
	  Former smoker
	  Ever-smoker
	  Current smoker
	Estrogen receptor-negative (*n* = 119)
	  Former smoker
	  Ever-smoker
	  Current smoker
		
		0.9 (0.6–1.4)
		0.95 (0.7–1.4)
		1.3 (0.8–2.0)
		
		1.9 (0.99–3.6)
		1.6 (1.00–2.7)
		1.3 (0.7–2.5)
			Cigarette smoking associated with increased risk of estrogen receptor-negative cancer; women aged 20–74 years; adjusted for menopausal status

	Former smoker
	Ever-smoker
	Current smoker
	Cigarettes/day
	  1–15
	  > 15
	Pack–years
	  1–< 5
	  5–< 14
	  14–< 25
	  ≥ 25
		1.04 (0.7–1.5)
		1.2 (0.9–1.5)
		1.4 (0.95–2.0)
		
		1.2 (0.7–1.9)
		1.6 (0.99–2.6)
		
		0.99 (0.6–1.6)
		1.1 (0.7–1.8)
		1.1 (0.7–1.8)
		1.6 (0.99–2.5)
			Adjusted for family history of breast cancer, practice of breast self-examination, history of benign breast disease, obesity, menopausal status and alcohol consumption
			
			p for trend = 0.088

Kato *et al.* (1989) Japan 1980–86	Ever-smoker	0.9 (0.7–1.02)	Adjusted for age, alcohol use, marital status, residence, occupation and family history of breast cancer

Meara *et al.* (1989) United Kingdom 1980–84	25–44 years
	  Former smoker
	  Current smoker
	    1–14 cigarettes/day
	    ≥ 15 cigarettes/day
	45–69 years
	  Former smoker
	  Current smoker
	    1–14 cigarettes/day
	    ≥ 15 cigarettes/day
	  Former smoker
	  Current smoker
	    1–14 cigarettes/day
	    ≥ 15 cigarettes/day
		
		0.9 (0.6–1.5)
		
		0.6 (0.3–0.95)
		1.2 (0.7–1.8)
		
		0.95 (0.7–1.3)
		
		0.8 (0.6–1.2)
		0.8 (0.6–1.1)
		0.99 (0.4–2.3)
		
		1.8 (0.7–4.7)
		2.9 (1.2–7.3)
			Adjusted for menopausal status, age at first full-term pregnancy, age at menarche, family history of breast cancer in first-degree relatives, duration of oral contraceptive use, alcohol use, Quetelet index and socioeconomic status
			
			p for trend < 0.05

Table 2.1.9.2 (contd)

Reference Country and years of study	Smoking categories	Relative risk (95% CI)	Comments
Schechter et al. (1989) Canada 1982–85 (prevalence) 1981–87 (incidence)	**Prevalent cases** Ever-smoker *Pack–years* 1–10 > 10–25 > 25 **Incident cases** Ever-smoker *Pack–years* 1–10 > 10–25 > 25	1.1 (0.9–1.5) 1.0 (0.6–1.5) 1.1 (0.7–1.7) 1.2 (0.8–1.7) 1.2 (0.9–1.6) 1.2 (0.9–1.8) 1.1 (0.8–1.7) 1.3 (0.9–1.9)	Adjusted for age at menarche, age at first live birth, parity, age at menopause, family history of breast cancer, history of benign breast disease, breast symptoms, oral contraceptive use, estrogen replacement, height, weight, skinfold thickness, ethnicity, marital status, education, centre, age, use of breast self-examination and number of previous mammograms
Chu et al. (1990) USA 1980–82	Former smoker Ever-smoker Current smoker *Cigarettes/day* < 15 15–24 ≥ 25 *Duration (years)* < 10 10–19 20–29 ≥ 30 *Age at starting smoking (years)* ≥ 23 20–22 17–19 < 17 *Pack–years* < 10 10–19 20–29 30–39 ≥ 40 *Years since quitting* 0–1 2–5 6–9 ≥ 10	1.1 (1.0–1.3) 1.2 (1.1–1.3) 1.2 (1.1–1.3) 1.1 (1.0–1.3) 1.2 (1.0–1.3) 1.2 (1.1–1.4) 1.1 (0.9–1.2) 1.3 (1.1–1.4) 1.2 (1.1–1.4) 1.1 (0.9–1.3) 1.3 (1.1–1.5) 1.2 (1.0–1.4) 1.2 (1.1–1.4) 1.1 (1.0–1.2) 1.1 (1.0–1.3) 1.1 (1.0–1.3) 1.1 (1.0–1.3) 1.3 (1.1–1.6) 1.1 (0.9–1.4) 1.2 (1.1–1.3) 1.2 (1.0–1.5) 1.3 (1.0–1.7) 1.1 (0.9–1.3)	Adjusted for age, parity, menopausal status, age at first birth, age at menarche, family history of breast cancer, history of benign breast disease and estrogen replacement therapy

Table 2.1.9.2 (contd)

Reference Country and years of study	Smoking categories	Relative risk (95% CI)	Comments
Ewertz (1990) Denmark 1983–84	Former smoker	1.0 (0.8–1.2)	Adjusted for age and place of residence
	Current smoker	0.9 (0.8–1.1)	
	Cigarettes/day		
	1–4	0.9 (0.7–1.3)	
	5–9	1.05 (0.8–1.4)	
	10–14	1.02 (0.8–1.3)	
	15–19	1.01 (0.8–1.4)	
	≥ 20	0.8 (0.6–1.00)	
	Duration (years)		
	< 10	0.8 (0.6–1.1)	
	10–19	0.9 (0.7–1.2)	
	20–29	0.99 (0.8–1.3)	
	30–39	0.99 (0.8–1.2)	
	≥ 40	0.95 (0.7–1.3)	
	Age at starting smoking (years)		
	≥ 30	0.8 (0.6–1.1)	
	25–29	0.97 (0.7–1.4)	
	20–24	0.9 (0.7–1.1)	
	15–19	0.99 (0.8–1.2)	
	< 15	1.1 (0.8–1.6)	
	Pack–years		
	1–< 5	0.8 (0.6–1.1)	
	5–< 14	1.1 (0.9–1.4)	
	14–< 25	0.9 (0.8–1.2)	
	≥ 25	0.9 (0.7–1.2)	
Palmer *et al.* (1991) Canada	Former smoker	1.0 (0.7–1.3)	Adjusted for age, age at menopause, age at menarche, age at first birth, parity, family history of breast cancer, history of fibrocystic breast disease, body-mass index, oral contraceptive use, alcohol use, years of education and geographical area
	Ever-smoker	1.0 (0.8–1.3)	
	Current smoker	1.1 (0.9–1.4)	
	Cigarettes/day		
	< 25	1.0 (0.8–1.2)	
	25–34	1.1 (0.8–1.5)	
	≥ 35	1.5 (0.9–2.5)	
USA 1982–86	Former smoker	1.1 (0.9–1.4)	
	Ever-smoker	1.2 (1.0–1.5)	
	Current smoker	1.3 (1.1–1.6)	
	Cigarettes/day		
	< 25	1.2 (1.0–1.5)	
	25–34	1.2 (0.8–1.9)	
	≥ 35	1.2 (0.9–1.8)	

Table 2.1.9.2 (contd)

Reference Country and years of study	Smoking categories	Relative risk (95% CI)	Comments
Field *et al.* (1992) USA 1982–84	Ever-smoker	1.03 (0.9–1.2)	Age-adjusted for birth-year and county of residence
	Cigarettes/day (approx.)		
	1–9	0.9 (0.7–1.1)	
	10–20	1.2 (1.00–1.4)	
	30	0.9 (0.7–1.1)	
	40	0.98 (0.7–1.4)	
	> 40	1.2 (0.7–2.0)	
	Duration (years)		
	1–9	1.00 (0.8–1.3)	
	10–19	1.2 (0.9–1.5)	
	20–29	0.9 (0.7–1.1)	
	30–39	1.04 (0.9–1.3)	
	≥ 40	1.04 (0.8–1.3)	
	Age at starting smoking (years)		
	≥ 30	0.9 (0.6–1.2)	
	20–29	1.1 (0.9–1.4)	
	< 20	1.00 (0.9–1.2)	
	Age at quitting (years)		
	< 30	1.05 (0.8–1.4)	
	30–39	1.2 (0.9–1.5)	
	40–49	0.98 (0.8–1.2)	
	50–59	1.03 (0.8–1.3)	
	≥ 60	0.9 (0.7–1.1)	
Smith *et al.* (1994) UK 1984–88	Ever-smoker	1.01 (0.8–1.3)	Adjusted for age at menarche, nulliparity, age at first full-term pregnancy, breastfeeding (ever/never), family history of breast cancer, total oral contraceptive use, biopsy for benign breast disease and total alcohol consumption at age 18
	Cigarettes/day		
	≤ 15	0.95 (0.7–1.2)	
	≥ 16	1.1 (0.8–1.5)	
	Duration (years)		
	1–9	1.1 (0.8–1.5)	
	≥ 10	0.97 (0.8–1.3)	
	Pack–years		
	< 1–10	1.00 (0.8–1.3)	
	≥ 10	1.02 (0.8–1.4)	
	Age at starting smoking (years)		
	≥ 17	0.9 (0.7–1.2)	
	≤ 16	1.1 (0.8–1.4)	
Ranstam & Olsson (1995) Sweden 1981–84	**Premenopausal**		Adjusted for age, age at menarche, age at first full-term pregnancy, parity and age at menopause
	Ever-smoker	1.0 (0.6–1.5)	
	Cigarettes/day		
	1–10	0.7 (0.3–1.4)	
	> 11	1.2 (0.7–2.1)	
	Postmenopausal		
	Ever-smoker	0.7 (0.4–1.2)	
	Cigarettes/day		
	1–10	0.7 (0.4–1.3)	
	> 11	0.8 (0.4–1.6)	

Table 2.1.9.2 (contd)

Reference Country and years of study	Smoking categories	Relative risk (95% CI)	Comments
Baron *et al.* (1996) USA 1988–91	Former smoker	1.1 (1.01–1.2)	Adjusted for age at menarche, age at first term birth, parity, history of lactation, family history of breast cancer, history of benign breast disease, alcohol intake and menopausal status
	Current smoker	1.0 (0.9–1.1)	
	Cigarettes/day		
	≤ 10	1.04 (0.95–1.1)	
	10–20	1.1 (0.98–1.2)	
	21–30	1.1 (0.9–1.2)	
	31–40	1.04 (0.9–1.2)	
	> 40	1.1 (0.8–1.5)	
	trend/10 cigarettes	0.99 (0.96–1.04)	
	Duration (years)		
	≤ 10	0.96 (0.8–1.1)	
	11–20	1.02 (0.9–1.2)	
	21–30	1.1 (1.00–1.3)	
	31–40	1.1 (1.00–1.3)	
	41–50	1.01 (0.9–1.2)	
	> 50	1.1 (0.8–1.4)	
	trend/10 years	1.03 (0.99–1.08)	
	Years since quitting		
	> 30	0.9 (0.8–1.1)	
	21–30	0.9 (0.8–1.1)	
	11–20	1.1 (0.95–1.2)	
	3–10	1.2 (1.1–1.4)	
	≤ 3	1.4 (1.1–1.7)	
	trend/10 years	0.9 (0.9–0.96)	
Braga *et al.* (1996) Italy 1991–94	Former smoker	1.1 (0.9–1.4)	Adjusted for age, centre, education, parity, body-mass index and reproductive factors
	Ever-smoker	0.9 (0.8–1.1)	
	Current smoker	0.8 (0.7–1.0)	
	Cigarettes/day		
	< 5	1.02 (0.8–1.3)	
	5–14	0.99 (0.8–1.2)	
	15–24	0.8 (0.6–1.0)	
	≥ 25	1.2 (0.8–1.7)	
	Duration (years)		
	< 20	0.97 (0.8–1.2)	
	20–29	0.9 (0.7–1.0)	
	≥ 30	0.99 (0.8–1.2)	
	Age at starting smoking (years)		
	≥ 25	0.95 (0.8–1.1)	
	19–24	0.9 (0.8–1.1)	
	16–18	0.9 (0.7–1.1)	
	< 16	0.97 (0.7–1.3)	
	Years since quitting		
	≥ 16	0.7 (0.5–1.1)	
	7–15	1.1 (0.9–1.6)	
	3–6	1.8 (1.3–2.5)	
	< 3	1.5 (0.9–2.3)	

Table 2.1.9.2 (contd)

Reference Country and years of study	Smoking categories	Relative risk (95% CI)	Comments
Haile *et al.* (1996) USA, Canada Up to 1989	1–20 pack–years > 20 pack–years *Family history of breast cancer (n = 63)* 1–20 pack–years > 20 pack–years *No family history (n = 78)* 1–20 pack–years > 20 pack–years	0.9 (0.5–1.6) 1.0 (0.5–2.1) 0.9 (0.3–2.2) 2.3 (0.7–8.1) 0.8 (0.3–2.0) 0.4 (0.1–1.4)	Cases of premenopausal bilateral breast cancer at < 50 years of age. Results adjusted for age, alcohol, oral contraceptive use, body-mass index and education
Morabia *et al.* (1996) Switzerland 1992–93	*Former smoker (cig/day)* 1–9 10–19 ≥ 20 *Ever-smoker (cig/day)* 1–9 10–19 ≥ 20 *Current smoker (cig/day)* 1–9 10–19 ≥ 20 *Pack–years* < 20 ≥ 20	3.3 (1.4–7.6) 3.6 (1.6–8.1) 3.7 (1.5–8.8) 2.2 (1.0–4.4) 2.7 (1.4–5.4) 4.6 (2.2–9.7) 1.5 (0.6–3.9) 2.1 (0.9–4.8) 5.1 (2.1–12.6) 2.1 (1.0–4.5) 2.9 (1.4–6.0)	Reference group comprised subjects not exposed to active or passive smoking.
Yoo *et al.* (1997) Japan 1988–92	*Ever-smoker* All Estrogen receptor-positive Estrogen receptor-negative	1.3 (1.1–1.5) 1.4 (1.0–1.9) 1.3 (0.9–2.0)	Results presented for progesterone receptor status were similar to estrogen receptor status. Adjusted for age at diagnosis, current occupation, family history of breast cancer among first-degree relatives, menstrual regularity, menopausal status, history of full-term pregnancy, alcohol use, age at menarche, age at menopause, age at first full-term pregnancy, number of full-term pregnancies and average months of breastfeeding per child.
Brunet *et al.* (1998) USA, Canada NS	Ever-smoker *Packs/week* < 5 ≥ 5 *Pack–years* ≤ 4 > 4	0.5 (0.3–0.8) 0.6 (0.4–1.1) 0.5 (0.3–0.8) 0.7 (0.4–1.2) 0.5 (0.3–0.8)	Adjusted for parity, age at first birth, age at last birth and geographical area

Table 2.1.9.2 (contd)

Reference Country and years of study	Smoking categories	Relative risk (95% CI)	Comments
Ghadirian et al. (1998) Canada 1989–93	Ever-smoker Untipped cigarettes	0.7 (0.6–0.98) 0.4 (0.2–0.7)	Adjusted for age, marital status, parity, age at first full-term pregnancy, history of benign breast disease and ovarian cancer, income and body-mass index
Gammon et al. (1998) USA 1990–92	Former smoker Ever-smoker Current smoker	0.99 (0.8–1.2) 0.9 (0.8–1.1) 0.8 (0.7–1.01)	Women < 45 years of age. Adjusted for age, centre, usual alcohol consumption, parity, age at first birth, age at menarche, breastfeeding, abortion, miscarriage, menopausal status, ever being married, education, income, race, body-mass index at age 20 years, body-mass index as an adult, oral contraceptive use, non-contraceptive hormone use, calorie intake, history of breast biopsy, family history of breast cancer

Millikan et al. (1998) USA 1993–96	Former smoker
	Current smoker
	Cigarettes/day
	  < 10
	  11–20
	  > 20
	Duration (years)
	  ≤ 10
	  11–20
	  > 20
	Years since quitting
	  ≥ 20
	  10–19
	  4–9
	  ≤ 3
		1.3 (0.9–1.8)
		1.0 (0.7–1.4)
		
		1.1 (0.8–1.6)
		1.3 (0.9–1.9)
		1.1 (0.7–1.7)
		
		1.0 (0.7–1.5)
		0.8 (0.5–1.2)
		1.6 (1.1–2.3)
		
		1.1 (0.7–1.9)
		0.8 (0.5–1.4)
		1.7 (1.0–3.0)
		2.2 (1.2–4.0)
			Adjusted for age, age at menarche, age at first full-term pregnancy, family history of breast cancer, benign breast biopsy and alcohol consumption

Gammon et al. (1999) USA 1996–92	*TP53-positive*
	  Former smoker
	  Current smoker
	TP53-negative
	  Former smoker
	  Current smoker
	Ratios of the odds ratios
	  Former smoker
	  Current smoker
		
		1.7 (1.02–2.7)
		1.3 (0.8–2.1)
		
		1.2 (0.8–1.8)
		0.7 (0.4–1.1)
		
		1.4 (0.8–2.4)
		2.0 (1.1–3.5)
			Cases with tissue studies, aged < 45 years. Adjusted for age, race, education, alcohol, body-mass index, age at first birth, parity, age at menarche, family history of breast cancer, prior breast biopsy, caloric intake and electric blanket use. Data available on intensity, duration, pack–years and age at start by *TP53* status for ever-smokers and current smokers

Table 2.1.9.2 (contd)

Reference Country and years of study	Smoking categories	Relative risk (95% CI)	Comments
Lash & Aschengrau (1999) USA 1983–86	Ever-smoker	2.0 (1.1–3.6)	Ever smoked compared with subjects not exposed to active or passive smoke. Current smokers defined as persons who had smoked within 5 years before diagnosis
	Current smoker	2.3 (0.8–6.8)	
	Cigarettes/day		
	≤ 20	2.1 (1.0–4.6)	
	> 20	1.6 (0.6–4.3)	
	Duration (years)		
	0–19	2.6 (1.2–5.5)	
	20–39	1.5 (0.7–3.2)	
	≥ 40	2.4 (1.1–5.5)	
	Age at starting smoking (years)		
	≥ 21	2.4 (1.0–5.7)	
	17–20	2.3 (1.0–5.5)	
	< 17	2.4 (0.8–7.2)	
	Years since quitting		
	> 15	2.2 (1.0–4.9)	
	5–15	3.9 (1.4–10)	
	< 5 or current	2.3 (0.8–6.8)	
Johnson *et al.* (2000) Canada 1994–97	**Premenopausal**		Referent groups were subjects not exposed to active or passive smoking.
	Former smoker	2.6 (1.3–5.3)	
	Ever-smoker	2.3 (1.2–4.5)	
	Current smoker	1.9 (0.9–3.8)	
	Postmenopausal		
	Former smoker	1.4 (0.9–2.1)	
	Ever-smoker	1.5 (1.0–2.3)	
	Current smoker	1.6 (1.0–2.5)	
Marcus *et al.* (2000) USA 1993–96	Former smoker	1.1 (0.8–1.3)	Women aged 20–74 years with focus on exposures during adolescence
	Current smoker	1.2 (0.9–1.5)	
	Cigarettes/day		
	< 20	1.0 (0.8–1.4)	
	≥ 20	1.1 (0.9–1.4)	
	Duration (years)		
	< 20	0.9 (0.7–1.2)	
	≥ 20	1.3 (1.1–1.8)	
	Age at starting smoking (years)		
	≥ 20	1.2 (0.8–1.5)	
	15–19	1.0 (0.8–1.3)	
	10–14	1.5 (0.9–2.5)	
Innes & Byers (2001) USA 1989–95	Smoking during pregnancy	3.1 (1.3–7.3)	Women aged 26–45 years. Adjusted for age, age at first birth, maternal education, maternal race and marital status

Table 2.1.9.2 (contd)

Reference Country and years of study	Smoking categories	Relative risk (95% CI)	Comments
Kropp & Chang-Claude (2002) Germany 1992–95 1999–2000	Former smoker	1.2 (0.8–1.7)	Women diagnosed by age 50 years.
	Ever-smoker	1.3 (0.9–1.9)	Never active/never passive smokers used
	Current smoker	1.5 (1.0–2.2)	as referent.
	Duration (years)		Adjusted for alcohol, total months of
	1–9	0.99 (0.6–1.6)	breastfeeding, education, family history of
	10–19	1.4 (0.9–2.2)	breast cancer, menopausal status and
	≥ 20	1.5 (1.0–2.2)	body-mass index
	Age at starting smoking (years)		*p* for trend = 0.047
	9–15	1.02 (0.6–1.7)	
	16–18	1.3 (0.8–1.9)	*p* for trend = 0.015
	≥ 19	1.5 (1.0–2.4)	
	Pack–years		
	≤ 10	1.2 (0.8–1.8)	
	11–20	1.8 (1.2–2.9)	
	≥ 21	1.1 (0.7–1.9)	
	Years since quitting		
	1–9	1.6 (0.98–2.8)	
	10–19	0.98 (0.6–1.6)	
	≥ 20	1.04 (0.6–1.9)	
	High exposure to active and passive smoking	1.8 (1.2–2.7)	

Table 2.1.9.3. Additional cohort studies on tobacco smoking and breast cancer: main characteristics of study design

Reference	Cohort sample	Cases/deaths identification	Comments
Bennicke et al. (1995) Denmark 1989–91	All women referred for mammography to the radiology department of a large public hospital, aged 15–92 years	Diagnosis of breast cancer from mammography and clinical examination	Former smokers were included in the 'smoker' category.
van den Brandt et al. (1995) Netherlands 1986–89	62 573 women aged 55–69 years (all menopausal); cases taken from entire cohort; controls taken from a subcohort of 1716 randomly sampled subjects	Incident cases	Case–control approach without matching; controls excluded cancers other than skin cancer.
Thomas et al. (1997) China 1989–91	267 040 women working in the Shanghai Textile Industry Bureau, recruited for a randomized trial of breast self-examination, born 1925–58	Cases identified primarily by trial workers during visits to the factory's medical clinic	
Million Women Study Group (1999) UK 1996–99	121 000 women aged 50–64 years recruited nationwide when invited for routine breast screening; response rate, 71%	Cases identified by linkage with screening centres	Study designed primarily to investigate use of hormone replacement therapy and risk of breast cancer

Table 2.1.9.4. Cohort studies on tobacco smoking and breast cancer

Reference Country and years of study	Name of study No. of subjects	No. of cases	Smoking categories	Relative risk (95% CI)	Comments
Hiatt & Fireman (1986) (USA) 1964–80	Kaiser Permanente Medical Care Program Study 84 172 women	1363 cases	Current smoker Former smoker Nonsmoker	Incidence rate 1.4 1.6 1.3	Annual age-adjusted rate per 1000 person–years Relative risks are comparable for pre- and post-menopausal women.
				RR	
			Former smoker	1.2 (1.0–1.4)	
			Current smoker		
			Light	1.0 (0.8–1.1)	
			Moderate	1.2 (1.1–1.4)	
			Heavy	1.2 (0.9–1.6)	
Vatten & Kvinnsland (1990) (Norway) 1974–88	Norwegian Screening Study 24 329 women	242 cases	*Cigarettes/day* 1–9 ≥ 10	Incidence rate ratio 1.2 (0.9–1.7) 0.9 (0.6–1.2)	Adjusted for age at entry, age at diagnosis, occupation and body-mass index
			Cases < 51 years 1–9 cigarettes/day ≥ 10 cigarettes/day	1.1 (0.7–1.7) 0.8 (0.5–1.2)	
			Cases ≥ 51 years 1–9 cigarettes/day ≥ 10 cigarettes/day	1.0 (0.6–1.7) 0.8 (0.5–1.3)	
Tverdal *et al.* (1993) (Norway) 1972–88	Norwegian Screening Study 24 535 women	70 deaths	Never-smoker Former smoker Current smoker 1–9 cigarettes/day ≥ 10 cigarettes/day	Mortality rate 19.9 18.8 28.0 29.4 24.8	Annual mortality rate per 100 000 women Adjusted for age and area

Table 2.1.9.4 (contd)

Reference Country and years of study	Name of study No. of subjects	No. of cases	Smoking categories	Relative risk (95% CI)	Comments
Calle et al. (1994) (USA) 1982–88	CPS II 604 412 women	880 deaths		Rate ratio	Adjusted for family history of breast cancer, body-mass index, education, alcohol consumption, breast cysts, age at first birth, age at menarche and age at menopause
			Former smoker	0.9 (0.7–1.03)	
			Ever-smoker	1.0 (0.9–1.19)	
			Current smoker	1.3 (1.1–1.5)	
			≥ 40 cigarettes/day	1.7 (1.2–2.6)	
			≥ 40 years	1.4 (1.1–1.8)	
			Age at starting smoking		
			< 16 years	1.6 (1.2–2.2)	
Bennicke et al. (1995) (Denmark) 1989–91	3240 women	230 cases	*Duration (years)*		Adjusted for age, parity, breastfeeding, family history of breast cancer and previous gynaecological surgery
			1–10	1.1 (0.6–2.4)	
			11–20	0.9 (0.5–1.7)	
			21–30	1.3 (0.8–2.1)	
			≥ 31	1.6 (1.1–2.3)	
Engeland et al. (1996) (Norway) 1966–93	Norwegian Cohort Study	41 138	Former smoker Current smoker	1.1 (0.8–1.5) 1.0 (0.8–1.2)	
Nordlund et al. (1997) (Sweden) 1964–89	Swedish Census Study	996	Former smoker	1.2 (0.9–1.7)	
			Current smoker	0.95 (0.8–1.1)	
			Cigarettes/day		
			1–7	0.9 (0.7–1.1)	
			8–15	1.04 (0.8–1.4)	
			≥ 16	1.07 (0.7–1.7)	
			Age at starting smoking (years)		
			20–23	0.99 (0.6–1.5)	
			< 19	1.2 (0.8–1.8)	*p* for trend = 0.35

Table 2.1.9.4 (contd)

Reference Country and years of study	Name of study No. of subjects	No. of cases	Smoking categories	Relative risk (95% CI)	Comments
Egan et al. (2002) (USA) 1976–96	Nurse's Health Study 78 206 women	3140 cases	Current smoker	1.0 (0.9–1.2)	Smoking status ascertained at baseline and updated biennially from 1978–94.
			Former smoker	1.1 (1.0–1.2)	Adjusted for current age, age at menarche, age at first birth and parity, history of benign breast disease, family history of breast cancer in mother or sister, menopausal status and age at menopause, weight at age 18 years, adult weight change, adult height, g alcohol/week, total carotenoid intake and menopausal hormone use (current, former, never)
			Age at starting smoking (years)		
			19–20	1.1 (1.0–1.2)	
			17–18	1.0 (0.9–1.1)	
			< 17	1.2 (1.0–1.4)	

CI, confidence interval

Table 2.1.9.5. Relative risk of breast cancer in ever- versus never-smokers by study design and country

Study (country) Reference	No. of cases/ controls	% ever smoked cases/controls	Relative risk of breast cancer in ever-versus never-smokers (standard error)
I. Cohort studies			
Nurses Health Study (USA) Willett *et al.* (1987)	1224/5599	49/49	1.01 (0.07)
Iowa Women's Health (USA) Gapstur *et al.* (1992)	679/2725	25/26	0.93 (0.10)
Canadian NBSS (Canada) Friedenreich *et al.* (1993)	181/662	35/35	1.25 (0.23)
Netherlands Cohort (Netherlands) van den Brandt *et al.* (1995)	119/504	27/30	0.89 (0.23)
American Cancer Society (CPS II) (USA) Thun *et al.* (1997)	213/922	34/33	1.07 (0.19)
Million Women Study (UK) (1999)	324/1291	50/44	1.24 (0.15)
Other Hiatt & Bawol (1984); Mills *et al.* (1989); Land *et al.* (1994); Thomas *et al.* (1997)	1932/7655	4/5	0.78 (0.12)
All cohort studies	**4663/19 398**	**25/26**	**1.00 (0.04)**
II. Case–control studies, population controls			
Brinton (USA) Harvey *et al.* (1987)	649/872	29/26	1.12 (0.14)
Rohan (Australia) Rohan & McMichael (1988)	188/213	35/32	1.06 (0.31)
CASH (USA) Chu *et al.* (1989)	1817/1821	49/43	1.28 (0.08)
Bain/Siskind (Australia) Siskind *et al.* (1989)	248/514	32/29	1.31 (0.26)
Clarke (Canada) Rosenberg *et al.* (1990)	114/211	40/42	0.88 (0.31)
(Denmark) Ewertz (1991)	227/198	59/57	0.88 (0.27)
Paul & Skegg (New Zealand) Sneyd *et al.* (1991)	538/1058	43/41	1.09 (0.13)
Yang & Gallagher (Canada) Yang *et al.* (1992)	505/517	48/44	1.15 (0.17)
Long Island (USA) Weinstein *et al.* (1993)	153/208	37/34	0.99 (0.32)

Table 2.1.9.5 (contd)

Study (country) Reference	No. of cases/ controls	% ever smoked cases/controls	Relative risk of breast cancer in ever-versus never-smokers (standard error)
Rookus & van Leeuwen (Netherlands) (1994)	247/247	52/51	0.90 (0.21)
UK studies (UK) Smith *et al.* (1994)	655/662	47/45	1.08 (0.13)
Daling (USA) White *et al.* (1994)	211/286	42/42	0.87 (0.21)
Four-state study (USA) Longnecker *et al.* (1995a)	1507/2247	39/39	1.07 (0.09)
Ross & Paganini-Hill (USA) Longnecker *et al.* (1995b)	578/590	53/52	1.02 (0.13)
(Slovenia) Primic-Zakelj *et al.* (1995)	115/128	29/30	0.67 (0.38)
Stanford/Habel (USA) Rossing *et al.* (1996)	152/181	52/49	0.79 (0.26)
WISH (USA) Swanson *et al.* (1997)	353/241	59/68	0.63 (0.21)
Bernstein (USA) Enger *et al.* (1999)	336/317	50/48	1.18 (0.20)
Magnusson (Sweden) Magnusson *et al.* (1999)	1311/1312	32/33	0.91 (0.08)
McCredie & Hopper (Australia) McCredie *et al.* (1998); Hopper *et al.* (1999)	774/518	38/36	1.03 (0.15)
Chang-Claude (Germany) Chang-Claude *et al.* (2000)	168/251	46/52	0.94 (0.25)
Johnson (Canada) Johnson *et al.* (2000)	974/1110	42/40	1.14 (0.11)
Other Lee *et al.* (1987); Adami *et al.* (1988); Yuan *et al.* (1988); Ursin *et al.* (1992); Wang *et al.* (1992); Morabia *et al.* (1996); Viladiu *et al.* (1996); Gao *et al.* (2000)	2851/3567	11/13	0.99 (0.12)
All case–control studies, population controls	**14 671/17 269**	**36/35**	**1.07 (0.03)**
III. Case–control studies, hospital controls			
Le Gerber & Clavel (France) Le *et al.* (1986); Richardson *et al.* (1989); Clavel *et al.* (1991)	492/923	18/24	0.82 (0.16)

Table 2.1.9.5 (contd)

Study (country) Reference	No. of cases/ controls	% ever smoked cases/controls	Relative risk of breast cancer in ever-versus never-smokers (standard error)
Franceschi (Italy) La Vecchia *et al.* (1987); Ferraroni *et al.* (1998)	831/1025	31/31	1.01 (0.12)
La Vecchia (Italy) La Vecchia *et al.* (1989)	980/1034	28/30	0.82 (0.10)
Vessey (UK) Meara *et al.* (1989)	154/171	44/53	0.71 (0.30)
Katsouyanni (Greece) Katsouyanni *et al.* (1994)	219/462	21/24	1.28 (0.29)
Other Ferraroni *et al.* (1993); Levi *et al.* (1996)	245/550	20/26	0.72 (0.25)
All case–control studies, hospital controls	**2921/4165**	**27/29**	**0.89 (0.06)**
All studies	**22 255/40 832**	**33/30**	**1.03 (0.02)**

From Collaborative Group on Hormonal Factors in Breast Cancer Study (2002)

References

Adami, H.O., Lund, E., Bergstrom, R. & Meirik, O. (1988) Cigarette smoking, alcohol consumption and risk of breast cancer in young women. *Br. J. Cancer*, **58**, 832–837

Baron, J.A., Newcomb, P.A., Longnecker, M.P., Mittendorf, R., Storer, B.E., Clapp, R.W., Bogdan, G. & Yuen, J. (1996) Cigarette smoking and breast cancer. *Cancer Epidemiol. Biomarkers Prev.*, **5**, 399–403

Bennicke, K., Conrad, C., Sabroe, S. & Sorensen, H.T. (1995) Cigarette smoking and breast cancer. *Br. med. J.*, **310**, 1431–1433

Braga, C., Negri, E., La Vecchia, C., Filiberti, R. & Franceschi, S. (1996) Cigarette smoking and the risk of breast cancer. *Eur. J. Cancer Prev.*, **5**, 159–164

van den Brandt, P.A., Goldbohm, R.A. & 't-Veer, P. (1995) Alcohol and breast cancer: Results from the Netherlands Cohort Study. *Am. J. Epidemiol.*, **141**, 907–915

Brinton, L.A., Schairer, C., Stanford, J.L. & Hoover, R.M. (1986) Cigarette smoking and breast cancer. *Am. J. Epidemiol.*, **123**, 614–622

Brownson, R.C., Blackwell, C.W., Pearson, D.K., Reynolds, R.D., Richens, J.W., Jr & Papermaster, B.W. (1988) Risk of breast cancer in relation to cigarette smoking. *Arch. intern. Med.*, **148**, 140–144

Brunet, .S., Ghadirian, P., Rebbeck, T.R., Lerman, C., Garber, J.E., Tonin, P.N., Abrahamson, J., Foulkes, W.D., Daly, M., Wagner-Costalas, J., Godwin, A., Olapade, I.I., Mosleti, R., Liede, A., Tutreal, P.A., Weber, B.A., Lenoir, G.M., Lynche, H.T. & Narod, S.A. (1998) Effect of smoking on breast cancer in carriers of mutant BRCA1 or BRCA2 genes. *J. natl Cancer Inst.*, **90**, 761–766

Calle, E.E., Miracle-McHill, H.L., Thun, M.J. & Heath, C.W. (1994) Cigarette smoking and risk of fatal breast cancer. *Am. J. Epidemiol.*, **139**, 1001–1007

Chang-Claude, J., Eby, N., Kiechle, M., Bastert, G. & Becher, H. (2000) Breastfeeding and breast cancer risk by age 50 among women in Germany. *Cancer Causes Control*, **11**, 687–695

Chu, S.Y., Lee, N.C., Wingo, P.A. & Webster, L.A. (1989) Alcohol consumption and the risk of breast cancer. *Am. J. Epidemiol,*. **130**, 867–877

Chu, S.Y., Stroup, N.E., Wingo, P.A., Lee, N.C., Peterson, H.B. & Gwinn, M.L. (1990) Cigarette smoking and the risk of breast cancer. *Am. J. Epidemiol.*, **131**, 244–253

Clavel, F., Andrieu, N., Gairard, B., Bremond, A., Piana, L., Lansac, J., Breart, G., Rumeau-Rouquette, C., Flamant, R. & Renaud, R. (1991) Oral contraceptives and breast cancer: A French case–control study. *Int. J. Epidemiol.*, **20**, 32–38

Collaborative Group on Hormonal Factors and Breast Cancer (2002) Alcohol, tobacco and breast cancer — Collaborative reanalysis of individual data from 53 epidemiological studies, including 58 515 women with breast cancer and 95 067 women without the disease. *Br. J. Cancer*, **87**, 1234–1245

Cooper, J.A., Rohan, T.E., Cant, E.L.McK., Horsfall, D.J. & Tilley, W.D. (1989) Risk factors for breast cancer by oestrogen receptor status: A population-based case–control study. *Br. J. Cancer*, **59**, 119–125

Egan, K.M., Stampfer, M.J., Hunter, D., Hankinson, S., Rosner, B.A., Holmes, M., Willett, W.C. & Colditz, G.A. (2002) Active and passive smoking in breast cancer: Prospective results from the Nurses' Health Study. *Epidemiology*, **13**, 138–145

Engeland, A., Andersen, A., Haldorsen, T. & Tretli, S. (1996) Smoking habits and risk of cancers other than lung cancer: 28 years' follow-up of 26 000 Norwegian men and women. *Cancer Causes Control*, 7, 497–506

Enger, S.M., Ross, R.K., Paganini-Hill, A., Longnecker, M.P. & Bernstein, L. (1999) Alcohol consumption and breast cancer oestrogen and progesterone receptor status. *Br. J. Cancer*, **79**, 1308–1314

Ewertz, M. (1990) Smoking and breast cancer risk in Denmark. *Cancer Causes Control*, **1**, 31–37

Ewertz, M. (1991) Alcohol consumption and breast cancer risk in Denmark. *Cancer Causes Control*, **2**, 247–252

Ferraroni, M., Gerber, M., Decarli, A., Richardson, S., Marubini, E., Crastes-de-Paulet, P., Crastes-de-Paulet, A. & Pujol, H. (1993) HDL-cholesterol and breast cancer: A joint study in northern Italy and southern France. *Int. J. Epidemiol.*, **22**, 772–780

Ferraroni, M., Decarli, A., Franceschi, S. & La Vecchia, C. (1998) Alcohol consumption and risk of breast cancr: A multicentre Italian case–control study. *Eur. J. Cancer*, **34**, 1403–1409

Field, N.A., Baptiste, M.S., Nasca, P.C. & Metzger, B.B. (1992) Cigarette smoking and breast cancer. *Int. J. Epidemiol.*, **21**, 842–848

Friedenreich, C.M., Howe, G.R. & Miller, A.B. (1993) A cohort study of alcohol consumption and risk of breast cancer. *Am. J. Epidemiol.*, **137**, 512–520

Gammon, M.D., Schoenberg, J.B., Teitelbaum, S.L., Brinton, L.A., Potischman, N., Swanson, C.A., Brogan, D.J, Coates, R.J., Malone, K.E. & Stanford, J.L. (1998) Cigarette smoking and breast cancer risk among young women (United States). *Cancer Causes Control*, 9, 583–590

Gammon, M.D., Hibshoosh, H., Terry, M.B., Bose, S., Schoenberg, J.B., Brinton, L.A., Bernstein, J.L. & Thompson, W.D. (1999) Cigarette smoking and other risk factors in relation to p53 expression in breast cancer among young women. *Cancer Epidemiol. Biomarkers Prev.*, **8**, 255–263

Gao, Y.T., Shu, X.O., Dai, Q., Potter, J.D., Brinton, L.A., Wen, W., Sellers, T.A., Kushi, L.H., Ruan, Z., Bostick, R.M. (2000) Association of menstrual and reproductive factors with breast cancer risk: Results from the Shanghai Breast Cancer Study. *Int. J. Cancer*, **87**, 295–300

Gapstur, S.M., Potter, J.D., Sellers, T.A. & Folsom, A.R. (1992) Increased risk of breast cancer with alcohol consumption in postmenopausal women. *Am. J. Epidemiol.*, **136**, 1221–1231

Ghadirian, P., Lacroix, A., Perret, C., Maisonneuve, P. & Boyle, P. (1998) Sociodemographic characteristics, smoking, medical and family history, and breast cancer. *Cancer Detect. Prev.*, **22**, 485–494

Haile, R.W., Witte, J.S., Ursin, G., Siemiatychi, J., Bertolli, J., Thompson, W.D. & Paganini-Hill, A. (1996) A case–control study of reproductive variables, alchol, and smoking in premenopausal bilateral breast cancer. *Breast Cancer Res.*, **37**, 49–56

Harvey, E.B., Schairer, C., Brinton, L.A., Hoover, R.N. & Fraumeni, J.F., Jr (1987) Alcohol consumption and breast cancer. *J. natl Cancer Inst.*, **78**, 657–661

Hiatt, R.A. & Bawol, R.D. (1984) Alcoholic beverage consumption and breast cancer incidence. *Am. J. Epidemiol.*, **120**, 676–683

Hiatt, R.A. & Fireman, B.H. (1986) Smoking, menopause, and breast cancer. *J. natl Cancer Inst.*, **76**, 833–838

Hopper, J.L., Chenevix-Trench, G., Jolley, D.J., Dite, G.S., Jenkins, M.A., Venter, D.J., McCredie, M.R. & Giles, G.G. (1999) Design and anlaysis issues in a population-based, case–control-family study of the genetic epidemiology of breast cancer and the Co-operative Family Registry for Breast Cancer Studies (CFRBCS). *Natl Cancer Inst. Monogr.*, **26**, 95–100

IARC (1986) *IARC Monographs on the Evaluation of the Carcinogenic Risk of Chemicals to Humans*, Vol. 38, *Tobacco Smoking*, Lyon, IARCPress

Innes, K.E. & Byers, T.E. (2001) Smoking during pregnancy and breast cancer risk in very young women (United States). *Cancer Causes Control*, **12**, 179–185

Johnson, K.C., Hu, J. & Mao, Y. for the Canadian Cancer Registries Epidemiology Search Group (2000) Passive and active smoking and breast cancer risk in Canada, 1994–97. *Cancer Causes Control*, **11**, 211–221

Kato, I., Tominata, S. & Terao, C. (1989) Alcohol consumption and cancers of hormone-related organs in females. *Jpn. J. clin. Oncol.*, **19**, 202–207

Katsouyanni, K., Trichopoulou, A., Stuver, S., Vassilaros, S., Papadiamantis, Y., Bournas, N., Skarpou, N., Mueller, N. & Trichopoulos, D. (1994) Ethanol and breast cancer: An association that may be both confounded and causal. *Int. J. Cancer*, **58**, 356–361

Kropp, S. & Chang-Claude, J. (2002) Active and passive smoking and risk of breast cancer by age 50 years among German women. *Am. J. Eidemiol.*, **156**, 616–626

La Vecchia, C., Decarli, A., Parazzini, F., Gentile, A., Negri, E., Cecchetti, G. & Franceschi, S. (1987) General epidemiology of breast cancer in northern Italy. *Int. J. Epidemiol.*, **16**, 347–355

La Vecchia, C., Negri, E., Parazzini, F., Boyle, P., Fasoli, M., Gentile, A. & Franceschi, S. (1989) Alcohol and breast cancer: Update from an Italian case–control study. *Eur. J. Cancer clin. Oncol.*, **25**, 1711–1717

Land, C.E., Hayakawa, N., Machado, S.G., Yamada, Y., Pike, M.C., Akiba, S. & Tokunaga, M. (1994) A case–control interview study of breast cancer among Japanese A-bomb survivors. Interactions with radiation dose. *Cancer Causes Control*, **5**, 167–176

Lash, T.L. & Aschengrau, A. (1999) Active and passive cigarette smoking and the occurrence of breast cancer. *Am. J. Epidemiol.*, **149**, 5–12

Le, M.G., Moulton, L.H., Hill, C. & Kramar, A. (1986) Consumption of dairy produce and alcohol in a case–control study of breast cancer. *J. natl Cancer Inst.*, **77**, 633–636

Lee, N.C., Rosero-Bixby, L., Oberle, M.W., Grimaldo, C., Whatley, A.S. & Rovira, E.Z. (1987) A case–control study of breast cancer and hormonal contraception in Costa Rica. *J. natl Cancer Inst.*, **79**, 1247–1254

Levi, F., Pasche, C., Lucchini, F. & La Vecchia, C. (1996) Alcohol and breast cancer in the Swiss Canton of Baud. *Eur. J. Cancer*, **32A**, 2108–2113

Longnecker, M.P., Paganini-Hill, A. & Ross, R.K. (1995a) Lifetime alcohol consumption and breast cancer risk among postmenopausal women in Los Angeles. *Cancer Epidemiol. Biomarkers Prev.*, **4**, 721–725

Longnecker, M.P., Newcomb, P.A., Mittendorf, R., Greenberg, E.R., Clapp, R.W., Bogdan, G.F., Baron, J., MacMahon, B. & Willett, W.C. (1995b) Risk of breast cancer in relation to lifetime alcohol consumption. *J. natl Cancer Inst.*, **87**, 923–929

Magnusson, C., Baron, J.A., Correia, N., Bergstrom, R., Adami, H.O. & Persson, I. (1999) Breast-cancer risk following long-term oestrogen- and oestrogen-progestin-replacement therapy. *Int. J. Cancer*, **81**, 339–344

Marcus, P.M., Newman, B., Millikan, R.C., Moorman, P.G., Day Baird, D. & Qaqish, B. (2000) The associations of adolescent cigarette smoking, alcoholic beverage consumption, environmental tobacco smoke, and ionizing radiation with subsequent breast cancer risk (United States). *Cancer Causes Control*, **11**, 271–278

McCredie, M.R., Dite, G.S., Giles, G.G. & Hopper, J.L. (1998) Breast cancer in Australian women under the age of 40. *Cancer Causes Control*, **9**, 189–198

McTiernan, A., Thomas, D.B., Johnson, L.K. & Roseman, D. (1986) Risk factors for estrogen receptor-rich and estrogen receptor-poor breast cancers. *J. natl Cancer Inst.*, **77**, 849–854

Meara, J., McPherson, K., Roberts, M., Jones, L. & Vessey, M. (1989) Alcohol, cigarette smoking and breast cancer. *Br. J. Cancer*, **60**, 70–73

Millikan, R.C., Pittman, G.S., Newman, B., Tse, C.K., Selmin, O., Rockhill, B., Xavitz, D., Moorman, P.G. & Bell, D.A. (1998) Cigarette smoking, N-acetyltransferases 1 and 2, and breast cancer risk. *Cancer Epidemiol. Biomarkers Prev.*, **7**, 371–378

Million Women Study Collaborative Group (1999) The Million Women Study: Design and characteristics of the study population. *Breast Cancer Res.*, **1**, 73–80

Mills, P.K., Beeson, W.L., Phillips, R.L. & Fraser, G.E. (1989) Prospective study of exogenous hormone use and breast cancer in Seventh-day Adventists. *Cancer*, **64**, 591–597

Morabia, A., Bernstein, M., Heritier, S. & Khatchatrian, N. (1996) Relation of breast cancer with passive and active exposure to tobacco smoke. *Am. J. Epidemiol.*, **143**, 918–928

Nordlund, L.A., Carstensen, J.M. & Pershagen, G. (1997) Cancer incidence in female smokers: A 26-year follow-up. *Int. J. Cancer*, **73**, 625–628

O'Connell, D.L., Hulka, B.S., Chambless, L.E., Wilkinson, W.E. & Deubner, D.C. (1987) Cigarette smoking, alcohol consumption, and breast cancer risk. *J. natl Cancer Inst.*, **78**, 229–234

Palmer, J.R., Rosenberg, L., Clarke, E.A., Stolley, P.D., Warshauer, M.E., Zauber, A.G. & Shapiro, S. (1991) Breast cancer and cigarette smoking: A hypothesis. *Am. J. Epidemiol.*, **134**, 1–13

Primic-Zakelj, M., Evstifeeva, T., Ravnihar, B. & Boyle, P. (1995) Breast-cancer risk and oral contraceptive use in Slovenian women aged 25 to 54. *Int. J. Cancer*, **62**, 414–420

Ranstam, J. & Olsson, H. (1995) Alcohol, cigarette smoking, and the risk of breast cancer. *Cancer Detect. Prev.*, **19**, 487–493

Richardon, S., de Vincenzi, I., Pujol, H. & Gerber, M. (1989) Alcohol consumption in a case–control study of breast cancer in southern France. *Int. J. Cancer*, **44**, 84–89

Rohan, T.E. & Baron, J.A. (1989) Cigarette smoking and breast cancer. *Am. J. Epidemiol.*, **129**, 36–42

Rohan, T.E. & McMichael, A.J. (1988) Alcohol consumption and risk of breast cancer. *Int. J. Cancer*, **41**, 695–699

Rookus, M.A. & van Leeuwen, F.E. for the Netherlands Oral Contraceptives and Breast Cancer Study Group (1994) Oral contraceptives and risk of breast cancer in women aged 20–54 years. *Lancet*, **344**, 844–851

Rosenberg, L., Schwingl, P.J,. Kaufman, D.W., Miller, D.R., Helmrich, S.P., Stolley, P.D., Schottenfeld, D. & Shapiro, S. (1984) Breast cancer and cigarette smoking. *New Engl. J. Med.*, **310**, 92–94

Rosenberg, L., Palmer, J.R., Miller, D.R., Clarke, E.A. & Shapiro, S. (1990) A case–control study of alcohol beverage consumption and breast cancer. *Am. J. Epidemiol.*, **131**, 6–14

Rossing, M.A., Stanford, J.L., Weiss, N.S. & Habel, L.A. (1996) Oral contraceptive use and risk of breast cancer in middle-aged women. *Am. J. Epidemiol.*, **144**, 161–164

Schechter, M.T., Miller, A.B. & Howe, G.R. (1985) Cigarette smoking and breast cancer: A case–control study of screening program participants. *Am. J. Epidemiol.*, **121**, 479–487

Schechter, M.T., Miller, A.B., Howe, G.R., Baines, C.J., Craib, K.J. & Wall, C. (1989) Cigarete smoking and breast cancer: Case–control studies of prevalent and incident cancer in the Canadian National Breast Screening Study. *Am. J. Epidemiol.*, **130**, 213–220

Siskind, V., Schofield, F., Rice, D. & Bain, C. (1989) Breast cancer and breastfeeding: Results from an Australian case–control study. *Am. J. Epidemiol.*, **130**, 229–236

Smith, E.M., Sowers, M.F. & Burns, T.L. (1984) Effects of smoking on the development of female reproductive cancers. *J. natl Cancer Inst.*, **73**, 371–376

Smith, S.J., Deacon, J.M. & Cilvers, C.E. for the UK National Case–Control Study Group (1994) Alcohol, smoking, passive smoking and caffeine in relation to breast cancer risk in young women. *Br. J. Cancer*, **70**, 112–119

Sneyd, M.J., Paul, C., Spears, G.F. & Skegg, D.C. (1991) Alcohol consumption and risk of breast cancer. *Int. J. Cancer*, **48**, 812–815

Standford, J.L., Szklo, M., Boring, C.C., Brinton, L.A., Diamond, E.A., Greenberg, R.S. & hoover, R.N. (1987) A case–control study of breast cancer stratified by estrogen receptor status. *Am. J. Epidemiol.*, **125**, 184–194

Stockwell, H.G. & Lyman, G.H. (1987) cigarette smoking and the risk of female reproductive cancer. *Am. J. Obstet. Gynecol.*, **157**, 35–40

Swanson, C.A. Coates, R.J., Malone, K.E., Gammon, M.D., Schoenberg, J.B., Brogan, D.J., McAdams, M., Potischman, N., Hoover, R.N. & Brinton, L.A. (1997) Alcohol consumption and breast cancer risk among women under age 45 years. *Epidemiology*, **8**, 231–237

Thomas, D.B., Gao, D.L, Self, S.G., Allison, C.J., Tao, Y., Mahloch, J., Ray, R., Quin, Q., Presley, R. & Porter, P. (1997) Randomized trial of breast self-examination in Shangai: Methodology and preliminary results. *J. natl Cancer Inst.*, **89**, 355–365

Thun, M.J., Peto, R., Lopez, A.D., Monaco, J.H., Henley, S.J., Heath, C.W. & Doll, R. (1997) Alcohol consumption and mortality among middle-aged and elderly US adults. *New Engl. J. Med.*, **337**, 1705–1714

Tverdal, A., Thelle, D., Stensvold, I., Leren, P. & Bjartveit, K. (1993) Mortality in relation to smoking history: 13 years' follow-up of 68,000 Norwegian men and women 35–49 years. *J. clin. Epidemiol.*, **46**, 475–487

US Department of Health and Human Services (DHHS) (2001) *Women and Smoking. A Report of the Surgeon General*, Rockville, MD [available at http://www.cdc.gov/tobacco/sgr/ sgr_forwomen/index]

Ursin, G. Aragaki, C.C., Paganini-Hill, A., Siemiatychi, J., Thompson, W.D. & Haile, R.W. (1992) Oral contraceptives and premenopausal bilateral breast cancer: A case–control study. *Epidemiology*, **3**, 414–419

Vatten, L.J. & Kvinnsland, S. (1990) Cigarette smoking and risk of breast cancer: A prospective study of 24,329 Norwegian women. *Eur. J. Cancer*, **26**, 830–833

Viladiu, P., Izquierdo, A., de Sanjose, S. & Bosch, F.X. (1996) A breast cancer case–control study in Girona, Spain. Endocrine, familial and lifestyle factors. *Eur. J. Cancer Prev.*, **5**, 329–335

Wang, Q.S., Ross, R.K., Yu, M.C., Ning, J.P., Henderson, B.E. & Kimm, H.T. (1992) A case–control study of breast cancer in Tianjin, China. *Cancer Epidemiol. Biomarkers Prev.*, **1**, 435–439

Weinstein, A.L., Mahoney, M.C., Nasca, P.C., Hanson, R.L., Leske, M.C. & Varma, A.O. (1993) Oestrogen replacement therapy and breast cancer risk: A case–control study. *Int. J. Epidemiol.*, **22**, 781–789

White, E., Malone, K.E., Weiss, N.S. & Daling, J.R. (1994) Breast cancer among young US women in relation to oral contraceptive use. *J. natl Cancer Inst.*, **86**, 505–514

Willett, W.C., Stampfer, M.J., Colditz, G.A., Rosner, B.A., Hennekens, C.H. & Speizer, F.E. (1987) Moderate alcohol consumption and the risk of breast cancer. *New Engl. J. Med.*, **316**, 1174–1180

Yang, C.P., Daling, J.R., Band, P.R., Gallagher, R.P., White, E. & Weiss, N.S. (1992) Noncontraceptive hormone use and risk of breast cancer. *Cancer Causes Control*, **3**, 475–479

Yoo, K.Y., Tajima, K., Miura, S., Takeuchi, T., Hirose, K., Risch, H. & Dubrow, R. (1997) Breast cancer risk factors according to combined estrogen and progesterone receptor status: A case–control analysis. *Am. J. Epidemiol.*, **146**, 307–314

Yuan, J.M., Yu, M.C., Ross, R.K., Gao, Y.T. & Henderson, B.E. (1988) Risk factors for breast cancer in Chinese women in Shangai. *Cancer Res.*, **48**, 1949–1953

2.1.10 Cervical cancer

A positive correlation between the incidence of cervical cancer and other cancers known to be related to cigarette smoking across populations prompted the hypothesis that smoking may affect the risk for cervical cancer (Winkelstein, 1977). Excess risk for cervical cancer among smokers has been observed in a number of case–control studies. However, the extent to which the relationship between smoking and cervical cancer reflected a causal association independent of infection with human papillomavirus (HPV) remained a cause for concern. It was believed that the association of smoking with cervical cancer may be causal, may reflect confounding or risk modification among women with HPV infection, or may even reflect causality via an effect of smoking on risk for HPV infection.

In the earlier IARC evaluation of tobacco smoking (IARC, 1986), the Working Group noted that the effect of smoking is confounded by sexual behaviour variables, but the data were not adequate to remove the confounding effect, and that a reasonable conclusion from the available studies of invasive cervical cancer is that the results, although they indicate a positive effect of smoking, are compatible with the residual effects of variables that play a fundamental role in the etiology of cervical cancer (IARC, 1986). At the time of the 1986 review, a specific causal agent had not been identified, but was proposed to be an infective agent related to sexual activity.

Infection with HPV is now recognized as the main etiological factor for invasive and pre-invasive cervical neoplasia worldwide (IARC, 1995). Persistent infection with certain high-risk types of HPV, i.e. HPV 16, 18, 31, 33, 45, 52 and 58, is considered to be a necessary cause of invasive cervical cancer (IARC, 1995). Using the most sensitive polymerase chain reaction-based assays, HPV DNA has been found in 99.7% of approximately 1000 cervical cancer specimens from 22 countries worldwide (Walboomers et al., 1995) and odds ratios close to 100.0 for high-risk HPV types have been obtained in numerous case–control studies (IARC, 1995). Co-factors acting in conjunction with HPV, however, could be important for the development of cervical neoplasia or invasive cervical cancer. In order to investigate the possibility that smoking acts as a co-factor in conjunction with HPV in the production of cervical cancer, it is important to account accurately for the presence of HPV infection. Less than 10% of invasive cervical cancers have a histology of adenocarcinoma or adenosquamous-cell carcinoma, whereas squamous-cell types account for over 90%. This review, therefore, focuses on squamous-cell invasive cervical cancer; data for adenocarcinoma and adenosquamous-cell carcinoma are used for comparative purposes.

Ten cohort studies and 31 case–control studies have provided information about the association of cigarette smoking with the incidence of invasive squamous-cell cervical cancer and six cohort studies and 22 case–control studies evaluated the association of tobacco smoking with preinvasive neoplasms (cervical intraepithelial neoplasia (CIN) and cervical cancer *in situ*). In addition, seven case–control studies evaluated the association of adenocarcinoma and adenosquamous-cell carcinoma with tobacco smoking. The characteristics of and the main results from these studies are shown in Tables 2.1.10.1–2.1.10.12 (see Tables 2.1, 2.1.10.1 and 2.1.10.2 for details on study design). These tables are organized by type of disease and level of control for HPV status. HPV status was controlled for in data analysis or by restriction of analyses to HPV-positive cases and controls. Twenty-eight of the earliest case–control studies of invasive squamous-cell cervical cancer and 25 case–control studies and one cohort study on the association of CIN with smoking did not control for HPV status (Tables 2.1.10.3–2.1.10.6). Four case–control studies of invasive cervical cancer (Peng *et al.*, 1991; Chichareon *et al.*, 1998; Ngelangel *et al.*, 1998; Lacey *et al.*, 2001), and one cohort study (Moscicki *et al.*, 2001) and four case–control studies (Muñoz et *al.*, 1993; Ho *et al.*, 1998; Yoshikawa *et al.*, 1999; Kjellberg *et al.*, 2000) of CIN controlled for HPV status by adjustment in the data analysis (Tables 2.1.10.7–2.1.10.9). More recent studies controlled for HPV status by restricting analyses to HPV-positive cases and controls. The results of eight case–control studies of invasive squamous-cell cervical cancer (Bosch *et al.*, 1992; Eluf-Neto *et al.*, 1994; Chaouki *et al.*, 1998; Chichareon *et al.*, 1998; Ngelangel *et al.*, 1998; Rolon *et al.*, 2000; Hildesheim *et al.*, 2001; Santos et al., 2001) and two case–control studies of CIN (Olsen *et al.*, 1998; Deacon *et al.*, 2000) are shown in Tables 2.1.10.10 and 2.1.10.11. In addition, the results of six case–control studies that examined the association of adenocarcinoma and adenosquamous-cell carcinoma with tobacco (Brinton *et al.*, 1986; Ursin *et al.*, 1996; Chichareon *et al.*, 1998; Ngelangel *et al.*, 1998; Lacey *et al.*, 2001; Madeleine *at al.*, 2001) are shown in Table 2.1.10.12.

In these studies, the association between cervical cancer and smoking was not eliminated, even though most studies controlled for several well-established risk factors for cervical cancer, including early age at first sexual intercourse, history of multiple sexual partners, low socioeconomic status and, in the recent studies, infection with HPV. Most studies in which the risk values were not adjusted for HPV infection reported a relative risk of approximately 2.0 among smokers compared with nonsmokers. Women who had smoked for a long period or at high intensity generally had the highest risk. In several studies, the relationship was restricted to, or strongest among, recent or current smokers. Some studies reported that the highest risk occurred among women who had started smoking late in life, but other studies reported the opposite effect, namely a higher risk among women who had begun smoking at young ages (La Vecchia *et al.*, 1986; Daling *et al.*, 1996). In the studies that assessed the association of adenocarcinoma and adenosquamous-cell carcinoma of the cervix with smoking, there was generally no significant association noted for adenocarcinoma or adenosquamous-cell carcinoma of the cervix.

Recent studies have chosen to control for the confounding effect of HPV as indicated by either the presence of HPV DNA in cervical cells or of anti-HPV serum antibodies in multivariate analytical models, or have restricted their analyses to HPV-positive cases and controls.

Several of the studies reviewed, including the IARC multicentre pooled analysis of 10 studies of invasive cervical cancer (Plummer *et al.*, 2003), examined tobacco smoking as a co-factor to HPV infection by restricting the analysis to HPV DNA-positive study participants, a decision justified by the necessity of HPV infection in the causation of invasive cervical cancer (Hildesheim *et al.*, 2001). The results from these analyses showed no significant alteration in risk whether or not the study participants were HPV DNA-positive. Similarly, other studies that investigated the effect of smoking among HPV-seropositive cases and controls found that the effect of smoking remained, and there was evidence of a dose–response relationship. The association between smoking and invasive cervical cancer was not notably reduced by adjustment for a woman's reported number of lifetime sexual partners, age at first sexual intercourse or other potential confounding factors (Hildesheim *et al.*, 2001). Thus, the effect of smoking is unlikely to represent a surrogate marker for a woman's sexual behaviour.

Cervical infection with HPV has not been found to be consistently associated with tobacco smoking in cross-sectional studies (Plummer *et al.*, 2003). Therefore, it would appear that HPV is not a significant confounding factor for the association between cervical cancer and smoking.

The detection of HPV DNA has a different meaning for cases and control participants. In cases, HPV DNA-positivity indicates a persistent HPV infection, whereas some control participants may have a transient HPV infection or have been infected with HPV in the past and have cleared their infection. Given that the ascertainment of overall HPV prevalence and the relative distribution of HPV types may differ according to status as case or control, careful account of the type of HPV infection (such as high-risk versus low-risk types) must be taken.

Persistent cervical infections with HPV have been shown to increase the risk of progression of cervical dysplasia (Remmink *et al.*, 1995). As there is currently no reliable marker of persistent HPV infection, case–control studies based on a cross-sectional measurement of HPV-DNA by polymerase chain reaction assays cannot distinguish between transient and persistent infections (Franco *et al.*, 1999). To improve the likelihood that the effect being examined is that of smoking among persistent HPV carriers, analyses by some investigators were limited to women who were HPV-DNA-positive for high-risk HPV types that are more likely to represent persistent infections than non-oncogenic types (Franco *et al.*, 2001). Increased rate ratios for smoking were observed in one study that conducted these analyses (Hildesheim *et al.*, 2001).

Table 2.1.10.1. Case–control studies on tobacco smoking and cervical cancer: main characteristics of study design

Reference[a] Country and years of study	Number of cases and controls	Criteria for eligibility and comments
Tokuhata (1967) USA Not specified	266 cases and 1463 controls	Population-based study Cases and controls selected from county death registry among women ever married and having died after 1950 Controls: breast cancer, heart and other non-cancerous diseases City and county directories used to identify next-of-kin Response rates ≥ 95% for both cases and controls
Thomas (1972) USA 1965–69	324 cases, aged 15–50 years, and 302 controls	Hospital-based study Cases histologically confirmed Controls: 1:30 probability sample of the 15–50-year-old white female residents of the county having at least one smear on record from 1965–69
Williams & Horm (1977); Williams et al. (1977) USA, Not specified	266 cases and 3198 controls	Cases and controls from the Third National Cancer Survey (57% of those selected for interview). Controls included all cases of cancer of other sites except lung, larynx, oral cavity, oesophagus and bladder [no matching].
Harris et al. (1980) UK 1974–79	237 cases and 422 controls	Hospital-based study at two Oxford hospitals Controls attended gynaecological clinics during a similar period to the cases; a few additional controls had received an initial cervical smear at the Abingdon Health Centre; excluding controls who had had hysterectomy or with history of cancer or severe mental illness
Stellman et al. (1980) USA 1974–77	332 cases and 1725 controls, aged 20–89 years	Hospital-based study Cases histologically confirmed Controls hospitalized for non-neoplastic diseases Analysis restricted to ever-married women, excluding former smokers
Wigle et al. (1980) Canada 1971–73	676 cases (168 ICC and 508 CIS) and 3644 controls, aged 20–64 years	Hospital-based study Cases histologically confirmed Controls comprised women with primary cancers unrelated to smoking and with benign breast neoplasms.

Table 2.1.10.1 (contd)

Reference[a] Country and years of study	Number of cases and controls	Criteria for eligibility and comments
Buckley et al. (1981) UK 1974–79	237 cases and 422 controls, aged 32–70 years	Hospital-based study Cases histologically confirmed Controls were women attending gynaecological care units for cervical smears, excluding those who had had hysterectomy or abnormal smear.
Clarke et al. (1982) Canada 1973–76	178 cases, aged 20–69 years, and 865 controls matched on age	Population-based study among residents of York County, Toronto Cases histologically confirmed Controls selected from the same neighbourhood as the cases
Berggren & Sjöstedt (1983) Sweden 1974–78	609 cases and 6090 controls, aged 15–65 years	Population-based study Cases histologically confirmed Controls were residents of the same geographical area as the cases, born on the same day as the cases or soon thereafter, excluding women with previous history of cervical cancer or abnormal smear.
Lyon et al. (1983) USA 1975–77	217 cases and 243 controls	Population-based study among residents of the metropolitan area of Utah Cases histologically confirmed Controls selected by random-digit dialling to give an age- and geographically stratified sample of the same population
Marshall et al. (1983) USA 1957–65	513 cases and 490 controls matched on age	Hospital-based study Cases histologically confirmed Controls selected from a pool of patients with non-neoplastic diseases of sites other than the genitourinary and gastrointestinal tracts
Trevathan et al. (1983) USA 1980–81	374 (194 mild/moderate dysplasia, 81 severe dysplasia, 99 in situ) cases, aged 17–55 years, and 288 controls	Hospital-based study Cases histologically confirmed Controls with negative Pap smears and no prior cervical biopsy selected from women attending the Family Planning Clinic
Martin & Hill (1984) South Africa 1950–74	257 case–control pairs, matched on age, number of children and home area (age range, 22–89 years)	Hospital- and population-based study [% of histologically confirmed cases not indicated Controls free of cancer (no information on selection of controls)]

Table 2.1.10.1 (contd)

Reference[a] Country and years of study	Number of cases and controls	Criteria for eligibility and comments
Clarke et al. (1985) Canada 1979–81	250 cases aged 20–59 years, and 500 controls matched on age, neighbourhood and type of dwelling	Population-based study among residents of the Toronto area Cases histologically confirmed Controls with intact uterus and no history of cancer identified from municipal records
Mayberry (1985) USA Not specified	210 cases and 317 controls (data from previous study on HSV-2 and *Chlamydiae trachomatis* and cervical cancer)	Hospital-based study Cases histologically confirmed Controls free of cervical abnormalities who attended gynaecological and birth control clinics at the University of California Medical Center in San Francisco
Baron et al. (1986) USA 1957–75	1174 cases aged 40–89 years, and 2128 controls	Hospital-based study Controls in the same age range, admitted during the same time period, with no diagnosis of cancer during hospitalization and no smoking-associated respiratory or circulatory diseases
Brinton et al. (1986) USA 1982–84	480 cases (incl. 63 adenocarcinoma or adenosquamous carcinoma), aged 20–74 years, and 797 controls, matched on telephone exchange, race and age	Population-based study in five cities reporting to the Comprehensive Cancer Patient Data System – Birmingham (AL), Chicago, Denver, Miami and Philadelphia Controls obtained by random-digit dialling
La Vecchia et al. (1986) Italy 1981–84	155 ICC (aged 22–74 years) and 169 controls 89 CIN (aged 19–71 years) and 118 controls Cases and controls matched on age	Hospital-based study in six wards of three major university hospitals in Milan Cases histologically confirmed Controls for ICC admitted for acute conditions other than malignant, hormonal or gynaecological disorders; controls for CIN were women with normal cervical smear from the same screening clinics
Peters et al. (1986) USA 1980–81	200 cases and 200 controls, matched on race, date of birth and language of interview	Population-based study Cases histologically confirmed Controls identified by an algorithm defining a sequence of houses in the neighbourhood where the case lived at diagnosis

Table 2.1.10.1 (contd)

Reference[a] Country and years of study	Number of cases and controls	Criteria for eligibility and comments
Celentano et al. (1987) USA 1982–85	153 cases and 153 controls, matched on age, race, residence within neighbourhood, intact uterus	Population-based study among Maryland residents referred to the Division of Gynecologic Oncology at John's Hopkins Hospital, MD Cases histologically confirmed Controls without history of cervical cancer obtained by case nomination (97), canvassing neighbourhood (49) and from senior citizen centres (7)
Ebeling et al. (1987) Germany 1983–85	129 cases and 275 controls	Hospital-based study Cases histologically confirmed Controls identified at the Skin Disease Hospital and at the Orthopaedic University Hospital, which drew patients from the same area as the gynaecological hospitals; women with venereal diseases, prior CIN and prior hysterectomy excluded
Nischan et al. (1988) Germany 1983–85	225 cases, aged 64 years or younger, and 435 controls, matched on age	Hospital-based study in four hospitals in Leipzig Cases histologically confirmed Controls, excluding women with venereal diseases, prior CIN and prior hysterectomy, identified at the Skin Disease Hospital and at the Orthopaedic University Hospital
Brock et al. (1989) Australia 1980–83	116 cases, aged 18–65 years, and 193 controls, matched on age	Population-based study within the Sydney metropolitan area Cases histologically confirmed Controls selected from the files of the family doctor or from a university-affiliated general practitioner from the same residential area
Herrero et al. (1989) Colombia, Costa Rica, Mexico, Panama 1986–87	667 cases, aged less than 70 years, and 1430 controls	Hospital- and community-based study Cases histologically confirmed Hospital controls selected from primary referral hospitals (Costa Rica and Panama); from eight tertiary level government hospitals (Bogota); and from three Social Security hospitals (Mexico City); all hospitals located in the area of residence of the cases Community controls randomly selected from current census listings of the corresponding case's county of residence
Slattery et al. (1989) USA 1984–87	266 cases, aged 20–59 years, and 408 controls, matched on age and residence	Population-based study in the urban areas of Utah Cases histologically confirmed Controls selected using random-digit dialling; women who had had a hysterectomy before 1984 excluded

Table 2.1.10.1 (contd)

Reference[a] Country and years of study	Number of cases and controls	Criteria for eligibility and comments
Licciardone et al. (1989) USA 1984–86	331 cases and 993 controls matched on age	Cancer registry-based study Cases histologically confirmed Controls randomly selected from other patients reported to the Missouri Cancer Registry during the same time period after exclusion of cancers at smoking- or alcohol-related sites
Cuzick et al. (1990) UK 1984–88	497 cases (110 CIN I, 103 CIN II, 284 CIN III), aged 18–39 years, and 833 controls	Population-based study in the London area Cases histologically confirmed Controls: randomly selected patients of local general practitioners or family planning clinics in the catchment area from which cases were drawn
Jones et al. (1990) USA 1982–84	293 cases, aged 20–74 years, and 801 controls, matched on race and age	Population-based study in Birmingham, Chicago, Denver, Miami and Philadelphia Controls ascertained using random–digit dialling
Peng et al. (1991) China 1987–88	101 cases, and 146 controls selected to provide a similar distribution of age and occupation	Hospital-based study in Chengdu, Sichuan Cases histologically confirmed Controls: patients admitted to the gynaecological ward/clinic, excluding women with abnormal cervical cytology, prior hysterectomy, or vulvar cancer
Bosch et al. (1992, 1993); Muñoz et al. (1992, 1993) Spain, 1985–87 Colombia, 1985–88	525 cases, aged less than 70 years, and 512 controls, matched on age, place of recruitment and date of cytology	Population-based study in nine provinces in Spain and in one city in Colombia (Cali) Cases histologically confirmed Controls with normal cytology or with inflammation only (Pap smear grades I and II) randomly selected from the population that generated the cases; included only those women who had not had previous treatment for cervical cancer or a hysterectomy.
Coker et al. (1992) USA 1987–88	103 cases (40 CIN II and 63 CIN III), aged 18–45 years, and 268 controls	Hospital-based study in North Carolina Cases histologically confirmed Controls: University of North Carolina Hospital Family Practice Center patients receiving routine Pap smear and having normal cervical cytology
Parazzini et al. (1992) Italy 1981–90	366 cases (58 CIN I, 70 CIN II, 238 CIN III), aged 18–59 years, and 323 controls with comparable age distribution	Hospital-based study in Milan Cases histologically confirmed Controls: women with normal cervical smears interviewed at the same screening clinic where cases were identified

Table 2.1.10.1 (contd)

Reference[a] Country and years of study	Number of cases and controls	Criteria for eligibility and comments
Becker et al. (1994) USA 1989–92	201 cases, aged 18–40 years, and 307 controls	Hospital-based study in the Albuquerque metropolitan area Cases histologically confirmed Frequency-matched controls, with normal cervical cytology, selected from the same clinics to which cases were referred for colposcopic examination
Eluf-Neto et al. (1994) Brazil 1990–91	199 cases, aged 25–79 years, and 225 controls, matched on age	Hospital-based study in seven hospitals in São Paulo City Cases histologically confirmed Controls selected from the same hospitals, excluding women with known risk factors for cervical neoplasia, treated for gynaecological conditions, or having had hysterectomy or conization
de Vet et al. (1994) Netherlands Not specified	257 cases, aged 20–65 years, and 705 controls, matched on age	Multicentre randomized clinical trial Cases histologically confirmed Controls: random sample of the female population of three cities and one neighbouring village for each city; subjects with recent pregnancy, diabetes mellitus or severe bowel or liver dysfunction excluded
Lazcano-Ponce et al. (1995) Mexico 1990–92	397 ICC, 233 CIN III and 1005 controls	Population-based study Cases histologically confirmed Controls: random sample from houses in the Mexico City metropolitan area
Stone et al. (1995) Costa Rica 1982–85	564 cases (415 carcinoma in situ, 149 invasive cancer), aged 25–59 years, and 764 controls, matched on age	Population-based study Cases histologically confirmed, identified through the Costa Rican National Tumor Registry Controls selected from a national multistage probability household survey
Cuzick et al. (1996) UK 1985–91	121 cases, aged 40 years or younger, and 241 controls, matched on age	Population-based study Cases histologically confirmed Controls drawn from the same general practitioner as the cases
Daling et al. (1996) USA 1986–92	314 cases, aged 18–74 years, and 672 controls, matched on age	Population-based study Cases histologically confirmed Controls identified using random-digit dialling

Table 2.1.10.1 (contd)

Reference[a] Country and years of study	Number of cases and controls	Criteria for eligibility and comments
Hirose et al. (1996) Japan 1988–93	556 cases, aged 18 years or older, and 26 751 controls	Hospital-based study Cases histologically confirmed Controls: first-visit outpatients with no prior diagnosis of cancer
Kjaer et al. (1996) Denmark 1987–88	645 cases (586 carcinoma in situ, 59 invasive cancer), aged 20–49 years, and 614 controls, matched on age	Population-based study among women living in greater Copenhagen Cases histologically confirmed Controls identified by random sampling using the computerized Danish Central Population Register
Ursin et al. (1996) USA 1977–91	195 cases and 386 controls, matched on age, race and neighbourhood	Population-based study in Los Angeles County, CA Cases histologically confirmed Controls identified by visiting houses in the cases' neighbourhood according to a predetermined algorithm
Chaouki et al. (1998) Morocco 1991–93	214 cases, aged 18–80 years, and 203 controls, matched on age	Hospital-based study in Rabat Cases histologically confirmed Controls from the same cancer hospital and a nearby general hospital, excluding women with a history of hysterectomy or conization, and conditions related to risk factors for cervical neoplasm (other anogenital cancers, cancers of the breast, oral cavity, oesophagus, lung, bladder and liver, cardiovascular diseases, chronic bronchitis, emphysema and sexually transmitted diseases)
Chichareon et al. (1998) Thailand 1990–93	338 cases (including 39 with adenocarcinoma/adenosquamous carcinoma) and 261 controls	Hospital-based study in Hat-Yai Cases histologically confirmed Age-stratified controls without anogenital tract cancers, cancers of the breast, endometrium, ovary, colon, benign genital tumours, tobacco-related diseases or history of conization or hysterectomy, selected from the same hospital
Ho et al. (1998) USA 1992–94	258 women with HPV infection (163 CIN I, 51 CIN II and 44 CIN III)	Hospital-based study in New York Cases histologically confirmed Reference population constituted of women with CIN I. Eligibility criteria included having had cervical biopsy and/or endocervical curettage on the day of recruitment, not being pregnant, no history of cancer and having an intact cervix

Table 2.1.10.1 (contd)

Reference[a] Country and years of study	Number of cases and controls	Criteria for eligibility and comments
Kanetsky et al. (1998) USA 1993–95	32 cases (12 CIN I, 10 CIN II, 9 CIN III/CIS, 1 ungradable CIN), aged 18 years and above, and 113 controls	Hospital-based study at the Harlem Hospital Center Cases histologically confirmed Controls: HIV-negative, black, non-Hispanic women with normal cervical cytology recruited from the gynaecology and family planning clinics
Ngelangel et al. (1998) The Philippines 1991–93	356 cases (including 33 with adenocarcinoma/adenosquamous carcinoma) and 381 controls matched on age	Hospital-based study in Manila Cases histologically confirmed Controls without diseases associated with known risk factors for cervical neoplasia and no history of conization or hysterectomy, selected from the same hospital
Olsen et al. (1998) Norway 1991–92	90 cases (10 CIN II, 80 CIN III), aged 20–44 years, and 216 controls	Population-based study in Oslo Cases histologically confirmed Controls without cervical dysplasia enrolled from an age-stratified random sample of women obtained through the Norwegian Central Population Register
Parazzini et al. (1998) Italy 1981–93	261 cases, aged less than 45 years, and 257 controls	Hospital-based study Cases histologically confirmed Controls aged less than 45 years, admitted to the same network of hospitals for acute conditions unrelated to cervical cancer risk factors, and belonging to the same catchment areas as cases
Hsieh et al. (1999) China, Province of Taiwan Not specified	183 cases and 293 controls, matched on age, marital status and residential area	Population-based study in Taipei Cases histologically confirmed Controls randomly selected from local household registration offices
Yoshikawa et al. (1999) Japan 1995–96	167 cases (94 CIN I, 40 CIN II, 33 CIN III), aged 55 years or younger, and 167 controls, matched on age and hospital	Hospital-based study in nine hospitals Cases histologically confirmed Controls selected from subjects with normal cervical cytology
Kjellberg et al. (2000) Sweden 1993–95	122 cases, aged 25–59 years, and 346 controls	Population-based study in northern Sweden Cases histologically confirmed

Table 2.1.10.1 (contd)

Reference[a] Country and years of study	Number of cases and controls	Criteria for eligibility and comments
Rolon et al. (2000) Paraguay 1988–90	113 cases, aged 18–85 years, and 91 controls, matched on age	Hospital-based study in Asunción Cases histologically confirmed Controls without cervical cancer and with no history of conization or hysterectomy selected from outpatient clinics at the same hospitals; exclusion criteria included diseases associated with cervical cancer risk factors, tobacco-related diseases and cancer of the breast, endometrium, ovary or colon)
Lacey et al. (2001) USA 1992–96	263 cases (124 adenocarcinoma, 139 squamous-cell carcinoma), aged 18–69 years, and 307 controls, matched on age, race and geographical region	Multicentre population-based study Cases histologically confirmed Controls identified through random-digit dialling, excluding women with hysterectomy
Madeleine et al. (2001) USA 1990–96	150 cases, aged 18–70 years, and 651 controls, matched on age	Population-based study Cases histologically confirmed, identified through the SEER Cancer Surveillance System Controls identified using random-digit dialling among residents at reference date of the 13-county area in western Washington state; women with an intact uterus, who spoke English
Santos et al. (2001) Peru 1996–97	198 cases (173 squamous-cell carcinomas and 25 adenocarcinoma/adenosquamous carcinomas) and 196 controls, matched on age	Hospital-based study in two hospitals in Lima Cases histologically confirmed Controls selected from women without cervical cancer or history of conization or hysterectomy, attending the same hospitals; exclusion criteria included diseases associated with known risk factors for cervical cancer (cancers of the anogenital tract, tobacco-related cancers and cancer of the breast, endometrium, ovary or colon)

[a] Studies published after 1986, or before 1986 but not included in Volume 38 of the *IARC Monographs* ICC, invasive cervical cancer; CIS, carcinoma *in situ*; CIN, cervical intraepithelial neoplasia

Table 2.1.10.2. Description of additional cohort studies on tobacco smoking and cervical cancer, cervical intraepithelial neoplasia (CIN) and carcinoma *in situ* (CIS) (with or without control for human papilloma virus (HPV) status)

Reference Country and years of study	Name of study	Cohort sample	Cases/deaths identification	Comments
Wright *et al.* (1978); Zondervan *et al.* (1996) UK 1968–77	Oxford Family Planning Association Study	17 032 women recruited in 17 large family planning clinics in England and Scotland, aged 25–39 years	Cases ascertained by follow-up in clinics	
Beral *et al.* (1988) UK 1968–87	Royal College of General Practitioners' Oral Contraception Study	47 000 women aged ≥ 15 years, half of whom were using oral contraceptives at recruitment	Cases ascertained by general practitioners	Study designed primarily to investigate oral contraceptive use and female genital cancer
Gram *et al.* (1992) Norway 1979–89	Tromsö Study	8143 women aged 20–49 years living in Tromsö with at least one negative test for CIN between 1977 and 1980	Cases ascertained by linkage to the Pathology Registry of the University Hospital	Participants were followed for development of CIN III or cervical cancer
Schiffman *et al.* (1993) USA 1989–90		21 146 women presenting for routine Pap smear screening	Cases diagnosed at the Kaiser Permanente clinic	Nested case–control study without matching; HPV-positive: 81% cases, 18% controls
Ylitalo *et al.* (1999) Sweden 1969–95		146 889 women born in Sweden and resident in Uppsala between 1969 and 1995, aged ≤ 50 years, and having had at least one smear test	Cases identified through National Cancer Registry	Nested case–control study; controls randomly selected among cohort, matched by date of entry into cohort (± 90 days), year of birth; with intact uterus and without history of prior in situ or invasive cervical carcinoma
Moscicki *et al.* (2001) USA 1990–2000		496 women examined at 2 family clinics with normal cytological findings at baseline and first follow-up excluding those testing HPV-negative at any time during follow-up	Cases ascertained at the clinics	Study designed primarily to investigate development of low-grade squamous intraepithelial lesions in HPV-infected women

Table 2.1.10.3. Case–control studies on tobacco smoking and invasive cervical cancer (ICC) (without control for human papillomavirus (HPV) status)

Reference Country and years of study	Relative risk (95% CI)				Adjustment factors	Comments
	Ever	Current	Former	By quantity/duration		
Tokuhata (1967) USA Not specified	1.2					Similar in white and black women
Williams & Horm (1977) USA Not specified				*Pack-years* **Invasive** ≥ 20 1.2 21–39 1.6 ≥ 40 1.8	After adjustment for race, no. of children, socioeconomic indicators, a 'mild' positive association remained.	266 cases
Stellman et al. (1980) USA 1974–77				Risk ratios for > 10 cigarettes/day ranged from 1.4 to 1.6 before adjustments and from 1.2 to 1.3 after adjustment for age and socioeconomic status, the value depending on the amount smoked. Smokers of < 10 cigarettes/day have a relative risk of < 1.		Socioeconomic status has little confounding effect; the reduction of relative risks after adjustment is due mainly to age.
Wigle et al. (1980) Canada 1971–73		Invasive, 2.0 CIS, 3.8	Invasive, 1.0 CIS, 1.3	*Pack-years* **Invasive** < 10 1.2 11–20 1.7 21–30 2.1 ≥ 31 2.7	No adjustment made for social or sexual variables	
Buckley et al. (1981) UK 1974–79		Combined risk (dysplasia, CIS, ICC) 7.0 7.8 3.2	2.8 3.7 2.7		No adjustment No. of sexual partners of husband Smoking of husband	Relative risk 35 among small series of multiple-partner women with husbands who smoked versus those with nonsmoking or formerly smoking husbands

Table 2.1.10.3 (contd)

Reference Country and years of study	Relative risk (95% CI)			By quantity/duration	Adjustment factors	Comments
	Ever	Current	Former			
Clarke et al. (1982) Canada 1973–76		2.3 (1.6–3.3)	1.7 (1.0–2.8)	< ½ pack/day > 1 pack/day	2.2 2.9	Age, education, age at first intercourse, sexual stability
Marshall et al. (1983) USA 1957–65		1.6 (1.2–2.1)	0.8 (0.5–1.4)	< ½ pack/day ½–1 packs/day 1–2 packs/day > 2 packs/day	1.7 (1.1–2.6) 1.7 (1.2–2.3) 1.0 (0.8–1.2) 0.4 (0.2–1.2)	
Baron et al. (1986) USA 1957–75				1–14 packs/year ≥ 15 packs/year	1.4 (1.1–1.7) 1.8 (1.5–2.2)	Age, marital status, no. of pregnancies
Brinton et al. (1986) USA 1982–84	1.5 (1.1–1.9)	1.5 (1.2–2.0)	1.3 (0.9–1.9)	*Years of smoking* < 10 10–19 20–29 30–39 ≥ 40 *Cigarettes/day* < 10 10–19 20–29 ≥ 40	1.1 (0.7–1.7) 1.6 (1.1–2.4) 1.3 (0.9–2.0) 1.5 (1.0–2.4) 2.2 (1.2–4.2) 1.1 (0.6–1.7) 1.3 (0.9–2.0) 1.5 (1.1–2.1) 2.4 (1.4–4.1)	Age, race, no. of sexual partners, age at first intercourse, education

$p < 0.001$

Table 2.1.10.3 (contd)

Reference Country and years of study	Relative risk (95% CI) Ever	Current	Former	By quantity/duration		Adjustment factors	Comments
La Vecchia et al. (1986) Italy 1981–84			0.8 (0.4–1.7)	*Current*		Age, marital status, education, social class, sexual partners, age at first intercourse, no. of sexual partners, parity, no. of abortions at menopause, no. of previous Pap smears, use of oral contraceptives and other use of female hormones and clinical history of other sexually transmitted diseases	
				< 15 cigarettes/day	1.7 (0.8–3.4)		
				≥ 15 cigarettes/day	1.8 (0.9–3.6)		
				Total duration of smoking (years)			
				< 10	1.3 (0.6–3.1)		
				10–19	1.0 (0.4–2.1)		
				20–29	1.4 (0.7–2.8)		
				30–39	1.5 (0.6–3.1)		
				≥ 40	7.8 (1.5–39.9)		$p = 0.05$
				Age at starting smoking (years)			
				> 24	1.4 (0.81–2.4)		
				18–24	1.2 (0.59–2.3)		
				< 18	1.9 (0.7–5.4)		
Peters et al. (1986) USA 1980–81				*Cigarettes/day*		Race, sex, date of birth and language of interview	
				0–5	1.0		
				6–19	1.5 (0.8–2.7)		
				≥ 20	3.7 (2.0–6.9)		
				Years of smoking			Women currently smoking > 5 cigarettes/day
				0–1 year	1.0		
				2–20 years	1.5 (0.8–2.8)		
				≥ 21 years	4.0 (2.0–7.8)		$p < 0.001$
Celentano et al. (1987) USA 1982–85				Years of smoking	1.0 (1.0–1.0)		

Table 2.1.10.3 (contd)

Reference Country and years of study	Relative risk (95% CI)				Adjustment factors	Comments
	Ever	Current	Former	By quantity/duration		
Eberling et al. (1987) Germany 1983–85	1.3 (0.8–2.3)				Age, no. of pregnancies, age at first pregnancy, number of sexual partners, age at first intercourse, history of discharge, months since last Pap smear	
Nischan et al. (1988) Germany 1983–85	1.2 (0.8–1.7)			Never 1.0 <10 years 0.7 10–19 years 1.3 20–29 years 1.7 ≥ 30 years 2.7 ($p < 0.05$)	Age, no. of sexual partners, age at first intercourse, no. of pregnancies, years since last screening test	
Herrero et al. (1989) Costa Rica, Colombia, Mexico, Panama 1986–87		1.0 (0.7–1.2)	1.0 (0.8–1.3)	*Cigarettes/day* < 10 1.0 (0.8–1.2) 10–19 1.0 (0.6–1.7) 20–29 1.0 (0.6–1.5) ≥ 30 1.1 (0.5–2.5) *Age at starting smoking (years)* > 30 1.7 (1.1–2.6) 21–30 0.9 (0.7–1.4) 16–20 0.8 (0.6–1.1) < 16 years 1.1 (0.7–1.6) *Duration of smoking (years)* < 10 1.0 (0.7–1.4) 10–19 1.0 (0.7–1.4) 20–29 1.1 (0.7–1.7) 30–39 0.6 (0.4–1.1) ≥ 40 1.5 (0.8–2.8)	Age, no. of sexual partners, alcohol consumption	$p = 0.8$ $p = 0.8$

Table 2.1.10.3 (contd)

Reference, Country and years of study	Relative risk (95% CI) Ever	Current	Former	By quantity/duration	Adjustment factors	Comments
Herrero et al. (1989) (contd)				**HPV negative**		
				Ever-smoker 0.9 (0.7–1.3)		
				Cigarettes/day		
				< 10 1.0 (0.7–1.5)		
				≥ 10 0.8 (0.5–1.3)		
				Age at starting smoking (years)		
				> 30 1.4 (0.7–2.9)		
				≤ 30 0.9 (0.6–1.2)		
				Duration of smoking (years)		
				< 10 1.0 (0.6–1.7)		
				10–19 1.0 (0.6–1.6)		
				> 20 0.9 (0.6–1.5)		
				HPV positive		
				Ever-smoker 6.3 (4.3–9.2)		
				Cigarettes/day		
				< 10 5.5 (3.5–8.3)		
				≥ 10 8.4 (4.4–16.2)		
				Age at starting smoking (years)		
				> 30 13.1 (5.7–29.0)		
				≤ 30 5.1 (3.4–7.8)		
				Duration of smoking (years)		
				< 10 5.7 (3.0–10.6)		
				10–19 5.9 (3.1–11.1)		
				> 20 6.6 (3.6–12.1)		
Licciardone et al. (1989) USA 1984–86			1.7 (1.0–2.9)	< 1 pack/day 2.2 (1.4–3.6)	Age, alcohol consumption, stage at diagnosis	
				≥ 1 pack/day 3.9 (2.7–5.6)		

Table 2.1.10.3 (contd)

Reference Country and years of study	Relative risk (95% CI)				Adjustment factors	Comments
	Ever	Current	Former	By quantity/duration		
Bosch et al. (1992) Spain, 1985–87 Colombia, 1985–88	1.5 (1.0–2.2)				Age, centre, HPV status by PCR, no. of sexual partners, education, age at first birth, previous cytology screening	
Eluf-Neto et al. (1994) Brazil 1990–91	1.5 (1.0–2.3)				Age and socioeconomic status	
Lazcano-Ponce et al. (1995) Mexico 1990–92				Never smoker 1.0 1st tertile 1.4 (0.96–2.1) 2nd tertile 1.2 (0.78–1.8) 3rd tertile 1.3 (0.81–1.9)	Age, socioeconomic status, age at sexual intercourse, no. of sexual partners	Tertiles of tobacco consumption
Stone et al. (1995) Costa Rica 1982–85	1.3 (0.9–1.3)				Age	
Cuzick et al. (1996) UK 1985–91		1.2 (0.7–2.3)	1.3 (0.7–2.6)	Pack-years 0.1–5: 1.3 (0.6–2.6) 6–10: 1.8 (0.8–4.1) 11–20: 0.9 (0.4–1.9) > 20: 1.7 (0.6–4.7)	No. of sexual partners, age at first intercourse	p for trend = 0.54

Table 2.1.10.3 (contd)

Reference, Country and years of study	Relative risk (95% CI)			By quantity/duration	Adjustment factors	Comments
	Ever	Current	Former			
Daling et al. (1996) USA 1986–92		2.5 (1.8–3.4)	1.5 (1.1–2.2)	Duration of smoking (years)	Age, no. of lifetime sexual partners	
		1.7 (1.1–2.6)	1.5 (1.0–2.5)	< 10 1.0 10–19 2.4 (1.1–5.3) ≥ 20 2.8 (1.1–6.9)	Age, no. of lifetime sexual partners, HSV-2 seropositivity, oral contraceptive use of 17 years or less, HPV 16 antibody status	
Hirose et al. (1996) Japan 1988–93		2.2 (1.8–2.7)		Cigarettes/day < 10 1.3 (0.8–2.1) ≥ 10 2.5 (2.0–3.1)	Age of first visit	
Kjaer et al. (1996) Denmark 1987–88	0.8 (0.4–1.5)	1.0 (0.5–1.9)	0.5 (0.1–1.9)	Duration of smoking (years) ≤ 4 0.9 (0.3–2.9) 5–14 1.0 (0.4–2.2) ≥ 15 0.9 (0.4–1.8) Age at starting smoking (years) ≥ 19 0.7 (0.2–2.1) 16–18 0.7 (0.7–1.7) ≤ 15 1.1 (0.5–2.2) Cigarettes/day < 10 0.5 (0.2–1.5) ≥ 10 1.0 (0.5–1.9)	Age, no. of sexual partners, use of barrier method of contraception	Crude estimates also available, showing a weak association that disappears after adjustment

Table 2.1.10.3 (contd)

Reference Country and years of study	Relative risk (95% CI)				Adjustment factors	Comments
	Ever	Current	Former	By quantity/duration		
Parazzini et al. (1998) Italy 1981–93		1.1 (0.8–1.7)	1.3 (0.6–2.8)	*Cigarettes/day* < 5 0.9 (0.4–2.3) 5–14 1.6 (0.8–2.9) ≥ 15 0.9 (0.5–1.5)	Age, education, calendar year, parity, no. of sexual partners, oral contraceptive use	Subjects aged < 45 years
Hsieh et al. (1999) China, Province of Taiwan Not specified	1.4 (0.4–5.3)				Age, educational level, monthly family income	

CI, confidence interval; CIS, carcinoma *in situ*; PCR, polymerase chain reaction; HSV, herpes simplex virus

Table 2.1.10.4. Cohort studies on tobacco smoking and invasive cervical cancer (ICC) (without control for human papillomavirus (HPV) status)

Reference Country and years of study	Name of study	No. of cases	Smoking categories	Relative risk (95% CI)	Adjustment factors/comments
Hirayama (1975) Japan 1965–73	Six-prefecture Study 142 857 women	288 deaths	Current smoker *Cigarettes/day* < 20 20–29	1.7 1.8 3.5	Standardized mortality ratio (SMR)
Garfinkel (1980) USA 1959–72	Cancer Prevention Study (CPS) I 590 562 women	308 deaths	Nonsmoker vs entire cohort	**SMR** 0.87	
Hirayama (1985) Japan 1965–81	Six-prefecture Cohort Study	Deaths (no. not specified)	*Cigarettes/day* 1–24 ≥ 25	**SMR** 1.6 1.9	*p* for trend < 0.0001
Beral et al. (1988) UK 1968–87	47 000 women	65 ICC	*Cigarettes/day* 0 1–14 > 15	5.4 1.1 0.9	Age, parity, smoking, social class, no. of previously normal cervical smears, history of sexually transmitted diseases
Tverdal et al. (1993) Norway 1972–88	Norwegian Screening Study 24 535 women	23 deaths	Nonsmoker Former smoker Current smoker *Cigarettes/day* 1–9 > 10	**Mortality rate** 5.1 5.2 11.4 **RR** 1.0 2.4 (1.0–5.5)	Age, area; annual mortality rate/100 000 women
Engeland et al. (1996) Norway 1966–93	Norwegian Cohort Study 14 269 women	86 cases	Current smoker *Cigarettes/day* < 5 5–9 ≥ 10	2.5 (1.6–3.9) 1.9 (1.0–3.6) 3.3 (1.9–5.8) 2.4 (1.2–4.8)	No significant difference was observed for age at start of smoking, type of cigarette or urban/rural residence.

Table 2.1.10.4 (contd)

Reference Country and years of study	Name of study	No. of cases	Smoking categories	Relative risk (95% CI)	Adjustment factors/comments
Zondervan et al. (1996) UK 10 years	17 000 women		*Cigarettes/day*		
			< 1 (nonsmoker)	1.0	
			1–4	0.8 (0.3–2.5)	
			> 15	3.1 (1.3–7.3)	
Nordlund et al. (1997) Sweden 1964–89	Swedish Census Study	138 cases	Former smoker	1.01 (0.4–2.8)	
			Current smoker	2.5 (1.7–3.7)	
			Cigarettes/day		
			1–7	2.3 (1.5–3.7)	
			8–15	2.4 (1.4–4.2)	
			≥ 16	4.0 (2.0–8.1)	
			Age at starting smoking (years)		
			20–23	0.6 (0.2–1.6)	
			< 19	1.9 (1.0–3.8)	*p* for trend = 0.06
Tulinius et al. (1997) Iceland 1968–95	Reykjavik Study 155 800 women	40 cases	Former smoker	1.2 (0.4–3.9)	Age
			Current smoker (cigarettes/day)		
			1–14	2.6 (1.2–5.7)	
			15–24	2.5 (1.0–5.8)	
			≥ 25	1.7 (0.2–13)	
Liaw & Chen (1998) China, Province of Taiwan 1982–94	Taiwanese Study	6 deaths	Current smoker	5.3 (0.6–46.8)	

CI, confidence interval

Table 2.1.10.5. Case–control studies on tobacco smoking and cervical intraepithelial neoplasia (CIN) and carcinoma *in situ* (CIS) (without control for human papilloma virus (HPV) status)

Reference Country and years of study	Type of disease	Relative risk (95% CI) by smoking status		By quantity/ duration	Relative risk (95% CI)	Adjustment factors	Comments
		Ever	Current	Former				
Thomas (1972) USA 1965–69	104 carcinoma, 105 dysplasia (as at biopsy)		Dysplasia, 1.2 Carcinoma, 0.8 Total, 1.1				13 variables, including age	Risk among users of oral contraceptives
Thomas (1973) USA 1965–69	209 CIS and dysplasia		CIS, 1.7 Dysplasia, 1.2 CIS, 1.5 Dysplasia, 1.1				Variety of social factors	'Cases and controls did not differ significantly by the proportion that had ever smoked regularly, the proportion that smoked when interviewed, amount smoked, or age at which smoking started.' (statement by authors)
Harris et al. (1980) UK 1974–79	Dysplasia/CIS				*Cigarettes/day* 0 1–15 15–19 ≥ 20	1.0 2.2 2.5 2.1	Age, no. of sexual partners, pregnancy outside marriage, years of oral contraceptive use	
Wigle et al. (1980) Canada 1971–73	168 invasive, 508 CIS		Invasive, 2.0 CIS, 3.8	Invasive, 1.0 CIS, 1.3	*Pack-years* < 10 11–20 21–30 ≥ 31	**CIS** 2.8 4.0 3.9 3.7	No adjustment made for social or sexual variables	*p* for trend = 0.003

(contd)

Table 2.1.10.5 (contd)

Reference, Country and years of study	Type of disease	Relative risk (95% CI) by smoking status — Ever	Current	Former	By quantity/duration	Relative risk (95% CI)	Adjustment factors	Comments
Buckley et al. (1981) UK 1974–79	17 preinvasive, 14 invasive reporting only; 1 sexual partner	3.2 (1.9–5.8)	7.0 / 7.8; 3.2 / 2.2	2.8 / 3.7; 2.7 / 2.0	Before adjustment / After adjustment		Matched; No. of sexual partners of husband; Smoking of husbands of cases	Relative risk 35 among a small series of multiple-partner women with husbands who smoke versus those with nonsmoking or formerly smoking husbands
Berggren & Sjöstedt (1983) Sweden 1974–78	609 preinvasive		2.7 (crude)		Age (years): 15–24, 25–29, 30–34, 35–39, 40–44, 45–49, 50–54, 55–59, ≥60	9.5 (4.0–22.4), 4.4 (2.9–6.8), 3.1 (2.1–4.5), 2.5 (1.7–3.6), 2.8 (1.7–4.7), 1.6 (0.9–2.8), 1.3 (0.6–3.2), 1.5 (0.5–4.2), 5.1 (1.1–23.4)	Geographical area (urban/rural)	Relative risk changes sharply with age
Lyon et al. (1983) USA 1975–77	CIS		3.5 (2.3–5.2)		Duration (years): 0, 1–19, ≥20	1.0, 1.4, 2.4	No. of lifetime partners, religion; No. of lifetime partners, age	
Trevathan et al. (1983) USA 1980–81	Mild to moderate dysplasia; Severe dysplasia; CIS	2.4 (1.6–3.7); 3.3 (1.9–5.8); 3.6 (2.1–6.2)	2.6 (1.7–4.1); 3.0 (1.6–5.6); 4.2 (2.7–7.5)	1.6 (0.8–3.6); 5.7 (2.4–13.5); 2.1 (0.8–5.6)	Cigarettes smoked (pack-years): <1, 1–3.9, 4–6.9, 7–11.9, ≥12	*In-situ*: 2.3, 2.4, 3.8, 9.1, 12.7; *Severe dysplasia*: 2.5, 2.4, 4.1, 12.7, 10.2; *Moderate dysplasia*: 0.7, 1.8, 3.3, 10.4, 11.3	Age, no. of sexual partners, age at first intercourse, socioeconomic status, oral contraceptive use	χ^2 for trend: all p values significant; strong dose–response relationship

Table 2.1.10.5 (contd)

Reference, Country and years of study	Type of disease	Relative risk (95% CI) by smoking status			By quantity/duration	Relative risk (95% CI)			Adjustment factors	Comments
		Ever	Current	Former						
Trevathan et al. (1983) (contd)					*Age at starting smoking (years)*				Age, no. of sexual partners, age at first intercourse, socio-economic status, oral contraceptive use, pack-years of cigarette smoking	
					Never	1.0	1.0	1.0		
					≥20	0.5	0.3	0.3		
					17–19	2.0	7.2	1.7		
					15–16	2.6	2.0	2.1		
					<15	4.8	5.8	3.1		
Martin & Hill (1984) South Africa 1950–74	257 cervical cancers	*Use of tobacco in any form* 1.5 1.3							Crude Alcohol consumption	p < 0.05 p > 0.05
Clarke et al. (1985) Canada 1979–81	Dysplasia		3.2 (p < 0.01)	1.3	*Cigarettes/day* 1–10 11–20 >20	3.1 2.7 3.4			Sexual stability, age at first intercourse, grade of education, use of oral contraceptives	
Mayberry (1985) USA Not specified	CIN	1.7 (1.2–2.4)	1.9 (1.3–2.7)	1.3 (1.1–1.5)	*Intensity (pack-day)* <1/2 1/2–1 1–2 >2	1.2 (0.7–2.0) 1.8 (1.1–2.9) 2.2 (1.4–3.7) 1.5 (0.5–4.6)			Age, marital status, education, social class, no. of sexual partners, age at first intercourse, no. of abortions, no. of previous Pap smears, oral contraceptive use, clinical history of other sexually transmitted diseases	Includes 35 women with severe dysplasia, 9 with CIS, and 10 with ICC
					Duration (years) <5 5–10 10–15 >15	1.0 (0.5–1.9) 1.8 (1.2–2.8) 2.1 (1.2–3.7) 1.9 (1.0–3.8)				
					Age at starting smoking (years) ≥20 17–19 <17	3.2 (1.6–6.6) 1.2 (0.8–2.0) 1.8 (1.2–2.8)				

Table 2.1.10.5 (contd)

Reference Country and years of study	Type of disease	Relative risk (95% CI) by smoking status			By quantity/ duration	Relative risk (95% CI)	Adjustment factors	Comments
		Ever	Current	Former				
La Vecchia et al. (1986) Italy 1981–84	CIN			2.5 (0.9–6.7)	*Cigarettes/day* < 15 ≥ 15 *Age at starting smoking (years)* Never > 24 18–24 < 18 *Duration (years)* < 10 10–19 ≥ 20	 0.9 (0.5–1.6) 2.7 (1.3–5.2) 1.0 1.2 (0.6–2.4) 1.6 (0.8–3.0) 3.3 (1.4–8.1) 1.4 (0.7–2.9) 1.7 (0.9–3.1) 1.7 (0.8–3.7)	Age, marital status, education, social class, age at first intercourse, no. of sexual partners, no. of abortions, age at menopause, no. of previous Pap smears, oral contraceptive use, clinical history of sexually transmitted disease	$p = 0.04$
Brock et al. (1989) Australia 1980–83	CIS		4.5 (2.2–9.1)	1.3 (0.6–3.0)	*Cigarettes/day* < 10 10–19 20–29 ≥ 30 *Duration (years)* < 5 5–9 10–14 ≥ 15	 2.3 (0.8–6.4) 2.0 (0.9–4.4) 3.8 (1.7–8.4) 5.1 (1.5–17.3) 2.2 (0.7–7.0) 2.2 (0.8–6.1) 3.8 (1.6–9.6) 1.8 (0.7–4.6)	Age at first intercourse, no. of sexual partners, use of oral contraceptives	$p = 0.05$
Slattery et al. (1989) USA 1984–87	CIS (and ICC)		3.4 (2.1–5.6)	1.4 (0.8–2.5)	*Cigarettes/day* None 1–15 > 15 *Pack-years* ≤ 5 > 5 *Age at starting smoking (years)* > 16 ≤ 16	 1.0 2.2 (1.3–3.7) 2.2 (1.3–3.6) 1.5 (0.9–2.6) 2.8 (1.7–4.6) 2.4 (1.4–3.7) 2.6 (1.5–4.3)	Age, church attendance, education, no. of sexual partners	Included 35 cases of ICC $p = 0.001$

Table 2.1.10.5 (contd)

Reference Country and years of study	Type of disease	Relative risk (95% CI) by smoking status			By quantity/ duration	Relative risk (95% CI)	Adjustment factors	Comments
		Ever	Current	Former				
Slattery et al. (1989) (contd)					*Duration (years)*			
					1–10	1.7 (1.0–2.8)		
					>10	2.2 (1.2–3.9)		
Cuzick et al. (1990) UK 1984–88	CIN (CIN I, CIN II, CIN III)	1.7 (1.2–2.4)	1.5 ($p < 0.05$)	1.0	*Pack-years*		Age, social class and sexual reproductive factors	
					0	1.0		
					0.01–2	0.8		
					2.01–4	1.1		
					4.01–8	1.5		
					8.01–12	2.2		
					>12	2.7 $p < 0.05$		
					Age at starting smoking (years)			
					Never	1.0		
					≥20	0.8		
					17–19	1.6		
					≤16	1.7 $p < 0.05$		
Jones et al. (1990) USA 1982–84	CIS	1.9 (1.3–2.7)		1.5 (1.0–2.4)	*Cigarettes/day*		Age, race, interval since last Pap smears, no. of abnormal smears, no. of lifetime partners, years of oral contraceptive use, years of diaphragm use, history of sexually transmitted diseases	
					<10	1.6 (0.8–2.9)		
					10–19	1.4 (0.9–2.3)		
					20–29	1.7 (1.1–2.6)		
					≥30	2.3 (1.4–3.8)		$p < 0.001$
					Age at starting smoking (years)			
					≥30	0.5 (0.1–1.6)		
					21–29	1.9 (1.1–3.3)		
					17–20	1.6 (1.1–2.4)		
					≤16	2.2 (1.4–3.4)		
					Duration (years)			
					<10	1.1 (0.7–1.9)		
					10–19	1.8 (1.2–2.9)		
					20–29	2.5 (1.6–4.1)		
					30–39	1.6 (0.8–3.2)		
					≥40	1.7 (0.6–4.7)		$p = 0.001$

Table 2.1.10.5 (contd)

Reference Country and years of study	Type of disease	Relative risk (95% CI) by smoking status			By quantity/ duration	Relative risk (95% CI)	Adjustment factors	Comments
		Ever	Current	Former				
Coker et al. (1992) USA 1987–88	CIN II, CIN III	1.7 (0.9–3.3)	3.4 (1.7–7.0)		*Duration (years)* 1–4 5–9 ≥ 10 *Age at starting smoking (years)* > 18 16–17 < 16	0.6 (0.2–1.7) 1.6 (0.6–4.0) 2.7 (1.1–6.9) 1.4 (0.6–3.2) 1.2 (0.5–3.2) 2.9 (1.1–8.0)	Age, race, education, no. of sexual partners, no. of Pap smears five years prior, genital warts	
Parazzini et al. (1992) Italy 1981–90	CIN I+II, CIN III		*CIN I+II* 2.2 (1.2–3.0) *CIN III* 2.5 (1.7–3.6) *CIN I+II* 1.8 (1.1–2.9) *CIN III* 2.0 (1.3–3.1)	*CIN I+II* 1.0 (0.4–2.5) *CIN I+II* 1.1 (0.4–2.9) *CIN III* 1.7 (0.8–3.5)	*CIN I+II* < 10 cigarettes/day ≥ 10 cigarettes/day *CIN III* < 10 cigarettes/day ≥ 10 cigarettes/day	2.3 (1.3–3.9) 2.2 (1.5–3.9) 2.6 (1.5–4.7) 2.6 (1.7–4.1)	Age Age at first birth, age at first intercourse, no. of partners, CIN grade in Milan (Italy), age, education, lifetime no. of Pap tests	χ^2 trend = 5.91 (p = 0.03) χ^2 trend = 22.12 (p = 0.001; former smokers excluded from trend calculation)
Becker et al. (1994) USA 1989–92	CIN II, CIN III	1.4 (1.0–2.1)	1.8 (1.2–2.8)	0.9 (0.5–1.5)	*Cigarettes/day* 1–9 10–19 ≥ 20 *Pack/years* < 2 2–5 ≥ 6 *Duration (years)* 0–1 1–4 5–9 ≥ 10	1.2 (0.7–1.8) 1.4 (0.8–2.4) 2.4 (1.3–4.2) 1.0 (0.6–1.7) 1.6 (1.0–2.6) 2.0 (1.2–3.5) 1.0 1.3 (0.8–2.2) 1.2 (0.7–2.1) 1.7 (1.0–2.8)	Ethnicity, age, age at first intercourse, no. of lifetime partners	

Table 2.1.10.5 (contd)

Reference Country and years of study	Type of disease	Relative risk (95% CI) by smoking status			By quantity/ duration	Relative risk (95% CI)	Adjustment factors	Comments
		Ever	Current	Former				
Becker et al. (1994) (contd)					*Use at menarche*			
					None	1.0		
					Before	2.2 (1.2–4.1)		
					After	1.3 (0.9–1.9)		
					1–9 cigarettes/day	1.9 (1.0–3.4)		
					for < 15 years	2.7 (1.2–6.4)		
					for ≥ 15 years	1.4 (0.5–3.4)		
					10–19 cigarettes/ day	1.6 (0.9–2.7)		
					for < 15 years	2.1 (1.1–4.0)		
					for ≥ 15 years	1.3 (0.7–2.6)		
					≥ 20 cigarettes/day	3.5 (2.1–5.9)		
					for < 15 years	7.0 (3.5–13.7)		
					for ≥ 15 years	2.2 (1.2–4.1)		
de Vet et al. (1994) The Netherlands not specified	Dysplasia			2.0 (1.1–3.4)			Age, education, no. of sexual partners, age at first intercourse, current frequency of intercourse, use of contraceptives, dietary intake of β-caro- tene, retinol, vitamin C and dietary fibre	
Stone et al. (1995) Costa Rica 1982–85	*In situ*		1.3 (1.0–1.7)				Age	

Table 2.1.10.5 (contd)

Reference Country and years of study	Type of disease	Relative risk (95% CI) by smoking status			By quantity/ duration	Relative risk (95% CI)	Adjustment factors	Comments
		Ever	Current	Former				
Kjaer et al. (1996) Denmark 1987–88	CIS	2.3 (1.6–3.2)	2.4 (1.7–3.4)	1.6 (1.0–2.7)	*Cigarettes/day*		Age, no. of sexual partners, percentage of sexual active life without use of barrier contraceptives, years with intrauterine devices, no. of births, age at first episode of genital warts	
					≤ 4	1.2 (0.6–2.3)		
					5–14	2.0 (1.4–2.9)		
					15–19	2.4 (1.6–3.6)		
					≥ 20	2.8 (1.9–4.1)		
					Age at starting smoking (years)			
					≥ 19	2.3 (1.4–3.7)		
					16–18	2.4 (1.6–3.5)		
					14–15	2.2 (1.5–3.2)		
					≤ 13	2.2 (1.4–3.6)		
					Duration (years)			
					≤ 4	1.4 (0.8–2.4)		
					5–14	2.7 (1.9–4.0)		
					15–19	2.1 (1.4–3.2)		
					≥ 20	2.3 (1.3–3.9)		
Madeleine et al. (2001) USA 1990–96	*In situ*	0.9 (0.6–1.3)	0.8 (0.5–1.3)	1.0 (0.6–1.5)			Age, no. of sexual partners	

CI, confidence interval; ICC, invasive cervical cancer; CIN II and CIN III define disease progression

Table 2.1.10.6. Cohort studies on tobacco smoking and cervical intraepithelial neoplasia (CIN) and carcinoma *in situ* (CIS) (without control for HPV status)

Reference Country and years of study	Subjects	Number of cases	Smoking categories	Relative risks	Adjustment factors	Comments
Cederlöf *et al.* (1975) Sweden 1963–72	26 467 women	178; not explicitly stated but must contain mainly CIS cases	Former smoker Current smoker *Cigarettes/day* 1–7 8–15 ≥ 16	1.4 3.0 2.8 3.0 3.4	Age-adjusted Place of residence, income	Little confounding
Wright *et al.* (1978) UK 1968–74	17 032 women	65 cases: 33 CIS, 6 invasive, 26 dysplasia	*Cigarettes/day* 1–14 ≥ 15	1.5 2.9	Significance unaltered by adjustment for contraceptive method	'In our view, it is unlikely that use of tobacco could have any direct effect on the cervix' (statement by authors)
Beral *et al.* (1988) UK 1968–87	47 000 women	207 CIS	*Cigarettes/day* 0 1–14 > 15	*In-situ* 4.8 3.6 1.3	Adjusted for age, parity, smoking, social class, no. of previously normal cervical smears, history of sexually transmitted diseases	

Table 2.1.10.6 (contd)

Reference Country and years of study	Subjects	Number of cases	Smoking categories	Relative risks	Adjustment factors	Comments
Gram *et al.* (1992) Norway 1980–89	6812 women	185 cases (177 CIN, 8 ICC)	Former smoker Current smoker *Cigarettes/day* 1–14 ≥ 15 *Duration (years)* 1–9 > 10 *Age at starting smoking (years)* ≥ 22 19–21 16–18 < 16	0.6 (0.4–1.1) 1.5 (1.0–2.2) 1.4 (0.9–2.1) 1.8 (1.1–3.0) (*p* = 0.02) 1.2 (0.7–1.9) 1.8 (1.2–2.8) (*p* = 0.01) 0.9 (0.4–1.9) 1.1 (0.6–2.0) 1.7 (1.1–2.7) 2.0 (1.1–3.5) (*p* < 0.01)	Adjusted for age, marital status, frequency of intoxication by alcohol	
Zondervan *et al.* (1996) UK 10 years	17 000 women	159 dysplasia 121 CIS	*Cigarettes/day* 1–14 > 15 1–14 > 15	**Dysplasia** 1.8 (1.2–2.7) 1.9 (1.2–2.9) **CIS** 1.9 (1.2–3.0) 1.8 (1.0–2.9)		
Ylitalo *et al.* (1999) Sweden 1969–95	146 889 women	105 cases, 168 controls	Former smoker Current smoker *Cigarettes/day* 1–4 5–9 10–14 ≥ 15	1.5 (0.9–2.3) 1.9 (1.3–2.9) 1.4 (0.9–2.4) 2.1 (1.3–3.2) 2.1 (1.3–3.6) 1.3 (0.7–2.4)	Education, marital status, age at first intercourse, no. of sexual partners, age at menarche, parity, oral contraceptive use HPV DNA	Nested case–control study

Table 2.1.10.6 (contd)

Reference Country and years of study	Subjects	Number of cases	Smoking categories	Relative risks	Adjustment factors	Comments
Ylitalo et al. (1999) (contd)			*Duration (years)*			
			1–9	1.7 (1.1–2.8)		
			10–19	1.8 (1.2–2.7)		
			≥ 20	1.8 (1.0–3.1)		
			Age at starting smoking (years)			
			12–15	2.1 (1.3–3.4)		
			16–17	1.4 (0.9–2.2)		
			18–19	2.0 (1.1–3.4)		
			≥ 20	1.7 (1.0–2.8)		
			Pack-years			
			< 1	1.3 (0.7–2.3)		
			2–3	2.2 (1.3–3.8)		
			4–5	2.1 (1.2–3.7)		
			6–7	2.6 (1.4–4.7)		
			8–11	1.5 (0.9–2.7)		
			≥ 12	1.5 (0.8–2.6)		
			Time since starting (years)			
			1–9	1.3 (0.6–2.7)		
			10–14	2.4 (1.4–4.4)		
			15–19	2.1 (1.3–3.5)		
			≥ 20	1.5 (0.9–2.4)		
			Years since quitting			
			≥ 10	1.9 (1.0–3.7)		
			1–9	1.5 (0.9–2.5)		
			0	1.9 (1.3–21.7)		

Table 2.1.10.7. Case–control studies on tobacco smoking and invasive cervical cancer (ICC) (adjusted for human papillomavirus (HPV) status)

Reference Country and years of study	Relative risk (95% CI) Ever	Comments
Peng *et al.* (1991) China 1987–88	1.2 (0.5–2.8)	Age, income, residence, HPV 16/33 DNA positivity
Chichareon *et al.* (1998) Thailand 1990–93	1.6 (0.7–3.3)	HPV DNA, age, education, age at first intercourse, no. of live births, lifetime no. of sexual partners, any venereal disease, use of hormonal contraceptives, time since last Pap smear
Ngelangel *et al.* (1998) The Philippines 1991–93	11.2 (3.9–32.0)	HPV, age, no. of household amenities, age at first intercourse, no. of live births, no. of sexual partners, use of oral contraceptives, time since last Pap smear

CI, confidence interval

Table 2.1.10.8. Case–control studies on tobacco smoking and cervical intraepithelial neoplasia (CIN) and carcinoma *in situ* (CIS) (with adjustment for human papillomavirus (HPV))

Reference Country and years of study	Type of disease	Relative risk (95% CI) by smoking status — Ever	Current	Former	By quantity/duration	Adjustment factors
Muñoz et al. (1993) Spain, 1985–87 Colombia, 1985–88	CIN III		1.3 (0.7–2.3) 2.0 (1.3–5.0)	0.9 (0.2–3.8) 1.8 (0.9–3.5)	*Pack–years* — *Spain* / *Colombia* 0.1–4.9: 0.5 (0.2–1.1) / 1.6 (0.9–2.9) 5–9.9: 3.4 (1.5–8.0) / 2.0 (0.8–5.1) 10–14.9: 3.6 (1.1–11.4) / 0.9 (0.8–2.3) ≥15: 2.2 (0.7–6.7) / 1.8 (0.8–4.2)	Adjusted for age, centre, HPV, no. of sexual partners, age at first intercourse, *Chlamydiae trachomatis*, husband's sexual partners
Ho et al. (1998) USA 1992–94	CIN I, II and III	CIN III compared with CIN I in HPV+ women	2.4 (1.1–5.2)	1.8 (0.6–5.2)	*Cigarettes/day* ≤10: 1.5 (0.6–3.7) >10: 3.4 (1.2–9.2) *Pack–years* None: 1.0 ≤5: 1.8 (0.7–4.3) >5: 2.7 (1.2–6.2)	Age, education, ethnicity, number of Pap smears in last 3 years, HPV status
Kanetsky et al. (1998) USA 1993–95	CIN I, II and III	1.7 (0.5–5.4)	1.8 (0.5–6.1)	1.3 (0.2–8.1)	*Age at starting smoking (years)* ≥17: 2.1 (0.6–7.8) ≤16: 1.1 (0.2–5.4) *Duration (years)* ≤14: 1.3 (0.3–5.1) ≥15: 2.4 (0.5–10.2) *Cigarettes/day* ≤9: 2.3 (0.6–9.6) ≥10: 1.3 (0.3–5.1) *Pack–years* ≤6: 1.4 (0.4–5.6) ≥7: 2.1 (0.5–8.8)	Age, education, medical coverage, time since last Pap smear and HPV infection
Yoshikawa et al. (1999) Japan 1995–96	CIN I, II and III	0.8 (0.2–2.2)		0.3 (0.1–1.3)		HPV DNA

Table 2.1.10.8 (contd)

Reference Country and years of study	Type of disease	Relative risk (95% CI) by smoking status			By quantity/duration		Adjustment factors
		Ever	Current	Former			
Kjellberg *et al.* (2000) Sweden 1993–95	CIN II and III	3.0 (1.9–4.7)	3.1 (1.8–5.2)	2.8 (1.5–5.2)	1–4 cigarettes/day	1.9 (0.6–6.0)	HPV-capsid, age
					5–14 cigarettes/day	2.4 (1.3–4.6)	
					≥ 15 cigarettes/day	6.0 (2.7–13.3)	
					Joint effect of smoking and HPV seropositivity		
					Seronegative		
					Never-smoker	1.0	
					Ever-smoker	5.2 (1.8–15.2)	
					Seropositive		
					Never-smoker	4.6 (1.6–12.9)	
					Ever-smoker	7.2 (2.5–20.6)	
					HPV DNA-positive		HPV DNA
					1–4 cigarettes/day	0.5 (0.1–1.9)	
					5–14 cigarettes/day	3.2 (1.2–8.4)	
					≥ 15 cigarettes/day	5.9 (1.7–19.4)	
					HPV DNA-negative		
					Never-smoker	1	
					Ever-smoker	3.8 (1.3–11.2)	
					HPV DNA-positive		
					Never-smoker	93 (31–280)	
					Ever-smoker	186 (62–556)	

CI, confidence interval

Table 2.1.10.9. Cohort studies on tobacco smoking and cervical intraepithelial neoplasia (CIN) and carcinoma *in situ* (CIS) (with control for human papillomavirus (HPV) status)

Reference Country and years of study	Cohort characteristics	No. of cases	Smoking categories	Relative risk (95% CI)	Adjustment
Schiffman *et al.* (1993) USA 1989–90	21 146 women; nested case–control study	500 cases of CIN III, CIN II, CIN I, condylomatous atypia; 500 controls	Current smoker Former smoker	1.2 (0.8–1.8) 1.0 (0.6–1.6)	Age
Moscicki *et al.* (2001) USA 1990–2000	496 HPV DNA-positive women attending family planning clinics	109 incident cases of low-grade squamous intraepithelial lesions	Smoking daily	1.7 (1.2–2.6)	

Table 2.1.10.10. Study populations used in analysis of associations of tobacco smoking and invasive cervical cancer and carcinoma *in situ* in human papillomavirus (HPV)-positive study subjects

Reference Country and years of study	ASR (world)	HPV tested		HPV-positive				Ever-smokers (%)		Cigarettes per day controls
		Cases	Controls	Cases	(%)	Controls	(%)	Cases	Controls	
Invasive cervical cancer (ICC)										
Bosch *et al.* (1992); Muñoz *et al.* (1992) Colombia 1985–88	32.9	110	126	86	(78.2)	22	(17.5)	42.4	28.1	11
Bosch *et al.* (1992); Muñoz *et al.* (1992) Spain 1985–87	7.2	159	136	131	(82.4)	8	(5.9)	20.4	14.3	10
Eluf-Neto *et al.* (1994) Brazil 1990–91	31.3	187	196	181	(96.8)	34	(17.3)	47.2	36	10
Chaouki *et al.* (1998) Morocco 1991–93	18.8	188	176	182	(96.8)	38	(21.6)	2.8	4.4	7
Chichareon *et al.* (1998) Thailand 1990–93	20.7	378	261	363	(96.0)	41	(15.7)	17.1	13	5
Ngelangel *et al.* (1998) The Philippines 1991–93	22.7	364	381	349	(95.9)	35	(9.2)	20.4	7.2	8

Table 2.1.10.10 (contd)

Reference Country and years of study	ASR (world)	HPV tested		HPV-positive				Ever-smokers (%)		Cigarettes per day controls
		Cases	Controls	Cases	(%)	Controls	(%)	Cases	Controls	
Rolon et al. (2000) Paraguay 1988–90	41.1	112	90	109	(97.3)	17	(18.9)	32.2	19	3
Santos et al. (2001) Peru 1996–97	39.9	196	175	186	(94.9)	31	(17.7)	9.6	3.6	7
Hildesheim et al. (2001) Costa Rica Population-based nested case–control study	40 ICC, 128 HSIL		843 HPV+			843 HPV+				
Carcinoma in situ										
Bosch et al. (1993); Muñoz et al. (1993) Columbia 1985–87		135	181	96	(71.1)	19	(10.5)	37.2	23.7	10
Bosch et al. (1993); Muñoz et al. (1993) Spain 1985–88		157	193	115	(73.2)	9	(4.7)	54.5	38.4	9
TOTAL		1986	1915	1798		254				

ASR, age-standardized rate; HSIL, high-grade squamous intra-epithelial lesions

Table 2.1.10.11. Studies on tobacco smoking and cervical intraepithelial neoplasia (CIN) and carcinoma *in situ* (CIS) in human papillomavirus (HPV)-positive subjects

Reference Country and years of study	Type of disease	Relative risk (95% CI) by smoking status				By quantity/duration		Adjustment factors	Comments
		HPV status	Never-smoker	Ever-smoker	Former smoker				
Olsen et al. (1998) Norway 1991–92	CIN II and III (90 cases, 216 controls)	HPV-16-seronegative	1.0	4.4 (1.8–10.9)				Age	Case–control study; controlled for HPV status. Jointly unexposed (HPV-16-negative never-smokers used as the referent to determine risk of CIN II and III in HPV-positive smokers and nonsmokers)
		HPV-16-seropositive	2.9 (0.7–11.0)	15.3 (5.3–44.1)					
		HPV-16 DNA-negative	1.0	2.2 (0.8–5.6)					
		HPV-16 DNA-positive	15.7 (3.2–76.5)	65.9 (22.3–194.3)					
	(60 cases, 14 controls)	HPV-16 DNA-positive	1.0	4.6 (0.9–22.9)	4.2 (0.5–37.9)	*Duration (years)*			
						0	1.0		
						1–9	2.1 (0.3–12.3)		
						≥ 10	7.5 (1.2–45.8)		
						Cigarettes/day			
						1–10	3.3 (0.5–10.8)		
						≥ 10	5.9 (1.0–35.6)		
	(31 cases, 34 controls)	HPV-16 capsid-positive	1.0	5.1 (1.5–17.7)	4.3 (0.8–23.2)	*Duration (years)*			
						0	1.0		
						1–9	4.3 (0.9–20.3)		
						≥ 10	5.3 (1.4–20.0)		
						Cigarettes/day			
						1–10	4.6 (1.1–20.4)		
						≥ 10	6.5 (1.4–30.1)		
Deacon et al. (2000) UK	CIN III	CIN III	2.2 (1.4–3.4)	1.7 (0.76–3.8)		*Cigarettes/day*		Age, age at first intercourse, total no. of sexual partners, years since last regular relationship, history of spontaneous abortion	Nested case–control study within the Manchester cohort (199 HPV-positive cases, 181 HPV-positive cases and 203 HPV-negative controls)
						1–10	1.4 (0.7–2.5)		
						11–16	2.2 (1.2–3.9)		
						≥ 17	3.1 (1.8–5.3)		
						Duration (years)			
						Never	1.0		
						1–9	1.8 (0.89–3.6)		
						10–19	2.0 (1.2–3.3)		
						≥ 20	3.1 (1.6–6.2)		

Table 2.1.10.12. Case-control studies on tobacco smoking and invasive cervical cancer (ICC) (adeno- and adenosquamous carcinoma)

Reference, Country and years of study	Relative risk (95% CI)				Adjustment factors
	Ever	Current	Former	By quantity/duration	
Brinton et al. (1986) USA 1982–84	1.1 (0.7–1.9)	1.2 (0.7–2.1)	0.8 (0.4–2.0)	*Cigarettes/day* <10 1.5 (0.7–3.1) 10–19 0.9 (0.4–2.1) 20–29 0.9 (0.4–1.9) >30 2.0 (0.6–6.0) *Duration (years)* <10 1.1 (0.4–2.8) 10–19 1.2 (0.5–2.5) 20–29 1.1 (0.6–2.1) >40 1.1 (0.3–3.7)	Education, income, weight gain from age 18 years to diagnosis, total no. of sexual partners, no. of sexual partners before age 20 years, duration of diaphragm use, history of stillbirths, known episodes of genital warts, use of oral contraceptives
Ursin et al. (1996) USA 1977–91		1.0 (0.5–1.9) [1.7 (1.1–2.6)]	1.2 (0.7–1.9) [1.5 (1.0–2.4)]	*Pack-years* <1300 1.7 (0.9–3.2) 1301–4000 1.0 (0.5–2.0) 4001–7500 0.6 (0.3–1.3) >7500 1.2 (0.6–2.3)	Life partners, HCV-2 seropositivity, oral contraceptive use at 17 years or less, HPV VLP antibody status HPV DNA adjusted HPV DNA restricted
Chichareon et al. (1998) Thailand 1990–93	1.9 (0.4–8.9) 1.0 (0.2–6.8)				Age, no. of household amenities, age at first intercourse, no. of live births, lifetime no. of sexual partners, use of hormonal contraceptives, time since last Pap smear Only 2 cases ever smoked. HPV DNA-adjusted HPV DNA-restricted
Ngelangel (1998) The Philippines 1991–93	0.9 (0.2–4.1) 4.7 (0.2–129.0) 13.6 (0.1–2599)				

Table 2.1.10.12 (contd)

Reference Country and years of study	Relative risk (95% CI)			By quantity/ duration	Adjustment factors
	Ever	Current	Former		
Lacey *et al.* (2001) USA 1992–96	**Adenocarcinomas**				Age, ethnicity, education, lifetime sexual partners and no. of Pap smears in the last 10 years, HPV
	0.8 (0.5–1.2)	0.6 (0.3–1.1)	1.0 (0.6–1.6)	<1 pack/day	0.9 (0.5–1.5)	
				≥1 pack/day	0.7 (0.4–1.3)	
					p for trend, 0.28	
				<5 pack–years	0.8 (0.4–1.6)	
				5–14 pack–years	0.9 (0.4–1.7)	
				≥15 pack–years	0.8 (0.41–1.6)	
					p for trend, 0.41	
				Duration (years)		
				≤10	0.7 (0.4–1.4)	
				11–20	0.9 (0.5–1.8)	
				≥20	0.8 (0.4–1.6)	
					p for trend, 0.5	
				Age at starting smoking (years)		
				≥21	0.7 (0.3–1.6)	
				18–20	1.0 (0.5–1.9)	
				16–17	0.8 (0.4–1.6)	
				11–15	0.6 (0.3–1.4)	
					p for trend, 0.51	
	Adenocarcinoma versus HPV+ controls only				Age, ethnicity
	0.7 (0.3–1.5)	0.5 (0.2–1.1)	1.0 (0.4–2.5)	<5 pack–years	1.1 (0.4–2.8)	
				5–14 pack–years	0.8 (0.3–2.1)	
				≥15 pack–years	0.5 (0.2–1.6)	
				Duration (years)		
				≤10	0.9 (0.4–2.1)	
				11–20	1.3 (0.4–4.0)	
				≥20	0.4 (0.1–1.2)	
				<1 pack/day	1.2 (0.5–2.9)	
				≥1 pack/day	0.4 (0.2–1.0)	

Table 2.1.10.12 (contd)

Reference Country and years of study	Relative risk (95% CI)			By quantity/ duration		Adjustment factors
	Ever	Current	Former			
	Squamous-cell carcinoma					
Lacey et al. (2001) (contd)	1.4 (0.8–2.3)	1.6 (0.9–2.9)	1.1 (0.6–2.1)	*Duration (years)*		Age, ethnicity, education, lifetime sexual partners, no. of Pap smear in the last 10 years, HPV
				≤ 10	1.0 (0.5–2.0)	
				11–20	1.9 (0.95–3.9)	
				≥ 20	1.5 (0.7–2.9)	
				Cigarettes/day		
				< 20	1.1 (0.6–1.9)	
				≥ 20	1.8 (1.0–3.3)	
				Age at starting smoking (years)		
				≥ 21	1.1 (0.4–2.6)	
				18–20	1.3 (0.6–2.7)	
				16–17	1.5 (0.7–2.9)	
				11–15	1.3 (0.6–2.6)	
				Pack-years		
				< 5	1.2 (0.6–2.4)	
				5–14	1.3 (0.7–2.6)	
				≥ 15	1.7 (0.9–3.2)	
Madeleine et al. (2001) USA (see data in Table 2.1.10.5)						

CI, confidence interval; HCV, hepatitis C virus; VLP, virus-like particles

References

Baron, J.A., Byers, T., Greenberg, E.R., Cummings, K.M. & Swanson, M. (1986) Cigarette smoking in women with cancers of the breast and reproductive organs. *J. natl Cancer Inst.*, **77**, 677–680

Becker, T.M., Wheeler, C.M., McGough, N.S., Parmenter, C.A., Stidley, C.A., Jamison, S.F. & Jordan, S.W. (1994) Cigarette smoking and other risk factors for cervical dysplasia in southwestern Hispanic and non-Hispanic white women. *Cancer Epidemiol. Biomarkers Prev.*, **3**, 113–119

Beral, V., Hannaford, P. & Kay, C. (1988) Oral contraceptive use and malignancies of the genital tract. Results from the Royal College of General Practitioners' Oral Contraception Study. *Lancet*, **ii**, 1331–1335

Berggren, G. & Sjostedt, S. (1983) Preinvasive carcinoma of the cervix uteri and smoking. *Acta obstet. gynecol. scand.*, **62**, 593–598

Bosch, F.X., Muñoz, N., de Sanjosé, S., Izarzugaza, I., Gili, M., Viladiu, P., Tormo, M.J., Moreo, P., Ascunce, N., Gonzalez, L.C., Tafur, L., Kaldor, J.M., Guerrero, E., Aristizabal, N., Santamaria, M., Alonso de Ruiz, P. & Shah, K. (1992) Risk factors for cervical cancer in Colombia and Spain. *Int. J. Cancer*, **52**, 750–758

Bosch, F.X., Muñoz, N., de Sanjose, S., Navarro, C., Moreo, P., Ascunce, N., Gonzalez, L.C., Tafur, L., Gili, M. & Larranaga, I. (1993) Human papillomavirus and cervical intraepithelial neoplasia grade III/carcinoma in situ: A case–control study in Spain and Colombia. *Cancer Epidemiol. Biomarkers Prev.*, **2**, 415–422

Brinton, L.A., Schairer, C., Haenzel, W., Stolley, P., Lehman, H.F., Levine, R. & Savitz, D.A. (1986) Cigarette smoking and invasive cervical cancer. *J. Am. med. Assoc.*, **255**, 3265

Brock, K.E., MacLennan, R., Brinton, L.A., Melnick, J.L., Adam, E., Mock, P.A. & Berry, G. (1989) Smoking and infectious agents and risk of in situ cervical cancer in Sydney, Australia. *Cancer Res.*, **49**, 4925–4928

Buckley, J.D., Harris, R.W., Doll, R., Vessey, M.P. & Williams, P.T. (1981) Case–control study of the husbands of women with dysplasia or carcinoma of the cervix uteri. *Lancet*, **ii**, 1010–1015

Cederlöf, R., Friberg, L., Hrubec, Z. & Lorich, U. (1975) *The Relationship of Smoking and Some Social Covariables to Mortality and Cancer Morbidity. A Ten Year Follow-up in a Probability Sample of 55000 Swedish Subjects Age 18–69, Part 1 and Part 2*, Stockholm, Karolinska Institute, Stockholm Dept Environmental Hygiene. p.

Celentano, D.D., Klassen, A.C., Weisman, C.S. & Rosenshein, N.B. (1987) The role of contraceptive use in cervical cancer: The Maryland Cervical Cancer Case–Control Study. *Am. J. Epidemiol.*, **126**, 592–604

Chaouki, N., Bosch, F.X., Munoz, N., Meijer, C.J., El Gueddari, B., El Ghazi, A., Deacon, J., Castellsague, X. & Walboomers, J.M. (1998) The viral origin of cervical cancer in Rabat, Morocco. *Int. J. Cancer.*, **75**, 546–554

Chichareon, S., Herrero, R., Munoz, N., Bosch, F.X., Jacobs, M.V., Deacon, J., Santamaria, M., Chongsuvivatwong, V., Meijer, C.J. & Walboomers, J.M. (1998) Risk factors for cervical cancer in Thailand: A case–control study. *J. natl Cancer Inst.*, **90**, 50–57

Clarke, E.A., Morgan, R.W. & Newman, A.M. (1982) Smoking as a risk factor in cancer of the cervix: Additional evidence from a case–control study. *Am. J. Epidemiol.*, **115**, 59–66

Clarke, E.A., Hatcher, J., McKeown-Eyssen, G.E. & Lickrish, G.M. (1985) Cervical dysplasia: Association with sexual behavior, smoking, and oral contraceptive use? *Am. J. Obstet. Gynecol.*, **151**, 612–616

Coker, A.L., Rosenberg, A.J., McCann, M.F. & Hulka, B.S. (1992) Active and passive cigarette smoke exposure and cervical intraepithelial neoplasia. *Cancer Epidemiol. Biomarkers Prev.*, **1**, 349–356

Cuzick, J., Singer, A., De Stavola, B.L. & Chomet, J. (1990) Case–control study of risk factors for cervical intraepithelial neoplasia in young women. *Eur. J. Cancer*, **26**, 684–690

Cuzick, J., Sasieni, P. & Singer, A. (1996) Risk factors for invasive cervix cancer in young women. *Eur. J. Cancer*, **32A**, 836–841

Daling, J.R., Madeleine, M.M., McKnight, B., Carter, J.J., Wipf, G.C., Ashley, R., Schwartz, S.M., Beckmann, A.M., Hagensee, M.E., Mandelson, M.T. & Galloway, D.A. (1996) The relation-ship of human papillomavirus-related cervical tumors to cigarette smoking, oral contraceptive use, and prior herpes simplex virus type 2 infection. *Cancer Epidemiol. Biomarkers Prev.*, **5**, 541–548

Deacon, J.M., Evans, C.D., Yule, R., Desai, M., Binns, W., Taylor, C. & Peto, J. (2000) Sexual behaviour and smoking as determinants of cervical HPV infection and of CIN3 among those infected: A case–control study nested within the Manchester cohort. *Br. J. Cancer*, **83**, 1565–1572

Ebeling, K., Nischan, P. & Schindler, C. (1987) Use of oral contraceptives and risk of invasive cervical cancer in previously screened women. *Int. J. Cancer*, **39**, 427–430

Eluf-Neto, J., Booth, M., Munoz, N., Bosch, F.X., Meijer, C.J. & Walboomers, J.M. (1994) Human papillomavirus and invasive cervical cancer in Brazil. *Br. J. Cancer*, **69**, 114–119

Engeland, A., Andersen, A., Haldorsen, T. & Tretli, S. (1996b) Smoking habits and risk of cancers other than lung cancer: 28 years' follow-up of 26,000 Norwegian men and women. *Cancer Causes Control*, **7**, 497–506

Franco, E.L., Villa, L.L., Sobrinho, J.P., Prado, J.M., Rouseau, M.C., Desy, M. & Rohan, T.E. (1999) Epidemiology of acquisition and clearance of cervical human papillomavirus infection in women from a high-risk area for cervical cancer. *J. infect. Dis.*, **180**, 1415–1423

Franco, E.L., Duarte-Franco, E. & Ferenczy, A. (2001) Cervical cancer: Epidemiology, prevention and the role of human papillomavirus infection. *Can. med. Assoc. J.*, **164**, 1017–1025

Garfinkel, L. (1980) Cancer mortality in nonsmokers: Prospective study by the American Cancer Society. *J. natl Cancer Inst.*, **65**, 1061–1066

Gram, I.T., Austin, H. & Stalsberg, H. (1992) Cigarette smoking and the incidence of cervical intra-epithelial neoplasia, grade III, and cancer of the cervix uteri. *Am. J. Epidemiol.*, **135**, 341–346

Harris, R.W., Brinton, L.A., Cowdell, R.H., Skegg, D.C., Smith, P.G., Vessey, M.P. & Doll, R. (1980) Characteristics of women with dysplasia or carcinoma in situ of the cervix uteri. *Br. J. Cancer*, **42**, 359–369

Herrero, R., Brinton, L.A., Reeves, W.C., Brenes, M.M., Tenorio, F., de Britton, R.C., Gaitan, E., Garcia, M. & Rawls, W.E. (1989) Invasive cervical cancer and smoking in Latin America. *J. natl Cancer Inst.*, **81**, 205–211

Hildesheim, A., Herrero, R., Castle, P.E., Wacholder, S., Bratti, M.C., Sherman, M.E., Lorincz, A.T., Burk, R.D., Morales, J., Rodriguez, A.C., Helgesen, K., Alfaro, M., Hutchinson, M., Balmaceda, I., Greenberg, M. & Schiffman, M. (2001) HPV co-factors related to the develop-ment of cervical cancer: Results from a population-based study in Costa Rica. *Br. J. Cancer*, **84**, 1219–1226

Hirayama, T. (1975) Prospective studies on cancer epidemiology based on census population in Japan. In: Buccalossi, P., Veronesi, U. & Cascinelli, N., eds, *Proceedings of the XIth Inter-*

national Cancer Congress, Florence, 1974, Vol. 3, *Cancer Epidemiology, Environmental Factors*, Amsterdam, Excerpta Medica, pp. 26–35

Hirayama, T. (1985) A cohort study on cancer in Japan. In: Blot, W.J., Hirayama, T. & Hoel, D.G., eds, *Statistical Methods in Cancer Epidemiology*, Hiroshima, Radiation Effects Research Foundation, pp. 73–91

Hirose, K., Tajima, K., Hamajima, N., Takezaki, T., Inoue, M., Kuroishi, T., Kuzuya, K., Nakamura, S. & Tokudome, S. (1996) Subsite (cervix/endometrium)-specific risk and protective factors in uterus cancer. *Jpn. J. Cancer Res.*, **87**, 1001–1009

Ho, G.Y., Kadish, A.S., Burk, R.D., Basu, J., Palan, P.R. , Mikhail, M. & Romney, S.L. (1998) HPV 16 and cigarette smoking as risk factors for high-grade cervical intraepithelial neoplasia. *Int. J. Cancer*, **78**, 281–285

Hsieh, C.Y., You, S.L., Kao, C.L. & Chen, C.J. (1999) Reproductive and infectious risk factors for invasive cervical cancer in Taiwan. *Anticancer Res.*, **19**, 4495–4500

IARC (1986) *IARC Monographs on the Evaluation of the Carcinogenic Risk of Chemicals to Humans*, Vol. 38, *Tobacco Smoking*, Lyon, pp. 37–375

IARC (1995) *IARC Monographs on the Evaluation of Carcinogenic Risks to Humans*, Vol. 64, *Human Papillomaviruses*, Lyon

Jones, C.J., Brinton, L.A., Hamman, R.F., Stolley, P.D., Lehman, H.F., Levine, R.S. & Mallin, K. (1990) Risk factors for in situ cervical cancer: Results from a case–control study. *Cancer Res.*, **50**, 3657–3662

Kanetsky, P.A., Gammon, M.D., Mandelblatt, J., Zhang, Z.F., Ramsey, E., Wright, T.C., Thomas, L., Matseoane, S., Lazaro, N., Felton, H.T., Sachdev, R.K., Richart, R.M. & Curtin, J.P. (1998) Cigarette smoking and cervical dysplasia among non-Hispanic black women. *Cancer Detect. Prev.*, **22**, 109–119

Kjaer, S.K., Engholm, G., Dahl, C. & Bock, J.E. (1996) Case–control study of risk factors for cervical squamous cell neoplasia in Denmark. IV: Role of smoking habits. *Eur. J. Cancer Prev.*, **5**, 359–365

Kjellberg, L., Hallmans, G., Ahren, A.M., Johansson, R., Bergman, F., Wadell, G., Angstrom, T. & Dillner, J. (2000) Smoking, diet, pregnancy and oral contraceptive use as risk factors for cervical intra-epithelial neoplasia in relation to human papillomavirus infection. *Br. J. Cancer*, **82**, 1332–1338

Lacey, J.V., Jr, Frisch, M., Brinton, L.A., Abbas, F.M., Barnes, W.A., Gravitt, P.E., Greenberg, M.D., Greene, S.M., Hadjimichael, O.C., McGowan, L. Mortel, R., Schwartz, P.E., Zaino, R.J. & Hildesheim, A. (2001) Associations between smoking and adenocarcinomas and squamous cell carcinomas of the uterine cervix (United States). *Cancer Causes Control*, **12**, 153–161

La Vecchia, C., Franceschi, S., Decarli, A., Fasoli, M., Gentile, A. & Tognoni, G. (1986) Cigarette smoking and the risk of cervical neoplasia. *Am. J. Epidemiol.*, **123**, 22–29

Lazcano-Ponce, E.C., Hernandez-Avila, M. , Lopez-Carrillo, L., Alonso-de-Ruiz, P., Torres-Lobaton, A., Gonzalez-Lira, G. & Romieu, I. (1995) [Reproductive risk factors and sexual history associated with cervical cancer in Mexico.] *Rev. Invest. clin.*, **47**, 377–385 (in Spanish)

Liaw, K.M. & Chen, C.J. (1998) Mortality attributable to cigarette smoking in Taiwan: A 12-year follow-up study. *Tob. Control*, **7**, 141–148

Licciardone, J.C., Wilkins, J.R., Brownson, R.C. & Chang, J.C. (1989) Cigarette smoking and alcohol consumption in the aetiology of uterine cervical cancer. *Int. J. Epidemiol.*, **18**, 533–537

Lyon, J.L., Gardner, J.W., West, D.W., Stanish, W.M. & Hebertson, R.M. (1983) Smoking and carcinoma in situ of the uterine cervix. *Am. J. public Health*, **73**, 558–562

Madeleine, M.M., Daling, J.R., Schwartz, S.M., Shera, K., McKnight, B., Carter, J.J., Wipf, G.C., Critchlow, C.W., McDougall, J.K., Porter, P. & Galloway, D.A. (2001) Human papillomavirus and long-term oral contraceptive use increase the risk of adenocarcinoma in situ of the cervix. *Cancer Epidemiol. Biomarkers Prev.*, **10**, 171–177

Marshall, J.R., Graham, S., Byers, T., Swanson, M. & Brasure, J. (1983) Diet and smoking in the epidemiology of cancer of the cervix. *J. natl Cancer Inst.*, **70**, 847–851

Martin, P.M. & Hill, G.B. (1984) Cervical cancer in relation to tobacco and alcohol consumption in Lesotho, southern Africa. *Cancer Detect. Prev.*, **7**, 109–115

Mayberry, R.M. (1985) Cigarette smoking, herpes simplex virus type 2 infection, and cervical abnormalities. *Am. J. public Health*, **75**, 676–678

Moscicki, A.B., Hills, N., Shiboski, S., Powell, K., Jay, N., Hanson, E., Miller, S., Clayton, L., Farhat, S., Broering, J. &. (2001) Risks for incident human papillomavirus infection and low-grade squamous intraepithelial lesion development in young females. *J. Am. med. Assoc.*, **285**, 2995–3002

Muñoz, N., Bosch, F.X., de Sanjose, S., Tafur, L., Izarzugaza, I., Gili, M., Viladiu, P., Navarro, C., Martos, C. & Ascunce, N. (1992) The causal link between human papillomavirus and invasive cervical cancer: A population-based case–control study in Colombia and Spain. *Int. J. Cancer*, **52**, 743–749

Muñoz, N., Bosch, F.X., de Sanjose, S., Vergara, A., Del Moral, A., Munoz, M.T., Tafur, L., Gili, M., Izarzugaza, I. & Viladiu, P. (1993) Risk factors for cervical intraepithelial neoplasia grade III/carcinoma in situ in Spain and Colombia. *Cancer Epidemiol. Biomarkers Prev.*, **2**, 423–431

Ngelangel, C., Muñoz, N., Bosch, F.X., Limson, G.M., Festin, M.R., Deacon, J., Jacobs, M.V., Santamaria, M., Meijer, C.J. & Walboomers, J.M. (1998) Causes of cervical cancer in the Philippines: A case–control study. *J. natl Cancer Inst.*, **90**, 43–49

Nischan, P., Ebeling, K. & Schindler, C. (1988) Smoking and invasive cervical cancer risk. Results from a case–control study. *Am. J. Epidemiol.*, **128**, 74–77

Nordlund, L.A., Carstensen, J.M. & Pershagen, G. (1997) Cancer incidence in female smokers: A 26-year follow-up. *Int. J. Cancer*, **73**, 625–628

Olsen, A.O., Dillner, J., Skrondal, A. & Magnus, P. (1998) Combined effect of smoking and human papillomavirus type 16 infection in cervical carcinogenesis. *Epidemiology*, **9**, 346–349

Parazzini, F., La Vecchia, C., Negri, E., Fedele, L., Franceschi, S. & Gallotta, L. (1992) Risk factors for cervical intraepithelial neoplasia. *Cancer*, **69**, 2276–2282

Parazzini, F., Chatenoud, L., La Vecchia, C., Negri, E., Franceschi, S. & Bolis, G. (1998) Determinants of risk of invasive cervical cancer in young women. *Br. J. Cancer*, **77**, 838–841

Peng, H.Q., Liu, S.L., Mann, V., Rohan, T. & Rawls, W. (1991) Human papillomavirus types 16 and 33, herpes simplex virus type 2 and other risk factors for cervical cancer in Sichuan Province, China. *Int. J. Cancer*, **47**, 711–716

Peters, R.K., Thomas, D., Hagan, D.G., Mack, T.M. & Henderson, B.E. (1986) Risk factors for invasive cervical cancer among Latinas and non-Latinas in Los Angeles County. *J. natl Cancer Inst.*, **77**, 1063–1077

Plummer, M., Herrero, R., Franceschi, S., Meijer, C.J.L.M., Snijders, P., Bosch, F.X., de Sanjosé, S. & Muñoz, N. (2003) Smoking and cervical cancer: Pooled analysis of the IARC multicentric case–control study. *Cancer Causes Control*, **14**, 805–814

Remmink, A.J., Walboomers, J.M., Helmerhorst, T.J., Voorhorst, F.J., Rozendaal , L., Risse, E.K., Meijer, C.J. & Kenemans, P. (1995) The presence of persistent high-risk HPV genotypes in dysplastic cervical lesions is associated with progressive disease: Natural history up to 36 months. *Int. J. Cancer*, **61**, 306–311

Rolon, P.A., Smith, J.S., Munoz, N., Klug, S.J., Herrero, R., Bosch, X., Llamosas, F., Meijer, C.J. & Walboomers, J.M. (2000) Human papillomavirus infection and invasive cervical cancer in Paraguay. *Int. J. Cancer*, **85**, 486–491

Santos, C., Munoz, N., Klug, S.J., Almonte, M., Guerrero, I., Alvarez, M., Velarde, C., Galdos, O., Castillo, M., Walboomers, J., Meijer, C. & Caceres, E. (2001) HPV types and cofactors causing cervical cancer in Peru. *Br. J. Cancer*, **85**, 966–971

Schiffman, M.H., Bauer, H.M., Hoover, R.N., Glass, A.G., Cadell, D.M., Rush, B.B., Scott, D.R., Sherman, M.E., Kurman, R.J. & Wacholder, S. (1993) Epidemiologic evidence showing that human papillomavirus infection causes most cervical intraepithelial neoplasia. *J. natl Cancer Inst.*, **85**, 958–964

Slattery, M.L., Robison, L.M., Schuman, K.L., French, T.K., Abbott, T.M., Overall, J.C. & Gardner, J.W. (1989) Cigarette smoking and exposure to passive smoke are risk factors for cervical cancer. *J. Am. med. Assoc.*, **261**, 1593–1598

Stellman, S.D., Austin, H. & Wynder, E.L. (1980) Cervix cancer and cigarette smoking: A case control study. *Am. J. Epidemiol.*, **111**, 383–388

Stone, K.M., Zaidi, A., Rosero-Bixby, L., Oberle, M.W., Reynolds, G., Larsen, S., Nahmias, A.J. , Lee, F.K., Schachter, J. & Guinan, M.E. (1995) Sexual behavior, sexually transmitted diseases, and risk of cervical cancer. *Epidemiology*, **6**, 409–414

Thomas, D.B. (1972) Relationship of oral contraceptives to cervical carcinogenesis. *Obstet. Gynecol.*, **40**, 508–518

Thomas, D.B. (1973) An epidemiologic study of carcinoma in situ and squamous dysplasia of the uterine cervix. *Am. J. Epidemiol.*, **98**, 10–28

Tokuhata, G.K. (1967) Epidemiology of cancer of the cervix. IV. Tobacco and cancer of the genitalia among married women. *Am. J. public Health*, **57**, 830–839

Trevathan, E., Layde, P., Webster, L.A., Adams, J.B., Benigno, B.B. & Ory, H. (1983) Cigarette smoking and dysplasia and carcinoma in situ of the uterine cervix. *J. Am. med. Assoc.*, **250**, 499–502

Tulinius, H., Sigfusson, N., Sigvaldason, H., Bjarnadottir, K. & Tryggvadottir, L. (1997) Risk factors for malignant diseases: A cohort study on a population of 22,946 Icelanders. *Cancer Epidemiol. Biomarkers Prev.*, **6**, 863–873

Tverdal, A., Thelle, D., Stensvold, I., Leren, P. & Bjartveit, K. (1993) Mortality in relation to smoking history: 13 years' follow-up of 68,000 Norwegian men and women 35–49 years. *J. clin. Epidemiol.*, **46**, 475–487

Ursin, G., Pike, M.C., Preston-Martin, S., d'Ablaing, G. & Peters, R.K. (1996) Sexual, repro-ductive, and other risk factors for adenocarcinoma of the cervix: Results from a population-based case–control study (California, United States). *Cancer Causes Control*, **7**, 391–401

de Vet, H.C., Sturmans, F. & Knipschild, P.G. (1994) The role of cigarette smoking in the etiology of cervical dysplasia. *Epidemiology*, **5**, 631–633

Walboomers, J.M., Husman, A.M., Snijders, P.J., Stel, H.V., Risse, E.K., Helmerhorst, T.J., Voorhorst, F.J. & Meijer, C.J. (1995) Human papillomavirus in false negative archival cervical smears: Implications for screening for cervical cancer. *J. clin. Pathol.*, **48**, 728–732

Wigle, D.T., Mao, Y. & Grace, M. (1980) Re: Smoking and cancer of the uterine cervix: Hypothesis. *Am. J. Epidemiol.*, **111**, 125–127

Williams, R.R. & Horm, J.W. (1977) Association of cancer sites with tobacco and alcohol consumption and socioeconomic status of patients: Interview study from the Third National Cancer Survey. *J. natl Cancer Inst.*, **58**, 525–547

Williams, R.R., Stegens, N.L. & Horm, J.W. (1977) Patient interview study from the Third National Cancer Survey: Overview of problems and potentials of these data. *J. natl Cancer Inst.*, **58**, 519–524

Winkelstein, W.J. (1977) Smoking and cancer of the uterine cervix: Hypothesis. *Am. J. Epidemiol.*, **106**, 257–259

Wright, N.H., Vessey, M.P., Kenward, B., McPherson, K. & Doll, R. (1978) Neoplasia and dysplasia of the cervix uteri and contraception: A possible protective effect of the diaphragm. *Br. J. Cancer*, **38**, 273–279

Ylitalo, N., Sorensen, P., Josefsson, A., Frisch, M., Sparen, P., Ponten, J., Gyllensten, U., Melbye, M. & Adami, H.O. (1999) Smoking and oral contraceptives as risk factors for cervical carcinoma in situ. *Int. J. Cancer*, **81**, 357–365

Yoshikawa, H., Nagata, C., Noda, K., Nozawa, S., Yajima, A., Sekiya, S., Sugimori, H., Hirai, Y., Kanazawa, K., Sugase, M., Shimizu, H. & Kawana, T. (1999) Human papillomavirus infection and other risk factors for cervical intraepithelial neoplasia in Japan. *Br. J. Cancer*, **80**, 621–624

Zondervan, K.T., Carpenter, L.M., Painter, R. & Vessey, M.P. (1996) Oral contraceptives and cervical cancer — Further findings from the Oxford Family Planning Association contraceptive study. *Br. J. Cancer*, **73**, 1291–1297

2.1.11   Endometrial cancer

A total of 27 case–control studies have examined the association between cigarette smoking and endometrial cancer. The principal design characteristics and results of these studies are summarized in Tables 2.1.11.1 and 2.1.11.2, respectively.

All but two case–control studies (Shu *et al.*, 1991; Weir *et al.*, 1994) reported an inverse association of cigarette smoking with endometrial cancer, and in the majority of these studies the decrease in risk was statistically significant (Weiss *et al.*, 1980; Lesko *et al.*, 1985; Baron *et al.*, 1986; Franks *et al.*, 1987; Levi *et al.*, 1987; Stockwell & Lyman, 1987; Kato *et al.*, 1989; Koumantaki *et al.*, 1989; Elliott *et al.*, 1990; Rubin *et al.*, 1990; Brinton *et al.*, 1993; Parazzini *et al.*, 1995; McCann *et al.*, 2000; Weiderpass & Baron, 2001). Quantitative measures of smoking in relation to endometrial cancer have been examined in 13 studies. Most studies showed a negative trend with increasing intensity (Lesko *et al.*, 1985; Levi *et al.*, 1987; Stockwell & Lyman, 1987; Parazzini *et al.*, 1995; Weiderpass & Baron, 2001), duration (Brinton *et al.*, 1993; Parazzini *et al.*, 1995) or pack–years (Williams & Horm, 1977; Baron *et al.*, 1986; Lawrence *et al.*, 1987). Only one study found a significantly elevated risk for endometrial cancer related to smoking. This was in pre-menopausal women who smoked 10–20 cigarettes/day, and no dose–response relationship was observed (Weir *et al.*, 1994). Also, one study found a significant positive trend between risk for endometrial cancer and amount smoked daily, but the effects of duration were not statistically significant (Shu *et al.*, 1991).

In studies that investigated the risk associated with smoking cessation, the effect was greater among current smokers than among former smokers (Lesko *et al.*, 1985; Levi *et al.*, 1987; Lawrence *et al.*, 1987, 1989; Rubin *et al.*, 1990; Austin *et al.*, 1993; Weiderpass & Baron, 2001) or was confined to current smokers (Tyler *et al.*, 1985; Elliott *et al.*, 1990; Brinton *et al.*, 1993), and the association weakened with time since smoking cessation (Weir *et al.*, 1994; Parazzini *et al.*, 1995).

Three studies (Lesko *et al.*, 1985; Brinton *et al.*, 1993; Weir *et al.*, 1994) examined results by menopausal status and showed that the reduced risk among smokers was restricted to women diagnosed with endometrial cancer after menopause.

Prospective cohort studies of smoking and endometrial cancer risk in which the problems of unbiased selection of study subjects and recall are minimized are scarce. The limited evidence that is available from prospective studies does not refute the existence of an inverse association between smoking and risk for endometrial cancer (Table 2.1.11.3).

Factors suggested as potential confounders in the evaluation of the association of endometrial cancer with exposure to cigarette smoke include estrogen replacement therapy, obesity, lack of physical activity and age at menopause. Several investigators have assessed whether the presence of selected risk factors could modify the relationship between smoking and risk for endometrial cancer. Some studies have noted a greater reduction in smoking-associated risk among obese women (Brinton *et al.*, 1993; Parazzini *et al.*, 1995). Others have reported a greater reduction in smoking–associated risk among women taking estrogen replacement therapy (Weiss *et al.*, 1980), but not all studies support the existence of such an effect (Brinton *et al.*, 1993).

The biological mechanisms that might underlie the reduced risk for endometrial cancer among smokers remain unclear. In the previous *IARC Monograph* on tobacco smoking (IARC, 1986), the Working Group noted that there was consistent evidence that menopause occurs 1–2 years earlier among cigarette smokers than in nonsmokers, indicating that smoking affects hormonal status, a factor known to be related to endometrial cancer. However, no conclusion was drawn regarding the observed reduction in endometrial cancer associated with tobacco exposure due to methodological problems with the interpretation of mortality studies.

Some researchers have suggested that exposure to tobacco may reduce estrogen production, a hypothesis that has received some support from findings that estriol excretion is reduced among postmenopausal smokers. Another theory is that smoking affects the metabolism, absorption or distribution of hormones. Recent studies have proposed a reduction in relative body weight and consequent decrease in levels of circulating estrogen and an earlier age at menopause as a possible mechanism (Terry *et al.*, 2002b).

Table 2.1.11.1 Case–control studies on smoking and endometrial cancer: main characteristics of study design

Reference Country and years of study	Cases and controls	Criteria for eligibility
Williams & Horm (1977) USA Early 1960s	358 cases and 3188 controls	Hospital-based study Cases and controls from the Third National Cancer Survey Controls with tobacco-related cancers (lung, larynx, mouth, oesophagus and bladder) excluded
Weiss et al. (1980) USA 1975–76	322 cases and 289 controls	Population-based study in western Washington Cases aged 50–74 years; 85% response rate Controls randomly selected from general population; aged 50–74 years; controls who had a hysterectomy > 1 year before interview and non-Caucasians excluded
Kelsey et al. (1982) USA 1977–79	167 cases and 903 controls	Hospital-based study in Connecticut Cases confirmed histologically; aged 45–74 years; 67% response rate Controls in same age group admitted to surgical departments; large variety of diagnoses, none of which accounted for more than 4%; hysterectomy excluded; 72% response rate
Smith et al. (1984) USA 1980–82	70 cases and 612 controls	Population-based study Cases identified through Cancer Registry of Iowa; stage of cancer reviewed; aged 20–54 years Controls frequency-matched for age; controls with previous cancer of reproductive organs excluded 95% response rate for cases and controls
Lesko et al. (1985) USA 1976–83	510 cases and 727 controls	Hospital-based study in the north-east of USA, conducted using interviews Cases histologically confirmed; median age, 59 years; 95% response rate; history of previous or concurrent malignant disease and bilateral oophorectomy excluded Controls with specific, non-tobacco-related cancers: colorectal cancer (40%), melanoma (38%), lymphoreticular neoplasia or cancer of thyroid or adrenal glands (22%); history of previous or concurrent malignant disease and bilateral oophorectomy excluded; median age, 52 years
Tyler et al. (1985) USA 1980–82	437 cases and 3200 controls	Population-based cancer and steroid hormone study conducted using interviews Cases confirmed histologically; 72% of cases interviewed; aged 20–54 years Controls selected by random-digit dialling; aged 20–54 years; frequency-matched on age (5-year groups); 83% response rate

Table 2.1.11.1 (contd)

Reference Country and years of study	Cases and controls	Criteria for eligibility
Baron et al. (1986) USA 1957–65	476 cases and 2128 controls	Hospital-based study in Buffalo, NY Cases aged 40–89 years Controls with benign conditions of the uterus, breast, gastrointestinal tract and skin; cancers and diseases of the respiratory or circulatory systems excluded; aged 40–89 years
Franks et al. (1987) USA 1980–82	79 cases and 416 controls	Population-based study in 6 areas Cases confirmed histologically; postmenopausal women aged 40–55 years; perimenopausal women excluded Controls selected through random-digit dialling in same areas as cases; aged 40–55 years
Lawrence et al. (1987) USA 1979–81	200 cases and 200 controls	Population-based study in New York conducted using interviews Cases confirmed histologically as stage IA (83) or IB (117); aged 40–69 years; 65% of eligible cases participated. Controls randomly selected through driver's licence files; individually matched by county of residence and year of birth; 71% of first selected controls participated.
Levi et al. (1987) Italy 1983–85	357 cases and 1122 controls	Hospital-based study in Milan conducted using interviews Cases histologically confirmed; aged 31–74 years Controls with traumatic conditions (32%), non-traumatic orthopaedic disorders (25%), surgical conditions (15%) and eye, nose, throat and dental disorders (28%); aged 25–74 years; malignant, hormonal, gynaecological and tobacco-related diseases and hysterectomy excluded 98% of eligible cases and controls participated.
Stockwell & Lyman (1987) USA 1981	1374 cases and 3921 controls	Population-based study Study population identified through Florida Cancer Data System; 28% with unknown smoking status Controls with non-tobacco-related cancers: colon cancer (62%) or rectal cancer (23%), melanoma (11%), or endocrine neoplasms (4%) (tobacco-related cancer sites excluded) Controls older than cases
Kato et al. (1989) Japan 1980–86	239 cases and 8920 controls	Hospital-based study at Aichi Cancer Centre Cases aged ≥ 20 years Controls with cancer of stomach (31%), large intestine (19%), uterus other than corpus (17%), lung (7%) and other sites; alcohol-related cancer and cancer of ill-defined sites excluded

Table 2.1.11.1 (contd)

Reference Country and years of study	Cases and controls	Criteria for eligibility
Koumantaki et al. (1989) Greece 1984	83 cases and 164 controls	Hospital-based study among Greek Caucasians conducted using interviews Cases confirmed by biopsy; aged 40–79 years; 80% of eligible cases participated. Controls with traumatic fractures (58%), other traumatic conditions (6%), rheumatoid arthritis (46%) and other orthopaedic conditions (10%); hysterectomy excluded; aged 40–79 years; 95% participation rate
Lawrence et al. (1989) USA 1979–81	84 cases and 168 controls	Population-based study conducted using interviews Cases histologically confirmed stage 2–4; aged 40–69 years; 84% of eligible cases participated. Controls randomly selected through driver's license registry, individually matched (2:1) for county of residence and year of birth; 69% response rate
Elliott et al. (1990) USA 1985–87	46 cases and 140 controls	Population-based study in Baltimore conducted using interviews Cases confirmed histologically; mean age, 62.2 years Controls selected through random digit dialling after frequency-matching for prefix of telephone number (as proxy for area of residence); hysterectomy excluded; mean age, 54.3 years; 58% participation rate
Rubin et al. (1990) USA 1980–82	196 cases and 986 controls	Population-based study in 8 geographical areas conducted using interviews Cases from cancer and steroid hormone study, histologically confirmed; aged 40–54 years; 73% participation rate Controls selected by random digit dialling, frequency-matched on age (5-year groups); hysterectomy excluded; 84% participation rate
Shu et al. (1991) China 1988–90	268 cases and 268 controls	Population-based study in Shanghai conducted using interviews Cases histologically confirmed; aged 18–74 years; 91% of eligible cases participated. Controls randomly selected from Shanghai population registry, individually matched for age (± 2 years); hysterectomy excluded; 96% participation rate
Austin et al. (1993) USA 1984–88	168 cases and 334 controls	Hospital-based study in Alabama conducted using interviews Cases confirmed histologically; aged 40–82 years; 93% participation rate Controls from university optometry clinic, frequency-matched by age and race; hysterectomy excluded; 77% participation rate

Table 2.1.11.1 (contd)

Reference Country and years of study	Cases and controls	Criteria for eligibility
Brinton et al. (1993) USA 1987–90	405 cases and 297 controls	Population-based study in 5 areas conducted using interviews Cases confirmed histologically; aged 20–74 years; 87% of eligible cases participated. Controls < 65 years selected through random digit dialling and controls ≥ 65 years through Health Care Financing Administration files; individually matched on age (5-year group), race and area of residence; 66% of eligible controls participated
Weir et al. (1994) Canada 1977–78	88 cases and 551 controls	Population-based study conducted using interviews Cases confirmed histologically; aged 40–74 years Controls individually matched by age (± 5 years), neighbourhood and type of dwelling; hysterectomy and history of cancer excluded
Parazzini et al. (1995) Italy 1983–92	726 cases and 1452 controls	Hospital-based study in Milan conducted using interviews Cases confirmed histologically; aged 31–74 years Controls with traumatic conditions (34%), non traumatic orthopaedic conditions (26%), surgical conditions (15%) and other illnesses (25%) 98% participation rate for cases and controls
Hirose et al. (1996) Japan 1988–93	145 cases and 26 751 controls	Hospital-based study at Aichi Cancer Centre conducted using a questionnaire; 98% participation rate Cases confirmed histologically; aged ≥ 18 years Controls aged ≥ 20 years; cancer diagnosis excluded
Goodman et al. (1997) Hawaii, USA, 1985–93	332 cases and 511 controls	Population-based study conducted using interviews Cases confirmed histologically; aged 18–84 years; 66% of eligible cases participated. Controls randomly selected from population rosters, individually matched 2:1 or 3:1 for ethnicity and age (± 2.5 years); hysterectomy excluded; 73% participation rate
Jain et al. (2000) Canada 1994–98	552 cases and 562 controls	Population-based study in Toronto, Peel, Halton and York conducted using interviews Cases identified through Ontario Cancer Registry, histologically confirmed; aged 30–79 years Controls randomly selected from property assessment lists, frequency-matched by age (5-year group) and geographical area; hysterectomy excluded; low participation rate

Table 2.1.11.1 (contd)

Reference Country and years of study	Cases and controls	Criteria for eligibility
McCann et al. (2000) USA 1986–91	232 cases and 639 controls	Population-based study conducted using interviews Cases confirmed histologically; aged 40–85 years; 51% response rate Controls < 65 years randomly selected from driver's licence lists and for controls ≥ 65 years from Health Care Financing Administration lists, frequency-matched on age and county of residence; hysterectomy excluded; 51% of eligible controls participated.
Parslov et al. (2000) Denmark 1987–94	237 cases and 538 controls	Population-based study; questionnaire Cases histologically confirmed; aged 25–49 years; 93% participation rate Controls randomly selected from Danish Central Person Registry, individually matched by age and geographical region; 91% participation rate
Weiderpass & Baron (2001) Sweden 1994–95	789 cases and 3368 controls	Population-based study among postmenopausal Swedish women residents with intact uterus Cases confirmed histologically; aged 50–74 years; 75% participation rate Controls randomly selected from Swedish population registry; aged 50–74 years; 80% participation rate

Table 2.1.11.2. Case–control studies on smoking and endometrial cancer

Reference Country and years of study	Exposure estimates	Relative risk (95% CI) Nonsmoker	Ever-smoker	Comments
Williams & Horm (1977) USA Early 1960s	*Pack–years* < 20 20–40 > 40	0.89 0.79 0.74		Adjusted for age and sex
Weiss et al. (1980) USA 1975–76	*Non-contraceptive estrogen use (years)* < 1 1–7 ≥ 8	1.0 2.6 (1.2–5.6) 14.9 (6.7–33.2)	0.4 (0.2–0.7)† 1.1 (0.5–2.5) 3.4 (1.6–7.4)	Adjusted for age, parity, weight, hypertension and estrogen use †$p < 0.05$
Kelsey et al. (1982); Baron (1984) USA 1977–79	Ever-smoker	0.83		Adjusted for age, parity, weight, menopausal status, education, oral contraceptive/estrogen use
Smith et al. (1984) USA 1980–82	Sporadic smoker Continuous smoker	0.7 (0.4–1.4) 0.8 (0.4–1.5)		Crude odds ratio
Lesko et al. (1985) USA 1976–83	Former smoker Current smoker *Cigarettes/day* 1–14 15–24 ≥ 25 *Smokers of ≥ 25/day†* Premenopausal Postmenopausal	0.9 (0.6–1.2) 0.7 (0.5–1.0) 0.8 (0.5–1.3) 1.0 (0.6–1.5) 0.5 (0.3–0.8) 0.9 (0.4–2.2) 0.5 (0.2–0.9)		Adjusted for age, body-mass index, duration of conjugated estrogen use †Compared with nonsmokers of the same category
Tyler et al. (1985) USA 1980–82	Ever-smoker Former smoker Current smoker	0.9 (0.7–1.1) 1.0 (0.7–1.4) 0.8 (0.7–1.1)		Adjusted for age, body weight, oral contraceptive use, alcohol consumption, menopausal status, hypertension and estrogen use

Table 2.1.11.2 (contd)

Reference Country and years of study	Exposure estimates	Relative risk (95% CI)	Comments
Baron et al. (1986) USA 1957–65	*Pack-years* 1–14 ≥15 p for trend	0.8 (0.5–1.1) 0.6 (0.4–0.9) 0.003	Adjusted for age, marital status, parity and body-mass index (Quetelet index)
Franks et al. (1987) USA 1980–82	Ever-smoker	0.5 (0.3–0.8)	Crude odds ratio Adjustment for age, age at menopause, race, Quetelet index, hypertension, diabetes, infertility, parity, history of contraceptive use and geographical regions did not appreciably alter risk estimates.
Lawrence et al. (1987) USA 1979–81	*Pack-years* ≤1 >1 p for trend	**Current**[†] / Former 0.7 / 1.02 0.5 / 0.6	[95% CI not reported] [†] p for trend < 0.025, one-sided
Levi et al. (1987) Italy 1983–85	Former smoker Current smoker *Cigarettes/day* <15 ≥15 p for trend	0.9 (0.5–1.5) 0.5 (0.3–0.7) 0.5 (0.3–0.8) 0.4 (0.2–0.9) <0.001	Odds ratios adjusted for age, marital status, education, social class, age at menarche, menopausal status, age at menopause, parity, number of live births, family history of gynaecological cancer, body-mass index, use of oral contraceptive and estrogen replacement therapy
Stockwell & Lyman (1987) USA 1981	Former smoker Current smoker *Cigarettes/day* <20 20–40 >40	0.6 (0.5–0.8) 0.5 (0.3–0.9) 0.9 (0.7–1.2) 0.7 (0.5–0.9) 0.5 (0.3–0.9)	Adjusted for age, race and marital status
Kato et al. (1989) Japan 1980–86	Ever-smoker	0.5 (0.3–0.8)	Adjusted for alcohol drinking, marital status, age, area of residence, occupation and family history of breast cancer

Table 2.1.11.2 (contd)

Reference Country and years of study	Exposure estimates	Relative risk (95% CI)		Comments
		Current	Former	
Koumantaki et al. (1989) Greece 1984	Smoker	0.5 (0.3–0.9)		Relative risk for 20 years of smoking Adjusted for age, parity, age at menarche, age at menopause, height and weight
Lawrence et al. (1989) USA 1979–81	*Packs/day* ≤ 1 > 1 *p* for trend	0.6 0.95 > 0.3	0.8 1.02 > 0.3	Matched analysis
Elliott et al. (1990) USA 1985–87	Former smoker Current smoker	1.2 (0.5–3.0) 0.2 (0.1–0.7)		Adjusted for age, waist to hip circumference ratio and parity; controls significantly older than cases
Rubin et al. (1990) USA 1980–82	Former smoker Current smoker	0.8 (0.5–1.2) 0.7 (0.5–1.0)		Crude odds ratio
Shu et al. (1991) China 1988–90	Current smoker *Cigarettes/day* ≤ 9 ≥ 10 *p* for trend *Age at starting smoking (years)* ≥ 31 ≤ 30 *Duration (years)* ≤ 19 ≥ 20 *p* for trend	1.7 (0.9–3.0) 1.3 (0.7–2.8) 2.3 (1.0–5.7) 0.05 1.6 (0.7–3.5) 1.7 (0.8–3.8) 1.7 (0.7–4.0) 1.6 (0.8–3.4) 0.11		Low prevalence of smoking (< 10%) Adjusted for age, number of pregnancies and weight

Table 2.1.11.2 (contd)

Reference Country and years of study	Exposure estimates	Relative risk (95% CI)		Comments
Austin et al. (1993) USA 1984–88	Former smoker Current smoker	0.8 (0.5–1.5) 0.7 (0.4–1.2)		Adjusted for age, race, education, body mass, use of replacement estrogens and number of pregnancies
Brinton et al. (1993) USA 1987–90	Ever-smoker Former smoker Current smoker	0.8 (0.5–1.1) 1.1 (0.7–1.6) 0.4 (0.2–0.7)		Adjusted for age, education, number of births, weight, use of oral contraceptives and use of hormone replacement therapy
	Cigarettes/day < 20 20–29 ≥ 30 *p* for trend	0.8 (0.5–1.2) 0.7 (0.4–1.2) 0.7 (0.4–1.4) 0.12		
	Age at starting smoking (years) ≥ 22 18–21 < 18	0.7 (0.4–1.2) 0.9 (0.6–1.5) 0.7 (0.4–1.1)		
	Duration (years) < 20 20–39 ≥ 40 *p* for trend	1.0 (0.5–1.7) 0.8 (0.5–1.3) 0.5 (0.3–0.9) 0.05		
		Premenopausal	Postmenopausal	
	Ever-smoker Former smoker Current smoker	1.8 (0.8–4.0) 3.0 (1.2–7.4) 0.5 (0.1–1.7)	0.6 (0.4–0.9) 0.8 (0.4–1.2) 0.4 (0.2–0.7)	
	Cigarettes/day < 20 20–29 ≥ 30	2.0 (0.7–5.5) 1.7 (0.6–5.2) 1.3 (0.2–7.1)	0.6 (0.3–0.9) 0.5 (0.3–0.9) 0.6 (0.3–1.3)	

Table 2.1.11.2 (contd)

Reference Country and years of study	Exposure estimates	Relative risk (95% CI)		Comments
Brinton et al. (1993) (contd)	*Age at starting smoking (years)*			
	≥ 22	2.7 (0.8–8.6)	0.4 (0.2–0.8)	
	18–21	1.3 (0.5–3.8)	0.8 (0.4–1.5)	
	< 18	1.7 (0.5–5.9)	0.5 (0.3–1.0)	
	Duration (years)			
	< 20	2.2 (0.9–5.5)	0.6 (0.3–1.3)	
	20–29	0.5 (0.1–2.4)	0.4 (0.2–0.9)	
	≥ 30	6.2 (0.9–42.3)	0.6 (0.4–1.0)	
	p for trend	0.15	0.02	
Weir et al.(1994) Canada 1977–78		Premenopausal (*n* = 14)	Postmenopausal (*n* = 74)	Adjusted for age, Quetelet index, estrogen use, age at menopause and education
	Ever-smoker	2.4 (0.7–8.9)	0.8 (0.5–1.4)	
	Current smoker	2.8 (0.7–11.3)	0.8 (0.5–1.5)	
	Cigarettes/day			
	< 10	0.6 (0.1–6.4)	0.8 (0.4–1.7)	
	10–20	6.4 (1.2–32.7)	1.0 (0.5–2.0)	
	≥ 21	2.1 (0.3–14.7)	0.6 (0.3–1.5)	
	Duration (years)			
	< 25	1.7 (0.3–9.7)	0.7 (0.3–1.6)	
	≥ 25	3.1 (0.7–13.1)	0.9 (0.5–1.6)	
	Years since quitting			
	≥ 10	–	0.9 (0.3–2.1)	
	< 10	1.8 (0.3–11.3)	0.8 (0.3–2.5)	

Table 2.1.11.2 (contd)

Reference Country and years of study	Exposure estimates	Relative risk (95% CI)	Comments
Parazzini *et al.* (1995) Italy 1983–92	Former smoker	0.6 (0.4–0.9)	Adjusted for age, education, parity, Quetelet index, menopausal status, diabetes, hypertension and use of oral contraceptives or estrogen replacement therapy [no trend calculated]
	Current smoker	0.8 (0.7–1.1)	
	Cigarettes/day		
	< 20	0.8 (0.6–1.1)	
	≥ 20	0.6 (0.4–0.9)	
	Duration (years)		
	< 20	1.0 (0.7–1.4)	
	≥ 20	0.5 (0.2–1.2)	
	Years since quitting		
	≥ 10	0.8 (0.5–1.4)	
	< 10	0.4 (0.2–0.8)	
Hirose *et al.* (1996) Japan 1988–93	Current smoker	0.7 (0.4–1.3)	Low smoking prevalence (13.3%) Adjusted for age and year of first visit
	Cigarettes/day		
	< 10	0.5 (0.1–2.1)	
	≥ 10	0.8 (0.4–1.5)	
Goodman *et al.* (1997) USA, Hawaii 1985–93	Ever-smoker	0.8 (0.6–1.2)	Adjusted for history of pregnancy, oral contraceptive use, unopposed-estrogen use, history of diabetes and body-mass index
Jain *et al.* (2000) Canada 1994–98	Ever-smoker	1.01 (0.8–1.3)	Low participation rate of controls Crude odds ratio

Table 2.1.11.2 (contd)

Reference Country and years of study	Exposure estimates	Relative risk (95% CI)		Comments
		Cases	**Controls**	
Parslov et al. (2000) Denmark 1987–94	Ever-smoker	56.5	64.7	Values represent percentages Difference not significant after adjustment for other variables [data not shown]
Weiderpass & Baron (2001) Sweden 1994–95	Former smoker	0.9 (0.7–1.1)		Adjusted for age, use of hormone replacement therapy, body-mass index, parity, age at menopause, age at last birth, use of oral contraceptives, diabetes mellitus
	Current smoker	0.6 (0.5–0.8)		
	Cigarettes/day			
	1–10	0.9 (0.7–1.1)		
	11–20	0.7 (0.5–0.9)		
	> 20	0.7 (0.4–1.3)		
	Duration (years)			
	1–14	0.7 (0.2–2.6)		
	15–30	0.6 (0.3–1.1)		
	31–45	0.6 (0.3–0.9)		
	> 45	0.94 (0.91–1.0)		

Table 2.1.11.3. Cohort studies on smoking and endometrial cancer

Reference Country and years of study	Study subjects	Cases	Exposure estimates	Relative risk (95% CI)	Comments
Cederlöf et al. (1975); Baron (1984) Sweden 1963–72	Swedish Census Study 27 732 women	80 cases, 33 deaths	*Ever-smoker* Case Death	0.7 1.9	Adjusted for age
Garfinkel (1980) USA 1959–72	Cancer Prevention Study (CPS) I 590 562 women	224	Regular smoker *vs.* entire cohort	~1[†]	Adjusted for age [†]Standardized mortality ratio for nonsmoker versus entire cohort is 96.
Engeland et al. (1996) Norway 1966–93	Norwegian Cohort Study 14 269 women 310 000 person–years	140	Former smoker Current smoker	1.2 (0.6–2.2) 1.1 (0.7–1.6)	Smoking habits recorded in 1964–65 Adjusted for attained age
Nordlund et al. (1997) Sweden 1964–89	Swedish Census Study 25 829 women	248	Former smoker Current smoker Cigarettes/day 1–7 8–15 ≥ 16 Age at starting smoking (years) 20–23 < 19	1.02 (0.5–2.0) 0.8 (0.6–1.2) 0.7 (0.4–1.1) 0.97 (0.6–1.6) 1.04 (0.4–2.5) 1.4 (0.6–3.0) 0.6 (0.2–1.5)	*p* for trend = 0.35

Table 2.1.11.3 (contd)

Reference Country and years of study	Study subjects	Cases	Exposure estimates	Relative risk (95% CI)	Comments
Tulinius et al. (1997) Iceland 1968–95	Reykjavik Study 11 580 women	98	Former smoker *Cigarettes/day* 1–14 15–24 ≥ 25	0.7 (0.4–1.3) 0.5 (0.3–1.0) 0.5 (0.3–1.1) 0.9 (0.2–3.8)	Adjusted for all variables significant at the 10% level in univariate analysis, i.e. body-mass index, body surface, body fat, lean body mass, weight, glycaemia, blood pressure (systolic and diastolic) and hypertension
Terry et al. (1999) Sweden 1968–95	Swedish Twin Registry study 11 659 women	133	Former smoker *Cigarettes/day* 1–10 ≥ 11	0.7 (0.3–2.0) 1.2 (0.6–2.3) 0.5 (0.1–2.0)	Low smoking prevalence (13%) Relative risks adjusted for age, physical activity, weight at enrolment and parity
Terry et al. (2002a) Canada 1980–93	70 591 women	403	Former smoker Current smoker *Cigarettes/day* 1–20 > 20 *p* for trend *Duration (years)* 1–20 > 20 *p* for trend *Pack–years* 1–20 > 20 *p* for trend *Years since quitting* ≥ 20 10–19 1–9 *p* for trend	0.99 (0.8–1.3) 0.8 (0.6–1.1) **Current** / **Former** 1.1 (0.8–1.6) / 1.04 (0.8–1.4) 0.6 (0.4–0.9) / 0.9 (0.6–1.3) 0.03 / 0.64 0.9 (0.5–1.6) / 0.9 (0.7–1.2) 0.8 (0.6–1.1) / 1.1 (0.8–1.6) 0.19 / 0.66 1.0 (0.7–1.5) / 0.95 (0.7–1.3) 0.7 (0.5–1.1) / 1.0 (0.7–1.5) 0.10 / 0.97 0.9 (0.7–1.2) 1.1 (0.6–1.8) 1.1 (0.7–1.8) 0.54	Adjusted for age, Quetelet index, education, physical activity, hormone replacement therapy, use of oral contraceptives, menopausal status, parity and alcohol consumption

References

Austin, H., Drews, C. & Partridge, E.E. (1993) A case–control study of endometrial cancer in relation to cigarette smoking, serum estrogen levels, and alcohol use. *Am. J. Obstet. Gynecol.*, **169**, 1086–1091

Baron, J.A. (1984) Smoking and estrogen–related disease. *Am. J. Epidemiol.*, *119*, 9–22

Baron, J.A., Byers, T., Greenberg, E.R., Cummings, K.M. & Swanson, M. (1986) Cigarette smoking in women with cancers of the breast and reproductive organs. *J. natl Cancer Inst.*, **77**, 677–680

Brinton, L.A., Barrett, R.J., Berman, M.L., Mortel, R., Twiggs, L.B. & Wilbanks, G.D. (1993) Cigarette smoking and the risk of endometrial cancer. *Am. J. Epidemiol.*, **137**, 281–291

Cederlöf, R., Friberg, L., Hrubec, Z. & Lorich, U. (1975) *The Relationship of Smoking and Some Social Covariables to Mortality and Cancer Morbidity. A Ten Year Follow-Up in a Probability Sample of 55, 000 Swedish Subjects, Age 18–69, Part 1 and Part 2*, Stockholm, Department of Environmental Hygiene, The Karolinska Institute

Elliott, E.A., Matanoski, G.M., Rosenshein, N.B., Grumbine, F.C. & Diamond, E.L. (1990) Body fat patterning in women with endometrial cancer. *Gynecol. Oncol.*, **39**, 253–258

Engeland, A., Andersen, A., Haldorsen, T. & Tretli, S. (1996) Smoking habits and risk of cancers other than lung cancer: 28 years' follow-up of 26,000 Norwegian men and women. *Cancer Causes Control*, **7**, 497–506

Franks, A.L., Kendrick, J.S. & Tyler, C.W., Jr and The Cancer and Steroid Hormone Study Group (1987) Postmenopausal smoking, estrogen replacement therapy, and the risk of endometrial cancer. *Am. J. Obstet. Gynecol.*, **156**, 20–23

Goodman, M.T., Hankin, J.H., Wilkens, L.R., Lyu, L.C., McDuffie, K., Liu, L.Q. & Kolonel, L.N. (1997) Diet, body size, physical activity, and the risk of endometrial cancer. *Cancer Res.*, **57**, 5077–5085

Hirose, K., Tajima, K., Hamajima, N., Takezaki, T., Inoue, M., Kuroishi, T., Kuzuya, K., Nakamura, S. & Tokudome, S. (1996) Subsite (cervix/endometrium)-specific risk and protective factors in uterus cancer. *Jpn. J. Cancer Res.*, **87**, 1001–1009

IARC (1986) *IARC Monographs on the Evaluation of the Carcinogenic Risk of Chemicals to Humans*, Vol. 38, *Tobacco Smoking*, Lyon, IARCPress

Jain, M.G., Howe, G.R. & Rohan, T.E. (2000) Nutritional factors and endometrial cancer in Ontario, Canada. *Cancer Control*, **7**, 288–296

Kato, I., Tominaga, S. & Terao, C. (1989) Alcohol consumption and cancers of hormone-related organs in females. *Jpn. J. clin. Oncol.*, **19**, 202–207

Kelsey, J.L., LiVolsi, V.A., Holford, T.R., Fischer, D.B., Mostow, E.D., Schwartz, P.E., O'Connor, T. & White, C. (1982) A case–control study of cancer of the endometrium. *Am. J. Epidemiol.*, **116**, 333–342

Koumantaki, Y., Tzonou, A., Koumantakis, E., Kaklamani, E., Aravantinos, D. & Trichopoulos, D. (1989) A case–control study of cancer of endometrium in Athens. *Int. J. Cancer*, **43**, 795–799

Lawrence, C., Tessaro, I., Durgerian, S., Caputo, T., Richart, R., Jacobson, H. & Greenwald, P. (1987) Smoking, body weight, and early-stage endometrial cancer. *Cancer*, **59**, 1665–1669

Lawrence, C., Tessaro, I., Durgerian, S., Caputo, T., Richart, R.M. & Greenwald, P. (1989) Advanced-stage endometrial cancer: Contributions of estrogen use, smoking, and other risk factors. *Gynecol. Oncol.*, **32**, 41–45

Lesko, S.M., Rosenberg, L., Kaufman, D.W., Helmrich, S.P., Miller, D.R., Strom, B., Schottenfeld, D., Rosenshein, N.B., Knapp, R.C., Lewis, J. & Shapiro, S. (1985) Cigarette smoking and the risk of endometrial cancer. *New Engl. J. Med.*, **313**, 593–596

Levi, F., La Vecchia, C. & Decarli, A. (1987) Cigarette smoking and the risk of endometrial cancer. *Eur. J. Cancer clin. Oncol.*, **23**, 1025–1029

McCann, S.E., Freudenheim, J.L., Marshall, J.R., Brasure, J.R., Swanson, M.K. & Graham, S. (2000) Diet in the epidemiology of endometrial cancer in Western New York (United States). *Cancer Causes Control*, **11**, 965–974

Nordlund, L.A., Carstensen, J.M. & Pershagen, G. (1997) Cancer incidence in female smokers: A 26-year follow-up. *Int. J. Cancer*, **73**, 625–628

Parazzini, F., La Vecchia, C., Negri, E., Moroni, S. & Chatenoud, L. (1995) Smoking and risk of endometrial cancer: Results from an Italian case–control study. *Gynecol. Oncol.*, **56**, 195–199

Parslov, M., Lidegaard, O., Klintorp, S., Pedersen, B., Jønsson, L., Eriksen, P.S. & Ottesen, B. (2000) Risk factors among young women with endometrial cancer: A Danish case–control study. *Am. J. Obstet. Gynecol.*, **182**, 23–29

Rubin, G.L., Peterson, H.B., Lee, N.C., Maes, E.F., Wingo, P.A. & Becker, S. (1990) Estrogen replacement therapy and the risk of endometrial cancer: Remaining controversies. *Am. J. Obstet. Gynecol.*, **162**, 148–154

Shu, X.O., Brinton, L.A., Zheng, W., Gao, Y.T., Fan, J. & Fraumeni, J.F., Jr (1991) A population-based case–control study of endometrial cancer in Shanghai, China. *Int. J. Cancer*, **49**, 38–43

Smith, E.M., Sowers, M.F. & Burns, T.L. (1984) Effects of smoking on the development of female reproductive cancers. *J. natl Cancer Inst.*, **73**, 371–376

Stockwell, H.G. & Lyman, G.H. (1987) Cigarette smoking and the risk of female reproductive cancer. *Am. J. Obstet. Gynecol.*, **157**, 35–40

Terry, P., Baron, J.A., Weiderpass, E., Yuen, J., Lichtenstein, P. & Nyrén, O. (1999) Lifestyle and endometrial cancer risk: A cohort study from the Swedish Twin Registry. *Int. J. Cancer*, **82**, 38–42

Terry, P., Miller, A.B. & Rohan, T.E. (2002a) A prospective cohort study of cigarette smoking and the risk of endometrial cancer. *Br. J. Cancer*, **86**, 1430–1435

Terry, P.D., Rohan, T.E., Franceschi, S. & Weiderpass, E. (2002b) Cigarette smoking and the risk of endometrial cancer. *Lancet Oncol.*, **3**, 470–480

Tulinius, H., Sigfússon, N., Sigvaldason, H., Bjarnadóttir, K. & Tryggvadóttir, L. (1997) Risk factors for malignant diseases: A cohort study on a population of 22,946 Icelanders. *Cancer Epidemiol. Biomarkers Prev.*, **6**, 863–873

Tyler, C.W., Jr, Webster, L.A., Ory, H.W. & Rubin, G.L. (1985) Endometrial cancer: How does cigarette smoking influence the risk of women under age 55 years having this tumor? *Am. J. Obstet. Gynecol.*, **151**, 899–905

Weiderpass, E. & Baron, J.A. (2001) Cigarette smoking, alcohol comsumption, and endometrial cancer risk: A population–based study in Sweden. *Cancer Causes Control*, **12**, 239–247

Weir, H.K., Sloan, M. & Kreiger, N. (1994) The relationship between cigarette smoking and the risk of endometrial neoplasms. *Int. J. Epidemiol.*, **23**, 261–266

Weiss, N.S., Farewall, V.T., Szekely, D.R., English, D.R. & Kiviat, N. (1980) Oestrogens and endometrial cancer: Effect of other risk factors on the association. *Maturitas*, **2**, 185–190

Williams, R.R. & Horm, J.W. (1977) Association of cancer sites with tobacco and alcohol consumption and socioeconomic status of patients: Interview study from the Third National Cancer Survey. *J. natl Cancer Inst.*, **58**, 525–547

2.1.12 *Prostate cancer*

In a review of prostate cancer and its relationship to smoking, Hickey *et al.* (2001) found that the relationship in cohort studies that examined only causes of death was stronger than that in studies in which the incidence of cancer was determined during the individuals' lives, which suggested to the reviewers that smoking might convert a relatively benign cancer into a more aggressive one. Alternatively, the small excesses observed in the mortality studies may have been caused by the diagnostic bias referred to as one of the problems with cohort studies in the General Remarks: namely, the effect of death in the course of a slowly progressive major disease, as prostate cancer may be, is attributed to the chronic disease when it actually occurred as a result of an acute disease related to smoking, such as bronchopneumonia or myocardial infarction. It is certain, from the many studies that have been reported, that any association with smoking is at most weak and the cohort studies in this review are consequently limited to those that reported cancer incidence rates. Their design is described in Tables 2.1 and 2.1.12.1. The results of 18 studies, including separately the two series reported by Hakulinen *et al.* (1997) are summarized in Table 2.1.12.2. One study included in the review of Hickey *et al.* (2001), namely that by Whittemore *et al.* (1984), has been omitted as 44% of the 243 cases were diagnosed only at death, thus causing it to share the potential bias of a mortality study.

Several of the incidence studies provide only rudimentary details about smoking behaviour as they were focused primarily on other factors. Of the 17 studies, two provided evidence of statistically significantly increased risks associated with smoking. Firstly, Adami *et al.* (1996) found some evidence of a dose–response relationship, with the risk increasing with the number of cigarettes smoked per day ($p = 0.04$), although the small number of heavy smokers (38) showed no excess incidence. Secondly, Cerhan *et al.* (1997) found a significantly increased risk of 2.7 (95% CI, 1.2–6.0) for the nine cigarette smokers in their series who smoked 20 or more cigarettes a day. Seven studies, however, found lower risks for current smokers than for nonsmokers, which was almost as many as the nine studies that found increased risks.

The results of 30 case–control studies have been reviewed by Levi and La Vecchia (2001). Two of the studies found some evidence of a positive relationship (Honda *et al.*, 1988; based on 216 cases; Schuman *et al.*, 1977; based on 48 cases) and a third found a significantly positive relationship with ever smoking, but no relationship with either dose or duration (van der Bulden *et al.*, 1994; based on 345 cases). In contrast, the larger study by Villeneuve *et al.* (1999; based on 1623 cases) found a non-significant inverse relationship. The rest found no association worth noting.

Table 2.1.12.1. Description of additional cohort studies on smoking and prostate cancer

Reference Country and years of study	Name of study Cohort sample	Cases/deaths	Comments
Le Marchand et al. (1994) Hawaii, USA 1975–89	Random sample among 20 316 men from the 5 main ethnic groups in Hawaii: Japanese, Caucasians, Filipino, Hawaiian/Part-Hawaiian, Chinese; aged ≥ 45 years	Cases identified by the Hawaiian Tumor Registry	Study investigating primarily animal fat intake and prostate cancer
Parker et al. (1999) USA 1986–95	1177 Iowa men aged 40–86 years	Cases ascertained by Iowa Cancer Registry	Cohort based on controls of a case–control study conducted in 1986–89; study investigating primarily farming activities and risk of prostate cancer
Cerhan et al., 1997 USA 1982–93	Iowa 65+ Rural Health Study 1050 non-institutionalized residents of rural counties in Iowa, aged 65–101 years	Cases ascertained by State Health Registry of Iowa's cancer database	Study investigating primarily body mass and physical activity as risks for prostate cancer
Thompson et al. (1989) USA 1972–87	Adult residents of an upper-middle-class community in southern California, aged 50–84 years	1) Incident cases and 2) cases diagnosed before entering cohort or listed on death certificate without prior reporting	[Results based on total cases cannot be considered prospective.]

Table 2.1.12.2. Cohort studies on smoking and prostate cancer

Reference Country and years of study	Name of study No. of men	No. of cases	Exposure related to nonsmokers	Relative risk (95% CI)
Mills et al. (1989) USA 1976–82	Adventists' Health Study approximately 14 000 men	172	Former smoker Current smoker	1.2 (0.9–1.7) 0.5 (0.2–1.6)
Severson et al. (1989) USA 1965–86	American Men of Japanese Ancestry Study 8006 men	174	Former smoker Current smoker	0.9 (0.6–1.3) 0.9 (0.6–1.2)
Thompson et al. (1989) USA 1972–87	1776 men	54	Current smoker	1.3 (0.8–2.3)
Ross et al. (1990) USA 1981–88	Leisure World Study 5106 retirees	138	Former smoker Current smoker	0.8 (NS) 0.9 (NS)
Hiatt et al. (1994) (USA) 1979–85	Kaiser Permanente Medical Care Program Cohort II 43 432 men	222	Former smoker Current smoker < 20 cigarettes/day ≥ 20 cigarettes/day	1.1 (0.8–1.5) 1.0 (0.6–1.6) 1.9 (1.2–3.1)
Le Marchand et al. (1994) USA 1975–89	8881 men	198	Cigarettes/day Low quartile Intermediate quartile (i) Intermediate quartile (ii) High quartile	1.0 0.9 (0.6–1.4) 1.0 (0.7–1.6) 1.0 (0.6–1.6)
Thune & Lund (1994) Norway 1972–91	Norwegian Screening Study 43 685 men	211	Per 10 cigarettes/day	1.1 (0.9–1.3)

Table 2.1.12.2 (contd)

Reference Country and years of study	Name of study No. of men	No. of cases	Exposure related to nonsmokers	Relative risk (95% CI)
Adami et al. (1996) Sweden 1971–91	Swedish Construction Worker Cohort 135 006 men	2368	Former smoker	1.1 (1.0–1.2)
			Current smoker	1.1 (1.0–1.2)
			Cigarettes/day	
			1–4	1.06 (0.93–1.20)
			5–14	1.10 (0.99–1.22)
			15–24	1.14 (0.99–1.31)
			≥25	1.00 (0.72–1.38)
				p for trend = 0.04
Engeland et al. (1996) Norway 1966–93	Norwegian Cohort Study 11 863 men	703	Former smoker	0.9 (0.7–1.1)
			Current smoker	1.1 (0.9–1.4)
Grönberg et al. (1996) Sweden 1959–89	Swedish Twin Registry Study 9680 men	406	Former smoker	0.9 (0.7–1.2)
			Current smoker	1.0 (0.7–1.4)
			Ever-smoker	
			Tobacco use (g/day)	
			1–9	1.1 (0.8–1.5)
			10–19	1.0 (0.7–1.4)
			≥20	0.7 (0.4–1.2)
Hakulinen et al. (1997) Finland 1962–93	Finnish Men's Cohort 4601 men	209	Never-smoker	SIR[a] 1.1
			Former smoker	0.9 [0.7–1.2]
			Current smoker	1.1 [0.9–1.4]
1972, 1977–93	11 373 men	109	Never-smoker	0.9
			Former smoker	1.1 [0.8–1.4]
			Current smoker	0.8 [0.6–1.1]

Table 2.1.12.2 (contd)

Reference Country and years of study	Name of study No. of men	No. of cases	Exposure related to nonsmokers	Relative risk (95% CI)
Cerhan *et al.* (1997) USA 1982–93	Iowa 65+ Rural Health Study 1050 men	71	Former smoker Current smoker (cigarettes/day) < 20 ≥ 20	1.2 (0.7–2.1) 1.8 (0.7–2.4) 2.7 (1.2–6.0)
Tulinius *et al.* (1997) Iceland 1968–95	Reykjavik Study 11 366 men	524	Compared with never-smokers differences for all smoking categories *p* ≥ 0.1	
Veierød *et al.* (1997) Norway 1977–92	Norwegian Screening Study 25 708 men	69	Former smoker Current smoker (cigarettes/day) < 10 ≥ 10	0.6 (0.3–1.1) 0.5 (0.3–1.1) 0.6 (0.3–1.2)
Giovannucci *et al.* (1999) USA 1986–94	Health Professionals Follow-up Study 47 781 men	1369	Former smoker stopped ≥ 10 years Former smoker stopped < 10 years Current smoker	0.9 (0.9–1.0) 1.0 (0.9–1.2) 1.1 (0.9–1.3)
Heikkilä *et al.* (1999) Finland 1972–91	Mobile Clinic Health Study 16 481 men	166	Current smoker vs entire cohort	0.76
Parker *et al.* (1999) USA 1986–99	1177 men	81	Former smoker Current smoker (cigarettes/day) < 20 ≥ 20	1.3 (0.8–2.2) 1.7 (0.8–3.8) 1.9 (0.8–4.5)

NS, not significant
[a] Standardized incidence ratio calculated using the rates for Finland as the reference

References

Adami, H.O., Bergström, R., Engholm, G., Nyren, O., Wolk, A., Ekbom, A., Englund, A. & Baron, J. (1996) A prospective study of smoking and risk of prostate cancer. *Int. J. Cancer*, **67**, 764-768

Cerhan, J.R., Torner, J.C., Lynch, C.F., Rubenstein, L.M., Lemke, J.H., Cohen, M.B., Lubaroff, D.M. & Wallace, R.B. (1997) Association of smoking, body mass, and physical activity with risk of prostate cancer in the Iowa 65+ Rural Health Study (United States). *Cancer Causes Control*, **8**, 229–238

Engeland, A., Andersen, A., Haldorsen, T. & Tretli, S. (1996) Smoking habits and risk of cancers other than lung cancer: 28 years' follow-up of 26,000 Norwegian men and women. *Cancer Causes Control*, **7**, 497–506

Giovannucci, E., Rimm, E.B., Ascherio, A., Colditz, G.A., Spiegelman, D., Stampfer, M.J. & Willett, W.C. (1999) Smoking and risk of total and fatal prostate cancer in United States health professionals. *Cancer Epidemiol. Biomarkers Prev.*, **8**, 277–282

Grönberg, H., Damber, L. & Damber, J.E. (1996) Total food consumption and body mass index in relation to prostate cancer risks. A case–control study in Sweden with prospectively collected exposure data. *J. Urol.*, **155**, 969–974

Hakulinen, T., Pukkala, E., Puska, P., Tuomilehto, J. & Vartiainen, E. (1997) Various measures of smoking as predictors of cancer of different types in two Finnish cohorts. In: Colditz, G.A., ed., *Proceedings of the RMA Consensus Conference on Smoking and Prostate Cancer, Brisbane, February 12–14, 1996*, Canberra, Repatriation Medical Authority

Heikkilä, R., Aho, K., Heliövaara, M., Hakama, M., Marniemi, H., Reunanen, A. & Knekt, P. (1999) Serum testosterone and sex hormone-binding globulin concentrations and the risk of prostate cancer. *Cancer*, **86**, 312–315

Hiatt, R.A., Armstrong, M.A., Klatsky, A.L. & Sidney, S. (1994) Alcohol consumption, smoking, and other risk factors and prostate cancer in a large health plan cohort in California (United States). *Cancer Causes Control*, **5**, 66–72

Hickey, K., Do, K.-A. & Green, A. (2001) Smoking and prostate cancer. *Epidemiol. Rev.*, **23**, 115–125

Honda, G.D., Bernstein, L., Ross, R.K., Greenland, S., Gerkins, V. & Henderson, B.E. (1988) Vasectomy, cigarette smoking, and age at first sexual intercourse as risk factors for prostate cancer in middle-aged men. *Br. J. Cancer*, **57**, 326–331

Le Marchand, L., Kolonel, L.N., Wilkens, L.R., Myers, B.C. & Hirohata, T. (1994) Animal fat consumption and prostate cancer: A prospective study in Hawaii. *Epidemiology*, **5**, 276–282

Levi, F. & La Vecchia, C. (2001) Tobacco smoking and prostate cancer: Time for an appraisal. *Ann. Oncol.*, **13**, 733–738

Mills, P.K., Beeson, W.L., Phillips, R.L. & Fraser, G.E. (1989) Cohort study of diet, lifestyle, and prostate cancer in Adventist men. *Cancer*, **64**, 598–604

Parker, A.S., Cerhan, J., Putnam, S.D., Cantor, K.P. & Lynch, C.F. (1999) A cohort study of farming and risk of prostate cancer in Iowa. *Epidemiology*, **10**, 452–455

Ross, R.K., Bernstein, L., Paganini-Hill, A. et al. (1990) Effects of cigarette smoking on 'hormone-related' diseases in a southern Californian retirement community. In: Wald, N. & Baron, J., eds, *Smoking and Hormone-related Disorders*, Oxford, Oxford University Press, pp. 32–54

Schuman, L.M., Mandel, J., Blackard, C., Bauer, H., Scarlett, J. & McHugh, R. (1977) Epidemiologic study of prostate cancer. Preliminary report. *Cancer Treat. Rep.*, **61**, 181–186

Severson, R.K., Nomura, A.M.Y., Grove, J.S. & Stemmermann, G.M. (1989) A prospective study of demographics, diet, and prostate cancer among men of Japanese ancestry in Hawaii. *Cancer Res.*, **49**, 1857–1860

Thompson, M.M., Garland, C., Barrett-Connor, E., Khaw, K.-T., Friedlander, N.J. & Wingard, D.L. (1989) Heart disease risk factors, diabetes, and prostatic cancer in an adult community. *Am. J. Epidemiol.*, **129**, 511–517

Thune, I. & Lund, E. (1994) Physical activity and the risk of prostate and testicular cancer: A cohort study of 53,000 Norwegian men. *Cancer Causes Control*, **5**, 549–556

Tulinius, H., Sigfusson, N., Sigvaldason, H., Bjarnadottir, K. & Tryggvadottir, L. (1997) Risk factors for malignant diseases: A cohort study on a population of 22,946 Icelanders. *Cancer Epidemiol. Biomarkers Prev.*, **6**, 863–873

Van der Bulden, J.W.J., Verbeek, A.L.M. & Kolk, J.J. (1994) Smoking and drinking habits in relation to prostate cancer. *Br. J. Urol.*, **73**, 182–189

Veierød, M.B., Laake, P. & Thelle, D.S. (1997) Dietary fat intake and risk of prostate cancer: a prospective study of 25,708 Norwegian men. *Int. J. Cancer*, **73**, 634–638

Villeneuve, P.J., Johnson, K.C., Kreiger, N. & Mao, Y. (1999) Risk factors for prostate cancer. Results from the Canadian National Enhanced Cancer Surveillance System. The Canadian Cancer Registries Epidemiology Research Group. *Cancer Causes Control*, **10**, 155–167

Whittemore, A.S., Paffenbarger, R.S., Jr, Anderson, K. & Lee, J.E. (1984) Early precursors of uro-genital cancers in former college men. *J. Urol.*, **132**, 1256–1261

2.1.13 Leukaemia

The study of the effects of smoking on leukaemia presents a problem, because leukaemia is not one disease with a specific etiology, but a combination of several diseases that have a pathological characteristic in common (namely, an abnormal number of white cells in the blood) and which may have — and in some respects certainly do have — different causes. In principle, it would be desirable to consider separately at least four diseases: namely, the acute myeloid, chronic myeloid, acute lymphoid and chronic lymphoid leukaemias of adults. For therapeutic purposes, the myeloid leukaemias may be subdivided further, but the number of cases in most of the categories would be small and they have not generally been considered separately in etiological studies. Indeed even the acute and chronic forms have seldom been studied separately (although chronic lymphoid leukaemia is sometimes distinguished and may be classed with lymphomas) and the data available in relation to smoking permit only the examination of leukaemia as a whole and of the myeloid and lymphoid categories separately.

It is clear, from the many studies that have been reported, that any association of leukaemia with smoking is weak, so that the most valid evidence is likely to be obtained from cohort studies rather than from case–control studies. Two types of leukaemia (acute myeloid and acute lymphoid leukaemia) are usually rapidly fatal and there is little likelihood that cause of death would be attributed incorrectly to these leukaemias rather than to independent concurrent disease. It is also usually clear whether death during the course of chronic myeloid leukaemia is attributable to the disease itself. Only in the case of chronic lymphoid leukaemia is there any appreciable risk of death being attributed to the disease when it was actually due to an independent smoking-related condition. Table 2.1.13.1 therefore summarizes the results of both incidence and mortality studies. Many of these are studies of leukaemia only. In others, however, leukaemia was only one of many cancers examined and the results of these need to be interpreted with caution when the numbers are small, as they may have been singled out for report because they appeared to be of interest. Two such small mortality studies have been excluded, because cigarette smokers were compared with non-cigarette smokers (including men who smoked only pipes and/or cigars) rather than with lifelong nonsmokers (Tverdal et al., 1993; Weir & Dunn, 1970).

The results provide some weak evidence of an association of smoking with leukaemia. The incidence data are conflicting. The largest study, based on 400 cases, provided no evidence of an increased risk (Adami et al., 1998), but most of the others did, including two that reported statistically significant excesses for the heaviest cigarette smokers, but were based on very small numbers (Mills et al., 1990; Tulinius et al., 1997). The mortality data, in contrast, mostly showed small and statistically significant excesses of the order of 30–50% among current smokers, including the data from the US Veterans' study (McLaughlin et al., 1989) and the data in men from the two studies carried out by the American Cancer Society (Garfinkel & Boffeta, 1990). Three of the four studies of men, moreover, showed positive dose–response relationships. The only one of the six sets of data not to show any excess risk in cigarette smokers was that for women in the first of the American Cancer Society's studies, which described the observations made between 1959 and 1965 when few women had been smoking for very many years.

Eight studies gave separate data for myeloid leukaemias; six of these also gave data for lymphoid leukaemias, including three that did not provide any data for all leukaemias combined (Paffenbarger *et al.*, 1978; Friedman, 1993; Doll *et al.*, 1994). Separate data for myeloid and lymphoid leukaemia are summarized in Table 2.1.13.2, but descriptions of the studies are not included in this table, as most of them are described in Table 2.1.13.1 (McLaughlin *et al.*, 1989; Garfinkel & Boffeta, 1990; Mills *et al.*, 1990; Linet *et al.*, 1991; Adami *et al.*, 1998). Three, however, are not listed in Table 2.1.13.1 and are described below. Doll *et al.* (1994) followed 34 000 male physicians in the United Kingdom, who had been sent questionnaires about their smoking habits at the end of October 1951 and subsequently in 1957, 1966, 1972, 1978 and 1990, and determined the causes of death of those who died before November 1991. Paffenbarger *et al.* (1978) followed 50 000 former students (all males) at Harvard and Pennsylvania State Universities, who had been given questionnaires on entry in 1916–50 and 1931–40, respectively, and determined the causes of death of those who had died by 1975. In a case–control study nested in this cohort, each person who had died was matched with four controls from the same area, born in the same year, and alive at the time the affected person had died. Friedman (1993) followed 61 704 men and 81 287 women with known smoking habits, who had attended two Kaiser Permanente Medical Centers in the USA, for a regular health appraisal, from the time of first attendance in 1964–72 to the end of 1988, death, or cessation of requested follow-up and determined the incidence of leukaemia from their clinical records. The incidence of leukaemia among nonsmokers and former smokers did not take into account data for smokers of cigars or pipe, but the data for current smokers did so. The results of all the studies were adjusted for age and (where necessary) for sex and, in some instances, also for additional characteristics, i.e. for calendar year of observation by Doll *et al.* (1994) and for area of residence by Nordlund *et al.* (1997).

There is strong evidence for an association of cigarette smoking with myeloid leukaemia. Six out of eight sets of data for men, or for men and women treated as a single group, showed excess relative risks for current cigarette smokers. All of the excess risks were more than 60% and all were associated with dose–response relationships. The exceptions were the data set of Adami *et al.* (1998) in Sweden and a small data set for white insurance policy-holders in the USA reported by Linet *et al.* (1991). Of the two data sets for women, one (the first obtained by the American Cancer Society) showed no association with smoking whereas the other (the second obtained by the American Cancer Society) suggested a weak association that was not statistically significant (Garfinkel & Boffetta, 1990).

The data for lymphoid leukaemia are very different. Only two of eight studies provide any evidence of an increased risk associated with smoking (Paffenbarger *et al.*, 1978; Linet *et al.*, 1991) and in neither case was the excess risk statistically significant.

Although the strongest evidence comes from cohort studies, some data are also available from case–control studies, details of which are not included in this review. It is worth noting, however, that when Brownson *et al.* (1993) undertook an overview of the published studies of cigarette smoking and adult leukaemia, they found that a pooled analysis of eight case–control series (including the study by Paffenbarger *et al.* (1978) as a case–control study) gave relative risks of 1.1 (95% CI, 1.0–1.2) for all leukaemias, 0.9 (95% CI, 0.8–1.1) for chronic lymphoid leukaemia, 1.2 (95% CI, 0.9–1.5) for chronic myelocytic leukaemia and 1.3 (95% CI, 1.1–1.5) for acute non-lymphoid leukaemia (equivalent to acute myeloid leukaemia in most studies).

Five subsequent studies provided inconsistent, but generally similar results when smokers were compared with nonsmokers. Mele *et al.* (1994) reported on 118 cases of acute myeloid leukaemia and 28 cases of acute lymphoid leukaemia in three Italian cities from 1987 to 1990. The relative risks obtained were 1.6 (95% CI 0.9–2.8) for acute myeloid leukaemia in current smokers [smokers with a history of consumption of more than 10 pack–years are at greater risk] and 0.6 (95% CI, 0.2–2.0) for acute lymphoid leukaemia in current smokers. Wakabayashi *et al.* (1994) reported on 75 cases of acute non-lymphoid leukaemia seen at the Hyogo College of Medicine in Japan from 1981 to 1990; a relative risk of 1.76 (95% CI, 0.96–3.23) was found for smokers. Kane *et al.* (1999) reported on 695 cases of acute myeloid leukaemia and 99 cases of acute lymphoid leukaemia seen in five areas of England from 1991 to 1996; the odds ratios for current smokers were 1.4 (95% CI, 1.1–1.8) for acute myeloid leukaemia and 1.3 (95% CI, 0.7–2.3) for acute lymphoid leukaemia. Bjork *et al* (2001) reported on 372 cases of acute myeloid leukaemia seen in southern Sweden; the relative risks obtained were greater than 1.0 when smoking had continued for more than 20 years for both light smokers (1–10 cigarettes per day: odds ratio, 1.1; 95% CI, 0.65–1.9) and moderate or heavy smokers (>10 cigarettes per day: odds ratio, 1.6; 95% CI, 1.0–2.4) but were less than 1.0 when smoking had continued for 20 years or less. However, Stagnaro *et al.* (2001) reported on 646 cases of leukaemia in 12 areas of Italy and found odds ratios of less than 1.0 for current smokers both for all leukaemia (0.88; 95% CI, 0.69–1.1) and acute myeloid leukaemia (0.93; 95% CI, 0.81–1.4) and an increased odds ratio for current smokers only for acute lymphoid leukaemia (1.2; 95% CI, 0.54–2.5).

For the most part, case–control studies and cohort studies show a difference in risk between myeloid and lymphoid leukaemias.

Characteristics of tobacco-related cases

In general, it has not been possible to link individual malignant neoplasms with specific causes. In the case of leukaemia, some evidence may be obtained from knowledge of the chemicals in tobacco smoke and their relationship to specific cytogenetic changes. For example, benzene, a well-known leukaemogen is known to be present in significant concentrations in tobacco smoke.

According to Korte *et al.* (2000), linear extrapolation from the known effects of high doses suggests that benzene may be responsible for 8–48% of smoking-induced cancer and a somewhat higher proportion (12–58%) of smoking-induced acute myeloid leukaemia. Specific increases in the frequency of partial loss of chromosomes 5 and 7 and translocations involving chromosomes 8 and 21 have been found in the lymphocytes of healthy Chinese workers occupationally exposed to benzene (Smith *et al.*, 1998; Zhang *et al.*, 1998) and similar chromosomal abnormalities have been noted in smokers in 5–10% of cases of adult acute myeloid leukaemia (Walker *et al.*, 1994; Grimwade *et al.*, 1998).

There have as yet been few detailed studies on the cytogenetics of acute myeloid leukaemia subdivided by the individuals' smoking habits, but some of them offer support for the concept of a specific effect of benzene in the smoker. Lebailly *et al.* (2002) divided 472 cases of acute myeloid leukaemia into six cytogenetic groups and found higher odds ratios among smokers than in nonsmokers in 32 cases with 8:21 translocations (ever-smokers, 4.77; 95% CI, 1.77–12.85; current smokers, 7.07; 95% CI, 2.64–18.95) and diminished odds ratios in 54 cases with 15:17 translocations (ever-smokers, 0.57; 95% CI, 0.32–1.00; current smokers, 0.41; 95% CI, 0.23–0.96), bearing out the earlier findings reported by Sandler *et al.* (1993) and Davico *et al.* (1998) from studies with smaller numbers. Among 155 cases of acute myeloid leukaemia with recognizable chromosomal aberrations, Sandler *et al.* (1993) found 19 8:21 translocations, giving an odds ratio for ever-smokers of 1.7 (95% CI, 0.60–5.13) and 26 with 15:17 translocations, giving an odds ratio of 0.42 (95% CI, 0.17–1.01), whereas among 26 cases of acute non-lymphoid leukaemia with recognizable chromosomal aberrations, Davico *et al.* (1998) found nine with aberrations of chromosome 8 (six 8+, two 8– and one 8:21 translocation), giving odds ratios of 4.1 (95% CI, 0.5–35.5) relative to patients with normal karyotypes for smokers of ≤ 10 cigarettes/day and 14.2 (95% CI, 1.4–142.3) for heavier smokers.

Only Bjork *et al.* (2001) failed to obtain similar results. Among 73 cases of acute myeloid leukaemia with recognizable chromosomal aberrations, 12 had 8+ aberrations, giving an odds ratio for ever versus never-smokers of 0.91 (95% CI, 0.25–3.30). Smoking, however, was light in this study, with a medium number of pack–years of 21 for all aberrations and 14 for 8+ aberrations.

Table 2.1.13.1. Cohort studies on tobacco smoking and leukaemias (all types)

Reference Country and years of study	Population studied	No. of cases	Smoking categories	Relative risk (95% CI)	Comments
Incidence studies					
Mills *et al.* (1990) USA 1976–82	Adventists' Health Study 34 198 men and women	45 men and women	Former smoker Current smoker *Cigarettes/day* 1–14 15–24 ≥ 25	2.0 (1.0–4.0) 2.1 (0.5–9.2) 1.0 (0.3–3.0) 2.4 (0.9–6.4) 3.0 (1.3–7.2)	*p* for trend = 0.09
Engeland *et al.* (1996) Norway 1966–93	Norwegian Cohort Study 11 863 men, 14 269 women	64 men 51 women	Former smoker Current smoker Former smoker Current smoker	0.9 (0.5–1.9) 0.6 (0.9–1.2) 0.3 (0.0–2.2) 1.3 (0.7–2.5)	
Nordlund *et al.* (1997) Sweden 1963–89	Swedish Census Study 26 032 women	110 women	Former smoker Current smoker *Cigarettes/day* 1–7 8–15 > 15	1.0 (0.3–3.3) 1.2 (0.7–2.1) 1.5 (0.8–2.9) 0.9 (0.3–2.7) 0.7 (0.1–5.0)	Adjusted for age and place of residence
Tulinius *et al.* (1997) Iceland 1968–1995	Reykjavik Study 11 366 men, 11 580 women	33 men and 26 women	No category of smoking Former smoker *Cigarettes/day* 1–14 15–24	(*p* < 0.10) 2.1 (0.7–6.4) 1.1 (0.3–3.8) 4.0 (1.5–10.3)	

Table 2.1.13.1 (contd)

Reference Country and years of study	Population studied	No. of cases	Smoking categories	Relative risk (95% CI)	Comments
Adami et al. (1998) Sweden 1971–91	Swedish Construction Workers Study 333 288 men	400 men	Former smoker	0.9 (0.6–1.1)	
			Current smoker	1.0 (0.8–1.2)	
			Cigarettes/day		
			1–14	1.1 (0.9–1.4)	
			≥ 15	≥ 1.0 (0.7–1.3)	
			Duration (years)		
			1–10	0.9 (0.5–1.5)	
			11–20	0.8 (0.5–1.2)	
			21–30	1.2 (0.9–1.7)	
			≥ 31	0.9 (0.7–1.2)	
Mortality studies					
McLaughlin et al. (1989), USA 1954–80	US Veterans' Study 293 916 men	1588 men	Nonsmoker	1.0	
		142	Ever smoker	1.3 ($p < 0.01$)	
		848	Former smoker	1.3 ($p < 0.01$)	
		299	Current smoker	1.3 ($p < 0.01$)	
		549	*Cigarettes/day*		
			< 10	1.1	
		82	10–20	1.3 ($p < 0.01$)	
		286	≥ 21	1.3 ($p < 0.01$)	*p* for trend < 0.001
		181			
Garfinkel & Boffetta (1990) USA 1959–65	Cancer Prevention Study I 437 197 men, 588 148 women	477 men and 339 women		*Men CI Women*	
			Former smoker	1.4* 0.9	*$p < 0.05$
			Current smoker	1.5* 0.8	
			Cigarettes/day		
			1–19	1.3* 0.8	*$p < 0.05$
			≥ 20	1.6* 0.8	

Table 2.1.13.1 (contd)

Reference Country and years of study	Population studied	No. of cases	Smoking categories	Relative risk (95% CI)		Comments
Garfinkel & Boffetta (1990) 1982–86	Cancer Prevention Study II 489 696 men, 622 488 women	327 men and 235 women	Former smoker	1.4*	1.3*	*p < 0.05
			Current smoker	1.5*	1.0	
			Cigarettes/day			
			1–19	1.6*	1.1	*p < 0.05
			≥ 20	1.4*	0.9	
Linet et al. (1991) USA 1966–86	17 633 men Lutheran Brotherhood Insurance Study	72 men	Any tobacco use	1.1 (0.6–1.9)		
			Cigarettes and other tobacco	1.3 (0.7–2.3)		
			Only cigarettes Ever-smoker	1.2 (0.6–2.6)		
			Cigarettes/day			
			≤ 10	0.9 (0.4–1.7)		
			11–20	1.3 (0.7–2.6)		
			> 20	1.8 (0.8–3.7)		*p* for trend < 0.05

Table 2.1.13.2. Cohort studies on tobacco smoking and myeloid and lymphoid leukaemias

Reference Country and years of study	Myeloid leukaemia				Lymphoid leukaemia			
	Sex	No. of cases	Status/quantity	Relative risk (95% CI)	Sex	No. of cases	Smoking categories	Relative risk (95% CI)
Incidence studies								
Mills et al. (1990) Adventists' Health Study	Men and women	12	Nonsmoker	1.0	No data			
		10	Former smoker	2.2 (0.9–5.5)				
		1	Current smoker	2.0 (0.3–16.7)				
			Cigarettes/day					
		4	1–14	1.9 (0.6–6.3)				
		2	15–24	1.5 (0.3–7.0)				
		5	≥ 25	3.6 (1.1–11.1)				
Friedman (1993)[a] Kaiser Permanente Medical Care Program Cohort I	Men	7	Nonsmoker	1.0	Men	71 (total)	Nonsmoker	1.0
		13	Former smoker	2.3 (0.9–5.7)			Former smoker	1.0 (0.5–1.8)
		26	Current smoker	2.8 (1.2–6.4)			Current smoker	0.8 (0.5–1.4)
			Cigarettes/day					
		7	< 20	Reference				
		14	20–40	1.4 (0.6–3.1)				
		5	> 40	1.6 (0.5–5.1)				
	Women	27	Nonsmoker	1.0	Women	46 (total)	Nonsmoker	1.0
		8	Former smoker	1.3 (0.6–2.8)			Fomer smoker	0.6 (0.2–1.7)
		14	Current smoker	0.9 (0.4–1.7)			Current smoker	0.6 (0.3–1.3)
Adami et al. (1998) Swedish Construction Workers Cohort	Men	58	Never-smoker	1.0	No data			
		30	Former smoker	0.7 (0.5–1.2)				
		83	Current smoker	1.0 (0.7–1.4)				
			Cigarettes/day					
		84	0	1.0				
		61	1–14	1.3 (0.9–1.7)				
		26	≥ 15	0.8 (0.5–1.3)				

Table 2.1.13.2 (contd)

Reference Country and years of study	Myeloid leukaemia Sex	No. of cases	Status/quantity	Relative risk (95% CI)		Lymphoid leukaemia Sex	No. of cases	Smoking categories	Relative risk (95% CI)	
Mortality studies										
Paffenbarger et al. (1978) Harvard Alumni Study	Men	41 (total)	Current smoker ≥ 10 cigarettes/day	2.4[b] 3.6[b]		Men	27 (total)	Current smoker ≥ 10 cigarettes/day	1.3 2.7	
McLaughlin et al. (1989) US Veterans' Study	Men	71 62 142	Nonsmoker Former smoker Current smoker *Cigarettes/day*[d]	1.0 1.3 1.6[b]			106 84 129	Nonsmoker Former smoker Current smoker *Cigarettes/day*	1.0 1.2 1.0	
		23 64 55	<10 10–20 >20	1.5 1.5[b] 2.0[b]			15 71 43	<10 10–20 >20	0.7 1.1 1.1	
				Men	**Women**				**Men**	**Women**
Garfinkel & Boffetta (1990) Cancer Prevention Study I	Men Women	Total 150 99	Former smoker Current smoker *Cigarettes/day*	2.2[b] 2.5[b]	0.4 0.7	Men Women	Total 130 86	Former smoker Current smoker *Cigarettes/day*	1.3 0.9	0.6 0.9
			1–19 ≥ 20	2.3[b] 2.9[b]	0.6 0.7			1–19 ≥ 20	0.8 1.0	0.9 0.8
Cancer Prevention Study II	Men Women	Total 147 124	Former smoker Current smoker *Cigarettes/day*	1.2 1.7[b]	1.3 1.2	Men Women	Total 93 59	Former smoker Current smoker *Cigarettes/day*	1.4 0.8	1.9 0.9
			1–19 ≥ 20	1.7 1.8	1.5 1.0			1–19 ≥ 20	0.9 0.7	0.7 1.1

Table 2.1.13.2 (contd)

Reference Country and years of study	Myeloid leukaemia				Lymphoid leukaemia			
	Sex	No. of cases	Status/quantity	Relative risk (95% CI)	Sex	No. of cases	Smoking categories	Relative risk (95% CI)
Linet et al. (1991) Lutheran Brotherhood Insurance Study	Men	8	Nonsmoker	1.0	Men	5	Nonsmoker	1.0
		22	Any tobacco use	0.8 (0.3–1.7)		24	Any tobacco use	1.4 (0.5–3.5)
		17	Cigarettes and other tobacco	1.0 (0.4–2.2)		15	Cigarettes and other tobacco	1.5 (0.6–4.2)
		2	Cigarettes only	0.3 (0.1–1.6)		8	Cigarettes only	2.7 (0.9–8.3)
			Cigarettes/day				Cigarettes/day	
		5	≤10	0.5 (0.2–1.6)		9	≤10	1.5 (0.5–4.6)
		8	11–20	0.8 (0.3–2.1)		9	11–20	1.7 (0.6–5.2)
		6	>20	1.3 (0.5–3.8)		4	>20	1.9 (0.5–7.2)
Doll et al. (1994) British Doctors' Study	Men	66	Former smoker	[2.0]	Men	98	Former smoker	[0.6]
			Current smoker	[1.8]			Current smoker	[0.9]
			Cigarettes/day[e]				Cigarettes/day	
			1–14	[0.8]			1–14	[1.1]
			15–24	[2.3]			15–24	[0.6]
			≥25	[2.5]			≥25	[0.9]

[a] Myeloid refers to acute non-lymphoid leukaemia and lymphoid to chronic lymphoid leukaemia.
[b] p < 0.05
[c] p < 0.01
[d] p for trend < 0.001
[e] p for trend < 0.05

References

Adami, J., Nyrén, O., Bergström, R., Ekbom, A., Engholm, G., Englund, A. & Glimelius, B. (1998) Smoking and the risk of leukemia, lymphoma, and multiple myeloma (Sweden). *Cancer Causes Control*, **9**, 49–56

Bjork, J., Albin, M., Mauritzson, N., Stromberg, U., Johansson, B. & Hagmar, L. (2001) Smoking and acute myeloid leukemia: Associations with morphology and karyotypic patterns and evaluation of dose–response relations. *Leuk. Res.*, **25**, 865–972

Brownson, R.C., Novotny, T.E. & Perry, M.C. (1993) Cigarette smoking and adult leukaemia. *Arch. intern. Med.*, **153**, 469–427

Davico, L., Sacerdote, C., Ciccone, G., Pegoraro, L., Kerim, S., Ponzio, G. & Vineis, P. (1998) Chromosome 8, occupational exposures, smoking, and acute nonlymphocytic leukemias: A population-based study. *Cancer Epidemiol. Biomarkers Prev.*, **7**, 1123–1125

Doll, R., Peto, R., Wheatley, K., Gray, R. & Sutherland, I. (1994) Mortality in relation to smoking: 40 years' observations on male British doctors. *Br. med. J.*, **309**, 901–911

Engeland, A., Andersen, A., Haldorsen, T. & Tretli, S. (1996) Smoking habits and risk of cancers other than lung cancer: 28 years' follow-up of 26,000 Norwegian men and women. *Cancer Causes Control*, **7**, 497–506

Friedman, G.D. (1993) Cigarette smoking, leukemia, and multiple myeloma. *Ann. Epidemiol.*, **3**, 425–428

Garfinkel, L. & Boffeta, P. (1990) Association between smoking and leukaemia in two American Cancer Society prospective studies. *Cancer*, **65**, 2356–2360

Grimwade, D., Walker, H., Oliver, F., Wheatley, K., Harrison, C., Harrison, G., Rees, J., Hann, I., Stevens, R., Burnett, A. & Goldstone, A. on behalf of the Medical Research Council Adult and Children's Leukaemia Working Parties (1998) The importance of diagnostic cytogenetics on outcome in AML: Analysis of 1,612 patients entered into the MRC AML 10 trial. *Blood*, **92**, 2322–2333

Kane, E.V., Roman, E., Cartwright, R., Parker, J. & Morgan, G. (1999) Tobacco and the risk of acute leukaemia in adults. *Br. J. Cancer*, **81**, 1228–1233

Korte, J.E., Hertz-Picciotto, I., Schulz, M.R., Ball, L.M. & Duell, E.J. (2000) The contribution of benzene to smoking-induced leukemia. *Environ. Health Perspect.*, **108**, 333–339

Lebailly, P., Willett, E.V., Moorman, A.V., Roman, E., Cartwright, R., Morgan, G.J. & Wild, C.P. (2002) Genetic polymorphisms in microsomal epoxide hydrolase and susceptibility to adult acute myeloid leukaemia with defined cytogenetic abnormalities. *Br. J. Haematol.*, **116**, 587–594

Linet, M.S., McLaughlin, J.K., Hsing, A.W., Wacholder, S., Co Chien, H.T., Schuman, L.M., Bjelke, E. & Blot, W.J. (1991) Cigarette smoking and leukaemia: Results from the Lutheran Brotherhood Cohort Study. *Cancer Causes Control*, **2**, 413–417

McLaughlin, J.K., Hrubec, Z., Linet, M.S., Heineman, E.F., Blot, W.J. & Fraumeni, J.F., Jr (1989) Cigarette smoking and leukemia. *J. natl Cancer Inst.*, **81**, 1262–1263

Mele, A., Szklo, M., Visani, G., Stazi, M.A., Castelli, G., Pasquini, P., Mandelli, F. & the Italian Leukemia Study Group (1994) Hair dye use and other risk factors for leukemia and pre-leukemia: A case–control study. *Am. J. Epidemiol.*, **139**, 609–619

Mills, P.K., Newell, C.R., Beeson, W.L., Fraser, G.E. & Phillips, R.L. (1990) History of cigarette smoking and risk of leukaemia and myeloma: Results from the Adventists Health Study. *J. natl Cancer Inst.*, **32**, 1832–1836

Nordlund, L.A., Carstensen, J.M. & Pershagen, G. (1997) Cancer incidence in female smokers: A 26-year follow-up. *Int. J. Cancer*, **73**, 625–628

Paffenbarger, R.S., Wing, A.L. & Hyde, R.T. (1978) Characteristics in youth predictive of adult-onset malignant lymphomas, melanomas, and leukaemias: Brief communication. *J. natl Cancer Inst.*, **60**, 89–92

Sandler, D.P., Shore, D.L., Anderson, J.R., Davey, F.R., Arthur, D., Mayer, R.J., Silver, R.T., Weiss, R.B., Moore, J.O., Schiffer, C.A., Wurster-Hill, D.H., McIntyre, R. & Bloomfield, C.D. (1993) Cigarette smoking and risk of acute leukemia: Associations with morphology and cytogenetic abnormalities in bone marrow. *J. natl Cancer Inst.*, **85**, 1994–2003

Smith, M.T., Zhang, L., Wang, Y., Hayes, R.B., Li, G., Wiemels, J., Dosemeci, M., Titenkno-Holland, N., Xi, L., Kolachana, P., Yin, S. & Rothman, N. (1998) Increased translocations and aneusomy in chromosomes 8 and 21 among workers exposed to benzene. *Cancer Res.*, **58**, 2176–2181

Stagnaro, E., Ramazzotti, V., Crosignani, P., Fontana, A., Masala, G., Miligi, L., Nanni, O., Neri, M., Rodella, S., Seniori Costantini, A., Tumino, R., Viganò, C., Vindigni, C. & Vineis, P. (2001) Smoking and hematolymphopoietic malignancies. *Cancer Causes Control*, **12**, 325–334

Tulinius, H., Sigfusson, N., Sigvaldason, H., Bjarnadottir, K. & Tryggvadottir, L. (1997) Risk factors for malignant diseases: A cohort study on a population of 22,946 Icelanders. *Cancer Epidemiol. Biomarkers Prev.*, **6**, 863–873

Tverdal, A., Thelle, D., Stensvold, I., Leren, P. & Bjartveit, K. (1993) Mortality in relation to smoking history: 13 years' follow-up of 68,000 Norwegian men and women 35–49 years. *J. clin. Epidemiol.*, **46**, 475–487

Wakabayashi, I., Sakamoto, K., Masui, H., Yoshimoto, S., Kanamaru, A., Kakishita, E., Hara, A., Shimo-Oka, M. & Hagai, K. (1994) A case–control study on risk factors for leukemia in a district of Japan. *Intern. Med.*, **33**, 198–203

Walker, H., Smith, F.J. & Betts, D.R. (1994) Cytogenetics in acute myeloid leukaemia. *Blood Rev.*, **8**, 30–36

Weir, J.M. & Dunn, J.E., Jr (1970) Smoking and mortality: A prospective study. *Cancer*, **25**, 105–112

Zhang, L., Rothman, N., Wang, Y., Hayes, R.B., Li, G., Dosemeci, M., Yin, S., Kolachana, P., Titenko-Holland, N. & Smith, M.T. (1998) Increased aneusomy and long arm deletion of chromosomes 5 and 7 in the lymphocytes of Chinese workers exposed to benzene. *Carcinogenesis*, **19**, 1955–1961

2.1.14   *Other organs*

The cancers reviewed in this section generally have low incidence and mortality rates and are not considered to be strongly associated with cigarette smoking. This raises the possibility of preferential reporting of positive associations in cohort studies.

(*a*)   *Cancer of the salivary gland*

A population-based case–control study on salivary gland cancer (based on 25 cases) from Puerto Rico (Hayes *et al.*, 1999) reported relative risks of 9.0 for men and 4.2 for women. Increasing number of cigarettes smoked per day showed a statistically significant trend for men (p = 0.02) and a statistically non-significant trend for women (p = 0.07). Two other case–control studies (Spitz *et al.*, 1990; Swanson & Burns, 1997), however, found no increase in risk for cancer of the salivary gland among cigarette smokers, or only for the highest category of smoking intensity ($\geq$ 80 pack–years).

(*b*)   *Cancer of the small intestine*

Results are available from three case–control studies on the association between smoking and cancer of the small intestine; two found a two- to fourfold increase in risk among smokers (Chen *et al.*, 1994; Wu *et al.*, 1997), and the third indicated a 90% increase in risk (Kaerlev *et al.*, 2002). In contrast, two other case–control studies, one conducted in the USA and the other in Italy, found no evidence for an effect of smoking on cancer of the small intestine (Chow *et al.*, 1993; Negri *et al.*, 1999).

(*c*)   *Cancers of the gallbladder and extra-hepatic bile ducts*

Cancers of the gallbladder and extra-hepatic bile ducts were considered in the previous *IARC Monograph* on tobacco smoking (IARC, 1986), but many more studies have been published since then. The results of the relevant cohort and case–control studies are summarized in Table 2.1.14.1.

In the US Veterans' Study, Chow *et al.* (1995) found marginally elevated relative risks in former smokers and significantly elevated risks in current smokers. Subjects who reported smoking more than 20 cigarettes per day also had significantly elevated relative risks. Starting smoking at a younger age (< 20 years) increased relative risks relative to subjects who had started smoking at a later age (> 20 years). Elevated, but non-significant risks were found in relation to duration of smoking.

Chow *et al.* (1994) studied 34 men and 30 women from Los Angeles county, CA, USA, with bile duct cancers, and 15 men and 26 women with cancer of the ampulla of Vater. These cases were compared with 97 men and 158 women chosen by random-digit dialling or from the Health Care Financing Administration files if over 65 years of age. All cases were histologically verified. Elevated, but non-significant risks were found in former smokers in all groups except for women with cancer of the ampulla of Vater.

Moerman *et al.* (1994) compared 114 cases of bile duct cancer with 487 population controls. After adjustment for age, sex and respondent status, former smokers were at a lower risk (0.7; 95% CI, 0.4–1.2) than current smokers (1.3; 95% CI, 0.8–2.2) and a non-significant trend in relative risks was observed in relation to the duration of smoking: 1.5 for current smokers at interview and 1.4, 1.1 and 1.2 in those who smoked for 2, 5 and 10 years, respectively, before the interview.

Yen *et al.* (1987) recruited 67 patients with bile duct cancer from 11 hospitals in Massachussets, USA, and 273 controls admitted with cancers unrelated to tobacco or alcohol consumption. After adjustment for age and sex, a negative association was found in relation to former smoking (odds ratio, 0.5), and in relation to current smoking (odds ratio, 0.4; *p* < 0.05).

Zatonski *et al.* (1992) compared 73 cases of gallbladder cancer with 186 controls in Opole, Poland. No significant association was found in relation to lifetime number of cigarettes smoked (odds ratio, 0.6 for < 197 100 cigarettes in lifetime; 1.1 for more).

Scott *et al.* (1999) compared the medical records of 68 cases of gallbadder cancer, all histologically verified, from six hospitals in Massachussets, USA, with 272 controls with gallstones or who underwent cholecystectomy. No significant associations between gall-bladder cancer and any smoking category (ever, current, former, years smoked or years since quitting) were found. A statistically non-significant fivefold increase in risk was found in relation to smoking after adjustment for age, sex, the presence/absence of gall-stones and history of gallstones.

[The Working Group noted that medical records are not necessarily a reliable source of information on tobacco smoking.]

Chalasani *et al.* (2000) compared 26 cases of cholangiocarcinoma to 87 controls from eight hospitals in the USA. After adjustment for age and duration of primary sclerosing cholangitis, no significant association was found in relation to former or current smoking.

Confounding

In considering cancer of the gallbladder and extra-hepatic bile ducts, particular attention has to be paid to potential confounders, namely body-mass index and gallbladder disease.

Chow *et al.* (1994) noted an increased risk for extrahepatic bile duct cancer in relation to body-mass index in both men (odds ratio, 4.0; 95% CI, 1.1–14.2) and women (odds ratio, 2.7; 95% CI, 0.8–9.4) in the highest body-mass index quartile. In addition, a history of gallbladder disease, gallstones and gallbladder inflammation was found to be an important risk factor for the development of gallbladder cancer. Gallbladder disease was also found to be an important risk factor in the study by Scott *et al.* (1999) (odds ratio, 17.2; 95% CI, 1.5–190), by Zatonski *et al.* (1992) and in a recent SEARCH case–control study on 196 cases and 1515 controls (odds ratio, 4.4 for gallbladder disease) (Zatonski *et al.*, 1997). The only study reviewed that was stratified by smoking and gallbladder disease and body-mass index was that of Zatonski *et al.* (1992) that did not find an association with tobacco smoking.

(d)   Soft-tissue sarcoma

One cohort study found an association between cigarette smoking and mortality from soft-tissue sarcoma after 26 years of follow-up, but no dose–response relationship was found with the number of cigarettes smoked per day, duration of smoking or number of pack–years (US Veterans' Study: Zahm et al., 1992). No effect of cigarette smoking was detected in an Italian hospital-based case–control study (Franceschi & Serraino, 1992).

(e)   Skin cancer

(i)   Melanoma

A number of case–control studies have found no difference in the prevalence of tobacco smoking between patients with malignant melanoma and controls (Østerlind et al., 1988; Siemiatycki et al., 1995; Westerdahl et al., 1996; Lear et al., 1998; de Hertog et al., 2001). An inverse association was found in one study (Green et al., 1999).

(ii)   Non-melanoma skin cancer

Tobacco smoking has been linked to the incidence of squamous-cell carcinoma in a prospective follow-up study of patients with prior skin cancer (Karagas et al., 1992) and in the Nurses' Health Study (Grodstein et al., 1995), as well as in several case–control studies (Aubry & MacGibbon, 1985; Lear et al., 1998; de Hertog et al., 2001). In contrast, neither cohort studies (Nurses' Health Study: Hunter et al., 1990; Skin Cancer Prevention Study: Karagas et al., 1992; Health Professionals' Follow-up Study: van Dam et al., 1999) nor case–control studies (Sahl et al., 1995; Lear et al., 1998; de Hertog et al., 2001) found an effect of smoking on the incidence of basal-cell carcinoma.

(f)   Ovarian cancer

Two studies have shown an association of smoking with ovarian cancer (British Doctors' Study: Doll et al., 1980; Green et al., 2001), but most studies were null (Smith et al., 1984; Stockwell & Lyman, 1987; Whittemore et al., 1988; Polychronopoulou et al., 1993; Norwegian Cohort Study: Engeland et al., 1996; Kuper et al., 2000). Recent interest in separating histological types of ovarian cancer has prompted researchers to report associations separately. Two studies have reported that smokers were at excess risk for mucinous epithelial ovarian cancer (Marchbanks et al., 2000; Green et al., 2001), but not for other histological types (Marchbanks et al., 2000), but a third study did not support these findings (Kuper et al., 2000).

(g)   Testicular cancer

No association has been found between cigarette smoking and risk for testicular cancer (Henderson et al., 1979; Coldman et al., 1982; UK Testicular Cancer Study Group, 1994; Siemiatycki et al., 1995). One study found an increased risk, but positive dose–response relationships for duration and intensity of smoking were seen only in patients from one of three hospitals (Brown et al., 1987).

(*h*)   *Cancer of the central nervous system*

The incidence of gliomas has been associated with smoking in men (Hurley *et al.*, 1996; Lee *et al.*, 1997), but not in women (Hurley *et al.*, 1996; Blowers *et al.*, 1997; Lee *et al.*, 1997) or in both sexes combined (Ryan *et al.*, 1992). One study reported increased risks for meningiomas associated with smoking (Ryan *et al.*, 1992). Another study found an association of brain tumours with smoking untipped cigarettes, but not with smoking filter-tipped cigarettes (Burch *et al.*, 1987). Other studies have shown a lack of association of tobacco use with tumours of the central nervous system (Hochberg *et al.*, 1990; US Veterans' Study: McLaughlin *et al.*, 1995).

(*i*)   *Thyroid cancer*

Three studies have reported an inverse association of smoking with risk for thyroid cancer (Galanti *et al.*, 1996; Kreiger & Parkes, 2000; Rossing *et al.*, 2000). Two studies have reported no association (Ron *et al.*, 1987; Kaiser Permanente Medical Care Program Study: Iribarren *et al.*, 2001) and two a positive association with smoking (Sokic *et al.*, 1994; Memon *et al.*, 2002).

(*j*)   *Cancer of the adrenal gland*

There are few data on risk factors for adrenal carcinoma. The US Veterans' Study reported a fivefold increase in risk among current cigarette smokers during 26 years of follow-up, with risk being particularly high among those who smoked most intensely (Chow *et al.*, 1996). Other forms of tobacco use were associated with a statistically non-significant increase in risk. A case–control study in the USA found a twofold increase in risk for adrenal cancer among heavy smokers in men, but not in women (Hsing *et al.*, 1996).

(*k*)   *Lymphoma*

(*i*)   *Non-Hodgkin lymphoma*

Six cohort studies have examined the association between non-Hodgkin lymphoma and smoking. In five of these, no increased risk among smokers was evident (British Doctors' Study: Doll *et al.*, 1994; US Veterans' Study: McLaughlin *et al.*, 1995; Swedish Construction Workers' Cohort: Adami *et al.*, 1998; Kaiser Permanente Medical Care Program Study: Herrinton & Friedman, 1998; Iowa Women's Health Study: Parker *et al.*, 2000). However, in one prospective study, men who had ever smoked cigarettes had a twofold increase in risk for non-Hodgkin lymphoma, and the risk was still higher among the heaviest smokers (Lutheran Brotherhood Insurance Study: Linet *et al.*, 1992). In general, data from case–control studies also fail to support a large effect of smoking on the incidence of non-Hodgkin lymphoma (reviewed by Peach & Barnett, 2001; Stagnaro *et al.*, 2001).

Only three studies have examined histological subtypes of non-Hodgkin lymphoma. In the Iowa Women's Health Study (37 336 women followed for 11 years), smoking was associated with increased risk for follicular non-Hodgkin lymphoma (Parker *et al.*, 2000). Similarly, two other studies reported a weak positive association between smoking and risk for follicular lymphoma, but no effect for other histological types (Herrinton & Friedman, 1998; Stagnaro *et al.*, 2001).

(ii) *Hodgkin lymphoma*

Three studies provided no support for the hypothesis that smoking increases risk for Hodgkin disease (Abramson *et al.*, 1978; Bernard *et al.*, 1987; Stagnaro *et al.*, 2001) and four studies found weak associations (Harvard Alumni Study: Paffenbarger *et al.*, 1977; US Veterans' Study: McLaughlin *et al.*, 1995; Siemiatycki *et al.*, 1995; Swedish Construction Workers Cohort: Adami *et al.*, 1998).

(*l*) *Multiple myeloma*

Nine studies suggested no association between smoking and risk of multiple myeloma. Support for this conclusion comes from a number of cohort studies (US Veterans' Study: Heineman *et al.*, 1992; Lutheran Brotherhood Insurance Study: Linet *et al.*, 1992; Kaiser Permanente Medical Care Program Study: Friedman, 1993; British Doctors' Study: Doll *et al.*, 1994; US Veterans' Study: McLaughlin *et al.*, 1995; Swedish Construction Workers' Cohort: Adami *et al.*, 1998) and case–control studies (Linet *et al.*, 1987; Brown *et al.*, 1992; Stagnaro *et al.*, 2001). Only the relatively small Adventists' Health Study reported an increased incidence of multiple myeloma among former and current smokers and statistically significant trends by number of cigarettes and duration of smoking (Mills *et al.*, 1990).

Table 2.1.14.1. Studies on tobacco smoking and cancers of the biliary tract and gallbladder

Reference Country and years of study	Subjects (cases and controls)	Smoking category	Relative risk (95% CI) (relative to never-smokers)				Comments
Cohort study							
Chow et al. (1995) USA 1954–80	US Veterans' Study 250 000 men; 303 biliary tract cancers	Former smoker	1.2 (0.8–1.8)				Adjusted for age and calendar time period; age at starting smoking and number of years of smoking also adjusted for cigarettes/day
		Current smoker	1.5 (1.1–2.0)				
		Cigarettes/day					
		< 10	1.6 (1.0–2.6)				
		10–20	1.2 (0.8–1.8)				
		≥ 21	1.8 (1.2–2.7)				
		Age at starting smoking (years)					
		< 20	1.8 (1.1–3.1)				
		20–24	1.6 (0.9–2.9)				
		> 24	1.4 (0.8–2.7)				
		Duration (years)					
		< 30	1.6 (0.8–3.3)				
		30–39	1.7 (0.9–2.9)				
		≥ 40	1.7 (1.0–2.9)				
Case–control studies							
Yen et al. (1987) USA 1975–79	67 extrahepatic bile duct cancers, 273 controls with other cancers	Former smoker	0.5 (0.3–1.0)				Adjusted for age and sex
		Current smoker	0.4 (0.2–0.9)				
		Packs/day					
		1	0.3 (1.0–0.9)				
		> 1	0.5 (0.2–1.2)				
			EBD		AV		
			Men	Women	Men	Women	
Chow et al. (1994) USA 1985–89	105 extrahepatic bile duct (EBD) and ampulla of Vater (AV) cancers, 255 population-based controls	Ever-smoker	1.7 (0.6–4.8)	1.6 (0.7–3.5)	4.7 (0.6–37.9)	0.7 (0.3–1.8)	Adjusted for age and ethnic origin
		Pack–years					
		1–50	1.1 (0.3–3.3)	1.0 (0.4–2.6)	4.9 (0.6–41.5)	0.4 (0.1–1.2)	
		> 50	2.2 (0.7–6.9)	3.1 (0.8–11.8)	4.3 (0.5–39.1)	2.9 (0.9–10.0)	

Table 2.1.14.1 (contd)

Reference Country and years of study	Subjects (cases and controls)	Smoking category	Relative risk (95% CI) (relative to never-smokers)	Comments
Scott et al. (1999) USA 1983–94	68 gallbladder cancers, 272 controls with gallstones	Ever-smoker Current smoker Former smoker Years of smoking Years since quitting	1.4 (p = 0.3) 0.9 (p = 0.8) 1.9 (p = 0.2) 1.0 (p = 0.4) 1.0 (p = 0.4)	Age-adjusted
Zatonski et al. (1992) Poland 1985–88	73 gallbladder cancers, 186 controls	*Lifetime no. of cigarettes smoked* < 197 100 ≥ 197 100	0.6 (0.2–1.7) 1.1 (0.4–3.1) p for trend = 0.9	Adjusted for age, sex and education
Moerman et al. (1994) Netherlands 1984–87	114 biliary tract cancers, 487 population controls	Former smoker Current smoker *Cigarette smoker* At interview 2 years before 5 years before 10 years before	0.7 (0.4–1.2) 1.3 (0.8–2.2) 1.5 (0.9–2.4) 1.4 (0.9–2.2) 1.3 (0.8–2.1) 1.2 (0.8–2.0)	Adjusted for age, sex and respondent type
Chalasani et al. (2000) USA 1991–98	26 cholangio-carcinomas with primary sclerosing cholangitis (PSC), 87 cancer-free controls with PSC	Ever-smoker	0.7 0.1–3.6)	Adjusted for duration of PSC and area

References

Abramson, J.H., Pridan, H., Sacks, M.I., Avitzour, M. & Peritz, E. (1978) A case–control study of Hodgkin's disease in Israel. *J. natl Cancer Inst.*, **61**, 307–314

Adami, J., Nyrén, O., Bergström, R., Ekbom, A., Engholm, G., Englund, A. & Glimelius, B. (1998) Smoking and the risk of leukemia, lymphoma, and multiple myeloma (Sweden). *Cancer Causes Control*, **9**, 49–56

Aubry, F. & MacGibbon, B. (1985) Risk factors of squamous cell carcinoma of the skin. A case–control study in the Montreal region. *Cancer*, **55**, 907–911

Bernard, S.M., Cartwright, R.A., Darwin, C.M., Richards, I.D.G., Roberts, B., O'Brien, C. & Bird, C.C. (1987) Hodgkin's disease: Case control epidemiological study in Yorkshire. *Br. J. Cancer*, **55**, 85–90

Blowers, L., Preston-Martin, S. & Mack, W.J. (1997) Dietary and other lifestyle factors of women with brain gliomas in Los Angeles County (California, USA). *Cancer Causes Control*, **8**, 5–12

Brown, L.M., Pottern, L.M. & Hoover, R.N. (1987) Testicular cancer in young men: The search for causes of the epidemic increase in the United States. *J. Epidemiol. Community Health*, **41**, 349–354

Brown, L.M., Everett, G.D., Gibson, R., Burmeister, L.F., Schuman, L.M. & Blair, A. (1992) Smoking and risk of non-Hodgkin's lymphoma and multiple myeloma. *Cancer Causes Control*, **3**, 49–55

Burch, J.D., Craib, K.J.P., Choi, B.C.K., Miller, A.B., Risch, H.A. & Howe, G.R. (1987) An exploratory case–control study of brain tumors in adults. *J. natl Cancer Inst.*, **78**, 601–609

Chalasani, N., Baluyut, A., Ismail, A., Zaman, A., Sood, G., Ghalib, R., McCashland, T.M., Reddy, K.R., Zervos, X., Anbari, M.A. & Hoen, H. (2000) Cholangiocarcinoma in patients with primary sclerosing cholangitis: A multicenter case–control study. *Hepatology*, **31**, 7–11

Chen, C.C., Neugut, A.I. & Rotterdam, H. (1994) Risk factors for adenocarcinomas and malignant carcinoids of the small intestine: Preliminary findings. *Cancer Epidemiol. Biomarkers Prev.*, **3**, 205–207

Chow, W.-H., Linet, M.S., McLaughlin, J.K., Hsing, A.W., Chien, H.T. & Blot, W.J. (1993) Risk factors for small intestine cancer. *Cancer Causes Control*, **4**, 163–169

Chow, W.-H., McLaughlin, J.K., Menck, H.R. & Mack, T.M. (1994) Risk factors for extrahepatic bile duct cancers: Los Angeles County, California (USA). *Cancer Causes Control*, **5**, 267–272

Chow, W.-H., McLaughlin, J.K., Hrubec, Z. & Fraumeni, J.F., Jr (1995) Smoking and biliary tract cancers in a cohort of US veterans. *Br. J. Cancer*, **72**, 1556–1558

Chow, W.-H., Hsing, A.W., McLaughlin, J.K. & Fraumeni, J.F., Jr (1996) Smoking and adrenal cancer mortality among United States veterans.*Cancer Epidemiol. Biomarkers Prev.*, **5**, 79–80

Coldman, A.J., Elwood, J.M. & Gallagher, R.P. (1982) Sports activities and risk of testicular cancer. *Br. J. Cancer*, **46**, 749–756

van Dam, R.M., Huang, Z., Rimm, E.B., Weinstock, M.A., Spiegelman, D., Colditz, G.A., Willett, W.C. & Giovannucci, E. (1999) Risk factors for basal cell carcinoma of the skin in men: Results from the Health Professionals Follow-up Study. *Am. J. Epidemiol.*, **150**, 459–468

Doll, R., Gray, R., Hafner, B. & Peto, R. (1980) Mortality in relation to smoking: 22 years' observations on female British doctors. *Br. med. J.*, **280**, 967–971

Doll, R., Peto, R., Wheatley, K., Gray, R. & Sutherland, I. (1994) Mortality in relation to smoking: 40 years' observation on male British doctors. *Br. med. J.*, **309**, 901–911

Engeland, A., Andersen, A., Haldorsen, T. & Tretli, S. (1996) Smoking habits and risk of cancers other than lung cancer: 28 years' follow-up of 26,000 Norwegian men and women. *Cancer Causes Control*, **7**, 497–506

Franceschi, S. & Serraino, D. (1992) Risk factors for adult soft tissue sarcoma in northern Italy. *Ann. Oncol.*, **3**, S85–S88

Friedman, G.D. (1993) Cigarette smoking, leukemia, and multiple myeloma. *Ann. Epidemiol.*, **3**, 425–428

Galanti, M.R., Hansson, L., Lund, E., Bergström, R., Grimelius, L., Stalsberg, H., Carlsen, E., Baron, J.H., Persson, I. & Ekbom, A. (1996) Reproductive history and cigarette smoking as risk factors for thyroid cancer in women: A population-based case–control study. *Cancer Epidemiol. Biomarkers Prev.*, **5**, 425–431

Green, A., McCredie, M., MacKie, R., Giles, G., Young, P., Morton, C., Jackman, L. & Thursfield, V. (1999) A case–control study of melanomas of the soles and palms (Australia and Scotland). *Cancer Causes Control*, **10**, 21–25

Green, A., Purdie, D., Bain, C., Siskind, V. & Webb, P.M. (2001) Cigarette smoking and risk of epithelial ovarian cancer (Australia). *Cancer Causes Control*, **12**, 713–719

Grodstein, F., Speizer, F.E. & Hunter, D.J. (1995) A prospective study of incident squamous cell carcinoma of the skin in the Nurses' Health Study. *J. natl Cancer Inst.*, **87**, 1061–1066

Hayes, R.B., Brabo-Otero, E., Kleinman, D.V., Brown, L.M., Fraumeni, J.F., Jr, Harty, L.C. & Winn, D.M. (1999) Tobacco and alcohol use and oral cancer in Puerto Rico. *Cancer Causes Control*, **10**, 27–33

Heineman, E.F., Zahm, S.H., McLaughlin, J.K., Vaught, J.B. & Hrubec, Z. (1992) A prospective study of tobacco use and multiple myeloma: Evidence against an association. *Cancer Causes Control*, **3**, 31–36

Henderson, B.E., Benton, B., Jing, J., Yu, M.C. & Pike, M.C. (1979) Risk factors for cancer of the testis in young men. *Int. J. Cancer*, **23**, 598–602

Herrinton, L.J. & Friedman, G.D. (1998) Cigarette smoking and risk of non-Hodgkin's lymphoma subtypes. *Cancer Epidemiol. Biomarkers Prev.*, **7**, 25–28

de Hertog, S.A., Wensveen, C.A., Bastiaens, M.T., Kielich, C.J., Berkhout, M.J., Westendorp, R.G. & Bouwes Bavinck, J.N. for the Leiden Skin Cancer Study (2001) Relation between smoking and skin cancer. *J. clin. Oncol.*, **19**, 231–238

Hochberg, F., Toniolo, P., Cole, P. & Salcman, M. (1990) Nonoccupational risk indicators of glioblastoma in adults. *J. Neurooncol.*, **8**, 55–60

Hsing, A.W., Nam, J.M., Co Chien, H.T., McLaughlin, J.K. & Fraumeni, J.F., Jr (1996) Risk factors for adrenal cancer: An exploratory study. *Int. J. Cancer*, **65**, 432–436

Hunter, D.J., Colditz, G.A., Stampfer, M.J., Rosner, B., Willett, W.C. & Speizer, F.E. (1990) Risk factors for basal cell carcinoma in a prospective cohort of women. *Ann. Epidemiol.*, **1**, 13–23

Hurley, S.F., McNeil, J.J., Donnan, G.A., Forbes, A., Salzberg, M. & Giles, G.G. (1996) Tobacco smoking and alcohol consumption as risk factors for glioma: A case–control study in Melbourne, Australia. *J. Epidemiol. Community Health*, **50**, 442–446

IARC (1986) *IARC Monographs on the Evaluation of the Carcinogenic Risk of Chemicals to Humans*, Vol. 38, *Tobacco Smoking*, Lyon, IARCPress

Iribarren, C., Haselkorn, T., Tekawa, I.S. & Friedman, G.D. (2001) Cohort study of thyroid cancer in a San Francisco Bay area population. *Int. J. Cancer*, **93**, 745–750

Kaerlev, L., Teglbjaerg, P.S., Sabroe, S., Kolstad, H.A., Ahrens, W., Eriksson, M., Guenel, P., Gorini, G., Hardell, L., Cyr, D., Zambon, P., Stang, A. & Olsen, J. (2002) The importance of smoking and medical history for development of small bowel carcinoid tumor: A European population-based case–control study. *Cancer Causes Control*, **13**, 27–34

Karagas, M.R., Stukel, T.A., Greenberg, E.R., Baron, J.A., Mott, L.A. & Stern, R.S. for the Skin Cancer Prevention Study Group (1992) Risk of subsequent basal cell carcinoma and squamous cell carcinoma of the skin among patients with prior skin cancer. *J. Am. med. Asooc.*, **267**, 3305–3310

Kreiger, N. & Parkes, R. (2000) Cigarette smoking and the risk of thyroid cancer. *Eur. J. Cancer*, **36**, 1969–1973

Kuper, H., Titus-Ernstoff, L., Harlow, B.L. & Cramer, D.W. (2000) Population based study of coffee, alcohol and tobacco use and risk of ovarian cancer. *Int. J. Cancer*, **88**, 313–318

Lear, J.T., Tan, B.B., Smith, A.G., Jones, P.W., Heagerty, A.H., Strange, R.C. & Fryer, A.A. (1998) A comparison of risk factors for malignant melanoma, squamous cell carcinoma and basal cell carcinoma in the UK. *Int. J. clin. Pract.*, **52**, 145–149

Lee, M., Wrensch, M. & Miike, R. (1997) Dietary and tobacco risk factors for adult onset glioma in the San Francisco Bay Area (California, USA). *Cancer Causes Control*, **8**, 13–24

Linet, M.S., Harlow, S.D. & McLaughlin, J.K. (1987) A case–control study of multiple myeloma in whites: Chronic antigenic stimulation, occupation, and drug use. *Cancer Res.*, **47**, 2978–2981

Linet, M.S., McLaughlin, J.K., Hsing, A.W., Wacholder, S., Co Chien, H.T., Schuman, L.M., Bjelke, E. & Blot, W.J. (1992) Is cigarette smoking a risk factor for non-Hodgkin's lymphoma or multiple myeloma? Results from the Lutheran Brotherhood Cohort Study. *Leuk. Res.*, **16**, 621–624

Marchbanks, P.A., Wilson, H., Bastos, E., Cramer, D.W., Schildkraut, J.M. & Peterson, H.B. (2000) Cigarette smoking and epithelial ovarian cancer by histologic type. *Obstet. Gynecol.*, **95**, 255–260

McLaughlin, J.K., Hrubec, Z., Blot, W.J. & Fraumeni, J.F., Jr (1995) Smoking and cancer mortality among US veterans: a 26-year follow-up. *Int. J. Cancer*, **60**, 190–193

Memon, A., Darif, M., Al-Saleh, K. & Suresh, A. (2002) Epidemiology of reproductive and hormonal factors in thyroid cancer: Evidence from a case–control study in the Middle East. *Int. J. Cancer*, **97**, 82–89

Mills, P.K., Newell, G.R., Beeson, W.L., Fraser, G.E. & Phillips, R.L. (1990) History of cigarette smoking and risk of leukemia and myeloma: Results from the Adventist health study. *J. natl Cancer Inst.*, **82**, 1832–1836

Moerman, C.J., Bueno de Mesquita, H.B. & Runia, S. (1994) Smoking, alcohol consumption and the risk of cancer of the biliary tract; a population-based case–control study in The Netherlands. *Eur. J. Cancer Prev.*, **3**, 427–436

Negri, E., Bosetti, C., La Vecchia, C., Fioretti, F., Conti, E. & Franceschi, S. (1999) Risk factors for adenocarcinoma of the small intestine. *Int. J. Cancer*, **82**, 171–174

Østerlind, A., Tucker, M.A., Stone, B.J. & Jensen, O.M. (1988) The Danish case–control study of cutaneous malignant melanoma. IV. No association with nutritional factors, alcohol, smoking or hair dyes. *Int. J. Cancer*, **42**, 825–828

Paffenbarger, R.S., Jr, Wing, A.L. & Hyde, R.T. (1977) Characteristics in youth indicative of adult-onset Hodgkin's disease. *J. natl Cancer Inst.*, **58**, 1489–1491

Parker, A.S., Cerhan, J.R., Dick, F., Kemp, J., Habermann, T.M., Wallace, R.B., Sellers, T.A. & Folsom, A.R. (2000) Smoking and risk of non-Hodgkin lymphoma subtypes in a cohort of older women. *Leuk. Lymphoma*, **37**, 341–349

Peach, H.G. & Barnett, N.E. (2001) Critical review of epidemiological studies of the association between smoking and non-Hodgkin's lymphoma. *Hematol. Oncol.*, **19**, 67–80

Polychronopoulou, A., Tzonou, A., Hsieh, C.C., Kaprinis, G., Rebelakos, A., Toupadaki, N. & Trichopoulos, D. (1993) Reproductive variables, tobacco, ethanol, coffee and somatometry as risk factors for ovarian cancer. *Int. J. Cancer*, **55**, 402–407

Ron, E., Kleinerman, R.A., Boice, J.D., Jr, LiVolsi, V.A., Flannery, J.T. & Fraumeni, J.F., Jr (1987) A population-based case–control study of thyroid cancer. *J. natl Cancer Inst.*, **79**, 1–12

Rossing, M.A., Cushing, K.L., Voigt, L.F., Wicklund, K.G. & Daling, J.R. (2000) Risk of papillary thyroid cancer in women in relation to smoking and alcohol consumption. *Epidemiology*, **11**, 49–54

Ryan, P., Lee, M.W., North, B. & McMichael, A.J. (1992) Risk factors for tumors of the brain and meninges: Results from the Adelaide Adult Brain Tumor Study. *Int. J. Cancer*, **51**, 20–27

Sahl, W.J., Glore, S., Garrison, P., Oakleaf, K. & Johnson, S.D. (1995) Basal cell carcinoma and lifestyle characteristics. *Int. J. Dermatol.*, **34**, 398–402

Scott, T.E., Carroll, M., Cogliano, F.D., Smith, B.F. & Lamorte, W.W. (1999) A case–control assessment of risk factors for gallbladder carcinoma. *Dig. Dis. Sci.*, **44**, 1619–1625

Siemiatycki, J., Krewski, D., Franco, E. & Kaiserman, M. (1995) Associations between cigarette smoking and each of 21 types of cancer: A multi-site case–control study. *Int. J. Epidemiol.*, **24**, 504–514

Smith, E.M., Sowers, M.F. & Burns, T.L. (1984) Effects of smoking on the development of female reproductive cancers. *J. natl Cancer Inst.*, **73**, 371–376

Sokic, S.I., Adanja, B.J., Vlajinac, H.D., Jankovic, R.R., Marinkovic, J.P. & Zivaljevic, V.R. (1994) Risk factors for thyroid cancer. *Neoplasma*, **41**, 371–374

Spitz, M.R., Fueger, J.J., Goepfert, H. & Newell, G.R. (1990) Salivary gland cancer. A case–control investigation of risk factors. *Arch. Otolaryngol. head neck Surg.*, **116**, 1163–1166

Stagnaro, E., Ramazzotti, V., Crosignani, P., Fontana, A., Masala, G., Miligi, L., Nanni, O., Neri, M., Rodella, S., Seniori Costantini, A., Tumino, R., Viganò, C., Vindigni, C. & Vineis, P. (2001) Smoking and hematolymphopoietic malignancies. *Cancer Causes Control*, **12**, 325–334

Stockwell, H.G. & Lyman, G.H. (1987) Cigarette smoking and the risk of female reproductive cancer. *Am. J. Obstet. Gynecol.*, **157**, 35–40

Swanson, G.M. & Brissette Burns, P. (1997) Cancers of the salivary gland: Workplace risks among women and men. *Ann. Epidemiol.*, **7**, 369–374

UK Testicular Cancer Study Group (1994) Social, behavioural and medical factors in the aetiology of testicular cancer: Results from the UK study. *Br. J. Cancer*, **70**, 513–520

Westerdahl, J., Olsson, H., Måsbäck, A., Ingvar, C. & Jonsson, N. (1996) Risk of malignant melanoma in relation to drug intake, alcohol, smoking and hormonal factors. *Br. J. Cancer*, **73**, 1126–1131

Whittemore, A.S., Wu, M.L., Paffenbarger, R.S., Sarles, D.L., Kampert, J.B., Grosser, S., Jung, D.L., Ballon, S. & Hendrickson, M. (1988) Personal and environmental characteristics related to epithelial ovarian cancer. II. Exposures to talcum powder, tobacco, alcohol, and coffee. *Am. J. Epidemiol.*, **128**, 1228–1240

Wu, A.H., Yu, M.C. & Mack, T.M. (1997) Smoking, alcohol use, dietary factors and risk of small intestinal adenocarcinoma. *Int. J. Cancer*, **70**, 512–517

Yen, S., Hsieh, C.C. & MacMahon, B. (1987) Extrahepatic bile duct cancer and smoking, beverage consumption, past medical history, and oral-contraceptive use. *Cancer*, **59**, 2112–2116

Zahm, S.H., Heineman, E.F. & Vaught, J.B. (1992) Soft tissue sarcoma and tobacco use: Data from a prospective study of United States veterans. *Cancer Causes Control*, **3**, 371–376

Zatonski, W.A., La Vecchia, C., Przewozniak, K., Maisonneuve, P., Lowenfels, A.B. & Boyle, P. (1992) Risk factors for gallbladder cancer: A Polish case–control study. *Int. J. Cancer*, **51**, 707–711

Zatonski, W.A., Lowenfels, A.B., Boyle, P., Maisonneuve, P., Bueno de Mesquita, H.B., Ghadirian, P., Jain, M., Przewozniak, K., Baghurst, P., Moerman, C.J., Simard, A., Howe, G.R., McMichael, A.J., Hsieh, C.C. & Walker, A.M. (1997) Epidemiologic aspects of gallbladder cancer: A case–control study of the SEARCH Program of the International Agency for Research on Cancer. *J. natl Cancer Inst.*, **89**, 1132–1138

2.2 Pipe, cigar, bidi and other tobacco smoking

2.2.1 Pipe and cigar smoking

(a) Introduction

Although cigar and pipe smoking are less common than cigarette smoking throughout much of the world, these products are used extensively in certain countries and sub-cultures. Furthermore, the resurgence in the use of premium cigars in the USA between 1993 and 1997 illustrates how aggressive marketing of a specific tobacco product can rapidly increase its usage, even in cultures where it appears to be no longer fashionable.

The data on cancer risk in relation to cigar and pipe smoking are more limited than those available from studies of cigarette smoking. Fewer people have exclusively smoked cigars and/or pipes than have exclusively smoked cigarettes. The published studies are generally based on men, even though women in certain countries smoke cigars and/or pipes. Most studies of smoking cessation have greater statistical power to examine ciga-rette smoking than smoking of cigars or pipes. The smaller number of exclusive cigar and/or pipe smokers limits the opportunity to examine cancer risk in relation to the amount and duration of smoking, or to assess interactions with alcohol consumption. Persons who smoke cigarettes in combination with cigars and/or pipes typically have a risk for tobacco-attributable cancers that is intermediate between those who smoke cigarettes only and those who exclusively smoke cigars or pipes. The analyses presented here pertain only to exclusive cigar and/or pipe smokers, excluding smokers who also smoked cigarettes. While the main characteristics of the case–control studies are presented together with the results of the studies, the reader is referred to the beginning of Section 2 for a description of the cohort studies presented.

The tables are subdivided between (a) studies on smokers of pipes only and cigars only and (b) studies on smokers of both pipes and cigars, and studies that combined pipe and/or cigar smokers in one category.

(b) Cancer of the lip, oral cavity and pharynx

(i) Cancer of the lip

Clinical reports as early as 1795 linked pipe smoking with carcinoma of the lip (ICD-9: 140) and tongue (ICD-9: 141) (Sömmering, 1795; Clemmesen, 1965) as noted by Doll (1998). These reports were not taken very seriously, however, and these carcinomas were generally attributed to the heat of the clay pipe stem rather than to any intrinsic carcino-genicity of tobacco (Doll, 1998). Several case series and case reports published since the 1920s have noted the association of lip cancer with various combinations of pipe smoking, sunlight, ionizing radiation, and/or alcohol consumption (Broders, 1920; Ahlbom, 1937; Ebenius, 1943; Bernier & Clark, 1951; Hämäläinen, 1955; Wynder et al., 1957).

Two large case–control studies of lip cancer provide information on the relationship of lip cancer with pipe and cigar smoking. Keller (1970) studied 314 male cases, repre-senting a 20% sample of patients discharged from all Veterans Administration hospitals in the USA from 1958 until 1962. Two control groups were identified by sampling — one of patients with cancers of the mucous membrane of the mouth and pharynx, the other of patients discharged during the same period with no oral or pharyngeal cancer. Smoking of pipes, cigars and cigarettes was significantly associated with lip cancer. [The Working Group noted that the data did not include the amount smoked or duration of smoking and that only frequencies of exposure were compared.]

Spitzer *et al.* (1975) studied all male cases of squamous-cell carcinoma of the lip occurring in Newfoundland, Canada, over an 11-year period (1961–71; 366 cases). Three control groups were selected: 132 patients with oral cavity cancer, 81 patients with squamous-cell carcinoma of the skin of the head and neck and 210 randomly selected population controls. In comparison with the population controls, the relative risk for lip cancer associated with pipe smoking, adjusted for age, was 1.5 ($p < 0.05$). [The Working Group noted that the study focused on risk for lip cancer related to the occupation of fishing and gave no other information on tobacco use.]

Subsequent case–control and prospective studies of oropharyngeal cancer have not been sufficiently large to examine lip cancer separately in relation to exclusive use of pipes and/or cigars.

(ii) *Oral and pharyngeal cancer*

Cohort studies

Table 2.2.1 presents the results from seven cohort studies that looked at cancers of the oral cavity and pharynx (ICD-9: 140–149) among men who smoked exclusively cigars and/or pipes (Hammond & Horn, 1958; Kahn, 1966; Doll & Peto, 1976; Carstensen *et al.*, 1987; Shanks & Burns, 1998; Iribarren *et al.*, 1999; Shapiro *et al.*, 2000).

The largest study was based on 12 years of follow-up of the Cancer Prevention Study I (CPS-I) cohort (Shanks & Burns, 1998). Twenty-five deaths from cancers of the oral cavity and pharynx were identified between 1959 and 1972 among the 15 191 men who reported current and exclusive smoking of cigars at the time of enrolment in the study. The age-standardized relative risk for death from cancer of the oral cavity and pharynx was 7.9 (95% CI, 5.1–11.7) among all cigar smokers, relative to lifelong nonsmokers and increased with the number of cigars smoked per day to 15.9 (95% CI, 8.7–26.8) in men who smoked five or more cigars per day. The corresponding estimate for men who reported current smoking of cigarettes exclusively was 8.2 (95% CI, 7.2–9.4). Mortality results were not reported for the 9623 men who smoked exclusively pipes at the time of enrolment in the study, or for former smokers of either cigars or pipes.

Iribarren *et al.* (1999) reported a higher incidence of cancer of the oral cavity and pharynx among 1546 men who reported current smoking of cigars only and no past cigarette smoking at the time of enrolment in the Kaiser Permanente Medical Care Program between 1964 and 1973 than in nonsmokers. Follow-up from 1971 until 1996 identified eight subjects with oral and pharyngeal cancer among the cigar smokers. The relative risk among cigar smokers compared with that of 16 228 men who had never smoked cigarettes and did not smoke a pipe at enrolment was 2.6 (95% CI, 1.2–5.8). Among cigar smokers, risk was higher among men who smoked five or more cigars per day (relative risk, 7.2; 95% CI, 2.4–21.2) than in those who smoked less than five cigars per day (relative risk, 1.3; 95% CI, 0.4–4.4). [The Working Group noted that the inclusion of former pipe smokers in the referent group in this analysis potentially underestimates the association between cigar smoking and cancer of the oral cavity and pharynx.]

Shapiro et al. (2000) examined death rates from cancers of the oral cavity and pharynx among 7888 current and 7868 former cigar smokers in the Cancer Prevention Study II (CPS-II), followed from 1982 to 1994. The relative risk was highest among men who reported smoking three or more cigars per day (relative risk, 7.6; 95% CI, 2.9–19.6) and those who had smoked cigars for ≥ 25 years (relative risk, 4.6; 95% CI, 1.6–13), relative to lifelong nonsmokers.

Case–control studies

The case–control studies published since 1986 have consistently shown an increased risk for cancer of the oral cavity and pharynx among men who exclusively smoke cigars or pipes (Table 2.2.2).

Zheng et al. (1990) identified 404 patients diagnosed with histologically confirmed oral cancer (ICD 141, 143–145) at participating hospitals in Beijing in 1988–89. An equal number of controls matched on age, sex and hospital were randomly selected from non-cancer patients attending hospital for minor surgery and other conditions judged to be of less than 1-year duration. Among pipe smokers, the odds ratio adjusted for alcohol consumption, years of education, sex and age was 5.7 (95% CI, 2.4–13.3) in men and 4.9 (95% CI, 1.5–16.0) in women. The corresponding estimates associated with cigarette smoking only were 1.6 (95% CI, 1.0–2.6) in men and 2.0 (95% CI, 0.9–4.4) in women.

La Vecchia et al. (1998) reported an association between exclusive cigar smoking and cancers of the upper aerodigestive tract from a hospital-based case–control study in Italy and Switzerland. The cases in this study included cancers of the oesophagus as well as tumours of the oral cavity and pharynx and overlap with those in an earlier study by Franceschi et al. (1990).

Four other case–control studies have combined cigar and pipe smokers to examine the relationship of tobacco and alcohol consumption with cancers of the oral cavity and pharynx (Blot et al., 1988; Franceschi et al., 1990, 1992; Fernandez Garrote et al., 2001). The largest of these studies is that by Blot et al. (1988), based on 762 cases of oropharyngeal cancer diagnosed in four population-based tumour registries in the USA and 837 controls. Trained interviewers collected the information on tobacco and alcohol consumption. The relative risk estimate for men who smoked 40 or more cigars per week was 16.7 (95% CI, 3.7–76.7) when compared with the risk in never-smokers. The corresponding estimate in men who smoked 40 or more pipes per week was 3.1 (95% CI, 1.1–8.7).

Franceschi et al. (1990, 1992) reported a strong association between ever smoking cigars or pipes and diagnosis of cancers of the oral cavity (all subsites combined) in a hospital-based case–control study in Italy (relative risk, 20.7; 95% CI, 5.6–76.3). The association was stronger for cancer of the mouth (relative risk, 21.9; 95% CI, 3.8–125.6) than for cancer of the tongue (relative risk, 3.4; 95% CI, 0.3–39.1).

Fernandez Garrote et al. (2001) examined the relationship between cigar or pipe smoking and incident cancer of the oral cavity and pharynx in a hospital-based study in Cuba. The relative risk estimate among men who smoked four or more cigars or pipes per day was 20.5 (95% CI, 4.7–89.7).

Table 2.2.3 presents the results of two studies that have stratified the analysis of cancer of the oral cavity and pharynx in relation to cigar and/or pipe smoking by levels of alcohol consumption (Blot et al., 1988; Iribarren et al., 1999). Men who smoked cigars and/or pipes and consumed three or more alcoholic drinks per day (Iribarren et al., 1999) or 30 or more alcoholic drinks per week (Blot et al., 1988) had a substantially higher risk than men who drank alcohol but abstained from smoking, or smoked pipe and/or cigar but drank alcohol only occasionally.

(c) Lung cancer

In most published cohort studies (Table 2.2.4) and case–control studies (Table 2.2.5), men who exclusively smoke cigars and/or pipes have a consistently higher risk for cancer of the trachea, lung and bronchus (ICD-162) than men who have never smoked any tobacco product.

Lung cancer risk increased with the number of cigars smoked per day in both the CPS-I (Shanks & Burns, 1998) and CPS-II (Shapiro et al., 2000) cohorts and in the Kaiser Permanente Medical Care Program cohort (Iribarren et al., 1999)

Lung cancer risk increased with the amount and/or duration of smoking in two large European multi-centre, hospital-based case–control studies (Lubin et al., 1984; Boffetta et al., 1999) and in a case–control study in China (Lubin et al., 1992).

In the case–control by Boffetta et al. (1999), lung cancer risk decreased with time since cessation of cigar or pipe smoking.

The relationship between depth of inhalation and lung cancer risk from cigar and/or pipe smoking has been examined in several studies (Lubin et al., 1984; Benhamou et al., 1986; Shanks & Burns, 1998; Boffetta et al., 1999; Shapiro et al., 2000). Lung cancer risk was generally highest in cigar smokers who report that they inhale the smoke, but cigar smokers who report no inhalation still have a lung cancer risk two to five times higher than that for lifelong nonsmokers (Boffetta et al., 1999; Shapiro et al., 2000). Men who had switched from cigarette smoking to pipes or cigars reported deeper inhalation of the smoke and had higher risks for lung cancer than men who had always smoked pipes or cigars (Wald & Watt, 1997).

There is some evidence that the risk for lung cancer from cigar smoking may have increased over time. The relative risk estimates in cohort studies from the 1950s and 1960s generally ranged from 1.5 to 2.0 for men who were current smokers of either pipes or cigars at the time of the study (Kahn, 1966). However, all of the cohort studies (Doll & Peto, 1976; Carstensen et al., 1987; Lange et al., 1992; Tverdal et al., 1993; Ben-Shlomo et al., 1994; Shanks & Burns, 1998; Iribarren et al., 1999; Shapiro et al., 2000) and case–control studies (Lubin & Blot, 1984; Benhamou *et al.*, 1986; Damber & Larsson, 1986; Boffetta *et al.*, 1999) published after 1975 have reported relative risk estimates of > 2.0, many with point estimates above 4.0.

(*d*) Laryngeal cancer

(i) Cohort studies

Cigar and pipe smoking were found to be strongly associated with increased risk for cancer of the larynx (ICD-9: 161) among men in three cohort studies (Table 2.2.6) (Kahn, 1966; Shanks & Burns, 1998; Shapiro *et al.*, 2000).

Kahn (1966) identified six deaths from laryngeal cancer among male US veterans who smoked exclusively cigars at the time of enrolment in the US Veterans' Study and were followed from 1954 until 1962. The age-adjusted relative risk estimate associated with current cigar smoking was 10.3 (95% CI, 2.6–41.3).

Death from laryngeal cancer was associated with cigar smoking in analyses based on a 12-year follow-up of men in the CPS-I cohort (Shanks & Burns, 1998). The age-adjusted relative risk associated with current cigar smoking was 10.0 (95% CI, 4.0–20.6), based on seven deaths from laryngeal cancer among cigar smokers. The relative risk estimate was increased to 26.0 (95% CI, 8.4–60.7) among men who smoked five or more cigars per day and to 53.3 (95% CI, 0.7–296) among those who reported moderate to deep inhalation. The increased risk for laryngeal cancer associated with current cigar smoking during the 12-year follow-up was similar to the increased risk associated with current cigarette smoking during the first four years of follow-up [relative risk, 10.0; 95% CI, 3.5–28.5] (US Department of Health and Human Services, 1989).

Seven deaths from laryngeal cancer were recorded in CPS-II during follow-up from 1982 until 1994 among men who exclusively smoked cigars (Shapiro *et al.*, 2000). Current cigar smoking was associated with an increased death rate from laryngeal cancer compared with never-smokers (relative risk, 10.3; 95% CI, 2.6–41.0). The corresponding age-adjusted estimate associated with current cigarette smoking was 10.5 (95% CI, 3.6–30.4) among men in CPS-II during the first 4 years of follow-up (1982–86) (US Department of Health and Human Services, 1989). In dose–response analyses based on a small number of cases, the relative risk associated with cigar smoking was higher in current smokers than in former smokers, in those who smoked more cigars per day, who reported smoking for 25 or more years and who reported inhaling the cigar smoke.

(ii) Case–control study

In a hospital-based case–control study in northern Italy, Franceschi *et al.* (1990) identified 162 incident cases of men with laryngeal cancer and 1272 controls between June 1986 and June 1989 (Table 2.2.7). Only one case exclusively smoked cigars or pipes, whereas 94% of cases and 76% of controls smoked cigarettes.

Several of the studies that examined the relation of cigar and/or pipe smoking to laryngeal cancer are not considered here, either because they included persons who also smoked cigarettes (Falk *et al.*, 1989; Muscat & Wynder, 1992) or because cigarette smokers were included in the referent group (Freudenheim *et al.*, 1992).

(e)   Oesophageal cancer

(i)   Cohort studies

Exclusive smoking of cigars and/or pipes has been associated with increased risk for cancer of the oesophagus (ICD-9: 150) in several cohort studies (Table 2.2.8) (Kahn, 1966; Carstensen *et al.*, 1987; Shanks & Burns, 1998; Shapiro *et al.*, 2000).

In the US Veterans' Study, 14 deaths from oesophageal cancer occurred between 1954 and 1962 among men who, at enrolment, reported currently or formerly smoking cigars exclusively (Kahn, 1966). Risk was higher among current cigar smokers (relative risk, 5.3; 95% CI, 2.4–12.1, based on 12 deaths), than in former cigar smokers (relative risk, 2.4; 95% CI, 0.5–10.9, based on two deaths). Few male veterans had smoked pipes exclusively. The association between current pipe smoking and oesophageal cancer was based on only three deaths (relative risk, 2.0; 95% CI, 0.6–7.1).

Pipe and cigar smoking were associated with similar increases in death rate from oesophageal cancer in a cohort of 25 129 Swedish men (Carstensen *et al.*, 1987). The Swedish Census Study cohort is unusual in that 27% of the men smoked a pipe, whereas only 5% smoked exclusively cigars and 32% cigarettes. The relative risk estimate associated with current pipe smoking was 3.6 (95% CI, 1.1–11.8, based on six deaths), whereas the association with current cigar smoking was 6.5 (95% CI, 1.3–33.5, based on two deaths).

The largest study of the association of oesophageal cancer with cigar smoking was based on CPS-I, in which 30 deaths from oesophageal cancer were identified among 15 191 men who reported exclusive cigar smoking at the time of enrolment (Shanks & Burns, 1998). The overall relative risk associated with current cigar smoking was 3.6 (95% CI, 2.2–5.6) relative to lifelong nonsmokers. Risk increased with the number of cigars smoked per day and with the self-reported depth of inhalation.

Shapiro *et al.* (2000) identified 17 deaths from oesophageal cancer among 15 756 men participating in CPS-II who reported current or former cigar smoking at the time of enrolment and were followed from 1982 through 1994. The relative risk estimate was slightly higher in current cigar smokers (relative risk, 1.8; 95% CI, 0.9–3.7) than in former cigar smokers (relative risk, 1.3; 95% CI, 0.6–2.8). Dose–response analyses based on nine deaths among current cigar smokers showed an increase in the risk of oesophageal cancer with the duration of smoking, but not with the number of cigars smoked per day or with depth of inhalation.

(ii)   Case–control studies

The case–control studies on smoking and oesophageal cancer are summarized in Table 2.2.9 (Franceschi *et al.*, 1990; Kabat *et al.*, 1993; La Vecchia *et al.*, 1998).

Kabat *et al.* (1993) examined the relationship of pipe and/or cigar smoking to specific histological types of oesophageal cancer in a hospital-based case–control study of 431 male cases and 4544 hospital controls in the USA. Eleven cases of squamous carcinoma of the oesophagus and nine cases of adenocarcinoma of the distal oesophagus or gastric cardia had smoked pipes and/or cigars only. The risk among pipe and/or cigar smokers was not significantly higher than that of lifelong nonsmokers for squamous carcinoma (relative risk, 1.8; 95% CI, 0.8–4.1) or adenocarcinoma (relative risk, 1.1; 95% CI, 0.5–2.3).

None of the studies of pipe and/or cigar smoking in relation to oesophageal cancer have been sufficiently large to assess the possible interactions between smoking and alcohol consumption.

(f) Stomach cancer

Pipe and/or cigar smoking were consistently associated with a small increase in incidence of stomach cancer (ICD-9: 151) in most cohort studies (Table 2.2.8) and case–control studies (Table 2.2.9), but the number of cases who smoked cigars and/or pipes exclusively was small and the 95% confidence intervals in these studies often included the null.

Chao et al. (2002) examined the relationship between tobacco smoking and death from stomach cancer among men who currently or formerly smoked cigars or pipes at the time of enrolment in CPS-II. Increased mortality from stomach cancer was associated with current cigar smoking (relative risk, 2.3; 95% CI, 1.5–3.5; 25 deaths) and pipe smoking (relative risk, 1.3; 95% CI, 0.8–2.2; 16 deaths). Relative risk estimates were highest in men who reported smoking five or more cigars per day (relative risk, 4.2; 95% CI, 2.3–7.6) and those who inhaled the smoke (relative risk, 3.9; 95% CI, 1.9–8.0).

(g) Colorectal cancer

Current pipe and/or cigar smoking were associated with an increased risk for cancer of the colon and/or rectum (ICD-9: 153–4) in several cohort studies (Table 2.2.10).

The largest analysis is based on follow-up of the US Veterans' Study from 1954 until 1980. Heineman et al. (1995) reported a higher death rate from both colon cancer (relative risk, 1.3; 95% CI, 1.1–1.4) and rectal cancer (relative risk, 1.4; 95% CI, 1.2–1.8) among men who exclusively smoked pipes and/or cigars compared with never-smokers. The relative risk for colon cancer increased significantly with the number of cigars smoked per day (p for trend = 0.004) and the relative risk for rectal cancer increased with the number of pipes smoked per day (p for trend = 0.007).

Current smoking of pipes and/or cigars was associated with an increased risk for colon or colorectal cancer in the British Doctors' Study (relative risk, 1.7; 95% CI not stated) (Doll & Peto, 1976), the Lutheran Brotherhood Insurance Study (relative risk, 1.6; 95% CI, 0.8–3.2) (Hsing et al., 1998) and the Finnish Mobile Clinic Health Examination Study (relative risk, 1.5; 95% CI, 0.8–2.6) (Knekt et al., 1998). Current cigar and/or pipe smoking was also significantly associated with increased mortality from colorectal cancer among men in the CPS-II who had smoked for 20 or more years (relative risk, 1.3; 95% CI, 1.1–1.6) (Chao et al., 2000).

The Working Group was aware of no published case–control studies of exclusive pipe and/or cigar smoking in relation to cancers of the colon and rectum.

(*h*)   *Cancer of the liver and intrahepatic bile ducts*

Carstensen *et al.* (1987) reported an association between current cigar smoking and increased death rates from cancer of the liver and biliary passages (ICD-9: 155–156) among 25 129 Swedish men followed from 1963 to 1979 (relative risk, 7.2; 95% CI, 2.2–23.4, based on four deaths) (Table 2.2.11).

Hsing *et al.* (1990a) reported an increased risk for primary liver cancer among current pipe and/or cigar smokers participating in the US Veterans' Study (relative risk, 3.1; 95% CI, 2.0–4.8).

(*i*)   *Cancer of the gallbladder and extrahepatic bile ducts*

Cancer of the extrahepatic bile ducts (ICD-O: 156.1) was also associated with cigar and/or pipe smoking in a population-based case–control study of 105 histologically confirmed cases and 255 controls in Los Angeles County, USA (Table 2.2.12) (Chow *et al.*, 1994). Two cases of cancer of the extrahepatic bile duct occurred among men who had ever smoked cigars or pipes exclusively (relative risk, 1.6; 95% CI, 0.3–9.9), compared with lifelong nonsmokers. Two additional cases involved the ampulla of Vater (relative risk, 7.6; 95% CI, 0.6–100.4).

(*j*)   *Cancer of the pancreas*

Pipe and/or cigar smoking were associated with an increased risk for pancreatic cancer (ICD-9: 157) in most of the cohort studies (Table 2.2.13) and case–control studies (Table 2.2.14).

(i)   *Cohort studies*

The largest study encompassed a 12-year follow-up of men in CPS-I (Table 2.2.13) (Shanks & Burns, 1998). The age-adjusted relative risk for death from pancreatic cancer among current exclusive cigar smokers, compared with lifelong nonsmokers, was 1.6 (95% CI, 1.2–2.1), based on 56 deaths. The risk for pancreatic cancer increased with the number of cigars smoked per day and with the depth of inhalation of the cigar smoke.

Higher risks for pancreatic cancer in current cigar smokers than in nonsmokers were also reported among men in the US Veterans' Study (relative risk, 1.5; 95% CI, 0.99–2.3, 27 deaths) (Kahn, 1966), in the Kaiser Permanente Medical Care Program Study (relative risk, 1.2; 95% CI, 0.5–2.9, 6 cases) (Iribarren *et al.*, 1999) and in CPS-II (relative risk, 1.3; 95% CI, 0.9–1.9, 28 deaths) (Shapiro *et al.*, 2000).

Current pipe smoking was significantly associated with increased risk for pancreatic cancer in the Swedish Census Study (relative risk, 2.8; 95% CI, 1.5–5.2) (Carstensen *et al.*, 1987).

(ii)   *Case–control study*

In the hospital-based case–control study reported by Muscat *et al.* (1997), men who ever smoked cigars exclusively had an increased risk for pancreatic cancer (relative risk, 3.1; 95% CI, 1.4–6.9) (Table 2.2.14). For ever smoking a pipe, the odds ratio for pancreatic cancer incidence was 1.8 (95% CI, 0.9–5.3).

(k)   *Cancer of the bladder and kidney*

Epidemiological studies of cigar and/or pipe smoking in relation to cancers of the urinary bladder (ICD-9: 188) and kidney (ICD-9: 189) are summarized in Table 2.2.15 (cohort studies) and Table 2.2.16 (case–control studies). Men who exclusively smoked pipes had a significantly increased risk for bladder cancer in the Swedish Census Study (relative risk, 4.0; 95% CI, 1.9–8.6), the largest prospective study to evaluate pipe smoking (Carstensen et al., 1987). Men who smoked more than three cigars daily had an increased risk for bladder cancer relative to that of lifelong nonsmokers in CPS-I (Shanks & Burns, 1998) and CPS-II (Shapiro et al., 2000).

Taken separately, none of the cohort or case–control studies included a sufficient number of cases who smoked pipes or cigars exclusively to evaluate dose–response relationships precisely. The largest study of bladder cancer was the pooled analysis of European case–control studies by Pitard *et al.* (2001). The risk for bladder cancer increased significantly with number of years of smoking for both pipes (p for trend = 0.006) and cigars (p for trend < 0.001).

The four studies on kidney cancer (Kahn, 1966; Jensen *et al.*, 1988; McLaughlin *et al.*, 1995; Iribarren *et al.*, 1999) had limited statistical power to assess associations between pipe or cigar smoking and cancers of the renal pelvis or parenchyma.

(l)   *Prostate cancer*

Men who exclusively smoked pipes or cigars had higher death rates from prostate cancer (ICD-9: 185) than lifelong nonsmokers during the first 8.5 years of follow-up of the US Veterans' Study (Kahn, 1966). Compared with lifelong nonsmokers, the relative risk estimate was 1.5 (95% CI, 0.98–2.4) for men who currently smoked pipes, and 1.5 (95% CI, 1.03–2.2) for current cigar smokers. Little association was seen between prostate cancer mortality and pipe and/or cigar smoking in the 26-year follow-up of the same cohort (Hsing *et al.*, 1991). [The Working Group noted that the information on smoking was not updated during either follow-up, so that misclassification of exposure could have attenuated the findings in the longer follow-up.]

Hsing *et al.* (1990b) also studied the much smaller Lutheran Brotherhood Insurance Study cohort (Table 2.2.17). Mortality from prostate cancer was higher among men who ever smoked pipes or cigars than in lifelong nonsmokers (relative risk, 1.6; 95% CI, 0.7–3.5), although the association was based on only nine deaths. No increase in risk for prostate cancer was seen among men who currently smoked pipes in the Norwegian Screening Study (Tverdal *et al.*, 1993) or among men who ever smoked pipes or cigars in a population based case–control study in Montreal, Canada (Table 2.2.18; Sharpe & Siemiatycki, 2001).

(m)   Cancer of the haematopoietic system

The cohort studies (Table 2.2.19) and case–control studies (Table 2.2.20) that have related cigar and/or pipe smoking to haematopoietic cancers are generally too small to be informative.

(n)   Cancer of other organs

The Norwegian Screening Study examined the relationship between pipe and/or cigar smoking and the risk for brain cancer (Tverdal *et al.*, 1993). The number of cases was too small to be informative (Table 2.2.21).

2.2.2   Bidi and other tobacco smoking

(a)   Introduction

This section covers smoking in forms practiced mainly in South Asia and in Africa. Most of the available studies have been conducted in India on the association of cancer with bidi smoking as well as, depending on the region studied, smoking of chillum (clay pipe), cheroot and chutta, including reverse chutta smoking. Other studies have reported on *khii yoo* smoking in Northern Thailand, kiraiku smoking in Kenya and reverse cigarette smoking.

Bidi smoking is the most common form of tobacco smoking in India. The bidi is an indigenous smoking stick 4–8 cm long, usually containing 0.15–0.25 g coarse tobacco flakes rolled in a rectangular piece of dried *temburni* leaf (*Diospyros melanoxylon*). The number of bidis produced and consumed in India is 7–8 times higher than the number of cigarettes, thus most studies on health risks to smokers in India have concentrated on bidi smoking. Moreover, cigarette smoking is common generally only in higher socioeconomic groups. Besides bidis and cigarettes, other smoking habits include various indigenous forms of pipe and cheroot smoking. Cheroots are small cigars made of heavy-bodied cured tobacco rolled in a dried tobacco leaf and tied with a thread. Chuttas are coarsely prepared cheroots. The length of chuttas varies from 5 to 12 cm. Chutta smoking is widespread in coastal areas of Andhra Pradesh, Tamil Nadu and Orissa. The hookah, or hooka, is a pipe that allows the tobacco smoke to pass through water before the smoker inhales it (water pipe). The chillum is a straight, conical clay pipe used for tobacco smoking.

When assessing the carcinogenic effects of smoking, it is necessary to consider several potentially confounding common habits such as chewing of betel quid with tobacco, chewing tobacco with or without lime, and drinking alcoholic beverages. Betel-quid chewing is the chewing of a quid made up of fresh betel leaves (*Piper betle*), areca nut (*Areca catechu*), slaked lime (calcium hydroxide) and almost always, tobacco. Various condiments are often added in small quantities. Other forms of smokeless tobacco include a powder or paste used to clean the teeth and snuff.

(b)   Cancer of the oral cavity and pharynx

Results of case–control studies on bidi and other tobacco smoking and cancer of the oral cavity and pharynx are presented in Table 2.2.22.

(i)   Cancer of the oral cavity

Three hospital-based case–control studies on cancers of subsites of the oral cavity (gingiva, tongue and floor of the mouth, buccal and labial mucosa) were conducted at the Regional Cancer Centre in Trivandrum, Kerala, a state in southern India, during 1983–84. Control patients, matched for age (within 5 years), sex and religion, were selected among outpatients who came for treatment to the Medical College in Trivandrum, with respiratory, intestinal and genitourinary infections or who came for a cancer check-up for sites other than the head and neck. Both cases and controls were interviewed by trained social workers to elicit sociodemographic information, history of habits and clinical details. All cancer cases were confirmed by biopsy. Chewing of betel quid with or without tobacco, bidi smoking, cigarette smoking, alcohol use and nasal snuff inhalation were the main habits practiced by the study population. These studies analysed only men for smoking and alcohol habits because few women practiced these habits.

The case–control study on carcinoma of the gingiva consisted of 187 cases and 895 matched controls (Sankaranarayanan *et al.*, 1989a). After using forward stepwise logistic regression on the four main habits of chewing of betel quid with tobacco, bidi smoking, alcohol drinking and snuff inhalation, the relative risk for smoking bidis for 20 years or less was 2.6 (95% CI, 0.7–9.9) and that for smoking bidis for more than 20 years was 2.1 (95% CI, 1.2–27.9).

The study on cancer of the tongue (n = 188) and floor of the mouth (n = 40) included 158 men and 70 women (Sankaranarayan *et al.*, 1989b). Two controls were selected for each case and matched for age (within 5 years), sex and religion. Forward stepwise logistic regression was used to estimate relative risk for chewing of betel quid with tobacco, bidi smoking, bidi–cigarette smoking and cigarette smoking. A relative risk of 7.5 (95% CI. 2.6–21.7) was noted for men who smoked 20 or more bidis per day.

The study of cancer of the buccal and labial mucosa included 413 cases and 895 controls (Sankaranarayan *et al.*, 1990a). When forward stepwise logistic regression was used to create a multivariate model of risk for cancer of the buccal and labial mucosa adjusted for other habits, bidi smoking had a relative risk of 2.9 (95% CI, 1.3–6.6) for a duration of the habit up to 20 years and 1.7 (95% CI, 1.1–2.6) for a habit that continued for 21 years or more.

A hospital-based case–control study was carried out during 1980–84 at the Tata Memorial Hospital, a cancer hospital in Mumbai (Bombay), India, on 713 men who were histopathologically diagnosed with oral cancer and 635 controls free from cancer, benign lesions or infectious diseases (Rao *et al.*, 1994). The average age of the case group was

50.4 years and that of the control group was 45.4 years. Those who smoked bidis had a relative risk of 1.6 (95% CI, 1.3–2.0) for oral cancer. Men who smoked hookah and chillum had a relative risk of 5.0 (95% CI, 1.4–22.0). The trends in relative risks by intensity and duration of bidi smoking were both statistically significant ($p < 0.001$). [The Working Group noted that the study had several deficiencies, particularly in the selection of controls that resulted in cigarette smoking apparently being protective for oral cancer. The data analysis seemed to be confined to univariate analysis.]

A hospital-based case–control study was undertaken on 647 male patients with tongue cancer at the Tata Memorial Hospital, in Mumbai, India, between 1980 and 1984 (Rao & Desai, 1998). During the same period, 635 men, the majority of whom had come to the hospital for a check-up and were found to be free of cancer, benign lesions and infection, were selected as unmatched controls. Habits included betel quid, areca nut, tobacco and lime, bidi, cigarettes and other forms of tobacco smoking. Bidi smoking was by far the most common smoking habit. Unconditional logistic regression was used to estimate relative risk after stratification by age and place of residence. Bidi smoking was a significant risk factor for cancer of the base of the tongue (relative risk, 5.9; 95% CI, 4.2–8.2). Bidi smoking did not pose a statistically significant relative risk for cancer of the anterior tongue at any level of smoking intensity, but the relative risks for cancer of the base of the tongue were statistically significant at all levels of smoking intensity and a statistically significant trend was observed. Duration of smoking was not a significant predictor of risk for cancer of the anterior tongue, but it was for cancer of base of the tongue, with a significant trend that peaked at 21–30 years (relative risk, 7.7; 95% CI, 4.8–13.0). A model created with unconditional logistic regression that included bidi smoking, alcohol drinking, illiteracy, non-vegetarian diet and tobacco chewing showed that the greatest risk for cancer of the base of the tongue came from smoking bidis (relative risk, 4.7; 95% CI, 3.5–6.3). Cancer of the anterior tongue was not associated with bidi smoking in this model.

A population-based case–control study of upper aerodigestive tract cancers was conducted in Bhopal, central India (Dikshit & Kanhere, 2000). Men who had cancers that had been recorded during 1986–92 by the Bhopal Population-Based Cancer Registry were potential cases. Those with tongue cancer (not otherwise specified) or registered from death certificate only were excluded. Only those subjects who gave complete information on tobacco use were included, giving 163 lung cancer patients, 247 oropharyngeal cancer patients and 148 oral cavity cancer patients (all squamous-cell carcinomas) as study cases. A total of 260 controls were randomly selected after age stratification of a sample of about 2500 men recruited during 1989–92 in a tobacco habit survey of a random sample of Bhopal voters. After adjustment for age and tobacco quid chewing, the relative risk for smokers (bidis and/or cigarettes) was 1.5 (95% CI, 0.9–2.4). Smoking for more than 30 years led to a significant relative risk for oral cavity cancer of 4.3 (95% CI, 2.0–9.1). The estimated relative risk for the highest of three levels of cumulative years of smoking was 6.0 (95% CI, 2.6–13.7).

A hospital-based case–control study of cancer of the oral cavity was conducted in three areas of southern India (Bangalore, Madras and Trivandrum) between 1996 and

1999 (Balaram *et al.*, 2002). A total of 591 incident cases were enrolled (309 men, 282 women). Control subjects were selected from the same hospitals (centres) as cases and were frequency-matched by centre, age and sex. In Madras and Bangalore, the controls were relatives and friends of other cancer patients. In Trivandrum, controls were selected from general medical outpatients or attendees of the cancer clinics who had been found free of malignancy. The control group included 292 men and 290 women. Odds ratios for men who smoked bidis were: for < 20 bidis per day, 2.0 (95% CI, 1.1–3.8); and for ≥ 20 per day, 2.5 (95% CI, 1.4–4.4).

(ii) *Pharyngeal cancer*

A hospital-based case–control study of oropharyngeal cancer was carried out in Nagpur, Maharashtra in Central India (Wasnik *et al.*, 1998). The cases were 123 patients newly diagnosed with oropharyngeal cancer, confirmed by histopathology. Each case was matched with two hospital controls on age and sex. For each case, one control was selected from non-cancer patients and the other from patients with cancer at sites other than head and neck. Unconditional logistic regression analysis was used with the major risk factors identified from an initial model. Odds ratios for tobacco smoking, predominantly in the form of bidi and/or chillum, were 2.3 (95% CI, 1.2–3.7) after adjusment for tobacco chewing and outdoor occupation. [The Working Group noted some problems with the data analysis.]

A case–control study was undertaken on 1698 men with pharyngeal and laryngeal cancers seen at the Tata Memorial Hospital, Mumbai from 1980 to 1984 (Rao *et al.*, 1999). There were 678 patients with cancer of oropharynx, 593 patients with cancer of the hypopharynx, and 427 patients with cancer of the larynx. A total of 635 controls were selected from male outpatients at the same hospital who had been found to be free from cancer, benign tumours and infectious disease. The estimated relative risk for bidi smoking was 5.6 (95% CI, 4.1–7.6) for cancer of the oropharynx and 2.0 (95% CI, 2.0–3.5) for cancer of the hypopharynx. A dose–response relationship was observed for intensity and duration of bidi smoking for both sites. When unconditional logistic regression was performed with adjustment for alcohol, illiteracy, diet and tobacco chewing, bidi smoking was the most important factor for both sites.

In the study by Dikshit and Kanhere (2000) (described in Section 2.2.2(*b*)(i)), a high relative risk for oropharyngeal cancer among subjects who smoked only bidis (odds ratio, 7.9; 95% CI, 5.1–12.4) and a positive relationship with intensity of bidi smoking were observed.

(iii) *Oral leukoplakia*

Case reports

A case of reverse cigarette smoking was reported from the Hospital 'De Tjongerschans', Heerenveen, the Netherlands, where a dentist had referred a 59 year-old woman who had smoked for 40 years with the glowing end inside the mouth, having learnt the habit from her mother who originated from Aruba in the Netherlands Antilles.

Oral examination revealed a thick, leathery palatal mucosa with burnt, charred areas. The buccal mucosa at both sides showed diffuse leukoplakic lesions. Biopsy of the palatal leukoplakia showed hyperkeratosis with slight to moderate epithelial dysplasia. After 4 years of follow-up, no malignant changes were noted (Hogewind et al., 1987).

A 69-year old immigrant from the Philippines was referred to the Department of Stomatology at the School of Dentistry, University of Manitoba in Winnipeg, Canada, with an unusual lesion of the hard palate. She reported having practiced reverse smoking for 10 years, having begun the habit in the Philippines. A white lesion covered her entire hard palate and near the mid-line there was an area of charred tissue. Minor salivary glands stood out as red spots, as in nicotine stomatitis. A biopsy of the hard palate revealed moderate hyperkeratinization without dysplasia. A 50-year-old woman who had emigrated from the Caribbean had a clinical history similar to that of the woman described above. She was diagnosed with hyperkeratinization without dysplasia (Stoykewych et al., 1992).

Cross-sectional and case–control studies (Table 2.2.23)

A cross section of villagers aged 21 years and above, in four villages in three districts of Andhra Pradesh where it was known that reverse chutta smoking was practised, was surveyed for palatal lesions (Van der Eb et al., 1993). A random sample of 758 persons was drawn from the electoral rolls and 480 of them (250 women, 230 men) were examined and interviewed by health professionals with special training. Many could not be examined due to bad weather, others due to emigration or death, but refusals were uncommon. Reverse chutta smokers constituted 33.3% of the sample, about two-thirds of which were women; conventional chutta smokers amounted to 12.5% (mainly men); bidi smokers, 4.2% (all men); cigarette smokers, 2.9%; tobacco chewers, 2.1 %; and those with mixed habits, 4.2%. Non-tobacco users constituted 33.5% of the sample, about two-thirds of which were women, and 7.3% were former smokers. Palatal lesions were found with all smoking habits, but were far more common and most severe in reverse smokers. The age and sex-standardized percentages of palatal lesions were as follows: 0.9% of the men and 3.9% of the women who were nonsmokers; 55% of the bidi smokers; 54.7% of the men and 63.3% of the women who were conventional chutta smokers; and 93.0 % of the men and 92.2 % of the women who practised reverse chutta smoking. Palatal lesions found in higher proportions in reverse smokers included preleukoplakia, leukoplakia and palatal keratosis. All but one of the atrophic areas were found in current and ex-reverse chutta smokers and all the nine carcinomas found were in current reverse chutta smokers.

A population-based case–control study of leukoplakia was carried out in Kenya by house-to-house survey using a cluster-sampling technique (Macigo et al., 1996). Individuals with leukoplakia found through oral examination (n = 85) were enrolled as cases. Controls (n = 141) were matched for sex, age and the cluster of origin. Tobacco was smoked in the form of cigarettes and *kiraiku* rolls, a type of local, handmade, smoking sticks, using cured, dried and crushed tobacco, rolled in any one of the following: dried banana leaves and stem peelings, dried corn husks, newspaper or other paper. The relative risk for oral leukoplakia in current cigarette smokers was 8.4 (95% CI, 4.1–17.4) and that for current *kiraiku* smokers was 10.0 (95% CI, 2.9–43.4). In former *kiraiku* smokers, the relative risk was 4.9 (95% CI, 2.3–10.4). Duration of smoking before cessation showed a trend towards greater risk with increasing duration. A gradual downward trend was seen for the number of years since quitting *kiraiku* smoking; however, the relative risk for an interval of more than 10 years since quitting was still significantly increased. [The Working Group noted that the study did not adequately control for possible confounding with cigarette smoking.]

Intervention studies

A large controlled prospective intervention trial for primary prevention of oral cancer was conducted in India in the districts of Ernakulam (Kerala), Bhavnagar (Gujarat) and Srikakulam (Andhra Pradesh). The intervention cohort consisted of over 12 000 tobacco users of 15 years of age and older in each of the three districts. Members of this cohort were interviewed about their tobacco use and examined for the presence of oral lesions. They took part in an educational programme on tobacco use through annual follow-ups during 1977–88. The control cohort consisted of over 17 000 persons, all tobacco users aged 15 and over in randomly selected villages in the same three districts, who were examined and followed up in a similar manner to that for the intervention cohort, but with minimal educational intervention during 1966–77 (Gupta *et al.*, 1986a). Eight annual follow-up surveys were conducted after the first 2 years, covering a 10-year period (1977–88). The analysis was restricted to tobacco users with an appropriate length of follow-up period. The results are discussed district by district, and are summarized in Table 2.2.24.

Bhavnagar District

The size of the intervention cohort in Bhavnagar was 12 221 and that of the control cohort was 3704, all subjects were men as very few women used tobacco in that area. Both bidis and clay pipes were commonly smoked by men in the Bhavnagar District. A small proportion of men practised chewing habits.

After five years of follow-up, the proportion of individuals re-examined at least once in the intervention cohort was 96.5% and in the control cohort, 83.5%. The proportions of individuals who quit their tobacco habits in the control and intervention cohorts were 9% and 13%, respectively. There was little difference in the incidence rate of leukoplakia between the two cohorts (Gupta *et al.*, 1986b).

Srikakulam District

The size of the intervention cohort in Srikakulam District was 12 038 and that of the control cohort was 7542. Smoking was the major tobacco habit, practised mostly in the form of reverse chutta smoking. Men also smoked chuttas in the conventional manner, and bidis. Women practised only reverse chutta smoking. The proportions of individuals who quit their tobacco habits in the control and intervention cohorts were 3.5% and 17%, respectively.

Incidence rates of oral precancerous lesions (mainly palatal lesions associated with reverse smoking) were substantially lower in the intervention cohort than in the control cohort for all tobacco habit groups. The 5-year age-adjusted incidence rates per 1000 for palatal changes for women who were reverse smokers were 513.9 in the control area and 292.0 in the intervention area and, among men, 427.7 and 163.3, respectively. The rate ratio for the protective effect of intervention on reverse smokers was 0.38 in men and 0.57 in women (Gupta et al., 1986b).

Ernakulam District

At baseline in the intervention cohort, the prevalence of leukoplakia was 2.9% in the intervention cohort and 2.7% in the control cohort (Mehta et al., 1982).

After eight years of follow-up, the expected number of cases of leukoplakia in the intervention cohort was calculated using age- and sex- specific incidence rates from the control cohort. The observed number of leukoplakia was only 41% of the expected number in men and only 28 % of the expected number in women (Gupta et al., 1990).

After 10 years of follow-up, 14.3% of tobacco users in the intervention cohort had discontinued their tobacco habit as compared with 4.5% in the control cohort. Among individuals who reported stopping bidi smoking, only one bidi-associated leukoplakia and one central papillary atrophy of the tongue were found, compared to the expected 5.8 leukoplakia, 6.0 central papillary atrophy and 27.1 other bidi-associated oral mucosal lesions (leukoedema, preleukoplakia and smokers' palate), based on the incidence rates among all other individuals. The differences in observed and expected rates were statistically significant ($p < 0.05$) (Gupta et al., 1992).

The relative risks for malignant transformation for the nodular form of leukoplakia were reported to be 3243.2, for ulcerated leukoplakia 43.8 and for homogeneous leukoplakia 25.6 when compared with individuals with a tobacco habit, but no oral precancerous lesions (Gupta et al., 1989).

[The Working Group noted the 10-year calendar time difference between the intervention and control cohorts.]

The educational intervention that was undertaken in these studies was helpful in reducing the use of tobacco in all areas and in increasing cessation rates in two of the three areas. Spontaneous regression rates of oral precancerous lesions were higher among individuals who reported stopping or reducing their tobacco use than in those who did not. The incidence rates of oral precancer were lower in the intervention cohorts in two of the areas (leukoplakia in Ernakulam and palatal changes in Srikakulam) than in the respective control cohorts.

(c)   Lung cancer

In northern Thailand, hand-rolled cigars called *khii yoo* are commonly smoked. In a hospital-based case–control study conducted in Chiang Mai, Thailand, the odds ratios for lung cancer for *khii yoo* smoking were 1.2 in men and 1.5 in women ($p > 0.05$) (Simarak et al., 1977).

In the case–control study by Dikshit & Kanhere (2000), described in Section 2.2.2(*b*)(i), the age-adjusted relative risk for lung cancer among smokers of bidis only was 11.6 (95% CI, 6.4–21.3) (Table 2.2.25).

A hospital-based case-control study of lung cancer was conducted in Chandigarh, northern India. A total of 235 men with cytologically or histologically confirmed lung cancer was recruited between January 1995 and June 1997. Four hundred and thirty-five male controls were selected from visitors and attendants of the patients. Results were presented both separately and combined for bidi, cigarette and hookah smoking. For the purpose of analysing smokers of different types of tobacco products, cigarette equivalents were calculated by applying a weight of 1 (= 1g of tobacco) to cigarettes, 0.5 to bidis, and 4 hookahs. The odds ratio for bidi smoking was 5.8 (95% CI, 3.4–9.7), and for hookah smoking, 1.9 (95% CI, 0.9–4.4). Risks by intensity of smoking bidis increased at successively higher intensities. The highest odds ratio for 9 pack–years was for bidi (3.9; 95% CI, 2.1–7.1), followed by hookah (1.9; 95% CI, 0.9–4.4) and cigarette (1.9; 95% CI, 0.9–4.4). There was a clear decreasing trend for years since quitting (Gupta *et al.*, 2001).

(*d*)   Laryngeal cancer

The case–control studies on bidi smoking and laryngeal and oesophageal cancer are summarized in Table 2.2.26.

In a hospital-based case–control investigation in Trivandrum, India, information on 190 men with squamous-cell carcinoma of the larynx confirmed by biopsy and 546 male controls was collected during 1983–84 (Sankaranarayanan *et al.*, 1990b). Unconditional logistic regression, sometimes with a forward stepwise approach, was used to produce estimates of relative risk adjusted for age and religion. Occasional users were excluded from the analyses of frequency, duration and age at starting smoking. All levels of intensity of bidi smoking were associated with significant relative risk estimates, ranging from 1.8 (95% CI, 1.1–2.9) to 5.1 (95% CI, 2.7–9.6), with a highly significant trend ($p < 0.001$). When duration of bidi smoking was tested in a forward stepwise logistic regression model adjusted for cigarette smoking, alcohol consumption and the combination of bidi with cigarette smoking, the relative risk for bidi smoking for more than 21 years was 7.1 (95% CI, 4.0–12.5), with a highly significant trend ($p < 0.001$). Daily intensity of bidi and cigarette smoking also exhibited a highly significant trend in this model ($p < 0.001$).

The case–control study described in the section on cancer of the pharynx (Rao *et al.*, 1999) also included 427 patients with cancer of larynx. A total of 635 controls were selected from male outpatients at the same hospital who had been found to be free from cancer, benign tumours and infectious disease. Cases and controls were stratified into four 5-year age groups and by place of residence. The estimated relative risk for bidi smoking was 2.3 (95% CI, 1.7–3.2). A dose–response relationship was observed for number of bidis smoked daily. When unconditional logistic regression was performed using five factors, bidi smoking was the most important risk factor.

(e)   Oesophageal cancer

A hospital-based case–control study of oesophageal cancer was carried out during 1983–84 at the Regional Cancer Centre, Trivandrum in Kerala, India (Sankaranarayanan et al., 1991). Among 267 cases recruited to the study, 67% were histopathologically confirmed and the remainder were radiologically diagnosed. From outpatients attending the centre and surrounding medical complex during this period, 895 controls with non-malignant or pre-malignant conditions were selected. Relative risks were adjusted for age and religion through unconditional logistic regression. Significant effects were noted in men for all levels of intensity of bidi smoking and for a duration of more than 20 years of bidi smoking (Table 2.2.26). The trends for intensity and for duration of smoking of bidis and of bidis and cigarettes were all significant. In a forward stepwise logistic regression model, duration of bidi smoking and daily frequency of bidi/cigarette smoking emerged as statistically significant factors.

A hospital-based case–control study investigated the risk for oesophageal cancer by subsite and histomorphology at the Kidwai Memorial Institute of Oncology, Bangalore, in Karnataka, India (Nandakumar et al., 1996). Of 549 patients (284 men, 265 women) diagnosed with oesophageal cancer between 1982 and 1985, data were collected on 343 (177 men, 166 women) using a structured questionnaire. Of these, 236 cases had a micros-copically confirmed diagnosis of squamous-cell carcinoma. For each case, two controls were randomly selected from a database of 1875 patients who were proven not to have cancer or benign tumours. They were matched on sex, 5-year age group, area of residence and calendar time of their hospital visit. Among the men, 12 cases and 15 controls predo-minantly smoked bidis but also smoked cigarettes, and were combined with the bidi smokers. Similarly, four men who predominantly smoked cigarettes but also smoked bidis were considered to be cigarette smokers. Women were not included in the analyses because few of them practised those habits. After adjusting for tobacco chewing, chewing of betel quid without tobacco, alcohol drinking and cigarette smoking, bidi smoking had an odds ratio of 4.0 (95% CI, 2.3–6.8) for cancer of the oesophagus. Bidi smoking resulted in a significantly elevated risk for all three segments of the oesophagus, but the highest was for the upper third (odds ratio, 7.1; 95% CI, 1.1–46.8), followed by the middle third (odds ratio, 6.0; 95% CI, 2.5–14.5) and the lower third (odds ratio, 3.9; 95% CI, 1.4–10.7).

In a case–control study conducted from February 1994 to March 1997 at the All India Institute of Medicine (AIIMS), New Delhi, 150 patients with histopathologically con-firmed oesophageal cancer were enrolled as cases (Nayar et al., 2000). An equal number of controls were selected from individuals accompanying patients to the same hospital, after matching for age (± 5 years), sex and socioeconomic status. Both cases and controls had to meet the criterion that they had not suffered from any major illness in the past that had caused them to change their dietary consumption pattern. Data were stratified on socioeconomic status into five groups. Using unconditional stepwise logistic regression, bidi smoking showed an odds ratio of 2.0 (95% CI, 1.2–3.3). This was adjusted for other risk factors in the model, such as chewing of betel leaf with tobacco and low consumption of vegetables other than leafy vegetables.

(f)   Stomach cancer

A hospital-based case–control study of stomach cancer was conducted at the Cancer Institute (WIA), Madras, located in south India, as part of a multi-centre study (Gajalakshmi & Shanta, 1996; see Table 2.2.27). Patients with stomach cancer confirmed by histology, endoscopy, barium meal or surgery were included in the study. The control pool was formed by cancer patients diagnosed at the Cancer Institute, excluding those with cancer of the oral cavity, pharynx, larynx, lung, urinary bladder, pancreas and gastro-intestinal tract. Each case was matched with a cancer patient from the control pool on age, sex, religion and mother tongue. Details collected on smoking habits included type of tobacco smoked, age at starting smoking, amount smoked per day, and age at cessation (more than 6 months prior to diagnosis of cancer). The odds ratio for stomach cancer for current smoking of any type of tobacco was 2.7 (95% CI, 1.8–4.1); for current bidi smoking the odds ratio was 3.2 (95% CI, 1.8–5.7); that for chutta smoking was 2.4 (95% CI, 1.2–4.9); that for having more than one smoking habit was 8.2 (95% CI, 1.7–38.9). The trend for increasing lifetime exposure to bidi smoking was highly significant ($p < 0.001$). A significant trend for increasing lifetime chutta smoking was also seen. In a multivariate model including tobacco habits, alcohol drinking and various dietary factors, as well as income, education and area of residence, the odds ratios for current smokers, former smokers and ever-smokers were not substantially different from those in the above models.

Table 2.2.1. Cohort studies on exclusive pipe and/or cigar smoking and cancer of the oral cavity and pharynx

Reference Study and years of study	Site ICD codes	Smoking category (cases or deaths)	Relative risk (95% CI)	Variables adjusted for/comments
Pipe only or cigar only				
Hammond & Horn (1958) American Cancer Society (9-State) Study 1952–55	Oral cavity, pharynx, larynx, oesophagus	Never-smoker (4) Ever pipe only (7) Ever cigar only (10)	1.0 3.5 [1.02–12.0] 5.0 [1.6–15.9]	Age
Kahn (1966) US Veterans' Study 1954–62	Oral cavity 140–144 (ICD-7)	Never-smoker (11) Former pipe only (1) Current pipe only (4) Former cigar only (2) Current cigar only (9)	1.0 2.5 [0.3–19.1] 3.1 [0.99–9.8] 3.0 [0.7–13.5] 4.1 [1.7–9.9]	Age
	Pharynx 145–148 (ICD-7)	Never-smoker (4) Former pipe only (0) Current pipe only (1) Former cigar only (1) Current cigar only (0)	1.0 – 2.0 [0.2–17.7] 3.7 [0.4–32.8] –	Age
Carstensen et al. (1987) Swedish Census Study 1963–79	Oral cavity, pharynx, larynx 140–146, 148, 161 (ICD-8)	Never-smoker (4) Current pipe only (3) Current cigar only (1)	1.0 1.4 [0.3–6.3] 0.6 [0.1–5.4]	Age, residence
Shanks & Burns (1998) Cancer Prevention Study I 1959–72	Oral cavity, pharynx, excluding salivary glands	Never-smoker (18) Current cigar only (25) 1–2 cigars/day 3–4 cigars/day > 5 cigars/day No inhalation Slight inhalation Moderate and deep inhalation	1.0 7.9 (5.1–11.7) 2.1 (0.4–6.2) 8.5 (3.7–16.8) 15.9 (8.7–26.8) 7.0 (4.1–11.0) 7.8 (1.6–22.9) 27.9 (5.6–81.5)	Age
	Pharynx	Never-smoker (10) Current cigar only (12) 1–2 cigars/day 3–4 cigars/day > 5 cigars/day	1.0 6.7 (3.5–11.8) 3.8 (0.8–11.1) 7.5 (2.0–19.3) 9.9 (3.2–23.2)	

Table 2.2.1 (contd)

Reference Study and years of study	Site ICD codes	Smoking category (cases or deaths)	Relative risk (95% CI)	Variables adjusted for/ comments
Shanks & Burns (1998) (contd)		No inhalation Slight inhalation Moderate and deep inhalation	6.9 (3.3–12.6) 5.0 (0.1–27.7) 15.5 (3.6–12.1)	
Iribarren et al. (1999) Kaiser Permanente Medical Care Program Study 1971–96	Oral cavity, pharynx	Never-smoker (39) Current cigar only (8) < 5 cigars/day (3) > 5 cigars/day (4)	1.0 2.6 (1.2–5.8) 1.3 (0.4–4.4) 7.2 (2.4–21.2)	Age, race, body-mass index, diabetes, alcohol, occupational exposures
	Oral cavity, pharynx, larynx, oesophagus	Never-smoker (57) Current cigar only (10) < 5 cigars/day (4) > 5 cigars/day (5)	1.0 2.0 (1.0–4.1) 1.1 (0.4–3.1) 5.2 (2.0–13.5)	
Shapiro et al. (2000) Cancer Prevention Study II 1982–94	Oral cavity, pharynx	Never-smoker (20) Former cigar only (4) Current cigar only (6) 1–2 cigars/day (0) > 3 cigars/day (6) < 25 years (0) ≥ 25 years (5) No inhalation (3) Inhalation (2)	1.0 2.4 (0.8–7.3) 4.0 (1.5–10.3) – 7.6 (2.9–19.6) – 4.6 (1.6–13.0) 3.2 (0.9–11.0) 6.5 (1.4–29.2)	Age, alcohol, use of smokeless tobacco
Pipe and cigar				
Doll & Peto (1976) British Doctors' Study 1951–71	Oral cavity (excluding nasopharynx), pharynx, larynx, trachea	Never-smoker Current pipe/cigar only	1.0 9.0	Age Includes former cigarette smokers
Chow et al. (1993) US Veterans' Study 1954–80	Nasopharynx	Never-smoker (5) Ever pipe/cigar only (2)	1.0 1.0 (0.2–5.2)	Age, year

Table 2.2.2. Case–control studies on exclusive pipe and/or cigar smoking and cancers of the oral cavity and pharynx

Reference Country and years of study	Study characteristics	Site ICD9 codes	Smoking category (cases/controls)	Relative risk (95% CI)	Variables adjusted for/comments
Pipe only or cigar only					
Zheng et al. (1990) China 1988–89	248 cases (men) 248 hospital controls, age 18–80 years, response rate 100/100%	Oral cavity 141,143–145	Never-smoker (58/105) Ever pipe only (47/13) < 8 g tobacco/day 8–15.2 g tobacco/day > 15.2 g tobacco/day	1.0 5.7 (2.4–13.3) 3.5 (1.2–10.1) 4.9 (2.0–12.1) 6.3 (2.6–15.2)	Hospital, age, alcohol, education
	156 cases (women) 156 hospital controls	Oral cavity 141,143–145	Never-smoker (104/140) Ever pipe only (26/5)	1.0 4.9 (1.5–16.0)	
La Vecchia et al. (1998) Italy/Switzerland 1984–97	59 cases (men) 801 hospital controls, age < 75 years, response rate 98/97%	Oral cavity, pharynx, oesophagus [codes not given]	Never-smoker (50/788) Current cigar only (7/5) Ever cigar only (9/13) Ever > 3 cigars/day (4/5)	1.0 14.9 (4.0–55.9) 6.8 (2.5–18.5) 8.9 (2.1–36.9)	Age, alcohol, education Same study population as Franceschi et al. (1990) (see below)
	36 cases (men) 23 cases (men)	Oral cavity, pharynx Oesophagus	Ever cigar only Ever cigar only	9.0 (2.7–30.0) 4.1 (0.7–23.0)	
Pipe and cigar					
Blot et al. (1988) USA 1984–85	762 cases (men) 837 population controls, age 18–79 years, median 63; response rate 75/76%	Oral cavity, pharynx 141,143–146; 148–149	Never-smoker (50/185) Ever pipe/cigar only (52/56) ≥ 40 cigars/week (14/1) ≥ 40 pipefuls/week (12/7)	1.0 1.9 (1.1–3.4) 16.7 (3.7–76.7) 3.1 (1.1–8.7)	Age, race, location, alcohol, respondent status (self/proxy)
Franceschi et al. (1990) Italy 1986–89	291 cases (men) 1272 hospital controls, age < 75 years, response rate 98/97%	Oral cavity 140–141, 143–145	Never-smoker (4/289) Ever pipe/cigar only (6/14)	1.0 20.7 (5.6–76.3)	Age, area
		Pharynx 146, 148, 161.1	Never-smoker (2/289) Ever pipe/cigar only (0/2)	—	

Table 2.2.2 (contd)

Reference Country and years of study	Study characteristics	Site ICD9 codes	Smoking category (cases/controls)	Relative risk (95% CI)	Variables adjusted for/ comments
Franceschi et al. (1992) Italy 1986–90	102 cases (men) 726 hospital controls 104 cases (men) age < 75 years, median 58, response rate 98/97%	Tongue 141 Mouth 143–145,149	Never-smoker (3/153) Current pipe/cigar only (1/6) Never-smoker (3/153) Current pipe/cigar only (5/6)	1.0 3.4 (0.3–39.1) 1.0 21.9 (3.8–125.6)	Age, area, occupation, alcohol Age, area, occupation, alcohol Same study population as as Franceschi et al. (1990) (see above)
Fernandez Garrote et al. (2001) Cuba 1996–99	200 cases (men/ women) 200 hospital controls, age 25–91 years, median 63; response rate 88/79%	Oral cavity, pharynx [codes not given]	Never-smoker (16/81) Current pipe/cigar only < 4 pipes/cigars/day (6/7) ≥ 4 pipes/cigars/day (11/3)	1.0 4.3 (1.1–16.4) 20.5 (4.7–89.7)	Age, sex, area, education, alcohol p for trend < 0.01

Table 2.2.3. Effect of interaction between pipe and/or cigar smoking and alcohol drinking on cancer of the oral cavity and pharynx

Reference Country and years of study	Study characteristics	Site ICD9 codes	Smoking/alcohol category (cases/deaths)	Relative risk (95% CI)	Variables adjusted for/comments
Pipe only or cigar only					
Iribarren et al. (1999) Kaiser Permanente Medical Care Program Study 1971–1996	17 774 men, 47 cases, age 30–85 years, median 46	Oral cavity, pharynx 140–149	Never-smoker/< 2 drinks/day (39) Never-smoker/> 3 drinks/day (1) Current cigar/< 2 drinks/day (4) Current cigar/> 3 drinks/day (4)	1.0 0.4 (0.1–2.8) 1.5 (0.5–4.3) 7.6 (2.7–21.6)	
Pipe and cigar					
Blot et al. (1988) USA 1984–85	762 cases (men) 837 population controls age 18–79 years, median 63	Oral cavity, pharynx 141, 143–146, 148–149	Never-smoker/< 1 drink/week Ever pipe/cigar/< 1 drink/week Ever pipe/cigar/1–4 drinks/week Ever pipe/cigar/5–14 drinks/week Ever pipe/cigar/15–29 drinks/week Ever pipe/cigar/≥ 30 drinks/week	1.0 0.6 1.0 3.7 4.7 23.0	Age, race, location, respondent status (self/ proxy)

Table 2.2.4. Cohort studies on exclusive pipe and/or cigar smoking and lung cancer

Reference Study and years of study	Smoking category (cases or deaths)	Relative risk (95% CI)	Variables adjusted for/comments
Pipe only or cigar only			
Hammond & Horn (1958) American Cancer Society (9-state) Study 1952–55	Never-smoker (15) Ever pipe only (18) Ever cigar only (7)	1.0 3.0 [1.5–6.0] 1.0 [0.4–2.5]	Age
Kahn (1966) US Veterans' Study 1954–62	Never-smoker (78) Former pipe only (7) Current pipe only (17) Former cigar only (5) Current cigar only (25)	1.0 2.4 [1.1–5.2] 1.8 [1.1–3.1] 1.0 [0.4–2.5] 1.6 [1.01–2.5]	Age
Carstensen et al. (1987) Swedish Census Study 1963–79	Never-smoker (23) Current pipe only (59) Current cigar only (11)	1.0 7.2 [4.4–11.7] 7.6 [3.7–15.6]	Age, residence; risk increased with grams of tobacco smoked per day.
Lange et al. (1992) Copenhagen City Heart Study 1976–89	Never-smoker (5) Current cigar/cheroot only (47) Current pipe only (16)	1.0 6.0 (2.2–17) 4.1 (1.4–13)	Men; age; 17% lung cancer deaths attributable to cigar/cheroot and pipe smoking
	Never-smoker (7) Current cigar/cheroot only (14)	1.0 4.9 (3.0–12)	Women; age; 10% lung cancer deaths attributable to cigar/cheroot smoking
Tverdal et al. (1993) Norwegian Screening Study 1973–88	Never-smoker (4) Current pipe only (19)	1.0 [13.0 (4.4–38.2)]	Age and area
Ben-Shlomo et al. (1994) Whitehall Study 1967–87	Never-smoker (24) Current pipe only (8) Current cigar only (1)	1.0 [4.0 (1.8–8.9)] [1.8 (0.2–13.3)]	Age
Wald & Watt (1997) BUPA Study 1975–93	Never-smoker (7) Current pipe/cigar only (6)	1.0 3.2 (1.1–9.5)	Age
Shanks & Burns (1998) CPS-I 1959–72	Never-smoker (191) Current cigar only (73) 1–2 cigars/day 3–4 cigars/day > 5 cigars/day No inhalation Slight inhalation Moderate and deep inhalation	1.0 2.1 (1.6–2.7) 0.9 (0.5–1.7) 2.4 (1.5–3.5) 3.4 (2.3–4.8) 2.0 (1.5–2.6) 1.9 (0.8–3.7) 4.9 (1.8–10.7)	Age

Table 2.2.4 (contd)

Reference Study and years of study	Smoking category (cases or deaths)	Relative risk (95% CI)	Variables adjusted for/comments
Iribarren *et al.* (1999) Kaiser Permanente Medical Care Program Study 1971–96	Never-smoker (54) Current cigar only (11) < 5 cigars/day (6) > 5 cigars/day (3)	1.0 2.1 (1.1–4.1) 1.6 (0.7–3.7) 3.2 (1.01–10.4)	Age, race, body-mass index, diabetes, alcohol, occupational exposures
Shapiro *et al.* (2000) CPS-II 1982–94	Never-smoker (269) Former cigar only (36) Current cigar only (88) 1–2 cigars/day (10) > 3 cigars/day (68) < 25 years (8) > 25 years (75) No inhalation (36) Inhalation (37)	1.0 1.6 (1.2–2.4) 5.1 (4.0–6.6) 1.3 (0.7–2.4) 7.8 (5.9–10.3) 2.1 (1.0–4.2) 5.9 (4.5–7.7) 3.3 (2.3–4.7) 11.3 (7.9–16.1)	Age, alcohol, smokeless tobacco
Pipe and cigar			
Doll & Peto (1976) British Doctors' Study 1951–71	Never-smoker Current pipe/cigar only	1.0 5.8	Age
Chow *et al.* (1992) Lutheran Brotherhood Insurance Study 1966–86	Never-smoker (6) Current pipe/cigar only (4) Former pipe/cigar only (1)	1.0 3.5 (1.0–12.6) 1.3 (0.2–10.5)	Age and occupation

Table 2.2.5. Case–control studies on exclusive pipe and/or cigar smoking and lung cancer

Reference Country and years of study	Study charac-teristics	Smoking category (cases/controls)	Relative risk (95% CI)	Variables adjusted for/comments
Pipe only or cigar only				
Lubin *et al.* (1984) 7 areas in Europe 1976–80	6920 cases (men) 13 460 hospital controls	Never-smoker (190/2616)	1.00	Age, study location, hospital
		Ever pipe only (39/197)	2.5 [1.8–3.7]	
		1–19 years (3/36)	1.1 [0.3–3.6]	
		20–29 years (3/43)	1.02 [0.3–3.3]	
		30–39 years (11/54)	2.5 [1.3–4.9]	
		≥ 40 years (22/64)	4.4 [2.7–7.4]	*p* for trend < 0.01
		1–3 pipes/day (14/49)	3.2 [1.8–6.0]	
		4–6 pipes/day (13/79)	2.2 [1.2–4.0]	
		≥ 7 pipes/day (12/68)	2.7 [1.4–5.1]	*p* for trend < 0.01
		Inhalation		
		Never inhaled	1.0	
		Moderately inhaled	1.3	
		Deeply inhaled	1.3	*p* for trend = 0.06 also adjusted for duration
		Current pipe only	1.0	
		1–4 years since quitting	2.0	
		> 5 years since quitting	0.9	*p* for trend = 0.33 also adjusted for duration
		Never-smoker (190/2616)	1.0	Age, study location, hospital
		Ever cigar only (37/145)	2.9 [2.0–4.3]	
		1–19 years (5/30)	2.4 [0.9–6.4]	
		20–29 years (10/29)	4.2 [2.0–8.8]	
		30–39 years (8/36)	2.4 [1.1–5.2]	
		≥ 40 years (14/50)	3.0 [1.6–5.5]	*p* trend < 0.01
		1–3 cigars/day (8/61)	1.6 [0.7–3.3]	
		4–6 cigars/day (12/59)	2.2 [1.2–4.1]	
		≥ 7 cigars/day (17/25)	8.9 [4.7–16.8]	*p* for trend < 0.01
		Inhalation		
		Never inhaled	1.0	
		Moderately inhaled	2.7	
		Deeply inhaled	9.5	*p* for trend < 0.01 also adjusted for duration
		Current cigar only	1.0	
		1–4 years since quitting	0.6	
		> 5 years since quitting	0.7	*p*-value for trend = 0.17 also adjusted for duration

Table 2.2.5 (contd)

Reference Country and years of study	Study characteristics	Smoking category (cases/controls)	Relative risk (95% CI)	Variables adjusted for/comments
Benhamou et al. (1986) France 1976–80	1529 cases (men) 2899 hospital controls [response rate not reported]	Never-smoker (36/650)	1.0	Age, hospital, interviewer
		Ever pipe only (5/56)	1.6 (0.5–4.5)	Same study population
		Inhalation		as Lubin et al. (1984)
		No inhalation (5/48)	1.9	
		Sometimes/rarely inhaled (0/6)	–	
		Usually/always inhaled (0/2)	–	
		Ever pipe only < 10 years (0/5)	1.0	
		Ever pipe only > 10 years (5/51)	1.17	
		Never-smoker (36/650)	1.0	Age, hospital,
		Ever cigar only (9/29)	5.6 (2.3–13.5)	interviewer
		Inhalation		
		No inhalation (6/28)	3.9	
		Sometimes/rarely inhaled (1/0)	–	
		Usually/always inhaled (2/1)	36.1	p for trend < 0.01
		Ever cigar only < 15 years (1/9)	1.0	
		Ever cigar only > 15 years (8/20)	3.6	
Damber & Larsson (1986) Sweden 1972–77	579 cases (men) 582 population controls (dead), response rate: 98/96%	Never-smoker (42/208)	1.0	Age; postal questionnaire —
		Ever pipe only (198/142)	6.9 [4.5–10.5]	answered by relatives
		< 100 g/week	4.7	of cases and or
		> 100 g/week	11.1	controls; risk increased
		Ever cigar only (7/7)	[5.0 (1.5–16.8)]	with years of smoking and decreased with years of cessation [odds ratios not given]
Qiao et al. (1989) China 1985	107 cases (men) 107 occupational controls, age 35–80 years, response rate: 100/100%	Never-smoker (3/5)	1.0	Age; participants were tin miners (1967–84); interviews with 10/6% proxy
		Ever water pipe only (24/23)	1.9 (0.4–9.4)	
Lubin et al. (1992) China 1984–88	544 cases (men) 1043 occupational and population controls, age 35–75 years, response rate: 92/91%	Never-smoker (9/72)	1.0	Age, type of control, proxy, years of work underground
		Ever pipe only (56/151)	1.8 (0.8–4.2)	
		1–150 g/month (18/41)	2.1 [0.9–5.1]	Smoking of water pipe
		200 g/month (4/18)	2.6 [0.7–9.3]	or Chinese long-stem
		250 g/month (25/44)	4.1 [1.8–9.6]	pipe (extension of
		≥ 300 g/month (9/47)	1.3 [0.5–3.5]	Qiao et al., 1989)
		1–29 years (7/21)	2.1 [0.7–6.3]	
		30–39 years (13/31)	2.7 [1.1–7.0]	
		40–49 years (24/70)	2.5 [1.1–5.8]	
		≥ 50 years (10/32)	2.1 [0.8–5.6]	

Table 2.2.5 (contd)

Reference Country and years of study	Study characteristics	Smoking category (cases/controls)	Relative risk (95% CI)	Variables adjusted for/comments
Boffetta *et al.* (1999) Germany, Italy, Sweden 1988–94	5621 cases (men) 7255 hospital controls, response rate 67/38% and above	**Pipe**		
		Nonsmoker (117/1750)	1.0	Age, study centre
		Ever pipe only (61/129)	7.9 (5.3–11.8)	
		< 20 years (3/33)	1.3 (0.4–4.5)	
		20.1–32 years (7/33)	3.4 (1.4–8.0)	
		32.1–44 years (21/33)	13.3 (7.2–24.9)	
		≥ 44.1 years (30/30)	19.1 (10.4–35.1)	*p* for trend < 0.0001
		< 3.5 g/day (2/10)	2.2 (0.5–10.4)	
		3.6–5.0 g/day (22/54)	7.9 (4.3–14.3)	
		5.1–10.7 g/day (6/18)	4.8 (1.9–12.6)	
		≥ 10.8 g/day (31/47)	12.4 (7.2–21.4)	*p* for trend = 0.1
		Age at start < 20 (27/48)	9.6 (5.6–16.7)	
		Age at start 20–26 (20/52)	6.3 (3.5–11.2)	
		Age at start ≥ 27 (14/29)	8.2 (4.1–16.3)	*p* for trend = 0.4
		Nonsmoker (117/1750)	1.0	Age, study centre
		Current pipe only	12.5 (7.7–20.2)	
		Former, quit 1–14 years ago	10.3 (5.1–20.5)	
		Former, quit > 15 years ago	1.4 (0.5–4.0)	
		Cigar/cigarillo		
		Nonsmoker (117/1750)	1.0	Age, study centre
		Ever cigar only (16/42)	5.6 (2.9–10.6)	
		Ever cigarillo only (21/31)	12.7 (6.9–23.7)	
		Ever cigar/cigarillo only (43/77)	9.0 (5.8–14.1)	
		< 13 years (4/21)	3.1 (1.0–9.4)	
		13.1–26 years (5/20)	4.3 (1.6–11.9)	
		26.1–39 years (12/17)	10.3 (4.7–22.7)	
		> 39.1 years (22/19)	20.7 (10.5–41.1)	*p* for trend = 0.0003
		< 5 g/day (5/22)	3.4 (1.3–9.5)	
		5.1–12 g/day (10/25)	6.2 (2.8–13.7)	
		12.1–15 g/day (5/11)	7.8 (2.6–23.4)	
		≥ 15.1 g/day (23/19)	21.1 (10.7–41.7)	*p* for trend = 0.01
		Age at start < 20 (20/20)	17.0 (8.6–33.4)	
		Age at start 20–26 (16/23)	10.5 (5.3–21.1)	
		Age at start > 27 (7/34)	3.4 (1.5–8.0)	*p* for trend = 0.002
		Inhalation		
		Non-inhaler	5.2 (2.7–10.0)	
		Inhaler	28.1 [9.5–83.6]	
		Nonsmoker (117/1750)	1.0	Age, study centre
		Current cigar/cigarillo only	10.6 (5.9–19.1)	
		Former, quit 1–14 years ago	8.8 (4.0–19.5)	
		Former, quit > 15 years ago	6.9 (3.1–15.1)	

Table 2.2.6. Studies on exclusive pipe and/or cigar smoking and cancer of the larynx

Reference Study and years of study	Smoking category (cases or deaths)	Relative risk (95% CI)	Variables adjusted for/ comments
Pipe only or cigar only			
Kahn (1966)	Never-smoker (3)	1.0	Age
US Veterans'	Former pipe only (0)	–	
Study	Current pipe only (0)	–	
1954–62	Former cigar only (0)	–	
	Current cigar only (6)	10.3 [2.6–41.3]	
Shanks & Burns	Never-smoker (4)	1.0	Age
(1998)	Current cigar only (7)	10.0 (4.0–20.6)	
CPS-I	1–2 cigars/day	6.5 (0.7–23.3)	
1959–72	3–4 cigars/day	–	
	> 5 cigars/day	26.0 (8.4–60.7)	
	No inhalation	10.6 (3.9–23.1)	
	Slight inhalation	–	
	Moderate and deep inhalation	53.3 (0.7–296.3)	
Shapiro et al.	Never-smoker (5)	1.0	Age, alcohol, smokeless
(2000)	Former cigar only (3)	6.7 (1.5–30.0)	tobacco use; excludes
CPS-II	Current cigar only (4)	10.3 (2.6–41.0)	cancer at baseline
1982–94	1–2 cigars/day (1)	6.0 (0.7–53.5)	
	> 3 cigars/day (3)	15.0 (3.4–65.9)	
	< 25 years (0)	–	
	> 25 years (4)	13.7 (3.4–54.5)	
	No inhalation (1)	4.2 (0.5–37.1)	
	Inhalation (3)	39.0 (8.4–180.1)	

Table 2.2.7. Case–control study on exclusive pipe and/or cigar smoking and cancer of the larynx

Reference Country and years of study	Study characteristics	Smoking category (cases/controls)	Relative risk (95% CI)	Variables adjusted for/ comments
Pipe and cigar				
Franceschi *et al.* (1990) Italy 1986–89	162 cases (men) 1272 hospital controls age < 75 years, response rate 98/97%	Never-smoker (8/289) Ever pipe/cigar only (1/14)	1.0 2.8 (0.3–26.1)	Age, area

Table 2.2.8. Cohort studies on exclusive pipe and/or cigar smoking and cancers of the oesophagus and stomach

Reference Name of study and years of study	Site	Smoking category (cases or deaths)	Relative risk (95% CI)	Variables adjusted for/comments
Pipe only or cigar only				
Hammond & Horn (1958) American Cancer Society (9-state) Study 1952–55	Stomach, pancreas, liver, colorectum	Never-smoker (100) Ever pipe only (41) Ever cigar only (63)	1.0 1.0 [0.7–1.4] 1.4 [1.1–1.8]	Age
Kahn (1966) US Veterans' Study 1954–62	Oesophagus	Never-smoker (11) Former pipe only (0) Current pipe only (3) Former cigar only (2) Current cigar only (12)	1.0 – 2.0 [0.6–7.1] 2.4 [0.5–10.9] 5.3 [2.4–12.1]	Age
	Stomach	Never-smoker (96) Former pipe only (4) Current pipe only (16 Former cigar only (8) Current cigar only (23)	1.0 1.1 [0.4–3.0] 1.4 [0.8–2.4] 1.3 [0.6–2.7] 1.2 [0.8–1.9]	
Carstensen et al. (1987) Swedish Census Study 1963–79	Oesophagus	Never smoker (5) Current pipe only (6) Current cigar only (2)	1.0 3.6 [1.1–11.8] 6.5 [1.3–33.5]	Age, residence
Tverdal et al. (1993) Norwegian Screening Study 1973–88	Stomach	Never-smoker (8) Current pipe only (4)	1.0 [1.5 (0.5–5.1)]	Age and area
Shanks & Burns (1998) CPS-I 1959–72	Oesophagus	Never-smoker (30) Current cigar only (19) 1–2 cigars/day 3–4 cigars/day > 5 cigars/day No inhalation Slight inhalation Moderate and deep inhalation	1.0 3.6 (2.2–5.6) 2.3 (0.7–5.3) 3.9 (1.4–8.6) 5.2 (2.2–10.2) 3.4 (1.9–5.6) 1.9 (0.0–10.6) 14.8 (3.0–43.5)	Age
Shapiro et al. (2000) CPS-II 1982–94	Oesophagus	Never-smoker (67) Former cigar only (8) Current cigar only (9) 1–2 cigars/day (4) > 3 cigars/day (5) < 25 years (1) > 25 years (8) No inhalation (5) Inhalation (1)	1.0 1.3 (0.6–2.8) 1.8 (0.9–3.7) 1.8 (0.6–5.0) 1.9 (0.8–4.9) 0.9 (0.1–6.4) 2.2 (1.0–4.7) 1.6 (0.7–4.1) 1.0 (0.1–7.2)	Age, alcohol, smokeless tobacco use

Table 2.2.8 (contd)

Reference Name of study and years of study	Site	Smoking category (cases or deaths)	Relative risk (95% CI)	Variables adjusted for/comments
Chao *et al.* (2002) CPS-II 1982–96	Stomach	Never-smoker	1.0	Age, race, education, family history of stomach cancer, use of aspirin and several dietary habits
		Former cigar only (13)	1.3 (0.7–2.2)	
		Current cigar only (25)	2.3 (1.5–3.5)	
		1–4 cigars/day (13)	1.7 (0.95–3.0)	
		≥ 5 cigars/day (12)	4.2 (2.3–7.6)	
		< 39 years of smoking (13)	2.4 (1.4–4.3)	
		≥ 40 years of smoking (10)	2.6 (1.3–4.9)	
		Age at starting		
		≥ 30 years (5)	1.6 (0.7–4.0)	
		20–29 years (12)	2.9 (1.6–5.2)	
		≤ 19 years (6)	2.4 (1.1–5.6)	
		No inhalation (15)	2.1 (1.2–3.6)	
		Inhalation (8)	3.9 (1.9–8.0)	
		Former pipe only (6)	0.7 (0.3–1.6)	
		Current pipe only (16)	1.3 (0.8–2.2)	
Pipe and cigar				
Doll & Peto (1976) British Doctors' Study 1951–71	Oesophagus	Never-smoker	1.0	Age
		Current pipe/cigar only	3.7	
Kneller *et al.* (1991) Lutheran Brotherhood Insurance Study 1966–86	Stomach	Never-smoker (8)	1.0	Age
		Tobacco but never cigarettes (6)	1.5 (0.5–4.4)	

Table 2.2.9. Case–control studies on exclusive pipe and/or cigar smoking and cancers of the oesophagus and stomach

Reference Country and years of study	Study characteristics	Site	Smoking category (cases/controls)	Relative risk (95% CI)	Variables adjusted for/comments
Pipe only or cigar only					
La Vecchia et al. (1998) Italy/Switzerland 1984–97	23 cases (men) 801 hospital controls age <75 years; response rate 98/97%	Oesophagus	Never-smoker (50/788) Ever cigar only	1.0 4.1 (0.7–23.0)	Age, alcohol consumption, education Same study population as Franceschi et al. (1990) below
Pipe and cigar					
Wu-Williams et al. (1990) USA 1975–82	137 cases (white men) 137 population controls, mean age 47 years, response rate 52% (matched design)	Stomach	Never-smoker (21/35) Ever pipe/cigar only (3/3)	1.0 1.8 (0.3–9.8)	Age, race, area
Franceschi et al. (1990) Italy 1986–89	288 cases (men) 1272 hospital controls age <75 years, response rate 98/97%	Oesophagus	Never-smoker (17/289) Ever pipe/cigar only (7/14)	1.0 6.3 (2.3–19.8)	Age, area
Kabat et al. (1993) USA 1981–90	431 cases (white men) 4544 hospital controls [response rate not reported]	SCCE AEC ADS	Never-smoker (15/1054) Ever pipe/cigar only (11/332) Never-smoker (25/1054) Ever pipe/cigar only (9/332) Never-smoker (23/1054) Ever pipe/cigar only (8/332)	1.0 1.8 (0.8–4.1) 1.0 1.1 (0.5–2.3) 1.0 1.0 (0.4–2.2)	Age, hospital, time period, education, alcohol consumption

SCCE, squamous-cell carcinoma of the oesophagus; AEC, adenocarcinoma of the oesophagus or cardia; ADS, adenocarcinoma of the distal stomach

Table 2.2.10. Cohort studies on exclusive pipe and/or cigar smoking and colorectal cancer

Reference Name of study and years of study	Site ICD code	Smoking category (cases or deaths)	Relative risk (95% CI)	Variables adjusted for/comments
Pipe only or cigar only				
Tverdal et al. (1993) Norwegian Screening Study 1973–88	Colon	Never-smoker (9)	1.0	Age and area
		Current pipe only (3)	[0.9 (0.2–3.2)]	
	Rectum	Never-smoker (7)	1.0	
		Current pipe only (4)	[1.6 (0.5–5.5)]	
Heineman et al. (1995) US Veterans' Study 1954–80	Colon	Never-smoker (782)	1.0	Age, calendar year, year of survey, socioeconomic status, sedentary job
		Current pipe/cigar only (576)	1.3 (1.1–1.4)	
		Current pipe < 5/day (22)	1.2 (0.8–1.9)	
		Current pipe 5–9/day (27)	1.2 (0.8–1.7)	
		Current pipe 10–19/day (11)	0.7 (0.4–1.2)	
		Current pipe > 20/day (15)	1.8 (1.1–2.9)	p for trend = 0.30
		Current cigar 1–2/day (50)	1.5 (1.1–1.9)	
		Current cigar 3–4/day (34)	0.9 (0.6–1.3)	
		Current cigar 5–8/day (44)	1.4 (1.1–1.9)	
		Current cigar > 9/day (15)	2.2 (1.3–3.7)	p for trend = 0.004
	Ascending 153.0	Never-smoker (67)	1.0	
		Current pipe/cigar only (48)	1.2 (0.8–1.7)	
	Transverse 153.1	Never-smoker (15)	1.0	
		Current pipe/cigar only (7)	0.8 (0.3–2.0)	
	Descending 153.2	Never-smoker (15)	1.0	
		Current pipe/cigar only (5)	0.6 (0.2–1.6)	
	Sigmoid 153.3	Never-smoker (67)	1.0	
		Current pipe/cigar only (54)	1.4 (1.0–2.0)	
	Rectum	Never-smoker (201)	1.0	
		Current pipe/cigar only (169)	1.4 (1.2–1.8)	
		Current pipe < 5/day (3)	0.6 (0.2–2.0)	
		Current pipe 5–9/day (11)	1.9 (1.0–3.5)	
		Current pipe 10–19/day (10)	2.3 (1.2–4.4)	
		Current pipe > 20/day (4)	1.8 (0.7–4.8)	p for trend = 0.007
		Current cigar 1–2/day (14)	1.6 (0.9–2.7)	
		Current cigar 3–4/day (13)	1.4 (0.8–2.4)	
		Current cigar 5–8/day (13)	1.6 (0.9–2.9)	
		Current cigar > 9/day (1)	0.6 (0.1–4.2)	p for trend = 0.12

Table 2.2.10 (contd)

Reference Name of study and years of study	Site ICD code	Smoking category (cases or deaths)	Relative risk (95% CI)	Variables adjusted for/comments
Iribarren et al. (1999) Kaiser Permanente Medical Care Program Study 1971–96	Colon and rectum	Never-smoker (332) Current cigar only (39)	1.0 1.1 (0.8–1.6)	Age, race, body-mass index, diabetes, alcohol, occupational exposure; excludes cancer of interest at baseline
Pipe and cigar				
Doll & Peto (1976) British Doctors' Study 1951–71	Rectum	Never-smoker Current pipe/cigar only	1.0 1.7	Age
Hsing et al. (1998) Lutheran Brotherhood Insurance Study 1966–86	Colon Colon and rectum	Never-smoker (16) Ever pipe/cigar only (16) Never-smoker (26) Ever pipe/cigar only (17)	1.0 1.6 (0.8–3.2) 1.0 1.0 (0.5–1.9)	Age, urban/rural, alcohol
Knekt et al. (1998) Finnish Mobile Clinic Health Examination Study 1966–94	Colon and rectum Colon Rectum	Never-smoker (264) Current pipe/cigar only (14) Never-smoker (144) Current pipe/cigar only (6) Never-smoker (120) Current pipe/cigar only (8)	1.0 1.5 (0.8–2.6) 1.0 1.5 (0.6–3.5) 1.0 1.5 (0.7–3.1)	Age, sex, body-mass index, area, occupation, marital status
Chao et al. (2000) CPS-II 1982–96	Colon and rectum	Never-smoker (2156) Current pipe/cigar only ≥ 20 years	1.0 1.3 (1.1–1.6)	Age, race, body-mass index, education, exercise, intake of aspirin, multivitamins, alcohol, fibre, vegetables and fatty meats, and family history of colorectal cancer

Table 2.2.11. Cohort studies on exclusive pipe and/or cigar smoking and cancer of the liver and intrahepatic bile ducts

Reference Name of study and years of study	Smoking category (cases or deaths)	Relative risk (95% CI)	Variables adjusted for/ comments
Pipe only or cigar only			
Carstensen *et al.* (1987) Swedish Census Study 1963–79	Never-smoker (9) Current pipe only (5) Current cigar only (4)	1.0 1.7 [0.6–5.1] 7.2 [2.2–23.4]	Age, residence
Hsing *et al.* (1990a) US Veterans' Study 1954–80	Nonsmoker (37) Current cigar/pipe smoker (47)	1.0 3.1 (2.0–4.8)	Age, year

Table 2.2.12. Case–control study on exclusive pipe and/or cigar smoking and cancer of the gallbladder and extrahepatic bile ducts

Reference Country and years of study	Study characteristics	Site	Smoking category (cases/controls)	Relative risk (95% CI)	Variables adjusted for/ comments
Pipe and cigar					
Chow et al. (1994) USA 1985–89	49 cases (white men) 97 population controls; age, 30–84 years; response rate: 76/84%	Extrahepatic bile duct	Never-smoker (6/25) Ever pipe/cigar only (2/7)	1.0 1.6 (0.3–9.9)	Adjusted for age and ethnicity (58% proxy for deceased cases)
		Ampulla of Vater	Never-smoker (1/25) Ever pipe/cigar only (2/7)	1.0 7.6 (0.6–100.4)	

Table 2.2.13. Cohort studies on exclusive pipe and/or cigar smoking and cancer of the pancreas

Reference Name of study and years of study	Smoking category (cases or deaths)	Relative risk (95% CI)	Variables adjusted for/ comments
Pipe only or cigar only			
Kahn (1966) US Veterans' Study 1954–62	Never-smoker (88) Former pipe only (2) Current pipe only (8) Former cigar only (5) Current cigar only (27)	1.0 0.6 [0.2–2.4] 0.7 [0.4–1.5] 0.9 [0.4–2.1] 1.5 [0.99–2.3]	Age
Carstensen et al. (1987) Swedish Census Study 1963–79	Never-smoker (20) Current pipe only (19) Current cigar only (1)	1.0 2.8 [1.5–5.2] 1.0 [0.1–7.5]	Age, residence
Tverdal et al. (1993) Norwegian Screening Study 1973–88	Never-smoker (5) Current pipe only (2)	1.0 [1.2 (0.2–6.2)]	Age and area

Shanks & Burns (1998)
CPS-I
1959–72
	Never-smoker (198)
	Current cigar only (56)
	  1–2 cigars/day
	  3–4 cigars/day
	  > 5 cigars/day
	  No inhalation
	  Slight inhalation
	  Moderate and deep inhalation
		1.0
		1.6 (1.2–2.1)
		1.2 (0.7–1.9)
		1.5 (0.9–2.5)
		2.2 (1.4–3.2)
		1.6 (1.1–2.1)
		2.2 (0.99–4.1)
		2.3 (0.5–6.6)
			Age

Iribarren et al. (1999) Kaiser Permanente Medical Care Program Study 1971–96	Never-smoker (46) Current cigar only (6)	1.0 1.2 (0.5–2.9)	Age, race, body-mass index, diabetes, alcohol, occupational exposures

Shapiro et al. (2000)
CPS-II
1982–94
	Never-smoker (327)
	Former cigar only (30)
	Current cigar only (28)
	  1–2 cigars/day (6)
	  > 3 cigars/day (18)
	  < 25 years (7)
	  > 25 years (19)
	  No inhalation (12)
	  Inhalation (12)
		1.0
		1.1 (0.7–1.6)
		1.3 (0.9–1.9)
		0.6 (0.3–1.4)
		1.6 (1.0–2.5)
		1.5 (0.7–3.3)
		1.1 (0.7–1.8)
		0.9 (0.5–1.5)
		2.7 (1.5–4.8)
			Age, alcohol, smokeless tobacco use

Pipe and cigar			
Doll & Peto (1976) British Doctors' Study 1951–71	Never-smoker Current pipe/cigar only	1.0 0.9	Age
Zheng et al. (1993) Lutheran Brotherhood Insurance Study 1966–86	Never-smoker (9) Ever pipe/cigar only (5)	1.0 0.8 (0.3–2.5)	Age, alcohol

Table 2.2.14. Case–control studies on exclusive pipe and/or cigar smoking and cancer of the pancreas

Reference Country and years of study	Study characteristics	Smoking category (cases/controls)	Relative risk (95% CI)	Variables adjusted for/comments
Pipe only or cigar only				
Muscat et al. (1997) USA 1985–93	290 cases (men) 572 hospital controls mean age 61 years; response rate 51/63%	Never-smoker (66/157) Ever pipe/cigar only (25/28)	1.0 2.1 (1.2–3.8)	Age, education; trained interviewer
		Nonsmoker (146/334) Ever pipe only (16/20)	1.0 1.8 (0.9–5.3)	Age, education; referent includes long-term quitters (> 20 years)
		1–20 years (6/7) > 20 years (10/13) 1–5 pipes/day (7/10) > 5 pipes/day (9/10)	1.8 (0.6–5.3) 1.6 (0.7–3.7) 1.4 (0.5–3.8) 1.4 (0.9–2.2)	
		Nonsmoker (146/334) Ever cigar only (15/12)	1.0 3.1 (1.4–6.9)	Age, education; referent includes long-term quitters (> 20 years)
		1–20 years (7/4) > 20 years (8/7) 1–4 cigars/day (8/11) > 4 cigars/day (7/1)	3.9 (1.2–13.6) 2.2 (0.8–7.3) 1.4 (0.6–3.6) 14.1 (1.7–115.7)	
Pipe and cigar				
Mack et al. (1986) USA 1976–81	490 cases (men/women) 490 population controls age < 65 years response rate 68/76%	Never-smoker (97/154) Ever pipe/cigar only (7/13)	1.0 0.9 (0.3–2.3)	Age, sex, race, neighbourhood
Partanen et al. (1997) Finland 1984–87	625 cases (men/women) 1700 hospital controls age 40–74 years [response rates not reported]	Never-smoker Ever pipe/cigar only Former pipe/cigar only Current pipe/cigar only	1.0 2.3 (1.3–4.4) 1.3 (0.8–2.0) 2.6 (1.4–4.9)	Adjusted for age and sex; smoking status in 1960; former smokers were those who had quitted before interview.
		Interaction with alcohol Never smoker/never drinker Never smoker/moderate drinker Never smoker/heavy drinker Ever pipe/cigar/never drinker Ever pipe/cigar/moderate drinker Ever pipe/cigar/heavy drinker	1.0 1.1 (0.7–1.6) 0.8 (0.2–3.0) 2.2 (0.8–6.0) 2.2 (0.8–6.0) 2.2 (0.4–12.2)	Adjusted for age and sex

Table 2.2.15. Cohort studies on exclusive pipe and/or cigar smoking and cancer of the bladder and kidney

Reference Name of study and years of study	Site	Smoking category (cases or deaths)	Relative risk (95% CI)	Variables adjusted for/ comments
Pipe only or cigar only				
Hammond & Horn (1958) American Cancer Society (9-State) Study 1952–55	Bladder, kidney, prostate	Never-smoker (38) Ever pipe only (21) Ever cigar only (19)	1.0 1.2 [0.7–2.0] 1.1 [0.6–1.8]	Age
Kahn (1966) US Veterans' Study 1954–62	Bladder	Never-smoker (52) Former pipe only (1) Current pipe only (8) Former cigar only (4) Current cigar only (10)	1.0 0.5 [0.1–3.5] 1.2 [0.6–2.5] 1.1 [0.4–3.0] 0.9 [0.5–1.9]	Age
	Kidney	Never-smoker (39) Former pipe only (1) Current pipe only (6) Former cigar only (2) Current cigar only (6)	1.0 0.7 [0.1–5.0] 1.3 [0.6–3.1] 0.8 [0.2–3.5] 0.8 [0.3–1.8]	
Carstensen et al. (1987) Swedish Census Study 1963–79	Bladder	Never-smoker (11) Current pipe only (16) Current cigar only (1)	1.0 4.0 [1.9–8.6] 1.9 [0.2–14.7]	Age, residence
Shanks & Burns (1998) CPS-I 1959–72	Bladder	Never-smoker (102) Current cigar only (25) 1–2 cigars/day 3–4 cigars/day > 5 cigars/day No inhalation Slight inhalation Moderate and deep inhalation	1.0 1.4 (0.9–2.0) 0.8 (0.3–1.7) 1.7 (0.8–3.2) 2.0 (0.97–3.7) 1.6 (1.00–2.4) – 1.5 (0.0–8.4)	Age
Iribarren et al. (1999) Kaiser Permanente Medical Care Program Study 1971–96	Bladder Kidney	Never-smoker (99) Current cigar only (10) Never-smoker (50) Current cigar only (5)	1.0 1.1 (0.6–2.0) 1.0 1.1 (0.4–2.7)	Age, race, body-mass index, diabetes, alcohol, occupational exposures
Shapiro et al. (2000) CPS-II, 1982–94	Bladder	Never-smoker (94) Former cigar only (10) Current cigar only (6) 1–2 cigars/day (0) > 3 cigars/day (6) < 25 years (0) > 25 years (5) No inhalation (2) Inhalation (4)	1.0 1.3 (0.7–2.5) 1.0 (0.4–2.3) – 1.9 (0.8–4.4) – 1.1 (0.4–2.7) 0.5 (0.1–2.1) 3.6 (1.3–9.9)	Age, alcohol, smokeless tobacco use

Table 2.2.15 (contd)

Reference Name of study and years of study	Site	Smoking category (cases or deaths)	Relative risk (95% CI)	Variables adjusted for/ comments
Pipe and cigar				
Doll & Peto (1976) British Doctors' Study 1951–71	Bladder	Never-smoker Current pipe/cigar only	1.0 1.6	Age
Steineck *et al.* (1988) Swedish Twin Registry Study 1967–82	Bladder	Never-smoker (8) Ever pipe/cigar only (16)	1.0 3.3 (1.5–7.4)	Age

Table 2.2.16. Case–control studies on exclusive pipe and/or cigar smoking and cancer of the bladder and kidney

Pipe only or cigar only

Reference Country and years of study	Study characteristics	Site	Smoking category (cases/controls)	Relative risk (95% CI)	Variables adjusted for/comments
Jensen et al. (1987) Denmark 1979–81	389 cases (men/ women), 787 population controls, response rate 94/75%	Bladder	Never-smoker (26/132) Ever pipe only (6/18) Ever cigar only (1/2) Ever cigarillo only (8/39) Ever mixed only (18/55)	1.0 1.9 (0.7–5.4) 2.5 (0.2–28.4) 1.0 (0.4–2.4) 1.9 (0.9–3.8)	Age, sex; mixed includes pipe, cigar and cigarillo combined; study included in Pitard et al. (2001)
Jensen et al. (1988) Denmark 1979–82	96 cases (men/women) 288 hospital controls age < 80 years, response rate 99/100%	Renal pelvis, ureter	Never-smoker (8/57) Ever pipe only (1/10) Ever cigar only (4/24) Ever pipe/cigar only (3/7)	1.0 2.2 (0.1–97) 1.3 (0.3–6.1) 6.5 (0.4–21.2)	Age, sex
McLaughlin et al. (1995) Australia, Europe, USA 1989–91	1774 cases 2359 controls age 20–79 years; response rate 72/75%	Renal cell	Never-smoker (585/846) Ever cigar only (18/34) Ever pipe only (19/29)	1.0 0.8 (0.4–1.4) 0.9 (0.5–1.7)	Age, sex, centre, body-mass index

Pitard et al. (2001) Europe 1980–95	2279 cases (men) 5268 controls age < 80 years Pooled analysis	Bladder	Never-smoker (154/1109)
			Ever pipe only (28/85)
			  1–39 years (11/52)
			  > 40 years (16/33)
			Ever cigar only (50/122)
			  1–29 years (15/62)
			  30–39 years (12/28)
			  > 40 years (22/32)
			  0.1–1.5 cigars/day (4/23)
			  > 1.5 cigars/day (8/34)
			Ever pipe/cigar only (10/46)
				1.0
				1.9 (1.2–3.1)
				1.4 (0.7–2.8)
				2.5 (1.3–4.9)
				2.3 (1.6–3.5)
				1.4 (0.8–2.6)
				2.7 (1.3–5.7)
				3.8 (2.1–7.1)
				1.3 (0.4–4.0)
				1.9 (0.8–4.4)
				1.3 (0.6–2.6)
					Age, centre, occupational exposures
					
					p for trend = 0.006
					
					p for trend < 0.001
					
					p for trend = 0.1

Table 2.2.17. Cohort studies on exclusive pipe and/or cigar smoking and prostate cancer

Reference Name of study and years of study	Smoking category (cases or deaths)	Relative risk (95% CI)	Variables adjusted for/comments
Pipe only or cigar only			
Kahn (1966) US Veterans' Study 1954–62	Never-smoker (117) Former pipe only (5) Current pipe only (23) Former cigar only (11) Current cigar only (36)	1.0 1.1 [0.4–2.6] 1.5 [0.98–2.4] 1.3 [0.7–2.5] 1.5 [1.03–2.2]	Age
Tverdal et al. (1993) Norwegian Screening Study 1973–88	Never-smoker (4) Current pipe only (1)	1.0 [0.7 (0.1–5.9)]	Age and area
Pipe and cigar			
Hsing et al. (1990b) Lutheran Brotherhood Insurance Study 1966–86	Never-smoker (19) Ever pipe/cigar only (9)	1.0 1.6 (0.7–3.5)	Age
Hsing et al. (1991) US Veterans' Study 1954–80	Never-smoker (1075) Current pipe/cigar only (497)	1.0 1.1 (0.99–1.2)	Age

Table 2.2.18. Case–control study on exclusive pipe and/or cigar smoking and prostate cancer

Reference Country and years of study	Study characteristics	Smoking category (cases/controls)	Relative risk (95% CI)	Variables adjusted for/ comments
Pipe and cigar				
Sharpe & Siemiatycki (2001) Canada 1979–85	399 cases (men) 476 population controls, age 45–70 years, response rate 81/72%	Never-smoker (47/76) Ever pipe only (6/6) Ever cigar only (6/7)	1.0 1.2 (0.4–4.1) 1.3 (0.4–4.5)	Age, ethnicity, respondent status, body-mass index, income, alcohol consumption

Table 2.2.19. Cohort studies on exclusive pipe and/or cigar smoking and cancer of the haematopoietic system

Reference Name of study and years of study	Site	Smoking category (cases or deaths)	Relative risk (95% CI)	Variables adjusted for/comments
Pipe only or cigar only				
Hammond & Horn (1958) American Cancer Society (9-state) Study 1952–55	Lymphoma, leukaemia	Never-smoker (31)	1.0	Age
		Ever pipe only (15)	1.3 [0.7–2.3]	
		Ever cigar only (10)	0.7 [0.4–1.5]	
Kinlen & Rogot (1988) US Veterans' Study 1954–69	Lymphatic leukaemia	Never-smoker (41)	1.0	Age
		Ever pipe only (3)	0.8 (0.2–2.4)	
		Ever cigar only (11)	2.0 (1.0–3.6)	
	Monocytic myeloid leukaemia	Never-smoker (60)	1.0	
		Ever pipe only (6)	1.2 (0.4–2.6)	
		Ever cigar only (14)	1.8 (1.0–3.0)	
	Acute leukaemia	Never-smoker (40)	1.0	
		Ever pipe only (3)	0.9 (0.2–2.5)	
		Ever cigar only (8)	1.5 (0.7–3.0)	
Heineman et al. (1992) US Veterans' Study 1954–80	Multiple myeloma	Never-smoker (141)	1.0	Age, calendar year, year of response
		Ever pipe/cigar only (95)	1.2 (0.9–1.5)	
		Ever pipe only		
		< 5 pipes/day (6)	1.9	
		5–9 pipes/day (2)	0.5	
		10–19 pipes/day (3)	1.0	
		> 20 pipes/day (1)	0.6	
		Ever cigar only		
		1–2 cigars/day (8)	1.3	
		3–4 cigars/day (8)	1.2	
		5–8 cigars/day (2)	0.4	
		> 9 cigars/day (2)	1.7	
Tverdal et al. (1993) Norwegian Screening Study 1973–88	Leukaemia	Never-smoker (6)	1.0	Age and area
		Current pipe only (3)	[1.5 (0.4–5.9)]	

Table 2.2.19 (contd)

Reference Name of study and years of study	Site	Smoking category (cases or deaths)	Relative risk (95% CI)	Variables adjusted for/comments
Pipe and cigar				
Garfinkel & Boffetta (1990) CPS-I, 1959–65	Lymphatic leukaemia	Never-smoker Ever pipe/cigar only	1.0 1.1	Age, men only
	Myeloid leukaemia	Never-smoker Ever pipe/cigar only	1.0 1.5	
CPS-II, 1982–86	Lymphatic leukaemia	Never-smoker Ever pipe/cigar only	1.0 1.2	
	Myeloid leukaemia	Never-smoker Ever pipe/cigar only	1.0 0.9	

Table 2.2.20. Case–control studies on exclusive pipe and/or cigar smoking and cancers of the haematopoietic system

Reference Country and years of study	Study characteristics	Site	Smoking category (cases/controls)	Relative risk (95% CI)	Variables adjusted for/ comments
Pipe and cigar					
Kabat et al. (1988) USA 1969–85	342 cases (men) 5862 hospital controls age 20–80 years, mean 51 years; response rate 95/95%	Leukaemia	Never-smoker (94/1320) Ever pipe/cigar only (23/416)	1.0 0.78 (0.49–1.24)	Not adjusted; relative risk for non-cancer controls
Brown et al. (1992a) USA 1981–84	578 cases (white men) 820 population controls age > 30 years; response rate 86/78%	Acute non-lymphocytic leukaemia	Never-smoker (29/197) Ever pipe/cigar only (4/40)	1.0 0.7 (0.2–2.1)	Age, state, alcohol
		Chronic myelogenous leukaemia	Never-smoker (8/197) Ever pipe/cigar only (1/40)	1.0 0.6 (0.1–5.1)	
		Chronic lymphocytic leukaemia	Never-smoker (40/197) Ever pipe/cigar only (13/40)	1.0 1.6 (0.8–3.2)	
		Acute lymphocytic leukaemia	Never-smoker (5/197) Ever pipe/cigar only (1/40)	1.0 0.8 (0.1–7.2)	
Brown et al. (1992b) USA 1981–84	622 cases (white men) 820 population controls; age > 30 years; response rate 89/78%	Non-Hodgkin lymphoma	Never-smoker (116/197) Ever pipe/cigar only (29/40)	1.0 1.2 (0.8–2.1)	Age, state
	173 cases (white men) 452 population controls; age > 30 years; response rate 84/78%	Multiple myeloma	Never-smoker (41/105) Ever pipe/cigar only (6/22)	1.0 0.6 (0.2–1.6)	Age

Table 2.2.21. Cohort study on exclusive pipe and/or cigar smoking and brain cancer

Reference Name of study and years of study	Smoking category (cases or deaths)	Relative risk (95% CI)	Variables adjusted for/comments
Tverdal *et al.* (1993) Norwegian Screening Study 1973–88	Never-smoker (11) Current pipe only (2)	1.0 [0.5 (0.1–2.5)]	Age and area

Table 2.2.22. Case–control studies on bidi and other tobacco smoking and cancer of the oral cavity and pharynx

Reference Country and years of study	Cancer site (ICD-9)	No. of cases	No. of controls	Smoking category	Relative risk (95% CI)	Comments
Oral cavity						
Sankaranarayanan et al. (1989a) India 1983–84	Gingiva (143.0, 143.1)			*No. of bidis/day*		Hospital-based; as very few women smoked, only men were analysed.
		54	402	Never-smoker	1.0	
		26	64	≤ 10	2.8 (1.6–4.8)	
		15	55	11–20	1.9 (1.0–3.6)	
		8	20	≥ 21	3.2 (1.3–7.7)	p for trend < 0.001
				Age at starting (years)		
		39	62	< 21	1.0	
		10	79	≥ 21	0.2 (0.1–0.4)	p for trend < 0.001 Multivariate analysis further adjusted for use of pan–tobacco, alcohol and snuff
				Duration (years)		
				Never	1.0	
				≤ 20	2.6 (0.7–9.9)	
				> 20	2.1 (1.2–27.9)	p for trend < 0.025
Sankaranarayanan et al. (1989b) India 1983–84	Tongue (141.1–141.4) and floor of mouth (144)			*Duration (years)*		Adjusted for age
		79	232	Never-smoker	1.0	
		17	12	≤ 20	3.9 (1.8–8.7)	
		60	67	≥ 21	2.7 (1.7–4.4)	p for trend < 0.001
				Lifetime exposure		
		79	232	Never-smoker	1.0	
		44	47	< 480	2.7 (1.6–4.5)	
		33	32	≥ 480	3.4 (1.8–6.2)	
					p for trend < 0.001	
				No. of bidis/day		Multivariate analysis adjusted for pan–tobacco chewing and bidi and cigarette smoking
				Never-smoker	1.0	
				< 10	5.2 (2.5–10.9)	
				11–20	4.1 (1.8–9.5)	
				> 20	7.5 (2.6–21.7)	p for trend < 0.001

Table 2.2.22 (contd)

Reference Country and years of study	Cancer site (ICD-9)	No. of cases	No. of controls	Smoking category	Relative risk (95% CI)	Comments
Sankaranarayanan et al. (1990a) India 1983–84	Buccal mucosa (145.0, 145.1, 145.6) and labial mucosa (140.3, 140.4)			*No. of bidis/day*		Hospital-based study; adjusted for age
		125	402	Never-smoker	1.0	
		51	64	≤ 10	2.4 (1.6–3.7)	
		43	55	11–20	2.5 (1.6–3.9)	
		17	20	≥ 21	2.8 (1.4–5.6)	*p* for trend < 0.001
				Lifetime exposure		
		125	402	Never-smoker	1.0	
		51	61	< 400	2.7 (1.7–4.1)	
		12	27	400–499	1.4 (0.7–2.9)	
		48	52	≥ 500	2.9 (1.8–4.5)	*p* for trend < 0.001
				Duration (years)		Multivariate analysis adjusted for pan– tobacco chewing, alcohol and snuff
				Never-smoker	1.0	
				≤ 20	2.9 (1.3–6.6)	
				≥ 21	1.7 (1.1–2.6)	*p* for trend < 0.01
Rao et al. (1994) India 1980–84	Oral cavity: lip, anterior tongue, upper and lower alveolus, buccal mucosa and hard palate, excluding base of the tongue (141.0) and soft palate (145.3)			*No. of bidis/day*		Hospital-based study
		407	440	Nonsmoker	1.0	
		163	95	1–10	1.9 (1.4–2.5)	
		64	41	11–20	1.7 (1.1–2.6)	
		66	52	21–30	1.4 (0.9–2.1)	
		10	6	≥ 31	1.8 (0.6–5.6)	*p* for trend < 0.001
				Duration (years)		
		407	440	Nonsmoker	1.0	
		61	64	1–10	1.0 (0.7–1.5)	
		61	48	11–20	1.4 (0.9–2.1)	
		86	39	21–30	2.4 (1.6–3.6)	
		96	43	≥ 31	2.4 (1.6–3.6)	*p* for trend < 0.001

Table 2.2.22 (contd)

Reference Country and years of study	Cancer site (ICD-9)	No. of cases	No. of controls	Smoking category	Relative risk (95% CI)	Comments
Rao et al. (1994) (contd)				*Cessation*		Stratified by 4 age groups and 3 areas of residence
		231	159	Current smoker	1.4 (1.0–1.8)	
		42	14	Quit 1 year before	2.1 (1.1–4.3)	
		10	3	Quit 2 years before	2.2 (0.5–12.0)	
		11	10	Quit > 2 years before	0.7 (0.2–1.9)	
		414	447	Nonsmoker	1.0	
Rao & Desai (1998) India 1980–84	Base of the tongue (141.0) and anterior tongue (141.1–141.4)	15	3	Hookah/chillum	5.0 (1.4–22.0)	Hospital-based study
				Base of tongue		
		91	337	Nonsmoker	1.0	[†]Includes smokers of both bidis and cigarettes.
		360	186	Bidi smoker	5.9 (4.2–8.2)	[‡]Includes smokers of cigarettes and other forms of tobacco
				No. of bidis/day[†]		
		129	438	Nonsmoker[‡]	1.0	
		141	79	1–10	4.3 (3.0–6.7)	
		94	54	11–20	5.2 (3.4–8.5)	
		107	56	21–30	4.8 (3.2–7.7)	
		24	4	≥ 31	14.3 (4.1–50.7)	
				Duration (years)[†]		
		129	438	Nonsmoker[‡]	1.0	
		30	63	1–10	2.2 (1.3–4.1)	
		64	48	11–20	4.5 (3.1–8.7)	
		123	39	21–30	7.7 (4.8–13.0)	
		149	43	≥ 31	5.1 (3.3–8.3)	
				Anterior tongue		
		73	337	Nonsmoker	1.0	
		53	186	Bidi smoker	1.1 (0.7–1.7)	
				No. of bidis/day[‡]		
		86	438	Nonsmoker[‡]	1.0	
		25	79	1–10	1.2 (0.7–2.2)	
		11	54	11–20	0.8 (0.8–1.8)	
		18	56	21–30	1.4 (0.7–2.7)	
		1	4	≥ 31	–	

Table 2.2.22 (contd)

Reference Country and years of study	Cancer site (ICD-9)	No. of cases	No. of controls	Smoking category	Relative risk (95% CI)	Comments
Rao & Desai (1998) (contd)				*Duration (years)*[†]		[†]Includes smokers of both bidis and cigarettes.
		86	438	Nonsmoker[‡]	1.0	[‡]Includes smokers of cigarettes and other forms of tobacco
		7	63	1–10	0.5 (0.2–1.3)	
		16	48	11–20	1.4 (0.7–2.7)	
		12	39	21–30	1.2 (0.6–2.8)	
		20	43	≥ 31	1.6 (0.8–3.4)	
				Bidi smoking		Adjusted for alcohol use, illiteracy, non-vegetarian diet and tobacco chewing
				Base of tongue	4.7 (3.5–6.3)	
				Anterior tongue	1.0 (0.6–1.5)	
				Tongue (base + anterior)	3.3 (2.6–4.3)	
Dikshit & Kanhere (2000) India 1986–92	Oral cavity (140, 141.1–141.5, 143, 144, 145.0–145.2, 145.5–145.9)	76	146	*Smoking status* Nonsmoker	1.0	Population-based; adjusted for age and tobacco-quid chewing
		72	114	Bidi/cigarette smoker[†]	1.5 (0.9–2.4)	[†]70–80% smoked only bidis.
Balaram *et al.* (2002) India 1996–99	Oral cavity			*No. of bidis/day* Nonsmoker	1.0	Hospital-based; frequency-matched for age and sex; adjusted for age, centre, education, alcohol use and chewing habits
		55	33	< 20	2.0 (1.1–3.8)	
		73	41	≥ 20	2.5 (1.4–4.4)	
Pharynx						
Wasnik *et al.* (1998) India [years of study not reported]	Oropharynx	72	112	Nonsmoker	1.0	Hospital-based; age- and sex-matched control patients — one cancer and one non-cancer
		5	16	Cigarette smoker	0.7 (0.3–1.9)	
		40	31	Bidi/chillum smoker	2.7 (1.6–4.5)	
		6	20	Bidi/cigarette smoker	3.1 (0.6–15.3)	

Table 2.2.22 (contd)

Reference Country and years of study	Cancer site (ICD-9)	No. of cases	No. of controls	Smoking category	Relative risk (95% CI)	Comments
Rao et al. (1999) India 1980–84	Oropharynx (141.0, 145.3, 146.9)			*No. of bidis/day*		Hospital-based
		193	445	Nonsmoker	1.0	
		188	77	1–10	4.3 (3.1–6.5)	
		124	52	11–20	4.9 (3.3–7.9)	
		141	53	21–30	4.7 (3.2–7.2)	
		31	4	≥ 31	12.2 (3.8–42.4)	
				Duration (years)		
		193	445	Nonsmoker	1.0	
		44	62	1–10	2.4 (1.5–4.1)	
		89	46	11–20	4.7 (3.4–8.6)	
		159	38	21–30	7.0 (4.5–11.4)	
		192	40	≥ 31	5.2 (3.4–8.1)	
				Bidi smoking		Adjusted for alcohol use, illiteracy, vegetarian/non-vegetarian diet and tobacco chewing
				Nonsmoker	1.0	
				Smoker	4.7 (3.6–6.3)	
Rao et al. (1999) India 1980–84	Hypopharynx (148)			*No. of bidis/day*		Hospital-based; alcohol as an additional risk factor
		242	445	Nonsmoker	1.0	
		126	77	1–10	2.1 (1.5–3.1)	
		81	52	11–20	2.5 (1.6–4.0)	
		112	53	21–30	3.5 (2.4–5.5)	
		25	4	≥ 31	8.3 (2.3–26.0)	
				Duration (years)		
		242	445	Nonsmoker	1.0	
		44	62	1–10	1.8 (1.1–3.1)	
		61	46	11–20	2.7 (1.8–4.9)	
		95	38	21–30	3.3 (2.2–5.7)	
		144	40	≥ 31	3.0 (1.9–4.7)	
				Bidi smoking		Adjusted for alcohol use, illiteracy, vegetarian/non-vegetarian diet and tobacco chewing
				Nonsmoker	1.0	
				Smoker	2.8 (2.1–3.7)	

Table 2.2.22 (contd)

Reference Country and years of study	Cancer site (ICD-9)	No. of cases	No. of controls	Smoking category	Relative risk (95% CI)	Comments
Dikshit & Kanhere (2000) India 1986–92	Oropharynx (posterior tongue, soft palate, uvula, nasopharynx, hypopharynx) (141.0, 141.6, 145.3, 145.4, 146, 147, 148.0–149.0)		NR	*Bidi smoking*		Population-based; adjusted for age and tobacco quid chewing
		59		No	1.0	
		188		Yes	7.3 (4.7–11.2)	
			NR	No. of bidis/day		
		59		1–10	4.1 (2.4–7.0)	
		63		11–20	11.4 (6.5–19.9)	
		84		> 20	17.0 (7.7–37.6)	$\chi^2_{\text{trend}} = 3.82$ (NS)
		41		Nonsmoker	1.0	
				Bidi smoker only	7.9 (5.1–12.4)	
				Cigarette smoker only	4.1 (2.0–8.4)	
				Bidi and cigarette smoker	6.2 (2.8–13.4)	

NR, not reported

Table 2.2.23. Cross-sectional studies on bidi and other tobacco smoking and oral lesions

Reference Country	Oral lesion	Smoking category	No. of lesions	Prevalence (%)	Total	Comments
Van der Eb et al. (1993) India	Palatal lesions	Nonsmoker	5	3	161	Randomly selected population sample; 9 carcinomas of the hard palate, all among reverse chutta smokers
		Chewing tobacco	0	0	10	
		Cigarette	3	21.4	14	
		Bidi	11	55.0	20	
		Conventional chutta	34	56.7	60	
		Ex-conventional chutta/bidi	6	42.9	14	
		Reverse chutta	139	86.9	160	
		Ex-reverse chutta	16	76.2	21	
		Mixed habits	11	55.0	20	
		Total	225	46.9	480	

Reference Country	Oral lesion	Smoking category	No. of cases	No. of controls	RR (95% CI)	Comments
Macigo et al. (1996) Kenya	Oral leukoplakia	**Kiraiku**[†]				Population-based [†]Home-processed hand-rolled products
		Never-smoker	42	120	1.0	
		Former smoker	29	17	4.9 (2.3–10.4)	
		Current smoker	14	4	10.0 (2.9–43.4)	
		Duration (years)				
		≤10	24	15	4.6 (2.1–10.2)	
		>10	5	2	7.1 (1.1–76.6)	
		Years since quitting				
		≥10	11	8	3.9 (1.4–11.6)	
		5–9	12	7	4.9 (1.7–14.9)	
		≤4	6	2	8.6 (1.4–88.7)	

Table 2.2.24. Intervention studies on tobacco use and oral lesions in India

Place Reference	Tobacco habit	Oral lesion	Sex	Intervention cohort		Control cohort		Rate ratio	Comments
				No.	Incidence rate/1000	No.	Incidence rate/1000		
Bhavnagar District									
Gupta et al. (1986b)	Bidi	Leukoplakia	Men	224	41.9	58	47.6	0.88	After 5 years of follow-up
Srikakulam District									
Gupta et al. (1986b)	Reverse smoking	Palatal lesions	Men	52	163.3	671	427.7	0.38	After 5 years of follow-up
			Women	428	292.0	1 167	513.9	0.57	
				Person–years	Incidence rate/1000	Person–years	Incidence rate/1000		
Gupta et al. (1994)	Reverse smoking	Palatal lesions	Men	7 341	1.1	7 718	6.2		After 10 years of follow-up
			Women	49 522	3.4	11 210	11.4		
				Observed	Expected				
Ernakulam District									
Gupta et al. (1990)	Bidi	Leukoplakia	Men	63	142.6			0.4	After 8 years of follow-up
			Women	0	2.6			0.0	
	Cigarette		Men	0	12.8			0.0	
			Women	0	0.0			–	

Table 2.2.24 (contd)

Place Reference	Tobacco habit	Oral lesion	Sex	Intervention cohort		Control cohort		Rate ratio	Comments
				Person-years	Incidence rate/1000	Person-years	Incidence rate/1000		
Gupta et al. (1992)	Bidi	Leukoplakia	Men	48 265	1.46	15 529	3.02	0.4	
			Women	1 444	–	199	5.86	0.0	
	Cigarette		Men	2 699	–	2 165	1.46	0.0	
			Women	6	–	0	0	–	

				Stopped			All others		Rate ratio
				Person-years	Observed	Expected	Person-years	Observed	
	Bidi	Oral lesions	Men	ca. 3000	8	42.3	ca. 40 000	601	0.15
						Incidence/100 000		Incidence/100 000	
						24		155	
		Leukoplakia			1			80	

Table 2.2.25. Case–control studies of bidi and other tobacco smoking and lung cancer

Reference Country and years of study	No. of cases	No. of controls	Smoking category	Relative risk (95% CI)	Comments
Dikshit & Kanhere (2000) India 1986–92	17	146	Nonsmoker	1.0	Population-based; adjusted for age
	100	81	Bidi smoker only	11.6 (6.4–21.3)	
	15	20	Cigarette smoker only	7.7 (3.2–18.4)	
	31	13	Bidi and cigarette smoker	24.1 (10.4–56.1)	
Gupta et al. (2001) India 1995–97	26	172	Nonsmoker	1.0	Hospital-based; males; relative risks adjusted for age and education
	208	261	Ever-smoker (any)	5.0 (3.1–8.0)	
	137	162	Bidi smoker	5.8 (3.4–9.7)	
	78	103	Cigarette smoker	3.9 (2.1–7.1)	
	12	31	Hookah smoker	1.9 (0.9–4.4)	
			Bidis		[†]Average consumption of cigarette equivalents (see text)
			Average no./day[†]		
	11	39	1–4	1.8 (0.8–4.0)	
	46	54	5–9	5.9 (3.2–10.8)	
	67	63	10–19	6.8 (3.9–12.1)	
	13	6	≥ 20	12.3 (4.2–36.1)	
			Duration (years)		
	23	45	0–24	3.7 (1.8–7.7)	
	48	36	25–34	9.6 (4.9–18.7)	
	30	48	35–44	3.7 (1.9–7.2)	
	37	33	≥ 45	6.4 (3.3–12.6)	
			Pack–years		
	41	71	0–9	3.9 (2.1–7.1)	
	57	54	10–19	6.5 (3.6–11.7)	
	26	23	20–29	6.9 (3.4–14.3)	
	13	14	≥ 30	5.3 (2.2–12.9)	
			Hookah		
			Average no./day[†]		
	12	31	1–4	1.9 (0.9–4.4)	
			Duration (years)		
	1	9	0–24	0.5 (0.1–4.4)	
	0	6	25–34	–	
	6	10	35–44	2.7 (0.9–8.5)	
	5	6	≥ 45	4.4 (1.2–16.4)	
			Pack–years		
	12	31	0–9	1.9 (0.9–4.4)	

Table 2.2.26. Case–control studies on bidi and other tobacco smoking and cancer of the larynx and oesophagus

Reference Country and years of study	No. of cases	No. of controls	Smoking category	Relative risk (95% CI)	Comments
Larynx					
Sankaranarayanan *et al.* (1990b)	101	402	*No. of bidis/day* None	1.0	Hospital-based
India	31	65	≤ 10	1.8 (1.1–2.9)	
1983–84	31	55	11–20	2.1 (1.3–3.5)	
	25	20	≥ 21	5.1 (2.7–9.6)	*p* for trend < 0.001 Adjusted for duration of cigarette smoking, frequency of bidi and cigarette smoking and duration of alcohol use
			Duration (years) Never	1.0	
			≤ 20	1.3 (0.3–6.4)	
			≥ 21	7.1 (4.0—12.5)	*p* for trend < 0.001
Rao *et al.* (1999)	203	445	*No. of bidis/day* Nonsmoker	1.0	Hospital-based
India	93	77	1–10	1.8 (1.2–2.8)	
1980–84	38	52	11–20	1.4 (0.8–2.4)	
	76	53	21–30	2.5 (1.7–4.1)	
	11	4	≥ 31	3.8 (0.9–14.1)	
	203	445	*Duration (years)* Nonsmoker	1.0	
	24	62	1–10	1.2 (0.7–2.3)	
	44	46	11–20	2.3 (1.4–4.3)	
	62	38	21–30	2.3 (1.4–4.1)	
	88	40	≥ 31	2.0 (1.3–3.2)	
			Bidi smoking Nonsmoker	1.0	Adjusted for alcohol use, illiteracy, vegetarian/non-vegetarian diet and tobacco chewing
			Smoker	2.1 (1.6–2.8)	

Table 2.2.26 (contd)

Reference Country and years of study	No. of cases	No. of controls	Smoking category	Relative risk (95% CI)	Comments
Oesophagus					
Sankaranarayanan et al. (1991)	88	402	*No. of bidis/day* None	1.0	Hospital-based
India	45	65	≤ 10	2.8 (1.8–4.5)	
1983–84	45	55	11–20	3.5 (2.2–5.5)	
	24	20	≥ 21	5.2 (2.7–10.0)	*p* for trend < 0.001
			Duration (years) Never	1.0	Adjusted for the number of bidis and cigarettes smoked daily, alcohol use and pan–tobacco chewing
			≤ 20	2.1 (0.8–5.9)	
			> 20	4.7 (2.8–7.9)	*p* for trend < 0.001
Nandakumar et al. (1996)	36	139	*All cases* Nonsmoker	1.0	Hospital-based; age- and sex-matched, adjusted for tobacco chewing, pan chewing without tobacco, alcohol drinking and cigarette smoking
India	115	144	Bidi smoker	4.0 (2.3–6.8)	
1982–85			*Upper third*		
	4	16	Nonsmoker	1.0	
	11	8	Bidi smoker	7.1 (1.1–46.8)	
			Middle third		
	14	76	Nonsmoker	1.0	
	60	73	Bidi smoker	6.0 (2.5–14.5)	
			Lower third		
	12	37	Nonsmoker	1.0	
	34	48	Bidi smoker	3.9 (1.4–10.7)	
Nayar et al. (2000),	83	112	*Bidi smoking* Never-smoker	1.0	Hospital-based; matched controls; adjusted for betel quid with tobacco and diet (other vegetables besides leafy greens)
India	66	37	Daily smoker	2.0 (1.2–3.3)	
1994–97					

Table 2.2.27. Case–control study of bidi and other tobacco smoking and stomach cancer

Reference Country and years of study	No. of cases	No. of controls	Smoking categories	Relative risk (95% CI)	Comments
Gajalakshmi & Shanta (1996) India 1988–90			*Current smoker*		Hospital-based; matched on age, sex, religion and mother tongue
	72	40	Bidi	3.2 (1.8–5.7)	
	43	33	Cigarette	2.0 (1.1–3.6)	
	31	22	Chutta	2.4 (1.2–4.9)	
	13	2	Combination	8.2 (1.7–38.9)	
			Bidis		
			Age at starting smoking (years)		
	10	5	> 30	3.6 (1.0–13.5)	
	27	16	21–30	2.7 (1.2–5.9)	
	35	19	≤ 20	3.7 (1.7–8.3)	*p* for trend < 0.001
			Lifetime exposure		
	21	17	Mild	2.0 (0.9–4.3)	
	17	11	Moderate	5.3 (1.6–18.3)	
	34	12	Heavy	4.5 (1.8–11.3)	*p* for trend < 0.001
			Chuttas		
			Age at starting smoking (years)		
	3	5	> 30	2.2 (0.3–13.5)	
	12	6	21–30	2.4 (0.8–7.2)	
	16	11	≤ 20	2.3 (0.9–6.0)	
			Lifetime exposure		
	12	12	Mild	2.8 (0.9–8.4)	
	8	7	Moderate	1.5 (0.5–4.6)	
	8	3	Heavy	4.4 (1.2–16.1)	*p* for trend < 0.05

References

Ahlbom, H.E. (1937) [Prädisponierende Faktoren für Plattenepithelkarzinome in Mund, Hals und Speiseröhre. Eine statistische Untersuchung am Material des Radiumhemmets, Stockholm]. *Acta Radiol.*, **18**, 163–185

Balaram, P., Sridhar, H., Rajkumar, T., Vaccarella, S., Herrero, R., Nandakumar, A., Ravichandran, K., Ramdas, K., Sankaranarayanan, R., Gajalakshmi, V, Munoz, N., & Franceschi, S. (2002) Oral cancer in southern India: The influence of smoking, drinking, paan-chewing and oral hygiene. *Int. J. Cancer*, **98**, 440–445

Benhamou, S., Benhamou, E. & Flamant, R. (1986) Lung cancer risk associated with cigar and pipe smoking. *Int. J. Cancer*, **37**, 825–829

Ben-Shlomo, Y., Smith, G.D., Shipley, M.J. & Marmot, M.G. (1994) What determines mortality risk in male former cigarette smokers? *Am. J. public Health*, **84**, 1235–1242

Bernier, J.L. & Clark, M.L. (1951) Squamous cell carcinoma of the lip: A critical statistical and morphological analysis of 835 cases. *Milit. Surg.*, **109**, 379–405

Blot, W.J., McLaughlin, J.K., Winn, D.M., Austin, D.F., Greenberg, R.S., Preston-Martin, S., Bernstein, L., Schoenberg, J.B., Stemhagen, A. & Fraumeni, J.F., Jr (1988) Smoking and drinking in relation to oral and pharyngeal cancer. *Cancer Res.*, **48**, 3282–3287

Boffetta, P., Pershagen, G., Jockel, K.H., Forastiere, F., Gaborieau, V., Heinrich, J., Jahn, I., Kreuzer, M. & Merletti, F., Nyberg, F., Rösch, F. & Simonato, L. (1999) Cigar and pipe smoking and lung cancer risk: A multicenter study from Europe. *J. natl Cancer Inst.*, **91**, 697–701

Broders, A.C. (1920) Squamous-cell epithelioma of the lip: A study of five hundred and thirty-seven cases. *J. Am. med. Assoc.*, **74**, 656–664

Brown, L.M., Gibson, R., Blair, A., Burmeister, L.F., Schuman, L.M., Cantor, K.P. & Fraumeni, J.F., Jr (1992a) Smoking and risk of leukemia. *Am. J. Epidemiol.*, **135**, 763–768

Brown, L.M., Everett, G.D., Gibson, R., Burmeister, L.F., Schuman, L.M. & Blair, A. (1992b) Smoking and risk of non-Hodgkin's lymphoma and multiple myeloma. *Cancer Causes Control*, **3**, 49–55

Carstensen, J.M., Pershagen, G. & Eklund, G. (1987) Mortality in relation to cigarette and pipe smoking: 16 years' observation of 25 000 Swedish men. *J. Epidemiol. Community Health*, **41**, 166–172

Chao, A., Thun, M.J., Jacobs, E.J., Henley, S.J., Rodriguez, C. & Calle, E.E. (2000) Cigarette smoking and colorectal cancer mortality in the Cancer Prevention Study II. *J. natl Cancer Inst.*, **92**, 1888–1896

Chao, A., Thun, M.J., Henley, S.J., Jacobs, E.J., McCullough, M.L. & Calle, E.E. (2002) Cigarette smoking, use of other tobacco products and stomach cancer mortality in US adults: The Cancer Prevention Study II. *Int. J. Cancer*, **101**, 380–389

Chow, W.H., Schuman, L.M., McLaughlin, J.K., Bjelke, E., Gridley, G., Wacholder, S., Chien, H.T. & Blot, W.J. (1992) A cohort study of tobacco use, diet, occupation, and lung cancer mortality. *Cancer Causes Control*, **3**, 247–254

Chow, W.H., McLaughlin, J.K., Hrubec, Z., Nam, J.M. & Blot, W.J. (1993) Tobacco use and naso-pharyngeal carcinoma in a cohort of US veterans. *Int. J. Cancer*, **55**, 538–540

Chow, W.H., McLaughlin, J.K., Menck, H.R. & Mack, T.H. (1994) Risk factors for extrahepatic bile duct cancers: Los Angeles County, California (USA). *Cancer Causes Control*, **5**, 267–272

Clemmesen, J. (1965) *Statistical Studies in Malignant Neoplasms. I. Review and Results*, Copenhagen, Munksgaard, pp. 59–116

Damber, L.A. & Larsson, L.G. (1986) Smoking and lung cancer with special regard to type of smoking and type of cancer. A case–control study in north Sweden. *Br. J. Cancer*, **53**, 673–681

Dikshit, R.P. & Kanhere, S. (2000) Tobacco habits and risk of lung, oropharyngeal and oral cavity cancer: A population-based case–control study in Bhopal, India. *Int. J. Epidemiol.*, **29**, 609–614

Doll, R. (1998) Uncovering the effects of smoking: Historical perspective. *Stat. Meth. med. Res.*, **7**, 87–117

Doll, R. & Peto, R. (1976) Mortality in relation to smoking: 20 years' observation on male British doctors. *Br. med. J.*, **ii**, 1525–1536

Ebenius, B. (1943) Cancer of the lip. A clinical study of 778 cases with particular regard to predisposing factors and radium therapy. *Acta radiol.*, **Suppl. 48**, 1–232

Falk, R.T., Pickle, L.W., Brown, L.M., Mason, T.J., Buffler, P.A. & Fraumeni, J.F., Jr (1989) Effect of smoking and alcohol consumption on laryngeal cancer risk in coastal Texas. *Cancer Res.*, **49**, 4024–4029

Fernandez Garrote, L., Herrero, R., Ortiz Reyes, R.M., Vaccarella, S., Lence Anta, J., Ferbeye, L., Munoz, N. & Franceschi, S. (2001) Risk factors for cancer of the oral cavity and oro-pharynx in Cuba. *Br. J. Cancer*, **85**, 46–54

Franceschi, S., Talamini, R., Barra, S., Baron, A.E., Negri, E., Bidoli, E., Serraino, D & La Vecchia, C. (1990) Smoking and drinking in relation to cancers of the oral cavity, pharynx, larynx, and esophagus in northern Italy. *Cancer Res.*, **50**, 6502–6507

Franceschi, S., Barra, S., La Vecchia, C., Bidoli, E., Negri, E. & Talamini, R. (1992) Risk factors for cancer of the tongue and the mouth. A case–control study from northern Italy. *Cancer*, **70**, 2227–2233

Freudenheim, J.L., Graham, S., Byers, T.E., Marshall, J.R., Haughey, B.P., Swanson, M.K. & Wilkinson, G. (1992) Diet, smoking and alcohol in cancer of the larynx: A case–control study. *Nutr. Cancer*, **17**, 33–45

Gajalakshmi, C.K. & Shanta, V. (1996) Lifestyle and risk of stomach cancer: A hospital-based case–control study. *Int. J. Epidemiol.*, **25**, 1146–1153

Garfinkel, L. & Boffetta, P. (1990) Association between smoking and leukemia in two American Cancer Society prospective studies. *Cancer*, **65**, 2356–2360

Gupta, P.C., Aghi, M.B., Bhonsle, R.B., Murti, P.R., Mehta, F.S., Mehta, C.R. & Pindborg, J.J. (1986a) An intervention study of tobacco chewing and smoking habits for primary prevention of oral cancer among 12 212 Indian villagers. In: Zaridze, D.G. & Peto, R., eds, *Tobacco: A Major International Health Hazard* (IARC Scientific Publications No.74), Lyon, IARCPress, pp. 307–318

Gupta, P.C., Mehta, F.S., Pindborg, J.J., Aghi, M.B., Bhonsle, R.B., Daftary, D.K., Murti, P.R., Shah, H.T. & Sinor, P.N. (1986b) Intervention study for primary prevention of oral cancer among 36 000 Indian tobacco users. *Lancet*, **i**, 1235–1239

Gupta, P.C., Bhonsle, R.B., Murti, P.R., Daftary, D.K., Mehta, F.S. & Pindborg, J.J. (1989) An epidemiologic assessment of cancer risk in oral precancerous lesions in India with special reference to nodular leukoplakia. *Cancer*, **63**, 2247–2252

Gupta, P.C., Mehta, F.S., Pindborg, J.J., Daftary, D.K., Aghi, M.B., Bhonsle, R.B., Murti, P.R. (1990) A primary prevention study of oral cancer among Indian villagers. Eight-year follow-up results. In: Hakama, M., Beral, V., Cullen, J.W. & Parkin, D.M., eds, *Evaluating Effectiveness of Primary Prevention of Cancer* (IARC Scientific Publications No.103), Lyon, IARC*Press*, pp. 149–156

Gupta, P.C., Mehta, F.S., Pindborg, J.J., Bhonsle, R.B., Murti, P.R., Daftary, D.K. & Aghi, M.B. (1992) Primary prevention trial of oral cancer in India: A 10-year follow-up study. *J. oral Pathol. Med.*, **21**, 433–439

Gupta, P.C., Mehta, F.S., Pindborg, J.J. & Aghi, M.B. (1994) A behavioural intervention study for primary prevention of oral cancer among reverse smokers of Srikakulam district, Andhra Pradesh. In: Verma, A.K., ed, *Oral Oncology,* Vol. IIIA, *Research* (3rd International Congress on Oral Cancer), Madras, MacMillan India, pp. 64–67

Gupta, D., Boffetta, P., Gaborieau, V. & Jindal, S.K. (2001) Risk factors of lung cancer in Chandigarh, India. *Indian J. med. Res.*, **113**, 142–150

Hämäläinen, M.J. (1955) Cancer of the lip. With specific reference to the predisposing influence of sunlight and other climatic factors. *Ann. Chir. Gynaecol. Fenn*, **44** (Suppl. 6), 1–159

Hammond, E.C. & Horn, D. (1958) Smoking and death rates — Report on forty-four months of follow-up of 187 783 men. II. Death rates by cause. *J. Am. med. Assoc.*, **166**, 1294–1308

Heineman, E.F., Hoar Zahm, S., McLaughlin, J.K., Vaught, J.B. & Hrubec, Z. (1992) A prospective study of tobacco use and multiple myeloma: Evidence against an association. *Cancer Causes Control*, **3**, 31–36

Heineman, E.F., Zahm, S.H., McLaughlin, J.K. & Vaught, J.B. (1995) Increased risk of colorectal cancer among smokers: Results of a 26-year follow-up of US veterans and a review. *Int. J. Cancer*, **59**, 728–738

Hogewind, W.F.C., Greebe, R.B. & Van der Wall, I. (1987) Reverse smoking in the Netherlands. *Int. J. oral Maxillofac. Surg.*, **16**, 500–504

Hsing, A.W., McLaughlin, J.K., Hrubec, Z., Blot, W.J. & Fraumeni, J.F., Jr (1990a) Cigarette smoking and liver cancer among US veterans. *Cancer Causes Control*, **1**, 217–221

Hsing, A.W., McLaughlin, J.K., Schuman, L.M., Bjelke, E., Gridley, G., Wacholder, S.G., Chien, H.T. & Blot, W.J. (1990b) Diet, tobacco use, and fatal prostate cancer: Results from the Lutheran Brotherhood cohort study. *Cancer Res.*, **50**, 6836–6840

Hsing, A.W., McLaughlin, J.K., Hrubec, Z., Blot, W.J. & Fraumeni, J.F., Jr (1991) Tobacco use and prostate cancer: 26-year follow-up of US veterans. *Am. J. Epidemiol.*, **133**, 437–441

Hsing, A.W., McLaughlin, J.K., Chow, W.-H., Schuman, L.M., Co Chien, H.T., Gridley, G., Bjelke, E., Wachholder, S. & Blot, W.J. (1998) Risk factors for colorectal cancer in a prospective study among US white men. *Int. J. Cancer*, **77**, 549–553

Iribarren, C., Tekawa, I.S., Sidney, S. & Friedman, G.D. (1999) Effect of cigar smoking on the risk of cardiovascular disease, chronic obstructive pulmonary disease, and cancer in men. *New Engl. J. Med.*, **340**, 1773–1780

Jensen, O.M., Wahrendorf, J., Blettner, M., Knudsen, J.B. & Sørensen, B.L. (1987) The Copenhagen case–control study of bladder cancer: Role of smoking in invasive and non-invasive bladder tumours. *J. Epidemiol. Commun. Health*, **41**, 30–36

Jensen, O.M., Knudsen, J.B,, McLaughlin, J.K. & Sorensen, B.L. (1988) The Copenhagen case–control study of renal pelvis and ureter cancer: Role of smoking and occupational exposures. *Int. J. Cancer*, **41**, 557–561

Kabat, G.C., Augustine, A. & Hebert, J.R. (1988) Smoking and adult leukemia: A case–control study. *J. clin. Epidemiol.*, **41**, 907–914

Kabat, G.C., Ng, S.K.C. & Wynder, E.L. (1993) Tobacco, alcohol intake, and diet in relation to adenocarcinoma of the esophagus and gastric cardia. *Cancer Causes Control*, **4**, 123–132

Kahn, H.A. (1966) The Dorn study of smoking and mortality among US veterans: Report on eight and one-half years of observation. In: Haenszel, W., ed., *Epidemiological Approaches to the Study of Cancer and Other Chronic Diseases* (Monograph 19), Bethesda, MD, US Department of Health, Education, and Welfare, National Cancer Institute, pp. 1–125

Keller, A.Z. (1970) Cellular types, survival, race, nativity, occupations, habits and associated diseases in the pathogenesis of lip cancers. *Am. J. Epidemiol.*, **91**, 486–499

Kinlen, L.J. & Rogot, E. (1988) Leukaemia and smoking habits among United States veterans. *Br. med. J.*, **297**, 657–659

Knekt, P., Hakama, M., Järvinen, R., Pukkala, E. & Heliövaara, M. (1998) Smoking and risk of colorectal cancer. *Br. J. Cancer*, **78**, 136–139

Kneller, R.W., McLaughlin, J.K., Bjelke, E., Schuman, L.M., Blot, W.J., Wacholder, S., Gridley, G., CoChien, H.T. & Fraumeni, J.F., Jr (1991) A cohort study of stomach cancer in a high-risk American population. *Cancer*, **68**, 672–678

La Vecchia, C., Bosetti, C., Negri, E., Levi, F. & Franceschi, S. (1998) Cigar smoking and cancers of the upper digestive tract (Letter). *J. natl Cancer Inst.*, **90**, 1670

Lange, P., Nyboe, J., Appleyard, M., Jensen, G. & Schnohr, P. (1992) Relationship of the type of tobacco and inhalation pattern to pulmonary and total mortality. *Eur. respir. J.*, **5**, 1111–1117

Lubin, J. & Blot, W. (1984) Assessment of lung cancer risk factors by histologic category. *J. natl Cancer Inst.*, **73**, 383–389

Lubin, J.H., Richter, B.S. & Blot, W.J. (1984) Lung cancer risk with cigar and pipe use. *J. natl Cancer Inst.*, **73**, 377–381

Lubin, J.H., Li, J.Y., Xuan, X.Z., Cai, S.K., Luo, Q.S., Yang, L.F., Wang, J.Z., Yang, L. & Blot, W.J. (1992) Risk of lung cancer among cigarette and pipe smokers in southern China. *Int. J. Cancer*, **51**, 390–395

Macigo, F.G., Mwaniki, D.L. & Guthua, S.W. (1996) Influence of dose and cessation of kiraiku, cigarettes and alcohol use on the risk of developing oral leukoplakia. *Eur. J. oral Sci.*, **104**, 498–502

Mack, T.M., Yu, M.C., Hanisch, R. & Henderson, B.E. (1986) Pancreas cancer and smoking, beverage consumption, and past medical history. *J. natl Cancer Inst.*, **76**, 49–60

McLaughlin, J.K., Lindblad, P., Mellemgaard, A., McCredie, M., Mandel, J.S., Schlehofer, B., Pommer, W. & Adami, H.O. (1995) International renal-cell cancer study. I. Tobacco use. *Int. J. Cancer*, **60**, 194–198

Mehta, F.S., Aghi, M.B., Gupta, P.C., Pindborg, J.J., Bhonsle, R.B., Jalnawalla, P.N. & Sinor, P.N. (1982) An intervention study of oral cancer and precancer in rural Indian populations: A preliminary report. *Bull. World Health Org.*, **60**, 441–446

Muscat, J.E. & Wynder, E.L. (1992) Tobacco, alcohol, asbestos and occupational risk factors for laryngeal cancer. *Cancer*, **69**, 2244–2251

Muscat, J.E., Stellman, S.D., Hoffmann, D. & Wynder, E.L. (1997) Smoking and pancreatic cancer in men and women. *Cancer Epidemiol. Biomarkers Prev.*, **6**, 15–19

Nandakumar, A., Anantha, N., Pattabhiraman, V., Prabhakaran, P.S., Dhar, M., Puttaswamy, K., Venugopal, T.C., Reddy, N.M.S., Rajanna, Vinutha, A.T. & Srinivas (1996) Importance of anatomical subsite in correlating risk factors in cancer of the oesophagus — Report of a case–control study. *Br. J. Cancer*, **73**, 1306–1311

Nayar, D., Kapil, U., Joshi, Y.K., Sundaram, K.R., Srivastava, S.P., Shukla, N.K. & Tandon, R.K. (2000) Nutritional risk factors in esophageal cancer. *J. Assoc. Physic. India*, **48**, 781–787

Partanen, T.J., Vainio, H.U., Ojajärvi, I.A. & Kauppinen, T.P. (1997) Pancreas cancer, tobacco smoking and consumption of alcoholic beverages: A case–control study. *Cancer Lett.*, **116**, 27–32

Pitard, A., Brennan, P., Clavel, J., Greiser, E., Lopez-Abente, G., Chang-Claude, J., Wahrendorf, J., Serra, C., Kogevina, M. & Boffetta, P. (2001) Cigar, pipe, and cigarette smoking and bladder cancer risk in European men. *Cancer Causes Control*, **12**, 551–556

Qiao, Y.L., Taylor, P.R., Yao, S.X., Schatzkin, A., Mao, B.L., Lubin, J., Rao, J.Y., McAdams, M., Xuan, X.Z. & Li, J.Y. (1989) Relation of radon exposure and tobacco use to lung cancer among tin miners in Yunnan Province, China. *Am. J. ind. Med.*, **16**, 511–521

Rao, D.N. & Desai, P.B. (1998) Risk assessment of tobacco, alcohol and diet in cancers of base tongue and oral tongue — A case–control study. *Indian J. Cancer*, **35**, 65–72

Rao, D.N., Ganesh B., Rao R.S. & Desai P.B. (1994) Risk assessment of tobacco, alcohol and diet in oral cancer — A case–control study. *Int. J. Cancer*, **58**, 469–473

Rao, D.N., Desai, P.B. & Ganesh, B. (1999) Alcohol as an additional risk factor in laryngo-pharyngeal cancer in Mumbai — A case–control study. *Cancer Detect. Prev.*, **23**, 37–44

Sankaranarayanan, R., Duffy, S.W., Padmakumary, G., Day, N.E. & Padmanabhan, T.K. (1989a) Tobacco chewing, alcohol and nasal snuff in cancer of the gingiva in Kerala, India. *Br. J. Cancer*, 60, 638–643

Sankaranarayanan, R., Duffy, S.W., Day, N.E., Nair, M.K. & Padmakumary, G. (1989b) A case–control investigation of cancer of the oral tongue and the floor of the mouth in southern India. *Int. J. Cancer*, **44**, 617–621

Sankaranarayanan, R., Duffy, S.W., Padmakumary, G., Day, N.E. & Nair, K. (1990a) Risk factors for cancer of the buccal and labial mucosa in Kerala, southern India. *J. Epidemiol. Community Health*, **44**, 286–292

Sankaranarayanan, R., Duffy, S.W., Nair, M.K., Padmakumary, G. & Day, N.E. (1990b) Tobacco and alcohol as risk factors in cancer of the larynx in Kerala, India. *Int. J. Cancer*, **45**, 879–882

Sankaranarayanan, R., Duffy, S.W., Padmakumary, G., Nair, S.M., Day, N.E. & Padmanabhan, T.K. (1991) Risk factors for cancer of the oesophagus in Kerala, India. *Int. J. Cancer*, **49**, 485–489

Shanks, T.G. & Burns, D.M. (1998) Disease consequences of cigar smoking. In: *Cigars — Health Effects and Trends* (Smoking and Tobacco Control, Monograph No. 9; NIH Publication No. 98-4302), Washington DC, US Department of Health and Human Services, National Institutes of Health, pp. 105–160

Shapiro, J.A., Jacobs, E.J. & Thun, M.J. (2000) Cigar smoking in men and risk of death from tobacco-related cancers. *J. natl Cancer Inst.*, **92**, 333–337

Sharpe, C.R. & Siemiatycki, J. (2001) Joint effects of smoking and body mass index on prostate cancer risk. *Epidemiology*, **12**, 546–551

Simarak, S., de Jong, U.W., Breslow, N., Dahl, C.J., Ruckphaopunt, K., Scheelings, P. & MacLennan, R. (1977) Cancer of the oral cavity, pharynx/larynx and lung in North Thailand: Case–control study and analysis of cigar smoke. *Br. J. Cancer*, **36**, 130

Sömmering, S. (1795) *De Morbis Vasorum Absorbentium Corporis Humani*, Frankfurt, Varrentrapp & Wenner

Spitzer, W.O., Hill, G.B., Chambers, L.W., Helliwell, B.E. & Murphy, H.B. (1975) The occupation of fishing as a risk factor in cancer of the lip. *New Engl. J. Med.*, **293**, 419–424

Steineck, G., Norell, S.E. & Feychting, M. (1988) Diet, tobacco and urothelial cancer. A 14-year follow-up of 16 477 subjects. *Acta oncol.*, **27**, 323–327

Stoykewych, A.A., DeBrouwere, R. & Curran, J.B. (1992) Reverse smoking and its effects on the hard palate: A case report. *J. Can. dent. Assoc.*, **58**, 215–216

Swanson, M.G. & Burns, P.B. (1997) Cancers of the salivary gland: Workplace risks among women and men. *AEP*, **7**, 369–374

Talamini, R., Franceschi, S., Barra, S. & La Vecchia, C. (1990) The role of alcohol in oral and pharyngeal cancer in non-smokers, and of tobacco in non-drinkers. *Int. J. Cancer*, **46**, 391–393

Talamini, R., La Vecchia, C., Levi, F., Conti, E., Favero, A. & Franceschi, S. (1998) Cancer of the oral cavity and pharynx in nonsmokers who drink alcohol and in nondrinkers who smoke tobacco. *J. natl Cancer Inst.*, **90**, 1901–1903

Thun, M.J. & Heath, C.W. (1997) Changes in mortality from smoking in two American Cancer Society prospective studies since 1959. *Prev. Med.*, **26**, 422–426

Tverdal, A., Thelle, D., Stensvold, I., Leren, P. & Bjartveit, K. (1993) Mortality in relation to smoking history: 13 years' follow-up of 68,000 Norwegian men and women 35–49 years. *J. clin. Epidemiol.*, **46**, 475–487

US Department of Health and Human Services (1989) *Reducing the Health Consequences of Smoking: 25 Years of Progress. A Report of the Surgeon General* (DHHS Publication No. (CDC) 89-8411), Rockville, MD, Public Health Service, Centres for Disease Control, Center for Chronic Disease Prevention and Health Promotion, Office on Smoking and Health

Van der Eb, M.M., Leyten, E.M., Gavarasana, S., Vandenbroucke, J.P., Kahn, P.M. & Cleton, F.J. (1993) Reverse smoking as a risk factor for palatal cancer: A cross-sectional study in rural Andhra Pradesh, India. *Int. J. Cancer*, **54**, 754–758

Wald, N.J. & Watt, H.C. (1997) Prospective study of effect of switching from cigarettes to pipes or cigars on mortality from three smoking-related diseases. *Br. med. J.*, **314**, 1860–1863

Wasnik, K.S., Ughade, S.N., Zodpey, S.P. & Ingole, D.L. (1998) Tobacco consumption practices and risk of oro-pharyngeal cancer: A case–control study in Central India. *S.E. Asian J. trop. Med. public Health*, **29**, 827–834

Wu-Williams, A.H., Yu, M.C. & Mack, T.M. (1990) Life-style, workplace and stomach cancer by subsite in young men of Los Angeles County. *Cancer Res.*, **50**, 2569–2576

Wynder, E.L., Bross, I.J. & Feldman, R.M. (1957) A study of the etiological factors in cancer of the mouth. *Cancer*, **10**, 1300–1323

Zheng, T.Z., Boyle, P., Hu, H.F., Duan, J., Jiang, P.J., Ma, D.Q., Shui, L.P., Niu, S.R. & MacMahon, B. (1990) Tobacco smoking, alcohol consumption, and risk of oral cancer: A case–control study in Beijing, People's Republic of China. *Cancer Causes Control*, **1**, 173–179

Zheng, W., McLaughlin, J.K., Gridley, G., Bjelke, E., Schuman, L.M., Silverman, D.T., Wacholder, S., Co Chien, H.T., Blot, W.J. & Fraumeni, J.F., Jr (1993) A cohort study of smoking, alcohol consumption, and dietary factors for pancreatic cancer (United States). *Cancer Causes Control*, **4**, 477–482

2.3 Synergistic carcinogenic effects of tobacco smoke and other carcinogens

2.3.1 *Introduction*

This section addresses the combined effects on cancer risk of cigarette smoking and other agents also associated with risk, excluding smokeless tobacco. The chapter is restricted to studies of smoking and exposures to single agents and does not address modification of risk by diet, whether by specific foods, nutrients or micronutrients.

For many cancers, including lung cancer, multiple causal factors are relevant and persons being exposed to more than one risk factor may be subject to risks beyond those anticipated from the individual agents acting alone. The terminology and methods used to characterize the combined effects of two or more agents have been poorly standardized with substantial blurring of concepts derived from toxicology, biostatistics and epidemiology (Greenland, 1993; Mauderly, 1993). Epidemiologists refer to *effect modification* if effects of multiple agents are interdependent whereas toxicologists assess whether the effects of multiple agents are *synergistic* (positive interdependence) or *antagonistic* (negative interdependence). Statisticians test whether there is *interaction* between independent determinants of cancer risk. For the purposes of this report, epidemiological concepts are followed, such that interdependence of effects is termed *effect modification*, and *synergism* and *antagonism* are used to describe the consequences of the interdependence of disease risk when both risk factors are present (Rothman & Greenland, 1998). The term *interaction* is reserved for the statistical approach for testing whether effect modification is present.

In a toxicological paradigm that extends from exposure through dose and finally to biological effects, there are a number of different points at which smoking might influence the effect of another risk factor. The 1985 Report of the US Surgeon General (US Department of Health and Human Services, 1985) set out a broad conceptual framework for considering the joint effect of smoking with an occupational agent, which can be extended more generally to other risk factors. The levels of potential interaction between agents are multiple, ranging from molecular to behavioural (Table 2.3.1). Current research on the molecular basis of carcinogenesis is improving the understanding of potential points of interaction at the mechanistic level, but approaches to assess effect modification remain largely empirical. Some of the potential points of interaction (Table 2.3.1) would have an impact on the level of exposure, others — including the exposure–dose relationship — on the dose–response relation of exposure with risk, either for smoking or for the modifying factor. Typically, epidemiological data do not provide evidence relevant for assessing each of these potential points of interaction of another risk factor with cigarette smoking. In assessing the presence of synergism or antagonism, a model is assumed to predict the combined effect from the individual effects; in the absence of sufficient biological understanding to be certain of the most appropriate model, the choice is often driven by convention or convenience. There is also a potential for the combined effects to vary over the life-span; as the carcinogenesis process advances, agents are cleared (e.g. chrysotile asbestos fibres are cleared or dissolve in the lung), or exposure to tobacco or the other agent ends. Epidemiological studies generally only capture combined effects over a single interval of time.

In a multi-stage formulation of carcinogenesis, inferences as to the stages at which agents act can be made based on patterns of effect modification, particularly if data are available on the timing of exposure (Doll, 1971; Whittemore, 1977; Thomas & Whittemore, 1988). Effect modification also has implications for prevention, as synergism may increase the disease burden beyond that anticipated from the risk of smoking alone and may place some people, e.g. occupationally exposed workers, at particularly high risk.

The identification of studies addressing effect modification is difficult as authors may not have noted that effect modification was examined and search terms are not sufficiently conclusive. It was also impossible to search all studies involving smoking and potential modifying factors. Consequently, targeted searches were used to find published articles that specifically mentioned interaction, synergism or antagonism. Summary reviews also could be used as a further source of references.

(a)   Epidemiological concepts

The effect of a risk factor for a disease may be estimated on an absolute scale or on a relative scale. In the absolute risk model, the risk $(r(x))$ of disease associated with some factor (x) can be expressed in a simple linear relationship as:

$r(x) = r_0 + \beta x$

while in a relative risk relationship, risk is given by:

$r(x) = r_0 \times (1 + \beta x) = r_0 + r_0 \beta x$

where r_0 is the background rate of disease in the absence of exposure and β describes the increment in risk per unit increment in exposure to x. Under a relative risk characterization of disease risk, the impact of an exposure on disease risk, $r_0 \beta x$, depends on the background rate. In the absolute risk model, the effect of exposure on disease risk, βx, does not depend on the level of r_0. The selection of the risk model (i.e. absolute or relative), has substantial implications for interpreting the combined effects of two agents and for extending risks observed in one population to another population that may not have comparable r_0 because of differing patterns of risk factors other than the exposure of interest.

These two models can be extended to address the effects of multiple causes of disease. In the example of two exposures, x_1 and x_2 (e.g. radon and smoking), disease risk $(r(x_1,x_2))$ under a relative risk model is given by:

Additive model: $r(x_1,x_2) = r_0 + r_0 \beta_1 x_1 + r_0 \beta_2 x_2$

Multiplicative model: $r(x_1,x_2) = r_0 \times (1 + \beta_1 x_1)(1 + \beta_2 x_2) =$
$r_0 + r_0 \beta_1 x_1 + r_0 \beta_2 x_2 + r_0 \beta_1 x_1 \beta_2 x_2 =$
$r_0 + r_0 \beta_1 x_1 + r_0 \beta_2 x_2(1 + \beta_1 x_1)$

Comparison of these two models highlights the differing dependence of the effect of x_2 on r_0 and x_1. In assessing the role of x_2 on disease risk, a multiplicative model implies that the effect of x_2 on disease risk depends not only on r_0, but also on the effect of x_1. In contrast, under the additive model, the effect of x_2 depends on r_0 but not on the effect of x_1.

Epidemiologists describe the effect of exposures in causing disease either as a difference on an absolute scale or as a ratio on a relative scale. The preference has been for ratio measures (e.g. the relative risk that compares risk in the exposed group to risk in a referent group, typically the unexposed group). Effect modification is considered to occur when the combined effect of two or more variables is larger or smaller than the anticipated effect predicted by the independent effects, based on the measure used (Greenland, 1993). Current analytical approaches compare the combined effect to predictions based on either additivity or multiplicativity of the individual effects, that is, using either the absolute risk or relative risk models described above. Thus, a factor may be an effect modifier in the additive model and not in the multiplicative model. Epidemiologists have recognized that the appropriate scale for assessing a combined effect depends on the intent of the analysis (Rothman *et al.*, 1980). For public health purposes, an effect greater than additive is considered as synergistic. Biological mechanisms, if sufficiently understood, may suggest an alternative scale for assessment.

Although epidemiological methods have been proposed for assessing effect modification, no strict criteria for determining its presence have been defined. Rothman (1976) developed a synergy index that quantifies departure from independence of effects. Statistical significance alone is recognized to be an insufficient criterion (Greenland, 1993), and the interpretation of patterns of interdependence remains subjective. Additionally, inadequate statistical power often limits the assessment of effect modification (Greenland, 1983) and interpretation of possible effect modification should also consider the consequences of exposure measurement error, which may differ in degree for smoking and the other agent(s).

The concern about limited power extends specifically to studies of smoking and disease. Particularly limiting is the small number of cases that occur among nonsmokers in the studies of occupational agents.

(b)   Statistical concepts

Statisticians have used the term 'interaction' to refer to interdependence as detected by a statistical approach or 'model'. Interaction, which is equivalent to the epidemiological concept of effect modification, has typically been assessed in a regression framework using product terms of the risk factors of interest to test for effect modification (Thomas & Whittemore, 1988; Rothman & Greenland, 1998). For example, interaction between two risk factors, x_1 (e.g. smoking) and x_2 (e.g. radon exposure) could be assessed using the following model:

$$r(x_1, x_2) = 1 + \beta_1 x_1 + \beta_2 x_2 + \beta_3 x_1 x_2$$

In this linear model, the product or interaction term, $\beta_3 x_1 x_2$, estimates the joint contribution of the two agents to the risk. The model provides an estimate of the value of β_3 and a test of the statistical significance of β_3 for the null hypothesis: $\beta_3 = 0$. This modelling approach inherently assumes a mathematical scale on which the interaction is characterized, the usual choices being additive or multiplicative. Most often, primarily because of computational convenience, the multiplicative scale is used. Alternative approaches for assessing interaction have been described (Thomas, 1981; Breslow & Storer, 1985; Lubin & Gaffey, 1988). These choices more flexibly estimate the combined effects of risk factors without imposing the rigidity of a particular scale. Imprecision and bias from measurement error may also limit estimates obtained from such modelling approaches.

(c)   Characterizing the burden of cancer attributable to smoking

In describing the burden of disease, epidemiologists use a quantity referred to as the attributable risk (Rothman & Greenland, 1998). The attributable risk indicates the burden of disease that could be avoided if exposure to the agent of concern were fully prevented. This measure has been widely used for cigarette smoking to estimate the burden of avoidable tobacco-caused disease.

One form of the attributable risk, the population attributable risk (PAR) describes the proportion of disease in a population associated with exposure to an agent. For a factor, x_1, having an associated relative risk RR_1, PAR is calculated as below, where I and I_0 and P_1 and P_0 are the disease rates and probabilities of exposure in the population under current conditions and under some counterfactual set of conditions of differing exposure (for smoking, generally the complete prevention of smoking), respectively:

$$PAR(x) = \frac{I - I_0}{I}$$

$$= \frac{P_1 I_1 + P_0 I_0 - I_0}{P_1 I_1 + P_0 I_0}$$

$$= \frac{P_1(RR_1 - 1)}{P_1(RR_1 - 1) + 1}$$

For diseases caused by several agents, the total burden of disease that is theoretically preventable may exceed the observed number of cases, or 100%, if there are synergistic patterns of effect modification on an additive scale. For example, an estimate of smoking-attributable lung cancer cases can be conceptualized as including those cases caused by smoking, and those caused by radon and smoking in smokers. In the above formula, the attributable risk figure for smoking includes those cases caused by smoking alone and radon and smoking acting together; similarly, the attributable risk figure for radon would include those cases caused by radon alone and those caused by radon acting together with smoking. Combining the attributable risk estimates for smoking and radon counts the jointly determined cases twice. This subtlety of the attributable risk statistic is not universally appreciated and there is widespread misperception that the attributable risk should add up to 100% when all the various causes of the cancer are considered.

For two factors, x_1 and x_2, the sum of the individual exposure-specific PAR estimates, PAR(x_1) and PAR(x_2), can exceed 100%. However, when evaluating two factors, these PARs are incorrectly determined by contamination of the referent groups; i.e. the subgroup of individuals with $x_1 = 0$ includes subjects for whom x_2 may be 0 or 1 and the subgroup of individuals with $x_2 = 0$ includes persons for whom x_1 may be 0 or 1.

For joint exposures to x_1 and x_2, PAR is defined as:

$$PAR_{(x1,x2)} = \frac{P_{1,1}(RR_{1,1} - 1) + P_{1,0}(RR_{1,0} - 1) + P_{0,1}(RR_{0,1} - 1)}{P_{1,1}(RR_{1,1} - 1) + P_{1,0}(RR_{1,0} - 1) + P_{0,1}(RR_{0,1} - 1) + 1}$$

The PAR for two exposures, e.g. smoking and radon, is the sum of components due to smoking in the absence of radon exposure, to radon exposure in the absence of smoking, i.e. in never-smokers, and to the combined effect of radon exposure and smoking. PAR(x_1,x_2), calculated with the above formula, cannot exceed 100%.

Finally, the definition of PAR can be generalized for a continuous exposure, x, with exposure distribution f, as

$$PAR(x) = \frac{I - I_0}{I}$$

$$= \frac{\int I(x)f(x)dx - I_0}{\int I(x)f(x)dx}$$

$$= \frac{\int RR(x)f(x)dx - 1}{\int RR(x)f(x)dx}$$

where RR(x) is the relative risk for exposure level x, relative to zero exposure.

2.3.2   Asbestos

Asbestos, a term referring to a group of fibrous silicates, has long been identified as a cause of lung cancer, and was classified by IARC as *carcinogenic to humans* (Group 1) (IARC, 1987). Many studies of asbestos-exposed workers have addressed the combined effect of asbestos and smoking on lung cancer risk. Data available at the time allowed the Working Group to establish that 'the relationship between asbestos exposure and smoking indicated a synergistic effect of smoking with regard to lung cancer' (IARC, 1987). There have been several recent comprehensive reviews on this topic (Erren *et al.*, 1999; Lee, 2001; Liddell, 2001), as well as several frequently-cited earlier reviews (Saracci, 1977; Vainio & Boffetta, 1994). The topic has also been addressed in several reviews on occupational carcinogens in general and smoking (Saracci, 1987; Saracci & Boffetta, 1994).

Tables 2.3.2 and 2.3.3 summarize the characteristics of the principal relevant case–control and cohort studies, respectively, reviewed by Lee (2001), together with one more recent study (Gustavsson *et al.*, 2002). These studies vary widely in design and in the quality and extent of information available on smoking and on asbestos exposure. In the cohort studies, exposure to asbestos was generally at levels that would be considered high in relation to today's occupational standards. Exposure estimates were based on available sources of information including measurements that were generally limited in scope. Types of information included: job and industry, judgement of industrial hygienists, and self-report. The extent of the available information on smoking was also variable and in many of the cohort studies information was collected only at the initiation of follow-up or some other single point in time. In the case–control studies, interviews with the participants or with a surrogate respondent for deceased persons were the principal source of information.

Tables 2.3.4 and 2.3.5, adapted from Lee (2001), provide the relative risks for the four strata created by dichotomous classification of smoking and asbestos exposure. The general pattern of the risk estimates indicated departure from additivity in many of the studies, although the findings of some studies did not indicate synergism (McDonald *et al.*, 1993; McDonald *et al.*, 1999). The extent of departure from additivity varied across studies, from only slightly greater than additive (Gustavsson *et al.*, 2002) to a multiplicative interaction (Hammond *et al.*, 1979).

The three recent reviews include quantitative summaries of the evidence on effect modification. [The Working Group did not attempt to replicate these analyses.]

Erren and colleagues (Erren *et al.*, 1999) identified 17 relevant reports published from 1966 to 1996. Of these, 12 were included in the analysis, which used Rothman's synergy index. The value of the synergy index exceeded unity in all of the 12 studies. After excluding one study and verifying the absence of significant heterogeneity between the studies, the weighted summary value of the synergy index was estimated as 1.66 (95% CI, 1.33–2.06).

Liddell (2001) focused on seven cohort studies and six case–control studies. He also calculated an index of effect modification, termed the relative asbestos effect (RAE), which exceeded unity if the effect was greater in nonsmokers than in smokers. For the cohort studies, the estimate of RAE was 2.04 (95% CI, 1.28–3.25), indicating that the relative risk for asbestos exposure in nonsmokers was twice that in smokers; for the case–control studies, the RAE estimate was 0.83 (95% CI, 0.53–1.30). Liddell set aside the case–control data as being of insufficient quality and found that the data from cohort studies were not consistent with a fully multiplicative interaction. [The Working group noted that Liddell did not test for departure from additivity].

Lee (2001) analysed data from 23 studies, testing for additivity and multiplicativity. The studies reviewed showed strong evidence for departure from additivity. A test of multiplicativity was used that was conceptually comparable to Rothman's synergy index. Although the value of this index varied substantially across studies, the summary value of the synergy index derived by meta-analysis was 0.90 (95% CI, 0.67–1.20), which was consistent with a multiplicative interaction.

The discrepancy between the analyses, findings and conclusions of Erren *et al.* (1999), Lee (2001) and Liddell (2001) lies in the selection of studies and the approaches used to abstract and analyse the evidence. All three reviews document the range of the evidence and the imprecision with which many of the studies assess effect modification.

The Working Group concluded that the evidence supports synergism between asbestos exposure and smoking in causing lung cancer, but notes that the degree of synergism remains uncertain.

2.3.3   *Radon and other ionizing radiation*

The combined effect of radon and smoking has been investigated in cohort studies of underground miners exposed to radon and radon progeny and in case–control studies of lung cancer and exposure to radon in homes. The Working Group for the *IARC Monograph* on radon 'considered that the epidemiological evidence [did] not lead to a firm conclusion concerning the interaction between exposure to radon decay products and tobacco smoking' (IARC, 1988a). The report of the US National Research Council's Biological Effects of Ionizing Radiation (BEIR) VI Committee provided an in-depth review of the combined effect of smoking and radon on lung cancer risk and the following section is largely based on this report (National Research Council, 1999). The cohort and case–control studies cited in that review, together with more recent studies, are included in Tables 2.3.6 and 2.3.7.

The BEIR VI Committee identified five cohort studies of underground miners that provided information on both smoking and exposure to radon progeny (Table 2.3.6). The extent of information available on smoking was variable and smoking was not systematically evaluated across the follow-up of any of the cohorts. Quantitative estimates of exposure to radon progeny were available for all participants. The data had been analysed by Lubin *et al.* (1994) using a mixture model that flexibly assessed effect modification. The two largest studies, the study of Colorado Plateau uranium miners and the study of Chinese tin miners, provided the strongest evidence of effect modification because of the size of the cohorts and the numbers of lung cancer deaths. Both studies provided evidence against the additive model, as did the overall estimate for the mixture parameter, which indicated a synergistic but submultiplicative interaction.

In modelling the risk for lung cancer, the BEIR VI Committee adopted this submultiplicative interaction. Relative to the overall effect of exposure to radon progeny on lung cancer risk, the risk estimate in ever-smokers was proportionally lower by a factor of 0.9 whereas the relative effect in never-smokers was proportionally higher by 1.9.

Hornung and colleagues (Hornung *et al.*, 1998) reported an analysis of the Colorado Plateau study that incorporated updated smoking information obtained in 1986 from surviving cohort members and next of kin of deceased members. The smoking histories, updated for about two-thirds of the original cohort, showed a substantial rise in the proportion of former smokers. Multiple analytical approaches were used to explore effect modification. The general finding was that the interaction between smoking and radon was submultiplicative, but there was no strong evidence against a multiplicative interaction.

Further evidence on smoking and exposure to radon progeny has come from a population-based case–control study conducted in Gejiu City, the site of the Yunnan Tin Corporation (Yao *et al.*, 1994). This study included 460 cases, of whom 368 had been miners, and 1043 controls. Tobacco was smoked by study participants as cigarettes or with water pipes or Chinese long-stem pipes; a mixed pattern of smoking was most common. In contrast to the cohort analysis of the Yunnan tin miners, the case–control data were consistent with a multiplicative model, although the best-fitting model was intermediate between additive and multiplicative.

The joint effect of smoking and exposure to radon progeny could plausibly vary with the sequence of the two exposures. Thomas and colleagues (Thomas *et al.*, 1994) analysed the Colorado Plateau data using a case–control approach to assess temporal modification of the interaction between radon progeny and smoking. They characterized the temporal sequence of the two exposures as: simultaneous; radon before smoking; and radon following smoking. Exposure to radon followed by smoking was associated with an essentially additive effect whereas smoking followed by exposure to radon was associated with a more than multiplicative effect on a relative risk scale. Thomas and colleagues interpreted this finding as suggesting that smoking could act to promote radon-initiated cells.

The data from the Colorado Plateau cohort and Yunnan tin miners cohort have been analysed with mechanistic carcinogenic models, based in the Moolgavkar, Venzon and Knudson two-mutation model (Moolgavkar *et al.*, 1993; Luebeck *et al.*, 1999; Hazelton *et al.*, 2001; Little *et al.*, 2002). Under the assumed models, inferences can be made as to the mutations affected by smoking and exposure to radon progeny. In the most recent analysis of the Colorado Plateau cohort data (Little *et al.*, 2002), the findings of a two-stage model implied action of both factors on the first mutation rate and an action of exposure to radon progeny on intermediate cell death or the differentiation rate. A two-stage model was applied by Hazelton *et al.* (2001) to the Yunnan tin miner cohort data, which included estimates of exposure to smoking, arsenic and radon progeny. Various models were fitted; all showed effects of each of the exposures; radon had the smallest effect and smoking the greatest.

Effect modification has also been assessed in case–control studies of lung cancer in the general population (Table 2.3.7). All studies made estimates of radon concentration in the current and past homes of persons with lung cancer and of appropriate controls. Information on smoking was obtained by interview with the index respondent or with a surrogate for deceased persons. Measurement error is an unavoidable limitation of these studies, as exposure to radon throughout the lifetime is considered relevant to risk for lung cancer in adulthood.

Because most cases of lung cancer occur in smokers, the case–control studies included few never-smokers and consequently effect modification cannot be characterized with great precision. The available studies do not provide evidence for effect modification, considered on the multiplicative scale. [The Working Group noted that the studies have not been systematically analysed for the presence of synergism, assessed as departure from additivity].

The combined effect of smoking and exposure to radiation has been assessed in a few populations exposed to low-linear energy transfer (LET) radiation. These populations included atomic bomb survivors (Prentice et al., 1983; Kopecky et al., 1986), persons receiving therapeutic irradiation for breast cancer (Kaldor et al., 1992; Neugut et al., 1994; Van Leeuwen et al., 1995), and workers subjected to mixed exposure to external gamma radiation and internal emitters (Petersen et al., 1990).

Of the cancer risks associated with exposure to radiation in atomic bomb survivors, relative risks for lung cancer are among the highest (Mabuchi et al., 1991). A series of studies conducted by the Radiation Effects Research Foundation have explored the effect of smoking on lung cancer in the atomic bomb survivors. Kopecky et al. (1986) reported an analysis of the combined effects of smoking and radiation in a selected cohort for which information was available on smoking. A total of 351 cases of lung cancer were reported in a cohort of 29 332 exposed survivors. Poisson regression models were used to assess the effects of exposure to radiation (using the T65 radiation dosimetry), and smoking, with control for other factors including age at the time of the bombing. Using an additive model for the excess relative risk, Kopecky et al. (1986) found that both exposure to radiation and cigarette smoking were determinants of lung cancer risk; an interaction term for the two exposures was not statistically significant ($p = 0.72$). While Kopecky et al. (1986) expressed a preference for the additive model based on these analyses, further analyses by the BEIR IV Committee (National Research Council, 1988) showed that the data were equally compatible with a multiplicative model.

Three studies have examined modification by cigarette smoking of the risk for lung cancer following therapeutic irradiation.

Neugut et al. (1994) conducted a case–control study of Connecticut women with a second primary cancer following an initial diagnosis of breast cancer. The cases ($n = 94$) were women with lung cancer as the second primary cancer whereas the controls ($n = 598$) had a second malignancy of a type not associated with smoking or radiation. The pattern of the increased risk associated with both smoking and radiation therapy for the initial breast cancer was consistent with a multiplicative interaction; however, the consistency of the data with different models was not formally assessed.

Van Leeuwen et al. (1995) used a nested case–control design to assess risk for lung cancer in relation to radiation and smoking in a cohort of 1939 patients who had received treatment for Hodgkin disease in the Netherlands. The 30 cases identified during an 18-year follow-up were matched to 82 controls. Radiation doses to the region of the lung where the case developed cancer were estimated and information on smoking was obtained from several sources. There was a significantly greater increase in risk among smokers in relation to estimated radiation dose than among nonsmokers. However, in reviewing the findings, Boivin (1995) showed that the pattern of combined effects was consistent with additivity of the excess relative risks. This study was limited by the small number of lung cancer cases and by the potential modifying effects of chemotherapy.

Therapy for small-cell carcinoma of the lung includes aggressive chemotherapy and radiation. Tucker *et al.* (1997) carried out a multi-centre study in North America of 611 persons treated for small-cell carcinoma of the lung and who remained cancer-free for at least two years after the therapy. The risks varied with smoking status with the highest risk being found in those who continued to smoke after the initial diagnosis of lung cancer (relative risk = 21); no second lung cancers were observed in the 13 never-smokers. The authors reported that the interaction was not statistically significant when a model was used to assess interaction.

2.3.4   *Arsenic*

The combined effect of smoking and arsenic on lung cancer risk has been examined in occupational groups exposed to arsenic through work in smelting or metal mining. Table 2.3.8 summarizes the studies included in two relevant reviews (Hertz-Picciotto *et al.*, 1992; Saracci & Boffetta, 1994).

Hertz-Picciotto *et al.* (1992) used data from six studies (Rencher *et al.*, 1977; Pershagen *et al.*, 1981; Enterline, 1983; Pershagen, 1985; Enterline *et al.*, 1987; Järup & Pershagen, 1991) to evaluate the pattern of joint effects. Although the data available from the different studies were not uniform, the analysis indicated a pattern of combined effects that was consistently greater than additive.

2.3.5   *Alcohol drinking*

The combined effects of smoking and alcohol consumption on cancers of the oral cavity, pharynx, larynx and oesophagus have been examined extensively, and to a lesser degree for cancer of the liver (Table 2.3.9). The studies varied in their methods and in the approaches used to assess effect modification, which ranged from descriptive to formal estimation of interaction terms in multivariate models.

(*a*)   *Cancers of the upper aerodigestive tract*

For cancers of the oral cavity and pharynx, the evidence comes entirely from case–control studies carried out in Asia, Australia, Europe and the United States. In the majority of the studies, evaluation of effect modification was descriptive, without formal assessment of interaction. Overall, however, the pattern of odds ratios for smoking, across categories of alcohol consumption, is consistent with synergism. In two studies with relatively large numbers of cases and controls, the pattern of increasing cancer risk with increasing alcohol consumption is strong (Mashberg *et al.*, 1993; Kabat *et al.*, 1994). In both studies, the pattern of odds ratios for men and women was consistent with synergism and a test for interaction was statistically significant for both sexes.

Seven case–control studies and one cohort study reported on joint effects of tobacco smoking and alcohol drinking on the risk for oesophageal cancer. Generally, the studies support a positive departure of joint effects from additivity. Since multiple logistic regression models were used for analysing most of these studies, some also were tested for departure from multiplicativity. These tests for interaction are inadequate to assess synergy as defined in this monograph.

Most of the case–control studies of laryngeal cancer provide strong evidence for synergism. The studies were carried out in a number of locations around the world. Only the study in Shanghai (Zheng et al., 1992) did not yield evidence consistent with synergism. In a number of studies, tests for interaction were carried out and reported to be 'non-significant.' These were tests for departure from the multiplicative models, typically multiple logistic regression models, used to analyze the case–control data, and not tests for departure from additivity.

Several studies reported on findings on cancer of the 'mixed upper aerodigestive tract', comprising studies of patients with squamous cell carcinomas, regardless of the specific site within the head and neck region. These studies also provided strong evidence for synergism.

(b)   Liver cancer

Alcohol consumption is an established cause of liver cancer (IARC, 1988b) and of hepatic injury, which may lead to hepatic cirrhosis. Six case–control studies were identified that included information on the joint effect of smoking and alcohol consumption on liver cancer risk. In three studies, odds ratios for smokers were greater if they were also in the higher category of alcohol consumption (Chen et al., 1991; Yu et al., 1991; Kuper et al., 2000). In one study (Kuper et al., 2000), there was a statistically significant and super-multiplicative interaction between heavy smoking and heavy drinking in causing liver cancer.

2.3.6   Infectious agents

(a)   Hepatitis B

Two case–control studies were identified that provided evidence on risk for liver cancer associated with smoking by serological status for hepatitis B infection (Table 2.3.10). The results are conflicting; the study conducted in Greece (Trichopoulos et al., 1987) showed generally lower odds ratios in subjects who were seropositive for hepatitis B surface antigen compared with those who were negative for the antigen, whereas the study from China, Province of Taiwan (Chen et al., 1991) showed greater risks in subjects who were positive for hepatitis B surface antigen.

(b)   Human papillomavirus

For cervical cancer (squamous-cell type), evidence suggests that human papillomavirus (HPV) is a necessary factor, and implies that the risk of smoking cannot be estimated in the absence of HPV infection. Because the absolute risk of cervical cancer in the absence of HPV infection, is hence by definition zero, the incremental risk associated with smoking is interpreted as indicating synergism (Table 2.3.11).

(c)   Helicobacter pylori

A case–control study of stomach cancer in Moscow examined the combined effect of smoking and *H. pylori* infection (Zaridze *et al.*, 2000). In non-infected persons, the odds ratio, comparing ever- to never-smokers was 1.2 (95% CI, 0.8–1.8) whereas in infected persons, the odds ratio was 1.6 (95% CI, 1.0–2.4). The odds ratios did not vary significantly with infection status. No other studies were identified.

2.3.7   Others

(a)   Nickel

Only one study addressed the combined effect of occupational exposure to nickel and cigarette smoking. Andersen and colleagues (Andersen *et al.*, 1996) reported the findings of a cohort study of workers (*n* = 4764) at the Falconbridge nickel refinery (Norway). Information on smoking was obtained primarily from medical records at the refinery and from co-workers. Assessment of effect modification was restricted to 1337 men who were in the same birth cohorts as a population comparison group. The results were consistent with a combined effect of nickel exposure and smoking that is multiplicative: the relative risk for unexposed smokers was 6.1; the relative risk for exposed never-smokers was 3.6; and relative risk for exposed smokers was 23.

(b)   Silica (silicon dioxide)

Exposure to silica is common among miners, sand-blasters and many other occupational groups. Crystalline silica has been classified by IARC as *carcinogenic to humans* (Group 1) (IARC, 1997) and is also known to cause silicosis, a fibriotic disorder of the lungs. Workers with silicosis have an increased risk for lung cancer that may be the direct consequence of the silica particles deposited in the lung, or an indirect consequence of the lung fibrosis.

Studies that have investigated the combined effect of smoking with silica exposure are summarized in Table 2.3.12 (Saracci & Boffetta, 1994). Both studies on silica exposure and on silicosis were included. No consistent patterns of effect modification were evident in either group of studies.

(c)   Chloromethyl ethers

The chloromethyl ethers include chloromethyl methyl ether and bis(chloromethyl)-ether; these compounds were used in the chemical industry as intermediates in organic synthesis and in the production of ion exchange resins. The strong association of exposure to this agent with lung cancer was first reported by Figueroa *et al.* (1973) who described 14 cases; three were in never-smokers and the histology for 13 of the cases showed that only one was not a small-cell carcinoma. On follow-up of workers in the plant, nonsmokers were found to comprise a higher proportion of cases than in the general population (Weiss *et al.*, 1979). In a small cohort ($n = 51$) apparently drawn from the same plant (Weiss, 1980), the standardized mortality rate for lung cancer death was markedly higher for never-smokers and former smokers together, compared with current smokers. The authors interpreted this analysis as indicating antagonism between smoking and exposure to chloromethyl ethers. [The Working Group noted the limited information available on the joint effect of smoking and exposure to chloromethyl ethers.]

Table 2.3.1. Examples of levels of interaction between smoking and another agent

Exposure
- Work assignments of smokers and nonsmokers are different.
- Absenteism rates differ for smokers and nonsmokers.

Exposure–dose relationships for the lung
- Differing patterns of physical activity and ventilation for smokers and nonsmokers
- Differing patterns of lung deposition and clearance in smokers and nonsmokers
- Differing morphometry of target cells in smokers and nonsmokers

Carcinogenesis
- Other carcinogens and tobacco smoke carcinogens act at the same or different steps in a multistage carcinogenic process.
- Smokers and non-smokers differ on other, unmeasured modifying factors.

Table 2.3.2. Characteristics of case–control studies on the combined effect of asbestos exposure and smoking in the causation of lung cancer

Reference[a]	Location	Years of study	Study type and population	Controls	No. of cases[b]	Source of diagnosis
Martischnig et al. (1977)	Gateshead, UK	1972–73	Hospital-based; shipbuilding area	Patients	201	Confirmed clinical
Blot et al. (1978, 1980, 1982)	Georgia, Virginia, Florida, USA	1970–78	Shipbuilding areas	Patients and decedents, no chronic obstructive pulmonary disease	1072	Death certificates, medical records
Rubino et al. (1979)	Balangero, Italy	1946–75	Nested case–control study in chrysotile miners and millers	Alive when case died	12	Death certificates, medical records
Pastorino et al. (1984)	Lombardy, Italy	1976–79	Industrial areas	Population	204	Confirmed clinical
Kjuus et al. (1986)	Telemark and Vestfold, Norway	1979–83	Hospital-based; industrial and shipbuilding areas	Patients, no chronic obstructive pulmonary disease, other diseases precluding employment in heavy industry	176	Medical records
Garshick et al. (1987)	USA	1981–82	Railroad workers	Decedent, no cancer, accident, suicide, unknown cause	1081	Death certificates
De Klerk et al. (1991)	Wittenoom, Australia	1979–86	Nested case–control study in crocidolite miners and millers	Alive, no asbestos-related disease	40	Death certificates, medical records
Minowa et al. (1991)	Yokosuka, Japan	1979–82	Shipbuilding area	Decedent, no cancer, pneumoconiosis, accident, suicide	96	Confirmed clinical or autopsy
Bovenzi et al. (1993)	Trieste, Italy	1979–81, 1985–86	Industrial and shipbuilding area	Decedent, no chronic obstructive pulmonary disease, smoking-related cancer	516	Autopsy records
Gustavsson et al. (2002)	Stockholm, Sweden	1985–90	All men aged 40–75 years, residents of Stockholm County	1. Alive 2. Decedent, no tobacco-related disease	1038	Regional cancer register

Adapted from Lee (2001)

[a] Reference from which main results were obtained

[b] Number of cases with data on smoking and asbestos exposure

Table 2.3.3. Characteristics of cohort studies on the combined effect of asbestos exposure and smoking in the causation of lung cancer

Reference[a]	Location	Follow-up period	Study population	No. of cases[b]	Source of diagnosis
Elmes & Simpson (1971)	Belfast, Northern Ireland	1940–66	Insulation workers	19	Death certificates, medical records
Selikoff & Hammond (1975)	New York and New Jersey, USA	1943–74	Insulation workers	47	Death certificates, medical records
Hammond et al. (1979)	USA and Canada	1967–76	Insulation workers	276	Death certificates, medical records
Selikoff et al. (1980)	New Jersey, USA	1961–77	Amosite asbestos factory workers	50	Death certificates, medical records
Acheson et al. (1984)	Uxbridge, UK	1947–79	Amosite asbestos factory workers	22	Death certificates
Berry et al. (1985)	East London, UK	1960–70, 1971–80	Asbestos factory workers	79	Death certificates
Hilt et al. (1985)	Telemark, Norway	1953–80	Workers in nitric acid production plant	127	Death certificates
Neuberger & Kundi (1990)	Vöcklabruck, Austria	1950–87	Asbestos cement products workers	49	Death certificates, medical records
Hughes & Weill (1991)	New Orleans, USA	1969–83	Asbestos cement products workers	26	Death certificates
Cheng & Kong (1992)	Tianjin, China	1972–87	Chrysotile asbestos products workers	21	Not given (death)
McDonald et al. (1993)	Quebec, Canada	1950–92	Chrysotile miners and millers	299	Death certificates
Zhu & Wang (1993)	8 factories, China	1972–86	Chrysotile asbestos products workers	57	Death certificates, medical records
Meurman et al. (1994)	North Savo, Finland	1953–91	Anthophyllite miners	55	Cancer registration
Oksa et al. (1997)	Finland	1967–94	(1) Asbestos sprayers	3	Cancer registry
			(2) Asbestosis patients	33	
			(3) Silicosis patients	15	

Adapted from Lee (2001)
[a] Reference from which main results were obtained.
[b] Number of cases with data on smoking and exposure to asbestos

Table 2.3.4. Case–control studies on the combined effect of exposure to asbestos and smoking in the causation of lung cancer

Reference	Definition and source of asbestos exposure	Definition of smoking exposure	Relative risk[a]				Inter-action[b]
			Not exposed to asbestos or smoking	Exposed to asbestos but not smoking	Exposed to smoking but not asbestos	Exposed to smoking and asbestos	
Martischnig et al. (1977)	Yes vs no: questionnaire on work history	≥ 15 vs 0–14 cigarettes/day	1	1.08	1.78	5.57	> M
Blot et al. (1978, 1980, 1982)	Ever vs never worked in shipbuilding: interview of patients or proxies about work history	Current or former < 10 years					
		Georgia (n = 458)	1	1.28	4.71	7.58	~ M
		Virginia (n = 319)	1	1.88	3.09	4.87	~ M
		Florida (n = 295)	1	1.80	6.01	7.79	
Rubino et al. (1979)	≥ 101 vs 100 fibre–years: work history, dust measurements	Smoker vs nonsmoker	0	0	1	2.32	
Pastorino et al. (1984)	Yes vs no: interview of patients or proxies about work history	≥ 10 vs 0–9 cigarettes/day	1	2.82	5.47	9.86	1
Kjuus et al. (1986)	Heavy or moderate vs uncertain or none: interview of patients about asbestos exposure	≥ 10 vs 0–9 cigarettes/day	1	2.41	5.41	19.86	~ M
Garshick et al. (1987)	Yes vs no: work history	> 50 pack–years vs never smoker[c]					
		age < 65 years	1	1.20	5.68	6.82	
		age ≥ 65 years	1	0.98	9.14	8.96	
De Klerk et al. (1991)	High vs low: work history, dust measurements	Current or former < 10 years vs nonsmoker or former ≥ 10 years	1	2.24	3.44	9.57	> M
Minowa et al. (1991)	Definite or suspected vs none: interview of proxies about work history	Current or former < 10 years vs never-smoker or former > 10 years	1	—[d]	3.38	8.28	

Table 2.3.4 (contd)

Reference	Definition and source of asbestos exposure	Definition of smoking exposure	Relative risk[a]				Inter-action[b]
			Not exposed to asbestos or smoking	Exposed to asbestos but not smoking	Exposed to smoking but not asbestos	Exposed to smoking and asbestos	
Bovenzi et al. (1993)	Definite or possible vs none: interview of proxies about work history	Ever- vs never-smoker	1	1.83	10.13	15.89	
Gustavsson et al. (2002)	≥ 2.5 fibre–years vs none: reported work histories evaluated by an industrial hygienist and linked to workplace measurements	Current smoker vs never-smoker	1	10.2	21.7	43.1	

Adapted from Saracci & Boffetta (1994); Lee (2001)

[a] 0 indicates no cases in this category; 1 indicates reference group.

[b] Interaction term taken from Saracci & Boffetta (1994); numbers in parentheses are based on the assumption of a relative risk due to smoking of 10;
A, additive; I, intermediate; M, multiplicative

[c] Fitted logistic regression assuming multiplicative model

[d] Not applicable because of zero division in odds ratio calculation

Table 2.3.5. Cohort studies on the combined effects of asbestos exposure and smoking in the causation of lung cancer

Reference	Definition and source of asbestos exposure	Definition of smoking exposure	Reference group[a]	Relative risk				Inter-action[c]
				Not exposed to asbestos or smoking	Exposed to asbestos but not smoking	Exposed to smoking but not asbestos[b]	Exposed to smoking and asbestos	
Elmes & Simpson (1971)	Study group: inferred from nature of population studied	Smoker vs nonsmoker	External	1	0[d]	(7.13)	112.94	
Selikoff & Hammond (1975)	Study group: inferred from nature of population studied	Ever vs never-smoker	External	1	8.44	(7.13)	73.71	(> M)
Hammond et al. (1979)	Study group: inferred from nature of population studied	Ever vs never-smoker	External	1	5.17	10.85	53.24	M
Selikoff et al. (1980)	Study group: inferred from nature of population studied	Ever vs never-smoker	External	1	25.00	(7.13)	33.44	I
Acheson et al. (1984)	Medium or heavy vs background: work history and dust measurements	Ever vs never-smoker	Internal External	0 1	1 6.07	0 (7.13)	2.57 15.53	(~ M)
Berry et al. (1985)	Severe vs low to moderate: work history	Ever vs never-smoker (1960–70) Men Women (1971–80) Men Women	Internal External	1 0 1 1	0 1 0 15.00	1.15 0 (7.13) (7.13)	1.93 2.26 19.33 33.97	(> M) (> M) (A) (I)
Hilt et al. (1985)	Exposed vs population controls: work history	Ever vs never-smoker	Internal	1	0	5.84	25.20	> M
Neuberger & Kundi (1990)	All workers: work history and dust measurements	Cigarettes/day smoked					[e]	
Hughes & Weill (1991)	Study group: work history and dust measurements	Ever vs never-smoker	External	1	0	(7.13)	~ 13	

Table 2.3.5 (contd)

Reference	Definition and source of asbestos exposure	Definition of smoking exposure	Reference group[a]	Relative risk				Interaction[c]
				Not exposed to asbestos or smoking	Exposed to asbestos but not smoking	Exposed to smoking but not asbestos[b]	Exposed to smoking and asbestos	
Cheng & Kong (1992)	Yes vs no: work history and dust measurements	Cigarette smoker vs nonsmoker	Internal	1	5.44	1.57	8.73	M
McDonald et al. (1993)	≥ 60 vs < 60 million particles per cubic foot × years: work history and dust measurements	Ever vs never-smoker	Internal External	1 1	1.65 4.07	4.46 (7.13)	4.51 11.13	
Zhu & Wang (1993)	Yes vs no: work history and dust measurements	Smoker vs nonsmoker	Internal	1	3.78	1.83	11.06	
Meurman et al. (1994)	Heavy vs moderate: work history	Cigarette smoker vs nonsmoker	Internal External	1 1	0.83 3.21	6.27 (7.13)	6.16 23.87	
Oksa et al. (1997)	Study group: medical interview	Ever-smoker vs never-smoker	External					
		Asbestos sprayers		1	0	(7.13)	74.77	
		Patients with asbestosis		1	0	(7.13)	81.72	
		Patients with silicosis		1	0	(7.13)	22.34	

Adapted from Saracci & Boffetta (1994); Lee (2001)

[a] Internal: internal data for all four comparison groups; external: external reference group for asbestos-exposed groups

[b] The value of 7.13, shown in parentheses, is a value assumed by Lee (2001) and taken from the British Doctors' Study (see Section 2.0).

[c] Interaction term taken from Saracci & Boffetta (1994); numbers in parentheses are based on the assumption of a relative risk due to smoking of 10; A, additive; I, intermediate; M, multiplicative

[d] Only five nonsmokers at risk

[e] Graph showing that the observed number of deaths was close to that expected according to the workers' smoking habits, indicating that 'exposure to chrysotile does not increase lung cancer'

Table 2.3.6. Cohort studies on the combined effect of smoking and exposure to radon progeny in the causation of lung cancer

Reference[a]	Place of study	Years of study	Study population	Total cases/cohort	Cases/cohort included	p value		Mixture	
						Multiplicative	Additive	λ	p value[b]
Radford & St Clair Renard (1984)	Sweden	1951–91	Iron miners	79/1294	51/1415	0.43	0.31	−0.3	0.38
Hornung & Meinhardt (1987)	Colorado, USA	1950–87	Uranium miners	329/3347	292/2205	0.58	0.04	0.7	0.49
Morrison et al. (1988)	Newfoundland, Canada	1950–84	Fluorspar miners	118/2088	25/1002	0.53	0.67	−0.1	0.85
Samet et al. (1991)	New Mexico, USA	1943–85	Uranium miners	69/3469	52/2602	0.15	0.11	0.4	0.16
Xuan et al. (1993)	Yunnan, China	1976–87	Tin miners	980/17 143	907/13 047	0.02	0.08	−0.3	0.39

Adapted from Lubin et al. (1994); NRC (1988)
[a] Most recent reference in 1994
[b] Refers to fit of mixture model versus full model.

Table 2.3.7. Case–control studies on the combined effect of smoking and radon exposure at home in the causation of lung cancer

Reference	Study location Years of study	No. of cases: Never-smoker/total	Findings
Axelson et al. (1988)	Sweden 1960–81	15/177	Increased risk for non- and occasional smokers vs. regular smokers in rural areas
Svensson et al. (1989)	Sweden 1983–85	35/210	Greater risk for smokers than never-smokers
Blot et al. (1990)	China 1985–87	123/308	Nonsignificantly greater risk in smokers ($p = 0.15$)
Schoenberg et al. (1990)	USA 1982–83	61/433	Exposure response strongest in light smokers; inverse in heaviest smokers
Ruosteenoja (1991)	Finland 1980–85	4/238	No pattern observed when heavier smokers compared with light smokers
Pershagen et al. (1994)	Sweden 1980–84	178/1360	Higher excess relative risk in current smokers than in never-smokers. Additivity rejected by data ($p = 0.02$)
Darby et al. (1998)	UK 1988–93	26/982	No evidence for heterogeneity of excess relative risk
Pisa et al. (2001)	Italy 1987–93	14/138	Interaction described as multiplicative, but analyses of interaction not significant
Wang et al. (2002)	China 1994–98	765/2009	No evidence for heterogeneity of excess relative risk

Adapted from NRC (1988)

Table 2.3.8. Studies on the combined effects of smoking and occupational exposure to arsenic on lung cancer

Reference Country and years of study	Study design	Source population	Exposure assessment (tobacco or arsenic)	No. of cases/ deaths	Smoking categories	Relative risks Exposure categories			Interaction/ excess risk (%)[a]	Comments
Rencher et al. (1977) USA 1959–69	Proportional mortality cohort	522 workers at Utah copper smelter who died in 1959–69	Smoking history obtained from work supervisors of deceased employees	31 deaths	Nonsmoker Smoker	*Mine* 1.0 4.7	*Concentrator* 1.1 4.7	*Smelter* 4.7 13.1	69	
Pershagen et al. (1981) Sweden 1928–77	Nested case–control	Cohort of 3958 workers at Ronnskar smelter employed for at least 3 months		76 deaths, 152 deceased controls	Nonsmoker Smoker	*No* 1.0 4.9	*Yes* 3.0 14.6		M; 131	Overlap of 41 cases with Pershagen (1985) and all 76 cases with Järup & Pershagen (1991)
Welch et al. (1982) USA 1938–77	Cohort	1800 workers from Anaconda, MT, smelter: heavy exposure and a 20% random sample of other exposure categories	Arsenic categories based on quantified exposure estimates for one point in time	80 deaths	Nonsmoker Smoker Nonsmoker Smoker	*Low* 1.0 1.3 *High* 3.0 3.8	*Medium* 0.9 3.3 *Very high* 6.6 8.5		M	Multiplicative interaction for (high + very high) vs low exposure
Pinto et al. (1978); Enterline (1983) USA 1949–73	Cohort	527 workers from Tacoma,WA, smelter who lived beyond age 65 and retired in 1949–73		32 deaths	Nonsmoker Smoker	*No* 1.0 7.2	*Yes* 5.1 20.7		(I); 91	

Table 2.3.8 (contd)

Reference, Country and years of study	Study design	Source population	Exposure assessment (tobacco or arsenic)	No. of cases/ deaths	Smoking categories	Relative risks — Exposure categories	Interaction/ excess risk (%)[a]	Comments
Pershagen (1985) Sweden 1961–79	Case–control	Residents in region where the Ronnskar smelter is located		212 deaths, 424 deceased controls	Nonsmoker Smoker	*None* 1.0 / *Residential* 2.3 8.3 / 17.5 *Mining* 10.4 / *Smelting* 8.4 35.2 / 26.2	Residential: 92 Mining: 105 Smelting: 71	Overlap of 52 cases with Järup & Pershagen (1991)
Enterline et al. (1987) USA 1949–80	Nested case–control	Cohort of 2288[b] workers employed at 6 copper smelters for ≥ 3 years in 1946–76, terminating employment at age > 44 and after 1949	Arsenic exposure very low compared with other smelters	55 cases, 126 controls	Nonsmoker Smoker for 20 years	*None* / *Mean exposure* 1.0 / 2.1 2.4 / 5.1	64	Included cases from study by Rencher et al. (1977). Fitted logistic model; mean exposure level over the six plants calculated as cumulative time-weighted average of 281.03 µg/m³-years.
Taylor et al. (1989) China 1971–84	Retrospective nested case–control	Past and present workers at Yunnan Tin Corporation	Arsenic categories based on quantified exposure estimates	107 cases, 107 controls	Light Medium Heavy	*Low* / *Medium* / *High* 1.0 / 3.2 / 5.0 1.0 / 4.9 / 4.4 1.4 / 8.9 / 4.9	~ A	Cases alive in 1985 Tobacco smoked in a water pipe; very few nonsmokers; interaction calculated for heavy vs light smokers and high vs low exposure
Tsuda et al. (1990) Japan 1972–89	Cohort	141 certified arsenic poisoning patients	Employment in arsenic mines	8 deaths	SMR Nonsmoker Smoker	*No* / *Yes* 0 / 264 0 / 1247	(> M)	Standardized mortality ratio using sex- and age-specific mortality rate of all Japanese in 1975, 1980 or 1985
Järup & Pershagen (1991) Sweden 1928–81	Nested case–control	Cohort of 3916 workers at Ronnskar smelter employed at least 3 months from 1928–67	Smokers of > 10 g tobacco/day; cumulative arsenic exposure	107 cases, 214 deceased controls excluding smoking-related causes	Nonsmoker Smoker	*Low* / *Medium* / *High* 1.0 / 1.4 / 5.6 40.1 / 9.4 / 29.2	Low: A Medium: ~ A High: I; 127	

Adapted from Hertz-Picciotto et al. (1992); Saracci & Boffetta (1994)

[a] Terms for interaction were taken from Saracci and Boffetta (1994); terms in parentheses are based on the assumption that the relative risk is 10. A, additive; I, intermediate; M, multiplicative; the numbers are the percentage by which observed exceeds predicted excess relative risk and are taken from Hertz-Picciotto et al. (1992).

[b] Original paper reported 5392 workers in the six plants considered.

Table 2.3.9. Studies with information on interaction of smoking and alcohol in the causation of cancer at various sites

Reference	Place, year	Study population	Definition of tobacco/alcohol exposure	Alcohol categories	Smoking categories	Relative risk (95% CI)	Comments
Oral cavity							
Choi & Kahyo (1991)	Seoul, Republic of Korea, 1986–89	Cases: 113 men, 44 women (oral cavity) Controls: 339 men, 132 women; hospital controls, matched on age, sex and admission date	Alcohol (soju) in mL/day: Light: < 8100 Medium: 8100–16 200 Heavy: > 16 200	Non-drinker	Nonsmoker ≤ 1 pack/day > 1 pack/day	1.0 0.5 1	Stratified analysis; ORs extrapolated from figure [no formal test for interaction]
				Light drinker	Nonsmoker ≤ 1 pack/day > 1 pack/day	0.1 0.5 1.1	
				Medium drinker	Nonsmoker ≤ 1 pack/day > 1 pack/day	1.5 1.5 1.8	
				Heavy drinker	Nonsmoker ≤ 1 pack/day > 1 pack/day	1 2 5.04	
Zheng et al. (1997)	Beijing, China, 1988–89	Cases: 111 cases (tongue) Controls: 111 hospital controls, matched by age and sex	Alcohol: lifetime consumption	Never-drinker	Nonsmoker ≤ 20 pack–years > 20 pack–years	1.0 1.2 7.6*	Logistic regression model; risk estimates adjusted for education level. *$p < 0.05$ [No formal test for interaction]
				≤ 255 kg	Nonsmoker ≤ 20 pack–years > 20 pack–years	1.9 1.6 23.3*	
				> 255 kg	Nonsmoker ≤ 20 pack–years > 20 pack–years	2.4 3.0 4.1	
Schlecht et al. (1999)	Brazil, 1986–89	Cases: 373 incident cases (oral cavity) Controls: 746 hospital controls, matched on hospital, trimester of admission, age and sex	Alcohol: lifetime consumption	0–10 kg	0–5 pack–years 6–42 pack–years > 42 pack–years	1.0 2.9 (1.2–6.8) 7.8 (2.9–21.0)	Logistic regression model that included an interaction term; risk estimates adjusted for race, beverage temperature, religion, wood stove use and consumption of spicy foods; no statistical evidence for effect modification [p not stated]
				11–530 kg	0–5 pack–years 6–42 pack–years > 42 pack–years	1.2 (0.4–3.4) 6.2 (2.7–14.1) 11.2 (4.8–26.3)	
				> 530 kg	0–5 pack–years 6–42 pack–years > 42 pack–years	2.3 (0.6–9.1) 19.5 (2.6–147) 20.3 (9.0–45.3)	
Pharynx							
Olsen et al. (1985)	Denmark, 1980–82	Cases: 32 incident cases (hypopharynx) Controls: 1141 population controls, matched on sex, residence and age	Tobacco: g of tobacco/week	< 150 g/week	< 10 g/week ≥ 10 g/week	1.0 3.0 (1.3–6.9)	Stratified analysis [no formal test for interaction]
				≥ 150 g/week	< 10 g/week ≥ 10 g/week	1.7 (0.5–5.9) 5.2 (2.0–13.6)	

Table 2.3.9 (contd)

Reference	Place, year	Study population	Definition of tobacco/alcohol exposure	Alcohol categories	Smoking categories	Relative risk (95% CI)	Comments
Choi & Kahyo (1991)	Seoul, Republic of Korea, 1986–89	Cases: 133 men, 19 women (pharynx) Controls: 399 men, 57 women; hospital controls, matched on age, sex and admission date	Alcohol (soju) in mL/day: Light: < 8100 Medium: 8100–16 200 Heavy: > 16 200	Nondrinker	Nonsmoker	1.0	Stratified analysis; ORs extrapolated from figure [no formal test for interaction]
					≤ 1 pack/day	0.8	
					> 1 pack/day	1.0	
				Light drinker	Nonsmoker	1.1	
					≤ 1 pack/day	0.9	
					> 1 pack/day	1.3	
				Medium drinker	Nonsmoker	1.0	
					≤ 1 pack/day	1.5	
					> 1 pack/day	1.2	
				Heavy drinker	Nonsmoker	1.0	
					≤ 1 pack/day	2.0	
					> 1 pack/day	6.7	
Schlecht et al. (1999)	Brazil, 1986–89	Cases: 217 incident cases (pharynx) Controls: 434 hospital controls, matched on hospital, trimester of admission, age and sex	Alcohol: lifetime consumption	0–10 kg	0–5 pack–years	1.0	Logistic regression model that included an interaction term; risk estimates were adjusted for race, beverage temperature, religion, wood stove use and consumption of spicy foods; interaction term statistically significant ($p = 0.007$)
					6–42 pack–years	2.4 (0.2–24.0)	
					> 42 pack–years	69.4 (6.9–694)	
				11–530 kg	0–5 pack–years	6.2 (0.7–56.6)	
					6–42 pack–years	21.7 (2.6–180)	
					> 42 pack–years	43.0 (4.9–340)	
				> 530 kg	0–5 pack–years	22.3 (2.1–238)	
					6–42 pack–years	66.3 (1.7–2556)	
					> 42 pack–years	77.3 (9.2–625)	

Table 2.3.9 (contd)

Oesophagus
Case–control studies

Reference	Place, year	Study population	Definition of tobacco/alcohol exposure	Alcohol categories	Smoking categories	Relative risk (95% CI)	Comments
Franceschi et al. (1990)	Northern Italy, 1986–89	Cases: 288 men, <75 years old Controls: men <75 years old, admitted to same hospitals for acute illness	*Tobacco:* Light: ex-smoker who quit ≥ 10 years ago or smoker of 1–14 cigs/day for < 30 years Moderate: 30–39 years duration regardless of amount, 15–24 cigs/day regardless of duration, 1–24 cigs/day for ≥ 40 yrs, or ≥ 15 cigs/day for < 30 yrs Heavy: ≥ 25 cigs/day for > 40 yrs *Alcohol:* 1 drink = 150 mL wine = 330 mL beer = 30 mL spirits	< 35 drinks/week 35–59 drinks/week ≥ 60 drinks/week	Nonsmoker Light smoker Moderate smoker Heavy smoker Nonsmoker Light smoker Moderate smoker Heavy smoker Nonsmoker Light smoker Moderate smoker Heavy smoker	1.0 1.1 2.7 6.4 0.8 7.9 8.8 11.0 7.9 9.4 16.7 17.5	Regression model; risk estimates adjusted for age, area of residence and years of education [no formal test for interaction]
Barón et al. (1993)	Italy, 1989–91	Cases: 271 men Controls: 1754 men, hospital controls, matched on age and area of residence	Tobacco: Light: ex-smoker who quit ≥ 10 years ago or smokers of 1–14 cigs/day for < 30 years Moderate: 15–24 cigs/day regardless of duration or 30–39 years duration regardless of amount, or ≥ 15 cigs/day for < 30 years Heavy: ≥ 25 cigs/day for ≥ 40 years	< 35 drinks/week 35–59 drinks/week ≥ 60 drinks/week	Nonsmoker Light smoker Moderate smoker Heavy smoker Nonsmoker Light smoker Moderate smoker Heavy smoker Nonsmoker Light smoker Moderate smoker Heavy smoker	1.0 2.1 4.4 8.4 2.2 4.4 9.7 18.5 2.6 5.5 11.4 21.8	Regression model; risk estimates adjusted for area of residence, age, education and profession [no formal test for interaction]

Table 2.3.9 (contd)

Reference	Place, year	Study population	Definition of tobacco/alcohol exposure	Alcohol categories	Smoking categories	Relative risk (95% CI)	Comments
Brown et al. (1994a)	Georgia, Michigan, New Jersey, USA, 1986–89	Cases: 373 men (squamous-cell carcinoma) (124 white, 249 black) Controls: 1364 men, community controls (750 white, 614 black)	Tobacco: Light: nonsmoker, former smoker or current smoker of < 1 pack/day Heavy: current smoker of ≥ 1 pack/day	White men 0–7 drinks/week	Light smoker Heavy smoker	1.0 3.3 (1.0–19.8)	Logistic regression model; risk estimates adjusted for age, geographical area and income. For both races, interaction between smoking and drinking was not significant [p value not provided]. Significant interaction ($p = 0.02$) between race and smoking/drinking variable
				8–14 drinks/week	Light smoker Heavy smoker	1.8 (0.5–6.1) 8.7 (2.4–32.4)	
				15–35 drinks/week	Light smoker Heavy smoker	4.6 (1.7–12.8) 22.1 (7.8–62.3)	
				36–84 drinks/week	Light smoker Heavy smoker	19.7 (7.2–53.4) 28.5 (10.1–80.2)	
				≥ 85 drinks/week	Light smoker Heavy smoker	29.0 (7.2–116.5) 35.4 (10.0–125.5)	
				Black men 0–7 drinks/week	Light smoker Heavy smoker	1.0 4.5 (1.4–14.6)	
				8–14 drinks/week	Light smoker Heavy smoker	5.7 (2.0–15.8) 14.2 (4.1–49.1)	
				15–35 drinks/week	Light smoker Heavy smoker	10.6 (4.1–27.2) 36.8 (13.9–97.2)	
				36–84 drinks/week	Light smoker Heavy smoker	39.5 (14.5–107.8) 42.1 (15.8–112.6)	
				≥ 85 drinks/week	Light smoker Heavy smoker	31.0 (9.8–98.5) 149.2 (39.2–567.4)	
Brown et al. (1994b)	Georgia, Michigan, New Jersey, USA, 1986–89	Cases: 174 white men (adenocarci-noma) Controls: 750 men, community controls, frequency-matched on age and race		< 8 drinks/week	< 1 pack/day ≥ 1 pack/day	1.0 2.4 (1.5–3.8)	Unconditional logistic regression model; risk estimates adjusted for age, area, and income; not possible to distinguish statistically between additive, multiplicative and intermediate models. [No formal test for interaction]
				≥ 8 drinks/week	< 1 pack/day ≥ 1 pack/day	2.4 (1.1–5.1) 3.8 (2.2–6.4)	

Table 2.3.9 (contd)

Reference	Place, year	Study population	Definition of tobacco/alcohol exposure	Alcohol categories	Smoking categories	Relative risk (95% CI)	Comments
Castelletto et al. (1994)	La Plata, Argentina, 1986–89	Cases: 131 incident cases Controls: 262 hospital controls, matched for age and hospital		0 mL/day	Nonsmoker 1–14 cigs/day ≥ 15 cigs/day	1.0 2.5 (0.4–16.5) 0.7 (0.1–6.5)	Logistic regression model; risk estimates adjusted for age, sex, hospital and education. Test for interaction between alcohol and tobacco not significant ($p = 0.45$)
				1–99 mL/day	Nonsmoker 1–14 cigs/day ≥ 15 cigs/day	1.6 (0.6–4.2) 4.3 (1.4–13.2) 3.7 (1.3–11.0)	
				100–199 mL/day	Nonsmoker 1–14 cigs/day ≥ 15 cigs/day	1.2 (0.1–12.0) 3.7 (1.3–11.0) 11.8 (3.7–37.7)	
				≥ 200 mL/day	Nonsmoker 1–14 cigs/day ≥ 15 cigs/day	5.7 (1.1–28.6) 5.0 (0.6–39.1) 19.0 (5.4–66.9)	
Hu et al. (1994)	Heilongjiang Province, China, 1985–1989	Cases: 196 incident cases Controls: 392 hospital controls (non-neoplastic, non-oesophageal disease), matched on age, gender and area of residence		≤ 57 L liquor/year	Nonsmoker 1–30 cigs/day ≥ 31 cigs/day	1.0 1.8 4.5	Regression model that does not assume multiplicative effects; synergistic effect that accounts for 38% of the excess risk [no formal test for interaction]; when using data in continuous form, interaction terms in the regression models were not significant.
				> 57 L liquor/year	Nonsmoker 1–30 cigs/day ≥ 31 cigs/day	1.0 5.3 7.9	
Zambon et al. (2000)	Northern Italy, 1992–97	Cases: 275 men (incident squamous-cell carcinoma) Controls: 593 men, hospital controls	Alcohol: 1 drink = 125 mL wine = 330 mL beer = 30 mL spirits	0–20 drinks/week	Nonsmoker 1–14 cigs/day 15–24 cigs/day ≥ 25 cigs/day	1.0 — —	Logistic regression model; risk estimates adjusted for area of residence, age and education; risk increase for the highest joint level of alcohol drinking and current smoking compatible with a multiplicative model (departure from multiplicativity β = 0.15, $p = 0.27$)
				21–34 drinks/week	Nonsmoker 1–14 cigs/day 15–24 cigs/day ≥ 25 cigs/day	2.1 (0.2–23.5) 18.9 (2.2–161.8) 35.3 (4.3–288.9) 44.1 (5.5–352.9)	
				35–59 drinks/week	Nonsmoker 1–14 cigs/day 15–24 cigs/day ≥ 25 cigs/day	8.9 (1.0–77.8) 36.5 (4.4–305.7) 57.2 (7.2–456.9) 66.8 (7.8–573.3)	
				≥ 60 drinks/week	Nonsmoker 1–14 cigs/day 15–24 cigs/day ≥ 25 cigs/day	56.1 (6.2–508.0) 40.3 (4.6–355.4) 117.6 (15.0–923.1) 130.3 (15.2–980.1)	

Table 2.3.9 (contd)

Reference	Place, year	Study population	Definition of tobacco/alcohol exposure	Alcohol categories	Smoking categories	Relative risk (95% CI)	Comments
Cohort study							
Kinjo et al. (1998)	Japan, 1966–81	Six-prefecture study (see Table 2.1) 440 deaths		≤ 3 times/week ≥ 4 times/week	Nonsmoker ≥ 1 cig/day Nonsmoker ≥ 1 cig/day	1.0 1.6 (1.1–2.1) 1.0 (0.4–2.0) 3.9 (2.7–5.4)	Risk estimates adjusted for attained age, prefecture, occupation and sex. Joint effect of alcohol drinking and smoking was more than additive. Data available for interaction of tobacco and alcohol stratified by tea consumption (hot/hot)
Larynx							
Wynder et al. (1976)	New York City, Houston, Los Angeles, Birmingham, Miami, New Orleans, USA, 1970–73	Cases: 258 men, 56 women Controls: 516 men, 168 women; hospital controls, matched on gender, year of interview, hospital status and age at diagnosis	*Tobacco:* 1 cigar = 5 cig. 1 pipe = 2.5 cig. *Alcohol:* 1 unit = 1 oz spirits = 4 oz wine = 6 oz beer	Men Nondrinker 1–6 units/day ≥ 7 units/day	Nonsmoker 1–15 cigs/day 16–34 cigs/day ≥ 35 cigs/day Nonsmoker 1–15 cigs/day 16–34 cigs/day ≥ 35 cigs/day Nonsmoker 1–15 cigs/day 16–34 cigs/day ≥ 35 cigs/day	1.0 3.0 (1.0–9.1) 6.0 (2.2–16.1) 7.0 (2.5–19.4) – 4.0 (1.0–15.6) 6.7 (2.3–19.7) 10.3 (3.6–29.8) – 3.3 (0.9–12.8) 13.8 (5.1–37.7) 22.1 (7.8–62.1)	Stratified analysis [no formal test for interaction]
Burch et al. (1981)	Ontario, Canada, 1977–79	Cases: 204 incident cases Controls: 204 community controls, matched on neighbourhood, sex and age	*Tobacco:* lifetime cigarette consumption *Alcohol:* lifetime oz ethanol consumption	0 oz < 10 000 oz 10 000–25 000 oz ≥ 26 000 oz	Nonsmoker < 150 000 cigs 150 000–299 000 cigs ≥ 300 000 cigs Nonsmoker < 150 000 cigs 150 000–299 000 cigs ≥ 300 000 cigs Nonsmoker < 150 000 cigs 150 000–299 000 cigs ≥ 300 000 cigs Nonsmoker < 150 000 cigs 150 000–299 000 cigs ≥ 300 000 cigs	1.0 2.0 3.9 7.6 2.0 3.5 6.3 11.1 3.9 6.3 10.1 16.3 7.7 11.2 16.3 23.7	Logistic regression model; coefficient for the interaction term (−0.10) not significant (SE = 0.11, $p = 0.177$)

Table 2.3.9 (contd)

Reference	Place, year	Study population	Definition of tobacco/alcohol exposure	Alcohol categories	Smoking categories	Relative risk (95% CI)	Comments
Flanders & Rothman (1982)	7 cities and 2 states in the USA, 1969–71	Cases: 87 men Controls: 956 men with cancers of other sites (excluding oral cavity, pharynx, oesophagus, stomach, lung, small intestine, colon, pancreas, bronchus, pleura, bladder and kidney)	Tobacco and alcohol: lifetime consumption in units 1 tobacco unit = 1 cigarette = 0.2 cigars = 0.4 pipefuls 1 alcohol unit = 1.5 oz spirits = 6 oz wine = 12 oz beer	0–49 units	0–49 units 50–549 units 550–899 units ≥ 900 units	Index of interaction[†] – – – –	[†]A value of 1.0 indicates no synergy.
				50–349 units	0–49 units 50–549 units 550–899 units ≥ 900 units	0.1 1.8 1.1	
				350–699 units	0–49 units 50–549 units 550–899 units ≥ 900 units	6.1 0.7 1.6	
				≥ 700 units	0–49 units 50–549 units 550–899 units ≥ 900 units	– 3.0 0.7 1.3	
			Daily consumption	0 units	0 unit 1–14 units 15–34 units ≥ 35 units	– – – –	
				1–9 units	0 unit 1–14 units 15–34 units ≥ 35 units	– 2.3 1.2 1.7	
				≥ 9 units	0 unit 1–14 units 15–34 units ≥ 35 units	– 1.8 3.0 3.9	
Herity et al. (1982)	Dublin, Ireland	Cases: 59 men Controls: 152 men, hospital controls		Non-/light drinker Heavy drinker	Non-/light smoker Heavy smoker Non-/light smoker Heavy smoker	1.0 3.3 (1.2–9.1) 4.0 (1.6–9.9) 14.0 (6.3–31.0)	Stratified analysis; synergistic effect between alcohol and tobacco, index of interaction = 2.5

Table 2.3.9 (contd)

Reference	Place, year	Study population	Definition of tobacco/alcohol exposure	Alcohol categories	Smoking categories	Relative risk (95% CI)		Comments
						LL	FL	
Walter & Iwane (1983)	7 cities and 2 states in the USA, 1969–71	Cases: 87 men Controls: 956 men with cancers of other sites (excluding oral cavity, pharynx, oesophagus, stomach, lung, small intestine, colon, pancreas, bronchus, pleura, bladder and kidney	Tobacco and alcohol: lifetime consumption in units 1 tobacco unit = 1 cigarette = 0.2 cigars = 0.4 pipefuls 1 alcohol unit = 1.5 oz spirits = 6 oz wine = 12 oz beer	0–49 units	0–49 units	1.0	1.0	Reanalysis of the data from Flanders and Rothman (1982); risk estimates adjusted for age LL = log linear model; FL = Flanders and Rothman model
					50–549 units	1.7	1.5	
					550–899 units	2.6	3.5	
					≥ 900 units	5.4	7.9	
				50–349 units	0–49 units	1.5	1.1	
					50–549 units	2.5	1.9	
					550–899 units	3.8	4.7	
					≥ 900 units	7.9	11.1	
				350–699 units	0–49 units	2.0	2.5	
					50–549 units	3.3	4.0	
					550–899 units	5.1	6.8	
					≥ 900 units	10.5	13.3	
				≥ 700 units	0–49 units	3.0	6.1	
					50–549 units	5.0	9.3	
					550–899 units	7.9	12.1	
					≥ 900 units	16.2	18.5	
Brownson & Chang (1987)	Missouri, USA, 1972–84	Cases: 63 white men Controls: 200 white men with colon cancer	Smoking (yes/no) Drinking (yes/no)	No alcohol	No smoking	1.0		Logistic regression model; risk estimates adjusted for age. Synergy index used to measure interaction between smoking and alcohol = 1.77 (77% greater than predicted additivity).
					Smoking	3.4		
				Alcohol	No smoking	2.4		
					Smoking	7.7		
De Stefani et al. (1987)	Uruguay, 1985–86	Cases: 107 men, aged 30–89 years Controls: 290 men, hospital controls		0–64 mL/day	0–15 cigs/day	1.0		Stratified analysis [no formal test for interaction]
					≥ 16 cigs/day	20.6		
				≥ 65 mL/day	0–15 cigs/day	16.7		
					≥ 16 cigs/day	123.4		

Table 2.3.9 (contd)

Reference	Place, year	Study population	Definition of tobacco/alcohol exposure	Alcohol categories	Smoking categories	Relative risk (95% CI)	Comments
Guénel et al. (1988)	Curie Institute, Paris, 1975–85	Cases: 411 men, ≥ 25 years old Controls: 4135 men, community controls, ≥ 25 years old	Tobacco: g tobacco/day	*Glottis (n = 197)* 0–39 g/day	0–9 g/day 10–19 g/day 20–29 g/day ≥ 30 g /day	1.0 0.4 (0.2–4.5) 9.3 (4.9-36.4) 19.2 (7.7-58.4)	Stratified analysis; risk estimates adjusted for age. To test deviation from the multiplicative model, a logistic model with cross-product
				40–99 g/day	0–9 g/day 10–19 g/day 20–29 g/day ≥ 30 g /day	1.6 (0.6-4.1) 2.9 (1.1-8.0) 12.3 (4.3-27.5) 27.4 (8.4-64.4)	variables alcohol × tobacco was compared to the simple multiplicative model: Glottis: chi-squared =10.2, p = 0.33 (9 degrees of freedom); Supraglottis:
				100–159 g/day	0–9 g/day 10–19 g/day 20–29 g/day ≥ 30 g /day	2.8 (1.2-15.2) 15.1 (5.2-43.4) 26.4 (7.8-62.3) 48.9 (16.9-132.8)	chi-squared = 4.78, p = 0.85 (9 degrees of freedom) [This indicated that the multiplicative model fits well.]
				≥ 160 g/day	0–9 g/day 10–19 g/day 20–29 g/day ≥ 30 g /day	5.1 (2.3-53.8) 40.9 (10.3-191.5) 125.3 (34.1-367.4) 289.4 (83.0-705.8)	
				Supraglottis (n = 214) 0–39 g/day	0–9 g/day 10–19 g/day 20–29 g/day ≥ 30 g /day	1.0 3.4 (0.6-20.9) 32.3 (4.4-82.1) 46.8 (6.7-152.6)	
				40–99 g/day	0–9 g/day 10–19 g/day 20–29 g/day ≥ 30 g /day	2.6 (0.3-10.4) 27.5 (2.1-49.8) 48.5 (6.7-101.0) 132.3 (16.6-283.8)	
				100–159 g/day	0–9 g/day 10–19 g/day 20–29 g/day ≥ 30 g /day	7.3 (1.6-57.3) 75.4 (8.4-187.0) 180.7 (27.3-415.2) 530.6 (77.7-1175.7)	
				≥ 160 g/day	0–9 g/day 10–19 g/day 20–29 g/day ≥ 30 g /day	50.6 (8.4-280.2) 115.5 (22.8-671.0) 647.7 (106.4-1749.1) 1094.2 (185.8-2970.7)	

Table 2.3.9 (contd)

Reference	Place, year	Study population	Definition of tobacco/alcohol exposure	Alcohol categories	Smoking categories	Relative risk (95% CI)	Comments
Tuyns et al. (1988)	France, Italy, Spain, Switzerland	Cases: 1147 men Controls: 3057 men, population controls, individually matched on area and frequency-matched on age		*Endolarynx* 0–40 g/day	0–7 cigs/day	1.0	Logistic regression model
					8–15 cigs/day	6.7	
					16–25 cigs/day	12.7	
					≥ 26 cigs/day	11.5	
				41–80 g/day	0–7 cigs/day	1.7	
					8–15 cigs/day	5.9	
					16–25 cigs/day	12.2	
					≥ 26 cigs/day	18.5	
				81–120 g/day	0–7 cigs/day	2.3	
					8–15 cigs/day	10.7	
					16–25 cigs/day	21.0	
					≥ 26 cigs/day	23.6	
				≥ 121 g/day	0–7 cigs/day	3.8	
					8–15 cigs/day	12.2	
					16–25 cigs/day	31.6	
					≥ 26 cigs/day	43.2	For multiplicative model, chi-squared = 5.8 (9 degrees of freedom)
				Hypopharynx/epilarynx 0–40 g/day	0–7 cigs/day	1.0	
					8–15 cigs/day	4.7	
					16–25 cigs/day	13.9	
					≥ 26 cigs/day	4.9	
				41–80 g/day	0–7 cigs/day	3.0	
					8–15 cigs/day	14.6	
					16–25 cigs/day	19.5	
					≥ 26 cigs/day	18.4	
				81–120 g/day	0–7 cigs/day	5.5	
					8–15 cigs/day	27.5	
					16–25 cigs/day	48.3	
					≥ 26 cigs/day	37.6	
				≥ 121 g/day	0–7 cigs/day	14.7	
					8–15 cigs/day	71.6	
					16–25 cigs/day	67.8	
					≥ 26 cigs/day	135.5	For multiplicative model, chi-squared = 14.5 (9 degrees of freedom)

Table 2.3.9 (contd)

Reference	Place, year	Study population	Definition of tobacco/alcohol exposure	Alcohol categories	Smoking categories	Relative risk (95% CI)	Comments
Falk et al. (1989)	Texas, USA, 1975–80	Cases: 151 living white men, aged 30–79 years; Controls: 235 living white men, community controls		< 4 drinks/week	Nonsmoker	1.0	Logistic regression model; risk estimates adjusted for age
					1–10 cigs/day	2.9 (2.2–3.9)	Goodness-of-fit for additive model:
					11–20 cigs/day	5.2 (2.5–10.7)	chi-squared = 4.44, p = 0.73
					21–39 cigs/day	8.0 (5.8–11.0)	Goodness-of-fit for multiplicative
					≥ 40 cigs/day	10.2 (8.6–12.2)	model: chi-squared = 4.09, p = 0.77
				≥ 4 drinks/week	Nonsmoker	1.8 (1.5–2.1)	
					1–10 cigs/day	4.6 (3.1–6.7)	
					11–20 cigs/day	6.5 (3.5–12.0)	
					21–39 cigs/day	10.5 (7.8–14.2)	
					≥ 40 cigs/day	15.4 (10.9–21.9)	
Franceschi et al. (1990)	Northern Italy, 1986–89	Cases: 162 men < 75 years old; Controls: Men < 75 years old admitted to same hospitals for acute illness	*Tobacco:* Light: ex-smoker who quit ≥ 10 years ago or smokers of 1–14 cigs/day for < 30 years; Moderate: 30–39 years duration regardless of amount, 15–24 cigs/day regardless of duration, 1–24 cigs/day for ≥ 40 years, or ≥ 15 cigs/day for < 30 years; Heavy: ≥ 25 cigs/day for > 40 years; *Alcohol:* 1 drink = 150 mL wine = 330 mL beer = 30 mL spirits	< 35 drinks/week	Nonsmoker	1.0	Regression model; risk estimates adjusted for age, area of residence and years of education. [No formal test for interaction]
					Light smoker	0.9	
					Moderate smoker	4.5	
					Heavy smoker	6.1	
				35–59 drinks/week	Nonsmoker	1.6	
					Light smoker	5.0	
					Moderate smoker	7.1	
					Heavy smoker	10.4	
				≥ 60 drinks/week	Nonsmoker	–	
					Light smoker	5.4	
					Moderate smoker	9.5	
					Heavy smoker	11.7	

Table 2.3.9 (contd)

Reference	Place, year	Study population	Definition of tobacco/alcohol exposure	Alcohol categories	Smoking categories	Relative risk (95% CI)	Comments
Choi & Kahyo (1991)	Seoul, Republic of Korea, 1986–89	Cases: 94 men, 6 women Controls: 282 men, 18 women; hospital controls, matched on age, sex and admission date	Alcohol (soju) in mL/day: Light: < 8100 Medium: 8100–16 200 Heavy: > 16 200	Non-drinker Light drinker Medium drinker Heavy drinker	Nonsmoker ≤ 1 pack/day > 1 pack/day Nonsmoker ≤ 1 pack/day > 1 pack/day Nonsmoker ≤ 1 pack/day > 1 pack/day Nonsmoker ≤ 1 pack/day > 1 pack/day	1.0 2 4 0.5 0.8 1.0 1.5 3 2.5 0.5 4 20.7	Stratified analysis; ORs extrapolated from figure [No formal test for interaction]
Freudenheim et al. (1992)	New York, USA, 1975–85	Cases: 250 incident (white) cases Controls: 250 (white) neighbourhood controls, matched on age	Alcohol: Drink-years = drinks/month multi-plied by number of years of drinking	≤ 1243 drink–years > 1243 drink–years	≤ 24 pack–years > 24 pack–years ≤ 24 pack–years > 24 pack–years	1.0 2.7 (1.4–5.2) 0.98 (0.5–2.1) 5.8 (3.3–10.4)	Logistic regression model; risk estimates adjusted for education; interaction between tobacco and alcohol [no formal test for interaction]
Zheng et al. (1992)	Shanghai, 1988–90	Cases: 201 incident cases Controls: 414 community controls, frequency-matched on sex and age	Alcohol lifetime consumption	Men Non-drinker < 300 kg 300–899 kg ≥ 900kg	0–9 pack–years 10–29 pack–years ≥ 30 pack–years 0–9 pack–years 10–29 pack–years ≥ 30 pack–years 0–9 pack–years 10–29 pack–years ≥ 30 pack–years 0–9 pack–years 10–29 pack–years ≥ 30 pack–years	1.0 3.1 (1.1–8.7) 35.7 (13.6–93.9) 1.0 (0.2–5.5) 3.8 (1.1–12.1) 12.1 (3.8–38.6) 7.5 (1.4–38.8) 3.7 (1.1–12.0) 23.2 (8.3–65.0) 2.5 (0.2–27.0) 7.4 (1.0–55.0) 25.1 (9.6–70.0)	Stratified analysis; risk estimates adjusted for age and education [no formal test for interaction]

Table 2.3.9 (contd)

Reference	Place, year	Study population	Definition of tobacco/alcohol exposure	Alcohol categories	Smoking categories	Relative risk (95% CI)	Comments
Barón et al. (1993)	Italy, 1989–91	Cases: 224 men Controls: 1754 men, hospital controls, matched on age and residence	Tobacco: Light: ex-smoker who quit ≥ 10 years ago or smokers of 1–14 cigs/day for < 30 years Moderate: 15–24 cigs/day regardless of duration or 30–39 years duration regardless of amount, or ≥ 15 cigs/day for < 30 years Heavy: ≥ 25 cigs/day for ≥ 40 years	< 35 drinks/week 35–59 drinks/week ≥ 60 drinks/week	Nonsmoker Light smoker Moderate smoker Heavy smoker Nonsmoker Light smoker Moderate smoker Heavy smoker Nonsmoker Light smoker Moderate smoker Heavy smoker	1.0 1.3 5.2 11.2 1.3 1.7 6.8 14.6 1.9 2.5 9.9 21.3	Regression model; risk estimates adjusted for area of residence, age, education and profession [no formal test for interaction]
Dosemeci et al. (1997)	Turkey, 1979–84	Cases: 832 men Controls: 829 men, hospital controls with selected cancers		Never-drinker 1–20 drink-years ≥ 21 drink-years	Nonsmoker 1–20 cigs/day ≥ 21 cigs/day Nonsmoker 1–20 cigs/day ≥ 21 cigs/day Nonsmoker 1–20 cigs/day ≥ 21 cigs/day	1.0 3.0 (2.2–4.1) 6.2 (3.9–9.9) – 5.6 (3.2–9.8) 6.0 (2.5–14.3) – 5.2 (1.9–15.1) 12.2 (3.1–57.6)	Stratified analysis; risk estimates also provided for glottis, supraglottis and other sites [no formal test for interaction]
Schlecht et al. (1999)	Brazil, 1986–89	Cases: 194 incident cases Controls: 388 hospital controls, matched on hospital, trimester of admission, age and sex	Alcohol: lifetime consumption	0–10 kg 11–530 kg > 530 kg	0–5 pack-years 6–42 pack-years > 42 pack-years 0–5 pack-years 6–42 pack-years > 42 pack-years 0–5 pack-years 6–42 pack-years > 42 pack-years	1.0 13.5 (2.7–66.8) 11.4 (2.1–62.0) 1.2 (0.1–14.4) 16.1 (3.4–76.2) 22.0 (4.5–107) 5.5 (0.4–71.5) 36.9 (0.7–1800) 43.1 (9.1–208)	Logistic regression model that included an interaction term; risk estimates adjusted for race, beverage temperature, religion, wood stove use and consumption of spicy foods. No statistical evidence for effect modification ($p = 0.945$)

Table 2.3.9 (contd)

Mixed upper aerodigestive tract (ADT)

Case–control studies

Reference	Place, year	Study population	Definition of tobacco/alcohol exposure	Alcohol categories	Smoking categories	Relative risk (95% CI)	Comments
Franceschi et al. (1990)	Northern Italy, 1986–89	Cases: 157 men < 75 years old Controls: 1272 men < 75 years old, admitted to same hospitals for acute illness	*Tobacco:* Light: ex-smoker who quit ≥ 10 years ago or smokers of 1–14 cigs/day for < 30 years Moderate: 30–39 years duration regardless of amount, 15–24 cigs/day regardless of duration, 1–24 cigs/day for ≥ 40 yrs, or ≥ 15 cigs/day for < 30 years Heavy: ≥ 25 cigs/day for > 40 yrs *Alcohol:* 1 drink = 150 mL wine = 330 mL beer = 30 mL spirits	< 35 drinks/week 35–59 drinks/week ≥ 60 drinks/week	Nonsmoker Light smoker Moderate smoker Heavy smoker Nonsmoker Light smoker Moderate smoker Heavy smoker Nonsmoker Light smoker Moderate smoker Heavy smoker	1.0 3.1 10.9 17.6 1.6 5.4 26.6 40.2 2.3 10.9 36.4 79.6	Logistic regression model; risk estimates adjusted for age, area of residence, education and occupation [no formal test for interaction]
Maier et al. (1992)	Germany, 1987–88	Cases: 200 men (squamous-cell cancer of the head and neck) Controls: 800 men, outpatient clinic controls	Tobacco: 1 tobacco-year = daily consumption of 20 cigarettes, 4 cigars, or 5 pipes for 1 year	< 25 g/day 25–75 g/day > 75 g/day	< 5 tobacco-years 5–50 tobacco-years > 50 tobacco-years < 5 tobacco-years 5–50 tobacco-years > 50 tobacco-years < 5 tobacco-years 5–50 tobacco-years > 50 tobacco-years	1.0 5.7 (1.9–17.3) 23.3 (6.6–82.5) 2.3 (0.6–8.8) 14.6 (4.8–43.9) 52.8 (15.8–176.6) 10.3 (1.9–55.8) 153.2 (44.1–532) 146.2 (37.7–566)	Logistic regression model; combined consumption of alcohol and tobacco increased the risk in a multiplicative manner. [No formal test for interaction]

Table 2.3.9 (contd)

Reference	Place, year	Study population	Definition of tobacco/alcohol exposure	Alcohol categories	Smoking categories	Relative risk (95% CI)	Comments
Barón *et al.* (1993)	Italy, 1989–91	Cases: 308 men (oral or pharyngeal cancer) Controls: 1754 men, hospital controls, matched on age and area of residence	Tobacco: Light: ex-smoker who quit ≥ 10 years ago or smokers of 1–14 cigs/day for < 30 years Moderate: 15–24 cigs/day regardless of duration or 30–39 years duration regardless of amount, or ≥ 15 cigs/day for < 30 years Heavy: ≥ 25 cigs/day for ≥ 40 years	< 35 drinks/week 35–59 drinks/week ≥ 60 drinks/week	Nonsmoker Light smoker Moderate smoker Heavy smoker Nonsmoker Light smoker Moderate smoker Heavy smoker Nonsmoker Light smoker Moderate smoker Heavy smoker	1.0 6.4 5.4 32.1 3.6 23.0 91.4 115.6 9.5 60.8 241.3 304.9	Regression model; risk estimates adjusted for area of residence, age, education and profession [no formal test for interaction]
Kune *et al.* (1993)	Melbourne, Australia, 1982	Cases: 41 men, incident cases (19 oral, 22 pharynx) Controls: 398 men, community controls		≤ 200 g/week > 200 g/week	Non/former smoker Current smoker Non/former smoker Current smoker	1.0 25.2 (3.1–204) 42.7 (5.5–330) 111.8 (15.5–865)	Logistic regression model; more than additive interaction [no formal test for interaction]

Table 2.3.9 (contd)

Reference	Place, year	Study population	Definition of tobacco/alcohol exposure	Alcohol categories	Smoking categories	Relative risk (95% CI)	Comments
Mashberg et al. (1993)	New Jersey, USA, 1972–83	Cases: 359 [men] (oral cavity-oropharynx) Controls: 2280 [men], hospital controls	Alcohol: 1 whisky equivalent (WE) = 10.24 g ethanol	0–1 WE/day	0–5 cigs/day	1.0	Logistic regression model; risk estimates adjusted for age; results suggest multiplicative interaction [no formal test for interaction] *$p < 0.05$
					6–15 cigs/day	10.8	
					16–25 cigs/day	7.6	
					≥ 36 cigs/day	–	
				2–5 WE/day	0–5 cigs/day	3.2	
					6–15 cigs/day	2.7	
					16–25 cigs/day	24.2*	
					26–35 cigs/day	29.7*	
					≥ 36 cigs/day	5.3	
				6–10 WE/day	0–5 cigs/day	10.2*	
					6–15 cigs/day	11.9	
					16–25 cigs/day	50.9*	
					26–35 cigs/day	28.9*	
					≥ 36 cigs/day	61.9*	
				11–21 WE/day	0–5 cigs/day	26.8*	
					6–15 cigs/day	12.5*	
					16–25 cigs/day	30.9*	
					26–35 cigs/day	44.8*	
					≥ 36 cigs/day	79.5*	
				≥ 22 WE/day	0–5 cigs/day	98.4*	
					6–15 cigs/day	8.3	
					16–25 cigs/day	27.5*	
					26–35 cigs/day	61.7*	
					≥ 36 cigs/day	70.3*	
						32.0*	

Table 2.3.9 (contd)

Reference	Place, year	Study population	Definition of tobacco/alcohol exposure	Alcohol categories	Smoking categories	Relative risk (95% CI)	Comments
Kabat et al. (1994)	8 cities in the USA, 1977–90	Cases: 1097 men, 463 women, incident cases (oral cavity, pharynx) Controls: 2075 men, 873 women; hospital controls		*Men* Nondrinker	Nonsmoker	1.0	Logistic regression model; risk estimates adjusted for age, years of schooling, race, time period and type of hospital
					Former smoker	1.1 (0.7–1.6)	
					1–20 cigs/day	1.5 (0.9–2.5)	
					21–30 cigs/day	2.2 (1.1–4.3)	
					≥ 31 cigs/day	2.0 (1.1–3.7)	
				1–3.9 oz/day	Nonsmoker	1.6 (0.9–2.7)	
					Former smoker	1.7 (1.1–2.6)	
					1–20 cigs/day	5.8 (3.7–9.1)	
					21–30 cigs/day	6.8 (3.6–12.7)	
					≥ 31 cigs/day	6.9 (3.9–12.4)	
				4–6.9 oz/day	Nonsmoker	1.2 (0.4–3.7)	
					Former smoker	3.1 (1.9–5.2)	
					1–20 cigs/day	5.9 (3.5–10.0)	
					21–30 cigs/day	15.8 (7.4–33.8)	
					≥ 31 cigs/day	18.8 (10.0–35.4)	
				≥ 7 oz/day	Nonsmoker	2.9 (1.1–8.1)	
					Former smoker	5.1 (3.3–7.8)	
					1–20 cigs/day	11.9 (7.7–18.4)	Test for interaction: chi-squared with 12 degrees of freedom = 24.6, p = 0.02
					21–30 cigs/day	13.5 (7.9–23.2)	
					≥ 31 cigs/day	20.1 (12.9–31.5)	
				Women Nondrinker	Nonsmoker	1.0	
					Former smoker	1.3 (0.9–2.0)	
					1–20 cigs/day	2.9 (1.9–4.3)	
					≥ 21 cigs/day	3.8 (2.3–6.2)	
				1–3.9 oz/day	Nonsmoker	0.7 (0.3–1.4)	
					Former smoker	2.1 (1.2–3.8)	
					≥ 21 cigs/day	5.8 (3.5–9.8)	
				≥ 4 oz/day	Nonsmoker	22.3 (9.6–51.8)	
					Former smoker	3.5 (0.9–13.4)	
					1–20 cigs/day	2.7 (0.95–7.9)	Test for interaction: chi-squared with 6 degrees of freedom = 18.7, p = 0.005
					≥ 21 cigs/day	17.6 (8.1–37.5)	
						26.7 (12.3–58.6)	

Table 2.3.9 (contd)

Reference	Place, year	Study population	Definition of tobacco/alcohol exposure	Alcohol categories	Smoking categories	Relative risk (95% CI)	Comments
André et al. (1995)	Doubs region, France, 1986–89	Cases: 299 men ≥ 35 years old (oral cavity, oropharynx and larynx) Controls: 645 men, population controls ≥ 35 years old	Tobacco: g of tobacco/day	0–40 g/day	0–7 g/day 8–19 g/day ≥ 20 g/day	1 7.1 (1.9–26.1) 10.9 (2.9–40.8)	Logistic regression model; risk estimates adjusted for age and environment [no formal test for interaction]
				41–100 g/day	0–7 g/day 8–19 g/day ≥ 20 g/day	4.9 (1.3–18.2) 25.3 (7.7–82.9) 42.8 (13.1–140)	
				> 100 g/day	0–7 g/day 8–19 g/day ≥ 20 g/day	62 (12.2–316) 194 (49.4–760) 199 (56.5–699)	
Muscat et al. (1996)	New York, Illinois, Michigan, Pennsylvania, 1981–90	Cases: 697 men, 322 women (oral neoplasia) Controls: 619 men, 304 women, hospital controls, matched on gender, age, race and date of admission	Tobacco: cumulative tar	*Men* 0 to < 1 drink/week	< 1.4 kg 1.4–3.5 kg > 3.5–6.8 kg > 6.8 kg	0.7 (0.3–1.8) 0.3 (0.1–1.1) 1.0 (0.5–2.6) 1.0 (0.4–2.8)	Reference category was never-smokers for all drinking categories. Logistic regression model; estimates adjusted for age and education; further modelling of data revealed a significant interaction between smoking and alcohol consumption for both men and women. [No formal test for interaction presented]
				Occasional drinker	< 1.4 kg 1.4–3.5 kg > 3.5–6.8 kg > 6.8 kg	0.9 (0.3–2.3) 0.5 (0.2–1.5) 1.2 (0.4–3.7) 1.6 (0.6–4.7)	
				1–4 drinks/day	< 1.4 kg 1.4–3.5 kg > 3.5–6.8 kg > 6.8 kg	1.0 (0.4–2.1) 1.5 (0.7–3.2) 1.8 (0.8–3.8) 2.5 (1.1–5.2)	
				> 4 drinks/day	< 1.4 kg 1.4–3.5 kg > 3.5–6.8 kg > 6.8 kg	2.1 (0.7–5.9) 2.7 (1.1–6.6) 4.7 (2.0–11.3) 6.1 (2.6–14.4)	
				Women 0 to < 1 drink/week	< 1.4 kg 1.4–3.5 kg > 3.5–6.8 kg > 6.8 kg	1.2 (0.6–2.4) 3.0 (1.3–7.0) 2.0 (1.0–4.0) 2.4 (0.8–6.9)	
				Occasional drinker	< 1.4 kg 1.4–3.5 kg > 3.5–6.8 kg > 6.8 kg	1.4 (0.5–4.3) 1.2 (0.4–3.6) 5.8 (1.7–20.3) 16.7 (1.8–152.6)	
				1–4 drinks/day	< 1.4 kg 1.4–3.5 kg > 3.5–6.8 kg > 6.8 kg	5.9 (1.7–20.5) 9.5 (2.8–32.0) 14.0 (4.1–48.5) 18.6 (4.0–86.8)	
				> 4 drinks/day	< 1.4 kg 1.4–3.5 kg > 3.5–6.8 kg > 6.8 kg	1.0 (0.01–27.9) 4.3 (0.1–116.9) 6.5 (0.1–174.2) 2.4 (0.0–55.1)	

Table 2.3.9 (contd)

Reference	Place, year	Study population	Definition of tobacco/alcohol exposure	Alcohol categories	Smoking categories	Relative risk (95% CI)	Comments
Lewin et al. (1998)	Sweden, 1988–90	Cases: 605 men (squamous-cell carcinoma of the head and neck) Controls: 756 men, population controls		< 10 g/day	Nonsmoker	1.0	Logistic regression model; risk estimates adjusted for age and health care area; joint effect of high alcohol intake and current smoking is nearly multiplicative. [No formal test for interaction]
					Former smoker	2.4 (1.4–4.1)	
					Current smoker	6.3 (3.7–10.5)	
				10–19 g/day	Nonsmoker	1.2 (0.5–3.1)	
					Former smoker	2.2 (1.2–4.1)	
					Current smoker	10.4 (5.9–18.3)	
				≥ 20 g/day	Nonsmoker	4.2 (1.8–9.7)	
					Former smoker	5.4 (2.8–10.2)	
					Current smoker	22.1 (13.0–37.8)	
Cohort study							
Chyou et al. (1995)	Hawaii, USA 1965–68	American Men of Japanese Ancestry Study (see Section 2.1.1) 92 incident cases of cancer of the upper aerodigestive tract		Non-drinker	Nonsmoker	1.0	Proportional hazards regression model; risk estimates adjusted for age; none of the tests for interaction were statistically significant (*p* > 0.05).
					≤ 20 cigs/day	3.0 (0.8–11.3)	
					> 20 cigs/day	3.2 (0.8–13.4)	
				< 14 oz/month	Nonsmoker	1.3 (0.3–6.3)	
					≤ 20 cigs/day	1.9 (0.5–7.7)	
					> 20 cigs/day	4.6 (1.2–17.8)	
				≥ 14 oz/month	Nonsmoker	6.5 (1.7–26.0)	
					≤ 20 cigs/day	10.7 (3.2–35.4)	
					> 20 cigs/day	14.4 (4.4–47.4)	
					Duration		
				Non-drinker	Nonsmoker	1.0	
					< 30 years	2.0 (0.4–8.8)	
					≥ 30 years	4.2 (1.1–15.5)	
				< 14 oz/month	Nonsmoker	1.3 (0.3–6.3)	
					< 30 years	2.4 (0.6–9.7)	
					≥ 30 years	3.3 (0.9–12.6)	
				≥ 14 oz/month	Nonsmoker	6.5 (1.6–25.9)	
					< 30 years	9.2 (2.7–31.9)	
					≥ 30 years	14.2 (4.4–46.3)	
Liver							
Austin et al. (1986)	Alabama, Florida, Massachussetts, North Carolina, Pennsylvania, USA	Cases: 85 cases Controls: 159 hospital controls, matched on gender, age and race		*HBsAg-negative subjects:* Nondrinker	Nonsmoker	1.0	Logistic regression model; information not provided on HBsAg-positive subjects. Test for interaction not statistically significant (*p* = 0.50)
					Former smoker	1.0	
					Current smoker	1.1	
				Occasional drinker	Nonsmoker	1.3	
					Former smoker	1.6	
					Current smoker	4.7	
				Regular drinker	Nonsmoker	3.2	
					Former smoker	1.0	
					Current smoker	3.4	

Table 2.3.9 (contd)

Reference	Place, year	Study population	Definition of tobacco/alcohol exposure	Alcohol categories	Smoking categories	Relative risk (95% CI)	Comments
Chen et al. (1991)	China, Province of Taiwan, 1985–87	Cases: 200 incident cases (men) Controls: 200 population controls		Not habitual drinker	Nonsmoker	1.0	Logistic regression model; interaction between smoking and drinking not significant under the multiplicative model [numbers not provided]
					1–10 cigs/day	1.0	
					11–20 cigs/day	1.8	
					> 20 cigs/day	2.7	
				Habitual drinker	Nonsmoker	2.9	
					1–10 cigs/day	3.2	
					11–20 cigs/day	6.2	
					> 20 cigs/day	11.7	
Yu et al. (1991)	Los Angeles County, USA, 1984–90	Cases: 74 incident cases Controls: 162 population controls		≤ 29 drink–years	Nonsmoker	1.0	Logistic regression model [no formal test for interaction]
					Former smoker	1.4 (0.3–6.0)	
					Current smoker	3.7 (0.9–15.5)	
				≥ 30 drink–years	Nonsmoker	4.2 (0.8–22.2)	
					Former smoker	4.8 (1.3–17.4)	
					Current smoker	5.4 (1.4–21.0)	
Tanaka et al. (1992)	Fukuoka, Japan, 1985–89	Cases: 168 men, 36 women Controls: 291 men, 119 women, hospital controls, frequency-matched on age and sex All subjects aged 40–69 years		< 9.8 drink–years	< 18.4 pack–years	1.0	Logistic regression model; risk estimates adjusted for sex, age, HBsAg status, history of blood transfusion and family history. Lowest drinking category used as reference. [No formal test for interaction]
					18.4–31.9 pack–years	1.0	
					≥ 32 pack–years	1.0	
				9.8–54.1 drink–years	< 18.4 pack–years	0.8	
					18.4–31.9 pack–years	1.2	
					≥ 32 pack–years	1.0	
				≥ 54.2 drink–years	< 18.4 pack–years	0.8	
					18.4–31.9 pack–years	2.1	
					≥ 32 pack–years	1.8	

Table 2.3.9 (contd)

Reference	Place, year	Study population	Definition of tobacco/alcohol exposure	Alcohol categories	Smoking categories	Relative risk (95% CI)	Comments
Mukaiya et al. (1998)	Sapporo, Japan, 1991–93	Cases: 104 men Controls: 104 men, hospital controls, matched on age	Alcohol: Nondrinker and ex-drinker for ≥ 10 years Current drinker and ex-drinker for < 10 years	Nondrinker Current drinker	Nonsmoker Former smoker Current smoker Nonsmoker Former smoker Current smoker	1.0 9.4 15.4 p for trend = 0.006 9.8 17.3 17.9 p for trend = 0.29	Stratified analysis [no formal test for interaction]
Kuper et al. (2000)	Athens, Greece, 1995–98	Cases: 333 incident cases Controls: 360 hospital controls		0–40 glasses/week ≥ 40 glasses/week	Nonsmoker < 3 packs/day ≥ 2 packs/day Nonsmoker < 3 packs/day ≥ 2 packs/day	1.0 2.1 (1.0–4.6) 1.7 (0.6–5.3) 4.2 (0.7–25.9) 2.4 (0.9–6.9) 10.9 (3.5–33.8)	Logistic regression model; risk estimates adjusted for age, gender, years of schooling and coffee drinking. Strong, statistically significant ($p = 0.0001$) and apparently super-multiplicative interaction between heavy smoking and heavy drinking in the causation of hepatocellular carcinoma. Effect stronger in HBV and/or HCV negative subjects, further confirmed by case–case analysis

Table 2.3.10. Studies on interaction of smoking and hepatitis B in the causation of cancer of the liver

Reference	Place, year	Study population	HBsAg categories	Smoking categories	Relative risk	Comments
Trichopoulos et al. (1987)	Athens, Greece, 1976–84	Cases: 194 incident hepatocellular carcinoma cases Controls: 456 hospital controls	HBsAg– subjects	Nonsmoker	1.0	Logistic regression model; risk estimates adjusted for age, sex, and alcohol consumption [nonsmokers used as reference group for both HBsAg subgroups]
				Former smoker	2.8	
				1–9 cigs/day	0.8	
				10–19 cigs/day	2.0	
				20–29 cigs/day	2.4	
				≥ 30 cigs/day	7.3	
			HBsAg+ subjects	Nonsmoker	1.0	
				Former smoker	1.3	
				1–9 cigs/day	1.2	
				10–19 cigs/day	2.2	
				20–29 cigs/day	1.2	
				≥ 30 cigs/day	2.0	
Chen et al. (1991)	China, Province of Taiwan, 1985–87	Cases: 200 incident cases (men) Controls: 200 population controls	HBsAg–, HBeAg–	Nonsmoker	1.0	Stratified analysis [no formal test for interaction]
				1–10 cigs/day	1.2	
				11–20 cigs/day	2.0	
				> 20 cigs/day	2.4	
			HBsAg+, HBeAg–	Nonsmoker	15.1	
				1–10 cigs/day	13.6	
				11–20 cigs/day	44.6	
				> 20 cigs/day	68.1	
			HBsAg+, HBeAg+	Nonsmoker	27.8	
				1–10 cigs/day	107.0	
				11–20 cigs/day	206.9	
				> 20 cigs/day	197.6	

Table 2.3.11. Studies on interaction of human papillomavirus (HPV) and smoking in the causation of cancer of the cervix

Reference	Study type	Place, year	Study population	HPV exposure	Smoking categories	Relative risk (95% CI)	Comments
Basu et al. (1991)	Cross-sectional study	New York, USA	75 women referred to a colposcopy clinic for abnormal Pap smear		Smoker HPV-positive	Cases vs non-cases (%) 53.5 vs 36.7 66.7 vs 53.3	Difference not statistically significant. Discrepancies between text and table for percentage of HPV-positive women among non-cases
Ylitalo et al. (1999)	Nested case–control (see Table 2.1.10.6)	Uppsala County, Sweden, 1965–95	Cohort: ~ 281 000 women Cases: 422 patients diagnosed with cervical carcinoma in situ Controls: 422 controls, matched on date of entry into cohort and birth year	HPV 16/18 DNA negative before diagnosis (n = 138) HPV 16/18 DNA positive before diagnosis (n = 178)	Nonsmoker Former smoker Current smoker 1–9 years of smoking 10–19 of smoking ≥ 20 of smoking 0.15–3.95 pack–years 4.00–7.95 pack–years ≥ 8.00 pack–years Nonsmoker Former smoker Current smoker 1–9 years of smoking 10–19 years of smoking ≥ 20 years of smoking 0.15–3.95 pack–years 4.00–7.95 pack–years ≥ 8.00 pack–years	1.0 1.5 (0.7–3.4) 1.8 (0.9–3.6) 1.5 (0.7–3.4) 1.7 (0.8–3.5) 2.0 (0.7–5.9) 1.4 (0.7–2.9) 2.7 (1.2–6.4) 1.6 (0.7–3.5) 1.0 2.1 (1.04–4.3) 2.3 (1.3–4.3) 2.3 (1.1–5.2) 2.5 (1.3–4.7) 1.8 (0.8–4.1) 2.3 (1.1–4.8) 3.4 (1.6–7.3) 1.6 (0.8–3.2)	Logistic regression models. Risk estimates adjusted for education, marital status, oral contraceptive use, age at sexual debut, number of sexual partners, age at menarche and parity. [No formal test for interaction]
Kjellberg et al. (2000)	Case–control	Northern Sweden, 1993–95	Cases: 137 women with high grade CIN Controls: 253 healthy population-controls, matched on age	HPV Ab– HPV Ab+	Never-smoker Ever-smoker Never-smoker Ever-smoker	1.0 5.6 (2.5–10.9) 5.2 (2.5–10.9) 10.5 (5.0–22.4)	Risk estimates adjusted for age [although matched on age]. No evidence of interaction. [No numbers provided]

Table 2.3.11 (contd)

Reference	Study type	Place, year	Study population	HPV exposure	Smoking categories	Relative risk (95% CI)	Comments
Hildesheim et al. (2001)	Cross-sectional	Costa Rica, 1993–94	Population: 989 HPV positive women Cases: 146 prevalent high-grade squamous intraepithelial lesions or cervical cancer Controls: women with or without low grade squamous intraepithelial lesions	All HPV positive	Never-smoker Former smoker Current smoker < 10 years smoking ≥ 10 years smoking 1–5 cigs/day ≥ 6 cigs/day	1.0 2.4 (1.2–5.1) 2.3 (1.3–4.3) 2.6 (1.2–5.3) 2.2 (1.2–4.2) 2.3 (1.3–3.9) 2.7 (1.1–6.7) p for trend = 0.0007	Logistic regression model. Risk estimates for overall analysis adjusted for age, HPV type, number of pregnancies and number of cigarettes/day. Risk estimates for high-risk analysis adjusted for age, number of pregnancies and number of cigarettes/day. No association was found between smoking habit of husband/live-in partner and high-grade squamous intraepithelial lesions/cancer among nonsmoking women. HPV testing for 44 different HPV types.
				High risk HPV types (16, 18, 31, 33, 35, 39, 45, 51, 52, 56, 58, 59, 68)	Never-smoker Former smoker Current smoker < 10 years smoking ≥ 10 years smoking 1–5 cigs/day ≥ 6 cigs/day	1.0 1.7 (0.8–4.0) 2.3 (1.2–4.3) 2.2 (1.0–4.8) 2.0 (1.0–3.8) 1.8 (0.99–3.3) 3.1 (2.2–7.9) p for trend = 0.003	

Table 2.3.12. Studies on the combined effect of tobacco smoking and silica exposure in the causation of lung cancer

Reference	Study design	Country, years of study	Source population	No. of cases and controls	Smoking categories (highest vs lowest exposure)	Silica exposure	Relative risk Non-smoker	Relative risk Smoker	Inter-action[a]	Comments
Forastiere et al. (1986)	Retrospective case-control	Italy, 1968-84	Male residents in region with pottery industry	72 deaths, 319 controls	Cigarettes per day 0; 1-20; > 20	Ceramic workers without silicosis with silicosis	1.5 0	4.1 1.8	~ M (> M)	Deceased cases and controls; all silicotics were ceramic workers.
Mastrangelo et al. (1988)	Case-control	Italy, 1978-80	Workers in quarrying and tunnelling	309 cases, 309 controls	Nonsmoker Ever-smoker	No silicosis Silicosis	1.3 5.3	0.9 1.7	~ A ~ A	Unadjusted analysis
Hessel et al. (1990)	Case-control	South Africa, 1975-79	Miners, mainly in gold mines, with silicosis	231 deaths, 318 controls	Cigarettes per day 0; 1-10; 11-20; ≥ 21	Hilar gland silicosis Parenchymal silicosis	1.1 1.6	0.8 0.9	(< A) (< A)	Unmatched odds ratios
Siemiatycki et al. (1990)	Case-control	Canada, 1979-85	Male residents of Montreal, aged 35-70 years	479 cases, 875 controls	Pack-years 0; 1-< 30; 30-< 60; ≥ 60	Substantial	2.6	1.5	1	Adenocarcinoma excluded; silica exposure estimated from job titles; adjusted for age, socio-economic status, job history, education, marital status and asbestos exposure
Chiyotani et al. (1990)	Cohort	Japan, 1979-83	3335 patients with pneumoconiosis qualifying for workmen's compensation (58% silicotics)	60 deaths	Nonsmoker Former smoker Current smoker	Pneumoconiosis	1.8	6.1	(> M)	
Amandus & Costello (1991)	Cohort	USA, 1959-75	9912 metal miners; white males	132 deaths	Nonsmoker Former smoker Current smoker	Silicosis Silicosis in low radon mines	2.2 5.1	1.3 1.7	~ A (~ A)	Adjusted for age; 'interaction between silicosis and cigarette smoking habits not a statistically significant factor related to lung mortality'
Hnizdo & Sluis-Cremer (1991)	Cohort	South Africa, 1968-86	2132 white gold miners with silicosis, aged 45-54 years	77 deaths	Pack-years ≥ 26 vs ≤ 25	≥ 31 vs ≤ 30 dust particle-years	1.4	1.9		'Combined effect of dust and smoking is more than additive.'

Table 2.3.12 (contd)

Reference	Study design	Country, years of study	Source population	No. of cases and controls	Smoking categories (highest vs lowest exposure)	Silica exposure	Relative risk		Interaction[a]	Comments
							Non-smoker	Smoker		
Amandus et al. (1991)	Cohort	USA, 1940–83	760 silicotics among dusty trades workers	33 deaths	Never-smoker Ever-smoker	Silicosis	SMR 1.7	SMR 3.4	(> M)	Standardized mortality ratios using US male population as reference group
Chia et al. (1991)	Cohort	Singapore, 1970–84	159 granite workers with silicosis	9 cases	Nonsmoker Smoker	Silicosis	1.3	2.2	(> M)	
Hnizdo et al. (1997)	Nested case–control	South Africa, 1970–86	2260 white gold miners, aged 45–54 years	78 cases, 386 controls	Pack–years: < 10; 10–29; ≥ 30	Without silicosis With silicosis	1.0 4.1	11.7 48.9		'Strong multiplicative combined effect of smoking and the presence of silicosis on the risk of lung cancer'
Hughes et al. (2001)	Nested case–control	USA, 1940–84	2670 male industrial sand workers	123 deaths, 219 controls	Nonsmoker Ever-smoker					'No indication of an interaction effect of cigarette smoking and cumulative exposure'

Adapted from Saracci & Boffetta (1994)
[a] Numbers in parentheses are based on the assumption that the relative risk due to smoking is 10; A, additive; I, intermediate; M, multiplicative

References

Acheson, E.D., Gardner, M.J., Winter, P.D. & Bennett, C. (1984) Cancer in a factory using amosite asbestos. *Int. J. Epidemiol.*, **13**, 3–10

Amandus, H. & Costello, J. (1991) Silicosis and lung cancer in US metal miners. *Arch. environ. Health*, **46**, 82–89

Amandus, H.E., Shy, C., Wing, S., Blair, A. & Heineman, E.F. (1991) Silicosis and lung cancer in North Carolina dusty trades workers. *Am. J. ind. Med.*, **20**, 57–70

Andersen, A., Berge, S.R., Engeland, A. & Norseth, T. (1996) Exposure to nickel compounds and smoking in relation to incidence of lung and nasal cancer among nickel refinery workers. *Occup. environ. Med.*, **53**, 708–713

André, K., Schraub, S., Mercier, M. & Bontemps, P. (1995) Role of alcohol and tobacco in the aetiology of head and neck cancer: A case–control study in the Doubs region of France. *Eur. J. Cancer*, **31B**, 301–309

Austin, H., Delzell, E., Grufferman, S., Levine, R., Morrison, A.S., Stolley, P.D. & Cole P. (1986) A case–control study of hepatocellular carcinoma and the hepatitis B virus, cigarette smoking, and alcohol consumption. *Cancer Res.*, **46**, 962–966

Axelson, O., Andersson, K., Desai, G., Fagerlund, I., Jansson, B., Karlsson, C. & Wingren, G. (1988) Indoor radon exposure and active and passive smoking in relation to the occurrence of lung cancer. *Scand. J. Work Environ. Health*, **14**, 286–292

Barón, A.E., Franceschi, S., Barra, S., Talamini, R. & La Vecchia, C. (1993) A comparison of the joint effects of alcohol and smoking on the risk of cancer across sites in the upper aero-digestive tract. *Cancer Epidemiol. Biomarkers Prev.*, **2**, 519–523

Basu, J., Palan, P.R., Vermund, S.H., Goldberg, G.L., Burk, R.D. & Romney, S.L. (1991) Plasma ascorbic acid and beta-carotene levels in women evaluated for HPV infection, smoking, and cervix dysplasia. *Cancer Detect. Prev.*, **15**, 165–170

Berry, G., Newhouse, M.L. & Antonis, P. (1985) Combined effect of asbestos and smoking on mortality from lung cancer and mesothelioma in factory workers. *Br. J. ind. Med.*, **42**, 12–18

Blot, W.J., Harrington, J.M., Toledo, A., Hoover, R., Heath, C.W., Jr & Fraumeni, J.F., Jr (1978) Lung cancer after employment in shipyards during World War II. *New Engl. J. Med.*, **299**, 620–624

Blot, W.J., Morris, L.E., Stroube, R., Tagnon, I. & Fraumeni, J.F., Jr (1980) Lung and laryngeal cancers in relation to shipyard employment in coastal Virginia. *J. natl Cancer Inst.*, **65**, 571–575

Blot, W.J., Davies, J.E., Brown, L.M., Nordwall, C.W., Buiatti, E., Ng, A. & Fraumeni, J.F., Jr (1982) Occupational and the high risk of lung cancer in northeast Florida. *Cancer*, **50**, 364–371

Blot, W.J., Xu, Z.Y., Boice, J.D., Jr, Zhao, D.Z., Stone, B.J., Sun, J., Jing, L.B. & Fraumeni, J.F., Jr (1990) Indoor radon and lung cancer in China. *J. natl Cancer Inst.*, **82**, 1025–1030

Boivin, J.F. (1995) Smoking, treatment for Hodgkin's disease and subsequent lung cancer risk. *J. natl Cancer Inst.*, **87**, 1502–1503

Bovenzi, M., Stanta, G., Antiga, G., Peruzzo, P. & Cavallieri, F. (1993) Occupational exposure and lung cancer risk in a coastal area of northeastern Italy. *Int. Arch. occup. environ. Health*, **65**, 35–41

Breslow, N.E. & Storer, B.E. (1985) General relative risk functions for case–control studies. *Am. J. Epidemiol.*, **122**, 149–162

Brown, L.M., Hoover, R.N., Greenberg, R.S., Schoenberg, J.B., Schwartz, A.G., Swanson, G.M., Liff, J.M., Silverman, D.T., Hayes, R.B. & Pottern, L.M. (1994a) Are racial differences in squamous cell esophageal cancer explained by alcohol and tobacco use? *J. natl Cancer Inst.*, **86**, 1340–1345

Brown, L.M., Silverman, D.T., Pottern, L.M., Schoenberg, J.B., Greenberg, R.S., Swanson, G.M., Liff, J.M., Schwartz, A.G., Hayes, R.B., Blot, W.J. & Hoover, R.N. (1994b) Adenocarcinoma of the esophagus and esophagogastric junction in white men in the United States: Alcohol, tobacco, and socioeconomic factors. *Cancer Causes Control*, **5**, 333–340

Brownson, R.C. & Chang, J.C. (1987) Exposure to alcohol and tobacco and the risk of laryngeal cancer. *Arch. environ. Health*, **42**, 192–196

Burch, J.D., Howe, G.R., Miller, A.B. & Semenciw, R. (1981) Tobacco, alcohol, asbestos, and nickel in the etiology of cancer of the larynx: A case–control study. *J. natl Cancer Inst.*, **67**, 1219–1224

Castelletto, R., Castellsague, X., Muñoz, N., Iscovich, J., Chopita, N. & Jmelnitsky, A. (1994) Alcohol, tobacco, diet, mate drinking, and esophageal cancer in Argentina. *Cancer Epidemiol. Biomarkers Prev.*, **3**, 557–564

Chen, C.J., Liang, K.Y., Chang, A.S., Chang, Y.C., Lu, S.N., Liaw, Y.F., Chang, W.Y., Sheen, M.C. & Lin, T.M. (1991) Effects of hepatitis B virus, alcohol drinking, cigarette smoking and familial tendency on hepatocellular carcinoma. *Hepatology*, **13**, 398–406

Cheng, W.N. & Kong, J. (1992) A retrospective mortality cohort study of chrysotile asbestos products workers in Tianjin 1972–1987. *Environ. Res.*, **59**, 271–278

Chia, S.E., Chia, K.S., Phoon, W.H. & Lee, H.P. (1991) Silicosis and lung cancer among Chinese granite workers. *Scand. J. Work Environ. Health*, **17**, 170–174

Chiyotani, K., Saito, K., Okubo, T. & Takahashi K. (1990) Lung cancer risk among pneumo-coniosis patients in Japan, with special reference to silicotics. In: Simonato, L., Fletcher, A.C., Saracci, R. & Thomas, T.L., eds, *Occupational Exposure to Silica and Cancer Risk* (IARC Scientific Publications No. 97), Lyon, IARC*Press*, pp. 95–104

Choi, S.Y. & Kahyo, H. (1991) Effect of cigarette smoking and alcohol consumption in the aetio-logy of cancer of the oral cavity, pharynx and larynx. *Int. J. Epidemiol.*, **20**, 878–885

Chyou, P.H., Nomura, A.M.Y. & Stemmermann, G.N. (1995) Diet, alcohol, smoking and cancer of the upper aerodigestive tract: A prospective study among Hawaii Japanese men. *Int. J. Cancer*, **60**, 616–621

Darby, S., Whitley, E., Silcocks, P., Thakrar, B., Green, M., Lomas, P., Miles, J., Reeves, G., Fearn, T. & Doll, R. (1998) Risk of lung cancer associated with residential radon exposure in South-West England: A case–control study. *Br. J. Cancer*, **78**, 394–408

De Klerk, N.H., Musk, A.W., Armstrong, B.K. & Hobbs M.S.T. (1991) Smoking, exposure to crocidolite, and the incidence of lung cancer and asbestosis. *Br. J. ind. Med.*, **48**, 412–417

De Stefani, E., Correa, P., Oreggia, F., Leiva, J., Rivero, S., Fernandez, G., Deneo-Pellegrini, H., Zavala, D. & Fontham, E. (1987) Risk factors for laryngeal cancer. *Cancer*, **60**, 3087–3091

Doll, R. (1971) The age distribution of cancer: Implications for models of carcinogenesis. *J. R. Stat. Soc.*, **A134**, 133–166

Dosemeci, M., Gokmen, I., Unsal, M., Hayes, R.B. & Blair, A. (1997) Tobacco, alcohol use, and risks of laryngeal and lung cancer by subsite and histologic type in Turkey. *Cancer Causes Control*, **8**, 729–737

Elmes, P.C. & Simpson, M.J.C. (1971) Insulation workers in Belfast. 3. Mortality 1940–66. *Br. J. ind. Med.*, **28**, 226–236

Enterline, P.E. (1983) Sorting out multiple causal factors in individual cases. In: Chiazze, L., Jr, Lundin, F.E. & Watkins, D., eds, *Methods and Issues in Occupational and Environmental Epidemiology*, Ann Arbor, MI, Ann Arbor Science, pp. 177–182

Enterline, P.E., Marsh, G.M., Esmen, N.A., Henderson, V.L., Callahan, C.M. & Paik, M. (1987) Some effects of cigarette smoking, arsenic and SO_2 on mortality among US copper smelter workers. *J. occup. Med.*, **29**, 831–838

Erren, T.C., Jacobsen, M. & Piekarski, C. (1999) Synergy between asbestos and smoking on lung cancer risks. *Epidemiology*, **10**, 405–411

Falk, R.T., Pickle, L.W., Brown, L.M., Mason, T.J., Buffler, P.A. & Fraumeni, J.F., Jr (1989) Effect of smoking and alcohol consumption on laryngeal cancer risk in coastal Texas. *Cancer Res.*, **49**, 4024–4029

Figueroa, W.G., Raszkowski, R. & Weiss, W. (1973) Lung cancer in chloromethyl methyl ether workers. *New Engl. J. Med.*, **288**, 1096–1097

Flanders, D.W. & Rothman, K.J. (1982) Interaction of alcohol and tobacco in laryngeal cancer. *Am. J. Epidemiol.*, **115**, 371–379

Forastiere, F., Lagorio, S., Michelozzi, P., Cavariani, F., Arca', M., Borgia, P., Perucci, C. & Axelson, O. (1986) Silica, silicosis and lung cancer among ceramic workers: A case–referent study. *Am. J. ind. Med.*, **10**, 363–370

Franceschi, S., Talamini, R., Barra, S., Barón, A.E., Negri, E., Bidoli, E., Serraino, D. & La Vecchia, C. (1990) Smoking and drinking in relation to cancers of the oral cavity, pharynx, larynx, and esophagus in northern Italy. *Cancer Res.*, **50**, 6502–6507

Freudenheim, J.L., Graham, S., Byers, T.E., Marshall, J.R., Haughey, B.P., Swanson, M.K. & Wilkinson, G. (1992) Diet, smoking, and alcohol in cancer of the larynx: A case–control study. *Nutr. Cancer*, **17**, 33–45

Garshick, E., Schenker, M.B., Muñoz, A., Segal, M., Smith, T.J., Woskie, S.R., Hammond, S.K. & Speizer, F.E. (1987) A case–control study of lung cancer and diesel exhaust exposure in railroad workers. *Am. Rev. respir. Dis.*, **135**, 1242–1248

Greenland, S. (1983) Tests for interaction in epidemiologic studies: A review and a study of power. *Stat. Med.*, **2**, 243–251

Greenland, S. (1993) Basic problems in interaction assessment. *Environ. Health Perspect.*, **101** (Suppl. 4), 59–66

Guénel, P., Chastang, J.F., Luce, D., Leclerc, A. & Brugère, J. (1988) A study of the interaction of alcohol drinking and tobacco smoking among French cases of laryngeal cancer. *J. Epidemiol. Community Health*, **42**, 350–354

Gustavsson, P., Nyberg, F., Pershagen, G., Schéele, P., Jakobsson, R. & Plato, N. (2002) Low-dose exposure to asbestos and lung cancer: Dose–response relations and interaction with smoking in a population-based case–referent study in Stockholm, Sweden. *Am. J. Epidemiol.*, **155**, 1016–1022

Hammond, E.C., Selikoff, I.J. & Seidman, H. (1979) Asbestos exposure, cigarette smoking and death rates. *Ann. N.Y. Acad. Sci.*, **330**, 473–490

Hazelton, W.D., Luebeck, E.G., Heidenreich, W.F. & Moolgavkar, S.H. (2001) Analysis of a historical cohort of Chinese tin miners with arsenic, radon, cigarette smoke, and pipe smoke exposures using the biologically based two-stage clonal expansion model. *Radiat. Res.*, **156**, 78–94

Herity, B., Moriarty, M., Daly, L., Dunn, J. & Bourke, G.J. (1982) The role of tobacco and alcohol in the aetiology of lung and larynx cancer. *Br. J. Cancer*, **46**, 961–964

Hertz-Picciotto, I., Smith, A.H., Holtzman, D., Lipsett, M. & Alexeeff, G. (1992) Synergism between occupational arsenic exposure and smoking in the induction of lung cancer. *Epidemiology*, **3**, 23–31

Hessel, P.A., Sluis-Cremer, G.K. & Hnizdo, E. (1990) Silica exposure, silicosis, and lung cancer: A necropsy study. *Br. J. ind. Med.*, **47**, 4–9

Hildesheim, A., Herrero, R., Castle, P.E., Wacholder, S., Bratti, M.C., Sherman, M.E., Lorincz, A.T., Burk, R.D., Morales, J., Rodriguez, A.C., Helgesen, K., Alfaro, M., Hutchinson, M., Balmaceda, I., Greenberg, M. & Schiffman, M. (2001) HPV co-factors related to the development of cervical cancer: Results from a population-based study in Costa Rica. *Br. J. Cancer*, **84**, 1219–1226

Hilt, B., Langård, S., Andersen, A. & Rosenberg, J. (1985) Asbestos exposure, smoking habits, and cancer incidence among production and maintenance workers in an electrochemical plant. *Am. J. ind. Med.*, **8**, 565–577

Hnizdo, E. & Sluis-Cremer, G.K. (1991) Silica exposure, silicosis, and lung cancer: A mortality study of South African gold miners. *Br. J. ind. Med.*, **48**, 53–60

Hnizdo, E., Murray, J. & Klempman, S. (1997) Lung cancer in relation to exposure to silica dust, silicosis and uranium production in South African gold miners. *Thorax*, **52**, 271–275

Hornung, R.W. & Meinhardt, T.J. (1987) Quantitative risk assessment of lung cancer in US uranium miners. *Health Phys.*, **52**, 417–430

Hornung, R.W., Deddens, J.A. & Roscoe, R.J. (1998) Modifiers of lung cancer risk in uranium miners from the Colorado Plateau. *Health Phys.*, **74**, 12–21

Hu, J., Nyrén, O., Wolk, A., Bergström, R., Yuen, J., Adami, H.O., Guo, L., Li, H., Huang, G., Xu, X., Zhao, F., Chen, Y., Wang, C., Qin, H., Hu, C. & Li, Y. (1994) Risk factors for oesophageal cancer in Northeast China. *Int. J. Cancer*, **57**, 38–46

Hughes, J.M. & Weill, H. (1991) Asbestosis as a precursor of asbestos related lung cancer: Results of a prospective mortality study. *Br. J. ind. Med.*, **48**, 229–233

Hughes, J.M., Weill, H., Rando, R.J., Shi, R., McDonald, A.D. & McDonald, J.C. (2001) Cohort mortality study of North American industrial sand workers. II. Case–referent analysis of lung cancer and silicosis deaths. *Ann. occup. Hyg.*, **45**, 201–207

IARC (1987) *IARC Monographs on the Evaluation of Carcinogenic Risks to Humans*, Suppl. 7, *Overall Evaluations of Carcinogenicity: An Updating of* IARC Monographs *Volumes 1 to 42*, Lyon, IARCPress

IARC (1988a) *IARC Monographs on the Evaluation of Carcinogenic Risks to Humans*, Vol. 43, *Man-made Mineral Fibres and Radon*, Lyon, IARCPress

IARC (1988b) *IARC Monographs on the Evaluation of Carcinogenic Risks to Humans*, Vol. 44, *Alcohol Drinking*, Lyon, IARCPress

IARC (1997) *IARC Monographs on the Evaluation of Carcinogenic Risks to Humans*, Vol. 68, *Silica, Some Silicates, Coal Dust and* para-*Aramid Fibrils*, Lyon, IARCPress

Järup, L. & Pershagen, G. (1991) Arsenic exposure, smoking, and lung cancer in smelter workers — A case–control study. *Am. J. Epidemiol.*, **134**, 545–551

Kabat, G.C., Chang, C.J. & Wynder, E.L. (1994) The role of tobacco, alcohol use, and body mass index in oral and pharyngeal cancer. *Int. J. Epidemiol.*, **23**, 1137–1144

Kaldor, J.M., Day, N.E., Bell, J., Clarke, E.A., Langmark, F., Karjalainen, S., Band, P., Pedersen, D., Choi, W., Blair, V., Henry-Amar, M., Prior, P., Assouline, D., Pompe-Kirn, V., Cartwright, R.A., Koch, M., Arslan, A., Fraser, P., Sutcliffe, S.B., Host, H., Hakama, M. & Stovall, M. (1992) Lung cancer following Hodgkin's disease: A case–control study. *Int. J. Cancer*, **52**, 677–681

Kinjo, Y., Cui, Y., Akiba, S., Watanabe, S., Yamaguchi, N., Sobue, T., Mizuno, S. & Beral, V. (1998) Mortality risks of oesophageal cancer associated with hot tea, alcohol, tobacco and diet in Japan. *J. Epidemiol.*, **8**, 235–243

Kjellberg, L., Hallmans, G., Åhren, A.M., Johansson, R., Bergman, F., Wadell, G., Ångström, T. & Dillner, J. (2000) Smoking, diet, pregnancy and oral contraceptive use as risk factors for cervical intra-epithelial neoplasia in relation to human papillomavirus infection. *Br. J. Cancer*, **82**, 1332–1338

Kjuus, H., Skjaerven, R., Langård, S., Lien, J.T. & Aamodt, T. (1986) A case–referent study of lung cancer, occupational exposures and smoking. II. Role of asbestos exposure. *Scand. J. Work Environ. Health*, **12**, 203–209

Kopecky, K.J., Nakashima, E., Yamamoto, T. & Kato, H. (1986) *Lung Cancer, Radiation, and Smoking among A-bomb Survivors, Hiroshima and Nagasaki* (Technical Report No. 13-86), [town?], Radiation Effects Research Foundation, pp. 1–32

Kune, G.A., Kune, S., Field, B., Watson, L.F., Cleland, H., Merenstein, D. & Vitetta, L. (1993) Oral and pharyngeal cancer, diet, smoking, alcohol, and serum vitamin A and β-carotene levels: A case–control study in men. *Nutr. Cancer*, **20**, 61–70

Kuper, H., Tzonou, A., Kaklamani, E., Hsieh, C.C., Lagiou, P., Adami, H.O., Trichopoulos, D. & Stuver, S.O. (2000) Tobacco smoking, alcohol consumption and their interaction in the causation of hepatocellular carcinoma. *Int. J. Cancer*, **85**, 498–502

Lee, P.N. (2001) Relation between exposure to asbestos and smoking jointly and the risk of lung cancer. *Occup. environ. Med.*, **58**, 145–153

Lewin, F., Norell, S.E., Johansson, H., Gustavsson, P., Wennerberg, J., Biörklund, A. & Rutqvist, L.E. (1998) Smoking tobacco, oral snuff, and alcohol in the etiology of squamous cell carcinoma of the head and neck: A population-based case–referent study in Sweden. *Cancer*, **82**, 1367–1375

Liddell, F.D. (2001) The interaction of asbestos and smoking in lung cancer. *Ann. occup. Hyg.*, **45**, 341–356

Little, M.P., Haylock, R.G.E. & Muirhead, C.R. (2002) Modelling lung tumour risk in radon-exposed uranium miners using generalizations of the two-mutation model of Moolgavkar, Venzon and Knudson. *Int. J. Radiat. Biol.*, **78**, 49–68

Lubin, J.H. & Gaffey, W. (1988) Relative risk models for assessing the joint effects of multiple factors. *Am. J. ind. Med.*, **13**, 149–167

Lubin, J.H., Boice, J.D., Jr, Edling, C., Hornung, R.W., Howe, G., Kunz, E., Kusiak, R.A., Morrison, H.I., Radford, E.P., Samet, J.M., Tirmarche, M., Woodward, A., Yao, S.X. & Pierce, D.A. (1994) *Radon and Lung Cancer Risk: A Joint Analysis of 11 Underground Miners Studies*, Bethesda, MD, US Department of Health and Human Services, Public Health Service, National Institutes of Health

Luebeck, E.G., Heidenreich, W.F., Hazelton, W.D., Paretzke, H.G. & Moolgavkar, S.H. (1999) Biologically based analysis of the data for the Colorado uranium miners cohort: Age, dose and dose–rate effects. *Radiat. Res.*, **152**, 339–351

Mabuchi, K., Land, C.E. & Akiba, S. (1991) *Radiation, Smoking and Lung Cancer. A Binational Study Provides New Insights into the Effects of Smoking and Radiation Exposure on Different Histological Types of Lung Cancer* (Update No. 3), [town?], Radiation Effects Research Foundation, pp. 7–8

Maier, H., Dietz, A., Gewelke, U., Heller, W.D. & Weidauer H. (1992) Tobacco and alcohol and the risk of head and neck cancer. *Clin. Invest.*, **70**, 320–327

Martischnig, K.M., Newell, D.J., Barnsley, W.C., Cowan, W.K., Feinmann, E.L. & Oliver, E. (1977) Unsuspected exposure to asbestos and bronchogenic carcinoma. *Br. med. J.*, **i**, 746–749

Mashberg, A., Boffetta, P., Winkelman, R. & Garfinkel, L. (1993) Tobacco smoking, alcohol drinking, and cancer of the oral cavity and oropharynx among US veterans. *Cancer*, **72**, 1369–1375

Mastrangelo, G., Zambon, P., Simonato, L. & Rizzi, P. (1988) A case–referent study investigating the relationship between exposure to silica dust and lung cancer. *Int. Arch. occup. environ. Health*, **60**, 299–302

Mauderly, J.L. (1993) Toxicological approaches to complex mixtures. *Environ. Health Perspect.*, **101** (Suppl. 4), 155–165

McDonald, J.C., Liddell, F.D.K., Dufresne, A. & McDonald, A.D. (1993) The 1891–1920 birth cohort of Quebec chrysotile miners and millers: Mortality 1976–88. *Br. J. ind. Med.*, **50**, 1073–1081

McDonald, J.C., McDonald, A.D. & Hughes, J.M. (1999) Chrysotile, tremolite and fibrogenicity. *Ann. occup. Hyg.*, **43**, 439–442

Meurman, L.O., Pukkala, E. & Hakama, M. (1994) Incidence of cancer among anthophyllite asbestos miners in Finland. *Occup. environ. Med.*, **51**, 421–425

Minowa, M., Hatano, S. & Ashizawa, M., Oguro, H., Naruhashi, H., Suzuki, M., Mitoku, K., Miwa, M., Wakamatsu, C., Yasuda, Y., Shirai, K. & Miura, H. (1991) A case–control study of lung cancer with special reference to asbestos exposure. *Environ. Health Perspect.*, **94**, 39–42

Moolgavkar, S.H., Luebeck, E.G., Krewski, D. & Zielinski, J.M. (1993) Radon, cigarette smoke, and lung cancer: A re-analysis of the Colorado plateau uranium miners' data. *Epidemiology*, **4**, 204–217

Morrison, H.I., Semenciw, R.M., Mao, Y. & Wigle, D.T. (1988) Cancer mortality among a group of fluorspar miners exposed to radon progeny. *Am. J. Epidemiol.*, **128**, 1266–1275

Mukaiya, M., Nishi, M., Miyake, H. & Hirata, K. (1998) Chronic liver diseases for the risk of hepatocellular carcinoma: A case–control study in Japan. Etiologic association of alcohol consumption, cigarette smoking and the development of chronic liver diseases. *Hepatogastroenterology*, **45**, 2328–2332

Muscat, J.E., Richie, J.P., Jr, Thompson, S. & Wynder, E.L. (1996) Gender differences in smoking and risk for oral cancer. *Cancer Res.*, **56**, 5192–5197

National Research Council (NRC) (1988) *Committee on the Biological Effects of Ionizing Radiations: Health Risks of Radon and Other Internally Deposited Alpha-Emitters: BEIR IV*, Washington DC, National Academy Press

National Research Council (NRC) (1999) *Committee on Health Risks of Exposure to Radon, Board on Radiation Effects Research and Commission on Life Sciences: Health Effects of Exposure to Radon: BEIR VI*, Washington DC, National Academy Press

Neuberger, M. & Kundi, M. (1990) Individual asbestos exposure: Smoking and mortality — A cohort study in the asbestos cement industry. *Br. J. ind. Med.*, **47**, 615–620

Neugut, A.I., Murray, T., Santos, J., Amols, H., Hayes, M.K., Flannery, J.T. & Robinson, E. (1994) Increased risk of lung cancer after breast cancer radiation therapy in cigarette smokers. *Cancer*, **73**, 1615–20

Oksa, P., Pukkala, E., Karjalainen, A., Ojajärvi, A. & Huuskonen, M.S. (1997) Cancer incidence and mortality among Finnish asbestos sprayers and in asbestosis and silicosis patients. *Am. J. ind. Med.*, **31**, 693–698

Olsen, J., Sabroe, S. & Ipsen, J. (1985) Effect of combined alcohol and tobacco exposure on risk of cancer of the hypopharynx. *J. Epidemiol. Community Health*, **39**, 304–307

Pastorino, U., Berrino, F., Gervasio, A., Pesenti, V., Riboli, E. & Crosignani, P. (1984) Proportion of lung cancers due to occupational exposure. *Int. J. Cancer*, **33**, 231–237

Pershagen, G. (1985) Lung cancer mortality among men living near an arsenic-emitting smelter. *Am. J. Epidemiol.*, **122**, 684–694

Pershagen, G., Wall, S., Taube, A. & Linnman, L. (1981) On the interaction between occupational arsenic exposure and smoking and its relationship to lung cancer. *Scand. J. Work Environ. Health*, **7**, 302–309

Pershagen, G., Åkerblom, G., Axelson, O., Clavensjö, B., Damber, L., Desai, G., Enflo, A., Lagarde, F., Mellander, H., Svartengren, M. & Swedjemark, G.A. (1994) Residential radon exposure and lung cancer in Sweden. *New Engl. J. Med.*, **330**, 159–164

Petersen, G.R., Gilbert, E.S., Buchanan, J.A. & Stevens, R.G. (1990) A case–cohort study of lung cancer, ionizing radiation, and tobacco smoking among males at the Hanford Site. *Health Phys.*, **58**, 3–11

Pinto, S.S., Henderson, V. & Enterline, P.E. (1978) Mortality experience of arsenic-exposed workers. *Arch. environ. Health*, **33**, 325–331

Pisa, F.E., Barbone, F., Betta, A., Bonomi, M., Alessandrini, B. & Bovenzi, M. (2001) Residential radon and risk of lung cancer in an Italian alpine area. *Arch. environ. Health*, **56**, 208–215

Prentice, R.L., Yoshimoto, Y. & Mason, M.W. (1983) Relationship of cigarette smoking and radiation exposure to cancer mortality in Hiroshima and Nagasaki. *J. natl Cancer Inst.*, **70**, 611–622

Radford, E.P. & St Clair Renard, K.G. (1984) Lung cancer in Swedish iron miners exposed to low doses of radon daughters. *New Engl. J. Med.*, **310**, 1485–1494

Rencher, A.C., Carter, M.W. & McKee, D.W. (1977) A retrospective epidemiological study of mortality at a large western copper smelter. *J. occup. Med.*, **19**, 754–758

Rothman, K.J. (1976) The estimation of synergy or antagonism. *Am. J. Epidemiol.*, **103**, 506–511

Rothman, K.J. & Greenland, S. (1998) *Modern Epidemiology*, 2nd Ed., Philadelphia, Lippincott-Raven Publishers

Rothman, K.J., Greenland, S. & Walker, A.M. (1980) Concepts of interaction. *Am. J. Epidemiol.*, **112**, 467–470

Rubino, G.F., Piolatto, G., Newhouse, M.L., Scansetti, G., Aresini, G.A. & Murray, R. (1979) Mortality of chrysotile asbestos workers at the Balangero Mine, northern Italy. *Br. J. ind. Med.*, **36**, 187–194

Ruosteenoja, E. (1991) *Indoor Radon and Risk of Lung Cancer: An Epidemiologic Study in Finland,* Doctoral Dissertation, Helsinki, Department of Public Health, University of Tampere, Finnish Government Printing Centre

Samet, J.M., Pathak, D.R., Morgan, M.V., Key, C.R., Valdivia, A.A. & Lubin, J.H. (1991) Lung cancer mortality and exposure to Rn progeny in a cohort of New Mexico underground U miners. *Health Phys.*, **61**, 745–752

Saracci, R. (1977) Asbestos and lung cancer: An analysis of the epidemiological evidence on the asbestos-smoking interaction. *Int. J. Cancer*, **20**, 323–331

Saracci, R. (1987) The interactions of tobacco smoking and other agents in cancer etiology. *Epidemiol. Rev.*, **9**, 175–193

Saracci, R. & Boffetta, P. (1994) Interactions of tobacco smoking and other causes of lung cancer. In: Samet, J.M., ed., *Epidemiology of Lung Cancer*, New York, Marcel Dekker, pp. 465–493

Schlecht, N.F., Franco, E.L., Pintos, J., Negassa, A., Kowalski, L.P., Oliveira, B.V. & Curado, M.P. (1999) Interaction between tobacco and alcohol consumption and the risk of cancers of the upper aero-digestive tract in Brazil. *Am. J. Epidemiol.*, **150**, 1129–1137

Schoenberg, J.B., Klotz, J.B., Wilcox, H.B., Nicholls, G.P., Gil del Real, M.T., Stemhagen, A. & Mason, T.J. (1990) Case–control study of residential radon and lung cancer among New Jersey women. *Cancer Res.*, **50**, 6520–6524

Selikoff, I.J. & Hammond, E.C. (1975) Multiple risk factors in environmental cancer. In: Fraumeni, J.F., Jr, ed., *Persons at High Risk of Cancer: An Approach to Cancer Etiology and Control*, New York, Academic Press, pp. 467–483

Selikoff, I.J., Seidman, H. & Hammond, E.C. (1980) Mortality effects of cigarette smoking among amosite asbestos factory workers. *J. natl Cancer Inst.*, **65**, 507–513

Siemiatycki, J., Gérin, M., Dewar, R., Lakhani, R., Begin, D. & Richardson, L. (1990) Silica and cancer associations from a multicancer occupational exposure case–referent study. In: Simonato, L., Fletcher, A.C., Saracci, R. & Thomas, T.L., eds, *Occupational Exposure to Silica and Cancer Risk* (IARC Scientific Publications No. 97), Lyon, IARCPress, pp. 29–42

Svensson, C., Pershagen, G. & Klominek, J. (1989) Lung cancer in women and type of dwelling in relation to radon exposure. *Cancer Res.*, **49**, 1861–1865

Tanaka, K., Hirohata, T., Takeshita, S., Hirohata, I., Koga, S., Sugimachi, K., Kanematsu, T., Ohryohji, F. & Ishibashi, H. (1992) Hepatitis B virus, cigarette smoking and alcohol consumption in the development of hepatocellular carcinoma: A case–control study in Fukuoka, Japan. *Int. J. Cancer*, **51**, 509–514

Taylor, P.R., Qiao, Y.L., Schatzkin, A., Yao, S.X., Lubin, J., Mao, B.L., Rao, J.Y., McAdams, M., Xuan, X.Z. & Li, J.Y. (1989) Relation of arsenic exposure to lung cancer among tin miners in Yunnan Province, China. *Br. J. ind. Med.*, **46**, 881–886

Thomas, D.C. (1981) General relative-risk models for survival time and matched case–control analysis. *Biometrics*, **37**, 673–686

Thomas, D.C. & Whittemore, A.S. (1988) Methods for testing interactions, with applications to occupational exposures, smoking, and lung cancer. *Am. J. ind. Med.*, **13**, 131–147

Thomas, D., Pogoda, J., Langholz, B. & Mack, W. (1994) Temporal modifiers of the radon–smoking interaction. *Health Phys.*, **66**, 257–262

Trichopoulos, D., Day, N.E., Kaklamani, E., Tzonou, A., Muñoz, N., Zavitsanos, X., Koumantaki, Y. & Trichopoulou, A. (1987) Hepatitis B virus, tobacco smoking and ethanol consumption in the etiology of hepatocellular carcinoma. *Int. J. Cancer*, **39**, 45–49

Tsuda, T., Nagira, T., Yamamoto, M. & Kume, Y. (1990) An epidemiological study on cancer in certified arsenic poisoning patients in Toroku. *Ind. Health*, **28**, 53–62

Tucker, M.A., Murray, N., Shaw, E.G., Ettinger, D.S., Mabry, M., Huber, M.H., Feld, R., Shepherd, F.A., Johnson, D.H., Grant, S.C., Aisner, J. & Johnson, B.E. for the Lung Cancer Working Cadre (1997) Second primary cancers related to smoking and treatment of small-cell lung cancer. *J. natl Cancer Inst.*, **89**, 1782–1788

Tuyns, A.J., Estève, J., Raymond, L., Berrino, F., Benhamou, E., Blanchet, F., Boffetta, P., Crosignani, P., del Moral, A., Lehmann, W., Merletti, F., Péquignot, G., Riboli, E., Sancho-Garnier, H., Terracini, B., Zubiri, A. & Zubiri, L. (1988) Cancer of the larynx/hypopharynx, tobacco and alcohol: IARC international case–control study in Turin and Varese (Italy), Zaragoza and Navarra (Spain), Geneva (Switzerland) and Calvados (France). *Int. J. Cancer*, **41**, 483–491

US Department of Health and Human Services (US DHHS) (1985) *The Health Consequences of Smoking — Cancer and Chronic Lung Disease in the Workplace. A Report of the Surgeon General*, Washington DC, US Government Printing Office

Vainio, H., & Boffetta, P. (1994) Mechanisms of the combined effect of asbestos and smoking in the etiology of lung cancer. *Scand. J. Work. Environ. Health*, **20**, 235–242

Van Leeuwen, F.E., Klokman, W.J., Stovall, M., Hagenbeek, A., van den Belt-Dusebout, A.W., Noyon, R., Boice, J.D., Jr, Burgers, J.M.V. & Somers, R. (1995) Roles of radiotherapy and smoking in lung cancer following Hodgkin's disease. *J. natl Cancer Inst.*, **87**, 1530–1537

Walter, S.D. & Iwane, M. (1983) Re: "Interaction of alcohol and tobacco in laryngeal cancer". *Am. J. Epidemiol.*, **117**, 639–641

Wang, Z., Lubin, J.H., Wang, L., Zhang, S., Boice, J.D., Jr, Cui, H., Zhang, S., Conrath, S., Xia, Y., Shang, B., Brenner, A., Lei, S., Metayer, C., Cao, J., Chen, K.W., Lei, S. & Kleinerman, R.A. (2002) Residential radon and lung cancer risk in a high-exposure area of Gansu Province, China. *Am. J. Epidemiol.*, **155**, 554–564

Weiss, W. (1980) The cigarette factor in lung cancer due to chloromethyl ethers. *J. occup. Med.*, **22**, 527–529

Weiss, W., Moser, R.L. & Auerbach, O. (1979) Lung cancer in chloromethyl ether workers. *Am. Rev. respir. Dis.*, **120**, 1031–1037

Welch, K., Higgins, I., Oh, M. & Burchfiel, C. (1982) Arsenic exposure, smoking, and respiratory cancer in copper smelter workers. *Arch. environ. Health*, **37**, 325–335

Whittemore, A.S. (1977) The age distribution of human cancer for carcinogenic exposures of varying intensity. *Am. J. Epidemiol.*, **106**, 418–432

Wynder, E.L., Covey, L.S., Mabuchi, K. & Mushinski, M. (1976) Environmental factors in cancer of the larynx: A second look. *Cancer*, **38**, 1591–1601

Xuan, X.Z., Lubin, J.H., Li, J.Y. & Blot, W.J. (1993) A cohort study in southern China of workers exposed to radon and radon decay products. *Health Phys.*, **64**, 120–131

Yao, S.X., Lubin, J.H., Qiao, Y.L., Boice, J.D., Jr, Li, J.Y., Cai, S.K., Zhang, F.M. & Blot, W.J. (1994) Exposure to radon progeny, tobacco use and lung cancer in a case–control study in southern China. *Radiat. Res.*, **138**, 326–336

Ylitalo, N., Sørensen, P., Josefsson, A., Frisch, M., Sparén, P., Pontén, J., Gyllensten, U., Melbye, M. & Adami, H.O. (1999) Smoking and oral contraceptives as risk factors for cervical carcinoma *in situ*. *Int. J. Cancer*, **81**, 357–365

Yu, M.C., Tong, M.J., Govindarajan, S. & Henderson, B.E. (1991) Nonviral risk factors for hepato-cellular carcinoma in a low-risk population, the non-Asians of Los Angeles County, California. *J. natl Cancer Inst.*, **83**, 1820–1826

Zambon, P., Talamini, R., La Vecchia, C., Dal Maso, L., Negri, E., Tognazzo, S., Simonato, L. & Franceschi, S. (2000) Smoking, type of alcoholic beverage and squamous-cell oesophageal cancer in northern Italy. *Int. J. Cancer*, **86**, 144–149

Zaridze, D., Borisova, E., Maximovitch, D. & Chkhikvadze, V. (2000) Alcohol consumption, smoking and risk of gastric cancer: Case–control study from Moscow, Russia. *Cancer Causes Control*, **11**, 363–371

Zheng, W., Blot, W.J., Shu, X.O., Gao, Y.T., Ji, B.T., Ziegler, R.G. & Fraumeni, J.F., Jr (1992) Diet and other risk factors for laryngeal cancer in Shanghai, China. *Am. J. Epidemiol.*, **136**, 178–191

Zheng, T., Holford, T., Chen, Y., Jiang, P., Zhang, B. & Boyle, P. (1997) Risk of tongue cancer asso-ciated with tobacco smoking and alcohol consumption: A case–control study. *Oral Oncol.*, **33**, 82–85

Zhu, H. & Wang, Z. (1993) Study of occupational lung cancer in asbestos factories in China. *Br. J. ind. Med.*, **50**, 1039–1042

3. Carcinogenicity Studies in Experimental Animals

3.1 Inhalation exposure: mainstream tobacco smoke

This section summarizes the information available on the effects of exposure to mainstream tobacco smoke and the occurrence of cancer in animals and includes data from the previous *IARC Monographs* on tobacco smoking (IARC, 1986) and subsequent publications to date (see Table 3.1).

Although the evidence for the carcinogenicity of tobacco smoke emerged first in humans, there was a need for an inhalation model in experimental animals in which the carcinogenicity of different types of tobacco and tobacco products could be studied. The availability of animal models also permits the investigation of various modifying factors in the development of cancer.

Early inhalation studies in rodents were reviewed by Wynder and Hoffmann (1967). From about 1960 onwards, the species of animal selected most often for carcinogenicity studies was the Syrian golden hamster, which has a low background incidence rate for spontaneous pulmonary tumours and is prone to few interfering respiratory infections. The discovery that inhalation of tobacco smoke caused carcinomas in the larynx of hamsters enabled the establishment of a model system in which the carcinogenicity of tobacco smoke for hamsters has been repeatedly confirmed (see below). Many bioassays have also been conducted in mice and rats and the results are summarized below.

To enable the responses of animals to tobacco smoke inhalation to be studied, it was necessary to develop methods and equipment to deliver smoke in a standardized, effective way. A number of devices have been employed, some involving whole-body exposure and some 'nose-only' exposure. Usually, in order to simulate human smoking patterns, a 2-s puff from a burning cigarette is diluted with air and forced into a chamber for a short period, followed by an air purge. However, animals that are being forced involuntarily to inhale the smoke suffer avoidance reactions and change their breathing patterns to shallow, hesitant inspirations with reduced minute volumes. This behaviour affects the doses delivered to the different parts of the respiratory system. Because rodents are obligatory nose-breathers and because rodents and dogs have more convoluted and intricate nasal turbinate patterns than humans, the dynamics of particle deposition in the upper respiratory tract might be expected to be different (see Wynder & Hoffmann, 1967;

Table 3.1. Selected studies of carcinogenicity in response to exposure to mainstream tobacco smoke in mouse, rat and hamster

Strain	Sex	No. of treated animals/group	Route	Type of exposure	Concentration of exposure agent	Exposure duration	Lung burden	Tumour incidence	Reference
Mouse									
C57BL	M	100	Nose-only	Mixture of fresh non-filter cigarette smoke/air (1/39, v/v)	Nicotine,0.1 mg/mL; CO, 0.064% (v/v)	12 min/day, lifetime	Nicotine, 14–17 µg	4/100 (alveologenic AdC) [p = 0.06], 0/100 (controls)	Harris & Negroni (1967)
	F	100						4/100 (alveologenic AdC) [p = 0.06], 0/100 (controls)	
C57BL	NG	126	Whole-body	Gas phase of 12 cigarettes puffed 2 s/min	NG	90 min/day, lifetime (~27 mo)	NG	7/126 (lung A) [NS], 3/90 (controls)	Otto & Elmenhorst (1967)
BLH	NG	126			NG		NG	40/126 (lung A) [NS], 19/60 (controls)	
Snell	M	160	Whole-body	Whole fresh cigarette smoke	NG	2 puffs, once/day, lifetime (26 mo)	Nicotine, 5 µg	7/107 (lung A), 8/106 (controls); 11/107 (lung AdC), 5/106 (controls)	Leuchtenberger & Leuchtenberger (1970)
	F	118						2/65 (lung A), 1/78 (controls); 5/65 (lung AdC), 3/78 (controls)	
	M	100		Gas phase of fresh cigarette smoke	NG		NG	1/44 (lung A), 8/106 (controls); 10/44 (lung AdC) (p = 0.005); 5/106 (controls)	
	F	89						3/44 (lung A), 1/78 (controls); 5/44 (lung AdC), 3/78 (controls)	
C57BL	M	100 (2×)	Nose-only	Mixture of fresh flue-cured or air cured cigarette smoke/air (1/39, v/v)	NG	12 min/day on alternate days; lifetime	NG	9/162[a] (flue-cured) [p = 0.07], 7/189[a] (air-cured) [p > 0.05], 3/160[a] (controls)	Harris et al. (1974)
	F	100 (2×)						7/164[a] (flue-cured) [p = 0.04], 0/173 (air-cured), 1/159[a] (controls)	
C57BL	M	100		Gas phase of flue-cured cigarette smoke	NG		NG	3/8[a] [p > 0.05], 3/160[a] (controls)	Harris et al. (1974)

Table 3.1 (contd)

Strain	Sex	No. of treated animals/group	Route	Type of exposure	Concentration of exposure agent	Exposure duration	Lung burden	Tumour incidence	Reference
(C57BL/Cum × C3H/Anf Cum)F$_1$	F	1014 and 2053	Nose-only	10% smoke from US reference cigarettes	NG	Smoke 20 s/min, 6–8 min/day, 5 days/wk, 110 wks	Particulate deposition, 125–200 μg	19/978 (alveolar AdC), 7/651 (sham-exposed controls); shorter latency of tumour occurrence in smoke-exposed group suggested ($p = 0.10$)	Henry & Kouri (1986)
Rat									
Wistar	F	408	Nose-only	Mixture of cigarette smoke/air (1/5)	NG	15 s/min, 2 × 11 min/day, 5 days/wk, lifetime (140 wks)	NG	4/408 (1 lung C + 3 lung neoplasms of uncertain malignancy), 0/104 (controls), 0/104 (sham treated controls)	Davis et al. (1975a)
Fischer 344	F	80	Nose-only	Mixture of non-filter cigarette smoke/air (1/10)	18.4 mg smoke particulate and 0.89 mg nicotine/cigarette	1 cigarette/h, 7 cigarettes/day, 5 days/wk, 128 wks termination at 160 wks	Particulate deposition, 1.75 mg/day	10/80 (1 nasal AdC, 1 nasal C, 5 pulmonary A, 1 pulmonary C, 2 alveologenic C) ($p < 0.05$), 3/93 (controls) 21/80 (subcutaneous sarcomas at forelimb ulceration sites) ($p < 0.05$), 0/93 (controls)	Dalbey et al. (1980)
CDF® (Fischer 344)/CrlBR	M, F	NG	Whole-body	Cigarette smoke/air	100 mg (LCS) or 250 mg (HCS) total particulate matter/m³	6 h/day, 5 days/wk, 126 wks		Males: 3/173 (lung tumours, LCS); 7/78 (HCS); 3/119 (filtered air) Females: 4/145 (LCS); 6/83 (HCS) [$p < 0.05$]; 0/113 (filtered air)	Finch et al. (1995)
Hamster									
Syrian golden	M + F	Group of 80 + 80	Whole-body	Mixture of German ref. cigarette smoke/air (1/15)	NG	Smoke of 30 cigarettes for 7–10 min: 1, 2 or 3 times/day, 5 days/wk, lifetime	NG	1/160, 17/160 and 9/160 (laryngeal C), 0/800 (controls)	Dontenwill et al. (1973)
	M + F	Group of 80 + 80		Mixture of dark air-cured cigarette smoke/air (1/15)	NG	Smoke of 30 cigarettes for 7–10 min: 2 times/day, 5 days/wk, lifetime	NG	2/160 (laryngeal C), 0/800 (controls)	Dontenwill et al. (1973)

Table 3.1 (contd)

Strain	Sex	No. of treated animals/ group	Route	Type of exposure	Concentration of exposure agent	Exposure duration	Lung burden	Tumour incidence	Reference
Inbred BIO 15.16	M	102	Whole-body	Mixture of US ref. cigarette smoke/air (1/5)	NG	8 puff cycles, twice/day, 5 days/wk, up to 100 wks	NG	9/84 (laryngeal tumour) and 2/84 (nasopharyngeal tumours), 0/42 (sham exposed controls), 0/40 (controls)	Bernfeld et al. (1974)
Inbred BIO 87.20	M	102	Whole-body	Mixture of German ref. cigarette smoke/air (1/15)	NG	Smoke of 30 cigarettes for 7–10 min: 1, 2, 2 or 3 times/day, 5 days/wk, lifetime	NG	2/87 (laryngeal tumour), 0/44 (sham exposed controls), 0/48 (controls)	Dontenwill et al. (1977a)
Syrian golden	M	80	Whole-body		1.5 mg nicotine, 0.173 mg phenol and 12.7 mL CO/cigarette		NG	0, 4, 6 and 11% (laryngeal C), 0% (controls)	Dontenwill et al. (1977a)
	F	80						0, 1, 2 and 7% (laryngeal C), 0% (controls)	
Inbred BIO 15.16	M	NG	Whole-body	11 or 22% smoke from commercial British filter cigarettes	NG	2 × 12 min/day, 7 days/wk, up to 74–80 wks	NG	3/44 (laryngeal C; 11% smoke) 27/57 (laryngeal C; 22% smoke) 0/36 (sham exposed controls) 0/50 (controls)	Bernfeld et al. (1979)

CO, carbon monoxide; AdC, adenocarcinoma; NG, not given; A, adenoma; NS, not significant; mo, month; wk, week; C, carcinoma; LCS, low cigarette smoke; HCS, high cigarette smoke
[a] Most of these lung tumours are adenomas.

Nagano *et al.*, 1982; Proctor & Chang, 1983; Reznik, 1983). Therefore, these exposure systems are not fully representative of the exposure pattern of smokers.

Under experimental conditions, the smoke in the chamber can be assayed for total particulate matter and carbon monoxide, and animals can be examined at intervals to determine the levels of carboxyhaemoglobin, nicotine or cotinine in their blood, and the deposition and retention of particulate matter in tissues, which gives some indication of the doses administered. In typical experiments, rodents were exposed to the smoke of seven to 10 cigarettes per day on 5–7 days per week (Dalbey *et al.*, 1980; Wehner *et al.*, 1981) and were found to have carboxyhaemoglobin levels of 20–40% (Bernfeld *et al.*, 1974).

3.1.1   *Mouse*

A number of early investigations of the effects of mainstream tobacco smoke on tumour development in mice were conducted using the C57BL strain. This strain is relatively resistant to the development of both spontaneous and chemically induced lung tumours (Shimkin & Stoner, 1975). [Therefore, the lack of tumour response in the first few investigations described below may have been due to the choice of this strain.]

Groups of 100 male and 100 female young adult C57BL mice were exposed (nose only) for 12 min/day to a mixture of fresh cigarette smoke and air (1/39, v/v) every other day for life. [The cigarettes were made from a composite blend of flue-cured tobaccos typical of the major brands of untipped cigarette smoked in the United Kingdom (Harris *et al.*, 1974).] The concentration of nicotine in the mixture was about 0.1 mg/mL and that of carbon monoxide, 0.064% (v/v). The nicotine content in the lungs of mice that died during exposure was 14–17 µg. Groups of 100 males and 100 females served as controls. No lung tumours, either adenomas or carcinomas, were found in control mice, but lung tumours (alveologenic adenocarcinomas) were found in 4/100 male and in 4/100 female mice exposed to tobacco smoke [$p = 0.06$]. Some of the adenocarcinomas were transplantable. Mice exposed to smoke often showed emphysema and marked peribronchial and perivascular infiltration with lymphocytes, independent of the presence of tumours (Harris & Negroni, 1967).

A total of 126 C57BL and 126 BLH mice [sex and initial group sizes unspecified] were exposed to the gas phase of 12 cigarettes [type unspecified] puffed for 2 s/min. The gas phase was generated by passing the smoke through a Cambridge filter that retained the particulate matter. The mice were exposed in a 200-L chamber for 90 min daily (approximately the maximal tolerated dose) until death (approximately 27 months). The survival rates for animals that received more than 12 months of treatment were not affected by treatment in either strain of mice [numbers not provided]. The percentages of mice with lung adenomas were 5.5% and 32% (7/126 and 40/126) in exposed C57BL and BLH mice and 3.4% and 22% (3/90 and 19/60) in C57BL and BLH controls, respectively. The percentages of BLH mice with lung adenomas that survived for at least 10 months were 37% of the treated group and 31% of the controls. The difference in incidence of adenoma between the control and treated groups was stated not to be statistically significant (Otto & Elmenhorst, 1967). [The Working Group noted the incomplete reporting of the experiment.]

A group of 50 male C57BL6/Mil mice, 6 weeks of age, was exposed to cigarette smoke from 85-mm unfiltered cigarettes [type unspecified] in a vacuum chamber for 15 min, five times per week, for 63 weeks. The nicotine content in the lungs of mice that were killed ranged from 14 to 27 μg. When the nasal cavity and respiratory tree were examined microscopically, the incidences of hyperplasia and metaplasia were found to be increased in exposed mice. These conditions were considered to be secondary to inflammation. No tumour was found (Wynder et al., 1968). [The Working Group noted the relatively short duration of the study.]

Groups of Snell's mice, 3–4 months of age at the start of treatment, were exposed to two puffs (15-mL puff volume, 2-s duration, 58-s interval between puffs) of either whole fresh cigarette smoke [type unspecified] (160 males and 118 females) or to the gas phase (100 males and 89 females); 117 males and 83 females served as controls. Animals were exposed in individual containers once a day (except during holidays and weekends) for life. When body weight loss was 4 g or more, animals were withdrawn from exposure treatment for periods varying from 2 days to 2 months. Two popular brands of unfiltered cigarettes were used; each cigarette was smoked to a butt length of 23 mm. The gas phase was produced by passing the smoke through a Cambridge filter. The efficiency of exposure was assessed by determining the carbon monoxide concentration in blood and the nicotine content of the lungs (about 5 μg). Survival after 12 months of age was distinctly reduced by treatment, being about 92% (184/200), 60% (172/278) and 40% (88/189) in the control, whole smoke-treated and gas phase-treated groups, respectively. After 12 months of age, the occurrence of pulmonary tumours was earlier in exposed mice than in controls. At the end of the experimental period (26 months), the numbers of mice that survived 12 months or more that had pulmonary adenomas were 8/106 and 1/78 male and female controls, 7/107 and 2/65, respectively ($p = 0.475$), male and female animals exposed to whole smoke and 1/44 and 3/44, respectively ($p = 0.15$), male and female animals exposed to the gas phase. The proportions of mice with pulmonary adenocarcinomas were 5/106 male and 3/78 female controls, 11/107 ($p = 0.15$) male and 5/65 ($p = 0.35$) female animals exposed to whole smoke and 10/44 ($p = 0.005$) male and 5/44 ($p = 0.15$) female animals exposed to the gas phase (Leuchtenberger & Leuchtenberger, 1970).

Groups of 100 male and 100 female C57BL mice, aged 14–18 weeks, were exposed (nose only) to a mixture of fresh cigarette smoke and air (1/39, v/v) for a 12-min period, generally on alternate days, for life. Groups were exposed to the whole smoke of two different types of cigarette, one made from flue-cured and the other from air-cured tobacco. The latter more closely resembled flue-cured cigarettes than typical air-cured cigarettes which contain, for example, burley tobacco. A further group of animals was exposed to the gas phase only of smoke from the flue-cured cigarette; this was generated by passing the whole smoke through a Cambridge filter to remove the particulate matter. A group of 200 males and 200 females served as controls. The experiments with whole smoke were repeated under similar conditions with another group of 100 male and 100 female mice. Mean survival time in eight of 10 groups of mice exposed to whole smoke was 4–14 weeks longer than that in controls. The incidences of lung tumours in controls were 3/160 males and 1/159 females; those in mice exposed to the whole smoke of cigarettes made from flue-cured tobacco were 9/162 males and 7/164 females [p = 0.07 and 0.04], respectively; the incidences in mice exposed to the gas phase of cigarettes made from flue-cured tobacco were 3/81 males [p > 0.05] and 2/88 females [p > 0.05]; and those in mice exposed to the whole smoke of cigarettes made from air-cured tobacco were 7/189 males [p > 0.05] and 0/173 females. The majority of the lung tumours were adenomas (Harris et al., 1974).

A group of 117 female BALB/c mice, 9 weeks of age, was exposed to smoke from 'high-tar'(16 mg tar, 1.1 mg nicotine) cigarettes diluted with air (7:1, air:smoke) for 7–8 min per day on 5 days per week for 95 weeks; the exposure was discontinued for 3 weeks starting between the 48th and 49th week of treatment. An untreated group of 130 females served as controls. Groups of approximately 16 control and 16 exposed mice were killed after 56, 64, 72 and 80 weeks of treatment. Twenty control and 10 exposed mice survived until termination of the experiment after 95 weeks. The incidence of bronchial adenomas was calculated by the authors to be 3.8 times higher in the exposed groups of mice than in the control groups after 83 weeks, but to be similar in the two groups after 95 weeks of exposure. The authors also reported an increase in the incidence of lymphomas after both 83 weeks (2.6 times) and 95 weeks (3.2 times) of exposure (Keast et al., 1981). [The Working Group noted that insufficient numerical data were provided in relation to the number of animals at risk.]

Two thousand and fifty-three (C57BL/Cum × C3H/AnfCum)F$_1$ mice were exposed (nose only) to cigarette smoke from University of Kentucky reference 2R1 cigarettes on 5 days/week for 110 weeks and observed until death. In addition, 1014 mice were sham-exposed and 449 mice were held as cage controls. The deposition of smoke particulates was estimated to be about 125–200 µg total particulate matter/lung/day. The only lung cancers observed were diagnosed as alveolar adenocarcinomas. These adenocarcinomas were observed in 19/978 smoke-exposed mice and 7/651 sham-exposed mice. The difference between the incidence in smoke- and sham-exposed groups was not significant, but the data suggested that the tumours occurred with a shorter latency in the smoke-exposed group (p = 0.10). Other changes associated with exposure to smoke were increased incidence of pigmented alveolar macrophages, otitis media and head and neck fibrosarcomas (Henry & Kouri, 1986). [The Working Group noted that both parent strains are relatively resistant to the development of spontaneous and chemically induced lung tumours.]

3.1.2   Rat

A group of 408 female Wistar rats, 10 weeks of age, was exposed (nose only) to a mixture of smoke and air in a ratio of 1:5 generated from T29 cigarettes (especially manufactured from a composite blend of flue-cured tobaccos, representing the major untipped cigarette brands smoked in the United Kingdom during 1967–68), for 15 s/min during

11 min, twice a day on 5 days per week for life. After 1 year, the rats received 5% carbon dioxide in air instead of air for 5 min before the start of each smoke exposure session and also for the 45-s/min interval during which smoke was not generated. Measurement of an arsenious sulfate tracer showed that 8.5% and 17.5% of the delivered tar was recovered in the lungs of rats subjected to the air and the air/carbon dioxide regimens, respectively. Two control groups of 102 animals were kept, one sham-exposed and one untreated. The smoke-exposed and sham-exposed animals had lower body weights than the untreated controls. About 25% of the treated rats were still alive at 100 weeks compared with 73% of 102 untreated controls and 66% of 102 sham-exposed controls. All treated animals had died by 140 weeks; the control animals had all died by 160 weeks. Three of the smoke-exposed rats had pulmonary squamous neoplasms of uncertain malignancy, and one had an invasive squamous-cell carcinoma of the lung. No lung tumour was observed in the sham-treated or untreated controls. The incidence of benign mammary tumours was lower in the smoke-exposed rats than in the sham-exposed or untreated controls (Davis *et al.*, 1975a). [The Working Group noted that the daily exposure period was very brief.]

A group of 18 female Wistar rats, 13–14 weeks of age, was exposed (nose only) to the gas phase of smoke (produced by passing the smoke through a Cambridge filter) from a standard British reference cigarette diluted 1:5 with air. Exposure took place for 15 s followed by exposure to air for 45 s during 11 min, twice daily on 5 days per week for life. A control group of 16 animals was kept. Average period of survival was 100 weeks for treated animals and 114 weeks for controls. No lung tumour was reported in either the exposed or the control rats (Davis *et al.*, 1975b). [The Working Group noted the small number of animals used and the short duration of the period of exposure each day.]

A group of 80 female Fischer 344 rats, 12–14 weeks of age, was exposed (nose only) to a mixture of smoke and air in a ratio of 1:10 for 28–30 s/min followed by air for 30 s during standard smoking of a US reference untipped cigarette (average, 8.4 periods of exposure/cigarette). The mean smoke particulate and nicotine levels recorded during chamber monitoring were 18.4 mg and 0.89 mg per cigarette, respectively. The animals were exposed to 1 cigarette/h, 7 cigarettes per day, on 5 days per week for 128 weeks, followed by observation for a further 6 months. The mean pulmonary particulate deposition during exposure was 0.25 mg/cigarette (total, 1.75 mg/rat per day). A group of 63 rats served as untreated controls and 30 rats were sham-exposed. The length of survival of smoke-treated, sham-treated and untreated controls was not significantly different, but smoke- and sham-treated animals had lower mean body weights. Because the tumour incidences in untreated and sham-treated controls were similar, the two groups were combined (93 animals). One alveologenic carcinoma was observed in one control rat and one pulmonary adenomatoid lesion in two other control rats. Ten respiratory tract tumours were observed in seven smoke-exposed rats: one nasal adenocarcinoma, one nasal squamous-cell carcinoma, five pulmonary adenomas, two alveologenic carcinomas and one squamous-cell carcinoma ($p < 0.05$). Of the smoke-exposed animals, 21 developed subcutaneous sarcomas at sites of ulceration on the forelimbs ($p < 0.05$), four rats developed benign tumours of the oral tissues ($p < 0.1$) and four developed adrenal gland tumours (one adenoma and three carcinomas) ($p < 0.1$). No such tumours occurred in controls. The incidences of tumours of the pituitary gland, uterus and ovary, haemato-lymphatic system and mammary gland were lower in smoke-exposed rats than in controls (Dalbey et al., 1980).

Three groups of 80 female Fischer 344 rats were exposed to a mixture of smoke and air in a ratio of 1:10. The smoke was generated from three research cigarettes [source not specified] containing 25.4 mg tar, 0.16 mg nicotine; 13.3 mg tar, 1.06 mg nicotine; or 25.7 mg tar, 1.91 mg nicotine, respectively (see also Griest et al., 1980). Each rat was exposed to smoke for 28 s/min followed by air for 30 s during standard smoking of the cigarettes, to provide 10–11 exposures/cigarette. The animals were exposed to eight ciga-rettes per day during a 16-h period, on 7 days per week for 96 weeks, at which time all survivors (50–70% of animals) were killed. Groups of 80 animals served as untreated and sham-treated controls. The occurrence of squamous metaplasia of the laryngeal and tracheal epithelium was significantly increased in smoke-exposed rats. One squamous-cell carcinoma of the lung was observed in a rat exposed to 'low-tar medium-nicotine' smoke; the incidences of other tumours were similar in treated and in control animals (Wehner et al., 1981). [The Working Group noted that, in contrast to the study described previously, all surviving animals were killed at 104 weeks of age and that the method for sampling for histopathology was not fully reported.]

In an experiment in which combined exposure of CDF®(Fischer 344)/CrlBR rats to mainstream tobacco smoke and ^{239}PuO$_2$ was studied, two groups of rats (6 weeks of age) were subjected to whole-body exposure for 6 h/day, 5 days per week, for 126 weeks to mainstream cigarette smoke diluted to concentrations of either 100 or 250 mg total parti-culate matter/m^3 (LCS and HCS groups). A significant increase in the occurrence of lung tumours was found in females exposed to smoke only but not in males. The incidences of benign and/or malignant lung tumours in female rats were 0/113, 4/145 (3%) and 6/83 (7%; $p < 0.05$; one-sided Yates test) in the groups treated with filtered air alone, and the LCS and HCS groups, respectively. The corresponding tumour incidences for males were 3/119 (2.5%), 3/173 (2%) and 7/78 (8%), respectively (Finch et al., 1995).

3.1.3   Syrian hamster

In a study involving 4440 hamsters, three groups of 80 male and 80 female Syrian golden hamsters, 8 weeks of age, were exposed to a mixture of smoke and air in a ratio of 1:15. The smoke was generated during a 7–10-min period from 30 German reference cigarettes, once, twice or three times a day on 5 days per week until death. Two groups of 80 males and 80 females were exposed either to the smoke of black (dark air-cured)-tobacco cigarettes twice a day, or to the vapour phase of German reference cigarettes, generated from 30 cigarettes during a 10-min period twice a day. Eight hundred animals served as untreated controls. The average length of survival was 52–65 weeks for treated males and 41–49 weeks for treated females. When compared with untreated controls, a shorter survival time and loss of body weight were noted in animals exposed to smoke. In all treated groups, 'the most remarkable and severe alterations' were observed in the larynx, and their severity depended on duration of treatment and dosage. The incidence of laryngeal leukoplakias ranged from an average of 11.3% in animals exposed to the reference cigarette for 10 min to 30.6% in those exposed for 30 min; the incidence in animals exposed to smoke from black-tobacco cigarettes was 10%, and slight leukoplakia was observed in 1–5% of control animals. The incidences of laryngeal carcinomas were 0.6–10.6% in animals exposed to smoke from the reference cigarette and 1.25% in animals exposed to smoke from black-tobacco cigarettes. No such tumour was observed in control animals or in those exposed to the vapour phase (Dontenwill et al., 1973).

Similar results were obtained in a study involving 2160 hamsters exposed to the smoke from German reference cigarettes or a modification thereof (Dontenwill et al., 1977a).

A modification of the method of Dontenwill (above) was used in a study of inbred Syrian golden hamsters. Groups of 102 male BIO® 87.20 and BIO® 15.16 hamsters (13 weeks of age) were exposed to smoke (1:5 in air) from University of Kentucky 1R1 reference cigarettes twice a day on 5 days per week for up to 100 weeks. Groups of 60 animals served as sham-exposed or cage controls for each strain. Exposure to smoke for up to 100 weeks had no effect on length of survival; however, a reduction in body weight was noted. Over 90% of the smoke-exposed animals of both strains showed hyperplastic or neoplastic changes in the larynx; and benign squamous-cell papillomas of the larynx were observed in both strains. Laryngeal cancer occurred nearly five times more frequently in strain BIO® 15.16, however, and two animals of this strain developed nasopharyngeal tumours. The incidences of tumours at locations other than the respiratory tract were similar in the two strains (Bernfeld et al., 1974).

Groups of 35–64 male BIO® 15.16 inbred Syrian golden hamsters, 60–70 days of age, were exposed to concentrations of 11% or 22% smoke from commercial British filter-tipped cigarettes or filter-tipped cigarettes composed of tobacco and Cytrel® (a tobacco substitute), or cigarettes made of 100% Cytrel® twice a day (12-min sessions of 27 smoke exposures/min) on 7 days per week for up to 74–80 weeks. Groups of 40 sham-exposed animals and 51 caged animals served as controls. Survival rates were markedly reduced in all groups after 59 weeks of age; a reduction in body weight was noted in treated animals when compared with controls. Laryngeal carcinomas occurred in 47.4% (27/57) of the animals exposed to smoke from the British filter-tipped cigarettes; the first tumours occurred after 59 weeks in the hamsters treated with the 22% smoke concentration. The incidence of this type of tumour was dose-related and decreased as the proportion of Cytrel® in the blends increased. No such tumour was observed in controls. Laryngeal papillomas, laryngeal epithelial hyperplasia and a few tracheal papillomas were also observed in treated animals. Histopathological findings at other sites did not appear to be related to smoke inhalation (Bernfeld et al., 1979).

A group of 51 male Syrian golden hamsters, 2 months of age, was exposed three times a day for 10 min, 5 days per week, for life, to smoke from University of Kentucky 1R1 reference cigarettes. Another group of 51 male hamsters served as sham-exposed controls. The smoke-exposed animals survived longer (mean, 19.6 months) than the sham-exposed animals (mean, 15.3 months). The smoke-exposed animals had significantly higher incidences of epithelial lesions of the larynx than the sham-exposed controls (22% versus 0%, $p < 0.01$) and also had a significantly higher total number of tumours than sham-exposed controls (28% versus 6%; $p < 0.05$). The laryngeal changes in the smoke-exposed group ranged from inflammatory conditions, with growth abnormalities of the epithelium, to squamous-cell papilloma formation (Wehner et al., 1974, 1975a,b, 1976).

3.1.4   Rabbit

Thirty rabbits were exposed daily in individual compartments to the smoke from 20 cigarettes (2 puffs/min, 2 cigarettes at each treatment period) for up to 66 months. No tumour that could be related to the exposure was observed in any of the exposed rabbits or in 31 controls that survived for 24 months or more (Holland et al., 1958, 1963). [The Working Group noted that details of the types of cigarettes, method of smoke generation and doses delivered were not provided.]

3.1.5   Dog

Groups of male beagle dogs, 1.7–3.3 years old, trained to inhale cigarette smoke through tracheostomata, were exposed to one of three different treatments: (1) smoke from seven untipped cigarettes containing 34.8 mg tar and 1.85 mg nicotine per day (62 dogs), (2) smoke from seven cigarettes containing the same tobacco, but with filter tips, containing 17.8 mg tar and 1.17 mg nicotine (12 dogs) or (3) smoke from 3.5 untipped cigarettes containing the same tobacco per day (12 dogs). Eight non-exposed tracheotomized dogs served as controls. The body weights of the dogs in the various groups did not differ significantly. Between day 57, when the training period ended, and day 876, when killing of the surviving dogs began, 28 dogs died: 24 in the first group, two in the second, two in the third and none in the control group. Extensive examination of the lungs and bronchial tree at autopsy and microscopically was carried out. Lesions of the lung (reported as tumours), described as 'bronchiolo-alveolar, invasive and noninvasive', were found in 23/62 of dogs in group 1; two of the lesion-bearing dogs in this group also had small bronchial lesions. Non-invasive bronchiolo-alveolar lesions were also found in 4/12 dogs in group 2, 7/12 dogs in group 3 and 2/8 control dogs. The bronchiolo-alveolar lesions tended to be multiple, with as many as 20 per lung lobe, and were found in 41 of the 203 lung lobes from the 29 dogs with such lesions. No distant metastasis was found (Auerbach et al., 1970; Hammond et al., 1970). [The Working Group noted that no data were given on specific smoking parameters or measures of exposure. They also noted the small number of control dogs used and the unusually high incidence of lung lesions in these animals; these are lesions that rarely occur spontaneously in dogs. The focal inflammatory lesions usually found in the lungs of animals exposed to smoke were not mentioned in the report of this study. Examination of the upper respiratory tract and other organ systems was not reported. The authors' interpretation of the photomicrographs as representing neoplasia was not considered to be entirely convincing.]

As part of a study on the combined effects of radon daughters or uranium ore dust and cigarette smoke on the induction of respiratory tumours (see below), 19 male and female beagle dogs, 24–30 months of age, were exposed to cigarette smoke only. The dogs were exposed to the smoke of 10 University of Kentucky 1R1 reference cigarettes per day (three in the morning, four at midday and three in the afternoon) on 7 days per week for 48–60 months; individual masks permitted smoke to be inhaled at every 10th breath. Eight dogs served as sham-exposed controls. Carboxyhaemoglobin levels in smoke-exposed dogs increased with the duration of the experiment, from 2% at 19 months to 4.7% after 50 months; the corresponding mean values for sham-exposed dogs were 1.4% and 1.8%, respectively. Smoke-exposed animals killed after 49 (six dogs), 60 (six dogs), 64 (six dogs) and 65 months (three dogs) were available for analysis. No significant respiratory lesion and no lung tumour was found in either group (Cross *et al.*, 1982). [The Working Group noted the small sizes of the groups and the limited evidence of smoke delivery.]

3.2   Inhalation exposure in conjunction with administration of known carcinogens and other agents

3.2.1   *Mouse*

(a)   4-(N-Nitrosomethylamino)-1-(3-pyridyl)-1-butanone

A 6-month bioassay in strain A/J mice was conducted to determine whether chronically inhaled mainstream cigarette smoke would either induce lung tumours or promote lung cancer induced by the tobacco-specific nitrosamine, 4-(*N*-nitrosomethylamino)-1-(3-pyridyl)-1-butanone (NNK). Groups of 20 female A/J mice were exposed to filtered air or cigarette smoke, injected with NNK, or exposed to both cigarette smoke and NNK. At 7 weeks of age, mice were given a single intraperitoneal injection of NNK at a dose of 100 mg/kg bw and, 3 days later, they were exposed to cigarette smoke for 6 h/day, 5 days per week, for 26 weeks at a mean concentration of 248 mg total particulate matter/m³. Animals were killed 5 weeks after cessation of exposure for gross and histopathological evaluation of lung lesions. No significant differences in survival between exposure groups were observed. A biologically significant level of exposure to cigarette smoke was achieved as indicated by the reductions in body weight, increases in lung weight and increases in carboxyhaemoglobin levels in blood of about 17%. Tumour incidences were similar between the groups exposed to cigarette smoke and filtered air, and the groups treated with NNK and with cigarette smoke + NNK. Incidences in either of the latter groups were higher than in the groups exposed to cigarette smoke and filtered air. Tumour multiplicity in tumour-bearing animals did not differ significantly between any of the three groups (filtered air, NNK, cigarette smoke + NNK) in which tumours were observed. Thus, exposure to cigarette smoke neither induced lung tumours nor promoted NNK-induced tumours (Finch *et al.*, 1996). [The Working Group noted that the animals were killed 5 weeks after cessation of exposure, which may have been an insufficiently long period to permit tumour development. See also Witschi *et al.* (1997).]

(b) Influenza virus

The possible interaction between various types of influenza virus and the inhalation of cigarette smoke in the induction of lung tumours in mice has been examined in a series of studies (Harris & Negroni, 1967; Harris *et al.*, 1974; Wynder *et al.*, 1968). No additive or synergistic effect was observed.

3.2.2 Rat

Selected studies are summarized in Table 3.2.

(a) Benzo[a]pyrene

A group of 84 female Wistar rats received a single intratracheal instillation of 2 mg benzo[*a*]pyrene (with infusine and carbon black) followed by exposure to cigarette smoke (cigarette T29, specially manufactured from a composite blend of tobacco representing the major plain cigarette brand smoked in the United Kingdom, diluted 1:5 with air), twice daily, five times per week for life. Three developed squamous-cell carcinomas of the lung. A squamous-cell carcinoma of the lung was observed in one of the 84 rats treated with the benzo[*a*]pyrene mixture alone, and four squamous-cell neoplasms (of which only one was clearly malignant) occurred among 408 rats exposed to cigarette smoke only. The mean survival times were 65 weeks for animals exposed to the smoke plus benzo[*a*]pyrene mixture, 63 weeks for animals exposed to smoke alone and 108 weeks for rats treated with the benzo[*a*]pyrene mixture alone. No lung tumour was observed in untreated or sham-exposed controls (Davis *et al.*, 1975a).

Groups of 35 male Wistar rats (weighing 50–70 g) were fed either vitamin A-deficient feed or a conventional diet and were exposed to three weekly intratracheal initiation doses of 20 mg benzo[*a*]pyrene mixed with ferric oxide during the 6th–8th week of the study, or subjected to cigarette smoke from the 2nd to 24th week or the 10th–24th week, or subjected to both types of treatment. The animals were exposed to five cigarettes, 1 h/day in 8.2-L chambers. Animals were killed after the 24th week. Inhalation of cigarette smoke during the initiation and post-initiation phases of carcinogenesis resulted in higher lung tumour multiplicity (2.14 tumours/animal) than that observed in rats exposed during the post-initiation phase only (1.33 tumours/animal) or in the rats treated with benzo[*a*]pyrene only (1.22 tumours/animal). This enhancement of tumour multiplicity was increased further by vitamin A deficiency (2.86 versus 1.67 or 1.83 tumours/animal, respectively). These tumours were classified histopathologically as squamous-cell carcinomas (Gupta *et al.*, 1990).

Table 3.2. Selected studies of carcinogenicity in response to exposure to mainstream tobacco smoke in conjunction with exposure to known carcinogens or other agents in rat and hamster

Strain	Sex	No. of treated animals/group	Agent co-administered	Type of exposure to cigarette smoke	Exposure duration	Tumour incidence	Reference
Rat							
Wistar	F	84–408	Benzo[a]pyrene (2 mg) + infusine + carbon black; intratracheally	British reference cigarette smoke/air (1/5)	1 cigarette, twice/day, 5 days/wk, lifetime	3/84 (lung C), 1/84 (lung C; benzo[a]pyrene alone), 4/408 (3 A + 1 malignant neoplasm; cigarette smoke only), 0/204 (controls + sham-exposed controls)	Davis et al. (1975a)
Wistar	M	35	Benzo[a]pyrene (20 mg) + Fe_2O_3; intratracheally (3 weekly doses) during 6th–8th wk of the study	Cigarette smoke (5 cigarettes/8.2 L air)	1 h/day, during 2nd–24th week or 10th–24th week of the study	Conventional diet: 2nd–24th wk, 2.14 lung C/animal; 10th–24th wk, 1.33 lung C/animal; benzo[a]pyrene control, 1.22 lung C/animal. Vitamin A-deficient diet: 2nd–24th wk, 2.86 lung C/animal; 10th–24th week, 1.67 lung C/animal; benzo[a]pyrene control, 1.83 lung C/animal	Gupta et al. (1990)
Sprague-Dawley	NG	28–50	Radon progeny (4000, 500 or 100 WLM)	French reference cigarette smoke (9 cigarettes/500 L air)	10–15 min session, 4 days/wk, 1 year	4000 WLM: 34/50 (lung C) [$p = 0.0015$]; 17/50 (lung C; radon progeny alone); 500 WLM: 8/30 (lung C); 2/28 (lung C; radon progeny alone); 100 WLM: 1/30 (lung C); 0/50 (radon progeny alone)	Chameaud et al. (1982)
CDF® (Fischer 344)/ CrlBR	M, F	NG	$^{239}PuO_2$ aerosol, 1 wk (6th wk of the study)	Cigarette smoke/air, 100 mg (LCS) or 250 mg (HCS) total particulate matter/m^3	6 h/day, 5 days/wk, 126 wks	49–61% (lung tumours, LCS + $^{239}PuO_2$) 72–74% (HCS + $^{239}PuO_2$) 20–33% ($^{239}PuO_2$) 2–3% (LCS) 7–8% (HCS)	Finch et al. (1995)

Table 3.2 (contd)

Strain	Sex	No. of treated animals/ group	Agent co-administered	Type of exposure to cigarette smoke	Exposure duration	Tumour incidence	Reference
Hamster							
Syrian golden/ M + F	M + F	(80 + 80)	DMBA (0.5 mg); intra-tracheally	German ref. cigarette smoke/air (1/15)	Smoke of 30 cigarettes for 7–10 min: twice/day, 5 days/wk, lifetime	32/160 (laryngeal C), 17/160 (laryngeal C; smoke only), 0/160 (DMBA alone)	Dontenwill et al. (1973)
Syrian golden	NG	20–40	DMBA (0.24 mg); intra-laryngeally	Cigarette smoke/air (1/7)	Cigarette smoke 2 × 10 min/day, 5 days/wk, 48 wks	3/40 (laryngeal C), 0/20 (smoke only), 0/20 (DMBA alone)	Hoffmann et al. (1979)
Syrian golden	M	10–30	NDEA (100 mg/kg bw); subcutaneously	Cigarette smoke/air (1/7)	Smoke of 30 cigarettes for 9 min: twice/day, 5 days/wk, 12 wks	Non-filter cigarettes (2.10 ± 1.74 P+H/animal) [$p < 0.01$] and filter cigarettes (1.93 ± 1.55 P + H/animal) [$p < 0.01$] versus sham-exposed (0.97 ± 1.03 P + H/animal)	Takahashi et al. (1992)
Syrian golden	M	30	NDEA (10 mg/hamster); subcutaneously (12 weekly doses)	Non-filter cigarette smoke/air (1/7)	Smoke of 30 cigarettes for 6 min: twice/day, 5 days/wk, 58 wks	14/30 (nasal cavity tumours) ($p < 0.05$), 5/30 (NDEA alone)	Harada et al. (1985)

C, carcinoma; A, adenoma; NG, not given; WLM, work-level-months; LCS, low cigarette smoke; HCS, high cigarette smoke; DMBA, 7,12-dimethylbenz[a]anthracene; NDEA, N-nitrosodiethylamine; P + H, epithelial hyperplasias and papillomas

(b)   Chrysotile

Yoshimura and Takemoto (1991) exposed male Wistar rats intratracheally to 15 mg asbestos (chrysotile) fibres. One month later, the rats were exposed to cigarette smoke in an exposure chamber (smoke from 10 cigarettes/day, 6 days per week, for 1 month). In the group exposed both to asbestos and to cigarette smoke, 4/29 rats developed lung carcinomas, as compared with 1/31 of the rats exposed to asbestos alone. No mesotheliomas were found in the rats treated with asbestos alone, whereas 2/29 rats exposed to a combination of asbestos and cigarette smoke developed mesotheliomas. [The Working Group noted the small numbers of animals per group.]

(c)   Radon progeny

Groups of 28–50 Sprague-Dawley rats were exposed to radon progeny at cumulative doses of 4000, 500 or 100 work-level-months (WLM)[1], with or without concurrent exposure to cigarette smoke by inhalation on 4 days per week for 1 year. Of the 50 rats exposed to 4000 WLM radon progeny without exposure to smoke, 17 developed carcinomas of the lung. In the same group, 34 carcinomas were seen in 50 rats exposed to radon and cigarette smoke. In the groups of rats exposed to 500 WLM radon progeny, two carcinomas of the lung were seen in the 28 rats exposed to radon only as compared with 8/30 rats exposed to radon and cigarette smoke. No lung tumour was observed in any of the 50 rats exposed to 100 WLM radon only, whereas one carcinoma was observed among 30 rats exposed to 100 WLM radon and cigarette smoke. Histopathological evaluation of the lung tumours indicated that approximately 75% were squamous-cell carcinomas, 20% were adenocarcinomas and the remainder were undifferentiated carcinomas (Chameaud et al., 1982).

(d)   Plutonium oxide

Beginning at 6 weeks of age, CDF®(Fischer 344)/CrlBR rats were subjected to whole-body exposure for 6 h/day, on 5 days per week, to either filtered air or mainstream cigarette smoke diluted to concentrations of either 100 or 250 mg total particulate matter/m^3 (LCS and HCS groups, respectively). At 12 weeks of age, rats were removed from the smoke exposure chambers and exposed nose-only to either filtered air or plutonium oxide (^{239}PuO$_2$) aerosol, and were returned to the smoke chambers 1 week later for 30 months of continued exposure to either filtered air or cigarette smoke. The incidences of lung tumours in animals exposed to cigarette smoke only are given in Section 3.1.2. In both sexes, there was a pronounced interaction between exposure to smoke and ^{239}PuO$_2$ in producing lung tumours. Tumour incidence reached 72–74% in HCS + ^{239}PuO$_2$-exposed rats and 49–61% in LCS + ^{239}PuO$_2$-exposed rats, whereas the incidence was 20–33%,

---

[1] WLM is defined as any combination of the short-lived radon daughters in 1 L of air that will result in an ultimate emission of 1.3×10^5 MeV of potential alpha energy in their decay through ^{214}Po. WLM is equivalent to 170 h of exposure to 1 WL.

2–3% and 7–8%, respectively, in rats exposed to $^{239}PuO_2$, LCS or HCS alone. The most prevalent malignant neoplasms were adenocarcinomas, followed by squamous-cell carcinomas and adenosquamous carcinomas. In groups exposed to both agents, there was increased tumour multiplicity, an increased proportion of neoplasms of the squamous phenotype, and several animals with airway-associated lung neoplasms (Finch *et al.*, 1995). [The Working Group noted the incomplete reporting of the study.]

3.2.3   *Syrian hamster*

Selected studies are summarized in Table 3.2.

(*a*)   *Benzo[a]pyrene*

A group of 40 Syrian golden hamsters received a single intratracheal administration of 5 mg benzo[*a*]pyrene mixed with ferric oxide, followed by exposure to cigarette smoke twice for 10 min daily, five times per week, for 48 weeks. Two papillomas of the larynx and three epithelial hyperplasias of the larynx were observed. No such lesion was observed in control groups of 20 hamsters that received benzo[*a*]pyrene plus ferric oxide or smoke alone, and no lung tumour was observed (Hoffmann *et al.*, 1979).

(*b*)   *Blue Cape asbestos*

Groups of 80 male and 80 female Syrian golden hamsters were exposed to a single intratracheal instillation of asbestos, followed by exposure to cigarette smoke twice daily, five times per week for life. No significant difference in the occurrence of laryngeal lesions or tumours was observed when compared with another group of hamsters exposed to cigarette smoke alone. No laryngeal tumour occurred in a control group exposed to a single dose of asbestos alone (Dontenwill *et al.*, 1973).

(*c*)   *7,12-Dimethylbenz[a]anthracene*

Three groups of 80 male and 80 female Syrian golden hamsters received 500 µg 7,12-dimethylbenz[*a*]anthracene (DMBA) intratracheally, followed by a 10-min exposure to cigarette smoke twice daily, five times per week for life, or were treated either with cigarette smoke or DMBA only. A total of 32 squamous-cell carcinomas of the larynx were observed in animals treated with both DMBA and cigarette smoke, in comparison with 17 in hamsters exposed to cigarette smoke only and none in hamsters treated with DMBA alone. A similar trend in the incidence of laryngeal leukoplakia was also observed. No increase was observed in the incidences of tumours at other sites in animals treated with both DMBA and cigarette smoke, when compared with animals treated with DMBA alone. Mean survival rates were comparable in all groups (Dontenwill *et al.*, 1973). Similar results were reported from other experiments in which Syrian golden hamsters were exposed to DMBA and cigarette smoke (Kobayashi *et al.*, 1974; Hoffmann *et al.*, 1979).

(d)   4-(N-Nitrosomethylamino)-1-(3-pyridyl)-1-butanone

Groups of 10 male and 9–10 female Syrian golden hamsters received a single subcutaneous injection of NNK at doses ranging from 1 to 10 mg, followed by exposure to University of Kentucky 1R1 reference cigarette smoke twice daily for 69 weeks. Tumours of the respiratory tract were observed in NNK-treated hamsters; their incidence was not affected by exposure to cigarette smoke (Hecht et al., 1983).

(e)   N-Nitrosobis(2-oxopropyl)amine

The influence of tobacco smoke on N-nitrosobis(2-oxopropyl)amine (NBOPA)-induced carcinogenesis of the pancreatic duct and respiratory tract was investigated using a two-stage carcinogenesis model in hamsters. Five-week-old male hamsters were divided into five groups. Group 1 ($n = 30$) was injected subcutaneously with NBOPA at a dose of 10 mg/kg bw once a week for 3 weeks for tumour initiation and exposed to cigarette smoke over the same period. Group 2 ($n = 30$) was exposed to cigarette smoke for 26 weeks after the NBOPA initiation. Group 3 ($n = 30$) was given NBOPA initiation alone and group 4 ($n = 10$), 26 weeks of exposure to cigarette smoke alone. Group 5 ($n = 10$) served as a sham-exposed negative control. The experiment was terminated 30 weeks after the first NBOPA injection. The incidence of pancreatic carcinomas was significantly decreased in group 1 (5/29, $p < 0.01$) relative to group 3 (17/30), whereas the incidence in group 2 (12/29) was not significantly less than that in group 3. In contrast, the incidence of proliferative lesions of the larynx and trachea (hyperplasias) was significantly higher in group 2 (11/29, $p < 0.01$) than in group 3 (2/30). The incidence of pulmonary hyperplasias was also higher in group 2 (13/29, $p < 0.05$) than in group 3 (5/30), although that of pulmonary adenomas or adenocarcinomas was lower in group 2 (14/29, $p < 0.01$) than in group 3 (24/30). Exposure to cigarette smoke in the NBOPA-initiation phase (group 1) did not affect the development of respiratory lesions. No animals in groups 4 or 5 developed any tumours of the pancreas or respiratory tract. These results suggest that exposure to cigarette smoke inhibits pancreatic carcinogenesis when given in the initiation phase, whereas it modulates (enhances or suppresses) the development of proliferative lesions in the respiratory tract if applied during the promotion stage to hamsters pre-treated with NBOPA (Nishikawa et al., 1994). [The Working Group noted the small size of the experimental groups and the short duration of the study.]

(f)   N-Nitrosodiethylamine

The potential short-term promoting effects of cigarette smoke on the development of tumours in the respiratory system were investigated in male Syrian golden hamsters. A dietary supplement of vitamin C (1%) was given to groups of 30 male Syrian hamsters exposed to cigarette smoke in air (1/7) from 30 unfiltered cigarettes for 6 min, twice a day, 5 days a week and also receiving 12 weekly subcutaneous injections of N-nitrosodiethyl-amine (NDEA) (total dose, 10 mg/hamster) to determine whether or not high doses of vitamin C could prevent the development of tumours by NDEA in the respiratory tract.

The experiment was terminated 58 weeks after initiation of the treatments. Treatment with NDEA resulted in the development of both benign and malignant tumours of the respiratory tract, and co-exposure to cigarette smoke potentiated the development of tumours in the nasal cavity (14/30 versus 5/30, $p < 0.05$) (Harada et al., 1985).

Three groups (1, 2 and 3) of 30 animals each received a single subcutaneous injection of 100 mg/kg bw NDEA and were then exposed to smoke from untipped cigarettes (NC), from filter-tipped cigarettes (FC) and sham smoke, respectively, from week 1 to week 12. In addition, groups 4, 5 and 6 (10 animals each) did not receive treatment with NDEA, but were exposed to the NC smoke, FC smoke or sham smoke, respectively, for the same time period. In the NDEA-treated groups, epithelial hyperplasias and/or papillomas were induced; in groups 1 and 2, the incidences and numbers of these lesions per animal were significantly higher than in group 3 (2.10 ± 1.74 and 1.93 ± 1.55 versus 0.97 ± 1.03, $p < 0.01$) (Takahashi et al., 1992).

3.2.4   Dog

Nineteen male and female beagle dogs, 24–30 months old, were exposed by inhalation to a combination of radon (105 nCi/L [3900 Bq/L]), radon progeny (605 WLM) and uranium ore dust (12.9 mg/m^3) for 4 h/day, on 5 days per week, for 54 months. A second group of 19 beagle dogs was exposed to the smoke from 10 cigarettes/day on 7 days per week at intervals between exposures to radon progeny and uranium ore dust. Lifespan was shorter in both groups than in controls. Eight dogs exposed to radon alone had nine respiratory tumours (two nasal carcinomas, six pulmonary carcinomas, one pulmonary fibrosarcoma); and 2/19 dogs in the group that received radon plus cigarette smoke had respiratory tumours (one nasal carcinoma and one pulmonary carcinoma) (Cross et al., 1982). [The Working Group noted the small sizes of the groups and the incomplete reporting.]

3.3   Administration of tobacco-smoke condensate[1]

Selected studies are summarized in Table 3.3.

Attempts to induce tumours with tobacco products were reported as early as 1911 (for a summary of early studies, see Wynder & Hoffmann, 1967). In the 1950s, Wynder et al. (1953) painted the skin of CAF$_1$ mice with cigarette-smoke condensate (CSC) suspended in acetone. After 24 months, 48/81 mice had developed skin papillomas and 36/81 had developed skin epidermoid carcinomas at the sites of application.

---

[1] The terms 'smoke condensate' and 'tar' are often used interchangeably. Cigarette-smoke condensates are produced by passing smoke through cold traps and recovering the material retained within them. This material is often washed from the traps with a volatile solvent, which is later removed, and unknown amounts of the volatile and semivolatile constituents are lost. Total particulate matter (TPM) is that material which is retained in a high-efficiency particulate filter. If this material is washed from the filter and concentrated as above, semivolatiles are lost. In the USA, the term 'tar' as used in official reports of tar yield is equivalent to TPM less nicotine and water.

Table 3.3. Selected studies of carcinogenicity in response to exposure to cigarette-smoke condensate in mouse, rat and rabbit

Strain	Sex	No. of treated animals/group	Type of exposure	Exposure dosage and duration	Tumour incidence	Reference
Mouse						
CAF1	M + F, 1:1	44–112	Skin painting (dorsal) of CSC	CSC/acetone solution (40 mg CSC/application), × 3/wk, lifetime	36/81 (skin epidermoid C, 0/30 (acetone controls)	Wynder et al. (1953)
ICR Swiss	F	5200	Skin painting (dorsal) of CSC	CSC/acetone solution (150 mg or 300 mg CSC/week), × 6/wk, 78 wks	482/5200 (skin C), 3/800 (acetone controls)[a]	Gargus et al. (1976)
ICR Swiss	F	4900	Skin painting (dorsal) of CSC	CSC/acetone solution (25 mg or 50 mg CSC/application), × 6/wk, 78 wks	1157/4900 (skin C), 0/800 (acetone controls)	Gori (1976)
ICR/Ha Swiss	F	100	Topical application with CSC to oral mucosa (lips and oral area)	CSC/acetone (26 mg CSC/application), × 5/wk, 15 months	52/81 (lung tumours)[b] (p < 0.0001), 20/89[b] (acetone controls)	DiPaolo & Levin (1965)
Initiation study						
ICR/Ha Swiss	F	30	Skin painting (dorsal) with CSC active fraction with or without subsequent painting of the skin with croton oil	CSC active fraction/acetone (2.5 mg of 0.6% CSC/application), 10 × on alternate days; Croton oil (2.5%) × 3/wk, up to 15 months, 10 days after last CSC active fraction application	After 12 and 15 months: 4/30 (skin C), 0/65 (croton oil controls)	Hoffman & Wynder (1971)
Promotion study						
Swiss	F	30–50	Skin painting (dorsal) of CSC with or without initiation by DMBA application	DMBA (75 μg); CSC/acetone (75 mg CSC/application, start: 1 wk after DMBA application), × 2–3/wk, 12 months – animals observed 3 months later	DMBA: 2/30 (skin C) (7 %); 2 × CSC: 1/40 (skin C) (3 %); DMBA + 2 × CSC: 8/30 (skin C) (27 %); 3 × CSC: 11/50 (skin C) (22 %); DMBA + 3 × CSC: 11/30 (skin C) (37 %)	Wynder & Hoffmann (1961)
Other tobacco						
Swiss albino	M	15	Oral gavage of Indian bidi smoke condensate	1 mg bidi smoke condensate/0.1 ml DMSO, 5 days/wk, 55 wks, termination 90 wks	4 hepatic haemangiomas, 1 stomach papilloma and C, and 1 oesophageal C/15 mice; 0/15 (untreated or DMSO-treated controls)	Pakhale et al. (1988)

Table 3.3 (contd)

Strain	Sex	No. of treated animals/ group	Type of exposure	Exposure dosage and duration	Tumour incidence	Reference
Rat						
Osborne Mendel	F	NG	Intrapulmonary administration of CSC pellet	CSC/beeswax:tricaprylin (24 mg CSC/injection), up to 107 wks after implantation	14/40[c] (lung squamous-cell C), 0/63[c] (beeswax:tricaprylin controls)	Stanton et al. (1972)
OM/NCR	F	120[d]	Intrapulmonary administration of CSC pellet	CSC/beeswax:tricaprylin (5, 10, 20 or 67 mg CSC/injection), 120 wks after implantation	4, 10, 20 and 42% pulmonary C prevalence; 0% C prevalence for 3 control groups of about 190 rats each	Dagle et al. (1978)
Rabbit						
Albino New Zealand	M + F	38	Skin painting of CSC (both ears)	CSC/acetone solution (100 mg CSC/ application/ear), × 5/wk, lifetime (4–6 yrs)	4/38 (2 skin C + 1 skin lipo- sarcoma + 1 skin fibrosarcoma), 0/7 (acetone controls)	Graham et al. (1957)

CSC, cigarette-smoke condensate; wk, week; C, carcinoma; DMBA, 7,12-dimethylbenz[a]anthracene; DMSO, dimethyl sulfoxide; NG, not given; yrs, years
[a] Skin papillomas
[b] Mostly adenomas
[c] Incidence in animals that died 43–107 weeks after injection
[d] 4 × 10 rats/group terminated before 120 weeks

During the next decade, methods of generating CSC and of treating animals were refined and standardized within and between laboratories. Currently, cigarettes are machine smoked, generally using a 35-mL puff drawn for 2 s each minute. The condensate is collected in glass vessels at low temperatures and removed using a volatile solvent, such as acetone, under reduced pressure. In some studies, animals have also been treated with a diluted suspension of CSC in a suitable solvent. Some of the variables that have not been standardized between different laboratories include choice of animal (or strain), dose and frequency of treatment, choice of solvent, conditions of storage of CSC, the puff profile of the smoking machine and the number of cigarettes that are puffed simultaneously.

Nevertheless, when mouse skin has been used as the test tissue in experiments carried out over the last 35 years, the results from various laboratories have been similar with respect to the overall degree of carcinogenic activity of CSC and to the major differences in activity between CSC from cigarettes of different design (Wynder *et al.*, 1957; Davies & Day, 1969; Dontenwill *et al.*, 1972; Bernfeld & Homburger, 1976; Gargus *et al.*, 1976; Gori, 1976; Dontenwill *et al.*, 1977b; Gori, 1977; Lee *et al.*, 1977; Gori, 1980). Subtle differences in smoking technique, CSC storage conditions and procedures for animal exposure do not appear to affect the results critically.

Animal studies conducted before 1964 provided a measure of support for the epidemiological demonstration that cigarette smoke is an important human carcinogen. Since that time, the mouse-skin studies have served primarily to determine whether differences in cigarette design affect the carcinogenic effects of CSC and whether these effects can be correlated with the chemical composition of the condensates. In addition, mouse-skin studies may help to elucidate the mechanisms through which CSC induces tumours in animal tissues. For example, it has been shown that CSC contains tumour initiators (Hoffmann & Wynder, 1971) and that CSC and some of its fractions and components can exhibit tumour-promoting activity (see, for example: Wynder & Hoffmann, 1961; Bock *et al.*, 1969; Hoffmann & Wynder, 1971; Lazar *et al.*, 1974; Van Duuren & Goldschmidt, 1976).

3.3.1   *Skin application*

(*a*)   *Mouse*

CSC produces both benign and malignant tumours on mouse skin. The carcinogenic potency of the CSC depends on tobacco variety, composition of cigarette paper and the presence of additives (see, for example, Wynder *et al.*, 1957; Davies & Day, 1969; Dontenwill *et al.*, 1972; Gargus *et al.*, 1976; Gori, 1976; Dontenwill *et al.*, 1977b; Gori, 1977, 1980). The tumours induced are usually of epidermal origin. Ohmori *et al.* (1981) reported a low, but significant incidence of mastocytomas in a series of experiments in which mouse skin was treated with CSC.

An example of mouse skin studies is given in a series of four publications (see Gargus *et al.*, 1976; Gori, 1976, 1977, 1980) that reported the results of skin-painting experiments in which more than 100 variables of CSC were tested in female ICR Swiss mice. These data permitted an evaluation of the overall carcinogenicity of CSC and of intralaboratory variation in bioassay results over time, because, in these studies, University of Kentucky 1R1 and SEB cigarettes stored at –20 °C were tested in four series of studies begun in 1970, 1972, 1974 and 1975, and the results (Table 3.4) are representative of the tumour response found in such studies. The purpose of the studies was to investigate possible relationships between biological activity and cigarette design as well as the chemical characteristics of cigarette smoke. The CSC derived from reference cigarettes and specially modified cigarettes was applied generally at two dose levels, usually 25 mg and 50 mg per 0.1-mL application, 6 days a week, for 78 weeks. Acetone was used as the solvent. In some instances, 3-, 6- and 12.5-mg doses were also given, and, for a single type of CSC, doses of 10 mg and 20 mg were given twice daily or five times a week for 78 weeks. Solvent-treated and untreated controls were kept. Test group sizes usually comprised 100 animals, but up to 800 controls were used; 6400–9200 mice were used for each of the four sets of experiments. A skin tumour was observed in 3/800 acetone-treated controls; otherwise, no tumours and no carcinomas were found in control animals. Skin tumours, frequently malignant, were found in every CSC-treated group. [These extensive studies reported differences in the activity of CSCs from cigarettes of different design. The Working Group of the *IARC Monographs* on tobacco smoking (IARC, 1986) noted that, although the trends of the differences were often consistent, different statistical procedures were used to analyse the data, and insufficient data were provided to permit a uniform analysis for quantitative comparison of these data.]

Cigar and pipe smoke condensates have also been tested on mouse skin. In one such study, a 1:1 (w/v) acetone solution of nicotine-free cigar or pipe tar was painted three

Table 3.4. Skin tumour[a] incidences in ICR Swiss mice after skin painting with smoke condensate from reference cigarettes[b,c]

Series	Date of start of study	Reference cigarette				
		1R1	SEBI	SEBII	SEBIII	SEBIV
I	1970	82/200	84/200	–	–	–
II	1972	98/200	115/200	383/800	–	–
III	1974	49/100	51/100	–	46/100	–
IV	1975	95/200	–	–	87/200	326/800

[a] Not corrected for interim deaths; tumours classified as 'papillomas' and 'carcinomas' in series I and II, as 'papillomas' and 'other malignancies' in series III, and as 'tumours' in series IV.
[b] From Gargus *et al.* (1976) and Gori (1976, 1977, 1980)
[c] Age of animals at start: 'approximately' 6 weeks in series I and II; 'at least' 6 weeks in III and IV.

times a week on the skin of female Swiss mice. A 1:1 acetone solution of whole CSC was also employed. At the end of 19 months, skin papillomas were produced in 65% and carcinomas in 41% of 46 mice treated with the nicotine-free cigar tar, papillomas in 69% and carcinomas in 33% of 45 mice treated with the nicotine-free pipe tar, and papillomas in 47% and carcinomas in 33% of 86 mice treated with CSC. No tumour was produced in 23 acetone-treated controls. At 9 months, when the first tumours appeared, 78% of the controls and 70–91% of the tar-treated animals were still alive (Croninger et al., 1958). [The Working Group recognized that the nicotine-free cigar and pipe tars were prepared in a manner that would cause unknown changes in their composition.]

(b)   Rat

McGregor (1976) and McGregor and Myers (1982) reported that CSC appeared to act as a co-carcinogen with β-irradiation on rat skin. CSC alone was reported to induce one benign tumour in 72 normal rats and six benign skin tumours in 78 rats in which the skin keratin layer had been removed before painting the skin. [The Working Group noted that the data, as presented, are not adequate to permit evaluation of these reports.]

(c)   Syrian hamster

Bernfeld and Homburger (1983) reported that Syrian golden hamster skin is not responsive to CSC applied alone. [The Working Group noted that only 16 of the 50 animals treated with CSC alone were observed for up to 46–47 weeks.]

(d)   Rabbit

CSC was applied using a brush to the inner surface of the ears of 38 rabbits five times a week as a 50% w/v suspension in acetone. On alternate weeks, the accumulated surface tar was removed using an acetone-soaked cotton ball or forceps. After 4–6 years of treatment, all of the rabbits had developed large papillomas, and four had skin cancer. Of seven control animals treated with acetone, none developed cancer, but five had small papillomas on the ears (Graham et al., 1957).

3.3.2   'Initiation–promotion' skin-painting studies

Mouse

A number of investigators have found that CSC and its fractions can act as co-carcinogens when applied together with other agents. In one assay for tumour-initiating activity, 50 μL of an acetone solution containing 2.5 mg of a CSC fraction (0.6% of the whole tar) was applied to the dorsal skin of female ICR/Ha Swiss mice during the second telogen phase of hair growth. This procedure was repeated on alternate days until a total of 10 doses had been applied. Ten days after the last initiating dose, the mice were painted three times a week with 2.5% croton oil in acetone. After 12 months, 67% (20/30) of mice had developed papillomas and 13% (4/30) had carcinomas; after 15 months, 73% (22/30) had papillomas and 13% (4/30) carcinomas The first tumour appeared within 4 months of start of initiating treatment. Sixty-five mice treated with croton oil only developed no tumours (Hoffmann & Wynder, 1971).

Groups of 30 female Swiss mice were painted twice weekly with 75 mg CSC (solution of 50% CSC in acetone) for 12 months. Of animals that had been treated first (one week before) with 75 µg DMBA, 13/30 (43%) developed skin papillomas and eight (27%) had carcinomas 15 months after initiation. In mice that did not receive DMBA treatment, only 4/40 (10%) had papillomas and one (3%) had a carcinoma. Of 50 mice painted three times weekly with CSC, 22 (44%) developed skin papillomas and 11 (22%) had carcinomas. Of 30 animals treated first (one week before) with a single dose of DMBA, 19 (63%) developed skin papillomas and 11 (37%) had carcinomas. Of mice treated with DMBA alone, 3/30 (10%) had skin papillomas and two (7%) had carcinomas. When a 10% solution of the phenolic fraction of CSC in acetone was applied three times weekly to 30 mice pre-treated with DMBA, nine animals (30%) developed papillomas, but no carcinomas. No tumour was seen in mice that had not received DMBA initiation (Wynder & Hoffmann, 1961). [The Working Group noted that the data do not establish that this effect was due to promotion or whether it represented an additive effect of two weak tumorigenic stimuli.]

3.3.3 Topical application to oral mucosa

Mouse

The lips and oral areas of groups of 100 ICR/Ha Swiss mice were painted five times a week for 15 months with approximately 26 mg CSC in an acetone suspension. Control groups of 100 mice were either untreated or treated with acetone alone. The study was terminated after 18–19 months, at which time 81–90% of the animals were still alive. Of the surviving mice in the experimental group, 64% (52/81, $p < 0.0001$) developed lung tumours, in contrast to 22% (20/89) in the control groups. In addition, 21% of the treated animals developed tumours of other organs, primarily lymphomas, in contrast to 3–8% in the two control groups (DiPaolo & Levin, 1965).

3.3.4 Intrapulmonary administration

(a) Rat

Stanton et al. (1972), following up the earlier studies of Blacklock (1961), injected 0.05 mL beeswax:tricaprylin (v/v) containing 24 mg CSC into the lungs of female Osborne Mendel pathogen-free rats after thoracotomy. The pellets thus formed were large enough to entrap bronchioles. The residues of the pellets could be recognized for more than 2 years after treatment. Fourteen of 40 rats that died between 43 and 107 weeks developed squamous-cell carcinomas. The non-polar constituents of CSC appeared to be an important, but not the sole contributor to this activity. Thus, when the beeswax:tricaprylin

mixture contained 12 mg of the heptane-soluble fraction of CSC, squamous-cell carcinomas developed in 5/18 rats. No tumour was seen in any of the 63 rats that died 43–107
weeks after injection with beeswax:tricaprylin alone.

These observations were confirmed by Dagle *et al.* (1978) using CSC from two different types of cigarette. They observed a dose-dependent incidence of lung carcinomas
when either condensate was injected in beeswax:tricaprylin. No carcinoma was induced
by beeswax:tricaprylin alone. With the highest dose of CSC (67 mg), the prevalence of
carcinoma reached 42% in 120 weeks. No difference was observed in tumour response to
the two CSCs.

Groups of Wistar rats were injected intratracheally with CSC or CSC fractions
without vehicle every 2 weeks for life. There was a dose-dependent increase in the mean
grade of squamous metaplasia in the groups treated with CSC and with several fractions
of CSC. After treatment with CSC and most fractions, no tumours were observed, but after
treatment with a fraction containing most of the polynuclear aromatic hydrocarbons of
cigarette smoke, 5/54 rats developed neoplastic lung lesions (Davis *et al.*, 1975c). [The
Working Group noted that the relatively infrequent dosage employed by Davis *et al.* may
have been less adequate as a stimulus than prolonged release of the material from a lipid
vehicle that persists at the injection site.]

(b)   Hamster

CSC and the 'nitromethane-soluble' fraction of CSC were found to be weak carcinogens when injected in beeswax directly into hamster lung (Ketkar *et al.*, 1979). The
method used was similar to that used by Stanton *et al.* (1972) in rats; 0.03 mL of a 1:1
beeswax: tricaprylin mixture was used as the solvent. A group of 31 hamsters injected
with 50 mg CSC developed one bronchogenic adenoma; two animals exhibited metaplasia. When 25 mg of the nitromethane fraction of CSC was given to another group of
31 animals, three developed bronchogenic adenomas and nine had metaplasia.

3.3.5   Gavage study

Mouse

The carcinogenicity of smoke condensates of Indian bidi [Indian sun-cured tobacco
wrapped in *tendu* leaf (*Diospyros melanoxylon* or *Diospyros ebenum)* and smoked] was
administered to male Swiss albino mice by oral gavage in suspensions of 1 mg conden-
sate/0.1 mg dimethyl sulfoxide, 5 days per week, for 55 weeks. Animals were killed when
moribund or 90 weeks after the beginning of treatment. Lung, liver, stomach and oesophagus were fixed in formalin and processed for histological examination. Four hepatic
haemangiomas, one stomach papilloma, one stomach carcinoma and one oesophageal
carcinoma were found in 15 mice that received bidi smoke condensate. No tumours were
seen in untreated controls (15 mice) or dimethyl sulfoxide controls (15 mice) (Pakhale
et al., 1988).

References

Auerbach, O., Hammond, E.C., Kirman, D. & Garfinkel, L. (1970) Effects of cigarette smoking on dogs. II. Pulmonary neoplasms. *Arch. environ. Health*, **21**, 754–768

Bernfeld, P. & Homburger, F. (1976) Mouse skin assay of condensate from smoking products other than tobacco. *J. natl Cancer Inst.*, **56**, 741–747

Bernfeld, P. & Homburger, F. (1983) Skin painting studies in Syrian hamsters. *Prog. exp. Tumor Res.*, **26**, 128–153

Bernfeld, P., Homburger, F. & Russfield, A.B. (1974) Strain differences in the response of inbred Syrian hamsters to cigarette smoke inhalation. *J. natl Cancer Inst.*, **53**, 1141–1157

Bernfeld, P., Homburger, F., Soto, E. & Pai, K.J. (1979) Cigarette smoke inhalation studies in inbred Syrian golden hamsters. *J. natl Cancer Inst.*, **63**, 675–689

Blacklock, J.W.S. (1961) An experimental study of the pathological effects of cigarette condensate in the lungs with special reference to carcinogenesis. *Br. J. Cancer*, **15**, 745–762

Bock, F.G., Swain, A.P. & Stedman, R.L. (1969) Bioassay of major fractions of cigarette smoke condensate by an accelerated technic. *Cancer Res.*, **29**, 584–587

Chameaud, J., Perraud, R., Chrétien, J., Masse, R. & Lafuma, J. (1982) Lung carcinogenesis during in vivo cigarette smoking and radon daughter exposure in rats. *Recent Results Cancer Res.*, **82**, 11–20

Croninger, A.B., Graham, E.A. & Wynder, E.L. (1958) Experimental production of carcinoma with tobacco products. V. Carcinoma induction in mice with cigar, pipe and all–tobacco cigarette tar. *Cancer Res.*, **18**, 1263–1271

Cross, F.T., Palmer, R.F., Filipy, R.E., Dagle, G.E. & Stuart, B.O. (1982) Carcinogenic effects of radon daughters, uranium ore dust and cigarette smoke in beagle dogs. *Health Phys.*, **42**, 33–52

Dalbey, W.E., Nettesheim, P., Griesemer, R., Caton, J.E. & Guerin, M.R. (1980) Chronic inhalation of cigarette smoke by F344 rats. *J. natl Cancer Inst.*, **64**, 383–390

Dagle, G.E., McDonald, K.E., Smith, L.G. & Stevens, D.L., Jr (1978) Pulmonary carcinogenesis in rats given implants of cigarette smoke condensate in beeswax pellets. *J. natl Cancer Inst.*, **61**, 905–910

Davies, R.F. & Day, T.D. (1969) A study of the comparative carcinogenicity of cigarette and cigar smoke condensate on mouse skin. *Br. J. Cancer*, **23**, 363–368

Davis, B.R., Whitehead, J.K., Gill, M.E., Lee, P.N., Butterworth, A.D. & Roe, F.J.C. (1975a) Response of rat lung to inhaled tobacco smoke with or without prior exposure to 3,4-benzpyrene (BP) given by intratracheal instillation. *Br. J. Cancer*, **31**, 469–484

Davis, B.R., Whitehead, J.K., Gill, M.E., Lee, P.N., Butterworth, A.D. & Roe, F.J.C. (1975b) Response of rat lung to inhaled vapour phase constituents (VP) of tobacco smoke alone or in conjunction with smoke condensate or fractions of smoke condensate given by intratracheal instillation. *Br. J. Cancer*, **31**, 462–468

Davis, B.R., Whitehead, J.K., Gill, M.E., Lee, P.N., Butterworth, A.D. & Roe, F.J.C. (1975c) Response of rat lung to tobacco smoke condensate or fractions derived from it administered repeatedly by intratracheal instillation. *Br. J. Cancer*, **31**, 453–461

DiPaolo, J.A. & Levin, M.L. (1965) Tumor incidence in mice after oral painting with cigarette smoke condensate. *J. natl Cancer Inst.*, **34**, 595–600

Dontenwill, W., Chevalier, H.-J., Harke, H.-P., Klimisch, H.-J., Lafrenz, O. & Reckzeh, G. (1972) [Experimental studies on tumorigenic activity of cigarette smoke condensate on mouse skin. IV.

Comparative studies of condensates from different reconstituted tobacco sheets, the effect of NaNO₃ as additive to tobacco or reconstituted tobacco sheets, the effect of volatile constituents of smoke, the effect of initial treatment with DMBA.] *Z. Krebsforsch.*, **78**, 236–264 (in German)

Dontenwill, W., Chevalier, H.-J., Harke, H.-P., Lafrenz, U., Reckzeh, G. & Schneider, B. (1973) Investigations on the effects of chronic cigarette-smoke inhalation in Syrian golden hamsters. *J. natl Cancer Inst.*, **51**, 1781–1832

Dontenwill, W., Chevalier, H.-J., Harke, H.-P., Klimisch, H.-J., Kuhnig, C., Reckzeh, G. & Schneider, B. (1977a) [Studies on the effect of chronic cigarette smoke inhalation in Syrian golden hamsters and the importance of vitamin A on morphological alterations after smoke exposure.] *Z. Krebsforsch.*, **89**, 153–180 (in German)

Dontenwill, W., Chevalier, H.-J., Harke, H.-P., Klimisch, H.-J., Reckzeh, G., Fleischmann, B. & Keller, W. (1977b) [Experimental investigations on the tumorigenic activity of cigarette smoke condensate on mouse skin. VII. Comparative studies of condensates from different modified cigarettes.] *Z. Krebsforsch.*, **89**, 145–151 (in German)

Finch, G.L., Nikula, K.J., Barr, E.B., Bechtold, W.E., Chen, B.T., Griffith, W.C., Hahn, F.F., Hobbs, C.H., Hoover, M.D., Lundgren, D.L. & Mauderly, J.L. (1995) Effects of combined exposure of F344 rats to radiation and chronically inhaled cigarette smoke. In: Bice, D.E., Hahn, F.F., Hoover, M.D., Neft, R.E., Thornton-Manning, J.R. & Bradley, P.L., eds, *Annual Report of the Inhalation Toxicology Research Institute* (ITRI-146), Albuquerque, NM, Inhalation Toxicology Research Institute, pp. 77–79

Finch, G.L., Nikula, K.J., Belinsky, S.A., Barr, E.B., Stoner, G.D. & Lechner, J.F. (1996) Failure of cigarette smoke to induce or promote lung cancer in the A/J mouse. *Cancer Lett.*, **99**, 161–167

Gargus, J.L., Powers, M.B., Habermann, R.T. & Everly, J.R. (1976) Mouse dermal bioassays of cigarette smoke condensates. In: Gori, G.B., ed., *Report No. 1. Toward Less Hazardous Cigarettes. The First Set of Experimental Cigarettes* (DHEW Publ. No. (NIH) 76-905), Washington DC, Department of Health, Education, and Welfare, Public Health Service, National Institutes of Health, National Cancer Institute, pp. 85–94

Gori, G.B. (1976) Report on the second set of experimental cigarettes. In: Gori, G.B., ed., *Report No. 2. Toward Less Hazardous Cigarettes. The Second Set of Experimental Cigarettes* (DHEW Publ. No. (NIH) 76-1111), Washington DC, Department of Health, Education, and Welfare, Public Health Service, National Institutes of Health, National Cancer Institute, pp. 4–15

Gori, G.B. (1977) Report on the third set of experimental cigarettes. In: Gori, G.B., ed., *Report No. 3. Toward Less Hazardous Cigarettes. The Third Set of Experimental Cigarettes* (DHEW Publ. No. (NIH) 77-1280), Washington DC, Department of Health, Education, and Welfare, Public Health Service, National Institutes of Health, National Cancer Institute, pp. 3–24

Gori, G.B. (1980) Report on the fourth set of experimental cigarettes. In: Gori, G.B., ed., *Report No. 4. Toward Less Hazardous Cigarettes. The Fourth Set of Experimental Cigarettes*, Washington DC, Department of Health, Education, and Welfare, Public Health Service, National Institutes of Health, National Cancer Institute, pp. 5–40

Graham, E.A., Croninger, A.B. & Wynder, E.L. (1957) Experimental production of carcinoma with cigarette tar. IV. Successful experiments with rabbits. *Cancer Res.*, **17**, 1058–1066

Griest, W.H., Guerin, M.R., Quincy, R.B., Jenkins, R.A. & Kubota, H. (1980) Chemical characterization of experimental cigarettes and cigarette smoke condensates in the fourth cigarette experiment. In: Gori, G.B., ed., Report No. 4. *Toward Less Hazardous Cigarettes. The Fourth Set of*

Experimental Cigarettes, Washington DC, Department of Health, Education and Welfare, Public Health Service, National Institutes of Health, National Cancer Institute, pp. 65–97

Gupta, M.P., Khanduja, K.L., Koul, I.B. & Sharma, R.R. (1990) Effect of cigarette smoke inhalation on benzo[*a*]pyrene-induced lung carcinogenesis in vitamin A deficiency in the rat. *Cancer Lett.*, **55**, 83–88

Hammond, E.C., Auerbach, O., Kirman, D. & Garfinkel, L. (1970) Effects of cigarette smoking on dogs. I. Design of experiment, mortality, and findings in lung parenchyma. *Arch. environ. Health*, **21**, 740–753

Harada, T., Kitazawa, T., Maita, K. & Shirasu, Y. (1985) Effects of vitamin C on tumor induction by diethylnitrosamine in the respiratory tract of hamsters exposed to cigarette smoke. *Cancer Lett.*, **25**, 163–169

Harris, R.J.C. & Negroni, G. (1967) Production of lung carcinomas in C57BL mice exposed to a cigarette smoke and air mixture. *Br. med. J.*, **iv**, 637–641

Harris, R.J.C., Negroni, G., Ludgate, S., Pick, C.R., Chesterman, F.C. & Maidment, B.J. (1974) The incidence of lung tumours in C57BL mice exposed to cigarette smoke:air mixtures for prolonged periods. *Int. J. Cancer*, **14**, 130–136

Hecht, S.S., Adams, J.D., Numoto, S. & Hoffmann, D. (1983) Induction of respiratory tract tumors in Syrian golden hamsters by a single dose of 4-(methylnitrosamino)-1-(3-pyridyl)-1-butanone (NNK) and the effect of smoke inhalation. *Carcinogenesis*, **4**, 1287–1290

Henry, C.J. & Kouri, R.E. (1986) Chronic inhalation studies in mice. II. Effects of long-term exposure to 2R1 cigarette smoke on (C57BL/Cum × C3H/AnfCum)F$_1$ mice. *J. natl Cancer Inst.*, **77**, 203–212

Hoffmann, D. & Wynder, E.L. (1971) A study of tobacco carcinogenesis. XI. Tumor initiators, tumor accelerators, and tumor promoting activity of condensate fractions. *Cancer*, **27**, 848–864

Hoffmann, D., Rivenson, A., Hecht, S.S., Hilfrich, J., Kobayashi, N. & Wynder, E.L. (1979) Model studies in tobacco carcinogenesis with the Syrian golden hamster. *Prog. exp. Tumor Res.*, **24**, 370–390

Holland, R.H., Wilson, R.H., Morris, D., McCall, M.S. & Lanz, H. (1958) The effect of cigarette smoke on the respiratory system of the rabbit. A preliminary report. *Cancer*, **11**, 709–712

Holland, R.H., Kozlowski, E.J. & Booker, L. (1963) The effect of cigarette smoke on the respiratory system of the rabbit. A final report. *Cancer*, **16**, 612–615

IARC (1986) *IARC Monographs on the Evaluation of the Carcinogenic Risk of Chemicals to Humans*, Vol. 38, *Tobacco Smoking*, Lyon, IARCPress

Keast, D., Ayre, D.J. & Papadimitriou, J.M. (1981) A survey of pathological changes associated with long-term high tar tobacco smoke exposure in a murine model. *J. Pathol.*, **135**, 249–257

Ketkar, M.B., Haas, H. & Althoff, J. (1979) Implantation of cigarette smoke condensate in the lungs of Syrian golden hamsters. *J. Cancer Res. clin. Oncol.*, **94**, 111–114

Kobayashi, N., Hoffmann, D. & Wynder, E.L. (1974) A study of tobacco carcinogenesis. XII. Epithelial changes induced in the upper respiratory tracts of Syrian golden hamsters by cigarette smoke. *J. natl Cancer Inst.*, **53**, 1085–1089

Lazar, P., Chouroulinkov, I., Izard, C., Moree-Testa, P. & Hemon, D. (1974) Bioassays of carcinogenicity after fractionation of cigarette smoke condensate. *Biomedicine*, **20**, 214–222

Lee, P.N., Rothwell, K. & Whitehead, J.K. (1977) Fractionation of mouse skin carcinogens in cigarette smoke condensate. *Br. J. Cancer*, **35**, 730–742

Leuchtenberger, C. & Leuchtenberger, R. (1970) Effects of chronic inhalation of whole fresh cigarette smoke and of its gas phase on pulmonary tumorigenesis in Snell's mice. In: Nettesheim,
P., Hanna, M.G., Jr & Deathevage, J.W., Jr, eds, *Morphology of Experimental Respiratory
Carcinogenesis. Proceedings of a Biology Division, Oak Ridge National Laboratory Conference*, US Atomic Energy Commission, pp. 329–346

McGregor, J.F. (1976) Tumor-promoting activity of cigarette tar in rat skin exposed to irradiation.
J. natl Cancer Inst., **56**, 429–430

McGregor, J.F. & Myers, D.K. (1982) Enhancement of skin tumorigenesis by cigarette smoke condensate following β-irradiation in rats. *J. natl Cancer Inst.*, **68**, 605–611

Nagano, K., Miyakawa, Y., Takahashi, M., Furukawa, F., Kokubo, T. & Hayashi, Y. (1982) Comparative studies on anatomical and histological structures of nasal cavity in rodents. *Natl
public Health Inst. Jpn*, **100**, 101–109

Nishikawa, A., Furukawa, F., Imazawa, T., Yoshimura, H., Ikezaki, S., Hayashi, Y. & Takahashi,
M. (1994) Effects of cigarette smoke on *N*-nitrosobis(2-oxopropyl)amine-induced pancreatic
and respiratory tumorigenesis in hamsters. *Jpn. J. Cancer Res.*, **85**, 1000–1004

Ohmori, T., Mori, H. & Rivenson, A. (1981) A study of tobacco carcinogenesis. XX. Mastocytoma
induction in mice by cigarette smoke particulates ('cigarette tar'). *Am. J. Pathol.*, **102**,
381–387

Otto, H. & Elmenhorst, H. (1967) [Experimental studies on tumour induction with the gas phase
of cigarette smoke.] *Z. Krebsforsch.*, **70**, 45–47 (in German)

Pakhale, S.S., Sarkar, S., Jayant, K. & Bhide, S.V. (1988) Carcinogenicity of Indian bidi and cigarette smoke condensate in Swiss albino mice. *Cancer Res. clin. Oncol.*, **114**, 647– 649

Proctor, D.F. & Chang, J.C.F. (1983) Comparative anatomy and physiology of the nasal cavity. In:
Reznik, G. & Stinson, S.F., eds, *Nasal Tumors in Animals and Man*, Vol. 1, *Anatomy, Physiology and Epidemiology*, Boca Raton, FL, CRC Press, pp. 1–33

Reznik, G. (1983) Comparative anatomy and histomorphology of the nasal and paranasal cavities
in rodents. In: Reznik, G. & Stinson, S.F., eds, *Nasal Tumors in Animals and Man*, Vol. 1, *Anatomy, Physiology and Epidemiology*, Boca Raton, FL, CRC Press, pp. 35–44

Stanton, M.F., Miller, E., Wrench, C. & Blackwell, R. (1972) Experimental induction of epidermoid
carcinoma in the lungs of rats by cigarette smoke condensate. *J. natl Cancer Inst.*, **49**, 867–877

Shimkin, M.D. & Stoner, G.D. (1975) The genetic basis of susceptibility to lung tumours in mice.
Adv. Cancer Res., **21**, 1–56

Takahashi, M., Imaida, K., Mitsumori, K., Okamiya, H., Shinoda, K., Yoshimura, H., Furukawa, F.
& Hayashi, Y. (1992) Promoting effects of cigarette smoke on the respiratory tract carcinogenesis of Syrian golden hamsters treated with diethylnitrosamine. *Carcinogenesis*, **13**,
569–572

Van Duuren, B.L. & Goldschmidt, B.M. (1976) Cocarcinogenic and tumor-promoting agents in
tobacco carcinogenesis. *J. natl Cancer Inst.*, **56**, 1237–1242

Wehner, A.P., Busch, R.H. & Olson, R.J. (1974) Effect of chronic exposure to cigarette smoke on
tumor incidence in the Syrian golden hamster. In: Karbe, E. & Park, J.F., eds, *Experimental
Lung Cancer. Carcinogenesis and Bioassays*, New York, Springer, pp. 360–368

Wehner, A.P., Busch, R.H., Olson, R.J. & Craig, D.K. (1975a) Chronic inhalation of nickel oxide
and cigarette smoke by hamsters. *Am. ind. Hyg. Assoc. J.*, **36**, 801–810

Wehner, A.P., Busch, R.H., Olson, R.J. & Craig, D.K. (1975b) Chronic inhalation of asbestos and
cigarette smoke by hamsters. *Environ. Res.*, **10**, 368–383

Wehner, A.P., Olson, R.J. & Busch, R.H. (1976) Increased life span and decreased weight in hamsters exposed to cigarette smoke. *Arch. environ. Health*, **31**, 146–153

Wehner, A.P., Dagle, G.E., Milliman, E.M., Phelps, D.W., Carr, D.B., Decker, J.R. & Filipy, R.E. (1981) Inhalation bioassay of cigarette smoke in rats. *Toxicol. appl. Pharmacol.*, **61**, 1–17

Witschi, H., Espiritu, I., Peake, J.L., Wu, K., Maronpot, R.R. & Pinkerton, K.E. (1997) The carcinogenicity of environmental tobacco smoke. *Carcinogenesis*, **18**, 575–586

Wynder, E.L. & Hoffmann, D. (1961) A study of tobacco carcinogenesis. VIII. The role of the acidic fractions as promoters. *Cancer*, **14**, 1306–1315

Wynder, E.L. & Hoffmann, D. (1967) *Tobacco and Tobacco Smoke. Studies in Experimental Carcinogenesis*, New York, Academic Press, pp. 225–231

Wynder, E.L., Graham, E.A. & Croninger, A.B. (1953) Experimental production of carcinoma with cigarette tar. *Cancer Res.*, **13**, 855–864

Wynder, E.L., Gottlieb, S. & Wright, G. (1957) A study of tobacco carcinogenesis. IV. Different tobacco types. *Cancer*, **10**, 1206–1209

Wynder, E.L., Taguchi, K.T., Baden, V. & Hoffmann, D. (1968) Tobacco carcinogenesis. IX. Effect of cigarette smoke on respiratory tract of mice after passive inhalation. *Cancer*, **21**, 134–153

Yoshimura, H. & Takemoto, K. (1991) Effect of cigarette smoking and/or *N*-bis(2-hydroxypropyl)-nitrosamine (DHPN) on the development of lung and pleural tumors in rats induced by administration of asbestos. *Jpn. J. ind. Health*, **33**, 81–93

4. Other Data Relevant to an Evaluation of Carcinogenicity and its Mechanisms

4.1   Absorption, distribution, metabolism and excretion

4.1.1   *Humans*

The Working Group attempted to provide extensive coverage of the published lite-rature since 1985, in some cases referring to recent reviews.

(*a*)   *Introduction*

Most carcinogens are enzymatically transformed to a series of metabolites as the exposed organism attempts to convert them to forms that are more readily excreted. The initial steps are usually carried out by cytochrome P450 (P450) enzymes that oxygenate the substrate (Guengerich, 1997). Other enzymes such as lipoxygenases, cyclooxyge-nases, myeloperoxidase and monoamine oxidases may also be involved, but less com-monly. If the oxygenated intermediates formed in these initial reactions are electrophilic, they may react with DNA or other macromolecules to form covalent binding products known as adducts. This process is called metabolic activation. Alternatively, these meta-bolites may undergo further transformations catalysed by glutathione S-transferases, uri-dine-5'-diphosphate (UDP)-glucuronosyltransferases, epoxide hydrolase (EH), N-acetyl-transferases (NATs) (Kadlubar & Beland, 1985), sulfotransferases and other enzymes (Armstrong, 1997; Burchell *et al.*, 1997; Duffel, 1997). Such reactions frequently, but not always, result in detoxification.

Figure 4.1 presents an overview of the metabolism of the six tobacco smoke carci-nogens for which the formation of DNA adducts has been demonstrated in human tissues, namely, benzo[*a*]pyrene (IARC, 1983a, 1987), 4-(*N*-nitrosomethylamino)-1-(3-pyridyl)-1-butanone (NNK) (IARC, 1985a; Hecht *et al.*, 1994), N-nitrosodimethylamine (NDMA) (IARC, 1978a; Shuker & Bartsch, 1994), N'-nitrosonornicotine (NNN) (IARC, 1985b; Hecht *et al.*, 1994), ethylene oxide (IARC, 1994a), and 4-aminobiphenyl (4-ABP) (IARC, 1972; Kadlubar, 1994). The major metabolic activation pathway of benzo[*a*]pyrene is con-version to a 7,8-diol-9,10-epoxide, which is highly carcinogenic and reacts with DNA to form adducts with the exocyclic N^2 of guanine (Cooper *et al.*, 1983). In competition with this process are detoxification pathways leading to phenols, diols and their conju-

Figure 4.1. Metabolism of six tobacco smoke carcinogens which produce DNA adducts that have been identified in the lungs of smokers

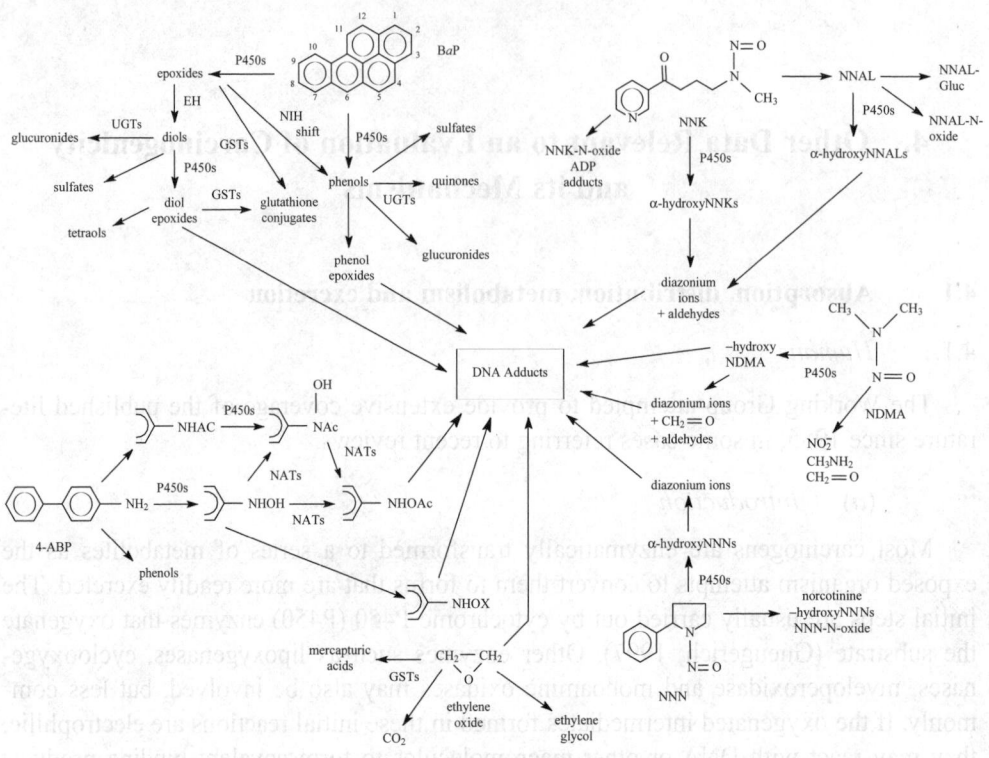

Clockwise from top left: benzo[*a*]pyrene (B*a*P), 4-(*N*-nitrosomethylamino)-1-(3-pyridyl)-1-butanone (NNK), *N*-nitrosodimethylamine (NDMA), *N'*-nitrosonornicotine (NNN), ethylene oxide and 4-aminobiphenyl (4-ABP) P450s, cytochrome P450s; EH, epoxide hydrolase; UGTs, uridine-5′-diphosphate-glucuronosyl transferases; GSTs, glutathione *S*-transferases; NNAL, 4-(*N*-nitrosomethylamino)-1-(3-pyridyl)-1-butanol; NATs, *N*-acetyl-transferases; gluc, glucuronide; 'NIH shift', phenomenon of hydroxylation-induced intramolecular migration; ADP, adenosine diphosphate; Ac, acetyl
In the 4-ABP scheme, X represents conjugates such as glucuronide or sulfate.
Adapted from Cooper *et al.* (1983); Preussmann & Stewart (1984); Kadlubar & Beland (1985); IARC (1994a); Hecht (1998, 1999)

gates as well as other metabolites. The major metabolic activation pathways of NNK and its main metabolite, 4-(*N*-nitrosomethylamino)-1-(3-pyridyl)-1-butanol (NNAL), involve hydroxylation of the carbons adjacent to the *N*-nitroso group (α-hydroxylation) which leads, via diazonium ions, to the formation of two types of DNA adduct: methyl adducts such as 7-methylguanine and *O⁶*-methylguanine (IARC, 1985a), and pyridyloxobutyl adducts (Hecht, 1998). Glucuronidation of NNAL and pyridine-*N*-oxidation of NNK and NNAL are detoxification pathways. The metabolic activation of NDMA occurs by α-hydroxylation leading, via methyl diazonium ions, to the formation of 7-methylguanine and O^6-methylguanine. Denitrosation, producing nitrite and methylamine, is considered to be a detoxification pathway (Preussmann & Stewart, 1984). Aldehydes are also formed in the metabolism of NNK and NDMA. Their role in carcinogenesis is unclear. α-Hydroxylation of NNN can lead to the formation of pyridyloxobutyl adducts whereas detoxification occurs by β-hydroxylation, pyridine-N-oxidation and denitrosation/oxidation to produce norcotinine (Hecht, 1998). Ethylene oxide reacts directly with DNA to form 7-(2-hydroxyethyl)guanine and other adducts. There are competing detoxification pathways involving glutathione conjugation (IARC, 1994b). 4-ABP is metabolically activated by N-hydroxylation. Conjugation of the resulting hydroxylamine with acetate or other groups such as sulfate ultimately produces nitrenium ions that react with DNA to produce adducts mainly at C-8 of guanine. Acetylation of 4-ABP can be a detoxification pathway if it is not followed by N-hydroxylation. Ring hydroxylation and conjugation of the phenols result in detoxification (Kadlubar & Beland, 1985).

The balance between metabolic activation and detoxification varies between individuals exposed to these genotoxic components of tobacco smoke and is likely to affect cancer risk because DNA adducts are absolutely central to the carcinogenic process induced by these agents (Hecht, 1999; Tang et al., 2001). DNA adducts, if unrepaired, can cause miscoding during replication resulting in permanent mutation.

Cells have DNA repair systems that can remove adducts and restore the DNA to its normal structure (Memisoglu & Samson, 2000; Pegg, 2000; Hanawalt, 2001; Norbury & Hickson, 2001). There are interindividual differences in their capacity for DNA repair that can affect cancer risk (Wei et al., 2000). Moreover, DNA repair systems are not completely efficient or error-free, and some adducts escape repair and persist in DNA. These persistent DNA adducts can cause miscoding. For example, when the O^6-position of guanine in DNA is methylated following metabolic activation of NNK, the resulting DNA adduct, O^6-methylguanine, is misread by DNA polymerases as adenine, and thymine is inserted during replication (Loechler et al., 1984). The consequence is the permanent conversion of a G:C base pair to an A:T base pair. This mutation and others can activate oncogenes such as KRAS or inactivate tumour-suppressor genes such as TP53. There are considerable data to indicate that mutations in KRAS and TP53 result directly from the reaction of these genes with metabolically activated carcinogens (Hecht, 1999). Many genetic abnormalities occur during the process of lung cancer induction. These include loss of heterozygosity, microsatellite alterations, mutations in RAS oncogenes, MYC amplification, BCL-2 expression, mutations in the TP53, RB, CDKN2A and FHIT tumour-suppressor genes, expression of telomerase activity and others (Figure 4.2) (Wistuba et al., 1997; Sekido et al., 1998). Although the temporal sequence of mutations is somewhat unclear, we do know that carcinogens can, through the process just described, cause irreversible damage to critical genes involved in the control of cellular growth. Smokers are subjected to a chronic barrage of metabolically activated carcinogens that cause these multiple changes (Figure 4.2). This constant assault on genes is entirely consistent with genetic derangements that lead to six proposed hallmarks of cancer:

— self-sufficiency in growth signals;

— insensitivity to anti-growth signals;
— evasion of apoptosis;
— tissue invasion and metastasis;
— sustained angiogenesis; and
— limitless replicative potential (Hanahan & Weinberg, 2000).

Figure 4.2. Scheme linking cigarette smoke carcinogens with genetic changes in lung and lung cancer development

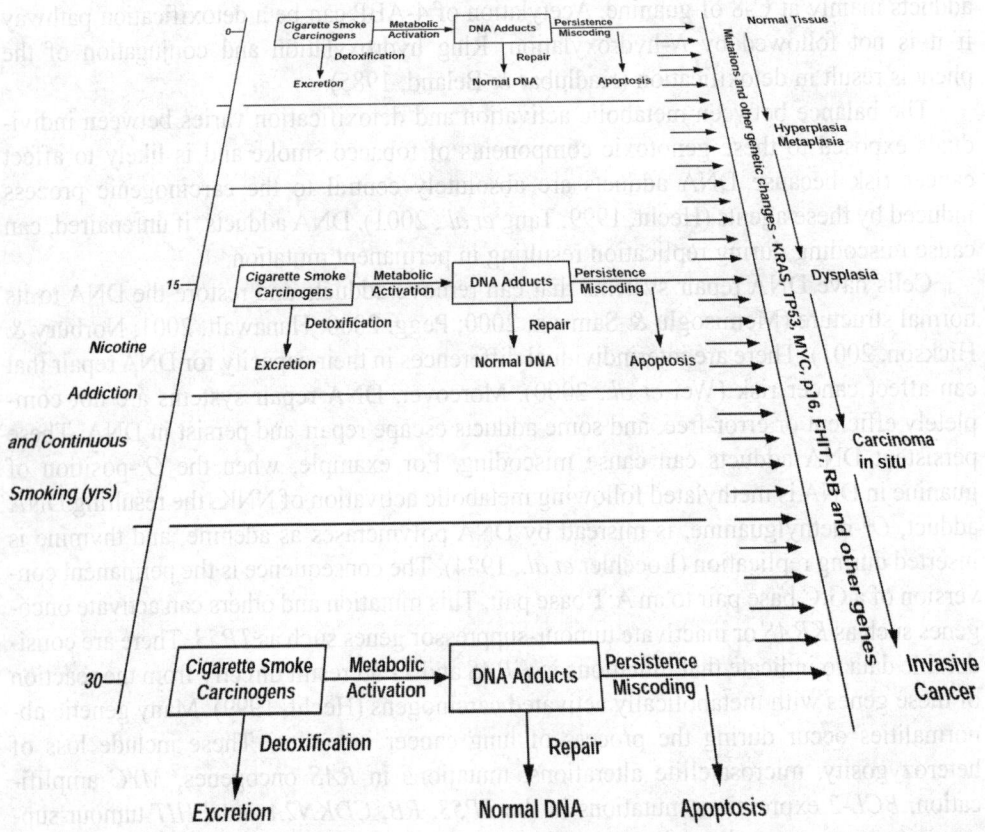

Adapted from Hecht (2002a)

This scheme may also apply to other cancers.

A key aspect is the chronic exposure of DNA to metabolically activated carcinogens resulting in the formation of DNA adducts and consequent genetic changes. This chronic barrage of DNA damage, taking place daily over a period of many years, is fully consistent with multiple genetic changes in lung cancer (it does not always take 30 years to get lung cancer; it may take only five years). Some cigarette smoke carcinogens may operate through other mechanisms. The time periods and sequence of genetic changes are uncertain. For further details see Sekido *et al.* (1998); Hecht (1999, 2002a).

Urinary carcinogen metabolites, carcinogen-protein adducts, and carcinogen-DNA adducts have been used as biomarkers to assess the uptake, metabolic activation and detoxification of tobacco carcinogens in humans. These are discussed in the following sections.

(b)   *Effects of tobacco smoke on human enzyme activities and metabolism*

(i)   *Enzyme induction*

In-vivo studies

The induction by tobacco smoke of several phase I and phase II enzymes in human tissues, including P4501A1, P4501A2, P4502E1 and some isoforms of UDP-glucuronosyltransferase has been widely reported (Anttila et al., 1991; Guengerich et al., 1991; Bock et al., 1994). Similarly, the pharmacological interactions between tobacco smoking and drugs, many of them as a consequence of enzyme induction, have been reviewed (Zevin & Benowitz, 1999). The consequences of this induction are evident in the altered rate of metabolism of many drugs and carcinogens (Zevin & Benowitz, 1999). For example, smoking decreases the activity of H_2-receptor antagonists in reducing nocturnal gastric secretion (Boyd et al., 1983). The metabolic enzymes are also induced by polycyclic aromatic hydrocarbons (PAHs), which may therefore be the components of tobacco smoke that are largely responsible for its enzyme-inducing activity. Cigarette smoke contains a variety of ligands that bind to the Ah receptor, which is known to mediate induction of P4501A1 and P4501A2 (Zevin & Benowitz, 1999).

Pulmonary P4501A1 activity (reflected by aryl hydrocarbon hydroxylase (AHH) activity) is elevated in smokers, and a highly significant correlation between enzyme activity and levels of PAH–DNA adducts has been reported (Geneste et al., 1991; Alexandrov et al., 1992). Among smokers, women with lung cancer had higher levels of *CYP1A1* mRNA and bulky DNA adducts than men with lung cancer (Mollerup et al., 1999).

Smoking results in induction of P450 activity in the human placenta. Evidence for this comes from in-vitro experiments in which placental microsomes were incubated with benzo[a]pyrene in the presence of calf thymus DNA; higher levels of DNA adducts result from incubation of microsomes of smokers than of those from nonsmokers (Kim et al., 1992). AHH activity is higher in placental microsomes from women who smoke than from women who do not, but EH activity is not (Vaught et al., 1979). Placental P450 activity, as measured by in-vitro oxidation of 7-ethoxyresorufin, was found to be 10- to 30-fold higher for female smokers than for nonsmokers (Manchester & Jacoby, 1981). In another study, placental microsomes from 32 female smokers were twice as active in benzo[a]pyrene metabolism as microsomes prepared from the placentas of 25 nonsmokers, but the in-vitro formation of DNA adducts in the presence of calf thymus DNA was not significantly higher in smokers (Sanyal et al., 1994). In a recent study, maternal smoking was found to be significantly associated with levels of placental *CYP1A1* mRNA ($p < 0.01$) but not with levels of PAH–DNA adducts measured by competitive enzyme-linked immunosorbent assay (ELISA) (Whyatt et al., 1998).

In humans, cigarette smoking significantly enhances CYP2E1 activity in alcoholic patients, as measured by increased metabolism of chlorzoxazone *in vivo* (Girre *et al.*, 1994). CYP2E1 bio-activates some substrates in tobacco smoke and other pro-carcinogens and several hepatotoxins (Guengerich *et al.*, 1991).

The levels of three enzymes involved in DNA repair in the peripheral blood cells of 20 smokers and 17 nonsmokers were compared. O^6-Alkylguanine–DNA–alkyltransferase activity was the same in both groups, but the activities of methylpurine (MeP) and 2,6-diamino-4-hydroxy-5N-formamidopyrimidine–DNA glycosylase were lower in non-smokers; the difference was statistically significant only for MeP (Hall *et al.*, 1993). Exposure of human buccal cell cultures to organic extracts of tobacco (bidi) smoke condensate and betel leaf decreased O^6-methylguanine–DNA methyltransferase activity (Liu *et al.*, 1997).

In-vitro studies

Although there have been many in-vitro studies of the properties of tobacco carcinogens, their effects are not always the same as those of the complex mixture of tobacco smoke. For example, exposure of human U937 cells (human [histiocytic] lymphoma cell line) to tobacco smoke increased the expression of haeme oxygenase-1 (HO-1) and inhibited the activity of nuclear factor-κB (NF-κB) (Favatier & Polla, 2001). However, the tobacco-specific nitrosamine NNK activates NF-κB and induces cyclooxygenase (COX)-1 expression in U937 cells (Rioux & Castonguay, 2000).

(ii)   *Enzyme inhibition*

In-vivo studies

Cigarette smoking has been demonstrated to reduce the level of monoamine oxidase B in the brain by about 40%, relative to the levels in nonsmokers or former smokers, although the effect is probably not caused by nicotine. This enzyme plays a key role in dopamine pharmacokinetics (Fowler *et al.*, 1996a). Measurable reductions in monoamine oxidase B were not observed when nonsmokers smoked only one cigarette, implying that the reduction seen in smokers requires chronic exposure and that it may be a gradual response (Fowler *et al.*, 1999). The activity of the enzyme was also significantly lower in the platelets of 23 heavy smokers (≥ 20 cigarettes/day) than in those of 41 non-smokers ($p < 0.001$) (Yong & Perry, 1986). Smoking cessation resulted in an increase in the activity of platelet monoamine oxidase B, which started after a week of abstinence and was approximately back to normal values after 4 weeks. Low baseline activity of mono-amine oxidase B is related to more intense withdrawal symptoms (Rose *et al.*, 2001). Similarly, the activity of monoamine oxidase A was markedly reduced (average, 28%) in the brains of smokers compared with nonsmokers (Fowler *et al.*, 1996b). The emerging view is that, whereas nicotine does not reduce monoamine (A and B) oxidase activity by itself, the reduction of this enzyme by other components of tobacco smoke may lead to the potentiation of nicotine's effect by slowing down the catabolism of certain neuro-transmitters, i.e. norepinephrine, dopamine and serotonin (Berlin & Anthenelli, 2001).

The activity of EH in human lung was measured in samples obtained from patients undergoing open chest surgery for lung cancer and non-neoplastic pulmonary disease. In 10 'non-recent' smokers (who had not smoked for > 1 month prior to surgery), levels of cytosolic EH activity, but not of microsomal EH activity, were significantly higher than in nine 'recent' smokers (who had smoked in the month prior to surgery). Cytosolic EH activity was positively correlated with the number of days since smoking cessation ($p < 0.05$) and was inversely correlated with the number of cigarettes smoked per day ($p < 0.01$) (Petruzzelli et al., 1992).

Emphysema is associated with decreased levels of α_1-antitrypsin, a plasma protease that inhibits neutrophil elastase activity. Cigarette smoking is associated with a decrease in neutrophil elastase inhibitory capacity in the lower respiratory tract, increasing the risk for the development of emphysema (Ogushi et al., 1991). Elastase activity in human leukocytes can be suppressed in vitro by cigarette smoke extract (Ejiofor et al., 1981). Serum antioxidant activity is significantly lower in smokers than in nonsmokers and, although there is a compensatory increase in ceruloplasmin levels, this increase is insufficient to prevent the suppression of elastase inhibitory capacity of α_1-antitrypsin by cigarette smoke extract (Galdston et al., 1984).

In-vitro studies

Numerous studies have reported enzyme inhibition in cultured cells treated with tobacco smoke, tobacco smoke condensate or extract, or known components of tobacco smoke.

A number of tobacco alkaloids, including N-n-octanoylnornicotine and N-(4-hydroxyundecanoyl) anabasine have been shown to inhibit aromatase activity in cultures of the human breast cancer cell lines, MDA-MB-231 and SK-BR-3, decreasing the estrogen biosynthesis (Kadohama et al., 1993). In cultured MA-10 Leydig tumour cells, tobacco alkaloids (nicotine, cotinine, anabasine) and aqueous extract of cigarette smoke inhibited progesterone synthesis and cell growth by a cytotoxic mechanism; this mechanism could reduce fertilization, implantation and early development of human embryos (Gocze & Freeman, 2000).

The activity of lecithin:cholesterol acyltransferase, which is believed to play a pivotal role in facilitating high-density lipoprotein-mediated removal of cholesterol from peripheral tissues such as arterial cells, is inhibited in human blood plasma by cigarette smoke extract and by a number of aldehydes present in tobacco smoke (i.e. acrolein (IARC, 1995a), hexanal, formaldehyde (IARC, 1995b), malonaldehyde (IARC, 1999a) and acetaldehyde (IARC, 1999b)). The inhibition of the enzyme activity is probably involved in the mechanism of smoking-induced atherosclerosis (Chen & Loo, 1995). There is evidence that the mechanism for this inhibition is based on the covalent modification of the two free cysteine residues (Cys-31 and Cys-184) of the enzyme (Bielicki et al., 1995). Further studies have shown that the activity of another enzyme implicated in protecting against atherosclerosis, plasma paraoxonase, is also inhibited through modification of its thiol groups by cigarette smoke extract (Nishio & Watanabe, 1997). However, exposure to gas-phase cigarette smoke from four cigarettes over an 8-h period did not inhibit para-oxonase in human plasma under conditions in which the activity of plasma leci-thin:cholesterol acyltransferase was inhibited by > 80% and platelet-activating factor acetylhydrolase by 50% (Bielicki *et al.*, 2001).

Thiol depletion by cigarette smoke may be induced by α,β-unsaturated aldehydes such as acrolein. The activation of respiratory burst by neutrophils stimulated by phorbol myristate acetate (PMA) was impaired by exposure to gas-phase cigarette smoke, either through depletion of cellular glutathione or by inhibition of NADPH oxidase activation. These effects also occurred when neutrophils were exposed to acrolein (Nguyen *et al.*, 2001). Subsequent experiments demonstrated that acrolein inhibits neutrophil apoptosis and that enzymes relevant to this process were either induced by acrolein, e.g. extracellular signal-regulated kinase (ERK) and p38 mitogen-activated protein kinases (p38 MAPKs), or their activation was prevented, e.g. caspase-3 (Finkelstein *et al.*, 2001). In human bronchial fibroblasts, reactive aldehydes such as acrolein have also been shown to be cytotoxic and to inhibit the DNA repair enzyme O^6-methylguanine–DNA methyltransferase, possibly by reacting with the cysteine thiol group at the active site of the enzyme; no effect on uracil–DNA glycosylase was observed (Krokan *et al.*, 1985).

The activity of aldehyde dehydrogenase (ALDH) in human blood cells *in vitro* was found to be inhibited by cigarette smoke condensate in a dose-dependent manner. This inhibition was associated with the non-volatile fraction of the condensate. The lower levels of ALDH activity observed in alcoholics could be due, in part, to smoking, as alco-holics are frequently also heavy smokers (Helander *et al.*, 1991).

Platelet-activating factor (PAF) (1-*O*-alkyl-2-acetyl-*sn*-glycero-3-phosphocholine) is a potent pro-inflammatory agent whose degradation is regulated by PAF acetyl hydrolase (PAF-AH), a plasma enzyme. The activity of this enzyme is inhibited in a dose-dependent manner by cigarette smoke extract, which may explain the increase in plasma PAF con-centration noted in smokers and may be relevant to the development of smoking-induced cardiovascular and pulmonary diseases (Miyaura *et al.*, 1992).

(c)   Biomarkers of tobacco smoke carcinogens

(i)   Urinary compounds

Urinary carcinogens and their metabolites are practical and useful biomarkers of the uptake of tobacco smoke constituents. They can provide important information about exposure to tobacco smoke carcinogens, carcinogen doses and mechanisms of carcino-genesis. The use of urinary compounds as biomarkers for investigating the links between tobacco and cancer has been reviewed (Hecht, 2002b). The structures of the compounds discussed below are illustrated in Figure 4.3.

Figure 4.3. Structures of compounds discussed in Section 4.1.1.(c)

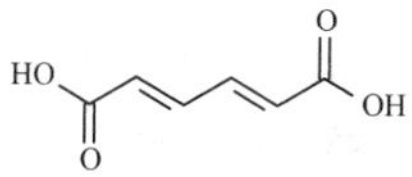

tt-MA

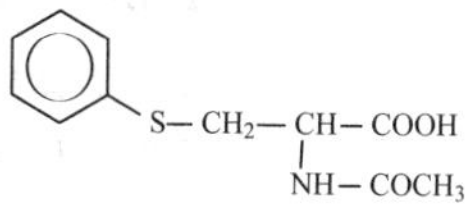

S-phenylmercapturic acid

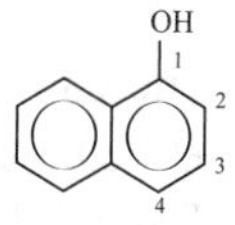

1-naphthol

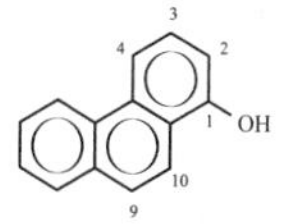

1-hydroxyphenanthrene

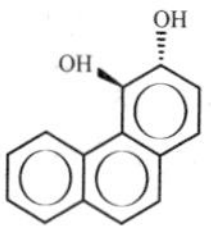

phenanthrene-3,4-dihydrodiol

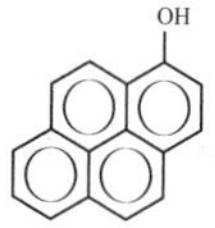

1-hydroxypyrene

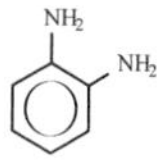

ortho-toluidine

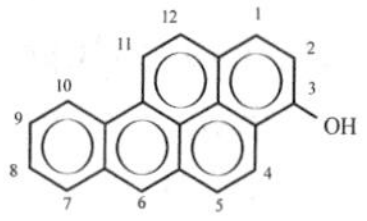

3-hydroxyB*a*P

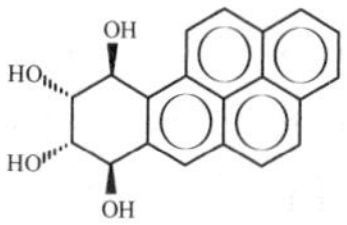

trans-anti-B*a*P-tetraol

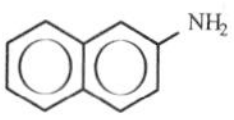

2-naphthylamine

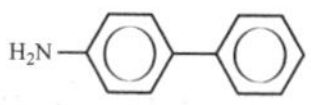

4-aminobiphenyl

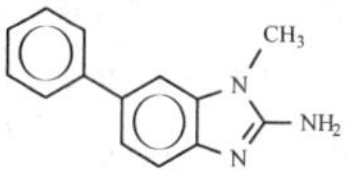

PhIP

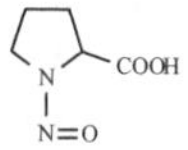

NPRO

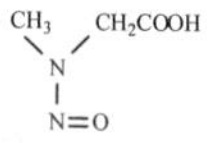

NSAR

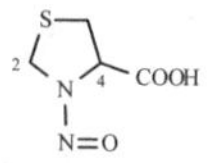

NTCA

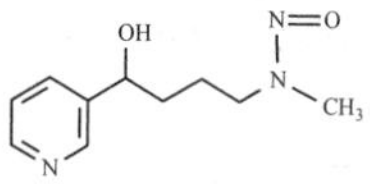

NNAL

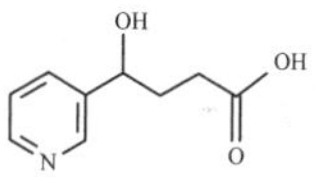

hydroxyacid
(4-hydroxy-4-(3-pyridyl)
butanoic acid)

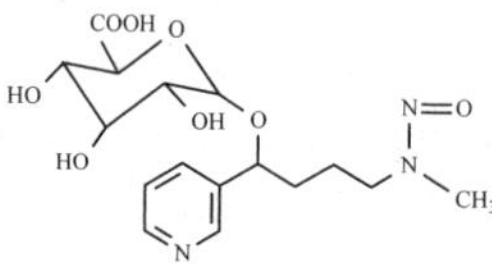

NNAL-*O*-Gluc

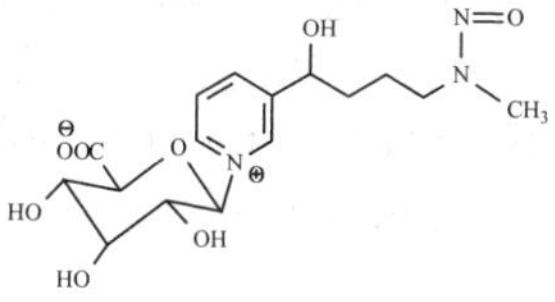

NNAL-*N*-Gluc

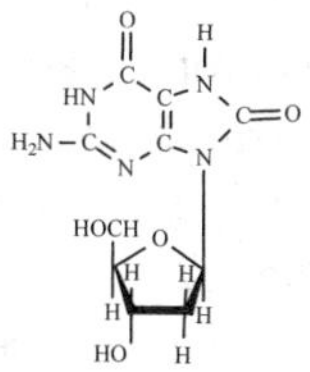

8-OHdG

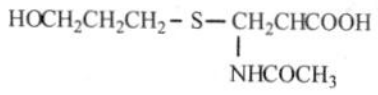

3-hydroxypropylmercapturic acid

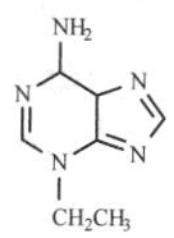

3-ethyladenine

From Hecht (2002b)

trans,trans-Muconic acid (*trans, trans*-2,4-hexadienedioic acid), *S*-phenyl-
mercapturic acid and other benzene metabolites

S-Phenylmercapturic acid (*S*-PMA) and *trans,trans*-muconic acid (*tt*-MA) are
believed to be the most sensitive biomarkers for exposure to low levels of benzene (IARC,
1982, 1987; Stommel *et al.*, 1989; van Sittert *et al.*, 1993; Boogaard & van Sittert, 1995,
1996; Qu *et al.*, 2000). A recent review has summarized the literature on this subject
(Scherer *et al.*, 1998). One pathway of benzene metabolism proceeds via ring oxidation
and ring cleavage to *trans, trans*-muconaldehyde and finally to *tt*-MA. This metabolite
has been widely used as a biomarker of benzene uptake. Significantly elevated levels of
tt-MA were found in the urine of smokers in 11 of 13 studies (Lee, B.L. *et al.*, 1993;
Melikian *et al.*, 1993; Lauwerys *et al.*, 1994; Melikian *et al.*, 1994; Ong *et al.*, 1994;
Rauscher *et al.*, 1994; Ghittori *et al.*, 1995; Ruppert *et al.*, 1995; Boogaard & van Sittert,
1996; Buratti *et al.*, 1996; Ghittori *et al.*, 1996; Kivistö *et al.*, 1997; Ruppert *et al.*, 1997).
The levels of *tt*-MA were 1.4–4.8 times higher in smokers than in nonsmokers and the
additional amount of *tt*-MA excreted by smokers ranged from 0.022 to 0.20 mg/g creatinine (Scherer *et al.*, 1998). However, sorbic acid (*trans, trans*-2,4-hexadienoic acid), a
widely used food preservative that can be transformed metabolically to *tt*-MA, can also
contribute to background levels of *tt*-MA, thereby decreasing its specificity as a benzene
biomarker (Scherer *et al.*, 1998; Pezzagno *et al.*, 1999).

S-PMA is formed by normal degradation of the glutathione conjugate of benzene
epoxide. Levels of *S*-PMA were reported to be significantly higher in smokers
(1.71 μmol/mol creatinine) than in nonsmokers (0.94 μmol/mol creatinine) whereas levels
of *tt*-MA in smokers and nonsmokers were not significantly different (Boogaard & van
Sittert, 1996).

Phenol (IARC, 1999c), hydroquinone (IARC, 1999d), catechol (IARC, 1999e) and
1,2,4-trihydroxybenzene are also urinary metabolites of benzene. Mixed results have been
obtained in studies of the relationship of the levels of these metabolites in urine to occupational exposure to benzene because background levels are high (Inoue *et al.*, 1988,
1989; Ong *et al.*, 1995, 1996; Qu *et al.*, 2000). There was no difference in levels of urinary
catechol between smokers and nonsmokers; diet being a major source of these metabolites, the contribution of smoking is comparatively small (Carmella *et al.*, 1982).

1- and 2-Naphthol

1-Naphthol and 2-naphthol (1- and 2-hydroxynaphthalenes) are metabolites of
naphthalene (IARC, 2002) that are excreted in urine as glucuronide and sulfate conjugates. The levels of these metabolites are higher in smokers than in nonsmokers (Hansen
et al., 1994; Heikkilä *et al.*, 1995; Jansen *et al.*, 1995; Andreoli *et al.*, 1999; Kim *et al.*,
1999; Yang, M. *et al.*, 1999; Nan *et al.*, 2001). For example, Nan *et al.* (2001) found levels
of 3.94 ± 1.89 μmol (geometric mean ± geometric standard deviation)/mol creatinine 2-
naphthol in smokers as opposed to 1.55 ± 2.19 μmol/mol creatinine in nonsmokers
($p < 0.01$). There is some indication that urinary naphthols may be particularly appropriate
as biomarkers of inhalation exposure to PAHs, possibly because of the high volatility of

naphthalene (Jansen *et al.*, 1995; Yang, M. *et al.*, 1999; Nan *et al.*, 2001). It has been proposed that urinary 2-naphthol is a better biomarker of inhalation exposure than urinary 1-naphthol (Nan *et al.*, 2001), because it correlated more closely with urinary cotinine level than did 1-naphthol (Yang, M. *et al.*, 1999). Levels of urinary 2-naphthol can be affected by genetic polymorphisms in carcinogen metabolizing enzymes such as *CYP2E1* and *GSTM1* (Yang, M. *et al.*, 1999; Nan *et al.*, 2001).

Polycyclic aromatic hydrocarbons

Hydroxyphenanthrenes and phenanthrene dihydrodiols

Phenanthrene (IARC, 1983b, 1987) is the simplest of the PAHs with a bay region and is a reasonable model for studies of the metabolism of carcinogenic molecules of PAHs with bay regions. Hydroxyphenanthrenes and phenanthrene dihydrodiols have been quantified in human urine. Heudorf and Angerer (2001), using high-performance liquid chromatography (HPLC) with fluorescence detection, reported highly significant differences in concentrations of 2-, 3- and 4-hydroxyphenanthrene between smokers and nonsmokers and dose–response relationships to cigarettes smoked per day, but such relationships were not found with 1-hydroxyphenanthrene. For example, the amounts of 3-hydroxyphenanthrene were 473 ± 302 ng (mean $\pm$ SD)/g creatinine in 100 smokers and 305 ± 209 ng/g creatinine in 288 nonsmokers ($p = 0.001$). Jacob *et al.* (1999) measured phenanthrene metabolites by gas chromatography–mass spectrometry (GC–MS). They found no significant differences in urinary concentrations of hydroxyphenanthrenes or phenanthrene dihydrodiols between 20 smokers and 10 nonsmokers. [The Working Group noted that the study size was small.] It should be noted that there are important sources of phenanthrene exposure other than smoking (Grimmer *et al.*, 1993; Angerer *et al.*, 1997; Grimmer *et al.*, 1997).

Jacob *et al.* (1999) found a lower ratio of phenanthrene-1,2-dihydrodiol to phenanthrene-3,4-dihydrodiol in the urine of smokers than in nonsmokers suggesting that smoking induces formation of phenanthrene-3,4-dihydrodiol via induction of P4501A2. Similar results were obtained by Heudorf and Angerer (2001) who found that the ratio of 1- plus 2-hydroxyphenanthrene to 3- plus 4-hydroxyphenanthrene decreased with increased number of cigarettes smoked per day. Both studies also reported a decreased ratio of phenanthrene metabolites to 1-hydroxypyrene with increased smoking, reflecting greater intake of pyrene than phenanthrene in smokers.

1-Hydroxypyrene

Pyrene (IARC, 1983c, 1987) is a non-carcinogenic component of all environmental mixtures of PAHs. The major urinary metabolite of pyrene is 1-hydroxypyrene glucuronide (Sithisarankul *et al.*, 1997). Jongeneelen and colleagues pioneered the development of a method for measurement of 1-hydroxypyrene in urine (Jongeneelen *et al.*, 1985). It has been measured in hundreds of studies of occupational and environmental exposure to PAHs. Several reviews of the data on the effects of smoking have been published (Jongeneelen, 1994; Van Rooij *et al.*, 1994; Levin, 1995; Heudorf & Angerer, 2001;

Jongeneelen, 2001). Most studies have measured significantly higher levels of 1-hydroxy-pyrene in smokers than in nonsmokers. Some representative data from recent investi-gations of urinary 1-hydroxypyrene are summarized in Table 4.1; these data are from non-occupationally exposed individuals. The levels of 1-hydroxypyrene in the urine of nonsmokers vary considerably and are likely to be influenced by environmental pollution and diet. In most studies, the concentrations of 1-hydroxypyrene in the urine of smokers are about twice as high as those in the urine of nonsmokers, although greater differences have been reported. These concentrations may be influenced by genetic polymorphisms in carcinogen metabolizing enzymes (Alexandrie et al., 2000; Nerurkar et al., 2000; Nan et al., 2001; van Delft et al., 2001).

Table 4.1. 1-Hydroxypyrene in the urine of smokers and nonsmokers: selected recent studies

Level of 1-hydroxypyrene[a]		Increase[b]	Reference
Nonsmoker	Smoker		
0.233 µg/g C[c]	0.408 µg/g C	1.8-fold	Roggi et al. (1997)
0.55 nmol/L urine	1.04 nmol/L urine	1.9-fold	Sithisarankul et al. (1997)
0.89 µmol/mol C	0.176 µmol/mol C (< 15 cig/day)	2.0-fold	Merlo et al. (1998)
	0.226 µmol/mol C (> 15 cig/day)	2.5-fold	
21.8 µg/24 h	60.3 µg/24 h	2.8-fold	Jacob et al. (1999)
0.25 µg/L urine	0.54 µg/L urine	2.3-fold	Pastorelli et al. (1999)
0.10 µmol/mol C[d]	0.17 µmol/mol C[d]	1.7-fold	Alexandrie et al. (2000)
0.02 µmol/mol C[d]	0.04 µmol/mol C[d]	2.0-fold	Dor et al. (2000)
0.04 µmol/mol C	0.20 µmol/mol C (light)	50.0-fold	Li, H. et al. (2000)
(average)	0.46 µmol/mol C (medium)	11.5-fold	
	1.16 µmol/mol C (heavy)	29.0-fold	
0.27 nmol/12 h	0.51 nmol/12 h	1.9-fold	Nerurkar et al. (2000)
0.157 µg/24 h	0.346 µg/24 h	2.2-fold	Scherer et al. (2000)
0.27 µmol/mol C	0.70 µmol/mol C	2.6-fold	van Delft et al. (2001)
0.03 µmol/mol C	0.05 µmol/mol C	1.7-fold	Kim, H. et al. (2001)
0.04 µmol/mol C[e]	0.05 µmol/mol C[e]	1.3-fold	Nan et al. (2001)
0.11 µmol/mol C	0.57 µmol/mol C	5.2-fold	Szaniszló & Ungváry (2001)

[a] Arithmetic mean unless otherwise stated
[b] All increases statistically significant, except for that in the study of Nan et al. (2001)
[c] C, creatinine
[d] Median
[e] Geometric mean

Benzo[a]pyrene metabolites

The concentrations of benzo[a]pyrene in cigarette smoke are quite low. In laboratory animals its metabolites are excreted mainly in the faeces. Therefore, benzo[a]pyrene metabolites are difficult to quantify in the urine of smokers.

3-Hydroxybenzo[*a*]pyrene is a major metabolite of benzo[*a*]pyrene *in vitro* and is excreted in urine as its glucuronide. Several methods for quantitation of 3-hydroxybenzo-[*a*]pyrene in human urine have been described (Grimmer *et al.*, 1997; Gündel & Angerer, 2000; Simon *et al.*, 2000). In occupationally exposed workers, the levels reported are quite low, ranging from about 1 to 14 (median value) ng/L urine. Limited data are available on the levels of 3-hydroxybenzo[*a*]pyrene in smokers. One small study reported 0.1–0.8 ng/L urine in three smokers as opposed to < 0.1–0.2 ng/L in three nonsmokers (Simon *et al.*, 2000). In workers in China occupationally exposed to coal smoke, elevated levels of 3-hydroxybenzo[*a*]pyrene and 9-hydroxybenzo[*a*]pyrene have been reported in the urine (Mumford *et al.*, 1995).

r-7,*t*-8,9,*c*-10-Tetrahydroxy-7,8,9,10-tetrahydrobenzo[*a*]pyrene (*trans-anti*-BaP-tetraol) is a hydrolysis product of *r*-7,*t*-8-dihydroxy-*t*-9,10-epoxy-7,8,9,10-tetrahydro-benzo[*a*]pyrene, the major established ultimate carcinogenic metabolite of benzo[*a*]-pyrene. This metabolite has been quantified in the urine of psoriasis patients treated with a coal-tar ointment and in coke-oven workers and smokers. Concentrations of *trans-anti*-BaP-tetraol in the urine of smokers were lower than in the other two groups, ranging from not detected to 0.2 fmol/μmol creatinine. It was detected in urine samples of nine out of 21 smokers (Simpson *et al.*, 2000).

Benzo[*a*]pyrene metabolites can be converted to benzo[*a*]pyrene by treatment with hydrogen iodide. This reaction has been employed as the basis for a technique to deter-mine urinary metabolites of benzo[*a*]pyrene and several other PAHs (Becher & Bjørseth, 1983; Becher *et al.*, 1984; Venier *et al.*, 1985; Haugen *et al.*, 1986; Buckley *et al.*, 1995). In individuals who were not exposed occupationally, the concentrations of benzo[*a*]-pyrene measured by this method ranged from 4 to 19 ng/mmol creatinine in nonsmokers (*n* = 5) and 18 to 102 ng/mmol creatinine in smokers (*n* = 4) (Becher *et al.*, 1984). The disadvantages of this method include different conversion rates for various metabolites and low analytical recoveries (Buckley *et al.*, 1995).

The presence of an unstable benzo[*a*]pyrene–DNA adduct, 7-(benzo[*a*]pyren-6-yl)-adenine, was reported in the urine of three out of seven smokers and measured in one as 0.6 fmol/mg creatinine (the concentrations were not quantifiable in the other two smokers) (Casale *et al.*, 2001).

Aromatic amines and heterocyclic aromatic amines

Aromatic amines, but not their metabolites, have been quantified in human urine. In one study, smokers excreted 6.3 ± 3.7 μg/24 h 2-toluidine (*ortho*-toluidine, see IARC, 2000), whereas the concentrations in the urine of nonsmokers were 4.1 ± 3.2 μg/24 h, a non-significant difference (El Bayoumy *et al.*, 1986). Another investigation reported higher concentrations of *ortho*-toluidine in the urine of smokers than in that of non-smokers (0.6 and 0.4 ng/L urine, respectively) (Riffelmann *et al.*, 1995). There appear to be important sources of human uptake of *ortho*-toluidine other than cigarette smoke. Smokers excreted amounts of 4-ABP (78.6 ± 85.2 ng/24 h) similar to those measured in nonsmokers (68.1 ± 91.5 ng/24 h) and the amounts of 2-aminonaphthalene (2-naphthylamine) (IARC, 1974, 1987) excreted by smokers (84.5 ± 102.7 ng/24 h) and nonsmokers (120.8 ± 279.2 ng/24 h) were also similar (Grimmer et al., 2000).

DNA adducts have been detected by ^{32}P-postlabelling in urinary bladder biopsies and in exfoliated urothelial cells isolated from the urine of smokers and nonsmokers. At least four adducts may have been related to smoking, one of which was qualitatively similar to the N-(deoxyguanosin-8-yl)-4-aminobiphenyl adduct (Talaska et al., 1991a,b).

Of the heterocyclic aromatic amines found in cigarette smoke, analyses of urinary metabolites have been carried out on only one, 2-amino-1-methyl-6-phenylimidazo-[4,5-b]pyridine (PhIP) (IARC, 1993a) (reviewed in Kulp et al., 2000). Most studies have focused on the effects of diet, but one found no effect of smoking on levels of PhIP in urine, after adjustment for ethnicity (Kidd et al., 1999).

N-Nitrosamines

N-*Nitrosoproline (IARC, 1978b, 1987) and other nitrosamino acids*

Ohshima and Bartsch (1981) demonstrated that N-nitrosoproline (NPRO) could be formed endogenously in humans after the ingestion of proline and nitrate. This finding led to the development of a test for endogenous nitrosation by measurement of NPRO in the urine of people who had ingested proline and nitrate, or proline alone with or without ascorbic acid, an inhibitor of nitrosation (Bartsch et al., 1989). The test is safe because NPRO is not metabolized and has not been shown to be carcinogenic. The NPRO test has been applied in several studies designed to compare endogenous nitrosation between smokers and nonsmokers. The results indicate that endogenous formation of NPRO occurs in smokers, and that thiocyanate catalysis may be important (Bartsch et al., 1989; Tsuda & Kurashima, 1991; Tricker, 1997). However, mixed results have been obtained in population-based studies (Tricker, 1997).

Several other nitrosamino acids are present in human urine. The major ones are N-nitrososarcosine (NSAR) (IARC, 1978c), N-nitrosothiazolidine 4-carboxylic acid (N-nitrosothioproline) (NTCA) and trans- and cis- isomers of N-nitroso-2-methylthiazolidine 4-carboxylic acid (NMTCA) (Bartsch et al., 1989; Tsuda & Kurashima, 1991). NTCA and NMTCA are formed by the reaction of formaldehyde or acetaldehyde with cysteine, followed by nitrosation. Some studies have demonstrated increased concentrations of urinary NTCA and NMTCA in smokers (Tsuda & Kurashima, 1991). Total nitrosamino acids correlated with urinary nicotine plus cotinine in smokers (Malaveille et al., 1989), but mixed results have been obtained in other studies (Tricker, 1997). Collectively, the available data support the concept that higher concentrations of nitrosamines can be formed endogenously in smokers than in nonsmokers under some conditions.

4-(N-nitrosomethylamino)-4-(3-pyridyl)butyric acid (iso-NNAC) was suggested as a potential monitor of the endogenous nitrosation of nicotine (Djordjevic et al., 1991). iso-NNAC was found in the urine of four of 20 cigarette smokers (at levels of 44, 65, 74 and 163 ng/day). However, no evidence for its formation after the oral administration of nicotine or cotinine to abstinent smokers could be found (Tricker et al., 1993).

Volatile nitrosamines

Low-molecular-weight nitrosamines such as NDMA and *N*-nitrosopyrrolidine (NPYR) (see IARC, 1978d, 1987) are extensively metabolized, but small amounts of the unchanged compounds have been quantified in urine (Tricker, 1997). One investigation found that smokers excreted higher levels of NDMA than nonsmokers (Conney *et al.*, 1986), but two other studies reported no effect of smoking on the amounts of volatile nitrosamines in urine (Mostafa *et al.*, 1994; van Maanen *et al.*, 1996).

4-(N-Nitrosomethylamino)-1-(3-pyridyl)-1-butanol, its glucuronides and other metabolites of 4-(N-nitrosomethylamino)-1-(3-pyridyl)-1-butanone (see Figure 4.1)

4-(*N*-Nitrosomethyl(amino)-1-(3-pyridyl)-1-butanol (NNAL), like NNK, is a pulmonary carcinogen with particularly strong activity in the rat (Hecht, 1998). Glucuronidation of NNAL at the pyridine nitrogen gives NNAL-*N*-Gluc while conjugation at the carbinol oxygen yields NNAL-*O*-Gluc (Carmella *et al.*, 2002). NNAL-*N*-Gluc and NNAL-*O*-Gluc both exist as a mixture of two diastereomers and each diastereomer is a mixture of *S*- and *R*-rotamers (Upadhyaya *et al.*, 2001). The NNAL glucuronides are collectively referred to as NNAL-Gluc.

NNAL and NNAL-Gluc can readily be determined in urine by gas chromatography–thermal energy analysis (GC–TEA) with nitrosamine-selective detection (Carmella *et al.*, 1993, 1995; Hecht *et al.*, 1999a). The presence of these metabolites in human urine has also been established by mass spectrometry methods, but these are less convenient and sensitive than GC–TEA (Carmella *et al.*, 1993; Parsons *et al.*, 1998; Carmella *et al.*, 1999; Hecht *et al.*, 2001). The amounts typically excreted are about 1 nmol NNAL/24 h and 2.2 nmol NNAL-Gluc/24 h (Hecht *et al.*, 1999a); unchanged NNK is not detected. The investigations of NNAL and NNAL-Gluc in the urine of smokers are summarized in Table 4.2. In all studies to date, these biomarkers have been found to be absolutely specific to tobacco exposure and have not been detected in the urine of nonsmokers unless they had been exposed to secondhand tobacco smoke. Because NNAL is not present in cigarette smoke (see Section 1), the NNAL and NNAL-Gluc in urine originate from the metabolism of NNK. Most investigations to date have demonstrated a correlation between NNAL plus NNAL-Gluc and cotinine. The ratio of NNAL-Gluc:NNAL varies at least 10-fold in smokers and, because NNAL-Gluc is a detoxification product of NNK whereas NNAL is carcinogenic, this ratio could be a potential indicator of cancer risk (Carmella *et al.*, 1995; Richie *et al.*, 1997). In human urine, (*R*)-NNAL-*O*-Gluc is the predominant diastereomer of NNAL-*O*-Gluc (68%) whereas (*R*)-NNAL is only slightly in excess (54%) over (*S*)-NNAL (Carmella *et al.*, 1999). (*R*)-NNAL is the more tumorigenic enantiomer of NNAL in A/J mouse lung in which it is as tumorigenic as NNK (Upadhyaya *et al.*, 1999). NNAL and NNAL-Gluc are released only slowly from the human body after smoking cessation (Hecht *et al.*, 1999a) and this finding has been linked to the particularly strong retention of (*S*)-NNAL (Upadhyaya *et al.*, 1999) [possibly at a receptor site].

Table 4.2. 4-(*N*-Nitrosomethylamino)-1-(3-pyridyl)-1-butanol (NNAL) and its glucuronides (NNAL-Gluc) in urine of smokers: biomarkers of 4-(*N*-nitroso-methylamino)-1-(3-pyridyl)-1-butanone (NNK) uptake

Study group	Main findings	Reference
11 smokers (9F)[a] 7 nonsmokers	NNAL (0.23–1 µg/24 h (1.1–4.8 nmol/24 h)) and 2 diastereomers of NNAL-*O*-Gluc (0.57–6.5 µg/24 h (1.5–17 nmol/24 h)) identified in urine of smokers, NNAL-GluC in 1/7[b] nonsmokers' urine. NNK not detected	Carmella *et al.* (1993)
61 smokers (31F)	NNAL and NNAL-*O*-Gluc: day-to-day levels stable in smokers' urine; NNAL-Gluc: NNAL ratios fairly stable, over a 4–5 day period; range of NNAL-Gluc:NNAL ratios 0.7–10.8	Carmella *et al.* (1995)
11 smokers (6F)	NNAL + NNAL-*O*-Gluc increased by 33.5% (*p* < 0.01) on days 2 and 3 when watercress was consumed compared with baseline period	Hecht *et al.* (1995)
19 smokers	NNAL-Gluc:NNAL ratio and NNAL plus NNAL-Gluc fairly stable over a 2-year period in one individual	Meger *et al.* (1996)
61 smokers (33F)	NNAL-Gluc:NNAL ratio higher in Caucasians than African Americans	Richie *et al.* (1997)
13 smokers (F)	Indole-3-carbinol caused significant decreases in levels of NNAL and NNAL-Gluc and increased NNAL-Gluc: NNAL ratio	Taioli *et al.* (1997)
30 smokers (18F)	Enantiomeric distribution of NNAL, 54% (*R*-NNAL); diastereomeric distribution of NNAL-Gluc, 68% (*R*-NNAL)	Carmella *et al.* (1999)
27 smokers (13F)	NNAL and NNAL-Gluc highly persistent after smoking cessation: 34.5% of baseline amount remained after 1 week, 15.3% after 3 weeks. No effect of nicotine patch use on levels or persistence of NNAL or NNAL-Gluc	Hecht *et al.* (1999a)
23 smokers (13F)	Reduction in smoking caused a significant decrease in NNAL-Gluc, but not NNAL	Hurt *et al.* (2000)
20 smokers (M)	Levels of NNAL and NNAL-Gluc were 1494 ± 1090 and 1724 ± 946 pmol/day (mean ± SD), respectively[c]	Meger *et al.* (2000)
10 smokers (4 F)	NNAL-*N*-Gluc identified in urine, comprises 50 ± 25% of total NNAL-Gluc	Carmella *et al.* (2002)

[a] Number and letter in parentheses represent number and sex of subjects; F, female; M, male
[b] One nonsmoker appeared to excrete NNAL-*O*-Gluc (~0.7 µg/24 h); the urine of all the other non-smokers were negative.
[c] [In the original paper, numbers given in the text and table were different; data given in the text are reported here.]

In rodents, NNK and NNAL undergo metabolic oxidation at the pyridine nitrogen giving NNK-*N*-oxide and NNAL-*N*-oxide, respectively. Both metabolites are less tumorigenic in rodents than NNK and NNAL (Hecht, 1998; Upadhyaya *et al.*, 1999). In humans, analysis of the urine of smokers for NNAL-*N*-oxide found that it was present at lower concentrations than NNAL; NNK-*N*-oxide was not detected in the urine of smokers. Thus, pyridine-*N*-oxidation is a relatively minor detoxification pathway of NNK and NNAL in humans (Carmella *et al.*, 1997).

4-Hydroxy-4-(3-pyridyl)butanoic acid (hydroxy acid) and 4-oxo-4-(3-pyridyl)butanoic acid (keto acid) are metabolites of NNK resulting from the α-hydroxylation metabolic activation pathway. These metabolites were investigated as potential biomarkers of NNK metabolic activation in humans, but they are also formed from nicotine, which is 1400–13 000 times more abundant in cigarette smoke than is NNK. Since hydroxy acid is chiral, it was thought possible that one enantiomer would be formed preferentially from NNK, whereas the other would be produced from nicotine. Studies in rats demonstrated that this was plausible (Trushin & Hecht, 1999). However, hydroxy acid is a more abundant nicotine metabolite in humans than in rats and consequently even the minor enantiomer, as formed from nicotine, was far greater in concentration than that which would be produced from NNK. Because of the abundant metabolism of nicotine to hydroxy acid and keto acid (see Section 4.1.1.e), these metabolites cannot be used as biomarkers of tobacco-specific nitrosamine metabolism in humans (Hecht *et al.*, 1999b; Trushin & Hecht, 1999).

Products of oxidative DNA damage

Cigarette smoke contains free radicals and induces oxidative damage (Pryor, 1997; Arora *et al.*, 2001). The gas phase of freshly generated cigarette smoke contains large amounts of nitric oxide (NO) and other unstable oxidants. The particulate phase is postulated to contain long-lived radicals which are an equilibrium mixture of semiquinones, quinones and hydroquinones that causes redox cycling (Pryor, 1997; Hecht, 1999). The presence of such free radicals and oxidants can lead to oxidative DNA damage resulting in the formation of products such as 8-oxo-7,8-dihydro-2′-deoxyguanosine (8-oxodG)[1], [8-hydroxy-2′-deoxyguanosine (8-OHdG)], thymine glycol, thymidine glycol and 5-hydroxymethyluracil. Repair of these modified DNA constituents ultimately leads to their being excreted in urine. 8-OHdG has been quantified frequently in the urine of smokers and nonsmokers and the results have been reviewed. Cigarette smoking usually results in modest increases in the levels of 8-OHdG in urine; 16–50% higher than those in non-smokers, although negative results have also been reported (Loft & Poulsen, 1998; Priemé *et al.*, 1998; Renner *et al.*, 2000; Besarati Nia *et al.*, 2001). Four weeks of smoking cessation caused a decrease in the excretion of 8-OHdG by 21% (Priemé *et al.*, 1998). A longitudinal study showed that intra-individual variation in the levels of urinary 8-OHdG

---

[1] There is an equilibrium (50–90%) between 8-oxo-dG and 8-OHdG. The compound will be called 8-OHdG throughout this document.

was greater than the increase due to smoking, suggesting that there may be a complex pattern of factors determining the levels of this biomarker in urine (Kasai *et al.*, 2001; Pilger *et al.*, 2001). No effect of smoking on urinary concentrations of 5-hydroxymethyl-uracil was observed (Pourcelot *et al.*, 1999).

Thioethers and mercapturic acids

Conjugation of electrophiles with glutathione ultimately results in the excretion of mercapturic acids (*N*-acetylcysteine conjugates) in the urine (van Doorn *et al.*, 1979, 1981). A method for determination of total thioethers in urine has been applied in nume-rous studies comparing smokers and nonsmokers reviewed by van Doorn *et al.* (1981), IARC (1986) and Scherer *et al.* (1996). Cigarette smokers excrete significantly higher levels of thioethers in urine than nonsmokers. There is considerable interindividual varia-tion when diet, a major source of sulfur-containing compounds, is not controlled (Aringer & Lidums, 1988; Scherer *et al.*, 1996). The assay of total thioethers in urine provides no information about the structure of the electrophiles which are ultimately detected in urine as conjugates.

More specific methods have been applied to investigate the presence of mercapturic acids in human urine (Scherer *et al.*, 2001a). 3-Hydroxypropylmercapturic acid, a likely detoxification product of acrolein, has been detected in the urine of smokers (Mascher *et al.*, 2001).

Alkyladenines and alkylguanines

Reaction of alkylating agents with DNA results in the formation of alkyladenines and alkylguanines among other products (Singer & Grunberger, 1983). Alkylation at the 3-position of deoxyadenosine or at the 7-position of deoxyguanosine weakens the glyco-sidic bond, which readily breaks either spontaneously or is cleaved by glycosylases, ulti-mately resulting in the excretion of 3-alkyladenines and 7-alkylguanines in urine. 3-Alkyladenines have been more extensively investigated as biomarkers of exposure to alkylating agents than 7-alkylguanines because background levels in urine are expected to be lower. However, substantial amounts of 3-methyladenine occur in the diet (Prévost *et al.*, 1993; Fay *et al.*, 1997). Nevertheless, two controlled studies have demonstrated increased excretion of 3-methyladenine in the urine of smokers compared with that of nonsmokers (Kopplin *et al.*, 1995; Prévost & Shuker, 1996). Background levels of 3-ethyladenine are lower than those of 3-methyladenine (Prévost *et al.*, 1993). Two studies demonstrated convincing increases in urinary concentrations of 3-ethyladenine in smokers, indicating the presence in cigarette smoke of an unidentified ethylating agent (Kopplin *et al.*, 1995; Prévost & Shuker, 1996). There was no effect of smoking on the concentration of 3-(2-hydroxyethyl)adenine in urine (Prévost & Shuker, 1996). One popu-lation-based study found greater amounts of both 3-methyladenine and 7-methylguanine in the urine of smokers than of nonsmokers (Stillwell *et al.*, 1991) while a second found no difference between 3-methyladenine concentrations in smokers and nonsmokers (Shuker *et al.*, 1991).

Metals

Large studies in Germany and the USA demonstrated that urinary cadmium increased with age and smoking (Hoffmann *et al.*, 2000; Paschal *et al.*, 2000). The study in the USA involved 22 162 participants in the Third National Health and Nutrition Examination survey (NHANES III 1988–94), and urine cadmium, expressed either as uncorrected (µg/L) or creatinine corrected (µg/g creatinine), increased with age and smoking (Paschal *et al.*, 2000). The German study, involving 4021 adults, found that active cigarette smoking was the predominant factor affecting cadmium concentrations in the blood and urine of adults. Environmental and occupational exposure to cadmium played only a minor role (Hoffmann *et al.*, 2000). These results are consistent with those of other studies of cadmium uptake in smokers (IARC, 1993b). The limited data available do not indicate consistent significant differences in levels of urinary nickel (IARC, 1990a), chromium (IARC, 1990b), or lead (IARC, 1980, 1987) between smokers and nonsmokers (Morimoto *et al.*, 1977; Schaller & Zober, 1982; Minoia *et al.*, 1988; Jin *et al.*, 1997; Huang *et al.*, 2000).

Conclusion

Representative levels (nmol/24 h) of eight urinary biomarkers discussed here are summarized in Table 4.3. The amounts of these compounds in urine are generally proportional to the levels of their parent compounds in cigarette smoke, with the possible exception of 8-OHdG and 3-ethyladenine, the precursors for which are not known. It should be noted that there are a number of established tobacco smoke carcinogens for which no urinary biomarkers have been validated. Examples include formaldehyde, acetaldehyde, 1,3-butadiene (IARC, 1999f), ethylene oxide and vinyl chloride (IARC, 1979, 1987; Hoffmann *et al.*, 2001).

Of the urinary biomarkers discussed here, the following are consistently higher in smokers than in nonsmokers: *tt*-MA, *S*-PMA, 1-naphthol, 2-naphthol, 1-hydroxypyrene, NNAL and NNAL-Gluc, 8-OHdG, 3-ethyladenine and cadmium. For all of these biomarkers, analytical methods with the requisite sensitivity and specificity are available, but only NNAL and NNAL-Gluc have high specificity as biomarkers of exposure to tobacco smoking because sources other than tobacco smoke, including environmental, dietary and occupational exposure, can contribute to the urinary concentration of the other possible biomarkers. Because NNAL and NNAL-Gluc are metabolites of the tobacco-specific nitrosamine NNK, they are not found in the urine of nonsmokers unless they have been exposed to environmental tobacco smoke (see the monograph on involuntary smoking, this volume). It is possible that other sources, such as nicotine replacement products, could, under certain conditions, contribute to the concentrations of urinary NNAL and NNAL-Gluc but this has not been demonstrated to date (Hecht *et al.*, 2000). Levels of NNAL plus NNAL-Gluc of less than 1 pmol/mL of urine have seldom been observed in smokers whereas the highest levels in nonsmokers exposed to environmental tobacco smoke seldom exceed 0.4 pmol/mL (Hecht *et al.*, 2001; Hecht, 2002b).

Table 4.3. Representative concentrations of biomarkers in urine of smokers

Biomarker	Amount: nmol/24h[a]	Precursor (see Section 1) [ng/cigarette smoke][a]	Reference
tt-MA	[1100] (153 µg/24 h)	[6000–70 000]; r = 0.65[b]	Scherer et al. (2001b)
2-Naphthol	[73[c]] (7.03 ng/mL) (8.49 µmol/mol creatinine)	[2000–4000]	Kim et al. (1999)
3-Hydroxyphenanthrene	[3.1] (598 ng/24 h)	[85–620]	Jacob et al. (1999)
1-Hydroxypyrene	1.6 (0.35 µg/24 h)	[50–270]	Scherer et al. (2000); Hecht (2002b)
trans-anti-BaP-tetraol	[0.0008] (0.5 fmol/mL)	[9]	Simpson et al. (2000)
NNAL + NNAL-Gluc	3.2[d]	[100–200]	Hecht et al. (1999a)
8-OHdG	25	?	Pilger et al. (2001)
3-Ethyladenine	[0.85] (16–139 ng/24 h)	?	Kopplin et al. (1995)

[a] [ ], Calculated by the Working Group, on the basis of data given in the cited reference;
[b] tt-MA excretion was significantly correlated with the number of cigarettes smoked per day.
[c] Estimate based on 1.5 L urine excreted per day
[d] NNAL/24 h = 944 pmol; NNAL-Gluc/24 h = 2200 pmol; NNAL + NNAL-Gluc = 3144 pmol/24 h = 3.2 nmol/24 h; correlation with nicotine, r = 0.44
tt-MA, trans,trans-muconic acid; BaP, benzo[a]pyrene; NNAL, 4-(N-nitrosomethylamino)-1-(3-pyridyl)-1-butanol; NNAL-Gluc, NNAL glucuronide; 8-OHdG, 8-hydroxy-2′-deoxyguanosine; ?, unknown

(ii) Protein adducts in human tissues (blood)

Although proteins are not the target molecules for mutagenic events, protein modifications can be useful biomarkers because of the greater abundance of proteins than of DNA and the fact that protein modifications are not subject to enzymatic repair. The rate of turnover of the proteins and/or of the cells that harbour them implies that carcinogen–protein adducts can provide evidence of exposure on a time-scale of up to several months. In theory, haemoglobin, serum albumin, histones and collagen are suitable proteins to study for this purpose (Skipper et al., 1994), but in practice only haemoglobin and albumin have been extensively studied as biomarkers of human exposure to environmental carcinogens.

Protein adducts are generally detected in one of three ways:

— mass spectrometric detection of the carcinogen moiety after its release from protein by mild acid or base hydrolysis, or release and detection of the modified N-terminal valine of haemoglobin;

— immunochemical analysis using antibodies raised against protein adducts; and

— HPLC with fluorescence detection of the released carcinogen (Phillips & Farmer, 1995).

The use of protein adducts as biomarkers of human exposure to carcinogens has been extensively reviewed elsewhere (Strickland *et al.*, 1993; Skipper *et al.*, 1994; Wild & Pisani, 1998; Poirier *et al.*, 2000).

The entire literature on smoking-related protein and DNA adducts in human tissues has been produced since the previous IARC evaluation of tobacco smoking (IARC, 1986). These studies are summarized below.

Adducts formed by aromatic amines

In an early study of 22 smokers and 24 nonsmokers, 4-ABP–haemoglobin adducts[1] were measured by GC–MS. The adduct levels of smokers were significantly higher than those of nonsmokers and there was a significant correlation with average number of packs smoked per day. It is noteworthy that the range of values for smokers (75–256 pg/g haemoglobin) did not overlap with that for nonsmokers (7–51 pg/g) (Perera *et al.*, 1987). The absence of overlap was also reported in another study involving 19 smokers (mean, 154 pg/g) and 26 nonsmokers (mean 28 pg/g); the difference between the two groups was highly significant ($p < 0.001$). The finding of detectable levels of adducts in all the non-smokers is consistent with the existence of environmental sources of 4-ABP other than tobacco smoking (Bryant *et al.*, 1987).

In a group of male volunteers from a case–control study of bladder cancer in Turin, Italy (Vineis *et al.*, 1984), haemoglobin adducts of 15 different aromatic amines were measured in nonsmokers and in smokers of blond- or black-tobacco cigarettes. The smokers of blond tobacco ($n = 40$) and black tobacco ($n = 18$), and three subjects who smoked both types, had significantly higher levels of 4-ABP adducts than 25 nonsmokers. Furthermore, adduct levels were significantly higher (40–50%) for smokers of black tobacco (mean, 288 pg/g) than for those of blond tobacco (mean, 176 pg/g). Adduct levels were found to be correlated with amount smoked per day for all smokers ($p = 0.0015$) and this correlation was also significant for smoking blond tobacco only ($p = 0.0074$). Of other aromatic amines, the levels of 3-ABP adducts were also significantly elevated in smokers ($p < 0.0001$) and associated with numbers of cigarettes smoked by the blond tobacco users ($p = 0.02$). The levels of adducts derived from a further five aromatic amines, 2-naphthylamine, *ortho*-toluidine, *para*-toluidine, 2-ethylaniline and 2,4-di-methylaniline, were significantly higher in the smokers, while those of *meta*-toluidine, 2,5-, 2,6-, 2,3-, 3,5- and 3,4-dimethylaniline and 3- and 4-ethylaniline were not (Bryant *et al.*, 1988). In a subsequent analysis, the authors sought explanations for variability observed between individuals. There appeared to be a distinct difference between the levels measured for the binuclear compounds and those obtained with the mononuclear compounds. Correlations between the levels of the three binuclear amines (2-naphthyl-amine, 4-ABP and 3-ABP) were significant ($p < 0.05$) and 49/54 of the correlations

---

[1] [Aminobiphenyls in tobacco have been implicated in bladder cancer etiology in smokers. 3- and 4-ABP–haemoglobin adduct levels are considered valid biomarkers of the internal dose of ABP to the bladder (Probst-Hensch *et al.*, 2000).]

between different mononuclear amines were significant, but only 2/33 correlations between a binuclear and a mononuclear amine were significant. These results suggest the existence of two distinct pathways of metabolic activation of aromatic amines and explain a part, but not all, of the interindividual variation in adduct levels observed (Ronco et al., 1990).

As part of a validation exercise in a study of 4- and 3-ABP–haemoglobin adducts in nonsmokers exposed to secondhand smoke (see the monograph on involuntary smoking, this volume), seven smokers who quit were monitored on the day they stopped smoking and again at least 2 months later. The mean levels of 4-ABP adducts fell by 75% from 130.4 pg/g at baseline to 33.3 pg/g and the mean level of 3-ABP fell by at least 80% (from 16.0 pg/g to a baseline of 1.7 pg/g) (in four cases levels of 3-ABP fell below the limit of sensitivity of the assay) (Maclure et al., 1989). A further study of smokers enrolled at a cessation clinic found that the 34 subjects starting the programme had a mean level of 4-ABP–haemoglobin of 120 ± 7 (SE) pg/g which declined to 82 ± 6 pg/g after 3 weeks. In the 15 smokers who remained abstinent after 2 months, the level was 34 ± 5 pg/g. The rate of decline was slightly more rapid than would be expected from the assumption that erythrocytes have a lifespan of 120 days. There was little correlation between plasma cotinine levels and haemoglobin adducts (Maclure et al., 1990). Similar findings were reported from another study of smoking cessation. The mean level of haemoglobin adducts at baseline was four-fold higher than the mean value 8 months later. Depending on the model used, the half-life of the adducts was estimated to be 7–12 weeks (Mooney et al., 1995).

In a study of 50 nonsmokers, 31 smokers of blond tobacco, 16 smokers of black tobacco and three pipe smokers, the relationship between smoking blond or black tobacco and 4-ABP–haemoglobin adduct levels was confirmed ($p = 0.0001$ in both tests). A linear relationship between adduct levels and the numbers of cigarettes smoked in the preceding 24 h was also observed. Furthermore, when the subjects were divided into slow and rapid acetylators (by measuring their urinary excretion of caffeine after administration of a test dose), it was found that the ratio of adduct levels in slow acetylators to that in rapid acetylators was 1.6 for nonsmokers, 1.3 for blond-tobacco smokers and 1.5 for black-tobacco smokers. This approximates to the estimated relative risk of the slow acetylator phenotype for bladder cancer of 1.3 (95% CI, 1.0–1.7) (Evans, 1986; Vineis et al., 1990). A further study of this group, as well as confirming these findings, also found that urinary mutagenicity was associated with the number of cigarettes smoked, but not with the acetylator phenotype (Bartsch et al., 1990). Subsequently, 4-ABP–haemoglobin adduct levels in 21 nonsmokers, 11 blond-tobacco smokers and seven black-tobacco smokers were found to correlate with the total amount of DNA adducts in exfoliated urothelial cells ($p = 0.03$) (Talaska et al., 1991b).

In a case–control study of lung cancer with 53 cases (23 smokers) and 56 controls (18 smokers) (33 with non-cancer pulmonary disease and 23 with non-pulmonary cancer), levels of 4-ABP–haemoglobin adducts were higher in smokers than in nonsmokers and reflected recent exposure to tobacco smoke. There was no association between adduct levels and lung cancer (Weston *et al.*, 1991). [The control group may have biased the results.] However, in a case–control study of bladder cancer, the mean adduct level in the cases (n = 13, all smokers) was significantly higher than in the controls (n = 13, all smokers) (103 ± 47 [SD] and 65 ± 44 pg/g haemoglobin, respectively; p = 0.04) (Del Santo *et al.*, 1991).

The levels of 4-ABP-haemoglobin adducts were also significantly higher in pregnant women who smoked (n = 15) than in those who did not (n = 40) (183 ± 108 and 22 ± 8 pg/g haemoglobin; $p < 0.001$), respectively, in a study in which levels of the adduct in fetal blood were also measured (see the monograph on involuntary smoking, this volume) (Coghlin *et al.*, 1991). Similarly, a study of 74 nonsmokers and an equal number of smokers measured paired maternal–fetal blood samples. The levels of 4-ABP-haemoglobin adducts were significantly higher in the smokers, and the ratios of adduct levels in maternal and fetal cord blood were found to be similar to those reported in the previous study. There was also a correlation between adduct levels in maternal blood and number of cigarettes smoked per day (Myers *et al.*, 1996).

In another study comparing 27 pregnant women who smoked with 78 who did not, significantly higher levels of haemoglobin adducts of 3-ABP ($p < 0.001$), 4-ABP ($p < 0.001$), *ortho*-toluidine ($p < 0.001$), *para*-toluidine ($p < 0.001$) and 2,4-dimethylaniline ($p < 0.05$) were found in smokers than in nonsmokers (Branner *et al.*, 1998).

A study of smokers and nonsmokers, in which an analysis of the haemoglobin adducts of several aromatic amines was made, revealed significantly higher levels in smokers of those adducts formed by 4-ABP ($p < 0.001$), 3-ABP ($p < 0.001$) and 2,4-dimethylaniline ($p < 0.05$), but not of those formed by aniline, *ortho*-toluidine, *meta*-toluidine, *para*-toluidine, 2-ethylaniline or *ortho*-anisidine (IARC, 1999g). For many of these comparisons, the number of subjects was small (4–22 smokers, 4–16 nonsmokers) (Falter *et al.*, 1994).

Comparisons of 3- and 4-ABP-haemoglobin adducts in three different racial groups (white, black and Asian) led, as expected, to the detection of higher levels of both adducts in 61 smokers than in 72 nonsmokers (these levels were highest in whites, intermediate in blacks and lowest in Asians). There was also a correlation with the numbers of cigarettes smoked per day ($p < 0.0005$). Subjects from all three ethnic groups with the slow acetylator phenotype had higher adduct levels than those in rapid acetylators (2.5-fold higher for 3-ABP, $p < 0.0005$; 1.2-fold higher for 4-ABP, p = 0.19) (Yu *et al.*, 1994).

Differences in the levels of 3- and 4-ABP–haemoglobin adducts between men and women have also been reported. When plotted against number of cigarettes smoked per day, the slopes of the linear regression lines of adduct levels were significantly steeper for women than for men in a cohort of 1514 patients with bladder cancer and 1514 matched controls ($p < 0.001$ and 0.006 for 3-ABP and 4-ABP, respectively) (Castelao *et al.*, 2001).

In a group of 55 smokers and four nonsmokers, the levels of 4-ABP–haemoglobin adducts were related to the number of cigarettes smoked, although saturation of adduct formation was apparent at > 30 cigarettes/day. *GSTM1* and *NAT2* polymorphisms did not affect the levels of haemoglobin adducts (Dallinga *et al.*, 1998). The same authors investigated other genetic polymorphisms in 67 smokers and found no overall effects of polymorphisms in *NAT1*, *NAT2*, *GSTM1* or *GSTT1* on 4-ABP–haemoglobin adduct levels, except that in smokers of < 25 cigarettes/day, *NAT2* slow acetylators had significantly higher adduct levels than fast acetylators ($p = 0.03$) (Godschalk *et al.*, 2001).

Another study also reported that *NAT2* slow acetylators had significantly higher levels of 4-ABP-haemoglobin adducts than rapid acetylators, but there was no association between the *NAT1**10 genotype and the levels of 3- or 4-ABP–haemoglobin adducts, after adjustment for NAT2 phenotype. As in previous studies, smokers had significantly higher levels of 3- and 4-ABP–haemoglobin adducts than nonsmokers and the levels increased with increasing numbers of cigarettes smoked per day ($p < 0.0001$) (82 smokers, 321 nonsmokers) (Probst-Hensch *et al.*, 2000).

Adducts formed by polycyclic aromatic hydrocarbons

In a study involving 87 mothers and their 87 children in which PAH–albumin adducts in the plasma were investigated as a biomarker of the children's exposure to secondhand smoke from smoking by their mothers (see the monograph on involuntary smoking, this volume), it was also noted that adduct levels were significantly higher in the mothers who smoked than in those who did not (Crawford *et al.*, 1994).

A GC–MS method was used to measure benzo[*a*]pyrene-diol epoxide (BPDE)–globin adducts in 10 smokers and 10 nonsmokers. Subjects were also monitored for formation of globin adducts of chrysene diol epoxide. In both cases the procedure involved measurement of the respective tetrols of PAHs released from globin by acid hydrolysis. Levels of BPDE adducts in smokers were 2.7-fold higher than those in nonsmokers ($p < 0.01$); although the levels of the chrysene diol epoxide adducts were 1.25-fold higher in smokers, this difference was not statistically significant ($p = 0.06$) (Melikian *et al.*, 1997).

BPDE adducts with both haemoglobin and serum albumin were determined by GC–MS of tetrols released by acid hydrolysis in a study of 44 men with incident lung cancer. Individuals who were positive for haemoglobin adducts ($n = 6$) all had detectable albumin adducts, but not vice versa (24 subjects were positive for albumin adducts). Those were carriers of a *CYP1A1* variant allele were more frequently positive for albumin adducts ($p = 0.03$) and those with two 'slow' *mEH* alleles had a lower frequency of these adducts (Pastorelli *et al.*, 1998).

In another study, 27 smokers were found to have significantly higher levels of BPDE–albumin adducts ($p < 0.05$) and non-significantly higher levels of BPDE–haemoglobin adducts than 42 nonsmokers (Scherer *et al.*, 2000) (see also the monograph on involuntary smoking, this volume).

Adducts formed by tobacco-specific nitrosamines (TSNA)

Treatment of NNK– or NNN–haemoglobin adducts with mild bases releases 4-hydroxy-1-(3-pyridyl)-1-butanone (HPB), which is derivatized to its pentafluoro-benzoate, which is detectable by GC–MS after purification. The mean value in 40 smokers was 79.6 ± 189 fmol HPB/g haemoglobin (undetectable in 11 individuals; limit of detection, 5 fmol/g), whereas that in 21 nonsmokers was 29.3 ± 25.9 fmol/g (undetectable in four individuals) [statistical significance not stated]. The HPB levels in 22 snuff dippers were 517 ± 538 fmol/g, i.e. significantly higher than those in smokers ($p < 0.0001$). No relationship was apparent between HPB levels in smokers and levels of plasma cotinine or number of cigarettes smoked (Carmella *et al.*, 1990).

In a comparison of 20 smokers and 15 nonsmokers, the HPB levels derived from haemoglobin were significantly higher in smokers (69.2 ± 43.9 versus 34.4 ± 16.0 fmol/g haemoglobin; $p < 0.005$) (Falter *et al.*, 1994).

In another study of 18 smokers and former smokers and 52 never-smokers, the levels of HPB–haemoglobin adducts were significantly higher in the smokers (26 ± 12 [SD] fmol HPB/g haemoglobin) than in never-smokers (19 ± 8 fmol/g) ($p = 0.02$). No differences were found between the sexes or between current smokers and former smokers [duration of smoking cessation not stated] (Atawodi *et al.*, 1998).

Significantly higher levels of haemoglobin adducts of TSNA ($p < 0.001$) were found in pregnant women who smoked than in pregnant women who did not smoke (Branner *et al.*, 1998).

Adducts formed by other compounds

Ethylene (IARC, 1994b) is a major gaseous constituent of tobacco smoke that converts, via ethylene oxide, the N-terminal valine of haemoglobin to N-(2-hydroxy-ethyl)valine (HOEtVal). The level of this adduct correlates linearly with the alkylating activity occurring in DNA: 10 pmol HOEtVal/g globin corresponds to 0.33 pmol adduct/g DNA (Farmer *et al.*, 1987; Bono *et al.*, 1999). In 11 smokers who smoked more than 20 cigarettes/day, the levels of HOEtVal in haemoglobin were in the range 217–690 pmol/g haemoglobin (mean ± SD, 389 ± 138), whereas in 14 nonsmokers the range was 27–106 pmol/g (58 ± 25). It is noteworthy that there was no overlap in values between the two groups (Törnqvist *et al.*, 1986). In a controlled experiment, two volunteers who were regular smokers (of 29 and 18 cigarettes/day, respectively) abstained from smoking for 7 days and then resumed. From the measurements of levels of HOEtVal before stopping, 7 days after stopping and 7 days after resuming, the investigators calculated that in the smoker of 29 cigarettes/day, each cigarette smoked increased the level of HOEtVal by 0.12 pmol/g globin. For the smoker of 18 cigarettes/day, the increase was 0.08 pmol/g (Granath *et al.*, 1994).

In a study of 26 smokers and 24 nonsmokers, the background levels of HOEtVal in the nonsmokers averaged 49.9 pmol/g haemoglobin (range, 22–106). In the smokers, the levels were significantly higher by an estimated 71 pmol/10 cigarettes/day (Bailey *et al.*, 1988).

As part of a maternal–fetal comparison of HOEtVal in haemoglobin (see the monograph on involuntary smoking, this volume), samples from 10 pregnant women who did not smoke and 13 pregnant women who smoked 15 or more cigarettes/day were analysed. In nonsmokers, 63 ± 20 (mean ± SD) pmol/g haemoglobin were measured, whereas in the smokers, the levels were 361 ± 107 pmol/g ($p < 0.01$) (Tavares *et al.*, 1994).

In a study of 146 adults (82 men and 64 women), 44 smokers were reported to have significantly higher levels of HOEtVal in haemoglobin than did 74 nonsmokers and 29 self-reported passive smokers (mean ± SD: 59.5 ± 53, 17 ± 21 and 17 ± 23 pmol/g haemoglobin, respectively). Linear regression analysis of adduct levels and the number of cigarettes smoked per day showed a highly significant correlation coefficient ($r = 0.63$, $p < 0.0001$). The adduct levels were also significantly higher in men than in women (mean value 2.2-fold higher, $p = 0.00001$) (Bono et al., 1999).

Ethylene oxide is a substrate for GSTT1. To determine whether polymorphisms in GSTT1 modulate HOEtVal formation, blood samples from 10 women (one smoker) and 17 men (five smokers) were analysed. The median level of the adduct was 5.6-fold higher in smokers than in nonsmokers, but no correlation with daily cigarette consumption was found. GSTM1 and GSTT1 genotypes did not influence the adduct levels in the smokers, although the GSTT1 genotype did influence the adduct levels in nonsmokers (a two-fold higher median HOEtVal value was detected in GSTT1-null individuals than in GSTT1-positive individuals) (Müller et al., 1998).

The effect of GSTT1 was also investigated in a study involving 14 nonsmokers, 16 smokers of one pack of cigarettes a day and 13 smokers of two packs a day. HOEtVal levels increased with increasing number of cigarettes smoked, and the differences between the three groups were statistically significant. In addition, levels of N-(2-cyanoethyl)valine (CEVal), which is formed from acrylonitrile, were also significantly correlated with increasing smoking in these subjects. HOEtVal and CEVal levels were found to be significantly correlated in smokers ($p = 0.003$). There was no effect of GSTM1 or GSTT1 genotypes on the levels of CEVal in any of the groups or of GSTM1 on HOEtVal levels; however, GSTT1-null individuals had higher levels of HOEtVal compared with GSTT1-positive individuals (slope of regression line 50% higher) (Fennell et al., 2000).

A study of the effects of exposure to acrylamide and acrylonitrile in laboratory workers (smokers and nonsmokers) included the measurement of ethylene oxide–haemoglobin adducts. The mean levels of adducts from acrylamide, acrylonitrile and ethylene oxide in 10 smokers were 116, 106 and 126 pmol/g, respectively; these levels were significantly higher than those in eight nonsmokers (31, < 2 and 17 pmol/g, respectively). In smokers, the levels of acrylamide, acrylonitrile and ethylene oxide adducts correlated with the number of cigarettes smoked per day (Bergmark, 1997).

Two other studies have reported on acrylonitrile–haemoglobin adducts in smokers. In the first, four smokers had 75–106 pmol CEVal/g haemoglobin (mean, 88) whereas in four nonsmokers the levels were all below the limit of detection of 20 pmol/g (Osterman-Golkar et al., 1994). In the second study, 13 mothers who smoked had adduct levels in the range 92.5–373 pmol/g haemoglobin (mean ± SD: 217 ± 85.1), but the levels in 10 nonsmoking mothers were below the limit of detection (1 pmol/g). In the smokers, there was a linear correlation with number of cigarettes smoked per day ($p = 0.02$) and also with the levels of the adducts in their newborn babies (see the monograph on involuntary smoking, this volume) (Tavares et al., 1996).

A study was conducted in 43 Chinese workers exposed to benzene and 44 unexposed controls. The haemoglobin and albumin adducts of two metabolites, benzene oxide and 1,4-benzoquinone, were measured in these subjects. Tobacco smoking was found to have an additive effect on 1,4-benzoquinone–albumin formation (p = 0.034), but not on benzene oxide–albumin formation (p = 0.23) (Yeowell-O'Connell et al., 2001).

Human haemoglobin contains relatively high background levels of N-methylvaline, which could limit its sensitivity as a biomarker of exposure to environmental carcinogens. However, in a study of 11 pairs of monozygotic twins discordant for tobacco smoking, both HOEtVal and N-methylvaline were found to be higher in the smokers than in the nonsmokers. In the smokers the levels of HOEtVal and N-methylvaline were 143 ± 24 (mean $\pm$ SE) and 268 ± 13 pmol/g haemoglobin, respectively, and in the nonsmokers 15.6 ± 1.9 and 225 ± 11 pmol/g, respectively. Thus, the levels of N-methylvaline adduct were significantly different between smokers and nonsmokers (p = 0.006) and there was a highly significant correlation with the number of cigarettes smoked per day (p < 0.001) (Törnqvist et al., 1992).

Similarly, levels of N-methylvaline were found to be higher in a group of 32 smokers than in a group of 37 nonsmokers (mean $\pm$ SD: 1546 ± 432 versus 1175 ± 176 pmol/g haemoglobin; p < 0.001); for the smokers there was also a linear correlation between adduct levels and the number of cigarettes smoked per day (p < 0.001). An increment of 42 pmol/g haemoglobin per cigarette per day was calculated. A significant difference between smokers and nonsmokers in levels of HOEtVal was also observed in this study (Bader et al., 1995).

Because cigarette smoke contains reactive species that can cause oxidative and nitrative damage in cellular macromolecules, samples of plasma protein from 52 lung cancer patients (24 smokers, 28 nonsmokers) and 43 control subjects (18 smokers, 25 never-smokers) were analysed for nitrotyrosine and carbonyl groups as markers of nitration and oxidation, respectively. The quantities of nitrated proteins were significantly higher in the patients than in the controls (p = 0.003), but were not related to smoking status. In contrast, the amounts of oxidized proteins were higher in smokers (p < 0.001), but were not related to disease status (Pignatelli et al., 2001).

(iii) DNA adducts and other types of DNA damage in human tissues

The induction of DNA damage, frequently in the form of chemically stable adduct formation, is an early and essential step in the sequence of events by which genotoxic carcinogens initiate the carcinogenic process. The detection of DNA adducts in human tissues is therefore a useful and appropriate means to assess human exposure to such agents and several different procedures have been used for this.

- ^{32}P-Postlabelling analysis, in which DNA is digested and the resultant carcinogen-modified nucleotides are radiolabelled enzymatically with [^{32}P]ortho-phosphate, provides a sensitive method that requires no prior knowledge of the structures of the adducts formed. A common feature of the postlabelled DNA obtained from cells or tissues exposed to complex mixtures of carcinogens, such as tobacco smoke, is the appearance of a diagonal radioactive zone (DRZ) seen when the material is resolved by two-dimensional thin-layer chromatography. Although the material in the DRZ has not been fully characterized, its properties are compatible with those of a complex mixture of aromatic and/or hydrophobic DNA adducts.

• Another method used to detect DNA adducts in human tissues employs antibodies raised against DNA or nucleotides modified by various carcinogens. Immuno-histochemistry allows locating of adducts within a tissue specimen and measure-ment of the intensity of fluorescent staining permits a semi-quantitative estimate of adduct levels.

• Fluorescence detection of adducts in DNA, or of products released from DNA by hydrolysis, has been used for carcinogens that have strongly fluorescent pro-perties, for example PAHs.

• Mass spectrometry has been used for the chemical-specific detection of certain adducts in DNA samples.

• Electrochemical detection has been used for some smaller DNA lesions, for example 8-OHdG, formed in DNA by oxidative processes.

The uses, strengths and limitations of the various techniques have been extensively described (Beach & Gupta, 1992; Strickland et al., 1993; Weston, 1993; Phillips, 1997; Kriek et al., 1998; Wild & Pisani, 1998; Poirier et al., 2000). Earlier studies of tobacco-related DNA adducts in human tissues have also been reviewed (Phillips, 1996).

Respiratory tract

Lung and bronchus

Many studies have been published comparing the levels and characteristics of DNA adducts in the lung and bronchus of smokers and nonsmokers. These studies are sum-marized in Table 4.4.

In most of these studies, significantly elevated levels of DNA adducts were detected in the peripheral lung, bronchial epithelium or in cells obtained by bronchial lavage of the smokers. This is the case for total bulky DNA adducts (as detected by the ^{32}P-postlabelling method) and for DNA adducts detected by more chemical-specific methods including HPLC/fluorescence and GC–MS. However, the levels of 4-ABP-DNA adducts in lung did not correlate with smoking status (Culp et al., 1997). In some studies in which smoking status was not known, but was inferred from plasma cotinine levels (indicating smoking habit at the time of death of the subjects), there was a poor correlation with the detection of only one specific type of adduct, such as 7-methyldeoxyriboguanosine (7-MedG) (Kato et al., 1995; Blömeke et al., 1996) or those formed by benzo[a]pyrene (Weston & Bowman, 1991; Kato et al., 1995).

Some studies have found a linear correlation between adduct levels and daily or life-time consumption of cigarettes (Phillips et al., 1988, 1990a; Dunn et al., 1991; Asami et al., 1997) but, in other studies, no such relationship was found (Godschalk et al., 1998;

Table 4.4. Studies of smoking-related DNA adducts in human lung and bronchus. Non-tumorous tissue was analysed except where indicated.

Study	Tissue	Method of analysis	Number of subjects	Outcome
Randerath et al. (1986)	Bronchus	^{32}P-Postlabelling	1 smoker 1 nonsmoker	Detection of DRZ from bronchial DNA in smoker only (> 1.5 packs/day for > 20 years, stopped smoking 3 months before his death)
Phillips et al. (1988)	Lung	^{32}P-Postlabelling	17 smokers 7 former smokers 5 nonsmokers	Adduct levels significantly higher in smokers. Linear relationship between levels and cigarettes smoked/day
Randerath et al. (1989)	Lung, bronchus	^{32}P-Postlabelling	7 smokers 3 former smokers 1 nonsmoker	DRZ detected in smokers' lungs in a dose-dependent manner (2/3 former smokers are tobacco chewers)
Weston et al. (1989a)	Lung (tumour and normal tissue)	Synchronous fluorescence spectroscopy	5 lung tumours and 4 matching normal tissues	Only 1/4 normal tissues positive for BPDE–DNA. Lung tumour tissues negative
Phillips et al. (1990a)	Bronchus	^{32}P-Postlabelling	37 smokers 8 former smokers 8 nonsmokers	Adduct levels in smokers significantly higher than in former and nonsmokers. Among smokers, correlation found between adduct levels and smoke exposure
Van Schooten et al. (1990a)	Lung (tumour and normal tissue)	^{32}P-postlabelling, ELISA	13 smokers 8 former smokers (5 tumorous; 16 non-tumorous tissues)	DRZ detected in all non-tumorous tissue and 4/5 tumours. BPDE–DNA adducts in 3 tumorous and 4 non-tumorous tissues. ELISA positive for 5 non-tumour tissues and 3 tumours. Poor correlation between adduct levels and smoking among current smokers
Dunn et al. (1991)	Bronchus	^{32}P-Postlabelling	28 smokers 40 former smokers 10 nonsmokers (biopsies of both tumour tissue and normal tissue available for 4 former smokers and 1 smoker)	DRZ observed in all smokers, 24/40 former smokers and 4/10 nonsmokers. Among smokers, levels correlated with smoke exposure. DRZ generally similar in tumorous and normal tissues except in 2 former smokers out of 5 for whom adduct levels were substantially higher in tumours

Table 4.4 (contd)

Study	Tissue	Method of analysis	Number of subjects	Outcome
Foiles et al. (1991)	Lung, tracheo-bronchus	GC–MS for 4-hydroxy-1-(3-pyridyl)-1-butanone after acid hydrolysis	9 smokers, 8 nonsmokers (lung); 4 smokers, 4 nonsmokers (bronchus)	TSNA–DNA adducts measured by HPB levels were higher in smokers for both tissues studied (lung, 11 ± 16 versus 0.9 ± 2.3 fmol/mg DNA, 7/9 positive versus 1/8 in nonsmokers; tracheobronchus, 16 ± 18 versus 0.9 ± 1.7, 2/4 positive versus 1/4).
Geneste et al. (1991)	Lung	^{32}P-Postlabelling	19 smokers 4 former smokers	Smokers had significantly higher adduct levels, which correlated with AHH inducibility
Izzotti et al. (1991)	Alveolar macrophages	Synchronous fluorescence spectroscopy	16 smokers 4 recent smokers 6 former smokers 13 nonsmokers	BPDE–DNA detected in 84.6% (11/13 pooled from the 16) smokers and 2/4 recent smokers, but not in former or nonsmokers
Weston & Bowman (1991)	Lung	Synchronous fluorescence spectroscopy	20 adults 5 infants	BPDE–DNA adducts detected in 6/25 samples; levels did not correlate with serum cotinine levels.
Alexandrov et al. (1992)	Lung	HPLC/fluorescence or ^{32}P-postlabelling	11 smokers 2 former smokers	BPDE–DNA detected in 9/11 smokers and 2/2 former smokers. Linear correlation noted between the 2 adduct methods
Routledge et al. (1992)	Lung	^{32}P-Postlabelling	16 smokers 7 former smokers 14 nonsmokers	Adduct levels significantly higher in smokers and former smokers than in nonsmokers
Gallagher et al. (1993a)	BAL cells	^{32}P-Postlabelling	5 smokers 11 nonsmokers	Adduct levels 1.7-fold higher in smokers
Mustonen et al. (1993)	Bronchus	^{32}P-Postlabelling	13 smokers 7 nonsmokers	7-Methylguanine–DNA adduct levels were significantly higher in smokers than in nonsmokers. For 5 smokers, lung adduct levels correlated with lymphocyte adduct levels.

Table 4.4 (contd)

Study	Tissue	Method of analysis	Number of subjects	Outcome
Schoket et al. (1993)	Bronchus	^{32}P-Postlabelling	45 smokers 37 former smokers 16 nonsmokers	Levels in smokers and short-term former smokers were significantly greater than in long-term former smokers and nonsmokers. Weak association found between adduct levels and daily cigarette consumption
Ryberg et al. (1994)	Lung	^{32}P-Postlabelling	49 smokers (38 male) 14 nonsmokers (7 male)	Significantly higher levels of adducts in smokers than nonsmokers. Women had higher levels than men after adjusting for smoke exposure. Linear regression analysis showed that adduct levels are inversely related to the number of years of smoking among male lung cancer patients.
Kato et al. (1995)	Lung	^{32}P-Postlabelling	90 autopsies	There was no correlation between levels of adducts (7-MedGMP or PAH-dGMP) and serum cotinine levels. Higher 7-MedGMP levels were associated with CYP2E1 minor alleles ($p = 0.05$) and CYP2D6 genotype ($p = 0.01$).
Sherman et al. (1995)	BAL cells	DNA single-strand breaks by fluorescence analysis of DNA alkaline unwinding	11 smokers 11 nonsmokers	Alveolar macrophages from smokers had $35 \pm 3\%$ double stranded DNA, as against $41 \pm 5\%$ for nonsmokers.
Wiencke et al. (1995)	Lung	^{32}P-Postlabelling	6 smokers 10 former smokers (≤ 1 year) 15 former smokers (> 1 year)	Correlation with adduct levels in blood mononuclear cells (mean value 2.5-fold higher in lung)

Table 4.4 (contd)

Study	Tissue	Method of analysis	Number of subjects	Outcome
Andreassen et al. (1996)	Lung	^{32}P-postlabelling or fluorescence	26 smokers 11 former smokers 2 nonsmokers (tumour and non-tumorous tissues from 39 lung cancer patients)	Heavy smokers (> 20 cigarettes/day) had significantly higher levels of adducts in DRZ than light smokers. Using ^{32}P, DRZ adducts were detected in 37 samples, and 33/37 samples had detectable adducts. Using fluorescence IAC, BPDE–DNA adducts were detected in 11/39 samples.
Blömeke et al. (1996)	Lung	^{32}P-Postlabelling	10 autopsies	Levels of 7-MedG adduct did not correlate with smoking exposure at time of death (plasma cotinine levels).
Petruzzelli et al. (1996)	BAL cells	^{32}P-Postlabelling	10 smokers 10 former smokers 10 nonsmokers	7-MedG was detected in 7/10 smokers, 2/10 former smokers and 2/10 nonsmokers. Levels of 7-MedG in smokers were significantly different ($p = 0.028$) from former smokers and nonsmokers. Adduct levels did not correlate with number of cigarettes smoked per day.
Asami et al. (1997)	Lung	HPLC/ECD	14 smokers 7 former smokers 9 nonsmokers	8-OHdG levels significantly higher in smokers than in nonsmokers; linear correlation with number of cigarettes smoked (daily and cumulative)
Culp et al. (1997)	Lung	^{32}P-Postlabelling, ELISA, GC/MS	14 smokers 11 former smokers	Levels of 4-ABP-DNA adducts in lung tissue did not correlate with smoking status.
Ryberg et al. (1997)	Lung	^{32}P-Postlabelling	70 smokers	Mean adduct levels increased significantly according to GSTP1 genotype AA<AG<GG ($n = 25, 35, 10$, respectively; $p = 0.01$, AA versus AG; $p = 0.02$, AA versus GG).
Godschalk et al. (1998)	BAL cells	^{32}P-Postlabelling	78 smokers 23 nonsmokers	Adduct levels in BAL cells did not correlate with smoking (pack–years) after correcting for age.

Table 4.4 (contd)

Study	Tissue	Method of analysis	Number of subjects	Outcome
Lodovici et al. (1998)	Lung	HPLC/fluorescence	12 smokers 6 former smokers 21 nonsmokers	BPDE–DNA adduct levels in smokers and former smokers significantly higher than in nonsmokers ($p < 0.05$)
Rojas et al. (1998)	Lung	HPLC/fluorescence	20 smokers	BPDE DNA adduct levels were higher in 2 individuals with GSTM1 null and CYP1A1 MspI variant genotypes.
Schoket et al. (1998)	Bronchus	^{32}P-Postlabelling	82 smokers 25 short-term former smokers (< 1 year) 20 long-term former smokers (> 1 year) 23 nonsmokers	Adduct levels significantly higher in current and short-term former smokers than in long-term former and nonsmokers. Adduct levels are the same in 66 male and 16 female current smokers. Apparent half-life of adducts ~1.7 years. Adduct levels did not correlate with daily cigarette dose or with GSTM1 or CYP1A1 MspI genotypes.
Butkiewicz et al. (1999)	Lung	^{32}P-Postlabelling	120 smokers 22 former smokers 23 nonsmokers	PAH adduct levels significantly higher in smokers than in former and nonsmokers. High adduct levels (upper quartile) significantly associated with CYP1A1 Ile-Val allele carriers in individuals who were GSTM1 null ($n = 86$)
Mollerup et al. (1999)	Lung	^{32}P-Postlabelling	122 smokers (29 women) 37 nonsmokers (13 women)	Adduct levels significantly higher in women than in men ($p = 0.047$ before adjustment for pack–years, $p = 0.0004$ after adjustment). Lung expression of CYP1A1 (15 women, 12 men) was significantly higher in women ($p = 0.016$) and in both sexes the correlation between CYP1A1 expression and adduct levels was significant ($p = 0.009$).

Table 4.4 (contd)

Study	Tissue	Method of analysis	Number of subjects	Outcome
Wiencke *et al.* (1999)	Lung	^{32}P-Postlabelling	57 smokers 79 former smokers 7 nonsmokers	Smokers had significantly higher adduct levels than former smokers. Age of commencing smoking was associated with adduct levels in former smokers, but not in current smokers. Good correlation noted between DNA adduct levels in blood mononuclear cells and lung tissues
Cheng *et al.* (2000)	Lung	^{32}P-Postlabelling	73 cancer cases (32 smokers, 38 nonsmokers) 33 non-cancer controls (11 smokers, 22 nonsmokers)	DNA adduct levels were significantly higher in cases than in controls, but not higher in smokers than in nonsmokers. Adduct levels not influenced by *CYP1A1 Msp*I or *GSTM1* genotypes.
Piipari *et al.* (2000)	BAL cells	^{32}P-Postlabelling	31 smokers 16 nonsmokers	PAH–DNA adduct levels 3-fold higher in smokers than in nonsmokers ($p < 0.001$) and correlated with number of cigarettes smoked daily. Smokers with high levels of *CYP3A* expression had higher adduct levels ($p < 0.002$).
Schoket *et al.* (2001)	Bronchus	^{32}P-Postlabelling	94 smokers and short-term former smokers ($\leq$ 1year)	Evidence for a weak influence of some combinations of *CYP* and *GST* genotypes on adduct levels

DRZ, diagonal radioactive zone; BPDE, benzo[*a*]pyrene diol epoxide; ELISA, enzyme-linked immunoassay; AHH, aryl hydrocarbon hydroxylase; GC–MS, gas chromatography/mass spectrometry; TSNA, tobacco-specific nitrosamines; HPB, 4-hydroxy-1-(3-pyridyl)-1-butanone; HPLC, high-performance liquid chromatography; BAL, bronchio-alveolar lavage; 7-MedGMP, 7-methyl-2'-deoxyriboguanosine-3'-monophosphate; PAH, polycyclic aromatic hydrocarbons; IAC, immunoaffinity chromatography; 7-MedG, 7-methyl-2'-deoxyriboguanosine; 4-ABP, 4-aminobiphenyl; ECD, electro-chemical detection; 8-OHdG, 8-hydroxydeoxyguanosine

Schoket *et al.*, 1998). In one study in a group of male smokers with lung cancer, a linear regression analysis showed that adduct levels were inversely related to the number of years of smoking (Ryberg *et al.*, 1994). Mean levels of adducts in former smokers (usually with an interval of at least 1 year since smoking cessation) were generally found to be intermediate between the levels found in smokers and in life-long nonsmokers. From these comparisons, the half-life of adducts in the lung is estimated to be 1.7 years in bronchial tissue from former smokers (Schoket *et al.*, 1998). This is somewhat longer than would be estimated from a consideration of the biochemical processes of DNA repair and the rate of cell turnover, and may be a consequence of the slow clearance of carcinogen-containing tar and particulate deposits from the lung, resulting in continued metabolic activation of tobacco carcinogens after smoking cessation.

In a study in Norway, adduct levels were higher in the lungs of women smokers than in those of men, a difference that was greater after adjustment for intensity of smoking (Ryberg *et al.*, 1994; Mollerup *et al.*, 1999). However, in a study in Hungary, adduct levels in male and female smokers with lung cancer were found to be the same (Schoket *et al.*, 1998).

Larynx

^{32}P-Postlabelling analysis of DNA from larynx mucosa revealed the presence of hydrophobic adducts (DRZ) in 21 smokers but not in four nonsmokers. The ability of both the nuclease P_1 digestion and the butanol extraction procedures to detect these adducts suggested that they were formed primarily by PAHs rather than aromatic amines. Adduct levels correlated with levels of P4501A1, 2C and 3A4, but not with levels of P4502E1 and 2A6 (Degawa *et al.*, 1994).

Another study compared adduct levels in laryngeal tumours with those in non-tumour tissue from 43 patients, 38 of whom were smokers. Adduct levels, as determined by ^{32}P-postlabelling, were higher in tumour tissue than in normal tissue, and the few non- or former smokers had lower levels than the smokers (differences were not significant) (Szyfter *et al.*, 1994). In a subsequent study, ^{32}P-postlabelling analysis was used to measure levels of 7-alkylguanine in DNA from laryngeal biopsies. In larynx tumour tissues, the levels reported in heavy smokers (> 40 cigarettes/day) were 2.5-fold higher than those in moderate smokers (~20 cigarettes/day) and 5.5-fold higher than in nonsmokers and former smokers. There was a significant correlation between 7-alkylguanine levels and aromatic/hydrophobic adduct levels in these tissue samples (Szyfter *et al.*, 1996).

An immunohistochemical study of laryngeal biopsies from 38 patients, using antibodies against 4-ABP–DNA adducts, included analyses of tumours (9), polyps (28) and surrounding tissue (1). The investigators noted a significantly higher staining intensity of polyps and surrounding tissue from smokers than of that from nonsmokers, but the differences between tumour tissue from smokers and nonsmokers were not significant [limited number of samples]. The study showed that 4-ABP–DNA adducts, related to smoking exposure, are formed in the larynx (Flamini *et al.*, 1998).

An analysis of laryngeal tumour biopsies from 33 patients was carried out by ^{32}P-post-labelling. DNA from tumour tissue, non-tumour tissue and the interarytenoid area was analysed separately. Large interindividual differences in adduct levels were reported, with highest levels in the interarytenoid area. Adduct levels were reported to be correlated with age (the highest levels in all tissues were noted in the 50–60-year and 60–70-year age groups), sex (28 of the patients were men, five were women; adduct levels were higher in the men), cigarette smoking (all patients were smokers, 19 smoked 20 cigarettes/day, 14 smoked 30–40) and stage of tumour progression (p values were not reported) (Banaszewski et al., 2000).

Sputum

DNA isolated from sputum, induced by inhalation of nebulized saline solution, was compared in a group of 20 smokers and 24 nonsmokers using the nuclease P_1 digestion method of ^{32}P-postlabelling analysis. All smokers, but only one nonsmoker, showed a DRZ in their adduct patterns, and adduct levels were significantly higher in smokers than in nonsmokers (3.1 ± 1.4 versus $0.6 \pm 0.8/10^8$ nucleotides; $p = 0.0007$) (Besarati Nia et al., 2000a). The same authors also found that the adduct levels in the induced sputum of nine smokers (monitored on three occasions) were significantly higher than those in nine non-smokers (monitored once) (Besarati Nia et al., 2000b). When immunohistochemical analysis of induced sputum was carried out, the cells of 20 smokers were found to have significantly greater intensity of staining when using antibodies against 4-ABP–DNA than the cells of 24 nonsmokers ($p = 0.001$), but not when BPDE–DNA antibodies were used ($p = 0.07$) (Besarati Nia et al., 2000c).

Oral and nasal cavities

In two early ^{32}P-postlabelling studies of DNA from oral mucosal cells, varying amounts of a variety of aromatic and/or hydrophobic adducts were seen in smokers and nonsmokers, but none of them were specific to exposure to tobacco smoke (Dunn & Stich, 1986; Chacko & Gupta, 1988).

DNA from clinically normal oral tissue (mucosa) from patients undergoing surgery for intraoral squamous-cell carcinoma was analysed by ^{32}P-postlabelling using both nuclease P_1 digestion and butanol extraction enhancement methods. Both the range and levels of adducts measured were greater with the latter method, and the mean level of adducts in the smokers ($n = 19 + 1$ pipe smoker) was statistically significantly higher than that in the four former smokers and nine nonsmokers combined (Jones et al., 1993). A comparison between DNA obtained from oral biopsies and from buccal mucosa from the same individuals showed that there was a good correlation between adduct levels from the two sources, with a significantly higher level of adducts in DNA from 20 smokers than that from 10 nonsmokers (Stone et al., 1995).

In a small study of nasal mucosal DNA from nine smokers, two former smokers and 10 nonsmokers, ^{32}P-postlabelling analysis detected the DRZ in eight of the smokers, one of the former smokers and one of the nonsmokers. The mean adduct level in smokers was significantly higher than that in the nonsmokers ($p < 0.01$; 4.8 versus $1.4/10^8$ nucleotides using the nuclease P_1 digestion) and a linear relationship between adduct levels and daily cigarette consumption was observed among the smokers (Peluso et al., 1997). In another study, the levels of DNA adducts detected by ^{32}P-postlabelling analysis in nasal cells from six smokers were also significantly higher than the levels in cells of 14 nonsmokers (mean value, 17.0 versus $6.8/10^8$ nucleotides) (Zhao et al., 1997).

Using a ^{32}P-postlabelling method to detect cyclic adducts such as 1,N^2-propanodeoxy-guanosine, possible products of the reaction of tobacco smoke constituents such as acrolein (A) and crotonaldehyde (C) with DNA, significantly higher levels of each of three such adducts (AdG, CdG1 and CdG2) were detected in the DNA of gingival tissue of 11 smokers than in that of 12 nonsmokers; the total levels of the adducts were 4.4-fold higher in smokers than in nonsmokers (Nath et al., 1998).

Using the alkaline comet (single-cell gel electrophoresis) assay to detect DNA strand breaks in exfoliated buccal cells, significantly higher DNA migration was found to occur in the cells of 11 smokers than in those of nine nonsmokers (Rojas et al., 1996).

A study of exfoliated oral cells from healthy volunteers used an immunohisto-chemical technique to stain cells with antibodies raised against BPDE–DNA adducts. The intensity of staining was significantly greater in cells from 33 smokers than in those from 64 nonsmokers, and increased intensity of staining was observed with increasing number of cigarettes smoked per day by the smokers (Romano et al., 1999a). Similar results were obtained in another study that used this technique. Both buccal cavity and mouth floor cells were investigated; staining intensity in both cell types was found to be significantly higher in 26 smokers than in 22 nonsmokers (Besarati Nia et al., 2000d). When antibodies to 4-ABP–DNA adducts were used, staining intensity was also found to be significantly higher in the exfoliated oral cells of 12 smokers than in those of 12 nonsmokers (Romano et al., 1997).

Immunohistochemical staining of human oral mucosal cells, using antibodies against BPDE–DNA adducts, revealed significantly higher intensities of staining in 16 smokers than in 16 matched nonsmokers (Zhang et al., 1995). A second study, using antibodies against BPDE–DNA adducts or against 4-ABP-modified DNA in exfoliated oral cells, showed significantly higher levels of DNA damage in 20 smokers than in 20 matched nonsmokers for both DNA adducts (Hsu et al., 1997). Subsequently, an analogous ana-lysis using antibodies to malonaldehyde–DNA adducts has demonstrated higher levels of this adduct, derived from lipid peroxidation, in the oral mucosal cells of 25 smokers than in 25 matched nonsmokers (Zhang et al., 2002).

Urogenital tissues

Bladder

Investigations of the presence of smoking-related DNA adducts in bladder cells have made use of autopsy and biopsy specimens and of exfoliated epithelial cells excreted in urine.

When the levels of DNA adducts were determined in bladder biopsy samples using ^{32}P-postlabelling with both butanol extraction and nuclease P_1 enhancement procedures, the mean levels of several specific adducts were higher in 13 smokers than in 20 former smokers and nine never-smokers; some adducts were present at similar levels in all groups and thus were not smoking-related. One of the smoking-related adducts was chromatographically identical to the major adduct formed in DNA by 4-ABP (Talaska et al., 1991a).

Exfoliated urothelial cells recovered from the urine of 39 of 73 individuals yielded sufficient DNA for ^{32}P-postlabelling analysis (21 from nonsmokers, 18 from current smokers). The DNA was found to contain several DNA adducts, of which at least four were present in the DNA of smokers at levels 2–20 times higher than those in the DNA of nonsmokers. One of these corresponded chromatographically to N-(deoxyguanosin-8-yl)-4-ABP (Talaska et al., 1991b). In a further study of the same subjects, two DNA adducts detected in exfoliated uroepithelial cells were found to be specifically associated with smoking and with the levels of 4-ABP–haemoglobin adducts (Vineis et al., 1996).

In a study of bladder biopsies of 20 bladder cancer patients and of exfoliated bladder cells of 36 healthy individuals, a dose–response relationship between smoking levels and adduct levels was found for both groups [statistics not given and the sizes of the groups studied were small]. The levels of adducts were not higher in the cases than in the controls (Talaska et al., 1994).

Bladder tissue samples taken at autopsy from 56 individuals were analysed by ^{32}P-postlabelling of DNA. A positive but weak association ($p = 0.09$) between adduct levels and tobacco smoking was found, and there was a correlation between the levels of adducts in lung and bladder ($p < 0.01$, Spearman rank correlation test) (Routledge et al., 1992) (see also Table 4.4).

A comparison of the adducts detected by ^{32}P-postlabelling in bladder biopsies from 30 smokers with those from 24 nonsmokers revealed that, overall, adduct levels were not significantly different between the two groups; 3–5-fold higher levels of adducts were detected by the butanol extraction procedure than by nuclease P_1 digestion, implying a preponderance of aromatic amine-like adducts over those formed by PAHs. In a more detailed analysis, however, the level of one minor DNA adduct was found to be twice as high in samples analysed from 17 smokers than in those from eight nonsmokers ($p < 0.005$, one-tailed) (Phillips & Hewer, 1993).

Biopsy samples from human bladder were subjected to immunohistochemical analysis with antibodies to 4-ABP–DNA adducts to determine the relationship between smoking history and intensity of staining. The adduct levels were significantly higher in 24 current smokers than in 22 nonsmokers ($p < 0.0001$). There was also a linear relationship between mean levels of adduct staining and number of cigarettes smoked per day (Curigliano et al., 1996). In another study using the same technique, higher levels of 4-ABP–DNA adducts were also observed in bladder specimens from 30 smokers than in those from 41 former smokers and 24 nonsmokers, but the statistical significance of this difference was borderline ($p = 0.07$) (Romano et al., 1999b).

Immunohistochemical staining of human exfoliated urothelial cells from urine, using antibodies to BPDE–DNA adducts or to 4-ABP–DNA adducts, revealed significantly higher ($p < 0.0005$) intensities of staining in 20 smokers than in 20 matched nonsmokers in both cases (Hsu *et al.*, 1997).

The presence of 3-alkyladenines in human urine was determined in two smokers who underwent a period of voluntary abstinence from smoking. In one subject, the excretion of 3-ethyladenine was significantly lower on nonsmoking days ($p < 0.01$). Smoking-dependent differences in levels of 3-methyladenine were apparent only when volunteers consumed a diet low in 3-alkyladenines during the study period. Thus, although both adducts are produced by alkylating agents in tobacco smoke, natural dietary levels of 3-methyladenine make this an insensitive biomarker of smoking (Prévost & Shuker, 1996).

In a study of depurinated adducts of benzo[*a*]pyrene in urine, detectable levels of BaP-6-N7 Ade[1] were found in the urine of three of seven smokers (not quantifiable but detectable up to 0.1–0.6 fmol/mg creatinine), but not in the urine from any of 13 non-smokers (Casale *et al.*, 2001).

The comet assay was used to analyse urinary bladder cells for DNA damage. A significant increase in comet tail moments for 18 smokers and former smokers was found as compared with 12 nonsmokers ($p < 0.03$) (Gontijo *et al.*, 2001).

In a study of oxidative DNA damage measured by 8-OHdG excretion in urine, 30 smokers were reported to have levels of the nucleoside that were 50% higher (corrected for body weight) than 53 nonsmokers (Loft *et al.*, 1992).

Taken together, the studies analysing DNA adducts in bladder tissue or exfoliated urothelial cells demonstrate that smoking-related formation of DNA adducts is detectable, but that some of the adducts present derive from other sources of environmental carcinogens.

Cervix

A pilot study of DNA isolated from cervical scrapes of 22 women and analysed by the butanol extraction enrichment procedure of ^{32}P-postlabelling showed the presence of the DRZ and higher levels of adducts in three of nine smokers than in 13 nonsmokers (Phillips *et al.*, 1990b). In a subsequent study, sufficient DNA was isolated from 33 of 38 cervical smear samples and subjected to ^{32}P-postlabelling analysis. Adduct levels were significantly higher in the DNA from 18 smokers than in that from 15 nonsmokers (Simons *et al.*, 1995).

Using DNA isolated from cervical biopsies, ^{32}P-postlabelling analysis with butanol extraction was carried out on samples from 39 women (11 smokers, seven former smokers and 21 never-smokers). Adduct levels were significantly higher in the smokers and former smokers than in the nonsmokers ($p = 0.048$). Exclusion of those women whose urinary cotinine levels did not confirm their self-reported nonsmoking status ($n = 7$) increased the differences in levels of adducts between smokers and nonsmokers ($p = 0.03$) (Simons *et al.*, 1993).

---

[1] N7-(benzo[*a*]pyrene-6-yl) adenine

A study of cervical biopsy samples from 35 women (19 smokers, five former smokers and 11 nonsmokers) found that DNA adduct levels, determined by ^{32}P-postlabelling analysis with the butanol extraction procedure, were significantly higher in the smokers than in the nonsmokers ($p = 0.002$), and an intermediate mean value was obtained for the former smokers (Phillips & Ni She, 1993). This study population was subsequently increased to 22 smokers, four former smokers and 14 nonsmokers and analysed by both butanol extraction and nuclease P_1 digestion procedures of ^{32}P-postlabelling. Adduct levels were significantly higher in smokers when the former procedure was used ($p = 0.005$), but not with the latter (Phillips & Ni She, 1994). The lack of a difference between smokers and nonsmokers using nuclease P_1 digestion was also reported in another small study in women not using oral contraceptives (15 smokers, eight nonsmokers) (King et al., 1994). However, in another larger study, ^{32}P-postlabelling analysis using nuclease P_1 digestion found significantly higher levels ($p = 0.07$) in DNA from histologically normal cervical biopsy tissue from 48 current smokers than in that from 48 non-current smokers (non-current smokers included nonsmokers, former smokers and passive smokers) (Ali et al., 1994).

Immunohistochemical analysis of human cervical cells, using antibodies against BPDE–DNA adducts, demonstrated significantly higher staining intensity ($p = 0.04$) in smears from 16 smokers than in smears from 16 nonsmokers (Mancini et al., 1999).

GC–MS analysis of BPDE–DNA adducts in cervical epithelial cells found that the level of adducts was approximately twofold higher in seven smokers than in seven nonsmokers and this difference was statistically significant ($p = 0.02$) (Melikian et al., 1999).

Other tissues

Breast

In a pilot study, a total of 31 samples of human breast tissue were analysed by ^{32}P-postlabelling using nuclease P_1 digestion to determine the levels of aromatic/hydrophobic DNA adducts. The breast tissues included samples from tumours and from tissues adjacent to tumours from 15 women with breast cancer and four samples from women who had had reduction mammoplasties. The characteristic DRZ was detected in tumorous and non-tumorous tissues from five of 15 cancer patients, all of whom were current smokers. None of the eight former smokers and nonsmokers displayed this pattern ($p < 0.01$) (Perera et al., 1995).

Another ^{32}P-postlabelling study using nuclease P_1 digestion of aromatic DNA adducts was conducted on normal (non-tumour) breast tissue from 87 breast cancer patients undergoing mastectomy and from 29 women who did not have cancer (controls) undergoing reduction mammoplasty. The characteristic DRZ was detected in 29 of 87 normal tissues from breast cancer patients (17/17 smokers, 5/8 former smokers, 4/52 nonsmokers, 3/10 with unknown smoking status), and in two of 10 control tissues. In addition, a benzo[a]-pyrene-like DNA adduct was observed in 36 normal adjacent breast tissue samples (27 of them from nonsmokers) from cancer patients and its presence was not significantly associated with smoking (Li et al., 1996).

Higher levels ($p = 0.0001$) of DNA adducts putatively derived from malonaldehyde and detected by ^{32}P-postlabelling using nuclease P_1 digestion were determined in tissue adjacent to tumours from 51 breast cancer patients than in tissue from 28 controls (undergoing reduction mammoplasty). The levels of these adducts were also associated with the previously detected benzo[a]pyrene-like DNA adduct (see above), but were significantly lower in smokers than in former smokers and in nonsmokers (Wang et al., 1996).

Immunohistochemical staining intensity of breast tumour tissue using antibodies against BPDE–DNA adducts was not significantly different between 35 smokers, 72 former smokers who had smoked one cigarette or more per day for 6 months or longer and 75 nonsmokers. However, among smokers and former smokers, there was a trend towards higher intensities of staining with greater levels of exposure or earlier age at starting smoking (Santella et al., 2000). Positive staining using antibodies against BPDE–DNA adducts was also obtained with tissue samples from 48 patients with breast tumours and tissue samples from 30 patients with benign disease (with higher adduct levels being found in tissues from patients with benign breast disease than in cancer tissues). This study was carried out on inhabitants of Upper Silesia, a region of Poland that has been subject to high levels of environmental pollution. However, in neither group of patients were staining intensities higher in smokers than in nonsmokers (Motykiewicz et al., 2001).

In a study of PAH–DNA adducts in breast tumour tissue from 119 cancer patients and from 108 patients with benign breast disease, immunohistochemical analysis indicated a significant association between adduct levels and breast cancer, but there was no relationship between smoking status, stage or tumour size and adduct levels (Rundle et al., 2000).

Pancreas

^{32}P-Postlabelling analysis of 20 pancreatic tumours and 13 samples of normal tissue adjacent to the tumour, using nuclease P_1 digestion, led to the detection of significantly higher levels of DNA adducts in the normal tissues surrounding the tumour than in either the tumour tissue or in normal pancreatic tissue from five patients with non-pancreatic cancer and 19 previously healthy organ donors who served as controls. Two novel clusters of adducts were observed: 11/13 in adjacent normal tissues from pancreatic cancer patients, 12/20 in tumour tissues and 2/24 in normal pancreatic tissues from controls. The presence of these adducts was positively correlated with smoking status (Wang et al., 1998).

Another study that used fluorescence spectral analysis for the presence of BPDE–DNA adducts in pancreatic samples revealed no detectable levels in any of 11 samples (six from smokers) (Alexandrov et al., 1996).

Colon

Fluorescence spectral analysis of samples of colon mucosa for the presence of BPDE–DNA adducts resulted in their detection in three of four samples from smokers and one of three samples from nonsmokers. Adduct levels were estimated to be in the range 0.2–1.0 adducts/10^8 nucleotides (Alexandrov *et al.*, 1996).

Stomach

Tumour DNA from 26 patients (18 smokers) with gastric cancer was analysed for DNA adducts using ^{32}P-postlabelling with butanol extraction. In men only, the numbers of DNA adducts were found to be significantly higher in the samples from 14 smokers than in that from four nonsmokers (Dyke *et al.*, 1992). [The Working Group noted that the number of nonsmokers was small.]

Placenta and fetal tissue

In the first study of placental DNA for the presence of DNA adducts, ^{32}P-postlabelling analysis and ELISA with antibodies against BPDE–DNA adducts were used. The use of the ELISA found a small but non-significant increase in adducts in placental tissue from smokers when compared with the numbers found in nonsmokers. Using ^{32}P-postlabelling analysis, one particular DNA adduct was found to be present in the DNA from 16 of 17 smokers, but in only three of 14 nonsmokers (Everson *et al.*, 1986). In a subsequent study using ^{32}P-postlabelling, up to seven different adducts were detected in 53 specimens of human placental tissue, three of these adducts were found 'almost exclusively' in smokers (Everson *et al.*, 1988).

The combined use of immunological, fluorescence spectroscopic and mass spectrometric methods has led to the detection and characterization of BPDE–DNA adducts in human placental DNA and also provided evidence for the presence of adducts formed by other PAHs (Weston *et al.*, 1989b; Manchester *et al.*, 1990). Synchronous fluorescence spectroscopy for the detection of BPDE–DNA adducts gave positive results in 10 of 28 human placental samples, but there was no correlation with smoking status (Manchester *et al.*, 1988). In a subsequent study, five of seven placentas from smokers and three of nine from nonsmokers gave positive results when analysed for these adducts (Manchester *et al.*, 1992).

Placental DNA from five smokers was found to contain adduct levels, detected as a DRZ by ^{32}P-postlabelling, 1.8-fold higher than that in placental DNA from five nonsmokers (4.3 ± 1.7 versus 2.3 ± 0.4 adducts/10^8 nucleotides) (Gallagher *et al.*, 1993a) [statistical significance not stated].

Using ^{32}P-postlabelling with nuclease P_1 digestion, DNA adducts were detected in DNA from placenta and umbilical cord regardless of whether or not the mothers were smokers. Adduct levels were significantly higher in maternal than in fetal tissue (and were higher in placenta than in umbilical cord) and, combining data for all tissues, total levels of DNA adducts were significantly higher in eight smokers than in 11 nonsmokers. Although individual tissues showed a trend towards increased levels of adducts in smokers, the differences were not statistically significant (Hansen *et al.*, 1992, 1993). DNA adducts derived from PAHs were detected by a competitive ELISA in six of 14 placentas and in five of 12 matched fetal lung samples from spontaneous abortions. None of the samples were from women who reported smoking during pregnancy; thus smoking was not a likely source of the adducts (Hatch *et al.*, 1990). However, in another study using ELISA with antibodies against BPDE–DNA adducts, a linear correlation was found between levels of adducts and levels of urinary cotinine for both placental DNA and umbilical cord DNA, the former tissue having the higher adduct levels. Overall, adducts were detected in 13 of 15 placental samples and 12 of 15 samples of umbilical cord blood from smokers and three of 10 placental samples and one of 10 samples of umbilical cord from nonsmokers (Arnould *et al.*, 1997).

When placental DNA was analysed both for bulky DNA adducts by ^{32}P-postlabelling with nuclease P_1 digestion and for 8-OHdG by electrochemical detection, neither method showed a difference between 11 smokers, 10 nonsmokers and nine nonsmokers who were exposed to secondhand smoke (Daube *et al.*, 1997).

Thus, although some studies indicate the presence of smoking-related DNA adducts in human placenta, overall the association between smoking status and adduct levels, determined by a variety of different methods, is weak. The results appear to indicate that there are significant sources of environmental carcinogens other than tobacco smoke that result in DNA adducts being formed in this tissue.

Sperm

In a study in which sperm DNA from 12 heavy smokers (> 20 cigarettes/day), 12 moderate smokers (1–19 cigarettes/day) and 12 nonsmokers was subjected to ^{32}P-postlabelling analysis, no discernible differences were observed between the patterns or levels of DNA adducts between the three groups of subjects (Gallagher *et al.*, 1993b).

However, immunohistochemical analysis of sperm, with antibodies against BPDE–DNA adducts showed significantly higher intensity of staining in the sperm of 11 smokers than in the sperm of 12 nonsmokers (Zenzes *et al.*, 1999a). Furthermore, in-vitro fertilization experiments using sperm from smokers and oocytes from nonsmoking partners suggested that there was transmission of benzo[*a*]pyrene-modified DNA to the embryos (Zenzes *et al.*, 1999b). In related studies, granulosa-lutein cells from women undergoing in-vitro fertilization were analysed. Immunostaining for BPDE–DNA adducts was confined to the nucleus and was significantly greater in cells from 14 smokers than in those from seven passive smokers and 11 nonsmokers (Zenzes *et al.*, 1998) (see also the monograph on involuntary smoking, this volume).

The sperm DNA of 28 smokers contained levels of 8-OHdG about 1.5 times higher than that of 32 age-matched nonsmokers, a difference that was statistically significant (6.19 ± 1.71 versus 3.93 ± 1.33 8-OHdG/10^5 dG, $p < 0.001$) (Shen *et al.*, 1997). The same authors reported a correlation between sperm defects and levels of 8-OHdG in sperm DNA, indicating that this lesion is useful for assessing sperm quality and male fertility (Shen *et al.*, 1999).

In another study, the sperm DNA of smokers ($n = 35$) was found to be more sensitive to acid-induced denaturation ($p < 0.02$) and to possess higher levels of DNA strand breaks ($p < 0.05$) than that of nonsmokers ($n = 35$) (Potts *et al.*, 1999).

Cardiovascular tissues

In a pilot study investigating the presence of DNA adducts by ^{32}P-postlabelling in a number of human tissues at autopsy, the DRZ characteristic of smoking-related DNA damage was observed in heart tissue from two smokers, but not in that of a nonsmoker who chewed tobacco. Moreover, of all the tissues examined, which included lung and bronchus, the levels of adducts were highest in heart tissue (Randerath *et al.*, 1989). A study comparing ^{32}P-postlabelling, HPLC-fluorescence detection of BPDE–DNA adduct hydrolysis products and synchronous fluorescence spectroscopy (SFS) detection of the same products demonstrated that all three methods were capable of detecting DNA adducts in atherosclerotic lesions in smooth muscle of human abdominal aorta. However, because of the limited number of samples investigated (four from smokers, three from former smokers), no conclusion could be drawn regarding the origins of the adducts detected (Izzotti *et al.*, 1995a). Another study measured DNA adducts by ^{32}P-postlabelling with nuclease P_1 digestion in the thoracic aorta of 133 victims of sudden or accidental death. Those with significant atherosclerotic changes and for whom atherosclerosis was classified as the main cause of death were designated as 76 cases, those with few athero-sclerotic changes as 57 controls. Smoking status was determined by measuring cotinine levels in plasma. Levels of bulky aromatic DNA adducts were significantly higher in the cases than in the controls, but when smokers and nonsmokers were compared, significant differences were observed in the controls, but not in the cases (Binková *et al.*, 2001).

Immunohistochemical staining of endothelial and smooth muscle cells of blood vessels using antibodies against BPDE–DNA adducts resulted in higher intensity of the endothelial cells. However, the correlation with smoking habits among the 33 subjects studied (samples from nine of 11 smokers showed positive staining, compared with 12 of 22 nonsmokers) was not statistically significant (Zhang *et al.*, 1998).

In a study of DNA from the right atrial appendage of 41 patients undergoing open heart surgery, the levels of aromatic DNA adducts detected by ^{32}P-postlabelling with nuclease P_1 digestion were significantly higher in 15 smokers than in 15 former smokers ($p < 0.01$) and in 11 nonsmokers ($p < 0.001$). A significant linear relationship between adduct levels and daily cigarette smoking was observed in the smokers (Van Schooten *et al.*, 1998).

Blood cells

Although nucleated peripheral blood cells are not generally considered to be target cells for tobacco-induced tumorigenesis, the relative ease with which they can be obtained from human subjects, when compared with many target organs, has led to a large number of studies exploring the differences between cells from smokers and nonsmokers. The studies in which smoking-related DNA adducts have been determined in blood cells are summarized in Table 4.5.

The picture that emerges from these many studies is an inconsistent one. Measurements made in the longer-lived cells (lymphocytes and monocytes) are more likely to reveal significant differences between smokers and nonsmokers than measurements made

Table 4.5. Studies of smoking-related DNA adducts in human blood cells

Study	Blood cells[a]	Method of analysis	Number of subjects	Outcome
Perera *et al.* (1987)	WBC	ELISA	22 smokers 24 nonsmokers	BPDE–DNA adducts detected in 5/22 smokers and 7/24 nonsmokers
Perera *et al.* (1989)	WBC	ELISA	81 lung cancer cases (38 smokers, 43 former and nonsmokers) 67 controls (19 smokers, 48 former and nonsmokers)	For cases, 19/38 smokers and 21/43 former and nonsmokers were positive for PAH–DNA adducts; for controls, 9/19 smokers and 27/48 former and nonsmokers were positive. Current smokers who were cases had higher (0.35) adduct levels than controls who smoked (0.14). But PAH–DNA adduct formation was unrelated to number of cigarettes smoked.
Holz *et al.* (1990)	Monocytes	^{32}P-Postlabelling + nuclease P_1 enhancement	5 smokers	In a controlled experiment, smoking caused the formation of DNA adducts. Not all adducts observed were smoking-related.
Jahnke *et al.* (1990)	Lymphocytes	^{32}P-Postlabelling	11 smokers 15 nonsmokers	Differences in distribution of lipophilic DNA adducts between smokers and nonsmokers not significant
Kiyosawa *et al.* (1990)	WBC	HPLC/ECD	10 smokers	10 minutes after smoking 2 cigarettes, 8-OHdG adduct levels in volunteers were increased 1.5-fold ($p < 0.05$).
Phillips *et al.* (1990a)	WBC	^{32}P-Postlabelling	31 smokers 20 nonsmokers	Adduct levels not significantly different in smokers and nonsmokers
Van Schooten *et al.* (1990b)	WBC	ELISA	44 controls	30% of controls had detectable BPDE–DNA adducts. Smokers had significantly higher adduct levels than nonsmokers (11/28 versus 2/16).
Savela & Hemminki (1991)	Lymphocytes, granulocytes	^{32}P-Postlabelling with nuclease P_1 enhancement	11 smokers 10 nonsmokers	DNA adducts in lymphocytes of smokers significantly higher ($p < 0.05$) than in those of nonsmokers. Differences in granulocytes not significant

Table 4.5 (contd)

Study	Blood cells[a]	Method of analysis	Number of subjects	Outcome
Mustonen & Hemminki (1992)	WBC, lymphocytes, granulocytes	^{32}P-Postlabelling	10 smokers 10 nonsmokers	DNA adduct levels as 7-methylguanine residues were significantly higher in smokers in all 3 cell populations. Adduct levels highest in lymphocytes and lowest in granulocytes
Santella et al. (1992)	Mononuclear[b] cells	ELISA	63 smokers 27 nonsmokers (all males)	BPDE–DNA adduct levels were higher in smokers (70%) than in nonsmokers (22%). DNA adduct levels in smokers did not correlate with number of cigarettes/day or pack–years.
Van Schooten et al. (1992)	WBC	^{32}P-Postlabelling, ELISA	39 lung cancer patients	Adduct levels were not significantly associated with smoking status, or with adduct levels in lung tissue (matching tissue for 20 subjects).
Gallagher et al. (1993a)	WBC, lymphocytes	^{32}P-Postlabelling	23 smokers 16 nonsmokers	Adduct levels 2.5-fold higher in smokers for both cell types ($p < 0.01$)
Holz et al. (1993)	Lymphocytes	Nick translation to detect DNA single strand breaks	5 smokers	Under controlled conditions, single-strand breaks increased in 4/5 smokers who smoked 24 cigarettes in 8 h, having refrained from smoking for 12 h prior to the test.
Mustonen et al. (1993)	Lymphocytes	^{32}P-Postlabelling	13 smokers 7 nonsmokers	7-Methylguanine DNA adduct levels significantly higher in smokers than in nonsmokers. In 5 smokers, lung adduct levels correlated with lymphocyte adduct levels.
Popp et al. (1993)	Lymphocytes	^{32}P-Postlabelling and alkaline elution	23 oral cancer patients 15 hospital controls 21 healthy nonsmokers	Significant correlation between smoking and DNA elution rates, but not DNA adduct levels

Table 4.5 (contd)

Study	Blood cells[a]	Method of analysis	Number of subjects	Outcome
Grinberg-Funes *et al.* (1994)	Mononuclear[b] cells	ELISA	63 male smokers	No relationship between smoking and PAH–DNA adduct levels observed previously (Santella *et al.*, 1992), but significant association of serum vitamin E and C observed among *GSTM1* null individuals with adduct levels
Ichiba *et al.* (1994)	WBC	^{32}P-Postlabelling + nuclear P1 digestion	26 chimney sweeps 14 controls	Smokers had 48% higher levels of aromatic DNA adducts than nonsmokers (statistically significant).
Rojas *et al.* (1994)	WBC	HPLC/fluorescence, ^{32}P-postlabelling + nuclease P$_1$ enrichment and ELISA	7 lung cancer patients (6 smokers); 3 controls (2 nonsmokers)	BPDE–DNA adducts detected in the 6 patients who smoked at substantially higher levels than in the controls who did not smoke. A good correlation was obtained with results from fluorometry and ^{32}P-postlabelling, but not from fluorometry and ELISA.
Binková *et al.* (1995)	WBC	^{32}P-Postlabelling with butanol enrichment	9 smokers 21 nonsmokers	In a study designed to investigate exposure of women working outdoors to PAH, no effect of smoking on adduct levels was observed.
Mooney *et al.* (1995)	WBC	ELISA	40 smokers	In a smoking cessation study, a 50–75% reduction in PAH–DNA adduct levels was observed 8 months after cessation, with similar reductions in 4-ABP–haemoglobin adduct levels.
Rojas *et al.* (1995)	Mononuclear[b] cells	HPLC/fluorescence	39 coke-oven workers 39 controls	Workers had higher levels of BPDE–DNA adducts than controls. In both groups, mean level in smokers was higher, but differences not statistically significant (large interindividual variation).

Table 4.5 (contd)

Study	Blood cells[a]	Method of analysis	Number of subjects	Outcome
Schell et al. (1995)	WBC, lymphocytes	^{32}P-Postlabelling	103 smokers 107 nonsmokers	In a study of several populations occupationally exposed to PAH and controls, no influence of smoking on adduct levels in WBC was evident, and only a weak trend in lymphocytes.
Tang et al. (1995)	WBC	ELISA	119 lung cancer cases (52 smokers, 58 former smokers, 9 nonsmokers) 98 controls (25 smokers, 34 former smokers, 39 nonsmokers)	Adduct levels were significantly higher in cases than in controls ($p < 0.01$) and higher in smokers and former smokers in both groups ($p < 0.05$). Adducts increased with number of cigarettes smoked in cases who were current smokers ($n = 51$), but not in control smokers. Adducts in WBC correlated with adducts in lung tumour tissue ($p < 0.05$, $n = 34$).
Wiencke et al. (1995)	Mononuclear cells	^{32}P-Postlabelling	6 smokers 10 former smokers (< 1 year) 15 former smokers (> 1 year)	Correlation of adduct levels in mononuclear cells with adduct levels in lung (value 2.6-fold higher in lung than in mononuclear cells)
Asami et al. (1996)	WBC	HPLC/ECD	10 smokers 10 former smokers 10 nonsmokers	Levels of 8-OH-guanine in DNA 1.88-fold higher in smokers than in nonsmokers ($p = 0.013$)
Mooney et al. (1997)	WBC	ELISA	159 smokers enrolled in a smoking cessation programme	PAH–DNA adduct levels 2-fold higher ($p < 0.03$) in individuals with CYP1A1 exon 7 Val allele[d] ($n = 10$). Association between plasma levels of β-carotene and adducts seen only in GSTM1 null subjects

Table 4.5 (contd)

Study	Blood cells[a]	Method of analysis	Number of subjects	Outcome
Van Schooten et al. (1997)	Lymphocytes	^{32}P-Postlabelling	54 smokers 21 nonsmokers	Aromatic DNA adduct levels significantly related to daily exposure to cigarette tar, with evidence of saturation at > 29 cigarettes/day. No significant correlation with adduct levels in BAL cells
Wang et al. (1997)	Lymphocytes	^{32}P-Postlabelling	94 smokers 98 nonsmokers	DNA adduct levels in smokers not significantly different from levels in nonsmokers. Plasma levels of β-carotene and α-tocopherol did not influence adduct levels significantly, nor did CYP1A1 or GSTM1 genotype.
Zhao et al. (1997)	WBC	^{32}P-Postlabelling	6 smokers 14 nonsmokers	Difference in adduct levels between smokers and nonsmokers of borderline significance ($p = 0.051$). No correlation between adducts and daily cigarette consumption
Arnould et al. (1998)	WBC	ELISA	58 smokers 20 nonsmokers	BPDE–DNA adducts not detected in nonsmokers. Adduct levels in smokers correlated with tobacco consumption ($p < 0.001$)
Dallinga et al. (1998)	Lymphocytes	^{32}P-Postlabelling	55 smokers 4 nonsmokers	DNA adduct levels correlated with cigarette and tar consumption, with evidence of saturation at higher smoking levels. No effect of GSTM1 genotype. Slow acetylators (NAT2) had significantly higher adduct levels ($p < 0.05$).

Table 4.5 (contd)

Study	Blood cells[a]	Method of analysis	Number of subjects	Outcome
Godschalk et al. (1998)	Lymphocytes, monocytes, granulocytes	^{32}P-Postlabelling	86 smokers 23 nonsmokers	Aromatic DNA-adduct levels significantly higher in lymphocytes and monocytes of smokers, but not granulocytes. Adduct levels in monocytes + lymphocytes of smokers ($n = 78$) linearly related to daily exposure to 'cigarette tar' but not cigarette consumption or pack–years
Pastorelli et al. (1998)	Lymphocytes	GC–MS	44 male lung cancer patients, all smokers	Significant correlation between levels of BPDE–DNA adducts and numbers of cigarettes smoked daily ($p = 0.02$) and pack–years ($p = 0.05$). No effect of CYP1A1, mEH or GSTM1 genotypes on levels of adducts
Rojas et al. (1998)	WBC	HPLC/fluorescence	20 smokers (coke-oven workers)	BPDE–DNA adduct levels higher in 1 individual with GSTM1 null and CYP1A1 2A/2A variant genotypes
Hou et al. (1999)	Lymphocytes	^{32}P-Postlabelling	179 lung cancer cases (36 smokers, 29 recent former smokers, 27 long-term former smokers, 87 never-smokers) 161 controls (46 smokers, 12 recent former smokers, 24 long-term former smokers, 79 never-smokers)	Aromatic DNA adduct levels significantly higher in smokers (cases + controls) than in long-term former smokers (> 2 years) and nonsmokers ($p = 0.0003$). No significant differences between cases and controls for any of the smoking categories
Pavanello et al. (1999)	Mononuclear cells	HPLC/fluorescence	130 subjects	Subjects were exposed to PAH from a variety of occupational and iatrogenic sources. Smoking did not influence BPDE–DNA adduct levels.

Table 4.5 (contd)

Study	Blood cells[a]	Method of analysis	Number of subjects	Outcome
Poli *et al.* (1999)	WBC	Comet assay	50 smokers 50 nonsmokers	Significant differences in DNA migration[c] between smokers and nonsmokers ($p < 0.001$)
Shinozaki *et al.* (1999)	Lymphocytes	Flow cytometry	40 smokers 35 nonsmokers	Mean level of BPDE–DNA adducts in smokers significantly higher than in nonsmokers. In smokers, adduct levels correlated with age, years of smoking and pack–years, but not with number of cigarettes/day.
Wiencke *et al.* (1999)	Mononuclear cells	^{32}P-Postlabelling	54 lung cancer patients	A significant correlation was observed between adduct levels in blood mononuclear cells and in lung ($r = 0.77$, $p < 0.001$)
van Zeeland *et al.* (1999)	WBC leukocytes	HPLC/ECD	57 smokers 16 former smokers 29 nonsmokers	Levels of 8-OHdG in DNA significantly lower in smokers than in nonsmokers ($p < 0.05$)
Besarati Nia *et al.* (2000b)	Lymphocytes	^{32}P-Postlabelling	9 smokers 9 nonsmokers	Lipophilic DNA adduct levels significantly higher in smokers than in nonsmokers ($p = 0.0001$). Levels of adducts in induced sputum higher than those in lymphocytes with adducts
Duell *et al.* (2000)	Mononuclear cells	^{32}P-Postlabelling	11 smokers 38 former smokers 11 nonsmokers	Polyphenol–DNA adducts showed a weak positive trend with the presence of *XRCC1* allele 399Gln. No association found with smoking. No effect of *ERCC2* polymorphism observed
Georgiadis *et al.* (2000)	Peripheral and cord WBC	Competitive repair assay	28 smokers 5 smokers	O^6-Methylguanine levels in DNA not influenced by smoking status
Jacobson *et al.* (2000)	Mononuclear[b] cells	ELISA	121 smokers	PAH–DNA and 8-OHdG adduct levels in smokers reduced by vitamin supplements, but differences from placebo group not significant

Table 4.5 (contd)

Study	Blood cells[a]	Method of analysis	Number of subjects	Outcome
Peluso et al. (2000)	WBC	^{32}P-Postlabelling	162 bladder cancer cases 104 hospital-based controls	No relationship between smoking and adduct levels found, although there was a strong association with case/control status. Adduct levels significantly reduced in subjects with higher fruit and vegetable consumption. Adduct levels influenced by NAT2 genotype, but not by GSTM1, GSTT1, GSTP1, COMT or NQO1 genotypes
Rojas et al. (2000)	WBC	HPLC/fluorescence	89 coke oven workers (35 smokers, 36 former smokers, 18 nonsmokers) 44 controls (all smokers)	BPDE–DNA adducts increased in smokers. GSTM1 genotype also influenced adduct levels, as did combinations of GSTM1 and CYP1A1 genotypes, but GSTT1 genotype did not.
Vulimiri et al. (2000)	Lymphocytes	^{32}P-Postlabelling	55 lung cancer cases (46 smokers, 6 former smokers, 3 nonsmokers) 58 controls (39 smokers, 6 former smokers, 13 nonsmokers)	Lung cancer cases had higher levels of aromatic adducts and 8-OHdG than controls regardless of smoking status; and among smokers, only higher levels of bulky adducts. No correlation was seen between levels of the two adduct types.
Besarati Nia et al. (2001)	Lymphocytes	HPLC/ECD for 8-OHdG; comet assay for oxidized pyrimidines	21 smokers 24 nonsmokers	Smokers had lower levels of 8-OHdG adduct than nonsmokers (38.6 versus 50.9 10^6 dG, $p = 0.05$). Levels of oxidized pyrimidines were lower (not statistically significant) than in nonsmokers.

Table 4.5 (contd)

Study	Blood cells[a]	Method of analysis	Number of subjects	Outcome
Godschalk et al. (2001)	Mononuclear cells[b]	^{32}P-Postlabelling + nuclease P₁ enrichment	67 smokers	A positive correlation was found between self-reported numbers of cigarettes smoked daily and aromatic-DNA adduct levels ($p = 0.04$). DNA adduct levels correlated with 4-ABP–haemoglobin adduct levels. Individuals with some combinations of GSTT1 or GSTM1 genotypes with NAT1 and NAT2 genotypes had significantly different adduct levels.
Hou et al. (2001)	Lymphocytes	^{32}P-Postlabelling + nuclease P₁ treatment	170 lung cancer cases 144 controls (113 smokers and recent former smokers, 201 long-term former smokers and nonsmokers)	Aromatic DNA adduct levels higher in smokers than in nonsmokers, especially in controls. Controls with the NAT2 slow genotype had higher adduct levels than controls with the rapid phenotype.
Matullo et al. (2001)	WBC	^{32}P-Postlabelling	81 smokers 92 former smokers 131 nonsmokers	No effect of smoking on adduct levels apparent, but within each group, polymorphisms in XRCC3 were associated with higher adduct levels. XRCC1 and XPD genotype affected adduct levels in nonsmokers only.
Tang et al. (2001)	WBC	^{32}P-Postlabelling	89 lung cancer cases (36 smokers, 36 former smokers, 16 nonsmokers) 173 controls (67 smokers, 72 former smokers, 32 nonsmokers)	In this prospective study, among current smokers, the mean level of adducts among cases was double that among the controls ($p = 0.03$). Smokers had higher levels of adducts than former and nonsmokers, but differences not significant.
van Delft et al. (2001)	Lymphocytes	^{32}P-Postlabelling TLC and HPLC	37 controls (18 smokers, 19 nonsmokers)	PAH–DNA adduct levels significantly higher in smokers by TLC method

Table 4.5 (contd)

Study	Blood cells[a]	Method of analysis	Number of subjects	Outcome
Whyatt et al. (2001)	WBC	^{32}P-Postlabelling, ELISA	160 mother/newborn infant pairs (16 smokers, 38 former smokers, 106 nonsmokers)	Cord blood of infants had higher aromatic DNA adduct levels than maternal WBC. When analysed by ELISA, PAH–DNA adduct levels were higher in 7/10 smoking mothers than in their infants ($p = 0.05$). Among mother/newborn pairs where blood samples were obtained concurrently ($n = 61$), aromatic DNA adducts were higher in the WBC of newborns than in the parental WBC in all groups except current smokers.
Hou et al. (2002)	Lymphocytes	^{32}P-Postlabelling	185 lung cancer cases (97 smokers, 88 never-smokers) 162 controls (83 smokers, 79 never-smokers)	Adduct levels similar in cases and controls, but increased in smokers and recent former smokers (statistically significant). Adduct levels significantly increased with increasing number of variant alleles in XPD exon 10 or exon 23

WBC, white blood cells; ELISA, enzyme-linked immunosorbent assay; BPDE, benzo[a]pyrene diol epoxide; PAH, polycyclic aromatic hydrocarbons; HPLC, high-performance liquid chromatography; ECD, electrochemical detection; 8-OHdG, 8-hydroxy-2'-deoxyguanosine; 4-ABP, 4-aminobiphenyl; BAL, bronchoalveolar lavage; GC–MS, gas chromatography–mass spectrometry; dG, deoxyguanosine; TLC, thin-layer chromatography

[a] White blood cells = leukocytes = granular + non-granular (lymphocytes and monocytes) cells

[b] Mononuclear cells: lymphocytes plus monocytes

[c] DNA migration = distance between the edge of comet head and end of tail

[d] Val allele = valine polymorphism

in whole white blood cell preparations (see Table 4.5). However, a study of adduct levels in smokers following cessation of the habit did show a decline over time (Mooney *et al.*, 1995). It is clear from studies of populations occupationally exposed to agents such as PAHs that there are many sources of exposure that result in DNA adducts in blood cells and whether or not the influence of tobacco smoking is discernible probably depends on the extent of the contribution of other occupational or environmental sources in particular study populations. There have also been reports of the influence of nutritional factors on levels of DNA adducts in blood cells in some studies (Grinberg-Funes *et al.*, 1994; Mooney *et al.*, 1997; Jacobson *et al.*, 2000), but not in others (Wang *et al.*, 1997). The modulating effects of genetic polymorphisms in xenobiotic metabolizing genes and DNA repair genes have been implicated in several studies. In general, these observations have been made on rather small numbers of subjects and the magnitude of the effects noted was not large. Confirmation of the findings from larger studies is required.

A few reports have suggested that the levels of adducts in the blood of smokers correlate with the levels of adducts in the lung (Tang *et al.*, 1995; Wiencke *et al.*, 1995, 1999). However, there are also conflicting studies in which no association was found between levels of blood BPDE–DNA adducts and levels of adducts in lung (Van Schooten *et al.*, 1992) or in cells obtained by bronchio-alveolar lavage (Van Schooten *et al.*, 1997).

A number of studies in lymphocytes have reported an increase in oxidative damage in the DNA of smokers (Kiyosawa *et al.*, 1990; Asami *et al.*, 1996). The magnitude of this increase, although significant, is generally small (less than twofold) and its biological significance is unclear. In contrast, there have been two reports in which smokers had lower levels of this lesion in DNA from their leukocytes or lymphocytes (van Zeeland *et al.*, 1999; Besarati Nia *et al.*, 2001).

Several studies that have compared smokers with cancer with smokers who are free of the disease have reported an approximately twofold higher level of lymphocyte adducts in the cases. This has been observed in two case–control studies of lung cancer (Perera *et al.*, 1989; Vulimiri *et al.*, 2000) and in one prospective study (Tang *et al.*, 2001), but not in another case–control study (Hou *et al.*, 1999). The effect was also observed in a case–control study of bladder cancer (Peluso *et al.*, 2000). These findings suggest that DNA adducts can be considered as biomarkers of risk in some populations, although the magnitude of the changes in levels is small when seen against a background of wide inter-individual variation, making the assessment of risk on an individual basis problematic.

Another approach to monitoring human exposure to carcinogens has been to detect the antigenic response to BPDE-DNA adducts in blood cells. Serum antibodies to these adducts have been detected in a number of groups of occupationally exposed workers, but in a study of smokers only four of 50 heavy smokers initially tested positive for the antibodies. Paradoxically, the frequency of positivity increased during a cessation programme in which 28 subjects quit smoking and 22 reduced cigarette consumption by 75% (Pulera *et al.*, 1997). Nevertheless, in a larger population study of 1345 individuals tested for the presence of detectable BPDE–DNA antibodies in serum, there was a positive association with smoking in 17.8% of nonsmokers, 21.5% of former smokers and 25.7% of smokers.

There was also a synergism between smoking and family history of lung cancer in deter-mining the prevalence of antibodies ($p = 0.02$) (Petruzzelli *et al.*, 1998).

(iv)   *Blood compounds*

Tobacco use is associated with increased levels of several carcinogens in blood. These compounds may prove useful as biomarkers of exposure to tobacco smoke when blood samples are collected in epidemiological studies.

Tobacco is a major source of exposure to cadmium in the general population and blood cadmium concentrations correlate positively with current tobacco smoking habits (WHO, 1992). Cadmium levels increase with the number of cigarettes smoked per day (Hoffmann *et al.*, 2000). Current smokers have, on average, levels of cadmium that are four to five times higher than those of never-smokers (Ellingsen *et al.*, 1997; Hoffmann *et al.*, 2000). Cigarette smoking or both sheesha (tobacco–fruit mixture cooked) and ciga-rette smoking lead to significantly higher blood cadmium levels than those observed in nonsmokers or in smokers of only sheesha (Al-Saleh *et al.*, 2000). Although smoking has less effect on lead levels than on those of cadmium, slightly higher levels of lead in blood have generally been reported for smokers than for nonsmokers or former smokers (Brockhaus *et al.*, 1983; Al-Saleh, 1995; Ellingsen *et al.*, 1997).

Many studies have shown that the levels of certain volatile organic compounds in blood were significantly higher in smokers than in nonsmokers (Ashley *et al.*, 1996). The mean levels of benzene and styrene in blood were significantly higher among smokers than nonsmokers. The concentrations of benzene in blood were significantly associated with the number of cigarettes smoked per day (Ashley *et al.*, 1995). The difference in the levels of benzene in blood persisted when comparisons between smokers and nonsmokers in the general public and in occupationally exposed groups were made (Brugnone *et al.*, 1999).

The levels of NNAL (a metabolite of NNK) has been measured in the blood (unhydro-lysed plasma) of smokers (Hecht *et al.*, 1999a). NNAL and its detoxification product, NNAL-glucuronide, can be detected in the blood plasma for up to 2 days after quitting tobacco use. Levels of NNAL and NNAL-glucuronide in blood are 18.8% and [4.1%] of those in urine, respectively (Hecht *et al.*, 2002).

(v)   *Breath compounds*

Exhaled carbon monoxide

The measurement of exhaled carbon monoxide (CO) has often been used as a tool for validation of self-reported cigarette consumption and smoking histories and to distinguish smokers from nonsmokers (Robertson *et al.*, 1987; Muranaka *et al.*, 1988; Morabia *et al.*, 2001).

The concentration of CO in exhaled air was significantly correlated with the self-reported number of cigarettes smoked per day. The average concentration of expired CO was 4.9 ppm (v/v) ($n = 20$) in nonsmokers and 18.5 ppm in smokers ($n = 20$; $p < 0.001$).

The concentration of expired CO in male smokers (n = 12) was 22.7 ppm and in female smokers was 12.0 ppm (n = 8; p < 0.05) (Muranaka *et al.*, 1988).

Various measures of exhaled CO as a marker of exposure to cigarette smoke were compared between 400 current regular male and female smokers. Cigarette consumption was categorized as moderate (< 15 cigarettes/day for at least 5 days per week for the last 2 years) or heavy (> 15 cigarettes/day for at least 2 years). Individuals with genetic variants of the *CYP2A6* gene (*CYP2A6*2* and *CYP2A6*A* genes) were not included in the analysis (n = 25). No difference was found in the number of cigarettes per day or levels of exhaled CO between the sexes among Caucasian smokers. Women smoked 19.3 cigarettes per day and exhaled 19.6 ppm (v/v) CO, whereas men smoked 19.8 cigarettes/day and exhaled 20.6 ppm CO. The ratio of nicotine:CO was determined using plasma nicotine levels. Women had significantly lower levels of nicotine in the blood than men (17.3 versus 20.9 ng/mL; p < 0.01). Although no significant difference was found in levels of CO in breath, women tended to smoke cigarettes with a lower nicotine content and their nicotine:CO ratios were lower than those measured in male smokers. Among other ethnic groups, there were no statistically significant gender differences in the number of cigarettes smoked per day, but men had higher concentrations of CO in exhaled air and higher concentrations of blood nicotine and cotinine (p < 0.01) than women (Zeman *et al.*, 2002).

The CO level measured in exhaled breath condensate was significantly higher in smokers (12.5 ppm) than in nonsmokers (3.4 ppm) and increased significantly to 19.6 ppm 30 min after exposure to tobacco smoke (Balint *et al.*, 2001).

At the time of delivery, pregnant women who smoked exhaled 8.42 ppm (v/v) CO corrected for inhaled air as opposed to 1.33 ppm exhaled by pregnant women who did not smoke (p < 0.0001) (Seidman *et al.*, 1999). The concentration of exhaled CO in mothers who smoked was strongly correlated with the number of cigarettes smoked per day (p < 0.000001). Within hours of delivery, the newborns of women smokers exhaled 10 ppm CO, whereas 1.74 ppm CO was exhaled by newborns of nonsmoking mothers (p < 0.0001). Maternal exhaled CO correlated strongly (p < 0.000001) with neonatal exhaled CO.

No differences in concentrations of exhaled CO were found between smokers of either three mentholated or three non-mentholated cigarettes with different nicotine content (the three cigarettes were smoked 45 min apart, in a single session) (Pickworth *et al.*, 2002). According to Clark *et al.* (1996), African American smokers had significantly higher levels of cotinine and CO per cigarette smoked and per millimetre of tobacco rod smoked than white American smokers (p < 0.001). After adjustment for race, number of cigarettes smoked per day and mean length of each cigarette smoked, the presence of menthol was associated with higher concentrations of cotinine (p = 0.03) and CO (p = 0.02).

A preliminary evaluation of a novel smoking system that employs electrical heating of tobacco (600 °C) instead of combustion (900 °C) (Accord®) was carried out by enrolling 10 smokers of 'light' cigarettes (≥ 10 cigarettes/day). The novel system limited users to eight puffs per cigarette instead of their usual 10–11 puffs. The levels of expired CO were lower in subjects using the novel system than when normal cigarettes were smoked (Buchhalter & Eissenberg, 2000).

Eclipse® is a novel nicotine delivery device that primarily heats, rather than burns, tobacco. In a cross-over study, the number of cigarettes smoked per day decreased from 19 at baseline to 2.1 after two weeks of using Eclipse® ($p < 0.001$), but exhaled CO concentrations increased from 21 ppm to 33 ppm ($p < 0.001$). During use of Eclipse®, the concentration of nicotine in blood remained fairly stable although it increased slightly from 16.8 ng/mL to 18.0 ng/mL (Fagerström et al., 2000).

Smoking fewer cigarettes may reduce exposure to toxins even if the smoker adopts a more intensive smoking behaviour to compensate for the reduced number of cigarettes. If consumption is reduced from an average of 37 cigarettes/day to an average of five cigarettes/day, the intake of tobacco toxins per cigarette increased roughly threefold and daily exposure to tar and CO declined by only 50% (Benowitz et al., 1986). The reduction of cigarette consumption from 40 cigarettes/day to 20 cigarettes/day was not followed by any consistent reduction in the levels of biomarkers of exposure to tobacco carcinogens (Hurt et al., 2000).

Exhaled nitric oxide

Nitric oxide (NO) is formed from L-arginine by the enzyme NO synthase (NOS). NO is a highly reactive molecule that can be oxidized or complexed with other biomolecules depending on the microenvironment. The stable oxidation products of NO metabolism are nitrite and nitrate. Cigarette smoking is associated with an increased risk for respiratory tract infection, chronic airway disease and cardiovascular diseases, all of which may be modulated by endogenous NO (which acts as an endogenous vasodilator). Cigarette smoking reduces the levels of NO exhaled by healthy subjects, but the mechanism for this is unclear (Schilling et al., 1994; Yates et al., 2001). In the study by Yates et al. (2001), the amount exhaled by active smokers was significantly less than the amounts of NO exhaled by subjects who were exposed to sham and passive smoking for the same length of time (49 ppb (v/v) after 15 min of active smoking, a 30.3% decrease from the baseline level of 71 ppb versus 115 ppb in subjects exposed to sham smoking and 102 ppb in subjects exposed to passive smoking). Schilling et al. (1994) reported the same trend, with concentrations of exhaled NO being lower in smokers than in nonsmokers exposed to secondhand smoke (mean, 16 ppb in women who smoked versus 21 ppb in women who did not smoke and 15 ppb in men who smoked versus 19 ppb in men who did not smoke). However, the absolute values were much lower than those reported by Yates et al. (2001). In a single-breath analysis, smokers exhaled about 20 ppb NO, healthy controls, 40 ppb and asthmatic patients, 60 ppb (Persson et al., 1994). Kharitonov et al. (1995) reported that smokers exhaled 42 ppb NO, whereas the concentration exhaled by nonsmokers was 88 ppb ($p < 0.01$). There was a significant relationship between the amount of exhaled NO and cigarette consumption ($r = -0.77$, $p < 0.001$).

Measurement of exhaled NO may yield information about the mechanisms underlying cigarette-induced lung damage. Balint *et al.* (2001) found that there was no difference between smokers and nonsmokers in the levels of nitrite, nitrite + nitrate, *S*-nitrosothiols and nitrotyrosine in the exhaled breath condensate at the baseline visit. Thirty minutes after smoking two cigarettes, the levels of nitrite + nitrate were significantly increased (from 20.2 to 29.8 µM, $p < 0.05$) and returned to the baseline within 90 min. There was no significant change in the levels of exhaled NO, nitrite, *S*-nitrosothiols or nitrotyrosine 30 and 90 min after smoking two cigarettes. There was no correlation between levels of exhaled NO and NO metabolites in breath condensate before and after smoking.

Benzene

Breath analysis under controlled conditions has been used to measure the exposure to benzene associated with active smoking (Jo & Pack, 2000). The mean benzene concentrations in exhaled breath measured 1 min after smoking 5.0 cm of a cigarette (to a remaining butt length of 3.3 cm) ranged from 58.1 to 81.3 µg/m^3, depending on the commercial cigarette brand, whereas benzene concentrations measured prior to smoking ranged from 15.9 to 19.2 µg/m^3. These post-exposure concentrations of benzene in breath were much higher than the mean concentrations of benzene in breath reported in some previous studies (e.g. 16 µg/m^3 among smokers versus 2.5 µg/m^3 among nonsmokers; $p < 0.001$) (Wallace & Pellizzari, 1986) in which the exposure conditions and post-sampling times were not controlled. The concentration of benzene in breath increases with the number of cigarettes smoked: from 9.4 µg/m^3 (no cigarettes) to 47 µg/m^3 (> 50 cigarettes/day). The increase in concentrations of benzene in breath after active smoking is due to benzene being absorbed through the lung while an individual is smoking. From direct measurements of benzene in mainstream smoke, it was calculated that a typical smoker (30 cigarettes/day) inhales 2 mg benzene daily, whereas a nonsmoker inhales 0.2 mg/day (Wallace *et al.*, 1987).

Volatile organic compounds

Volatile organic compounds (VOC) other than benzene are often measured in expired breath to determine the exposure to cigarette smoke. Among 20 VOC analysed by Wallace and Pellizzari (1986), the levels of *meta* + *para*-xylene, ethylbenzene, *ortho*-xylene, styrene and octane were found to be statistically significantly higher ($p < 0.05$) in smokers ($n = 198$) than in nonsmokers ($n = 322$). Significant increases in the concentration in breath with number of cigarettes smoked were noted for styrene, ethylbenzene and *meta* + *para*-xylene (Wallace *et al.*, 1987).

Gordon (1990) analysed VOC in the exhaled breath of 26 smokers and 43 non-smokers to identify possible biochemical markers of exposure to cigarette smoke. Among 230 GC–MS peaks, 2,5-dimethylfuran was found to have sufficient discriminatory power to allow almost complete distinction to be made between smokers and nonsmokers. Several other compounds could also be used to distinguish between the two groups with a high level of accuracy. However, the half-lives of these compounds must be determined before they can be exploited as practical indicators of exposure to smoking.

Ethane, often used routinely as a marker of lipid peroxidation, has the potential to be a non-invasive marker of free-radical activity. Ethane levels in exhaled air were found to be higher in active smokers than in former smokers and nonsmokers (2.9 pmol/min/kg versus 1.55 and 1.11 pmol/min/kg, respectively), reflecting the presence of ethane in cigarette smoke (Habib *et al.*, 1995).

The levels of isoprene in exhaled breath increased on average by 70% after smoking one cigarette. The concentration of acetone increased by 22%, whereas that of ethanol decreased by 28% after smoking one cigarette (Senthilmohan *et al.*, 2001).

(vi)   *Other*

Polycyclic aromatic hydrocarbons

Several studies have quantified PAHs in lung tissue (Tomingas *et al.*, 1976; Seto *et al.*, 1993; Tokiwa *et al.*, 1993; Lodovici *et al.*, 1998). In a recent investigation, the quantities of 11 PAHs were measured in 70 lung tissue samples from 37 smokers and 33 nonsmokers (defined by serum cotinine concentration). The sum of PAH concentrations was higher in smokers and there was a dose–response relationship for smoking characterized by increasing serum cotinine (Goldman *et al.*, 2001).

Benzo[a]pyrene

Benzo[a]pyrene and several of its metabolites were detected in the cervical mucus of both smokers and nonsmokers (Melikian *et al.*, 1999).

N-Nitrosamines

The tobacco-specific nitrosamine, NNK, was detected in 16 samples of cervical mucus from 15 women who were smokers at concentrations of 11.9–115 ng/g (mucus) (two samples were collected from one smoker at different times) and in nine of 10 samples from nonsmokers at concentrations of 4.1–30.8 ng/g (mucus), but the concentrations of NNK in specimens from cigarette smokers were significantly higher than in those obtained from nonsmokers (Prokopczyk *et al.*, 1997). Further studies demonstrated that human cervical tissue can metabolize NNK by both α-hydroxylation and carbonyl reduction (Prokopczyk *et al.*, 2001).

NNK was detected in 15 of 18 samples of pancreatic juice from smokers at concentrations of 1.4–604 ng/mL and in six of nine samples from nonsmokers (range of concentrations, 1.13–97 ng/mL), and the levels were significantly higher in smokers than in nonsmokers. NNAL was present in 11 of 17 samples from smokers and in 3/9 from nonsmokers. NNN was found in two of 17 samples from smokers (68 and 242 ng/mL) (Prokopczyk *et al.*, 2002).

Particulate matter (tar)

A problem in the analysis of exposure to tobacco smoke is that there is no direct marker for tar uptake (exposure). The biomarkers most frequently used for measuring the uptake of tobacco smoke (nicotine and cotinine) reflect the exposure to particulate-phase constituents.

Russel *et al.* (1986) and Woodward and Tunstall-Pedoe (1992) used an indirect measure, based on the assumption that the intake of different smoke components relative to one another is proportional to their concentration in the smoke, to evaluate the exposure of smokers in large population studies. Two tar indices were calculated:

- tar index (CO) = eCO × tar yield/CO yield; and
- tar index(cot) = serum cotinine × tar yield/nicotine yield

where the 'yields' were the values obtained by standard machine-smoking methods and expired CO (eCO) and serum cotinine were the individual's values. An average tar index was calculated as a weighted mean of the two indices for each individual, using the inverse standard deviations as the weights. This approach was validated by testing its ability to predict the levels of one marker by use of another. For example, using blood carboxyhaemoglobin (COHb) concentrations and CO:nicotine yield ratio of the cigarettes, the mean concentration of nicotine in the blood of smokers of low-tar cigarettes was predicted to be 31.9 ng/mL, whereas the measured mean was 31.8 ng/mL. Based on the measurements of the concentrations of cotinine, nicotine and COHb in blood and the calculated tar indices for 392 smokers (255 women and 137 men) of 'middle-tar' (17–22 mg), 'low-to-middle' (11–16 mg) and 'low-tar' (< 11 mg) cigarettes, Russell *et al.* (1986) concluded that despite substantial compensatory increases in inhalation, the low-tar smokers took in about 25% less tar, 15% less nicotine and 10% less CO than smokers of middle- and low-to-middle tar cigarettes. Similar outcomes were reported by Woodward and Tunstall-Pedoe (1992). They evaluated the exposure of 1133 male and 1621 female smokers of the three groups of cigarettes (low tar [< 13 mg/cigarette], middle tar [14–15 mg] and high tar [> 15 mg]) in the Scottish Heart Health Study by measuring the expired CO, serum thiocyanate and serum cotinine and calculating the indices of tar consumption. Expired CO and cotinine were found to peak in the middle-tar group. Tar consumption increased with tar yield of the cigarette smoked, but the increase in consumption was much lower than would be expected. This finding led to the conclusion that the tar yield of a cigarette is not an accurate guide to the amount of smoke components consumed by the smoker.

The atherogenic potential of mainstream smoke is associated with the particulate and vapour-phase components and not with CO. The thrombogenic potential is also associated with the particulate matter and vapour phase (Smith & Fisher, 2001).

Nicotine and its metabolites as markers of exposure to tobacco smoke

Nicotine is the principal alkaloid present in tobacco. Nicotine is also the main addictive constituent of tobacco products. It also has other pharmacological activities and toxic effects (Domino, 1999). Manufactured cigarettes contain 1–7% nicotine by weight

(6–12 mg nicotine/cigarette) and, of this, 15–25% enters the mainstream smoke while 75% is emitted into the air as sidestream smoke (Benowitz, 1999a). Nicotine is also found in exhaled smoke (Curvall & Enzell, 1986; IARC, 1986; California Environmental Protection Agency, 1997) (see Section 1).

An overview of the pathways of nicotine metabolism is presented in Figure 4.4. Nicotine is hydroxylated at the 5′-position by cytochromes P450 to yield an unstable intermediate, 5′-hydroxynicotine (**5**; see Figure 4.4), which exists in equilibrium with $\Delta^{1'(5')}$ iminium ion (**6**). 5′-Hydroxynicotine is oxidized by aldehyde oxidase to cotinine (**8**). Cotinine, in turn, is metabolized further to cotinine–glucuronide (cotinine–Gluc, **9**), *trans*-3′-hydroxycotinine (**12**) and *trans*-3′-hydroxycotinine–glucuronide (*trans*-3′-hydroxycotinine–Gluc, **13**) (Gorrod & Schepers, 1999). 2′-Hydroxylation of nicotine, mediated by cytochromes P450, gives 2′-hydroxynicotine (**4**), which spontaneously yields $\Delta^{1'(2')}$ iminium ion (**3**) and 4-(methylamino)-1-(3-pyridyl)-1-butanone (aminoketone, **7**), also known as pseudooxynicotine. Aminoketone (**7**) is then converted to 4-oxo-4-(3-pyridyl)butyric acid (keto acid, **11**) and 4-hydroxy-4-(3-pyridyl)butyric acid (hydroxy acid, **14**) (Hecht *et al.*, 2000).

The major urinary metabolite of nicotine in smokers is *trans*-3′-hydroxycotinine (**12**) (about 40% of total urinary nicotine and metabolites). This is followed by cotinine (**8**) and cotinine–Gluc (**9**) (12–15% of each), *trans*-3′-hydroxycotinine–Gluc (**13**) (10%), hydroxy acid (**14**) (8%) and keto acid (**11**) (2%). Unchanged nicotine (8% of total urinary nicotine plus metabolites) and nicotine–Gluc (**2**) (2–3%) also occur (Byrd *et al.*, 1992; Benowitz *et al.*, 1994; Hecht *et al.*, 1999b).

Since the mid-1980s, studies that have measured exposure to tobacco smoke and its biological effects have predominantly used nicotine and its metabolite cotinine determined in blood, urine or saliva as biological markers of exposure and uptake of tobacco smoke (IARC, 1986; National Research Council, 1986; US Department of Health and Human Services, 1986; Environmental Protection Agency, 1993; California Environmental Protection Agency, 1997). The main advantage of using nicotine and, consequently that of cotinine, as a marker compound over other markers is their specificity for tobacco and tobacco smoke. The measurements of all the metabolites in Figure 4.4 provides a more complete assessment of nicotine uptake.

The half-life of nicotine in the body is short, approximately 2 h in nonsmokers (IARC, 1986; Benowitz, 1996; Benowitz & Jacob, 1997; Benowitz, 1999b). Nicotine concentration can therefore reflect only acute exposure. This limits its use as a biomarker (IARC, 1986; US Environmental Protection Agency, 1993; Benowitz, 1996). The concentrations of nicotine in blood or plasma are higher in smokers than in nonsmokers, but vary considerably, mainly depending on the number of cigarettes smoked recently. Other variables, such as the tar content, yield of nicotine, average number of cigarettes smoked per day or type of filter, have been found to be poor predictors of nicotine concentrations in the blood (IARC, 1986).

The concentrations of cotinine can be measured in blood, urine or saliva samples. Because of its specificity and the availability of sensitive methods for reliable measure-

Figure 4.4. Pathways of mammalian nicotine metabolism initiated by 5′-hydroxyl-ation and 2′-hydroxylation

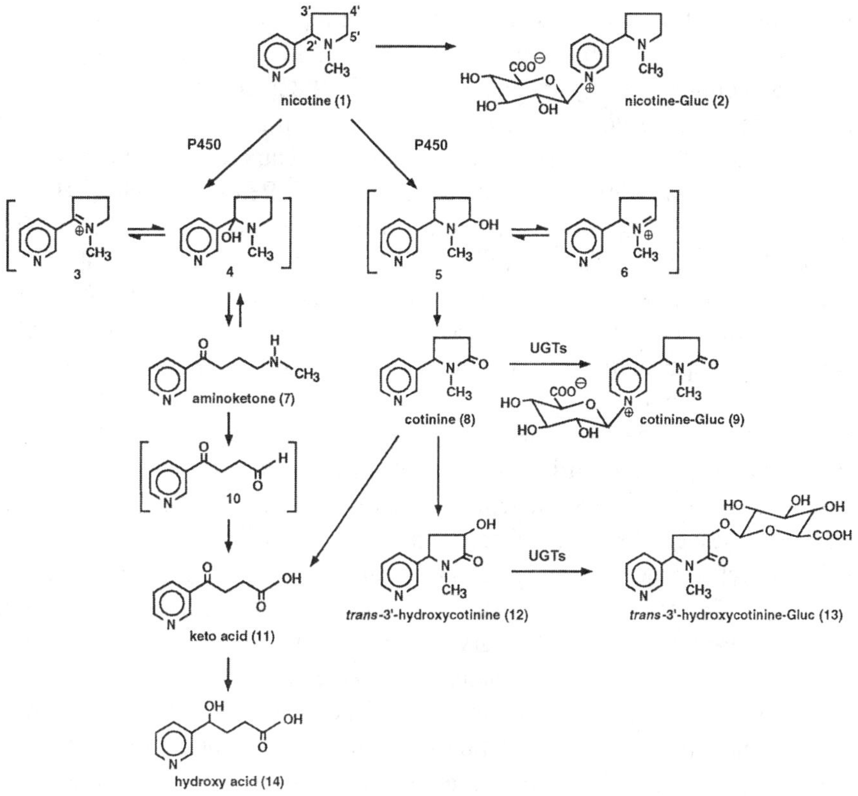

Other pathways not shown include *N*-oxidation, *N*-demethylation and *N*-methylation.
P450, cytochrome P450; UGTs, UDP-glucuronosyl transferases
Adapted from Hecht *et al.* (2000)

ments, cotinine, regardless of the body fluid, is currently the most widely used biomarker for measuring tobacco smoke uptake (reviewed in IARC, 1986; National Research Council, 1986; Jarvis *et al.*, 1987; Muranaka *et al.*, 1988; Etzel, 1990; US Environmental Protection Agency, 1993; Benowitz, 1996, 1999b). It has a sensitivity of 96–97% and a specificity of 99–100% (Jarvis *et al.*, 1987). The half-life of cotinine in smokers is longer than that of nicotine, on average about 16–20 h, with a range of approximately 10–40 h (US Environmental Protection Agency, 1993; Benowitz & Jacob, 1994; Benowitz, 1996; Pérez-Stable *et al.*, 1998; Benowitz, 1999a,b). Cotinine concentrations are a good measure of average daily exposure to tobacco smoke and reflect the exposure to tobacco smoke over the past 2–3 days (IARC, 1986; National Research Council, 1986; US Environmental Protection Agency, 1993). Cotinine concentration, however, is not suitable for measuring more long-term exposure, although it may serve as a surrogate measure for that purpose.

The main determinant of cotinine levels in smokers and nonsmokers, like that of nicotine, is exposure to tobacco smoke (reviewed in IARC, 1986; National Research Council, 1986; US Environmental Protection Agency, 1993; Benowitz, 1996, 1999a) and also exposure from use of products designed for nicotine replacement therapy (Leyden *et al.*, 1999). However, some variability due to individual differences in uptake, metabolism, distribution and elimination occurs (Benowitz *et al.*, 1982; Benowitz, 1996; Benowitz & Jacob, 1997; Benowitz *et al.*, 1999, 2002). The amount of nicotine converted to cotinine in humans varies, and this variability is attributable to dietary, environmental and genetic factors (Benowitz *et al.*, 1996; Benowitz & Jacob, 1997; Benowitz, 1999a; Hecht *et al.*, 1999b; Sellers *et al.*, 2000). Differences in the metabolism of nicotine and cotinine have been reported to occur between various racial and ethnic groups (Wagenknecht *et al.*, 1993; Caraballo *et al.*, 1998; Pérez-Stable *et al.*, 1998; Benowitz *et al.*, 1999; Kwon *et al.*, 2001). These differences have been associated with slower metabolism and lower uptake of nicotine in some populations (Benowitz *et al.*, 1999, 2002), whereas in others uptake may be higher (Caraballo *et al.*, 1998).

Many studies have demonstrated that cotinine levels are clearly higher in smokers than in nonsmokers, leading to increased levels of cotinine being detected in the urine, serum and/or saliva of smokers. Generally, urinary cotinine concentrations are more than one hundred times greater in smokers than those in nonsmokers (e.g. IARC, 1986; National Research Council, 1986; US Department of Health and Human Services, 1986; Jarvis *et al.*, 1987; Etzel, 1990; Tunstall-Pedoe *et al.*, 1991; Environmental Protection Agency, 1993; Pirkle *et al.*, 1996; Jarvis *et al.*, 2001). The large studies have been consistent in showing a positive correlation between cotinine levels and number of cigarettes smoked per day regardless of the body fluid in which cotinine was measured; however, the magnitude of the correlation varies to some extent (IARC, 1986; National Research Council, 1986; US Department of Health and Human Services, 1986; US Environmental Protection Agency, 1993; Law *et al.*, 1997a; Etter *et al.*, 2000).

Carboxyhaemoglobin and thiocyanate

The uptake of tobacco smoke constituents from the gaseous and particulate phases of mainstream smoke, inhaled by smokers, and of secondhand smoke, breathed in by nonsmokers, was investigated by Scherer *et al.* (1990). Tobacco smoke uptake was quantified by measuring COHb in erythrocytes and measuring nicotine and cotinine in plasma and urine, and the data obtained were correlated with urinary excretion of thioethers (biomarkers of electrophilic mainstream smoke carbonyls such as acrolein) and with mutagenic activity. An increase in all biochemical parameters was observed in smokers who inhaled the whole smoke of 24 cigarettes over a period of 8 h, whereas, after smoking the gas phase of mainstream smoke under the same conditions, only an increase of COHb and, to a minor degree, in urinary thioethers was found.

Serum thiocyanate has often been used for the validation of smoking histories as well as for the assessment of passive exposure to cigarette smoke. There was a significant increase ($p < 0.01$) in serum thiocyanate with increased smoking. The concentrations of serum thiocyanate in plasma were positively associated with moderate and heavy smoking, but could not distinguish between nonsmokers, light smokers and passive smokers. Fourteen smokers enrolled in this study had serum thiocyanate concentrations higher than 70 µM. The complementary assay of exhaled CO was helpful in confirming nonsmoking status. Using a combination of serum thiocyanate and exhaled CO levels, nonsmoking status was confirmed in 98% of the cases (Robertson et al., 1987).

Genetic factors affecting the metabolism of nicotine to cotinine

Genetic factors are among the major determinants of the variation in the metabolism of nicotine to cotinine. Poor metabolism of nicotine with lack of cotinine formation has been seen and shown to have a genetic basis (Benowitz et al., 1995). Many P450 enzymes are involved in the oxidative metabolism of nicotine; they include P4502A6, P4502B6, P4502D6, P4502E1, P4501A2, P4503A4 and P4501A1 (Yamazaki et al., 1999), but, in contrast to the findings reported from earlier studies, P4502D6 probably plays only a minor role (Benowitz et al., 1996; Nakajima et al., 1996; Yamazaki et al., 1999). According to present data, the most important and rate-limiting gene in 5′-hydroxylation [c-oxydation] of nicotine to cotinine is P4502A6 (Nakajima et al., 1996; Messina et al., 1997; Yamazaki et al., 1999). In addition, there are data indicating that P4502A6 is involved in 2′-hydroxylation of nicotine potentially leading to endogenous formation of NNK. This was reported to occur in human liver microsomes incubated with nicotine at a rate of about 6% of that of cotinine formation (Hecht et al., 2000).

P4502A6 enzyme activity can be lost as a result of a genetic polymorphism that can give rise to homozygosity for the inactive alleles of CYP2A6. In addition, individuals who are carriers of alleles with an inactivating mutation in a heterozygous condition and/or carry defective alleles of decreased enzyme activity are deficient in metabolizing nicotine to cotinine. Subjects with low P4502A6 enzyme activity have significantly lower levels of cotinine, as seen in smokers and in those administered nicotine via another route (Fernandez-Salguero et al., 1995; Oscarson et al., 1998; Kitagawa et al., 1999; Nunoya et al., 1999; Oscarson et al., 1999; Nakajima et al., 2000; Kwon et al., 2001; Nakajima et al., 2001; Yang et al., 2001; Xu et al., 2002). The prevalence of the homozygous genotypes with two inactive alleles varies in different populations. They are very rare among Caucasians and Japanese populations, but have been reported to be somewhat more common in the Chinese population (Yokoi & Kamataki, 1998; Kitagawa et al., 1999; Oscarson et al., 1999). More than 95% of members of Caucasian populations who show the CYP2D6 poor-metabolizer phenotype can be diagnosed by gene analysis, whereas about 20–30% of poor metabolizers can be diagnosed by the known mutant alleles in the Japanese population. Subsequently to this finding, a new mutation, CYP2D6 J9 was found in the Japanese population (Yokoi & Kamataki, 1998). In addition, a gene duplication genotype associated with increased plasma cotinine has recently been reported to occur at a low frequency in Caucasians (Rao et al., 2000). It has been proposed that CYP2A6 polymorphism may be a major determinant of an individual's smoking behaviour and may lead to less desire to smoke (Pianezza et al., 1998; Sellers et al., 2000).

In addition to the individual and racial variation that occurs in the oxidative metabolism of nicotine, variation in the glucuronide conjugation of nicotine and cotinine also
exists (Benowitz et al., 1999). Both nicotine and cotinine are metabolized by N-glucuronidation catalysed by uridine-5′-diphosphate-glucuronosyltransferase (UGT) enzymes
(see Figure 4.4; Byrd et al., 1992; Benowitz et al., 1994). Although the specific UGTs
involved in these metabolic steps are so far not known, it has been observed that N-glucuronidation of nicotine and cotinine is polymorphic, with evidence of slow and fast N-glucuronidation (Benowitz et al., 1999). Environmental factors may influence N-glucuronidation, but with current data indicating that many of the genes encoding UGTs are polymorphic (Burchell et al., 2000; Mackenzie et al., 2000), genetic polymorphism may also
be involved. Distribution of slow and fast glucuronidation has been found to vary according to ethnicity; the extent of N-glucuronidation is generally less in blacks than in whites
(Benowitz et al., 1999).

4.1.2   Experimental systems

(a)   Effects of tobacco smoke on enzyme activities

In-vivo studies

Most investigations of the effects of tobacco smoke on enzyme activities in animals
have measured changes in levels of phase I, phase II and antioxidant enzymes in the lung
and liver of mice and rats (Table 4.6). Some studies have also measured its effects on
enzyme activities in other organs such as the kidney, stomach, heart and brain.

Enzyme effects

The induction of several phase I enzymes, including P4501A1 (aryl hydrocarbon
hydroxylase), P4501A2, P4502B, P4502C, P4502D and P4502E1 by tobacco smoke in
mouse lung and liver has been reported (Table 4.6). An increase of at least twofold in the
activity of most of these enzymes is induced within a few days after initial exposure of
the mice to tobacco smoke, and the enzyme levels usually remain elevated throughout
exposure. It is probable that the induction of these enzymes can be attributed to the
presence of many carcinogens and toxins in tobacco smoke. P4502E1 appears to be
induced to a greater extent (5–13-fold) than other phase I enzymes both in the lungs and
liver of mice (Villard et al., 1994, 1998a,b). Similarly, P4502E1 is strongly induced by
tobacco smoke in mouse kidney (Seree et al., 1996). To investigate the role of nicotine in
the induction of CYP2E1, rats were treated once daily with saline or nicotine bitartrate
(0.1, 0.3 and 1.0 mg/kg bw, subcutaneously) for 7 days. After nicotine administration,
immunostaining for CYP2E1 was increased in the centrilobular region of the liver.
Western-blot analyses revealed that hepatic levels of CYP2E1 were increased 1.3–1.7-
fold by nicotine. In-vitro analysis of the metabolism of chlorzoxazone (i.e. 6-hydroxyl-
ation) showed that V_{max} values were higher than those measured in saline-treated rats
when hepatic microsomes from nicotine-treated rats were used (2.35 ± 0.04 versus
1.32 ± 0.55 nmol/mg/min, $p < 0.005$), with no change in affinity. The magnitude of the

Table 4.6. Effects of tobacco smoke on enzyme activities

Species	Strain/sex	Enzyme affected	Effect (tissue)	Reference
Mouse	C57BL/M	Aryl hydrocarbon hydroxylase	+ (lung)	Gairola (1987)
	NMRI/M	P450 1A1 P450 2B P450 2C P450 2D P450 2E1 P450 3A	+ (lung, liver) + (liver) + (liver) + (liver) + (lung, liver) + (liver)	Villard et al. (1994)
	NMRI/M	P450 1A1 P450 2B P450 3A P450 2E1	ND (kidney) ND (kidney) ND (kidney) + (kidney)	Seree et al. (1996)
	NMRI/M	P450 1A1 P450 1A2 P450 2B P450 2E1 P450 3A UDP-glucuronosyl-transferase	– (lung) + (liver) + (lung) + (lung, liver) + (lung, liver, kidney) + (liver) + (lung, liver)	Villard et al. (1998a)
	NMRI/M	P450 1A1 P450 2B P450 2E1 P450 3A	± (lung) – (liver) + (lung) ± (liver) + (lung, liver) + (liver)	Villard et al. (1998b)
Rat	S-D/M	Aryl hydrocarbon hydroxylase	+ (lung)	Gairola (1987)
	Wistar/M	Ethoxyresorufin-O-deethylase	+ (lung, liver)	Godden et al. (1987)
	S-D/M	Aryl hydrocarbon hydroxylase N-Nitrosodimethylamine demethylase	+ (lung, liver) NE	Pasquini et al. (1987)
	S-D/M	Aryl hydrocarbon hydroxylase Ethoxyresorufin-O-deethylase	+ (lung) + (liver)	Bagnasco et al. (1992)
	S-D/F	Catalase Glutathione peroxidase	NE (lung) NE (lung)	Wurzel et al. (1995)

Table 4.6 (contd)

Species	Strain/sex	Enzyme affected	Effect (tissue)	Reference
Rat	Albino/M	Glutathione reductase	– (kidney)	Anand et al. (1996)
		Gluathione peroxidase	+ (kidney)	
		Catalase	– (kidney)	
	Albino/M	Aniline 4-hydroxylase	+ (lung) NE (liver)	Eke et al. (1996)
		7-Ethoxyresorufin-O-deethylase	+ (lung) + (liver)	
		para-Nitroanisole O-demethylase	+ (lung) + (liver)	
		Glutathione-S-transferase	– (lung) ± (liver)	
		Aminopyrine N-demethylase	NE (lung) + (liver)	
	Fischer 344/M	P450 1A1	+ (lung, liver, nasal mucosa)	Wardlaw et al. (1998)
		P450 1A2	– (lung) + (liver, nasal mucosa)	
		P450 2B1/2B2	– (lung) + (liver) – (nasal mucosa)	
	Albino/M	Catalase	+ (lung, liver, kidney)	Baskaran et al. (1999)
		Superoxide dismutase	+ (lung, liver, kidney)	
		Glutathione peroxidase	+ (lung, liver, kidney)	
		Glutathione-S-transferase	+ (lung, liver, kidney, brain)	
	S-D (sex not specified)	Nitric oxide synthase-1	NE (lung)	Wright et al. (1999)
		Nitric oxide synthase-2	+ (lung)	
		Nitric oxide synthase-3	+ (lung)	
	Wistar/M	Nitric oxide synthase-2	+ (lung)	Chang et al. (2001)
		NF-κB	+ (lung)	
		Mitogen-activated protein kinases (Mek1, Erk2)	+ (lung)	
		Protein kinase C, Mekk1, Jnk, p38, c-Jun, c-Myc	NE (lung)	
Guinea-pig	Hartley/M	Aryl hydrocarbon hydroxylase	NE (lung)	Gairola (1987)
	Not specified	Collagenase	+ (lung)	Selman et al. (1996)

M, male; F, female; +, induced; –, decreased; ±, some studies report an increase, others a decrease; ND, not detected; UDP, uridine-5′-diphosphate; S-D, Sprague-Dawley; NE, no effect; NF-κB, nuclear factor-κB

enhancement of metabolism by microsomes from nicotine-treated animals is consistent with the observed increase in CYP2E1 protein as measured by immunoblot analysis. The data suggest that nicotine may increase CYP2E1-induced toxicity (Howard *et al.*, 2001). Although not detectable in mouse lung, P4503A is induced by tobacco smoke in mouse liver (Villard *et al.*, 1994). Some investigations have reported conflicting results on the extent of phase I enzyme induction by tobacco smoke. For example, in one study, P4501A1 was induced in the liver of NMRI mice exposed to tobacco smoke (Villard *et al.*, 1994) whereas, in another study in the same laboratory, P4501A1 activity was either reduced or not detected in the liver of NMRI mice (Villard *et al.*, 1998b). These opposing results might be explained by the length of the exposure period: P4501A1 was induced in mice exposed to tobacco smoke for 4 or 8 days, and was reduced in mice exposed for 30 days. In one report on the effects of tobacco smoke on phase II enzyme activity in the tissues of mice exposed to tobacco smoke, UGT was induced in the lung and liver, but not in the kidney (Villard *et al.*, 1998a).

The induction of phase I and phase II enzymes in rats has been thoroughly investigated (Table 4.6). An early study demonstrated a three- to fourfold induction of Ahh in lung microsomes of Sprague-Dawley rats exposed daily to either mainstream or sidestream whole smoke for 16 weeks (Gairola, 1987). The magnitude of Ahh induction in animals exposed to mainstream and sidestream smoke was similar, although the dose of smoke particulates received from rats exposed to sidestream smoke was significantly less than the amount inhaled by the corresponding group exposed to mainstream smoke. In another study, Ahh was induced in both the lung and liver of Sprague-Dawley rats given intraperitoneal injections of condensates of mainstream and sidestream smoke. The induction of the enzyme in the lung exceeded that in the liver, and the sidestream-smoke condensate was a more effective inducer than the mainstream-smoke condensate. The activity of lung and liver NDMA demethylase was unaffected by treatment with either condensate (Pasquini *et al.*, 1987). Ethoxyresorufin *O*-deethylase (associated with P4501A1/2) activity was induced to a similar extent in both the lung and liver of Wistar rats after a single, short exposure to cigarette smoke (Godden *et al.*, 1987). In another study, Sprague-Dawley rats were exposed to mainstream smoke produced by a commercial filter-tipped cigarette for 8 consecutive days, amounting to a cumulative exposure to 75 cigarettes. The most pronounced changes in enzyme expression consisted of a 2.6-fold induction of Ahh in the lung and an eightfold induction of ethoxyresorufin *O*-deethylase in the liver (Bagnasco *et al.*, 1992). In addition to Ahh and ethoxyresorufin *O*-deethylase, other phase I enzymes that were induced by tobacco smoke in either the lung or liver of rats included aniline 4-hydroxylase, *para*-nitroanisole *O*-demethylase, and aminopyrine *N*-demethylase (Eke *et al.*, 1996). With the exception of aniline 4-hydroxylase, the inducibility of these enzymes in the lung and liver was similar in rats ranging in age from 20 days to 360 days. Aniline 4-hydroxylase was induced in the lung and liver of 20-day-old rats, but not in 360-day-old rats (Eke *et al.*, 1997). A more recent study in Fischer 344 rats reported on the inducibility by tobacco smoke of P4501A1, P4501A2 and P4502B1/2 in the nasal mucosa, lung and liver. Rats were exposed to mainstream cigarette smoke or to filtered air for 2 or 8 weeks. The inducibility of the three enzymes varied significantly: P4501A1 levels were increased in all three tissues; P4501A2 was increased slightly in nasal mucosa and liver and decreased in lung; and P4502B1/2 was increased in liver and decreased in nasal mucosa and lung (Wardlaw *et al.*, 1998). These and other data suggest that the regulation of xenobiotic-metabolizing enzymes varies from one rodent tissue to another.

In a study of the effects of tobacco smoke on the activity of phase II enzymes in rat tissues, liver glutathione *S*-transferase (GST) activity with regard to ethacrynic acid was increased by tobacco smoke whereas that with regard to 1,2-epoxy-3-(*para*-nitrophenoxy)-propane was decreased (Eke *et al.*, 1996). Hepatic GST activities against 1-chloro-2,4-dinitrobenzene or 1,2-dichloro-4-nitrobenzene were unaltered. In the lung, however, the activity of GST against all substrates was decreased by tobacco smoke. These results indicate that the regulation of hepatic and pulmonary GSTs is differentially influenced by tobacco smoke. Cigarette smoke has the potential to depress severely the detoxification capacity of the lung.

The effects of tobacco smoke on the activities of the antioxidant enzymes catalase, superoxide dismutase, glutathione peroxidase and glutathione reductase in rat tissues have been investigated (Table 4.6). In one study in which Sprague-Dawley rats were exposed to mainstream cigarette smoke for 65 weeks, oxidative stress was increased whereas the activities of catalase and glutathione peroxidase in the lung were not significantly altered by exposure to smoke (Wurzel *et al.*, 1995). In another study, the activities of glutathione reductase and catalase were reported to be decreased in the kidney of rats exposed to tobacco smoke for 3 months, whereas the activity of glutathione peroxidase and lipid peroxide levels were increased. The excretion of glutathione and lipid peroxides in urine was also increased. The authors concluded that the reduced activity of glutathione reductase and the increased activity of glutathione peroxidase may perturb the ratio of reduced glutathione:oxidized glutathione, which in turn could lead to the increased levels of lipid peroxide in the kidney and urine seen in chronic exposure to tobacco smoke (Anand *et al.*, 1996). In a more recent study, the activities of catalase, superoxide dismutase and glutathione peroxidase were increased in the lung, liver and kidney of albino rats exposed to tobacco smoke for 2 × 15 min per day for 30 days. The activity of GST was also increased in the lung, liver and kidney. Interestingly, the activities of the antioxidant enzymes were unchanged in the brain and heart of the animals, but GST was increased in the brain. The authors concluded that tobacco smoke induces lipid peroxidation in the lung, liver and kidney, and the levels of the antioxidant enzymes are enhanced to protect these tissues against the deleterious effects of oxygen-derived free radicals (Baskaran *et al.*, 1999).

Nitric oxide synthase (Nos) catalyses the production of NO which, through its conversion to peroxynitrite, can cause damage to cellular macromolecules. The effects of tobacco smoke on *Nos* gene expression and protein production have been examined in the lung of rats exposed to tobacco smoke either once only or daily and killed after 1, 2, 7 or 28 days of exposure. *Nos1*, *Nos2* (inducible Nos (iNos)) and *Nos3* mRNAs in whole lung were quantified using reverse transcription polymerase chain reaction, and Nos protein levels were determined by Western blotting. Neither *Nos1* gene expression nor protein levels were altered by exposure to tobacco smoke. Levels of *Nos2* expression were more than doubled in animals exposed to smoke on day 1 and had decreased to control values by 28 days, whereas protein levels did not change. *Nos3* expression was increased by approximately 35% after 2 days of exposure and remained at this level to 28 days, whereas protein levels were increased by approximately 60% at day 7 and remained elevated to 28 days. In-situ hybridization showed that *Nos2* was diffusely expressed in the lung parenchyma, airways and vessels, and that *Nos3* was strongly expressed in vascular endothelium. The authors concluded that tobacco smoke could directly and rapidly affect *Nos* expression, and thus potentially affect the function of the pulmonary vasculature (Wright *et al.*, 1999). In another study, the expression of Nos2, NF-κB, the mitogen-activated protein kinases Mek1 (mitogen-activated extracellular kinase 1) and Erk2 (extracellular signal-regulated kinase 2), phosphotyrosine protein and c-Fos was increased in the terminal bronchioles of rats exposed to gas-phase tobacco smoke in association with an increase in lipid peroxidation. In contrast, the levels of protein kinase C, Mekk1, Jnk, p38, c-Jun and c-Myc in the terminal bronchioles were unchanged. The authors concluded that exposure to tobacco smoke results in oxidative stress (NOx and ROS) that leads to the induction of Nos2 (iNos) and c-Fos together with the induction of transduction signalling proteins, protein tyrosine phosphorylation and Mek1/Erk2 which, in turn, may promote lung pathogenesis (Chang *et al.*, 2001).

The effects of tobacco smoke on enzyme activities have also been investigated to a limited extent in guinea-pigs. In contrast to the results obtained in mice and rats, daily exposure of Hartley strain guinea-pigs to either mainstream or sidestream tobacco smoke for 16 weeks did not result in an increase in Ahh activity in the lung (Gairola, 1987). In another study, however, tobacco smoke-induced emphysema in the lungs of guinea-pigs was associated with an increase in the activity of a proteolitic enzyme–collagenase activity in the alveolar walls and interstitium (Selman *et al.*, 1996).

(b)   Biomarkers of tobacco smoke carcinogens

(i)   Urinary compounds

Urinary compounds are useful markers of the uptake of tobacco smoke constituents (Hecht, 2002b). Most, if not all, of the compounds detected in the urine of human smokers have also been found in the urine of animals exposed to mainstream tobacco smoke. Since 1985, however, there have been relatively few reports of the identification and quantitation of urinary compounds in animals exposed to tobacco smoke (Table 4.7). Rats exposed to four dilutions of cigarette smoke over a period of 4 weeks had a lower output of hydroxyproline (relative to creatinine) for all dilutions of smoke and showed a negative dose–response relationship (Read & Thornton, 1985). *cis*-3′-Hydroxycotinine was detected as a nicotine metabolite in the urine of human smokers as well as in the urine of rats and hamsters dosed with nicotine. This was the first report of the identification of *cis*-

Table 4.7. Biomarkers affected by exposure to mainstream tobacco smoke

Species	Strain/sex	Biomarker affected	Effect (tissue)	Reference
		Metabolites		
Rat	(ex Charles River)/M	Hydroxyproline	− (urine)	Read & Thornton (1985)
	S-D/M	cis-3′-Hydroxycotinine	+ (urine)	Voncken et al. (1990)
	Not specified	4-(Methylnitrosamino)-4-(3-pyridyl)-butyric acid	+ (urine)	Pachinger et al. (1993)
Hamster	Syrian/M	cis-3′-hydroxycotinine	+ (urine)	Voncken et al. (1990)
		DNA adducts		
Mouse	C57BL/6/M DBA/2/M	BPDE–DNA	ND (lung, liver) ND (lung, liver)	Bjelogrlic et al. (1989)
	A/J/F	O^6-MeG (reduced by tobacco smoke)	− (lung, liver)	Brown et al. (1999)
	B6C3F$_1$/M	Smoke-related	+ (lung, heart)	Brown et al. (1997)
Rat	Fischer 344/ N/M&F	Smoke-related	+ (lung)	Bond et al. (1989)
	S-D/M	Smoke-related	+ (nasal mucosa, lung) ND (liver)	Gupta et al. (1989)
	S-D/M	Smoke-related	+ (tracheal epithelial cells)	Izzoti et al. (1995b)
	BD6/F	Smoke-related	+ (lung, heart) ND (oesophagus, liver) + (oesophagus with ethanol)	Izzoti et al. (1998)
	S-D/M	Smoke-related	+ (heart, lung, trachea, larynx, bladder)	Gupta et al. (1999)
Guinea-pig	Not specified	Smoke-related	+ (lung)	Gupta et al. (1999)

M, male; F, female; S-D, Sprague-Dawley; BPDE, benzo[a]pyrene diol epoxide; O^6-MeG, O^6-methyl-guanine; +, significant increase; −, decrease; ND, not detected

3′-hydroxycotinine as a urinary metabolite of nicotine (Voncken et al., 1990). The compound 4-(methylnitrosamino)-4-(3-pyridyl)-butyric acid (iso-NNAC) was identified in the urine of rats exposed to tobacco smoke and in the urine of human smokers (Pachinger et al., 1993).

(ii)   *DNA adducts in animal tissues*

Mouse

There have been several reports of the detection of DNA adducts in tissues of mice exposed to tobacco smoke (Table 4.7). Synchronous fluorescence spectrophotometry was used to investigate the formation of the BPDE–DNA adducts in the lung and liver of genetically responsive C57BL/6 and non-responsive DBA/2 mice exposed to cigarette smoke for 3–16 days. Interestingly, BPDE–DNA adducts were not detected in the lung and liver of either mouse strain, although Ahh activity, an indicator of benzo[*a*]pyrene metabolism, was clearly induced in the lungs of C57BL/6 mice. Thus, there appeared to be no clear correlation between Ahh activity and the formation of BPDE–DNA adducts (Bjelogrlic *et al.*, 1989).

The effect of tobacco smoke on the formation of promutagenic O^6-methyldesoxyguanosine (O^6-MeG) adducts from the TSNA NNK, in the lungs and liver of A/J mice has been investigated. Mice were exposed to smoke generated from Kentucky 1R4F reference cigarettes at 0, 0.4, 0.6 or 0.8 mg wet total particulate matter per litre of air for 2 h, and a single intraperitoneal injection of NNK (0, 3.75 or 7.5 μmol/mouse) was administered midway through the exposure. Tobacco smoke alone did not yield detectable levels of O^6-MeG but NNK did form this adduct. The number of O^6-MeG adducts following intraperitoneal injection of NNK during cigarette smoke exposure was significantly ($p < 0.05$) reduced in both lung and liver. The same effect was seen in mice co-exposed to NNK and cotinine. The authors hypothesized that the reduction of O^6-MeG in liver and lung results from competitive inhibition by cotinine of the cytochrome P450 enzyme system for NNK activation (Brown *et al.*, 1999). The effect of exposure to tobacco smoke on the formation of DNA adducts in the lungs and heart of B6C3F$_1$ mice was determined using the ^{32}P-postlabelling assay. Mice were exposed for 1 h per day, 5 days per week for a period of 4 weeks to mainstream smoke at concentrations of 0, 0.16, 0.32 and 0.64 mg total particulate matter per litre of air. There was an exposure-dependent increase in the numbers of DNA adducts in lung and heart at all three concentrations; increases found in the mid- and high-exposure groups were significant ($p < 0.05$) (Brown *et al.*, 1997).

Mainstream-smoke condensate and sidestream-smoke condensate were applied topically to mouse skin, and DNA adducts were quantified in skin, lung, kidney, liver and bladder tissues by ^{32}P-postlabelling. Mainstream-smoke condensate produced higher levels of DNA adducts in mouse heart and bladder than sidestream-smoke condensate (but the difference was not statistically significant). However, sidestream-smoke condensate produced higher adduct levels in mouse skin, lung and kidney than mainstream smoke (Carmichael *et al.*, 1993).

Rat

The effect of mainstream tobacco smoke on the formation of DNA adducts in various tissues of rats has been investigated extensively by use of ^{32}P-postlabelling and SFS (Table 4.7). The formation of DNA adducts in the nasal cavity, lung and liver of Sprague-

Dawley rats exposed daily to fresh smoke from a University of Kentucky reference cigarette (2R1) for up to 40 weeks was examined by ^{32}P-postlabelling (Gupta *et al.*, 1989). The amount of total particulate matter inhaled with the smoke was 5–5.5 mg per animal per day. The average concentration of COHb in blood was 5.5%. Mainstream smoke induced at least four new DNA adducts in the nasal mucosa of rats and the amount of these adducts increased with length of exposure. In the lung, smoke induced an accumulation of one DNA adduct, which upon cessation of exposure for 19 weeks was reduced by about 75%. Smoke-related adducts were not detected in the liver. Selective chromatography and butanol extractability suggested that the DNA adducts in all tissues examined were aromatic and/or lipophilic. In a more recent study, Gupta *et al.* (1999) reported increases in the levels of DNA adducts in various tissues of Sprague-Dawley rats exposed to both mainstream and sidestream tobacco smoke, but not in liver. Mean total adduct levels in the various tissues ranked from heart > lung > trachea > larynx > bladder. Izzotti *et al.* (1995b) employed ^{32}P-postlabelling analysis to evaluate the effect of *N*-acetyl-L-cysteine (NAC) on the formation of carcinogen–DNA adducts in tracheal epithelial cells of Sprague-Dawley rats exposed (whole-body) to mainstream tobacco smoke for either 40 or 100 consecutive days. DNA adducts were observed after 40 days of exposure and no further increase was noted after 100 days. NAC, given by gavage in the 40-day study and in the drinking-water in the 100-day study, reduced the formation of smoke-related carcinogen–DNA adducts in the tracheal epithelium to the levels seen in sham-exposed control rats. These results indicate the considerable efficacy of oral NAC, a chemopreventive agent, in inhibiting the formation of smoke-related carcinogen–DNA adducts (Izzotti *et al.*, 1995b).

[32]P-Postlabelling was also used to investigate the effects of exposure mode, sex and time (adduct persistence) on the level of DNA adducts in tissues of Fischer 344 rats (Bond *et al.*, 1989). Rats were exposed to tobacco smoke for 6 h per day, 5 days per week for 22 days by intermittent nose-only, continuous nose-only or continuous whole-body exposure. The animals were killed at either 18 h or 3 weeks after the 22-day exposure period and DNA adducts in lung tissues were quantified. Significant ($p < 0.05$) increases in the levels of DNA adducts were observed in both male and female rats exposed to tobacco smoke. No significant effects of exposure mode or sex on the induction of lung DNA adducts were observed. Significantly fewer clearly resolved DNA adducts were found in the lungs of rats killed 3 weeks after exposure, suggesting that smoke-induced adducts were repaired by DNA repair mechanisms. A single unidentified adduct accounted for about 20% of the total resolved lung DNA adducts and occurred at levels nine- to 14-fold higher than those in control animals (Bond *et al.*, 1989). It is not certain whether this adduct is the same one as that described in the lung of Sprague-Dawley rats by Gupta *et al.* (1989) or in the skin of mice by Randerath *et al.* (1986). Izzotti *et al.* (1998) used ^{32}P-postlabelling to investigate the effects of tobacco smoke and alcohol consumption on DNA adduct levels in the oesophagus, lung, liver and heart of BD6 rats. Groups of female rats were exposed to ethanol (5% in drinking-water for 8 consecutive months) and/or whole-body to mainstream tobacco smoke (1 h per day, 5 days per week for 8 months). As

expected, ingestion of alcohol alone did not affect the levels of DNA adducts in any of the four organs studied. Exposure to tobacco smoke induced formation of DNA adducts in the lung and heart, but not in the oesophagus or liver. Combined exposure to alcohol and smoke, however, resulted in the significant formation of smoke-related DNA adducts in the oesophagus and in a further increase in the number of adducts in the heart. Therefore, a likely interpretation is that ethanol may solubilize water-insoluble smoke components in the upper aerodigestive tract, thereby determining a first-pass effect in the oesophagus (Izzotti *et al.*, 1998). Another important mechanism may be the induction by ethanol of CYP2E1-dependent microsomal monooxygenases that catalyse the metabolism of a variety of xenobiotics (Tsutsumi *et al.*, 1993; Gonzalez & Gelboin, 1994).

The formation of smoke-related DNA adducts and their chemoprevention were investigated in tissues of Sprague-Dawley rats by SFS which, as mentioned above, can detect BPDE–DNA adducts (Izzotti *et al.*, 1992). Animals were exposed (whole-body) to mainstream cigarette smoke once daily for up to 40 consecutive days. No adduct was detected in liver DNA, whereas smoke-related DNA adducts were detectable in the lung from the day 8 of exposure and continued to increase until the study ended at day 40. The levels of adducts in heart DNA were even higher than those found in the lung. The daily administration of NAC by gavage significantly inhibited the occurrence of the same adducts in both heart and lung DNA, as measured by ^{32}P-postlabelling of DNA adducts in tracheal epithelial cells (Izzotti *et al.*, 1995b).

It is currently not clear why rats exposed to cigarette smoke form lung DNA adducts when previous studies have not demonstrated smoke-induced pulmonary carcinogenesis in rats. However, it is possible that the previous studies failed to demonstrate smoke-induced cancer because:

— a smaller dose of particulate matter was delivered per gram of lung tissue than in human heavy smokers;

— less than lifetime exposures were used; and

— the experimental groups used were too small in number (Bond *et al.*, 1989).

Interspecies comparison

^{32}P-Postlabelling has also been used to detect and quantify DNA adducts in the lung of guinea-pigs and mice exposed to mainstream and sidestream tobacco smoke. DNA adducts were identified in lung, but less DNA-adduct formation was seen in guinea-pigs than in either mice or rats at the same level of exposure to tobacco smoke (Gupta *et al.*, 1999).

(iii)   *DNA damage in cultured human lung cells*

In cultured human lung cells, bubbling cigarette smoke through phosphate-buffered saline was found to induce DNA single-strand breaks and formation of 8-OHdG in DNA. Evidence was presented that this was mediated, in part, by the formation of reactive oxygen species (Leanderson, 1993). It was shown that cigarette tar promotes neutrophil-induced DNA damage in cultured human lung cells and that this activity is further enhanced by iron and inhibited by catalase (Leanderson & Tagesson, 1994).

Treatment of human fetal lung cells with the TSNAs NNN and NNK caused single-strand breaks in DNA. Inhibition of this effect by oxygen radical scavengers suggested that the hydroxyl radical was an important intermediate in the process (Weitberg & Corvese, 1993).

DNA damage, as measured by the alkaline single-cell gel microelectrophoresis (Comet) assay, has also been shown to be induced in human embryo lung cells treated with water-soluble compounds from cigarette smoke (Wang, Q. *et al.*, 2000).

Treatment of tracheobronchial epithelial cells with gas-phase cigarette smoke caused DNA strand breakage that was accompanied by increases in the levels of a number of DNA lesions, including 8-OHdG, xanthine and hypoxanthine. These latter lesions can arise from the deamination of guanine and adenine by a mechanism involving reactive nitrogen species. Thus, DNA damage induced by cigarette smoking may be mediated by both reactive oxygen species and reactive nitrogen species (Spencer *et al.*, 1995).

(c)   Other data

(i)   Effects on particle clearance

Cigarette smoking induces a variety of carcinogenic and non-carcinogenic effects in humans and laboratory animals. An issue of concern is the extent to which smoking might influence pulmonary responses to other inhaled toxic materials. This influence can take the form of a direct alteration of the deposition or clearance of another inhaled agent. For example, it has been reported that cigarette smoking delays the pulmonary clearance of inhaled, insoluble particles in humans (Bohning *et al.*, 1982) and in laboratory animals (Mauderly *et al.*, 1989).

Finch *et al.* (1995) investigated the influence of cigarette smoke exposure of Fischer 344 rats on the pulmonary clearance of inhaled, relatively insoluble radioactive tracer particles. Following 13 weeks of whole-body exposure to air or mainstream tobacco smoke for 6 h per day, 5 days per week at concentrations of 0, 100 or 250 mg/m^3 total particulate matter, rats were acutely exposed pernasally to ^{85}Sr-labelled fused aluminosilicate (^{85}Sr-FAP) tracer particles; exposure to air or smoke was then resumed. A decreased clearance of ^{85}Sr-FAP from the lungs, which was smoke concentration-dependent, was observed. By 180 days after exposure to the tracer aerosol, about 14, 20 and 40% of the initial activity of the tracer was detected in the control, 100-mg/m^3 and 250-mg/m^3 groups, respectively. Exposure to mainstream smoke produced lung lesions that contained increased numbers of pigmented alveolar macrophages throughout the parenchyma, and focal collections of enlarged alveolar macrophages with concomitant alveolar hyperplasia. The severity of lesions increased with duration of exposure. These data confirm previous findings that exposure to cigarette smoke decreases the ability of the lung to clear inhaled materials. In a subsequent publication, Finch *et al.* (1998) reported that chronic exposure to cigarette smoke containing 100 or 250 mg/m^3 total particulate matter increased the pulmonary retention and radiation dose of ^{239}plutonium inhaled as ^{239}PuO$_2$ in two groups of Fischer 344 rats. Assuming a linear dose–response relationship between radiation dose and the incidence of lung neoplasms, the exposure to ^{239}PuO$_2$ was predicted to increase the incidence of lung tumours relative to that in controls by 20% or 80%, depending upon the concentration of total particulate matter in smoke.

(ii)   *Carboxyhaemoglobin*

There have been several reports on the relationship between levels of exposure to carbon monoxide from tobacco smoke and levels of COHb adducts in the blood of animals. For example, Attolini *et al.* (1996) exposed male NMRI mice to tobacco smoke for 2, 4, 8 or 31 days. The levels of COHb in blood increased significantly after 4 or 8 days of exposure and decreased after 31 days to a level which remained higher than the level of the controls. Two hypotheses were proposed to explain the decrease in COHb levels at 31 days.

(1) The mice may develop a state of tolerance against compounds in tobacco smoke: the increase in respiratory rhythm leads to hyperventilation and to a concomitant decrease in the quantity of CO fixed to haemoglobin.

(2) Chronic exposure to tobacco smoke increases the thickness of the airway epithelium and alveolar septae, as well as mucus hypersecretion and ciliostasis, which increases the barrier to smoke constituents, reducing their accessibility to the blood circulation and therefore decreasing the level of CO fixed to haemoglobin.

Loennechen *et al.* (1999) exposed Sprague-Dawley rats to CO at 100 ppm for 1 week or to 100 ppm CO for 1 week followed by 200 ppm for 1 week. The formation of COHb was found to be dependent upon the amount of CO exposure; COHb was approximately 13% in the group exposed to the low level of CO and 23% in the group exposed to the higher level. Exposure to a high level of CO increased the expression of endothelin-1 mRNA by more than 50% in both the left and right ventricles of the heart. The authors concluded that chronic exposure to CO leading to COHb levels similar to those observed in smokers increases endothelin-1 gene expression and induces myocardial hypertrophy in the rat.

4.2   Toxic effects

4.2.1   *Humans*

(a)   *Nicotine addiction*

Cigarette smoking is the single largest avoidable cause of premature death and disability. Many smokers express a desire to stop smoking, and many have made one or more unsuccessful attempts to quit, supporting the evidence that tobacco smoking is addictive. Research has been focused on nicotine because it is the most addictive constituent of tobacco products (see also Section 4.1.1(*c*)(vi)). Therefore, cigarette smoking should be understood as a manifestation of nicotine addiction. This topic has been extensively reviewed (Benowitz, 1988; US Department of Health and Human Services, 1988; Moxham, 2000).

Nicotine is an addictive drug and smoking of tobacco rapidly delivers a dose of nicotine to receptors in the brain. The effects on the central nervous system are more important than those on the peripheral nervous system (Le Houezec & Benowitz, 1991). With repeated experience, consolidation into physiological and psychological addiction is reinforced by pronounced withdrawal symptoms.

To achieve a psychoactive impact, nicotine must be delivered rapidly to the brain which is best achieved by inhalation of tobacco smoke. The speed of nicotine delivery is a fundamental difference between cigarettes and products aimed at nicotine replacement. The nicotine-replacement products deliver nicotine at lower, subaddictive rates and are only effective in reducing cravings and withdrawal symptoms from tobacco-delivered nicotine dependence.

It is far from clear that the benefits attributed to nicotine use, such as stress relief, improved mood and enhanced cognitive performance, are real. Many of the perceived benefits are actually attributable to the relief of nicotine withdrawal symptoms (Le Houezec & Benowitz, 1991).

The addictive properties of nicotine imply that analytical measurements of tar and nicotine yields from cigarettes do not reflect the true exposure to tar and nicotine experienced by smokers. Smokers adjust the way they smoke in order to self-administer a satisfactory dose of nicotine (Benowitz, 1995).

(b)   *Health effects other than cancer*

Besides its carcinogenic effects, tobacco smoke has a number of other pathogenic properties. Causal associations have been established between active smoking and a number of specific diseases.

(i)   *Effects on the cardiovascular system*

Cigarette smoking is a major independent risk factor for coronary heart disease and the most important risk factor for atherosclerotic peripheral vascular disease. There is a dose–response relationship between cigarette smoking and cardiovascular disease: the risk increases with the number of cigarettes smoked daily, the total number of years for which a person has smoked, the degree of inhalation and earlier age of initiation of the smoking habit. Cigarette smoking has been found to elevate significantly the risk for sudden death (US Department of Health and Human Services, 1983, 1989). Cigarette smoking accounts for about half of deaths from coronary disease in women during middle age. It has been shown that premenopausal women have lower rates of heart disease than postmenopausal women. This protection is presumed to be provided by the presence of circulating estrogens, but it is unknown whether estrogens have the same protective effect in women who smoke (Villablanca et al., 2000). A synergistic effect between smoking and the use of oral contraceptives has also been reported (US Department of Health and Human Services, 1983). In female smokers who take oral contraceptives, particularly those over the age of 35 years, there is a well-established increase in risk of myocardial infarction and cerebrovascular disease (Villablanca *et al.*, 2000).

Cigarettes that nominally deliver less tar or nicotine have not consistently been shown to reduce the risk of cardiovascular disease (reviewed by Burns *et al.*, 2001).

(ii) *Effects on the cerebrovascular system*

Cigarette smoking is a major cause of cerebrovascular disease (ischaemic stroke). It is estimated that as many as 25% of all strokes can be attributed to smoking. The relative risk of stroke is similar in male and female smokers and is maximal near middle age (Hankey, 1999). Although nicotine has strong and potentially harmful effects on cerebral and peripheral vascular tissues, it is not certain whether and how these effects are related to stroke (Hawkins *et al.*, 2002).

(iii) *Effects on the respiratory system*

Cigarette smoking is the most important cause of cough, sputum production, chronic bronchitis and asthma (Hargreave & Leigh, 1999; Maestrelli *et al.*, 2001; Ulrik & Lange, 2001). It increases the risk for dying from chronic bronchitis and pulmonary emphysema (US Department of Health and Human Services, 1984; Aubry *et al.*, 2000; Seagrave, 2000; Fraig *et al.*, 2002).

(iv) *Gastrointestinal effects*

Smoking increases the risk for peptic ulcer and mortality from this disease (Ma *et al.*, 1998). It delays peptic ulcer healing and increases the risk of recurrence after healing (Ashley, 1997). Nicotine has been shown to potentiate aggressive gastric factors and to attenuate defensive ones; it also increases acid and pepsin secretions, gastric motility, duodenogastric reflux of bile salts, the risk of *Helicobacter pylori* infection, levels of free radicals and platelet-activating factor, endothelium generation and vasopressin secretion (Endoh & Leung, 1994). Although the mechanisms by which smoking or nicotine adversely affect the gastric mucosa have not been fully elucidated, the available evidence supports the hypothesis that nicotine is harmful to the gastric mucosa (Endoh & Leung, 1994). Smoking is also a risk factor for Crohn disease in both men and women, but the excess risk is higher among female smokers. There is growing evidence that smoking is inversely related to ulcerative colitis (Westman *et al.*, 1995; Rubin & Hanauer, 2000) and some evidence that it is a risk factor for gallstones (Ashley, 1997).

(v) *Neurological disorders*

The relationship between smoking and some neurological diseases has been controversial. A number of epidemiological studies have found a significant, negative association between cigarette smoking and Parkinson or Alzheimer disease, the risk among nonsmokers being approximately twice that of smokers (Fratiglioni & Wang, 2000). However, whereas a community-based longitudinal study of elderly people found a higher risk of Alzheimer disease in smokers than in nonsmokers (Merchant *et al.*, 1999), an analysis based on a comparison of persons with Alzheimer dementia with their unaffected siblings suggests that smoking does not decrease the risk for the disease (Debanne *et al.*, 2000). Both retrospective and prospective epidemiological studies have demonstrated an inverse association between cigarette smoking and Parkinson disease, leading to theories that smoking and nicotine may be neuroprotective. Coffee and caffeine consumption have been reported to have a similar effect (Ross & Petrovitch, 2001; Hernan *et al.*, 2002).

(vi)   *Other inverse associations of smoking with health effects*

Some studies suggest that there may be inverse associations of smoking with uterine fibroids and endometriosis, and protective effects against hypertensive disorders and vomiting during pregnancy are likely. Inverse associations of smoking with venous thrombosis after myocardial infarction are probably not causal, but indications of positive effects with regard to recurrent aphthous ulcers and control of body weight may reflect a genuine benefit. A variety of mechanisms for the potentially beneficial effects of smoking have been proposed; of these three predominate:

— the anti-estrogenic effect of smoking;
— alterations in prostaglandin production; and
— stimulation of nicotinic cholinergic receptors in the central nervous system.

It should be noted that even established inverse associations cannot be used as a rationale to encourage cigarette smoking because overall effects on health and mortality are clearly negative (Baron, 1996).

4.2.2   *Animals*

(a)   *Nicotine addiction/dependence*

(i)   *Studies with animal models*

Various animal models have been described that mimic nicotine dependence and withdrawal syndromes. In one such model, dependence is induced in rats by continuous subcutaneous infusion of nicotine (3 or 9 mg/kg bw per day as nicotine hydrogen tartrate) over 7 days by the use of implanted osmotic minipumps. The nicotine is absorbed quickly and almost completely. Abstinence is initiated through termination of infusion or by injection of nicotine antagonists. The resulting abstinence syndrome involves a pattern of behaviour somewhat resembling opiate abstinence, with weight gain and reduced locomotor activity. The model has been replicated in a number of laboratories. It is sensitive to various abstinence-alleviating therapeutic approaches, such as nicotine replacement and the administration of nitric oxide synthase inhibitors and serotonergic compounds. A strong reduction of abstinence symptoms was seen with bupropion and acetyl-L-carnitine, both of which are used clinically as part of smoking cessation regimens (Malin, 2001).

Nicotine has also been given orally to experimental animals either in liquid diets or in drinking fluids, or by forced oral administration (rats show an aversion to the taste of nicotine). When nicotine is given orally, it is absorbed slowly by the gastrointestinal tract and the concentrations in blood remain considerably lower than those observed after subcutaneous infusion (Le Houezec et al., 1989).

In another experimental model, mice were given drinking-water containing gradually increasing concentrations (50–500 µg/mL) of nicotine for 7 weeks. After replacement of the nicotine solutions with tap-water, a significantly higher fluid intake was seen in the nicotine-treated mice than in control animals, but this effect disappeared within 1 week. Plasma nicotine concentrations in the treated mice were found to be similar to those reported in heavy smokers. The results of a pharmacological study with this mouse model suggested that the effects of nicotine in striatal dopamine metabolism are critical for its stimulating and reinforcing effects (Pietilä & Ahtee, 2000).

(ii)   *Studies with genetically modified mice*

Numerous studies have shown that nicotine is likely to be responsible for the addictive properties of tobacco. In addition, nicotine has effects on locomotion, cognition, affect and sensitivity to pain. In recent studies with transgenic mice, molecular biology has been combined with pharmacology, electrophysiology and behavioural analysis to elucidate the specific role of nicotine in these phenomena. The physiological effects of nicotine are mediated by binding to and activation of nicotine acetylcholine receptors. These receptors are pentamers made up of subunits with distinct expression patterns in different neurons. More than 10 different neuronal receptor subunits have been identified, and for seven of these subunits, knock-out mice lacking one receptor subunit have been constructed. These mice are being used in studies to identify the receptor subtypes responsible for the different effects of nicotine. As an example, nicotine self-administration is abolished in mice lacking the β2 subunit of the receptor, which implies that this subunit is a component of the receptor that mediates nicotine reinforcement (Marubio & Changeux, 2000; Picciotto et al., 2000).

(b)   *Other effects in experimental animals*

(i)   *Effects on the cardiovascular system*

To determine whether chronic exposure to tobacco smoke for less than 2 months alters cardiovascular regulation, male Sprague-Dawley rats were exposed to tobacco smoke from low-nicotine cigarettes (1 mg/cigarette) for 4–6 weeks, and a second group served as sham controls receiving only puffs of room air. Reflex adjustments in mean arterial blood pressure after bilateral common carotid occlusion were compared between the two groups. In the anaesthetized control state, there was no significant difference between the cardiovascular parameters measured in the two groups. However, the increase in mean arterial blood pressure after carotid occlusion was significantly greater in the smoke-treated than in the control animals ($p < 0.05$). In addition, the time required to reach maximum arterial blood pressure after carotid occlusion was significantly less ($p < 0.05$) for the smoke-treated animals (8.5 ± 0.2 s) than in the controls (11.2 ± 0.3 s). The results show that chronic exposure to tobacco smoke in experimental animals for periods as short as 4–6 weeks alters the reflex regulation of the cardiovascular system (Bennett & Richardson, 1990).

To determine whether exposure to sidestream cigarette smoke promotes atherogenesis in a mouse model of human atherosclerosis, female ApoE-deficient mice, fed a western diet, were exposed to sidestream smoke in a whole-body exposure chamber for a total of 6 h/day, 5 days per week, for 7, 10 and 14 weeks. Animals exposed to filtered ambient air served as controls. Elevated concentrations of blood COHb and pulmonary CYP1A1 were indicative of effective exposure. There were no consistent changes in serum concentrations of cholesterol between control and exposed mice. Morphometric assessment of grossly discernible lesions covering the intimal area of the aorta showed remarkable increases in exposed mice, at all three durations of exposure studied. Increases in the area of the lesion were accompanied by higher levels of esterified and unesterified cholesterol in the aortic tissues of exposed mice. The results clearly demonstrate promotion of the development of atherosclerotic lesions by tobacco smoke in an atherosclerosis-susceptible mouse model (Gairola et al., 2001).

(ii)   Effects on the cerebrovascular system

Initial investigations with a rat model of nicotine exposure in adolescents have demonstrated that the vulnerable developmental period for nicotine-induced brain cell damage extends into adolescence. The effect of nicotine on cholinergic systems in adolescent male and female rats was investigated with a nicotine-infusion protocol designed to produce nicotine plasma concentrations similar to those measured in human smokers or in users of transdermal nicotine patches. Choline acetyltransferase activity (ChAT), a static marker that closely reflects the density of cholinergic innervation, and binding of [³H]hemicholinium-3 (HC-3), which labels the presynaptic high-affinity choline transporter, were monitored in the midbrain (the region most closely involved in reward and addiction pathways), as well as in the cerebral cortex and hippocampus. During nicotine treatment and for 1 month after termination of treatment, ChAT activity was significantly reduced and HC-3 binding was significantly increased in the midbrain, but not in the other regions. The levels returned to normal immediately after cessation of nicotine exposure and subsequently showed a transient suppression of activity. Although the cerebral cortex showed little or no change in HC-3 binding during or after nicotine administration, activity was persistently reduced in the hippocampus. The regionally selective effects of nicotine treatment of adolescent rats on cholinergic systems support the concept that adolescence is a vulnerable developmental period for determining ultimate effects on behaviour (Trauth et al., 2000).

(iii)   Effects on the respiratory system

To study the role of transforming growth factor-β1 (TGF-β1) in the pathogenesis of chronic bronchitis and emphysema, an animal model was used in which hamsters were exposed by chronic inhalation of cigarette smoke. The expression of TGF-β1 mRNA and protein in the pulmonary tissue was measured. In a parallel experiment, bronchial epithelium was stimulated with cigarette smoke extract *in vitro* and the expression of TGF-β1 was determined. After 3 months of exposure, the animals developed chronic bronchitis and emphysema. The increase in TGF-β1 immunoreactivity in the pulmonary tissue and in the cultured bronchial epithelial cells was significantly higher than in the controls ($p = 0.001$). The expression of TGF-β1 mRNA was also increased in the pulmonary tissue of exposed animals. The results indicate that exposure to cigarette smoke can induce over-expression of TGF-β1 in bronchial epithelia; this may be one of the mechanisms for smoking-induced chronic bronchitis and emphysema (Li *et al.*, 2002).

To assess induction of emphysema in the rodent lung, B6C3F$_1$ mice and Fischer 344 rats were exposed, whole-body, to cigarette smoke at a concentration of 250 mg/m^3 total particulate matter for 6 h per day, 5 days per week, for either 7 or 13 months. Morphometry included measurements of parenchymal air-space enlargement and tissue loss. In addition, centriacinar intra-alveolar inflammatory cells were counted to assess species differences in the type of inflammatory response associated with the exposure. In mice, significant differences in many of the morphometric parameters indicating emphysema were noted between smoke-exposed and control animals. In rats exposed to cigarette smoke, only some of the parameters differed significantly from control values. Morphological evidence of tissue destruction in the mice included alveoli that were irregular in size and shape and alveoli with multiple foci of septal discontinuities and isolated septal fragments. There were more morphometric anomalies in the mice at 13 months than at 7 months, suggesting a progression of the disease. Inflammatory lesions in the lungs of mice contained significantly more neutrophils than these lesions in rats. These results suggest that B6C3F$_1$ mice are more susceptible than Fischer 344 rats to the induction of emphysema by this exposure regimen and that the emphysema may be progressive in mice. Furthermore, the type of inflammatory response may be a determining factor for species differences in susceptibility to the induction of emphysema by exposure to cigarette smoke (March *et al.*, 1999).

The hypothesis was tested that variations in α1-antitrypsin expression modulate the pattern of emphysema and functional consequences in mice exposed to cigarette smoke. The effects of cigarette smoke were investigated in C57BL/6J (C57) mice and in low-α1-antitrypsin, C57BL/6J *pa$^+$/pa$^+$* (pallid) mice. After 4 months of exposure, a significant increase in the extent of emphysema was seen in pallid mice, but not in C57 mice. After 6 months, mechanical properties of lung, the extent and type of emphysema, and the cellular inflammatory response were measured. C57 mice and pallid mice had similar degrees of emphysema, whereas pallid mice, but not C57 mice, had developed a T-cell inflammation in the alveolar wall ($p < 0.01$). Although lung compliance was not changed in C57 mice after exposure to smoke, it increased significantly in pallid mice over the 6 months of exposure ($p < 0.0082$). In summary, exposure to cigarette smoke induced emphysema in C57 and pallid mice, but the emphysema, inflammatory infiltrate and the resulting physiological abnormalities were substantially different in the two strains, with the C57 and pallid mice exhibiting features similar to centrilobular and panlobular emphysema, respectively (Takubo *et al.*, 2002).

To determine whether smoking affects the clearance of asbestos fibres, guinea-pigs were given amosite asbestos by intratracheal instillation. They were divided into groups that received (a) no further treatment, (b) were exposed to tobacco smoke after asbestos instillation, or (c) were exposed to smoke both before and after asbestos instillation. The numbers and sizes of the asbestos fibres were measured in respiratory tract tissue and in lavage samples at 1 week and 1 month after exposure. During this time, the asbestos burden in the first group decreased sixfold on average, whereas no significant decrease was seen in either of the smoke-exposed groups. The mean length of retained fibres increased in the first group (asbestos only), but decreased in both the smoke-exposed groups. This phenomenon was seen in tissue samples and lavage samples, although the fibres in the lavage fluid were consistently shorter than those in tissue. The authors concluded that, in this model, cigarette smoking impeded asbestos clearance, largely by increasing retention of short fibres. This increased pulmonary fibre burden may be important in the increased rate of parenchymal fibrosis and carcinoma of the lung seen in asbestos workers who smoke (McFadden *et al.*, 1986).

(iv)   *Neurological disorders*

In view of the suggested inverse relationship in humans between cigarette smoking and the risk for Parkinson and Alzheimer disease, which are both characterized by enhanced oxidative stress, the antioxidant potential of nicotine was investigated in rats. Initial chromatographic studies suggested that nicotine can affect the formation of the neurotoxin 6-hydroxydopamine resulting from the addition of dopamine to Fenton's reagent (i.e. Fe^{2+} and hydrogen peroxide). Under certain circumstances, nicotine can strongly affect the course of the Fenton reaction. In in-vivo studies, adult male rats treated with nicotine showed greater memory retention than controls in a water-maze task. However, neurochemical analysis of neocortex, hippocampus and neostriatum from these animals revealed that nicotine had no effect on the formation of reactive oxygen species or on lipid peroxidation in any brain region studied. In an in-vitro study with rat neocortical homogenates, there were no differences in lipid peroxidation between nicotine-treated rats and controls. The results of these studies suggest that the beneficial/protective effects of nicotine in both Parkinson disease and Alzheimer disease may result, at least partly, from antioxidant mechanisms (Linert *et al.*, 1999).

The effects of nicotine on the central nervous system are mediated by the activation of neuronal heteromeric acetylcholine-gated ion channel receptors (also termed nicotinic acetylcholine receptors). The neuroprotective effects of nicotine were studied in two animal models of parkinsonism: diethyldithiocarbamate-induced enhancement of 1-methyl-4-phenyl-1,2,3,6-tetrahydropyridine toxicity in mice and methamphetamine-induced neurotoxicity in rats and mice. The neuroprotective effect of nicotine was very similar to that of the non-competitive *N*-methyl-D-aspartate receptor antagonist, MK-801. In parallel experiments, nicotine was shown to induce the basic fibroblast growth factor-2 (FGF-2) and the brain-derived neurotrophic factor in rat striatum. The effect on the induction of FGF-2 was prevented by the nicotinic acetylcholine receptor antagonist, mecamylamine, whereas MK-801 induced FGF-2 in the striatum. As trophic factors have been reported to be neuroprotective for dopaminergic cells, these data suggest that the increase in neurotrophic factors is a possible mechanism by which nicotine provides protection from experimental parkinsonism (Maggio *et al.*, 1998).

(v)   *Effects on the immune system*

Five groups of 2-month-old male Syrian golden hamsters were exposed to cigarette smoke for three 10-min periods per day, on 5 days per week, for the duration of their lives. Three of the groups were also chronically exposed to aerosols of chrysotile asbestos, cobalt oxide or nickel oxides. The fourth group was exposed to smoke and sham dust and was compared with the control group exposed to sham smoke and sham dust. The fifth group received 12 weekly injections of 0.25 mg of *N*-nitrosodiethylamine. Each cigarette smoke-exposed group was compared with the group exposed to sham smoke and the respective aerosol treatment. The cigarette smoke-exposed groups lived significantly ($p < 0.01$) longer than the sham-exposed groups and the untreated controls. Their mean body weights were significantly ($p < 0.01$) lower than those of the sham-exposed groups. The delayed onset of amyloidosis and the lower body weight in the smoke-exposed hamsters may have been responsible for their increased lifespans. The results suggest that cigarette smoke affects the immune system of the animals, resulting in retardation of amyloidosis, a frequent cause of death in hamsters (Wehner *et al.*, 1976).

In rats, chronic inhalation of cigarette smoke preferentially inhibited the plaque-forming cell response of lung-associated lymph nodes (LALN) to sheep erythrocytes rather than anatomically distant lymph nodes. Inhibition of the antibody response in LALN of smoke-exposed animals was first detected after 21 weeks of smoke inhalation and was well established by the 27th week of exposure to smoke. After prolonged exposure (> 34 weeks) to cigarette smoke, similar changes in the plaque-forming cell response were also observed in other lymphoid tissues. Cigarette smoke affected the response of LALN cells to sheep erythrocytes, a T cell-dependent antigen, but did not alter the relative percentages of W3/13-positive (T cells) or Ig-positive (B cells) cells, or those of T-cell subsets as scored by their surface phenotypes, i.e. T helper (W3/25⁺) or T suppressor/cytotoxic (OX-8⁺) cells. The percentage of phagocytic cells and the accessory cell functions of macrophages remained comparable between sham-exposed and smoke-exposed animals. Exposure to cigarette smoke did not significantly alter the response of LALN cells to T-cell mitogens (concanavalin A and phytohaemagglutinin). However, response to trinitrophenyl *Brucella abortus*, a T-cell-independent antigen, was also significantly reduced. The results show that exposure to cigarette smoke results in a decreased antibody response in the rat, primarily affecting the B-cell function (Sopori *et al.*, 1989).

Chronic exposure of mice and rats to cigarette smoke affects T-cell responsiveness which may account for the decreased T-cell proliferative and T-dependent antibody responses in humans and animals exposed to cigarette smoke. However, the mechanism by which cigarette smoke affects the T-cell function is not clearly understood. Chronic exposure of rats to nicotine has been shown to inhibit the antibody-forming cell response, to impair the antigen-mediated signalling in T cells and to induce T-cell anergy. To study cigarette smoke-induced immunosuppression and to compare it with the effects of chronic nicotine exposure, rats were exposed to diluted, mainstream cigarette smoke for up to 30 months or to nicotine (1 mg/kg bw per day) by osmotic minipumps for 4 weeks, and were evaluated for immunological function *in vivo* and *in vitro*. The T cells from rats subjected to long-term exposure to cigarette smoke showed decreased antigen-mediated prolife-ration and constitutive activation of protein tyrosine kinase and phospholipase C-γ1 acti-vities. Moreover, spleen cells from smoke-exposed and nicotine-treated animals had depleted inositol-1,4,5-trisphosphate-sensitive Ca^{2+} stores and a decreased ability to raise intracellular Ca^{2+} concentrations in response to T-cell antigen receptor ligation. The results suggest that chronic smoking causes T-cell anergy by impairing the antigen recep-tor-mediated signal transduction pathways and depleting the inositol-1,4,5-trisphosphate-sensitive Ca^{2+} stores. Moreover, nicotine may be responsible for or contribute to the immunosuppressive properties of cigarette smoke (Kalra *et al.*, 2000).

(vi)   *Toxic effects of kreteks*

Kreteks are a type of small cigarette containing approximately 60% tobacco and 40% ground clove buds (Stratton *et al.*, 2001). The typical chemical composition of main-stream smoke per kretek is total particulate matter, 52.3 mg; nicotine, 2.4 mg; and CO, 23.7 mg. In the several inhalation studies that have looked specifically at exposure of rats and hamsters to kreteks smoke, few signs of toxicity (focal alveolitis, bronchiolar epi-thelial hyperplasia, alveolar haemorrhage) were observed after 1 or 14 days' exposure (LaVoie *et al.*, 1986; Clark, 1989, 1990), but the routes and methods of exposure used do not replicate human exposure (Guidotti, 1989).

4.3   Reproductive and hormonal effects

4.3.1   *Humans*

(*a*)   *Reproductive effects*

Cigarette smoking has clearly been associated with a wide range of adverse effects on reproduction, some of which may have implications for cancer risk.

(i)   *Effects on female fertility*

Women who smoke cigarettes have an increased risk for both primary and secondary infertility, with an odds ratio of 1.6 (95% CI, 1.3–1.9) (Augood *et al.*, 1998 (meta-analysis of 12 studies); US Department of Health and Human Services, 2001). The resulting decrease in parity could have implications for risk for cancers of the breast, endometrium and ovary. There is also evidence that women who smoke cigarettes are more likely to be subfertile, and to take longer to get pregnant than women who do not smoke (Baird, 1992; Hughes & Brennan, 1996; Jensen *et al.*, 1998, Hull *et al.*, 2000; US Department of Health and Human Services, 2001).

(ii)   *Effects on pregnancy*

The use of tobacco products by pregnant women is associated with placenta praevia, placental abruption, premature rupture of membranes, pre-term birth, intrauterine growth restriction and sudden infant death syndrome (Castles *et al.*, 1999; Andres & Day, 2000; US Department of Health and Human Services, 2001). The association between smoking and pre-term delivery appears to be more pronounced for older women (US Department of Health and Human Services, 2001). There is also a relatively modest increase in the risk for spontaneous abortion and stillbirth among women who smoke during pregnancy (Windham *et al.*, 1999). Smoking may be responsible for 15% of all pre-term births, 20–30% of all infants of low birth weight, and for a 1.5-fold increase in overall perinatal mortality (Andres & Day, 2000).

Women who smoke cigarettes during pregnancy have been observed to have a decreased risk for various pregnancy-related disorders, including hypertension of pregnancy and pre-eclampsia, even after control for relevant covariates (Castles *et al.*, 1999; US Department of Health and Human Services, 2001).

Pre-eclampsia is caused by damage to the placenta and develops in the second half of pregnancy, usually in the last few weeks, or immediately after delivery. Initially, the main symptoms are raised blood pressure and the presence of protein in the urine of the mother, and a slower-than-normal growth of the unborn child. In rare cases, women can go on to develop fits, known in pregnancy as eclampsia. Cigarette smoking has been associated with a lower rate of pre-eclampsia among women who were pregnant for the first time, independent of other maternal factors (Newman *et al.*, 2001). For pre-eclampsia, however, dose–response relationships have not regularly been found (US Department of Health and Human Services, 2001). The limited data available regarding the association between cigarette smoking and the risk of eclampsia are mixed (US Department of Health and Human Services, 2001).

(iii)   *Effects on menopause*

Cigarette smoking has repeatedly been found to be associated with an earlier menopause. Current female smokers are about twice as likely to reach menopause at an earlier age as nonsmokers; the relative risk increases with the average number of cigarettes smoked. When the effect is expressed as a difference in the median (or mean) age at menopause, women who smoke reach menopause about 0.8 to 1.7 years earlier than never-smokers, again with a greater effect among heavier smokers. Women who have stopped smoking reach menopause at an age similar to that of never-smokers, or somewhat later (Midgette & Baron, 1990; US Department of Health and Human Services, 2001).

The association between smoking and earlier age-at-menopause has been very consistently found in studies from Asia (Kato *et al.*, 1988), northern Europe (Andersen *et al.*, 1982; Luoto *et al.*, 1994; Torgerson *et al.*, 1994), southern Europe (Parazzini *et al.*, 1992; Meschia *et al.*, 2000) and the USA (Jick *et al.*, 1977). Studies using various designs have reported this association, including cross-sectional surveys of patient populations (Jick *et al.*, 1977), population-based surveys (Andersen *et al.*, 1982; McKinlay *et al.*, 1985; Luoto *et al.*, 1994; Gold *et al.*, 2001), retrospective cohort studies (Kaufman *et al.*, 1980) or prospective cohort studies (Willett *et al.*, 1983; Bromberger *et al.*, 1997; Kato *et al.*, 1998). In a study from Nigeria, the effect of smoking on age-at-menopause could not be demonstrated because of the small numbers of female smokers in that country, where smoking by women is a social taboo (Okonofua *et al.*, 1990).

The mechanisms underlying this association are not entirely clear. However, at least in animals, the PAHs contained in cigarette smoke are toxic to ovarian follicles (Mattison & Thorgeirsson, 1978) and the human ovary probably contains the microsomal mono-oxygenases required to convert toxic chemicals into reactive species that affect oocytes. Smoking has been implicated in the increased rate of follicular atresia in women (Matisson, 1982). The higher concentrations of follicle-stimulating hormone in premenopausal smokers than in premenopausal nonsmokers are consistent with ovarian toxicity (Velasco *et al.*, 1990; Cooper *et al.*, 1995; Cooper & Thorp, 1999; Cramer *et al.*, 2002). The occurrence of a diminished ovarian reserve is significantly higher among women who smoke, as was shown in studies of infertile women undergoing assisted reproduction (Sharara *et al.*, 1994; El-Nemr *et al.*, 1998). Premenopausal women who smoke may have fewer ovarian follicles than nonsmokers (Westhoff *et al.*, 2000), although the data are conflicting. One study reported that smoking is associated with smaller ovarian volume (Syrop *et al.*, 1995), whereas another failed to demonstrate this association (Flaws *et al.*, 2000).

(iv)   *Effects on male reproductive potential*

Cigarette smoking has repeatedly been associated with modest reductions in sperm density, motility and morphology (Vine *et al.*, 1994; Wong *et al.*, 2000). It has also been associated with increases in the levels of estrone, estradiol, testosterone and free testosterone in serum (Vine, 1996; Trummer *et al.*, 2002). This effect may be mediated in part by constituents of seminal plasma. In one study, exposure of spermatozoa from non-smokers to seminal plasma from smokers was associated with decreased viability. On the other hand, when spermatozoa from smokers were incubated in seminal plasma from non-smokers, an improvement in the quality of semen was seen (Zavos *et al.*, 1998). Despite the relatively clear effects of smoking on sperm parameters and the possible delay in conception, smoking by the male partner has not been found to have a consistent impact on fertility (Bolumar *et al.*, 1996; Curtis *et al.*, 1997; Hull *et al.*, 2000).

(b)   *Hormonal effects*

(i)   *Sex hormones*

Estrogens

Smoking is thought to exert an 'antiestrogenic' effect in women (Baron *et al.*, 1990; US Department of Health and Human Services, 2001). This is based on the observation that smoking increases the risk for estrogen-deficiency disorders, and decreases the risk for many disorders associated with estrogen-excess. Generally, this effect seems more pronounced in postmenopausal women. Of the estrogen-deficiency disorders, smoking has been found to be associated with an increased risk for hip fracture (Law & Hackshaw, 1997; Law et al., 1997; US Department of Health and Human Services, 2001). Of the estrogen-excess disorders, smoking has been found to be inversely associated with endometrial cancer, uterine fibroids, endometriosis, vomiting during pregnancy and hypertensive disorders of pregnancy (Baron et al., 1990; US Department of Health and Human Services, 2001).

Cigarette smoking does not seem to affect endogenous levels of the major estrogens in either premenopausal (Lucero et al., 2001; Manson et al., 2001) or postmenopausal women (Baron et al., 1990; Law et al., 1997; Verkasalo et al., 2001) although there are reasons for predicting such effects: nicotine or smoke-associated PAHs may inhibit aromatase, an enzyme that is required for estrogen production, in granulosa cells (Barbieri et al., 1986). This lack of effect indicates that smoking alters estrogen-related processes in women in ways other than through direct modulation of endogenous estrogen levels. Nevertheless, among postmenopausal women who take oral estrogens, cigarette smoking has been shown to reduce circulating levels of estradiol (Jensen et al., 1985; Jensen & Christiansen, 1988; Bjarnason & Christiansen, 2000), unbound estradiol (not bound to sex hormone-binding globulin) (Cassidenti et al., 1990) and estrone (Jensen et al., 1985; Jensen & Christiansen, 1988; Geisler et al., 1999). During oral estrogen therapy, estrone sulfate accounts for a higher proportion of circulating total estrogens in smokers than in nonsmokers (Geisler et al., 1999; Cassidenti et al., 1990). With lower-dose regimens, smokers seem to have higher levels of follicle-stimulating hormone than nonsmokers (Bjarnason & Christiansen, 2000).

On the other hand, smoking does not affect the estradiol or estrone levels in plasma of women treated with parenteral (transdermal) estrogens (Jensen & Christiansen, 1988), at least in the dose-range studied. However, plasma levels of estrone sulfate may be reduced during parenteral estrogen therapy, although not significantly (Geisler et al., 1999). This difference from the findings after oral treatment suggests that cigarette smoking induces the hepatic enzymes that affect hormone metabolism in a 'first pass' manner.

The biological mechanisms that may explain an anti-estrogenic effect of smoking are not clear. Changes in body weight and age at menopause caused by smoking do not seem sufficient by themselves to provide an explanation. Some of the potentially anti-estrogenic effects occur in premenopausal women and adjustment for body weight and age at menopause does not greatly affect the observed associations. Smoking-related changes in adrenal androgens are also insufficient to explain the effects observed (Thomas et al., 1993) (see below). A smoking-induced shift in estrogen metabolism towards 2-hydroestrogens and catechol estrogens with weak estrogenic potency may play a role (Michnovicz et al., 1986, 1988). A recently described molecular mechanism may also be relevant. Cigarette smoking is a rich source of PAHs and other ligands for the aryl hydrocarbon receptor. The ligand–receptor complex has the capacity to bind to response elements in the promoter region of estrogen-regulated genes, thereby serving as a transcription repressor. This inhibition of estrogen may explain the lack of estrogen stimulation in women with normal estradiol and estrone levels (Safe *et al.*, 1998, 2001; Safe & McDougal, 2002).

Androgens

In women, the most potent circulating androgen, testosterone, derives both from the ovary (predominantly in premenopausal women) and the adrenal gland. Androstenedione and dihydroepiandrosterone, which have an adrenal origin, are much less potent as androgens, but may serve as precursors for other, more potent hormones, such as dihydroepiandrosterone sulfate (DHEAS). Circulating levels of testosterone, androstenedione and perhaps DHEAS have been associated with cancers of the breast and endometrium (Dorgan *et al.*, 1997; Zeleniuch-Jacquotte *et al.*, 1997; Akhmedkhanov *et al.*, 2001; Endogenous Sex Hormones and Breast Cancer Collaborative Group, 2002).

In postmenopausal women, cigarette smoking clearly increases serum concentrations of the adrenal androgens, androstenedione and DHEAS (Law *et al.*, 1997). In premenopausal women who smoke, DHEAS levels are significantly increased (Manson *et al.*, 2001); for androstenedione, findings are consistent with an increase, but the relevant studies are small and the results of individual studies are not statistically significant (Longcope & Johnston, 1988; Ruiz *et al.*, 1992; Thomas *et al.*, 1993).

The levels of the major circulating androgen, testosterone, seem unaffected by smoking in women. For example, Law *et al.* (1997) found that testosterone concentrations in postmenopausal women seem not to be substantially affected. Studies in premenopausal women have generally been small and have yielded conflicting results. Nevertheless, one larger investigation (of > 600 women) reported higher testosterone concentrations in the serum of female smokers than in nonsmokers (Sowers *et al.*, 2001), whereas an earlier study had reported a decreased free testosterone index (Ortego-Centeno *et al.*, 1994).

(ii)   *Diabetes mellitus and insulin resistance*

Diabetes mellitus is a risk factor for endometrial and breast cancers and possibly also for colorectal cancer (Giovannucci, 2001; Gupta *et al.*, 2002). Epidemiological data on type 2 diabetes suggest that cigarette smoking is a risk factor for this common disease. Type 2 diabetes, generally incident among children or young adults, has strong immunological and genetic determinants, and has essentially not been studied with respect to possible associations with tobacco use.

Recent cohort studies have shown a modest association of smoking with risk for incident type 2 diabetes mellitus, though typically the increased risks were found only in the heaviest smokers and in those who start smoking at a younger age (Feskens & Kromhout, 1989; Rimm *et al.*, 1993, 1995; Kawakami *et al.*, 1997; Manson *et al.*, 2000). The association was still observed after adjustment for multiple covariates, including body mass index and alcohol intake.

The biological plausibility of these findings is supported by the results from other investigations showing that cigarette smoking can induce insulin resistance (Facchini *et al.*, 1992; Hautanen & Adlercreutz, 1993; Zavaroni *et al.*, 1994; Eliasson *et al.*, 1997). Smokers have also been observed to have higher concentrations of glycosylated haemoglobin (HbA_1 and HbA_{1C}) than nonsmokers, indicating a tendency to higher glucose levels (Modan *et al.*, 1988; Simon *et al.*, 1989; Nilsson *et al.*, 1995; Sargeant *et al.*, 2001).

There are some hormonal mechanisms that might explain an association of smoking with an increased risk for diabetes. Smoking increases secretion of catecholamines, glucocorticoids and probably growth hormone; these are all 'counter-regulatory' hormones, i.e. they counteract the effects of insulin in glucose metabolism.

(iii) *Body weight and obesity*

Cigarette smoking distorts the normal association between leanness and health because current cigarette smokers weigh less than never-smokers and have a lower body mass index (Klesges *et al.*, 1989; Perkins, 1993; Flegal *et al.*, 1995; US Department of Health and Human Services, 2001). The relationship is 'U-shaped'; moderately heavy smokers weigh less than nonsmokers and also less than heavy smokers. The weight differences are larger for women and become more pronounced with age (Klesges *et al.*, 1989; Williamson *et al.*, 1991; Perkins, 1993; Rasky *et al.*, 1996; Molarius *et al.*, 1997; US Department of Health and Human Services, 2001). Initiation of smoking seems not to lead to weight loss — rather, continued smoking probably suppresses age-related weight gain (US Department of Health and Human Services, 2001).

It is clear that smoking cessation leads to weight gain, such that former smokers weigh more than current smokers of the same age (and smoking duration before cessation) (Williamson *et al.*, 1991; Perkins, 1993; Flegal *et al.*, 1995; US Department of Health and Human Services, 2001). The weight gain following cessation has generally been found to be greater in women than in men (Flegal *et al.*, 1995; O'Hara *et al.*, 1998; US Department of Health and Human Services, 2001).

The mechanisms underlying these effects have been studied extensively. The lower body weights of current smokers are not the result of taking more exercise or of lower caloric intake: if anything, smokers tend to consume more calories and be less active than never-smokers (Klesges *et al.*, 1989; Grunberg, 1990; US Department of Health and Human Services, 2001). After smoking cessation, there seems to be a transient increase in caloric intake, but this is not sufficient to explain the weight gain (Perkins, 1993). Metabolic studies, however, have repeatedly shown that smoking acutely increases energy expenditure, particularly in individuals who are not at rest (Perkins, 1993). Animal experiments and studies of individuals who use nicotine replacement as an aid to stop smoking suggest that nicotine is responsible for the weight differences (Grunberg, 1990). This may be due to the release of catecholamine associated with smoking (US Department of Health and Human Services, 1983).

In addition to its effects on body weight, cigarette smoking also affects the distribution of body weight. Although body weight is lower, the waist-to-hip ratio, an index of abdominal obesity associated with an increased risk for cardiovascular disease, is higher in smokers. As for body weight, this association also appears to be stronger among women than among men (Duncan *et al.*, 1995; Croft *et al.*, 1996; Ishizaki *et al.*, 1999; US Department of Health and Human Services, 2001).

(iv)   *Growth hormone, insulin-like growth factors and insulin-like growth factor-binding proteins*

Growth hormone is secreted by the pituitary gland; most of its effects are mediated through insulin-like growth factors (IGFs) that are synthesized under the influence of growth hormone in a variety of tissues. Relatively heavy exposures to tobacco smoke (e.g. smoking of two or more cigarettes in succession) acutely increase the levels of circulating growth hormone, at least in men (Cryer *et al.*, 1976; Winternitz & Quillen, 1977; Wilkins *et al.*, 1982). In women, data are limited, but are consistent with a similar effect. The increase in growth hormone concentration is similar in obese and lean female smokers (Szostak-Wegierek *et al.*, 1996).

Under the control of growth hormone, the liver synthesizes IGFs that are secreted into the circulation. High serum concentrations of IGF1 have been associated with cancers of the breast, prostate, colorectum and lung (Chan *et al.*, 1998; Ma *et al.*, 1999; Yu & Rohan, 2000; Kaaks *et al.*, 2000; Toniolo *et al.*, 2000; Giovannuci, 2001; Fürstenberger & Senn, 2002). The data regarding circulating IGF1 levels and cigarette smoking are conflicting. Although the studies on growth hormone have suggested that IGF1 levels might be increased by smoking (Eliasson *et al.*, 1993; Kaklamani *et al.*, 1999), a few studies have reported decreased IGF1 levels in smokers (Landin-Wilhelmsen *et al.*, 1994; Probst-Hensch *et al.*, 2001) and other investigations have found no association (Goodman-Gruen & Barrett-Connor, 1997; Ma *et al.*, 1999; Lukanova *et al.*, 2001). One study calculated free IGF1 levels and reported lower values in ever-smokers than in non-smokers, but this result is biased by the inclusion of former smokers with current smokers, and by the apparent lack of adjustment for covariates (Janssen *et al.*, 1998).

Research in this area is complicated by the presence of IGF-binding proteins, which can alter the availability and effects of the IGFs. There are few data regarding the effect of smoking on the binding proteins and some have suggested that smoking may decrease the levels of IGFBP3, the principal binding protein for IGF1 (Kaklamani *et al.*, 1999; Lukanova *et al.*, 2001), although other studies have found no association (Yu *et al.*, 1999; Probst-Hensch *et al.*, 2001).

(v)   *Vitamin D*

Vitamin D is well known as a family of hormones that regulate calcium, magnesium, phosphorus and bone metabolism. Vitamin D also has important effects on cell differentiation and proliferation, and may be inversely related to the risks for cancers of the breast, prostate and colorectum (Schwartz & Hulka, 1990; Martinez & Willett, 1998; Lipkin & Newmark, 1999; Bretherton-Watt *et al.*, 2001; Polek & Weigel, 2002).

Cigarette smoking has repeatedly been associated with reductions in serum levels of 25-hydroxyvitamin D (25-OH vitamin D), the compound that best reflects vitamin D status. A number of studies have reported that smokers have lower serum concentrations of 25-OH vitamin D than nonsmokers (Mellstrom *et al.*, 1993; Brot *et al.*, 1999; Harris *et al.*, 2000; Rapuri *et al.*, 2000; Chapurlat *et al.*, 2001; Need *et al.*, 2002). Most of these investigations adjusted for several covariates such as bone mineral density, vitamin D intake and exposure to sunlight (Brot *et al.*, 1999; Harris *et al.*, 2000; Rapuri *et al.*, 2000). 1,25-Dihydroxyvitamin D (1,25-$(OH)_2$ vitamin D) levels are tightly regulated and do not reflect vitamin D status except under conditions of obvious deficiency or excess. Nevertheless, in some studies (Brot *et al.*, 1999; Need *et al.*, 2002), but not all (Rapuri *et al.*, 2000), serum concentrations of this hormone have been found to be decreased in smokers.

The data reviewed in this section can be summarized as follows:

- Cigarette smoking has widespread and serious effects on reproductive function in women. Some of these effects may have implications for cancer risks in women.
- Cigarette smoking has important hormonal and metabolic effects that may be related to cancer risk at several sites. Smokers have an increased risk for type 2 diabetes, which may, in turn, increase the risk for cancer at several sites. Smokers also have a lower average body weight than nonsmokers, and smoking cessation has been associated with weight gain. Although this weight gain is admittedly a negative outcome, the benefits of smoking cessation still far exceed it.
- The 'anti-estrogenic' effect of cigarette smoking may be relevant to the development of cancers at several anatomical sites in women, and the effects of smoking on vitamin D status may be involved in the carcinogenic effects of tobacco.
- The implications of the findings regarding the association between smoking, insulin-like growth factors and adrenal androgens are not clear.

4.3.2   *Animals*

(*a*)   *Reproductive and perinatal effects*

(i)   *Effects on embryonic growth and malformations*

A study was conducted to determine whether chronic treatment of gestating monkeys with nicotine alters the concentrations of known regulators of energy balance in the newborn offspring. Gestating rhesus monkeys were treated with nicotine tartrate (1.5 mg/kg bw per day) starting on day 26 of gestation and were maintained until day 160 of gestation. Exposure to nicotine had no significant effect on absolute birth weights of the monkeys, although there was a 10% reduction in birth weights in animals exposed to nicotine when normalized to maternal weight. Plasma leptin concentrations on postnatal day 1 were lower by about 50% in the nicotine-treated group than those in controls, suggesting that the infant monkeys exposed to nicotine may also have lower body-fat levels. These data suggest that exposure to nicotine during gestation may increase energy expenditure in the developing fetus through actions on hypothalamic systems, resulting in lower birth weights and body-fat levels (Grove *et al*, 2001).

Gestating C57BL or mutant 'curly tail' mice were exposed to tobacco smoke in a smoking machine for 10 min, three times a day, either on the day of conception (day 0) and days 1 and 2, on days 3, 4 and 5, or from day 0 until day 17. After the first two treatments, embryonic development was subsequently assessed on day 9. Both these periods of exposure were associated with a dose-related retardation in embryonic growth, but the retardation was more marked in embryos exposed on days 0, 1 and 2. It would seem, therefore, that even brief episodes of maternal smoking are detrimental to the very early embryo, and even if smoking is stopped, the effects persist at least for some days and there is no immediate catch-up growth. In mice exposed continuously for 17 days, the fetuses were studied on day 18: a significant reduction in fetal body weight was observed in both strains of mice. There was also a reduction in the number of skeletal ossification centres, showing that developmental delay also occurred. In C57BL mice, one rib abnormality occurred, but no major congenital malformations were seen. However, in the curly tail mutants, 60% of which normally have a curly tail or an open neural tube defect, there was a modest increase in the frequency of open spina bifida and exencephaly; a few minor rib abnormalities also occurred, and one case of cleft lip with cleft palate. These results indicate that tobacco smoke, although detrimental to the developing fetus, is not a potent teratogen in the mouse, but may have minor effects in those individuals genetically predisposed to an abnormality. These results may explain the generally inconclusive findings regarding congenital malformations in the children of women who smoked during pregnancy. In all experiments, the detrimental effects were seen with both higher-tar cigarettes (tar and nicotine yields, 12.9 and 1.19 mg/cigarette, respectively) and lower-tar cigarettes (4.8 and 0.54 mg/cigarette, respectively), indicating that tobacco modification is not beneficial to the developing fetus (Seller & Bnait, 1995).

(ii)   Effects on the fetal respiratory system

Exposure of fetal rats to nicotine gives rise to increased mortality when animals are challenged postnatally with hypoxia. In one study, gestating rats received nicotine infusions simulating the plasma nicotine concentrations of smokers. At 1–2 days postpartum, the nicotine-treated group displayed normal heart rates, electrocardiogram waveforms and respiratory rates under normal oxygen conditions. With hypoxia (5% O_2, for 10 min), controls showed initial tachycardia and a subsequent slight decline in heart rate. Atrioventricular conduction was gradually impaired and repolarization abnormalities also appeared. The group exposed to nicotine showed no tachycardia and their heart rate declined rapidly and precipitously within a few minutes after the start of hypoxia. Changes in respiration were identical in the two groups: initial tachypnoea and subsequent decline. These results suggest that prenatal exposure to nicotine affects sinoatrial reactivity to hypoxia without impairing cardiac conduction *per se*. These mechanisms would explain the increased hypoxia-induced mortality noted in animals exposed to nicotine prenatally, and could contribute to increased morbidity, mortality and sudden infant death syndrome in humans (Slotkin *et al.*, 1997).

Rats were exposed to cigarette smoke or room air from days 2–22 of gestation. Immunoblots of dorsocaudal brainstem lysates at day 2 postpartum revealed no differences in protein kinase C (PKC) (α and β) or endothelial NOS expression. However, the immunoreactivities of PKC-γ, PKC-δ and neuronal NOS were reduced in the smoke-exposed group. The results indicate that smoking during gestation is associated with selective reductions in PKC and NOS isoforms within the dorsocaudal brainstem, which could decrease respiratory drive and lead to enhanced vulnerability to hypoxia in infants of mothers who smoke. These conditions are implicated in sudden infant death syndrome (Hasan et al., 2001).

Gestating rats received either nicotine (6 mg/kg bw per day) or vehicle administered continuously with an osmotic minipump from day 6 of gestation to days 5 or 6 postpartum. On days 5 or 6 postpartum, pups were either exposed to a single period of hypoxia (97% N_2; 3% CO_2) and their time to last gasp was determined, or exposed repeatedly to hypoxia and their ability to autoresuscitate from primary apnoea was determined. Perinatal exposure to nicotine did not alter the time to last gasp, but it did impair the ability of pups to autoresuscitate from primary apnoea. In the control group, pups were able to autoresuscitate from 18 ± 1 (SD) periods of hypoxia, whereas, after exposure to nicotine, the treated pups were able to autoresuscitate from only 12 ± 2 periods ($p < 0.001$) of hypoxia. These data provide evidence that perinatal exposure to nicotine impairs the ability of newborn rats to autoresuscitate from primary apnoea during repeated exposure to hypoxia, such as may occur during episodes of prolonged sleep apnoea (Fewell & Smith, 1998).

(iii)   *Mutagenic effects in the embryo*

Long-term chronic exposure to tobacco smoke is believed to be necessary for carcinogenesis. An investigation was conducted into the relationship between short-term exposure to smoke and the frequency of deletions in the mouse embryo. Deletions and other genome rearrangements are associated with carcinogenesis and inheritable diseases. The pink-eyed unstable (p^{un}) mutation in C57BL/6J mice is the result of internal duplication of 70 kb of DNA within the p gene. Spontaneous reversion events in homozygous p^{un}/p^{un} mice occur by deletion of one copy of the duplicated sequence. Reversion events occurring in the embryonic premelanocytes of the developing fetus give rise to black spots on the grey fur of the offspring after birth. The effects of exposure of pregnant p^{un} mice to cigarette smoke and cigarette-smoke condensate on the frequency of black spots occurring in the offspring were investigated. Gestating dams were exposed (whole body) to smoke generated by either filtered or unfiltered cigarettes for 4 h, or alternatively, mice were given a 15-mg/kg bw dose of cigarette-smoke condensate during day 10 of gestation. The concentrations of total particulate matter, CO, plasma nicotine and cotinine were determined to characterize the smoke exposure. There was a significant increase in the number of DNA deletions in the embryo as indicated by spotted offspring in both of the smoke-exposed groups and in the condensate-exposed group. The results suggest that embryos are highly sensitive to the genotoxic activity of cigarette smoke following a single exposure of only 4 h (Jalili *et al.*, 1998).

(iv)   *Effects on the postnatal brain*

The effects of prenatal exposure to CO, a major component of cigarette smoke, on the structural and neurochemical development of the postnatal brain at 1 and 8 weeks were studied alone or in combination with postnatal hyperthermia. Gestating guinea-pigs ($n = 11$) were exposed to 200 ppm CO for 10 h per day from mid-gestation until term (68 days), whereas control dams ($n = 10$) breathed room air. On postnatal day 4, neonates from the control and CO-exposed groups were exposed to hyperthermia (35 °C) for 75 min or remained at ambient temperature (23 °C). Semiquantitative immunohisto-chemical techniques revealed the following neurotransmitter alterations in the medulla after 1 week: a decrease in met-enkephalin-immunoreactivity following postnatal hyper-thermia and an increase in 5-hydroxytryptamine immunostaining following a combination of exposure to CO and hyperthermia. No alterations were observed in substance P- or tyrosine-hydroxylase staining in animals subjected to any of the treatments. At 8 weeks of age, the combination of prenatal exposure to CO followed by a brief hyperthermic stress postnatally resulted in lesions throughout the brain and an increase in immunoreactivity of glial fibrillary acidic protein in the medulla. Such effects on brain development could be of relevance in cardiorespiratory control in the neonate and could have implications for the etiology of sudden infant death syndrome, in which smoking and hyperthermia are major risk factors (Tolcos *et al.*, 2000).

Because the identity of the teratogenic agent in cigarette smoke remains controversial, a study was conducted to investigate whether nicotine can cause neural dysmorphology and, hence, act as a nervous system teratogen in cultured rat embryos. This in-vitro study confirmed the conclusion of previous reports on in-utero exposure that nicotine leads to growth retardation and impaired development of the nervous system, particularly of the forebrain and the branchial arches. This could lead to microcephaly and cleft palate in term fetuses. Cellular disruption and necrosis occurred in the neuroepithelium and under-lying mesenchyme; the effect was dose-dependent. There was severe disruption of cell and organelle membranes, and many healthy cells were found to contain engulfed, whole condensed or remnants of dead cells. The results show that nicotine acts as a nervous system teratogen leading to gross and cellular dysmorphology. This could be explained by a direct effect of this highly lipid-soluble compound on the membranes, or by an indirect effect through oxidative membrane damage (Joschko *et al.*, 1991).

(b)   *Hormonal effects*

(i)   *Estrogens*

Two groups of female rats (aged 2.5–3 months and 6 months) were exposed to main-stream cigarette smoke for 2 h per day for 3 weeks or 3 months. Exposure to tobacco smoke did not induce any changes in uterine weight or estrous cycle, but led to a decrease in the estradiol (E2) concentration in uterine tissue, in particular in the 6-month-old rats and in the young rats after 3 months of exposure. No signs of aneuploidy were found in the uterus of the smoke-exposed animals. Flow cytometry analysis showed that both the cell proliferation index and the proportion of cells in S-phase were increased by 3 weeks of exposure and both were decreased by 3 months of exposure (Berstein *et al.*, 1999)

(ii) Glucose tolerance, insulin

Cigarette smoking is a major risk factor for coronary heart disease. The effect of nicotine on blood pressure and glucose tolerance was studied in adult male Sprague-Dawley rats randomly assigned to receive either nicotine or placebo pellets as subcutaneous implants. Body-weight gain was controlled by pair-feeding, and was not significantly different between nicotine-treated and placebo-treated animals. Blood pressure increased throughout a 3-week treatment period in nicotine-treated animals and was significantly higher ($p < 0.05$) than in placebo-treated rats; it returned to normal within 1 week following exhaustion of the pellets. Oral glucose tolerance tests conducted at 2.5 weeks after implantation showed similar glucose, insulin and free fatty acid profiles in both groups. The results show that exposure to nicotine leads to sustained but reversible hypertension in rats without deterioration of glucose tolerance or insulin action, under conditions of controlled body-weight gain. Smokeless nicotine adversely affects the coronary risk profile by increasing blood pressure (Swislocki *et al.*, 1997).

(iii) Vitamin D

The effects of 2 months of nicotine treatment on bone formation and resorption were studied in adult female rats. In addition, the concentrations of calciotropic hormones, including parathyroid hormone, calcitonin, 25-OH vitamin D and 1,25-(OH)$_2$ vitamin D were determined. Groups of seven animals received either saline or nicotine at 3.0 or 4.5 mg/kg bw per day, delivered by subcutaneously implanted osmotic minipumps, for 2 months. Serum, right tibia, left femur and lumbar vertebrae (3–5) were collected to determine hormonal concentrations as well as histomorphometric parameters, bone-mineral density, bone-mineral content and vertebral strength. Although nicotine-treated rats had a lower level of 25-OH vitamin D (54.4 ± 3.1 ng/mL for the lower-dose group and 55.8 ± 2.8 ng/mL for the higher-dose group (mean $\pm$ SEM)) than the controls (74.8 ± 2.8 ng/mL) ($p < 0.01$), no significant difference could be detected between the levels of the remaining hormones. Similarly, no statistical differences were detected in histomorphometric parameters, bone-mineral density, bone-mineral content or vertebral strength between nicotine-treated and control rats. The results indicate that exposure to nicotine for 2 months causes a 30% reduction in serum concentration of 25-OH vitamin D, but no alteration in bone mass, strength or formation and resorption (Fung *et al.*, 1998).

(iv) Effects on the hypothalamus–hypophysis–adrenal hormones

The possible long-term effects of postnatal exposure to cigarette smoke were studied in male Sprague-Dawley rats exposed to the smoke from two Kentucky reference IR-1 type cigarettes every morning from day 1 after birth for a period of 5, 10 or 20 days. The rats were killed 24 h (for exposure periods of 5, 10 and 20 days), 1 week (for 20 days of exposure) or 7 months (for 20 days of exposure) after termination of the last exposure. Catecholamine levels and changes in catecholamine utilization in discrete hypothalamic regions were analysed by quantitative histofluorimetry. Serum prolactin, luteinizing hormone, thyroid-stimulating hormone and corticosterone concentrations were determined by radioimmunoassay. In the postnatal period, serum levels of luteinizing hormone were significantly increased 24 h after a 10-day or 20-day period of exposure to cigarette smoke. A highly significant increase in serum prolactin concentrations was observed in adults who had been exposed postnatally to cigarette smoke for a 20-day period, although the levels had been unaltered by this exposure when measured during the postnatal period. Twenty-four hours following a 20-day postnatal exposure, catecholamine utilization was increased in the medial palisade zone of the median eminence and was substantially reduced in the parvocellular and magnocellular parts of the paraventricular hypothalamic nucleus. Following 20 days of postnatal exposure to cigarette smoke, measurements made 1 week and 7 months later revealed no alterations in levels or utilization of catecholamine in various hypothalamic areas including the median eminence. No alteration in the development of body weight was observed with any of the above changes. The results indicate that marked but temporary increases in the secretion of luteinizing hormone occur 24 h after postnatal exposure to cigarette smoke, whereas increases in prolactin secretion develop only in adult life, when maturation of the brain and/or the anterior pituitary gland is complete. Changes in levels and utilization of catecholamine have been found in discrete hypothalamic nerve terminal networks, but do not play a major role in mediating the above changes in anterior pituitary function and are probably the result of a withdrawal phenomenon (Jansson et al., 1992).

Male rats were exposed to the smoke of 1–4 Kentucky reference IR-1 type cigarettes. Catecholamines in the diencephalon were measured by quantitative histofluorimetry in discrete dopamine (DA) and noradrenaline (NA) nerve terminal systems. Blood concentrations of thyroid-stimulating hormone, prolactin, luteinizing hormone, follicle-stimulating hormone, adrenocorticotropic hormone, vasopressin and corticosterone were determined by radioimmunoassays. Exposure to unfiltered, but not to glass fibre-filtered cigarette smoke resulted in dose-dependent reductions of NA levels in the various hypothalamic NA nerve terminal systems, and in dose-dependent increases of amine turnover in the various DA and NA nerve terminal systems in the hypothalamus. The decrease that was observed in secretion of thyroid-stimulating hormone, luteinizing hormone and prolactin after exposure to unfiltered smoke was probably induced by nicotine activating the lateral and medial tubero-infundibular DA neurons. Furthermore, unfiltered cigarette smoke produced a dose-related increase in corticosterone secretion (Andersson et al., 1985).

4.4   Genetic and related effects

This topic was reviewed previously by DeMarini (1983) and Obe (1984) and sum-marized in the first *IARC Monograph* on tobacco smoking (IARC, 1986). The present monograph provides only a brief overview of work prior to 1986 and, instead, summarizes work published since then.

4.4.1   *Humans*

(*a*)   *Mutagenicity, sister chromatid exchange,* HPRT *mutation and other effects*

(i)   *Urinary mutagenicity*

Urinary mutagenicity in smokers was detected first by Yamasaki and Ames (1977) by testing the XAD/acetone-extractable organic compounds from urine in the *Salmonella* (Ames) mutagenicity assay. Several years later, studies using essentially the same methods confirmed and clarified this original observation (Putzrath *et al.*, 1981; Kriebel *et al.*, 1985). The general approach to these studies has remained similar over the years. It involves concentration of the organic compounds from the urine by means of a solid-phase resin followed by elution with an organic solvent and then testing the resulting concentrate, after its fractional analysis by HPLC, in the *Salmonella* (Ames) mutagenicity assay in the presence of rat liver S9 mix for metabolic activation.

A comparison of three types of resin (C18, XAD-2 and CN) followed by elution with acetone showed that the highest levels of urinary mutagenicity were detected using C18 resin. This study found that urinary genotoxicity was higher in smokers of black tobacco than in smokers of blond tobacco (Kuenemann-Migeot *et al.*, 1996). A study of the stability of stored urine samples showed that no significant loss of mutagenic activity occurred in urine stored frozen for as long as 175 days, although near significance was reached, as a result of decreasing mutant response as storage time increased, for two of the higher doses tested (Williams *et al.*, 1990). A *Salmonella* microsuspension assay is generally more sensitive at detecting urinary mutagens from smokers than the standard plate-incor-poration assay (Kado *et al.*, 1983; Nylander & Berg, 1991). Peak mutagenic activity of the urine occurred 4–5 h after the beginning of smoking and decreased to pre-smoking levels 12 h after the cessation of smoking in occasional smokers and after 18 h in heavy smokers (Kado *et al.*, 1985). This study suggested that the mutagens are absorbed rapidly (3–5 h) and are eliminated from the body following first-order kinetics; the excretion rate constant for the occasional smoker was ~0.1 h^{-1}, and the half-life ($T_{1/2}$) was ~7 h. A study in which the SOS Chromotest was used as the indicator assay showed that urine from smokers that was mutagenic in *Salmonella typhimurium* TA98 was not mutagenic in the SOS Chromotest; this test is therefore not suitable for assaying urinary mutagens (De Méo *et al.*, 1988). Urine concentrates from subjects who both smoked tobacco and chewed areca nuts induced sister chromatid exchange and chromosomal aberrations in Chinese hamster ovary cells (Trivedi *et al.*, 1993, 1995).

The urine of smokers who smoked cigarettes that heated, but did not burn tobacco had levels of urinary mutagenicity similar to those of nonsmokers (Doolittle *et al.*, 1989; deBethizy *et al.*, 1990; Smith *et al.*, 1996). However, the urine of occupationally exposed bidi tobacco rollers was mutagenic (Bhisey & Govekar, 1991), suggesting that exposure to tobacco *per se* rather than tobacco pyrolysate products may be sufficient to produce mutagenic urine. Urinary mutagenicity generally correlated with the number, but not the tar level, of cigarettes smoked (Tuomisto *et al.*, 1986; Kuenemann-Migeot *et al.*, 1996). Interestingly, the urine of smokers of black tobacco was twice as mutagenic as the urine from smokers of blond tobacco, and there was a higher risk for bladder cancer in smokers of black tobacco than in smokers of blond tobacco (Vineis *et al.*, 1984; Bryant *et al.*, 1988; Malaveille *et al.*, 1989; see also Section 2.1.2.(*a*)(iii)). One study of bladder cancer patients showed that there was no association between levels of urinary mutagenicity and tumour status or recurrence of the bladder tumours (Kanaoka *et al.*, 1990).

Although consumption of fried meat can also produce mutagenic urine, experiments with subjects eating controlled diets showed that the higher urinary mutagenicity in smokers compared with nonsmokers was not the result of enhanced mutagenicity caused by diet-related heterocyclic amine mutagens in their urine (Doolittle *et al.*, 1990a). Although not reviewed exhaustively here, smoking was generally a potential factor in studies investigating urinary mutagenicity of occupational exposures, such as inks and pharmaceuticals (Dolara *et al.*, 1981), tyres (Crebelli *et al.*, 1985), coke or graphite-electrodes (Ferreira *et al.*, 1994), steel and coal processing (De Méo *et al.*, 1987) and benzidine (DeMarini *et al.*, 1987).

Indirect evidence suggests that the chemicals responsible for smoking-related urinary mutagenicity are primarily aromatic amines and/or heterocyclic polyaromatic amino compounds. For example, the urine of smokers was much more mutagenic in strain YG1024 of *Salmonella*, which overproduces *O*-acetyltransferase, than in strains with less of this activity (e.g. TA98) or that overproduce nitroreductase (YG1021) (Einistö *et al.*, 1990; Camoirano *et al.*, 2001). One study in which the urine of smokers was fractionated by reversed-phase HPLC and the fractions were then evaluated for their ability to induce chromosomal aberrations in Chinese hamster ovary cells concluded that clastogenic agents were present in the urine of smokers. This clastogenic activity was reduced by the addition of catalase or superoxide dismutase, suggesting that the activity of these agents may result from the production of active oxygen species (Dunn & Curtis, 1985).

Urinary mutagenicity has been shown to correlate with the levels of a 4-ABP–DNA adduct[1] in exfoliated urothelial cells from smokers (Talaska *et al.*, 1991b). However, the levels of a 4-ABP-haemoglobin adduct[2] showed a more complex association with urinary mutagenicity (Bartsch *et al.*, 1990). Chemical analysis of urine from a smoker with exceptionally high urinary mutagenicity revealed the presence of the mutagen 2-amino-7-naphthol, which is a metabolite of the bladder carcinogen 2-aminonaphthalene (β-naphthyl-

---

[1] 4-ABP–DNA adduct: *N*-(deoxyguanosin-8-yl)-4-aminobiphenyl–DNA adduct
[2] 4-ABP–haemoglobin adduct: *N*-(deoxyguanosin-8-yl)-4-aminobiphenyl–haemoglobin adduct

amine), a component of cigarette smoke (Connor *et al.*, 1983). Chemical fractionation of mutagenic urine from smokers indicated that much of the mutagenic activity may be due to PAHs and/or heterocyclic amines (Mure *et al.*, 1997). Although the concentration of urinary nicotine plus its metabolites correlated with urinary mutagenicity in smokers (Rahn *et al.*, 1991; Granella *et al.*, 1996), nicotine and its metabolites were not responsible for the mutagenicity. The absence of urinary mutagens in subjects who smoke cigarettes in which tobacco is heated but not burned has been demonstrated, although large quantities of nicotine and cotinine were found in the urine of such subjects (Curvall *et al.*, 1987; Rahn *et al.*, 1991).

(ii)   HPRT *mutations*

Several reviews (Cole & Skopek, 1994; Robinson *et al.*, 1994; Curry *et al.*, 1999) have noted that smoking generally increases the hypoxanthine-guanine phosphoribosyl-transferase (*HPRT*) (also called *HGPRT*) mutant frequency in peripheral blood lymphocytes by ~50%. However, the increases did not reach statistical significance in some studies because of the large interindividual variability of *HPRT* mutant frequencies. Using the autoradiographic *HPRT* assay, some elevated portion of the *HPRT* mutant frequency was shown to reflect recent exposure to tobacco smoke rather than the cumulative effect of past exposure. The two categories of smoker (light and heavy) had frequencies of mutant cells significantly different from each other and both were significantly higher than those of nonsmokers and former smokers (Ammenheuser *et al.*, 1997). Most importantly, *HPRT* mutant frequencies were similar in patients with lung cancer and in controls with the same smoking status, indicating that lung cancer *per se* has little if any effect on *HPRT* mutant frequency in lymphocytes. However, when cases and controls were combined, the *HPRT* mutant frequency was significantly higher in ever-smokers than in never-smokers (Hou *et al.*, 1999). Although some analyses have found no difference in the mutation spectrum at the *HPRT* locus between smokers and nonsmokers (Curry *et al.*, 1999), an increase in transversions, in particular, GC→TA, has been frequently noted among smokers (Burkhart-Schultz *et al.*, 1996; Podlutsky *et al.*, 1999; Hackman *et al.*, 2000). This is the primary class of base substitution induced by those PAHs that form bulky DNA adducts giving rise to transversion mutations. An excess of this class of mutation in the *HPRT* mutation spectrum of smokers would be consistent with exposure to the PAHs in cigarette smoke.

(iii)   *Genotoxic effects in reproductive tissues/fluids and in children of smokers*

Pregnant women who smoke not only had elevated *HPRT* mutant frequencies themselves, but analysis of cord blood indicated that their children also had elevated frequencies (Ammenheuser *et al.*, 1994, 1998). Sequencing of *HPRT* mutants in cord blood from mothers who smoke indicated that most (85.7%) of the mutations were illegitimate V(D)J recombinase activity-associated exon 2-3 deletions (Bigbee *et al.*, 1999). V(D)J recombinase is an enzyme system that mediates genomic rearrangements of germline-encoded variable (V), diversity (D) and junctional (J) regions responsible for gene-rating T-cell receptor and immunoglobulin gene diversity for antigen-specific recognition. These genomic *HPRT* deletions are an illegitimate recombination event associated with haematopoietic malignancies in early childhood (Gu *et al.*, 1992). In-utero exposure to tobacco smoke increased translocation frequencies in the newborn, and a significant asso-ciation was found between the *CYP1A1 MspI* polymorphism (variant genotypes of *CYP1A1*) and frequencies of chromosomal aberration in the newborns (Pluth *et al.*, 2000). Evidence has been obtained to suggest that smoking by the mother may cause detectable DNA strand breaks and alkali-labile damage in the lymphocytes of newborns detected by single-cell gel electrophoresis; the percentage of damaged cells increased with the fre-quency of smoking (Sardas *et al.*, 1995).

Smoking was shown to induce aneuploidy in sperm for certain chromosomes, inclu-ding 1, 13, and YY disomy (Rubes *et al.*, 1998; Härkönen *et al.*, 1999; Shi *et al.*, 2001), but not for others, such as XX, XY, 7 or 8 (Robbins *et al.*, 1997; Rubes *et al.*, 1998; Härkönen *et al.*, 1999). Smoking also appeared to induce oxidative damage to sperm DNA as indi-cated by higher levels of 8-OHdG in sperm DNA of smokers than in that of nonsmokers (Shen *et al.*, 1997). Consistent with this was the finding of higher levels of DNA strand breaks in the sperm from smokers than in that from nonsmokers (Potts *et al.*, 1999).

In investigations on the effects of smoking on oocytes, smokers were found to have fewer retrieved oocytes than nonsmokers, a finding consistent with the known reduction in their fertility (Zenzes *et al.*, 1995). The oocytes with diploid complements of chromosomes were more frequent in smokers than in nonsmokers. This diploidy probably resulted from the prevention of first polar body extrusion, which indicates meiotic immaturity. The pro-portion of diploid oocytes was strongly associated with the number of cigarettes smoked per day (Zenzes *et al.*, 1995). In addition, triploid zygotes occurred more frequently among smokers than nonsmokers, suggesting that digynic fertilization is an important mechanism leading to triploidy among smokers (Zenzes *et al.*, 1995). These results strongly indicated that cigarette smoking is hazardous to the viability and function of developing oocytes and their resulting embryos, and a recent study suggested that expression of the aromatic hydro-carbon receptor-driven *Bax* gene is required for premature ovarian failure caused by expo-sure of mice to PAHs. This ovarian damage caused by PAHs was prevented by aromatic hydrocarbon receptor Ah2 or *Bax* inactivation. Oocytes in human ovarian biopsies grafted into immunodeficient mice also accumulated Bax and underwent apoptosis after exposure to PAHs *in vivo* (Matikainen *et al.*, 2001). These data also suggest that the early onset of menopause in women smokers is caused, at least in part, by the pro-apoptotic action of tobacco smoke-derived PAHs in human oocytes.

The cervical mucus of smokers was more mutagenic than that of nonsmokers when tested in the *Salmonella* (Ames) mutagenicity assay (Holly *et al.*, 1986), and XAD/ace-tone extracts of amniotic fluid from mothers who smoke induced a higher number of sister chromatid exchanges in Chinese hamster ovary cells than did extracts from nonsmokers (Lähdetie *et al.*, 1993). This is consistent with the finding that cervical epithelial cells from smokers had higher numbers of micronuclei than those from nonsmokers (Cerqueira *et al.*, 1998).

As noted in the reviews by Sastry (1991) and Zenzes (2000), smoking causes numerous reproductive problems, as well as effects on meiotic spindle function, DNA damage (oxidative damage as well as PAH adducts) to spermatozoa and oocytes, in addition to gametic and placental transmission of genetic damage. As discussed above, smoking is also associated with second-generation effects. Together, these data provide suggestive evidence for paternal and possible maternal gametic transmission of genetic damage as well as indirect support for the possibility that tobacco smoke may be a germ-cell mutagen.

(iv)   *Cytogenetic effects*

Micronuclei

Bonassi *et al.* (2003) reviewed many studies that examined the influence of smoking on the frequency of micronuclei in peripheral lymphocytes. However, mixed results have been obtained. A pooled re-analysis of 24 databases from the Human MicroNucleus (HUMN) international collaborative project showed that smokers did not have an overall increase in the frequency of micronuclei in their lymphocytes. However, when the interaction with occupational exposure was considered, smokers of 30 cigarettes or more per day had a significantly higher frequency of micronuclei than did nonsmokers (Bonassi *et al.*, 2003). An increased frequency of micronuclei in smokers has been observed to occur preferentially in B lymphocytes and suppressor/cytotoxic T8 lymphocytes (Larramendy & Knuutila, 1991). Elevated frequencies of micronuclei have also been found in the tracheobronchial epithelium of smokers (Lippman *et al.*, 1990). Workers exposed to tobacco while making bidi cigarettes also had an elevated frequency of micronuclei in buccal epithelium (Bagwe & Bhisey, 1993).

Sister chromatid exchange

In contrast to micronuclei, the frequency of sister chromatid exchange in peripheral lymphocytes was generally higher in smokers than in nonsmokers. Numerous studies of the frequencies of sister chromatid exchange in peripheral lymphocytes in environmentally or occupationally exposed or unexposed populations have found that cigarette smoking induces sister chromatid exchange and can be a confounding factor in occupational studies (Sarto *et al.*, 1985; Stenstrand, 1985; Nagaya & Toriumi, 1985; Wulf *et al.*, 1986; Husgafvel-Pursiainen, 1987; Perera *et al.*, 1987; Bender *et al.*, 1988; Kelsey *et al.*, 1988; Reidy *et al.*, 1988; Thompson *et al.*, 1989; Nordic Study Group, 1990; Brinkworth *et al.*, 1992; Górecka & Gorski, 1993; Lazutka *et al.*, 1994; Rajah & Ahuja, 1995; Anderson *et al.*, 1997; Lemasters *et al.*, 1997; Bukvic *et al.*, 1998; Cebulska-Wasilewska *et al.*, 1999; Rowland & Harding, 1999). Of all the cytogenetic end-points, sister chromatid exchange is the most sensitive to the effect of smoking. One study even demonstrated that smoking was associated with higher frequency of sister chromatid exchange in peripheral lymphocytes than in bone marrow. An explanation of this finding

may be that circulating lymphocytes, with an average lifespan of 4.4 years, may accumulate more DNA damage than bone-marrow cells because they have a shorter lifespan
(Kao-Shan *et al.*, 1987). However, among healthy adults, smoking may account for only
19% of the variation in frequencies of sister chromatid exchange between individuals
(Husum *et al.*, 1986). There was a decrease in sister chromatid exchange in former
smokers during the first 78 days after stopping smoking; the decrease then was much
slower from the 78th to the 233rd day after cessation (Sarto *et al.*, 1987). The mechanism
by which smoking induced sister chromatid exchange does not appear to involve extra-
cellularly generated free radicals (Lee *et al.*, 1989).

The smoking of various types of tobacco product, including bidis (Ghosh & Ghosh,
1987; Murthy *et al.*, 1997; Yadav & Thakur, 2000a) and hookah (Yadav & Thakur, 2000b)
also induced sister chromatid exchange.

Chromosomal aberrations

Studies of large populations using classical cytogenetic banding techniques for chromosomal aberrations have given mixed results. One study found that the frequencies of
chromosomal aberrations were not increased by smoking (Bender *et al.*, 1988), whereas
another found that smoking caused a 10–20% increase in such aberrations (Nordic Study
Group, 1990). The results of smaller studies have also been mixed although several have
found significantly higher frequencies of chromosomal aberrations in lymphocytes from
smokers than in those from nonsmokers (Littlefield & Joiner, 1986; Sinués *et al.*, 1990;
Tawn & Whitehouse, 2001). Molecular cytogenetic techniques, such as fluorescence in-
situ hybridization, have also yielded mixed results. Some studies found that smoking:
— did not increase the frequency of stable or unstable aberrations, but did increase
  the frequency of hyperploidy (van Diemen *et al.*, 1995);
— produced a marginal increase in translocation frequency (Pressl *et al.*, 1999); or
— caused a significant increase in stable aberrations (translocations and insertions)
  (Ramsey *et al.*, 1995).
Chromosomal aberration frequencies were found to be elevated among workers in a
bidi tobacco plant who were exposed to tobacco particles and volatile constituents by the
cutaneous and nasopharyngeal routes (Mahimkar & Bhisey, 1995).

Mechanistic considerations include the observation that smokers had lower levels of
folic acid in their red cells than nonsmokers and this decrease in folic acid may play a role
in the higher levels of chromosomal aberrations detected in smokers relative to those in
nonsmokers, probably as a result of induction of common fragile sites (Chen *et al.*, 1989).
Various studies have found that exposure of peripheral lymphocytes from smokers to
various mutagens such as radiations or chemical compounds *in vitro* resulted in higher
frequencies of chromosomal aberrations than such types of exposure caused in lymphocytes from nonsmokers (Au *et al.*, 1991; Ban *et al.*, 1995; Strom *et al.*, 1995; Wang,
L.-E. *et al.*, 2000; Paz-y-Miño *et al.*, 2001). The levels of methylpurine–DNA glycosylase
and 2,6-diamino-4-hydroxy-5N formamidopyrimidine (FaPy)–DNA glycosylase were
higher in the peripheral blood leukocytes of smokers than in those of nonsmokers (Hall

et al., 1993). Collectively, these studies suggested that the cells of smokers, especially those from men, were less able to repair DNA damage and that DNA repair enzyme levels, fragile sites and telomeric associations can be affected by recent exposure.

A large international study showed that an elevated frequency of chromosomal aberrations in lymphocytes predicted the risk for cancer independently of exposure to carcinogens, including cigarette smoke (Bonassi *et al.*, 2000). However, many studies have demonstrated an association between smoking and certain genetic changes specifically predictive of various types of tumour. For example, in comparison with those of nonsmokers, the lymphocytes of smokers had higher frequencies of fragile sites and metaphases with extensive breakage, as well as elevated expression of fragile sites at cancer break-points and oncogene sites (Kao-Shan *et al.*, 1987). Analysis of normal bronchial epithelium from smokers using fluorescence in-situ hybridization found a considerable percentage of cancer-free tobacco smokers with trisomy 7 (Lechner *et al.*, 1997), and the frequence of loss of heterozygosity involving microsatellite DNA at three specific loci-chromosomes was significantly elevated at chromosomal sites containing putative tumour-suppressor genes in histologically normal bronchial epithelium from chronic smokers (Mao *et al.*, 1997). Perhaps most importantly, the fractional allelic loss or gain occurred at a much higher frequency in lung tumours from smokers (48%) than in those from nonsmokers (11%), suggesting that lung cancer in smokers resulted from genetic alterations distinct from those resulting in lung cancer in nonsmokers (Sanchez-Cespedes *et al.*, 2001).

Other genetic changes

Microsatellite instability in colon tumours (Slattery *et al.*, 2000) and chromosome 9 alterations in bladder tumours (Zhang *et al.*, 1997) have been associated with cigarette smoking. Smoking has also been associated with mutagen sensitivity of lymphocytes as a predictor of upper aerodigestive tract cancer (Spitz *et al.*, 1993). In another study, smoking was found not to be significantly associated with mutagen sensitivity of lymphocytes as an indication of predisposition to oral premalignant lesions (Wu *et al.*, 2002). Various cytogenetic changes and smoking have been associated with risk for leukaemia and other myelodysplastic syndromes (Sandler *et al.*, 1993; Davico *et al.*, 1998; Björk *et al.*, 2000, 2001; Moorman *et al.*, 2002).

DNA strand breaks and oxidative damage

A higher frequency of DNA strand breaks detected by the single-cell gel electrophoresis 'comet' assay has been found in lymphocytes (Einhaus *et al.*, 1994; Piperakis *et al.*, 1998; Poli *et al.*, 1999), buccal cells (Rojas *et al.*, 1996) and urothelial cells (Gontijo *et al.*, 2001) of cigarette smokers than in those of nonsmokers. Smoking also increased the level of F(2)-isoprostanes (one of the lipid peroxidation biomarkers), an index of oxidant stress (Dietrich *et al.*, 2002).

The role of smoking-induced oxidative DNA damage is discussed elsewhere in this monograph (see Section 4.1.1(*c*)).

(v)   *Chemoprevention of the formation of smoking-associated biomarkers of genotoxicity*

In humans, the administration of *N*-acetylcysteine to smokers significantly reduced the level of urinary mutagenicity (De Flora *et al.*, 1996) as well as the frequency of micronuclei in the mouth floor and in the soft palate cells (Van Schooten *et al.*, 2002). Administration of vitamins C and E as antioxidants to smokers also reduced the frequency of micronuclei in blood lymphocytes (Schneider *et al.*, 2001). Higher intakes of vitamin A and selenium were associated with a reduced frequency of sister chromatid exchange in smokers (Cheng *et al.*, 1995). However, administration to smokers of the anti-carcinogenic dithiolethione, oltipraz, had no influence on the levels of urinary mutagenicity (Camoirano *et al.*, 2001). Similarly, supplementary niacin (nicotinic acid precursor of NAD+, a substrate for the DNA repair-related enzyme poly(ADP-ribose)polymerase (PARP)) did not decrease the frequencies of *HPRT* variants or micronuclei in peripheral blood lymphocytes in smokers. However, sister chromatid exchange was increased in these cells after the same supplementation (Hageman *et al.*, 1998). Thus, the levels of smoking-associated urinary mutagenicity and micronuclei can be reduced by appropriate chemoprevention.

(b)   *Mutations in* TP53, K-RAS *and related genes*

Smoking is associated with cancer of various organs, and mutations in these smoking-associated tumours have been identified in both oncogenes and tumour-suppressor genes. The gene most frequently found to be mutated in smoking-associated lung tumours is *TP53*, and the studies of this observation have been extensively reviewed (Hernandez-Boussard & Hainaut, 1998; Hainaut & Pfeifer, 2001; Hussain *et al.*, 2001). Briefly, *TP53* mutations are more common in smokers than in nonsmokers, and the frequency of *TP53* mutations shows a direct correlation with the number of cigarettes smoked. *TP53* mutations are found in preneoplastic lesions of the lung, indicating that they are early events that are linked temporally to DNA damage caused by smoking.

The *TP53* mutation spectrum in lung tumours of smokers contains 30% GC→TA transversions, whereas only 10% of the *TP53* mutations in nonsmokers or other tumours are of this type. This percentage in lung exceeds 75% only after exposure resulting from the use of a PAH-rich smoky coal in poorly ventilated homes (DeMarini *et al.*, 2001). The elevated frequency of GC→TA transversion in smokers reflects the type of DNA damage and resulting mutations produced by PAHs, which are important carcinogenic components of cigarette smoke. There is a precise correspondence between the mutational hot spots and the sites of DNA adducts remaining after cells exposed to BPDE and other diol epoxides have undergone a period of DNA repair (Denissenko *et al.*, 1996; Smith *et al.*, 2000). These mutations are targeted at methylated CpG sites. There is a bias for most of the mutated guanines of the GC→TA mutations to be in the nontranscribed DNA strand in lung tumours from smokers. This bias results from the preferential binding and slow repair of BPDE adducts formed on the nontranscribed strand at mutational hot spot sites in the *TP53* gene and therefore the preferential repair of DNA adducts on the transcribed strand (Denissenko *et al.*, 1998). Taken together, these and other data indicate strongly that the *TP53* mutations in lung tumours of smokers are a result of direct DNA damage caused by the carcinogens in cigarette smoke. Although one report argued that *TP53* mutations in smoking-associated lung cancer were not induced by mutagens in cigarette smoke, but were pre-existing mutations selected by physiological, non-genotoxic stress (Rodin & Rodin, 2000), subsequent analysis has refuted this proposal (Hainaut & Pfeifer, 2001).

Mutations at the *K-RAS* or (*KRAS* 2) gene (codons 12, 13 or 61) occur in ~30% of the lung adenocarcinomas of smokers and are primarily GC→TA transversions as seen in *TP53* (Slebos *et al.*, 1991; Husgafvel-Pursiainen *et al.*, 1993; Westra *et al.*, 1993; Gealy *et al.*, 1999; Ahrendt *et al.*, 2001). These mutations are associated with smoking and occur less frequently in nonsmokers (Marchetti *et al.*, 1998; Gealy *et al.*, 1999).

Mutations in *TP53* and other genes, such as *FHIT*[1], *BCL-2* and *BAX*, loss of heterozygosity at specific chromosomal locations and gene overexpression (*TP53*, MDM_2) have also been characterized in smoking-associated tumours, including those of the bladder, oral cavity and breast (Spruck *et al.*, 1993; Schreiber *et al.*, 1997; Sozzi *et al.*, 1997; Baral *et al.*, 1998; Kaur *et al.*, 1998; Dosaka-Akita *et al.*, 1999; Gealy *et al.*, 1999; Tseng *et al.*, 1999; LaRue *et al.*, 2000; Hirao *et al.*, 2001; Conway *et al.*, 2002). Collectively, these observations are consistent with the mutagenic effects of cigarette smoke condensate and tobacco smoke as demonstrated in experimental systems.

> (c) *Influence of polymorphisms in carcinogen-metabolizing genes on smoking-associated biomarkers*

Numerous polymorphisms have been studied for their modulating effect on smoking-associated biomarkers, such as urinary mutagenicity or *HPRT* mutant frequency. However, much of this literature reports studies using small populations, and many studies have either not been repeated, or conflicting results have been obtained in repeated studies (Vineis *et al.*, 1999). Where effects were observed, they were frequently quite modest. Because of the incomplete and/or conflicting nature of this literature, firm conclusions cannot be drawn regarding the modulating effects of polymorphisms on smoking-associated biomarkers.

---

[1] FHIT: fragile histidine triad, a gene coding for a dinucleoside $5',5'''$-P^1,P^3-triphosphate hydrolase, a putative tumour-suppressor protein

4.4.2   *Experimental systems*

(a)   *Genotoxic effects, mutagenicity of cigarette-smoke condensate,*
       urinary mutagenicity and mutation spectra

As reviewed previously (IARC, 1986), cigarette-smoke condensate (CSC) is mutagenic in a variety of systems. Most studies have used condensate generated from various
reference cigarettes, such as K1R4F, which was developed jointly by the US National
Cancer Institute, the US Department of Agriculture and the University of Kentucky
Tobacco and Health Research Institute (Steele *et al.*, 1995). The average mutagenicity of
cigarette-smoke condensates of mainstream smoke from US commercial brands and
K1R4F reference cigarettes in the *Salmonella* mutagenicity assay (on a revertants/mg condensate or revertants/cigarette basis) was not significantly different between cigarettes
representing > 70% of the US cigarette market (Steele *et al.*, 1995). Similar results were
recently obtained in the studies of the K1R5F cigarette (Chepiga *et al.*, 2000), indicating
that these reference cigarettes are acceptable standards with which to compare mutagenicity of cigarettes typically purchased in the USA.

More recent studies have confirmed and extended the initial observations showing
that cigarette-smoke condensate is mutagenic in *Salmonella* and SOS assays (Morin *et al.*,
1987; Ong *et al.*, 1987; Chen & Lee, 1996), induces micronuclei in *Vicia faba* root tips (Ji
& Chen, 1996), deletions at the $Tk^{+/-}$ locus in mouse lymphoma cells (Cobb *et al.*, 1989),
Hprt mutants in Chinese hamster ovary cells (Jongen *et al.*, 1985), and can transform
human endocervical cells in culture to a malignant line with up-regulated levels of *B-Myb*,
p53 and *WAF*$_1$ genes (Yang *et al.*, 1997). Comparisons with wood-smoke condensate or
liquid smoke food flavourings have shown that some flavourings are more cytotoxic than
cigarette-smoke condensate. Nevertheless none of the liquid smoke food flavourings or
wood-smoke condensates was mutagenic in an assay using *S. typhimurium* TA98 and only
some of the liquid smoke food flavourings tested were positive with strain TA100, while
cigarette-smoke condensate was mutagenic in both strains (Putnam *et al.*, 1999).
However, the levels of exposure must be considered in evaluating the risk posed by such
substances (Fitzgerald, 2001; Smith *et al.*, 2001). The relative mutagenic potencies of
organic extracts of cigarette-smoke condensate and other combustion emissions rank
similarly in *Salmonella*, mouse lymphoma $Tk^{+/-}$ and mouse skin tumour-initiation assays,
suggesting that the results obtained using these different systems are reasonably comparable (Williams & Lewtas, 1985).

Most of the sister chromatid exchange-inducing ability of cigarette-smoke condensate
appears to reside in its neutral and highly polar, acidic/neutral fractions (Curvall *et al.*,
1985; Salomaa *et al.*, 1988); the sister chromatid exchange response of the acidic/neutral
fraction was observed only after metabolic activation, suggesting that the PAHs and acidic
compounds in cigarette-smoke condensate are responsible for this activity. Also, the acidic
fraction was the most potent direct-acting fraction that induced mutations involving deletions and/or chromosomal loss by non-disjunction in mammalian A_L hybrid cells of CHO-
K1, a Chinese hamster ovary cell containing one human chromosome 11 (Matsukura *et al.*,

1991). The acid fraction included phenolic compounds such as catechol and hydroquinone (Jansson *et al.*, 1986) that may generate free radicals (quinone and oxygen radicals) that could have produced the clastogenic effects observed. Reconstruction of a mixture containing the primary PAHs in cigarette-smoke condensate failed to reproduce the mutagenic activity of the condensate, suggesting that PAHs were not the primary cause of the activity (Asita *et al.*, 1991).

Nicotine and its metabolites were not mutagenic in *Salmonella*, did not induce sister chromatid exchange in Chinese hamster ovary cells in a study by Doolittle *et al.* (1995) and nicotine did not produce mutagenic urine in rats (Doolittle *et al.*, 1991). However, nicotine was reported to induce sister chromatid exchange in Chinese hamster ovary cells (Trivedi *et al.*, 1990). Although cigarette-smoke condensate contains a wide variety of agents of varying toxicity (Smith & Hansch, 2000), varying the amounts of 333 ingredients (e.g. casing materials, volatile top flavourings and menthol) added to typical commercially blended test cigarettes did not add significantly to the overall mutagenicity, cytotoxicity or inhalation toxicity of the resulting cigarettes (Carmines, 2002; Roemer *et al.*, 2002).

Several lines of evidence indicate that the primary source of mutagenic activity of cigarette-smoke condensate in the *Salmonella* mutagenicity assay is the aromatic amine and heterocyclic amine protein pyrolysate products. As reviewed previously (DeMarini, 1983; Obe, 1984; IARC, 1986), most of the mutagenic activity of this condensate resides in the basic or base/neutral fraction (Austin *et al.*, 1985; Salomaa *et al.*, 1988), which contains the aromatic amines and heterocyclic amines. The removal of protein and peptides from flue-cured or burley tobacco using water extraction followed by protease digestion reduced the mutagenicity of the resultant condensate by ~80% in *S. typhimurium* TA98 and ~50% in *S. typhimurium* TA100 (Clapp *et al.*, 1999). Condensates produced from tobacco smoke aerosols generated at temperatures below 400 °C or 475 °C were not mutagenic in TA98 or TA100, respectively, but those produced above those temperatures were (White *et al.*, 2001). Heterocyclic amine pyrolysate products from proteins are formed only at high temperatures, and the fact that mutagenic activity is found only in cigarette-smoke condensate produced at high temperatures indicates that such compounds are important contributors to this mutagenic effect. Exposure of hamsters to cigarette smoke enhanced the ability of their livers to convert heterocyclic amines to mutagens, suggesting that cigarette smoke, like heterocyclic amines themselves, induces cytochrome P4501A2. Therefore, this induced isoform metabolizes heterocyclic amines (Mori *et al.*, 1995).

Heterocyclic amines are much more mutagenic in *S. typhimurium* TA98 than in TA100. This probably explains the greatly reduced mutagenic activity of cigarette-smoke condensate in TA98 relative to TA100 when protein was removed from the tobacco prior to combustion (Clapp *et al.*, 1999). In addition, some of the activity detected in TA100 may be due to PAHs, which are more mutagenic in TA100 than in TA98. At the molecular level, the mutation spectrum of cigarette-smoke condensate in TA98 was identical to that of the heterocyclic amine Glu-P-1 (2-amino-6-methyldipyrido[1,2-a:3′,2′-*d*]imidazole),

suggesting that this class of compound was primarily responsible for the frameshift mutagenic activity of the condensate detected in TA98 (DeMarini *et al.*, 1995). In contrast,
most of the mutations (78%) induced by CSC in TA100 were GC→TA transversions; this
most closely resembled the mutation spectrum of a model PAH, benzo[*a*]pyrene
(DeMarini *et al.*, 1995). GC→TA transversions are not only the primary class of base-
substitution induced by cigarette-smoke condensate in TA100, but are also a primary class
of base-substitution found in lung tumours of cigarette smokers (see Section 4.4.1(*b*)).

(*b*)   *Cytogenetic effects of cigarette smoke and its condensate* in vitro

Data reviewed previously (IARC, 1986) and confirmed by Rutten and Wilmer (1986)
have shown that cigarette smoke and its condensate induced sister chromatid exchange in
mammalian cells in culture. Tobacco particulate matter has also been shown to induce
structural and numerical chromosomal aberrations (Lafi & Parry, 1988) and micronuclei
(Jones *et al.*, 1991) in cultured mammalian cells. Based on the lack of association between
micronuclei induction and DNA adducts, Jones *et al.* (1991) suggested that the micronuclei were not induced by aromatic compounds but, perhaps, by a direct-acting agent that
may induce small alkylations or damage caused by radicals in DNA. Jansson *et al.* (1986,
1988) and Curvall *et al.* (1985) showed that the neutral fractions and weakly acidic, semivolatile components of cigarette-smoke condensate were the most potent inducers of sister
chromatid exchange in cultured human lymphocytes. They identified a number of
potential candidate compounds, most of which were alkylphenols and benzaldehydes
(benzenes having vicinal oxygenation or a conjugated double bond), that may be
responsible for this activity. Whole smoke also induced micronuclei in Chinese hamster
V79 cells without a metabolic activation system (S9) (Massey *et al.*, 1998). In another
study based on immunocytochemical antikinetochore staining, which allowed differentiation between the clastogenic and aneugenic action of cigarette smoke, V79 cells
exposed to cigarette smoke appeared to be kinetochore-positive, suggesting that the
micronuclei formed were due to aneuploidy rather than clastogenicity (Veltel &
Hoheneder, 1996).

(*c*)   *Cytogenetic effects of cigarette smoke* in vivo

As noted in the earlier review (IARC, 1986), exposure of rodents to cigarette smoke
has generally produced sister chromatid exchange in the bone marrow. However, studies
on the induction of chromosomal aberrations in pulmonary alveolar macrophages by
exposure of rodents to cigarette smoke have produced some negative results (Lee, C.K.
et al., 1992, 1993) and one positive result (Rithidech *et al.*, 1989). Exposure of rodents to
cigarette smoke has consistently produced micronuclei in polychromatic erythrocytes of
the bone marrow (Balansky *et al.*, 1987; Mohtashamipur *et al.*, 1987; Balansky *et al.*,
1988; Mohtashamipur *et al.*, 1988; Stoichev *et al.*, 1993; Nersessian & Arutyunyan, 1994;
Balansky *et al.*, 1999), in normochromatic erythrocytes in peripheral blood (Balansky
et al., 1988, 1999) and in pulmonary alveolar macrophages (Balansky *et al.*, 1999).

(*d*)   *DNA strand breaks*

Several studies have demonstrated that both cigarette smoke and its condensate can induce DNA strand breaks either in rodents, mammalian cells in culture or in DNA *in vitro* (Nakayama *et al.*, 1985; Willey *et al.*, 1987; Fielding *et al.*, 1989; Leanderson & Tagesson, 1990; Bermudez *et al.*, 1994; Leanderson & Tagesson, 1994; Spencer *et al.*, 1995; Seree *et al.*, 1996; Yoshie & Ohshima, 1997; Liu *et al.*, 1999; Yang, Q. *et al.*, 1999). Cigarette smoke also induced nuclear accumulation of TP53 protein in mouse cells in culture, providing an indirect indication of DNA damage (Hess & Brandner, 1996). Collectively, these studies are consistent with the demonstrated clastogenicity of cigarette smoke and its condensate in experimental systems and humans. Several of these studies have indicated that reactive oxygen or nitrogen species formed in cigarette smoke and its condensate are the primary cause of the strand breaks.

(*e*)   *Studies on cigarettes that primarily heat but not burn tobacco, and modified cigarettes*

Although cigarettes that primarily heat rather than burn tobacco (Borgerding *et al.*, 1998) are not generally available commercially, studies generally found that their smoke condensate was not mutagenic in *Salmonella* and did not induce sister chromatid exchange, chromosomal aberrations or *Hprt* mutations in Chinese hamster ovary cells or unscheduled DNA synthesis in rat cells (Doolittle *et al.*, 1989; deBethizy *et al.*, 1990; Doolittle *et al.*, 1990b; Bombick, B.R. *et al.*, 1997). Whole smoke from such cigarettes was also either non-mutagenic or only slightly mutagenic in *Salmonella* and a weak inducer of sister chromatid exchange in Chinese hamster ovary cells, and it was negative in rat bone marrow for chromosomal aberrations, micronuclei and sister chromatid exchange. The relative cytotoxic and genotoxic potential observed in Chinese hamster ovary cells exposed to the whole smoke from these cigarettes is likely to reside in the vapour phase (Lee *et al.*, 1990a,b; Bombick *et al.*, 1998). Humans who smoked these cigarettes produced urine that was ~70% less mutagenic than the urine of smokers of standard cigarettes (Doolittle *et al.*, 1990b; Smith *et al.*, 1996; Bowman *et al.*, 2002).

In 1990, ~20% of the ~5200 deaths from fires in the USA occurred in those started by cigarettes (Brunnemann *et al.*, 1994). The smoke condensate from an experimental cigarette that has low-ignition propensity, and is therefore less likely than regular cigarettes to ignite surrounding material, was as mutagenic as that of reference cigarettes (Brunnemann *et al.*, 1994). An experimental carbon filter that reduces the amounts of certain vapour-phase components of tobacco smoke relative to charcoal filters currently used in commercial cigarettes produced whole smoke that was less mutagenic in *Salmonella* and induced less sister chromatid exchange in Chinese hamster ovary cells than smoke from cigarettes with the usual type of charcoal filter; however, the genotoxicity of the resulting smoke condensate was not significantly different from that of the condensate from standard cigarettes (Bombick, D.W. *et al.*, 1997).

Masheri, a pyrolysed tobacco product mainly used in India to clean the teeth, induced chromosomal aberrations, sister chromatid exchange and micronuclei in bone-marrow cells of mice and *Hprt* mutations in Chinese hamster lung fibroblast V79 cells as well as mutations in *Salmonella* (Kulkarni *et al.*, 1987).

(f)   Transplacental effects

Exposure of gestating mice to cigarette smoke showed that fetal liver, and peripheral blood and liver of newborn mice had elevated levels of micronuclei (Balansky & Blagoeva, 1989), and such exposure also induced sister chromatid exchange in mouse fetal liver (Karube *et al.*, 1989). Therefore, tobacco smoke contains clastogens that cross the mouse placental barrier and cause chromosomal damage in erythroblasts in fetal liver. Both tobacco smoke and its condensate have been shown to induce DNA deletions (reversion of the pink-eye unstable mutation) in the embryo of exposed mice (Jalili *et al.*, 1998).

(g)   Modulation of genotoxicity of tobacco smoke and cigarette-smoke condensate

Many studies have examined the ability of various agents to modulate the genotoxicity of tobacco smoke or its condensate *in vitro* or in experimental animals. Studies in rodents exposed to tobacco smoke (De Flora *et al.*, 2003) or those in *Salmonella* exposed to cigarette-smoke condensate (Camoirano *et al.*, 1994; Romert *et al.*, 1994) have identified a variety of agents that either inhibit or modulate the genotoxicity of tobacco smoke and/or its condensate. Such agents include *N*-acetylcysteine, chlorophyllin, phenolic compounds, isothiocyanates, dithiocarbamates, indoles, tetrapyroles and flavonoids. As noted in Section 4.4.1(*a*)(v), some of these agents have been shown to modulate the formation of smoking-associated biomarkers in humans.

4.5   Mechanistic considerations

Classically, tobacco smoke has been described as acting both as a tumour initiator and a tumour promoter (IARC, 1986). In the light of recent developments in the understanding of the molecular effects of tobacco smoke, this knowledge can be extended to describe how genetic and epigenetic changes cooperate in tobacco-induced carcinogenesis.

The modern synthesis of molecular biology and cancer biology identifies at least six major pathways that must be disrupted for a normal cell to become a tumour cell. These include self-sufficiency in growth signals, insensitivity to anti-growth signals, evasion of apoptosis, tissue invasion and metastasis, sustained angiogenesis and limitless replicative potential. Disruption of these major pathways can occur through genetic or genomic alterations in well-defined genes or through a number of epigenetic processes, including methylation of DNA, post-translational modifications of proteins and modification of gene expression patterns (Hanahan & Weinberg, 2000). There is evidence that smoking is associated with some of the genetic and epigenetic changes affecting these major pathways (Heusch & Maneckjee, 1998; Aoshiba *et al.*, 2001; Brandau & Bohle, 2001; Chang *et al.*, 2001; Forgacs *et al.*, 2001; Hittelman, 2001; Jull *et al.*, 2001; Kang & Park, 2001; Kim, D.H. *et al.*, 2001; Wistuba *et al.*, 2001). Some of these genetic and epigenetic changes have also been observed in smoking-associated diseases other than cancer, such as atherosclerosis and rheumatoid arthritis, indicating that these diseases share common pathways with cancer, and that these pathways are disrupted by tobacco smoke (Chen & Loo, 1995; Albano *et al.*, 2001; Wang, H. *et al.*, 2001).

Conceptually, the effects of tobacco smoke as a carcinogen can be viewed as the result of both genetic and epigenetic changes. Although epigenetic changes can trigger a complex, suppressive cellular stress response, genetic changes may endow some cells with a capacity to escape normal immunosuppression. Thus, the changes in the cellular environment inflicted by tobacco smoke may produce a selection procedure that favours the emergence of cells that have acquired the capacity to undergo clonal expansion. This phenomenon can occur simultaneously at several sites within an exposed tissue field, resulting in multifocal lesions, some of which can progress to cancer (field carcinogenesis).

Moreover, there is a remarkable convergence between the molecular changes induced by tobacco smoke summarized here, such as DNA damage and mutation, and recent experimental evidence for mechanisms of carcinogenesis. Collectively, these data support a multistep model of carcinogenesis in which the components of tobacco smoke are the direct cause of the cellular changes that accumulate to drive the carcinogenenic process.

The previous *IARC Monographs* on tobacco smoking (IARC, 1986) provided convincing evidence of the carcinogenicity of tobacco smoke. The present volume extends this evidence and provides compelling molecular data that explain some of the mechanisms by which tobacco smoke is carcinogenic. Most importantly, these data have largely been obtained from studies in humans, rather than in experimental animals. Thus, their relevance cannot be denied, and their explanatory powers cannot be easily dismissed.

References

Ahrendt, S.A., Decker, P.A., Alawi, E.A., Zhu, Y.-R., Sanchez-Cespedes, M., Yang, S.C., Haasler, G.B., Kajdacsy-Balla, A., Demeure, M.J. & Sidransky, D. (2001) Cigarette smoking is strongly associated with mutation of the K-*ras* gene in patients with primary adenocarcinoma of the lung. *Cancer*, **92**, 1525–1530

Akhmedkhanov, A., Zeleniuch-Jacquotte, A. & Toniolo, P. (2001) Role of exogenous and endogenous hormones in endometrial cancer: Review of the evidence and research perspectives. *Ann. N.Y. Acad. Sci.*, **943**, 296–315

Albano, S.A., Santana-Sahagun, E. & Weisman, M.H. (2001) Cigarette smoking and rheumatoid arthritis. *Semin. Arthritis Rheum.*, **31**, 146–159

Alexandrie, A.-K., Warholm, M., Carstensen, U., Axmon, A., Hagmar, L., Levin, J.O., Östman, C. & Rannug, A. (2000) CYP1A1 and GSTM1 polymorphisms affect urinary 1-hydroxypyrene levels after PAH exposure. *Carcinogenesis*, **21**, 669–676

Alexandrov, K., Rojas, M., Geneste, O., Castegnaro, M., Camus, A.M., Petruzzelli, S., Giuntini, C. & Bartsch, H. (1992) An improved fluorometric assay for dosimetry of benzo(a)pyrene diol-epoxide-DNA adducts in smokers' lung: Comparisons with total bulky adducts and aryl hydrocarbon hydroxylase activity. *Cancer Res.*, **52**, 6248–6253

Alexandrov, K., Rojas, M., Kadlubar, F.F., Lang, N.P. & Bartsch, H. (1996) Evidence of anti-benzo[*a*]pyrene diolepoxide–DNA adduct formation in human colon mucosa. *Carcinogenesis*, **17**, 2081–2083

Ali, S., Astley, S.B., Sheldon, T.A., Peel, K.R. & Wells, M. (1994) Detection and measurement of DNA adducts in the cervix of smokers and nonsmokers. *Int. J. Gynecol. Cancer*, **4**, 188–193

Al-Saleh, I.A. (1995) Lead exposure in Saudi Arabia and its relationship to smoking. *Biometals*, **8**, 243–245

Al-Saleh, I., Shinwari, N., Basile, P., Al-Dgaither, S. & Al-Mutairi, M. (2000) Exposure to cadmium among sheesah smokers and how do they compare to cigarrete smokers. *J. trace Elements exp. Med.*, **13**, 381–388

Ammenheuser, M.M., Berenson, A.B., Stiglich, N.J., Whorton, E.B. & Ward, J.B. (1994) Elevated frequencies of *hprt* mutant lymphocytes in cigarette-smoking mothers and their newborns. *Mutat. Res.*, **304**, 285–294

Ammenheuser, M.M., Hastings, D.A., Whorton, E.B. & Ward, J.B. (1997) Frequencies of *hprt* mutant lymphocytes in smokers, non-smokers, and former smokers. *Environ. mol. Mutag.*, **30**, 131–138

Ammenheuser, M.M., Berenson, A.B., Babiak, A.E., Singleton, C.R. & Whorton, E.B. (1998) Frequencies of *hprt* mutant lymphocytes in marijuana-smoking mothers and their newborns. *Mutat. Res.*, **403**, 55–64

Anand, C.V., Anand, U. & Agarwal, R. (1996) Anti-oxidant enzymes, gamma-glutamyl transpeptidase and lipid peroxidation in kidney of rats exposed to cigarette smoke. *Indian J. exp. Biol.*, **34**, 486–488

Andersen, F.S., Transbol, I. & Christiansen, C. (1982) Is cigarette smoking a promotor of the menopause? *Acta med. scand.*, **212**, 137–139

Anderson, D., Hughes, J.A., Nizankowska, E., Graca, B., Cebulska-Wasilewska, A., Wierzewska, A. & Kasper, E. (1997) Factors affecting various biomarkers in untreated lung cancer patients and healthy donors. *Environ. mol. Mutag.*, **30**, 205–216

Andersson, K., Fuxe, K., Eneroth, P., Mascagni, F. & Agnati, L.F. (1985) Effects of acute intermittent exposure to cigarette smoke on catecholamine levels and turnover in various types of hypothalamic DA and NA nerve terminal systems as well as on the secretion of adenohypophyseal hormones and corticosterone. *Acta physiol. scand.*, **124**, 277–285

Andreassen, Å., Kure, E.H., Nielsen, P.S., Autrup, H. & Haugen, A. (1996) Comparative synchronous fluorescence spectrophotometry and ^{32}P-postlabeling analysis of PAH–DNA adducts in human lung and the relationship to *TP53* mutations. *Mutat. Res.*, **368**, 275–282

Andreoli, R., Manini, P., Bergamaschi, E., Mutti, A., Franchini, I. & Niessen, W.M.A. (1999) Determination of naphthalene metabolites in human urine by liquid chromatography-mass spectrometry with electrospray ionization. *J. Chromatogr.*, **A847**, 9–17

Andres, R.L. & Day, M.-C. (2000) Perinatal complications associated with maternal tobacco use. *Semin. Neonatol.*, **5**, 231–241

Angerer, J., Mannschreck, C. & Gündel, J. (1997) Biological monitoring and biochemical effect monitoring of exposure to polycyclic aromatic hydrocarbons. *Int. Arch. occup. environ. Health*, **70**, 365–377

Anttila, S., Hietanen, E., Vainio, H., Camus, A.-M., Helboin, H.V., Park, S.S., Heikkilä, L., Karjalainen, A. & Bartsch, H. (1991) Smoking and peripheral type of cancer are related to high levels of pulmonary cytochrome P450IA in lung cancer patients. *Int. J. Cancer*, **47**, 681–685

Aoshiba, K., Tamaoki, J. & Nagai, A. (2001) Acute cigarette smoke exposure induces apoptosis of alveolar macrophages. *Am. J. Physiol. Lung cell. mol. Physiol.*, **281**, L1392–L1401

Aringer, L. & Lidums, V. (1988) Influence of diet and other factors on urinary levels of thioethers. *Int. Arch. occup. environ. Health*, **61**, 123–130

Armstrong, R.N. (1997) Glutathione transferases. In: Guengerich, F.P., ed., *Comprehensive Toxicology*, Vol. 3, *Biotransformation*, New York, Elsevier Science, pp. 307–327

Arnould, J.P., Verhoest, P., Bach, V., Libert, J.P. & Belegaud, J. (1997) Detection of benzo[*a*]pyrene–DNA adducts in human placenta and umbilical cord blood. *Hum. exp. Toxicol.*, **16**, 716–721

Arnould, J. P., Hermant, A., Levi-Valensi, P. & Belegaud, J. (1998) Detection of benzo[*a*]pyrene-DNA adducts from leukocytes from heavy smokers. *Pathol. Biol.*, **46**, 787–790

Arora, A., Willhite, C.A. & Liebler, D.C. (2001) Interactions of β-carotene and cigarette smoke in human bronchial epithelial cells. *Carcinogenesis*, **22**, 1173–1178

Asami, S., Hirano, T., Yamaguchi, R., Tomioka, Y., Itoh, H. & Kasai, H. (1996) Increase of a type of oxidative DNA damage, 8-hydroxyguanine, and its repair activity in human leukocytes by cigarette smoking. *Cancer Res.*, **56**, 2546–2549

Asami, S., Manabe, H., Miyake, J., Tsurudome, Y., Hirano, T., Yamaguchi, R., Itoh, H. & Kasai, H. (1997) Cigarette smoking induces an increase in oxidative DNA damage, 8-hydroxydeoxyguanosine, in a central site of the human lung. *Carcinogenesis*, **18**, 1763–1766

Ashley, M.J. (1997) Smoking and diseases of the gastrointestinal system: An epidemiological review with special reference to sex differences. *Can. J. Gastroenterol.*, **11**, 345–352

Ashley, D.L., Bonin, M.A., Hamar, B. & McGeehin, M.A. (1995) Removing the smoking confounder from blood volatile organic compounds measurements. *Environ. Res.*, **71**, 39–45

Ashley, D.L., Bonin, M.A., Cardinali, F.L., McCraw, J.M. & Wooten, J.V. (1996) Measurement of volatile organic compounds in human blood. *Environ. Health Perspect.*, **104**, 871–877

Asita, A.O., Matsui, M., Nohmi, T., Matsuoka, A., Hayashi, M., Ishidate, M., Jr, Sofuni, T., Koyano, M. & Matsushita, H. (1991) Mutagenicity of wood smoke condensates in the *Salmonella*/microsome assay. *Mutat. Res.*, **264**, 7–14

Atawodi, S.E., Lea, S., Nyberg, F., Mukeria, A., Constantinescu, V., Ahrens, W., Brueske-Hohlfeld, I., Fortes, C., Boffetta, P. & Friesen, M.D. (1998) 4-Hydroxy-1-(3-pyridyl)-1-butanone–hemoglobin adducts as biomarkers of exposure to tobacco smoke: Validation of a method to be used in multicenter studies. *Cancer Epidemiol. Biomarkers Prev.*, **7**, 817–821

Attolini, I.., Gantenbein, M., Villard, P.H., Lacarelle, B., Catalin, J. & Bruguerolle, B. (1996) Effects of different exposure times to tobacco smoke intoxication on carboxyhemoglobin and hepatic enzymate activities in mice. *J. pharmacol. toxicol. Meth.*, **35**, 211–215

Au, W.W., Walker, D.M., Ward, J.B., Whorton, E., Legator, M.S. & Singh, V. (1991) Factors contributing to chromosome damage in lymphocytes of cigarette smokers. *Mutat. Res.*, **260**, 137–144

Aubry, M.C., Wright, J.L. & Myers, J.L. (2000) The pathology of smoking-related lung diseases. *Clin. Chest Med.*, **21**, 11–35

Augood, C., Duckitt, K. & Templeton, A.A. (1998) Smoking and female infertility: A systematic review and meta-analysis. *Hum. Reprod.*, **13**, 1532–1539

Austin, A.C., Claxton, L.D. & Lewtas, J. (1985) Mutagenicity of the fractionated organic emissions from diesel, cigarette smoke condensate, coke oven, and roofing tar in the Ames assay. *Environ. Mutag.*, **7**, 471–487

Bader, M., Lewalter, J. & Angerer, J. (1995) Analysis of N-alkylated amino acids in human hemoglobin: Evidence for elevated N-methylvaline levels in smokers. *Int. Arch. occup environ. Health*, **67**, 237–242

Bagnasco, M., Bennicelli, C., Camoirano, A., Balansky, R.M. & De Flora, S. (1992) Metabolic alterations produced by cigarette smoke in rat lung and liver, and their modulation by oral N-acetylcysteine. *Mutagenesis*, **7**, 295–301

Bagwe, A.N. & Bhisey, R.A. (1993) Occupational exposure to tobacco and resultant genotoxicity in bidi industry workers. *Mutat. Res.*, **299**, 103–109

Bailey, E., Brooks, A.G.F., Dollery, C. T., Farmer, P.B., Passingham, B.J., Sleightholm, M.A. & Yates, D.W. (1988) Hydroxyethylvaline adduct formation in haemoglobin as a biological monitor of cigarette smoke intake. *Arch. Toxicol.*, **62**, 247–253

Baird, D.D. (1992) Evidence for reduced fecundity in female smokers. In: Poswillo, D. & Alberman, E., eds, *Effects of Smoking on the Fetus, Neonate, and Child*, Oxford, Oxford University Press, pp. 5–22

Balansky, R.M. & Blagoeva, P.M. (1989) Tobacco smoke-induced clastogenicity in mouse fetuses and in newborn mice. *Mutat. Res.*, **223**, 1–6

Balansky, R.M., Blagoeva, P.M. & Mircheva, Z.I. (1987) Investigation of the mutagenic activity of tobacco smoke. *Mutat. Res.*, **188**, 13–19

Balansky, R.M., Blagoeva, P.M. & Mircheva, Z.I. (1988) The mutagenic and clastogenic activity of tobacco smoke. *Mutat. Res.*, **208**, 237–241

Balansky, R.M., D'Agostini, F. & De Flora, S. (1999) Induction, persistence and modulation of cytogenetic alterations in cells of smoke-exposed mice. *Carcinogenesis*, **20**, 1491–1497

Balint, B., Donnelly, L.E., Hanazawa, T., Kharitonow, S.A. & Barnes, P.J. (2001) Increased nitric oxide metabolites in exhaled breath condensate after exposure to tobacco smoke. *Thorax*, **56**, 456–461

Ban, S., Cologne, J.B. & Neriishi, K. (1995) Effect of radiation and cigarette smoking on expression of FUdR-inducible common fragile sites in human peripheral lymphocytes. *Mutat. Res.*, **334**, 197–203

Banaszewski, J., Szmeja, Z., Szyfter, W., Szyfter, K., Baranczewski, P. & Möller, L. (2000) Analysis of aromatic DNA adducts in laryngeal biopsies. *Eur. Arch. Otorhinolaryngol.*, **257**, 149–153

Baral, R.N., Patnaik, S. & Das, B.R. (1998) Co-overexpression of p53 and c-myc proteins linked with advanced stages of betel- and tobacco-related oral squamous cell carcinomas from eastern India. *Eur. J. oral Sci.*, **106**, 907–913

Barbieri, R.L., McShane, P.M. & Ryan, K.J. (1986) Constituents of cigarette smoke inhibit human granulosa cell aromatase. *Fertil. Steril.*, **46**, 232–236

Baron, J.A. (1996) Beneficial effects of nicotine and cigarette smoking: The real, the possible and the spurious. *Br. med. Bull.*, **52**, 58–73

Baron, J.A., La Vecchia, C. & Levi, F. (1990) The antiestrogenic effect of cigarette smoking in women. *Am. J. Obstet. Gynecol.*, **162**, 502–514

Bartsch, H., Ohshima, H., Pignatelli, B. & Calmels, S. (1989) Human exposure to endogenous *N*-nitroso compounds: Quantitative estimates in subjects at high risk for cancer of the oral cavity, oesophagus, stomach and urinary bladder. *Cancer Surv.,* **8**, 335–362

Bartsch, H., Caporaso, N., Coda, M., Kadlubar, F., Malaveille, C., Skipper, P., Talaska, G., Tannenbaum, S.R. & Vineis, P. (1990) Carcinogen hemoglobin adducts, urinary mutagenicity, and metabolic phenotype in active and passive cigarette smokers. *J. natl Cancer Inst.*, **82**, 1826–1831

Baskaran, S., Lakshmi, S. & Prasad, P.R. (1999) Effect of cigarette smoke on lipid peroxidation and antioxidant enzymes in albino rat. *Indian J. exp. Biol.*, **37**, 1196–1200

Beach, A.C. & Gupta, R.C. (1992) Human biomonitoring and the ^{32}P-postlabeling assay. *Carcinogenesis*, **13**, 1053–1074

Becher, G. & Bjørseth, A. (1983) Determination of exposure to polycyclic aromatic hydrocarbons by analysis of human urine. *Cancer Lett.*, **17**, 301–311

Becher, G., Haugen, A. & Bjørseth, A. (1984) Multimethod determination of occupational exposure to polycyclic aromatic hydrocarbons in an aluminum plant. *Carcinogenesis*, **5**, 647–651

Bender, M.A., Preston, R.J., Leonard, R.C., Pyatt, B.E., Gooch, P.C. & Shelby, M.D. (1988) Chromosomal aberration and sister-chromatid exchange frequencies in peripheral blood lymphocytes of a large human population sample. *Mutat. Res.*, **204**, 421–433

Bennett, C.H. & Richardson, D.R. (1990) Time-dependent changes in cardiovascular regulation caused by chronic tobacco smoke exposure. *J. appl. Physiol.*, **68**, 248–252

Benowitz, N.L. (1988) Pharmacologic aspects of cigarette smoking and nicotine addiction. *New Engl. J. Med.*, **319**, 1318–1330

Benowitz, N.L. (1995) Clinical pharmacology of transdermal nicotine. *Eur. J. Pharm. Biopharm.*, **41**, 168–174

Benowitz, N.L. (1996) Cotinine as a biomarker of environmental tobacco smoke exposure. *Epidemiol. Rev.*, **18**, 188–204

Benowitz, N.L. (1999a) Biomarkers of environmental tobacco smoke exposure. *Environ. Health Perspect.*, **107** (Suppl. 2), 349–355

Benowitz, N.L. (1999b) Nicotine addiction. *Prim. Care*, **26**, 611–631

Benowitz, N.L. & Jacob, P. (1994) Metabolism of nicotine to cotinine studied by a dual stable isotope method. *Clin. Pharmacol. Ther.*, **56**, 483–493

Benowitz, N.L. & Jacob, P., III (1997) Individual differences in nicotine kinetics and metabolism in humans. In: Rapaka, R.S., Chiang, N. & Martin, B.R., eds, *Pharmacokinetics, Metabolism, and Pharmaceutics of Drugs of Abuse* (NIDA Research Monograph No. 173), Rockville, MD, National Institute on Drug Abuse, Division of Clinical Research, pp. 48–64

Benowitz, N.L., Jacob, P., III, Jones, R.T. & Rosenberg, J. (1982) Interindividual variability in the metabolism and cardiovascular effects of nicotine in man. *J. Pharmacol. exp. Ther.*, **221**, 368–372

Benowitz, N.L., Jacob, P., III, Kozlowski, L.T. & Yu, L. (1986) Influence of smoking fewer cigarettes on exposure to tar, nicotine, and carbon monoxide. *New Engl. J. Med.*, **315**, 1310–1313

Benowitz, N.L., Jacob, P., III, Fong, I. & Gupta, S. (1994) Nicotine metabolic profile in man: Comparison of cigarette smoking and transdermal nicotine. *J. Pharmacol. exp. Ther.*, **268**, 296–303

Benowitz, N.L., Jacob, P., III & Sachs, D.P. (1995) Deficient C-oxidation of nicotine. *Clin. Pharmacol. Ther.*, **57**, 590–594

Benowitz, N.L., Jacob, P., III & Perez-Stable, E. (1996) CYP2D6 phenotype and the metabolism of nicotine and cotinine. *Pharmacogenetics*, **6**, 239–242

Benowitz, N.L., Pérez-Stable, E.J., Fong, I., Modin, G., Herrera, B. & Jacob, P., III (1999) Ethnic differences in *N*-glucuronidation of nicotine and cotinine. *J. Pharmacol. exp. Ther.*, **291**, 1196–1203

Benowitz, N.L., Pérez-Stable, E.J., Herrera, B. & Jacob, P., III (2002) Slower metabolism and reduced intake of nicotine from cigarette smoking in Chinese-Americans. *J. natl Cancer Inst.*, **94**, 108–115

Bergmark, E. (1997) Hemoglobin adducts of acrylamide and acrylonitrile in laboratory workers, smokers and nonsmokers. *Chem. Res. Toxicol.*, **10**, 78–84

Berlin, I. & Anthenelli, R.M. (2001) Monoamine oxidases and tobacco smoking. *Int. J. Neuropsychopharmacol.*, **4**, 33–42

Bermudez, E., Stone, K., Carter, K.M. & Pryor, W.A. (1994) Environmental tobacco smoke is just as damaging to DNA as mainstream smoke. *Environ. Health Perspect.*, **102**, 870–874

Berstein, L.M., Tsyrlina, E.V., Gamajunova, V.B., Bychkova, N.V., Krjukova, O.G., Dzhumasultanova, S.V., Kovalenko, I.G. & Kolesnik, O.S. (1999) Study of tobacco smoke influence on content of estrogens and DNA flow cytometry data in uterine tissue of rats of different age. *Horm. metab. Res.*, **31**, 27–30

Besarati Nia, A., Maas, L.M., Van Breda, S.G.J., Curfs, D.M.J., Kleinjans, J.C.S., Wouters, E.F.M. & Van Schooten, F.J. (2000a) Applicability of induced sputum for molecular dosimetry of exposure to inhalatory carcinogens: ^{32}P-Postlabeling of lipophilic DNA adducts in smokers and nonsmokers. *Cancer Epidemiol. Biomarkers Prev.*, **9**, 367–372

Besarati Nia, A., Maas, L.M., Brouwer, E.M.C., Kleinjans, J.C.S. & Van Schooten, F.J. (2000b) Comparison between smoking-related DNA adduct analysis in induced sputum and peripheral blood lymphocytes. *Carcinogenesis*, **21**, 1335–1340

Besarati Nia, A., Van Straaten, H.W.M., Kleinjans, J.C.S. & Van Schooten, F.-J. (2000c) Immunoperoxidase detection of 4-aminobiphenyl- and polycyclic aromatic hydrocarbons–DNA adducts in induced sputum of smokers and nonsmokers. *Mutat. Res.*, **468**, 125–135

Besarati Nia, A., Van Straaten, H.W.M., Godschalk, R.W.L., Van Zandwijk, N., Balm, A.J.M., Kleinjans, J.C.S. & Van Schooten, F.J. (2000d) Immunoperoxidase detection of polycyclic aromatic hydrocarbon–DNA adducts in mouth floor and buccal mucosa cells of smokers and nonsmokers. *Environ. mol. Mutag.*, **36**, 127–133

Besarati Nia, A., Van Schooten, F.J., Schilderman, P.A.E.L., De Kok, T.M.C.M., Haenen, G.R., Van Herwijnen, M.H.M., Van Agen, E., Pachen, D. & Kleinjans, J.C.S. (2001) A multi-biomarker approach to study the effects of smoking on oxidative DNA damage and repair and antioxidative defense mechanisms. *Carcinogenesis*, **22**, 395–401

deBethizy, J.D., Borgerding, M.F., Doolittle, D.J., Robinson, J.H., McManus, K.T., Rahn, C.A., Davis, R.A., Burger, G.T., Hayes, J.R., Reynolds, J.H. & Hayes, A.W. (1990) Chemical and biological studies of a cigarette that heats rather than burns tobacco. *J. clin. Pharmacol.*, **30**, 755–763

Bhisey, R.A. & Govekar, R.B. (1991) Biological monitoring of bidi rollers with respect to geno-toxic hazards of occupational tobacco exposure. *Mutat. Res.*, **261**, 139–147

Bielicki, J.K., Forte, T.M. & McCall, M.R. (1995) Gas-phase cigarette smoke inhibits plasma leci-thin-cholesterol acyltransferase activity by modification of the enzyme's free thiols. *Biochim. biophys. Acta*, **1258**, 35–40

Bielicki, J.K., Knoff, L.J., Tribble, D.L. & Forte, T.M. (2001) Relative sensitivities of plasma leci-thin:cholesterol acyltransferase, platelet-activating factor acetylhydrolase, and paraoxonase to in vitro gas-phase cigarette smoke exposure. *Atherosclerosis*, **155**, 71–78

Bigbee, W.L., Day, R.D., Grant, S.G., Keohavong, P., Xi, L., Zhang, L. & Ness, R.B. (1999) Impact of maternal lifestyle factors on newborn *HPRT* mutant frequencies and molecular spectrum — Initial results from the Prenatal Exposures and Preeclampsia Prevention (PEPP) Study. *Mutat. Res.*, **431**, 279–289

Binková, B., Lewtas, J., Míšková, I., Lenícek, J. & Šrám, R. (1995) DNA adducts and personal air monitoring of carcinogenic polycyclic aromatic hydrocarbons in an environmentally exposed population. *Carcinogenesis*, **16**, 1037–1046

Binková, B., Strejc, P., Boubelík, O., Stávková, Z., Chvátalová, I. & Šrám, R.J. (2001) DNA adducts and human atherosclerotic lesions. *Int. J. Hyg. environ. Health*, **204**, 49–54

Bjarnason, N.H. & Christiansen, C. (2000) The influence of thinness and smoking on bone loss and response to hormone replacement therapy in early postmenopausal women. *J. clin. Endo-crinol. Metab.*, **85**, 590–596

Bjelogrlic, N., Iscan, M., Raunio, H., Pelkonen, O. & Vahäkangas, K. (1989) Benzo[*a*]pyrene–DNA-adducts and monooxygenase activities in mice treated with benzo[*a*]pyrene, cigarette smoke or cigarette smoke condensate. *Chem.-biol. Interact*, **70**, 51–61

Björk, J. Albin, M., Mauritzson, N., Stromberg, U., Johansson, B. & Hagmar, L. (2000) Smoking and myelodysplastic syndromes. *Epidemiology*, **11**, 285–291

Björk, J., Albin, M., Mauritzson, N., Stromberg, U., Johansson, B. & Hagmar, L. (2001) Smoking and acute myeloid leukemia: Associations with morphology and karyotypic patterns and eva-luation of dose–response relations. *Leuk. Res.*, **25**, 865–872

Blömeke, B., Greenblatt, M.J., Doan, V.D., Bowman, E.D., Murphy, S.E., Chen, C.C., Kato, S. & Shields, P.G. (1996) Distribution of 7-alkyl-2′-deoxyguanosine adduct levels in human lung. *Carcinogenesis*, **17**, 741–748

Bock, K.W., Schrenk, D., Forster, A., Griese, E.U., Morike, K., Brockmeier, D. & Eichelbaum, M. (1994) The influence of environmental and genetic factors on CYP2D6, CYP1A2 and UDP-glucuronosyltransferases in man using sparteine, caffeine, and paracetamol as probes. *Pharmacogenetics*, **4**, 209–218

Bohning, D.E., Atkins, H.L. & Cohn, S.H. (1982) Long-term particle clearance in man: Normal and impaired. *Ann. occup. Hyg.*, **26**, 259–271

Bolumar, F., Olsen, J., Boldsen, J. & the European Study Group on Infertility and Subfecundity (1996) Smoking reduces fecundity: A European multicenter study on infertility and sub-fecundity. *Am. J. Epidemiol.*, **143**, 578–587

Bombick, B.R., Murli, H., Avalos, J.T., Bombick, D.W., Morgan, W.T., Putnam, K.P. & Doolittle, D.J. (1997) Chemical and biological studies of a new cigarette that primarily heats tobacco. Part 2. *In vitro* toxicology of mainstream smoke condensate. *Food chem. Toxicol.*, **36**, 183–190

Bombick, D.W., Bombick, B.R., Ayres, P.H., Putnam, K.P., Avalos, J., Borgerding, M.F. & Doolittle, D.J. (1997) Evaluation of the genotoxic and cytotoxic potential of mainstream whole smoke and smoke condensate from a cigarette containing a novel carbon filter. *Fundam. appl. Toxicol.*, **39**, 11–17

Bombick, D.W., Ayres, P.H., Putnam, K., Bombick, B.R. & Doolittle, D.J. (1998) Chemical and biological studies of a new cigarette that primarily heats tobacco. Part 3. *In vitro* toxicity of whole smoke. *Food chem. Toxicol.*, **36**, 191–197

Bonassi, S., Hagmar, L., Strömberg, U., Montagud, A.H., Tinnerberg, H., Forni, A., Heikkilä, P., Wanders, S., Wilhardt, P., Hansteen, I.-L., Knudsen, L.E. & Norppa, H. (2000) Chromosomal aberrations in lymphocytes predict human cancer independently of exposure to carcinogens. European Study Group on Cytogenetic Biomarkers and Health. *Cancer Res.*, **60**, 1619–1625

Bonassi, S., Neri, M., Lando, C., Ceppi, M., Lin, Y.-P., Chang, W.P., Holland, N., Kirsch-Volders, M., Zeiger, E., Fenech, M. & the HUMN Collaborative Group (2003) Effect of smoking habit on the frequency of micronuclei in human lymphocytes: Results from the Human Micro-Nucleus Project. *Mutat. Res.*, **543**, 155–166

Bond, J.A., Chen, B.T., Griffith, W.C. & Mauderly, J.L. (1989) Inhaled cigarette smoke induces the formation of DNA adducts in lungs of rats. *Toxicol. appl. Pharmacol.*, **99**, 161–172

Bono, R., Vincenti, M., Meineri, V., Pignata, C., Saglia, U., Giachino, O. & Scursatone, E. (1999) Formation of *N*-(2-hydroxyethyl)valine due to exposure to ethylene oxide via tobacco smoke: A risk factor for onset of cancer. *Environ. Res.*, **81**, 62–71

Boogaard, P.J. & van Sittert, N.J. (1995) Biological monitoring of exposure to benzene: A comparison between *S*-phenylmercapturic acid, *trans,trans*-muconic acid, and phenol. *Occup. environ. Med.*, **52**, 611–620

Boogaard, P.J. & van Sittert, N.J. (1996) Suitability of *S*-phenyl mercapturic acid and *trans-trans*-muconic acid as biomarkers for exposure to low concentrations of benzene. *Environ. Health Perspect.*, **104** (Suppl. 6), 1151–1157

Borgerding, M.F., Bodnar, J.A., Chung, H.L., Mangan, P.P., Morrison, C.C., Risner, C.H., Rogers, J.C., Simmons, D.F., Uhrig, M.S., Wendelboe, F.N., Wingate, D.E. & Winkler, L.S. (1998) Chemical and biological studies of a new cigarette that primarily heats tobacco. Part 1. Chemical composition of mainstream smoke. *Food chem. Toxicol.*, **36**, 169–182

Bowman, D.L., Smith, C.J., Bombick, B.R., Avalos, J.T., Davis, R.A., Morgan, W.T. & Doolittle, D.J. (2002) Relationsip between FTC 'tar' and urine mutagenicity in smokers of tobacco-burning or Eclipse cigarettes. *Mutat. Res.*, **521**, 137–149

Boyd, E.J., Wilson, J.A. & Wormsley, K.G. (1983) Smoking impairs therapeutic gastric inhibition. *Lancet*, **i**, 95–97

Brandau, S. & Bohle, A. (2001) Bladder cancer. I. Molecular and genetic basis of carcinogenesis. *Eur. Urol.*, **39**, 491–497

Branner, B., Kutzer, C., Zwickenpflug, W., Scherer, G., Heller, W.-D. & Richter, E. (1998) Haemoglobin adducts from aromatic amines and tobacco-specific nitrosamines in pregnant smoking and non-smoking women. *Biomarkers*, **3**, 35–47

Bretherton-Watt, D., Given-Wilson, R., Mansi, J.L., Thomas, V., Carter, N. & Colston, K.W. (2001) Vitamin D receptor gene polymorphisms are associated with breast cancer risk in a UK Caucasian population. *Br. J. Cancer*, **85**, 171–175

Brinkworth, M.H., Yardley-Jones, A., Edwards, A.J., Hughes, J.A. & Anderson, D. (1992) A comparison of smokers and nonsmokers with respect to oncogene products and cytogenetic parameters. *J. occup. Med.*, **34**, 1181–1188

Brockhaus, A., Freier, I., Ewers, U., Jermann, E. & Dolgner, R. (1983) Levels of cadmium and lead in blood in relation to smoking, sex, occupation, and other factors in an adult population of the FRG. *Int. Arch. occup. environ. Health*, **52**, 167–175

Bromberger, J.T., Matthews, K.A., Kuller, L.H., Wing, R.R., Meilahn, E.N. & Plantinga, P. (1997) Prospective study of the determinants of age at menopause. *Am. J. Epidemiol.*, **145**, 124–133

Brot, C., Jørgensen, N.R. & Sørensen, O.H. (1999) The influence of smoking on vitamin D status and calcium metabolism. *Eur. J. clin. Nutr.*, **53**, 920–926

Brown, B.G., Lee, C.K., Bombick, B.R., Ayres, P.H., Mosberg, A.T. & Doolittle, D.J. (1997) Comparative study of DNA adduct formation in mice following inhalation of smoke from cigarettes that burn or primarily heat tobacco. *Environ. mol. Mutag.*, **29**, 303–311

Brown, B.G., Chang, C.J., Ayres, P.H., Lee, C.K., & Doolittle, D.J. (1999) The effect of cotinine or cigarette smoke co-administration on the formation of O^6-methylguanine adducts in the lung and liver of A/J mice treated with 4-(methylnitrosamino)-1-(3-pyridyl)-1-butanone (NNK). *Toxicol. Sci.*, **47**, 33–39

Brugnone, F., Perbellini, L., Romeo, L., Cerpelloni, M., Bianchin, M. & Tonello, A. (1999) Benzene in blood as a biomarker of low level occupational exposure. *Sci. total Environ.*, **235**, 247–252

Brunnemann, K.D., Hoffmann, D., Gairola, C.G. & Lee, B.C. (1994) Low ignition propensity cigarettes: Smoke analysis for carcinogens and testing for mutagenic activity of the smoke particulate matter. *Food chem. Toxicol.*, **32**, 917–922

Bryant, M.S., Skipper, P.L., Tannenbaum, S.R. & Maclure, M. (1987) Hemoglobin adducts of 4-aminobiphenyl in smokers and nonsmokers. *Cancer Res.*, **47**, 602–608

Bryant, M.S., Vineis, P., Skipper, P.L. & Tannenbaum, S.R. (1988) Hemoglobin adducts of aromatic amines: Associations with smoking status and type of tobacco. *Proc. natl Acad. Sci. USA*, **85**, 9788–9791

Buchhalter, A.R. & Eissenberg, T. (2000) Preliminary evaluation of a novel smoking system: Effects on subjective and physiological measures and on smoking behavior. *Nicotine Tob. Res.*, **2**, 39–43

Buckley, T.J., Waldman, J.M., Dhara, R., Greenberg, A., Ouyang, Z. & Lioy, P.J. (1995) An assessment of a urinary biomarker for total human environmental exposure to benzo[*a*]pyrene. *Int. Arch. occup. environ. Health*, **67**, 257–266

Bukvic, N., Bavaro, P., Elia, G., Cassano, F., Fanelli, M. & Guanti, G. (1998) Sister chromatid exchange (SCE) and micronucleus (MN) frequencies in lymphocytes of gasoline station attendants. *Mutat. Res.*, **415**, 25–33

Buratti, M., Fustinoni, S. & Colombi, A. (1996) Fast liquid chromatographic determination of urinary trans,trans-muconic acid. *J. Chromatogr.*, **B677**, 257–263

Burchell, B., McGurk, K., Brierley, C.H. & Clarke, D.J. (1997) UDP-glucuronosyltransferases. In: Guengerich, F.P., ed., *Comprehensive Toxicology*, Vol. 3, *Biotransformation*, New York, Elsevier Science, pp. 401–435

Burchell, B., Soars, M., Monaghan, G., Cassidy, A., Smith, D. & Ethell, B. (2000) Drug-mediated toxicity caused by genetic deficiency of UDP-glucuronosyltransferases. *Toxicol. Lett.*, **112–113**, 333–340

Burkhart-Schultz, K.J., Thompson, C.L. & Jones, I.M. (1996) Spectrum of somatic mutation at the hypoxanthine phosphoribosyltransferase (*HPRT*) gene of healthy people. *Carcinogenesis*, **17**, 1871–1883

Burns, D.M., Major, J.M., Shanks, T.G., Thun, M.J. & Samet, J.M. (2001) Smoking lower yield cigarettes and disease risks. In: *Risks Associated with Smoking Cigarettes with Low Machine-Measured Yields of Tar and Nicotine* (Smoking and Tobacco Control Monograph No. 13; NIH Publication No. 02-5074), Bethesda, MD, US Department of Health and Human Services, National Institutes of Health, pp. 65–158

Butkiewicz, D., Cole, K.J., Phillips, D.H., Harris, C.C. & Chorazy, M. (1999) *GSTM1, GSTP1, CYP1A1* and *CYP2D6* polymorphisms in lung cancer patients from an environmentally polluted region of Poland: Correlation with lung DNA adduct levels. *Eur. J. Cancer Prev.*, **8**, 315–323

Byrd, G.D., Chang, K.M., Green, J.M. & deBethizy, J.D. (1992) Evidence for urinary excretion of glucuronide conjugates of nicotine, cotinine and *trans*-3′-hydroxycotinine in smokers. *Drug. Metab. Dispos.*, **20**, 192–197

California Environmental Protection Agency (1997) *Field Notes. Our World* (http://www.calepa.cahwnet.gov/oehha)

Camoirano, A., Balansky, R.M., Bennicelli, C., Izzotti, A., D'Agostini, F. & De Flora, S. (1994) Experimental databases on inhibition of the bacterial mutagenicity of 4-nitroquinoline 1-oxide and cigarette smoke. *Mutat. Res.*, **317**, 89–109

Camoirano, A., Bagnasco, M., Bennicelli, C., Cartiglia, C., Wang, J.-B., Zhang, B.-C., Zhu, Y.-R., Qian, G.-S., Egner, P.A., Jacobson, L.P., Kensler, T.W. & De Flora, S. (2001) Oltipraz chemoprevention trial in Qidong, People's Republic of China: Results of urine genotoxicity assays as related to smoking habits. *Cancer Epidemiol. Biomarkers Prev.*, **10**, 775–783

Caraballo, R.S., Giovino, G.A., Pechacek, T.F., Mowery, P.D., Richter, P.A., Strauss, W.J., Sharp, D.J., Eriksen, M.P., Pirkle, J.L. & Maurer, K.R. (1998) Racial and ethnic differences in serum cotinine levels of cigarette smokers. Third National Health and Nutrition Examination Survey, 1988–1981. *J. Am. med. Assoc.*, **280**, 135–139

Carmella, S., LaVoie, E.J. & Hecht, S.S. (1982) Quantitative analysis of catechol and 4-methyl-catechol in human urine. *Food chem. Toxicol.*, **20**, 587–590

Carmella, S.G., Kagan, S.S., Kagan, M., Foiles, P.G., Palladino, G., Quart, A.M., Quart, E. & Hecht, S.S. (1990) Mass spectrometric analysis of tobacco-specific nitrosamine hemoglobin adducts in snuff dippers, smokers, and nonsmokers. *Cancer Res.*, **50**, 5438–5445

Carmella, S.G., Akerkar, S. & Hecht, S.S. (1993) Metabolites of the tobacco-specific nitrosamine 4-(methylnitrosamino)-1-(3-pyridyl)-1-butanone in smokers' urine. *Cancer Res.*, **53**, 721–724

Carmella, S.G., Akerkar, S., Richie, J.P., Jr & Hecht, S.S. (1995) Intraindividual and interindividual differences in metabolites of the tobacco-specific lung carcinogen 4-(methylnitrosamino)-1-(3-pyridyl)-1-butanone (NNK) in smokers' urine. *Cancer Epidemiol. Biomarkers Prev.*, **4**, 635–642

Carmella, S.G., Borukhova, A., Akerkar, S.A. & Hecht, S.S. (1997) Analysis of human urine for pyridine-*N*-oxide metabolites of 4-(methylnitrosamino)-1-(3-pyridyl)-1-butanone, a tobacco-specific lung carcinogen. *Cancer Epidemiol. Biomarkers Prev.*, **6**, 113–120

Carmella, S.G., Ye, M., Upadhyaya, P. & Hecht, S.S. (1999) Stereochemistry of metabolites of a tobacco-specific lung carcinogen in smokers' urine. *Cancer Res.*, **59**, 3602–3605

Carmella, S.G., Le K.-A., Upadhyaya, P. & Hecht, S.S. (2002) Analysis of *N*- and *O*-glucuronides of 4-(methylnitrosamino)-1-(3- pyridyl)-1-butanol (NNAL) in human urine. *Chem. Res. Toxicol.*, **15**, 545–550

Carmichael, P.L., Hewer, A., Jacob, J., Grimmer, G. & Phillips, D.H. (1993) Comparison of total DNA adduct levels induced in mouse tissues and human skin by mainstream and sidestream cigarette smoke condensates. In: Phillips, D.H., Castegnaro, M. & Bartsch, H., eds, *Post-labelling Methods for Detection of DNA Adducts* (IARC Scientific Publications No. 124), Lyon, IARC*Press*, pp. 321–326

Carmines, E.L. (2002) Evaluation of the potential effects of ingredients added to cigarettes. Part 1: Cigarette design, testing approach, and review of results. *Food chem. Toxicol.*, **40**, 77–91

Casale, G.P., Singhal, M., Bhattacharya, S., RamaNathan, R., Roberts, K.P., Barbacci, D.C., Zhao, J., Jankowiak, R., Gross, M.L., Cavalieri, E.L., Small, G.J., Rennard, S.I., Mumford, J.L. & Shen, M. (2001) Detection and quantification of depurinated benzo[*a*]pyrene-adducted DNA bases in the urine of cigarette smokers and women exposed to household coal smoke. *Chem. Res. Toxicol.*, **14**, 192–201

Cassidenti, D.L., Vijod, A.G., Vijod, M.A., Stanczyk, F.Z. & Lobo, R.A. (1990) Short-term effects of smoking on the pharmacokinetic profiles of micronized estradiol in postmenopausal women. *Am. J. Obstet. Gynecol.*, **163**, 1953–1960

Castelao, J.E., Tuan, J.-M., Skipper, P.L., Tannenbaum, S.R., Gago-Dominguez, M., Crowder, J.S., Ross, R.K. & Yu, M.C. (2001) Gender and smoking-related bladder cancer risk. *J. natl Cancer Inst.*, **93**, 538–545

Castles, A., Adams, E.K., Melvin, C.L., Kelsch, C. & Boulton, M.L. (1999) Effects of smoking during pregnancy. Five meta-analyses. *Am. J. prev. Med.*, **16**, 208–215

Cebulska-Wasilewska, A., Wierzewska, A., Nizankowska, E., Graca, B., Hughes, J.A. & Anderson, D. (1999) Cytogenetic damage and *ras* p21 oncoprotein levels from patients with chronic obstructive pulmonary disease (COPD), untreated lung cancer and healthy controls. *Mutat. Res.*, **431**, 123–131

Cerqueira, E.M., Santoro, C.L., Donozo, N.F., Freitas, B.A., de Braganca Pereira, C.A., Bevilacqua, R.G. & Machado-Santelli, G.M. (1998) Genetic damage in exfoliated cells of the uterine cervix. *Acta cytol.*, **42**, 639–649

Chacko, M. & Gupta, R.C. (1988) Evaluation of DNA damage in the oral mucosa of tobacco users and non-users by ^{32}P-adduct assay. *Carcinogenesis*, **9**, 2309–2313

Chan, J.M., Stampfer, M.J., Giovannucci, E., Gann, P.H., Ma, J., Wilkinson, P., Hennekens, C.H. & Pollak, M. (1998) Plasma insulin-like growth factor-I and prostate cancer risk: A prospective study. *Science*, **279**, 563–566

Chang, W.-C., Lee, Y.-C., Liu, C.-L., Hsu, J.-D., Wang, H.-C., Chen, C.-C. & Wang, C.-J. (2001) Increased expression of iNOS and c-fos via regulation of protein tyrosine phosphorylation and MEK1/ERK2 proteins in terminal bronchiole lesions in the lungs of rats exposed to cigarette smoke. *Arch. Toxicol.*, **75**, 28–35

Chapurlat, R.D., Ewing, S.K., Bauer, D.C. & Cummings, S.R. (2001) Influence of smoking on the antiosteoporotic efficacy of raloxifene. *J. clin. Endocrinol. Metab.*, **86**, 4178–4182

Chen, C.-C. & Lee, H. (1996) Genotoxicity and DNA adduct formation of incense smoke condensates: Comparison with environmental tobacco smoke condensates. *Mutat. Res.*, **367**, 105–114

Chen, C. & Loo, G. (1995) Inhibition of lecithin:cholesterol acyltransferase activity in human blood plasma by cigarette smoke extract and reactive aldehydes. *J. biochem. Toxicol.*, **10**, 121–128

Chen, A.T.L., Reidy, J.A., Annest, J.L., Welty, T.K. & Zhou, H.G. (1989) Increased chromosome fragility as a consequence of blood folate levels, smoking status, and coffee consumption. *Environ. mol. Mutag.*, **13**, 319–324

Cheng, T.-J., Christiani, D.C., Xu, X., Wain, J.C., Wiencke, J.K. & Kelsey, K.T. (1995) Glutathione *S*-transferase μ genotype, diet, and smoking as determinants of sister chromatid exchange frequency in lymphocytes. *Cancer Epidemiol. Biomarkers Prev.*, **4**, 535–542

Cheng, Y.-W., Chen, C.-Y., Lin, C.-P., Huang, K.H., Lin, T.-S., Wu, M.-H. & Lee, H. (2000) DNA adduct level in lung tissue may act as a risk biomarker of lung cancer. *Eur. J. Cancer*, **36**, 1381–1388

Chepiga, T.A., Morton, M.J., Murphy, P.A., Avalos, J.T., Bombick, B.R., Doolittle, D.J., Borgerding, M.F. & Swauger, J.E. (2000) A comparison of the mainstream smoke chemistry and mutagenicity of a representative sample of the US cigarette market with two Kentucky reference cigarettes (K1R4F and K1R5F). *Food chem. Toxicol.*, **38**, 949–962

Clapp, W.L., Fagg, B.S. & Smith, C.J. (1999) Reduction in Ames *Salmonella* mutagenicity of mainstream cigarette smoke condensate by tobacco protein removal. *Mutat. Res.*, **446**, 167–174

Clark, G.C. (1989) Comparison of the inhalation toxicity of kretek (clove cigarette) smoke with that of American cigarette smoke. I. One day exposure. *Arch. Toxicol.*, **63**, 1–6

Clark, G.C. (1990) Comparison of the inhalation toxicity of kretek (clove cigarette) smoke with that of American cigarette smoke. II. Fourteen days exposure. *Arch. Toxicol.*, **64**, 515–521

Clark, P.I., Gautam, S. & Gerson, L.W. (1996) Effect of menthol cigarettes on biochemical markers of smoke exposure among black and white smokers. *Chest*, **110**, 1194–1198

Cobb, R.R., Martin, J., Korytynski, E., Monteith, L. & Hughes, T.J. (1989) Preliminary molecular analysis of the *TK* locus in L5178Y large- and small-colony mouse lymphoma cell mutants. *Mutat. Res.*, **226**, 253–258

Coghlin, J., Gann, P.H., Hammond, S.K., Skipper, P.L., Taghizadeh, K., Paul, M. & Tannenbaum, S.R. (1991) 4-Aminobiphenyl hemoglobin adducts in fetuses exposed to the tobacco smoke carcinogen in utero. *J. natl Cancer Inst.*, **83**, 274–280

Cole, J. & Skopek, T. (1994) Somatic mutation frequency, mutation rates and mutation spectra in the human population in vivo. *Mutat. Res.*, **304**, 33–106

Conney, A.H., Garland, W.A., Rubio, F., Kornychuk, H., Norkus, E.P. & Kuenzig, W. (1986) Factors influencing the urinary excretion of nitrosodimethylamine and nitrosoproline in human beings. In: Hoffmann, D. & Harris, C.C., eds, *Mechanisms in Tobacco Carcinogenesis* (Banbury Report 23), Cold Spring Harbor, NY, Cold Spring Harbor Laboratory, pp. 21–32

Connor, T.H., Ramanujam, V.M., Ward, J.B. & Legator, M.S. (1983) The identification and characterization of a urinary mutagen resulting form cigarette smoke. *Mutat. Res.*, **113**, 161–172

Conway, K., Edmiston, S.N., Cui, L., Drouin, S.S., Pang, J., He, M., Tse, C.-K., Geradts, J., Dressler, L., Liu, E.T., Millikan, R. & Newman, B. (2002) Prevalance and spectrum of *p53* mutations associated with smoking in breast cancer. *Cancer Res.*, **62**, 1987–1995

Cooper, G.S. & Thorp, J.M., Jr (1999) FSH levels in relation to hysterectomy and to unilateral oophorectomy. *Obstet. Gynecol.*, **94**, 969–972

Cooper, C.S., Grover, P.L. & Sims, P. (1983) The metabolism and activation of benzo[*a*]pyrene. In: Bridges, J.W. & Chasseaud, L.F., eds, *Progress in Drug Metabolism*, Vol. 7, London, Wiley & Sons, pp. 295–396

Cooper, G.S., Baird, D.D., Hulka, B.S., Weinberg, C.R., Savitz, D.A. & Hughes, C.L., Jr (1995) Follicle-stimulating hormone concentrations in relation to active and passive smoking. *Obstet. Gynecol.*, **85**, 407–411

Cramer, D.W., Barbieri, R.L., Fraer, A.R. & Harlow, B.L. (2002) Determinants of early follicular phase gonadotrophin and estradiol concentrations in women of late reproductive age. *Hum. Reprod.*, **17**, 221–227

Crawford, F.G., Mayer, J., Santella, R.M., Cooper, T.B., Ottman, R., Tsai, W.-Y., Simon-Cereijido, G., Wang, M., Tang, D. & Perera, F.P. (1994) Biomarkers of environmental tobacco smoke in preschool children and their mothers. *J. natl Cancer Inst.*, **86**, 1398–1402

Crebelli, R., Paoletti, A., Falcone, E., Aquilina, G., Fabri, G. & Carere, A. (1985) Mutagenicity studies in a tyre plant: In vitro activity of workers' urinary concentrates and raw materials. *Br. J. ind. Med.*, **42**, 481–487

Croft, J.B., Freedman, D.S., Keenan, N.L., Sheridan, D.P., Macera, C.A. & Wheeler, F.C. (1996) Education, health behaviors, and the black-white difference in waist-to-hip ratio. *Obes. Res.*, **4**, 505–512

Cryer, P.E., Haymond, M.W., Santiago, J.V. & Shah, S.D. (1976) Norepinephrine and epinephrine release and adrenergic mediation of smoking-associated hemodynamic and metabolic events. *New Engl. J. Med.*, **295**, 573–577

Culp, S.J., Roberts, D.W., Talaska, G., Lang, N.P., Fu, P.P., Lay, J.O., Jr, Teitel, C.H., Snawder, J.E., Von Tungeln, L.S. & Kadlubar, F.F. (1997) Immunochemical, ^{32}P-postlabeling, and GC/MS detection of 4-aminobiphenyl-DNA adducts in human peripheral lung in relation to metabolic activation pathways involving pulmonary N-oxidation, conjugation, and peroxidation. *Mutat. Res.*, **378**, 97–112

Curigliano, G., Zhang, Y.-J., Wang, L.-Y., Flamini, G., Alcini, A., Ratto, C., Giustacchini, M., Alcini, E., Cittadini, A. & Santella, R.M. (1996) Immunohistochemical quantitation of 4-aminobiphenyl-DNA adducts and p53 nuclear overexpression in T1 bladder cancer of smokers and nonsmokers. *Carcinogenesis*, **17**, 911–916

Curry, J., Karnaoukhova, L., Guenette, G.C. & Glickman, B.W. (1999) Influence of sex, smoking and age on human *hprt* mutation frequencies and spectra. *Genetics*, **152**, 1065–1077

Curtis, K.M., Savitz, D.A. & Arbuckle, T.E. (1997) Effects of cigarette smoking, caffeine consumption, and alcohol intake on fecundability. *Am. J. Epidemiol.*, **146**, 32–41

Curvall, M. & Enzell, C.R. (1986) Monitoring absorption by means of determination of nicotine and cotinine. *Arch. Toxicol.*, **9**, 88–102

Curvall, M., Jansson, T., Pettersson, B., Hedin, A. & Enzell, C.R. (1985) In vitro studies of biological effects of cigarette smoke condensate. I. Genotoxic and cytotoxic effects of neutral, semivolatile constituents. *Mutat. Res.*, **157**, 169–180

Curvall, M., Romert, L, Norlén, E. & Enzell, C.R. (1987) Mutagen levels in urine from snuff users, cigarette smokers and non tobacco users — A comparison. *Mutat. Res.*, **188**, 105–110

Dallinga, J.W., Pachen, D.M.F.A., Wijnhoven, S.W.P., Breedijk, A., van't Veer, L., Wigbout, G., van Zandwijk, N., Maas, L.M., van Agen, E., Kleinjans, J.C. & van Schooten, F.J. (1998) The use of 4-aminobiphenyl hemoglobin adducts and aromatic DNA adducts in lymphocytes of smokers as biomarkers of exposure. *Cancer Epidemiol. Biomarkers Prev.*, **7**, 571–577

Daube, H., Scherer, G., Riedel, K., Ruppert, T., Tricker, A.R., Rosenbaum, P. & Adlkofer, F. (1997) DNA adducts in human placenta in relation to tobacco smoke exposure and plasma antioxidant status. *J. Cancer Res. clin. Oncol.*, **123**, 141–151

Davico, L., Sacerdote, C., Ciccone, G., Pegorano, L., Kerim, S., Ponzio, G. & Vineis, P. (1998) Chromosome 8, occupational exposures, smoking, and acute nonlymphocytic leukemias: A population-based study. *Cancer Epidemiol. Biomarkers Prevent.*, **7**, 1123–1125

Debanne, S.M., Rowland, D.Y., Riedel, T.M.& Cleves, M.A. (2000) Association of Alzheimer's disease and smoking: The case for sibling controls. *J. Am. Geriatr. Soc.*, **48**, 800–806

De Flora, S., Camoirano, A., Bagnasco, M., Bennicelli, C., van Zandwijk, N., Wigbout, G., Qian, G.S., Zhu, Y.R. & Kensler, T.W. (1996) Smokers and urinary genotoxins: Implications for selection of cohorts and modulation of endpoints in chemoprevention trials. *J. Cell Biochem.*, **25** (Suppl.), 92–98

De Flora, S., D'Agostini, F., Balansky, R., Camoirano, A., Bennicelli, C., Bagnasco, M., Cartiglia, C., Tampa, E., Longobardi, M.G., Lubet, R.A. & Izzotti, A. (2003) Modulation of cigarette smoke-related end-points in mutagenesis and carcinogenesis. *Mutat. Res.*, **523–524**, 237–252

Degawa, M., Stern, S.J., Martin, M.V., Guengerich, F.P., Fu, P.P., Ilett, K.F., Kaderlik, R.K. & Kadlubar, F.F. (1994) Metabolic activation and carcinogen–DNA adduct detection in human larynx. *Cancer Res.*, **54**, 4915–4919

van Delft, J.H.M, Steenwinkel, M.-J.S.T., van Asten, J.G., de Vogel, N., Bruijntjes-Rozier, T.C.D.M., Schouten, T., Cramers, P., Maas, L., Van Herwijnen, M.H., van Schooten, F.-J. & Hopmans, P.M.J. (2001) Biological monitoring the exposure to polycyclic aromatic hydrocarbons of coke oven workers in relation to smoking and genetic polymorphisms for *GSTM1* and *GSTT1*. *Ann. occup. Hyg.*, **45**, 395–408

Del Santo, P., Moneti, G., Salvadori, M., Saltutti, C., Delle Rose, A. & Dolara, P. (1991) Levels of the adducts of 4-aminobiphenyl to hemoglobin in control subjects and bladder carcinoma patients. *Cancer Lett.*, **60**, 245–251

DeMarini, D.M. (1983) Genotoxicity of tobacco smoke and tobacco smoke condensate. *Mutat. Res.*, **114**, 59–89

DeMarini, D.M., Brooks, L.R., Bhatnagar, V.K., Hayes, R.B., Eischen, B.T., Shelton, M.L., Zenser, T.V., Talaska, G., Kashyap, S.K., Dosemeci, M., Kashyap, R., Parikh, D.J., Lakshmi, V., Hsu, F., Davis, B.B., Jaeger, M. & Rothman, N. (1987) Urinary mutagenicity as a biomarker in workers exposed to benzidine: Correlation with urinary metabolites and urothelial DNA adducts. *Carcinogenesis*, **18**, 981–988

DeMarini, D.M., Shelton, M.L. & Levine, J.G. (1995) Mutation spectrum of cigarette smoke condensate in *Salmonella*: Comparison to mutations in smoking-associated tumors. *Carcinogenesis*, **16**, 2535–2542

DeMarini, D.M., Landi, S., Tian, D., Hanley, N.M., Li, X., Hu, F., Roop, B.C., Mass, M.J., Keohavong, P., Gao, W., Olivier, M., Hainaut, P. & Mumford, J.L. (2001) Lung tumor *KRAS* and *TP53* mutations in nonsmokers reflect exposure to PAH-rich coal combustion emissions. *Cancer Res.*, **61**, 6679–6681

De Méo, M.P., Duménil, G., Botta, A.H., Laget, M., Zabaloueff, V. & Mathias, A. (1987) Urine mutagenicity of steel workers exposed to coke oven emissions. *Carcinogenesis*, **8**, 363–367

De Méo, M.P., Miribel, V., Botta, A., Laget, M. & Duménil, G. (1988) Applicability of the SOS Chromotest to detect urinary mutagenicity caused by smoking. *Mutagenesis*, **3**, 277–283

Denissenko, M.F., Pao, A., Tang, M.-S. & Pfeifer, G.P. (1996) Preferential formation of benzo[*a*]pyrene adducts at lung cancer mutational hotspots in *P53*. *Science*, **274**, 430–432

Denissenko, M.F., Pao, A., Pfeifer, G.P. & Tang, M.-S. (1998) Slow repair of bulky DNA adducts along the nontranscribed strand of the human *p53* gene may explain the strand bias of transversion mutations in cancers. *Oncogene*, **16**, 1241–1247

van Diemen, P.C., Maasdam, D., Vermeulen, S., Darroudi, F. & Natarajan, A.T. (1995) Influence of smoking habits on the frequencies of structural and numerical chromosomal aberrations in human peripheral blood lymphocytes using the fluoresence *in situ* hybridization (FISH) technique. *Mutagenesis*, **10**, 487–495

Dietrich, M., Block. G., Hudes, M., Morrow, J.D., Norkus, E.P., Traber, M.G., Cross, C.E. & Packer, L. (2002) Antioxidant supplementation decreases lipid peroxidation biomarker F_2-isoprostanes in plasma of smokers. *Cancer Epidemiol. Biomarkers Prev.*, **11**, 7–13

Djordjevic, M.V., Sigountos, C.W., Brunnemann, K.D. & Hoffmann, D. (1991) Formation of 4-(methylnitrosamino)-4-(3-pyridyl)butyric acid in vitro and in mainstream cigarette smoke. *J. agric. Food Chem.*, **39**, 209–213

Dolara, P., Mazzoli, S., Rosi, D., Buiatti, E., Baccetti, S., Turchi, A. & Vannucci, V. (1981) Exposure to carcinogenic chemicals and smoking increases urinary excretion of mutagens in humans. *J. Toxicol. environ. Health*, **8**, 95–103

Domino, E.F. (1999) Pharmacological significance of nicotine. In: Gorrod, J.W. & Jacob, P., III, eds, *Analytical Determination of Nicotine and Related Compounds and their Metabolites*, New York, Elsevier, pp. 1–11

Doolittle, D.J., Rahn, C.A., Burger, G.T., Davis, R., deBethizy, J.D., Howard, G., Lee, C.K., McKarns, S.C., Riccio, E., Robinson, J., Reynolds, J. & Hayes, A.W. (1989) Human urine mutagenicity study comparing cigarettes which burn or only heat tobacco. *Mutat. Res.*, **223**, 221–232

Doolittle, D.J., Rahn, C.A., Riccio, E., Passananti, G.T., Howard, G., Vesell, E.S., Burger, G.T. & Hayes, A.W. (1990a) Comparative studies of the mutagenicity of urine from smokers and non-smokers on a controlled non-mutagenic diet. *Food chem. Toxicol.*, **28**, 639–646

Doolittle, D.J., Lee, C.K., Ivett, J.L., Mirsalis, J.C., Riccio, E., Rudd, C.J., Burger, G.T. & Hayes, A.W. (1990b) Comparative studies on the genotoxic activity of mainstream smoke condensate from cigarettes which burn or only heat tobacco. *Environ. mol. Mutag.*, **15**, 93–105

Doolittle, D.J., Rahn, C.A. & Lee, C.K. (1991) The effect of exposure to nicotine, carbon monoxide, cigarette smoke or cigarette smoke condensate on the mutagenicity of rat urine. *Mutat. Res.*, **260**, 9–18

Doolittle, D.J., Winegar, R., Lee, C.K., Caldwell, W.S., Hayes, A.W. & deBethizy, J.D. (1995) The genotoxic potential of nicotine and its major metabolites. *Mutat. Res.*, **344**, 95–102

van Doorn, R., Bos, R.P., Leijdekkers, C.-M., Wagenaas-Zegers, M.A.P., Theuws, J.L.G. & Henderson, P.T. (1979) Thioether concentration and mutagenicity of urine from cigarette smoker. *Int. Arch. occup. environ. Health*, **43**, 159–166

van Doorn, R., Leijdekkers, C.M., Bos, R.P., Brouns, R.M.E. & Henderson, P.T. (1981) Detection of human exposure to electrophilic compounds by assay of thioether detoxication products in urine. *Ann. occup. Hyg.*, **24**, 77–92

Dor, F., Haguenoer, J.-M., Zmirou, D., Empereur-Bissonnet, P., Jongeneelen, F.J., Nedellec, V., Person, A., Ferguson, C.C. & Dab, W. (2000) Urinary 1-hydroxypyrene as a biomarker of polycyclic aromatic hydrocarbons exposure of workers on a contaminated site: Influence of exposure conditions. *J. occup. environ. Med.*, **42**, 391–397

Dorgan, J.F., Stanczyk, F.Z., Longcope, C., Stephenson, H.E., Jr, Chang. L., Miller, R., Franz, C., Falk, R.T. & Kahle, L. (1997) Relationship of serum dehydroepiandrosterone (DHEA), DHEA sulfate, and 5-androstene-3beta,17beta-diol to risk of breast cancer in postmenopausal women. *Cancer Epidemiol. Biomarkers Prev.*, **6**, 177–181

Dosaka-Akita, H., Katabami, M., Hommura, H., Fujioka, Y., Katoh, H. & Kawakami, Y. (1999) Bcl-2 expression in non-small cell lung cancers: Higher frequency of expression in squamous cell carcinomas with earlier pT status. *Oncology*, **56**, 259–264

Duell, E.J., Wiencke, J.K., Cheng, T.-J., Varkonyi, A., Zuo, Z.F., Ashok, T.D.S., Mark, E. J., Wain, J. C., Christiani, D.C. & Kelsey, K.T. (2000) Polymorphisms in the DNA repair genes *XRCC1* and *ERCC2* and biomarkers of DNA damage in human blood mononuclear cells. *Carcinogenesis*, **21**, 965–971

Duffel, M.W. (1997) Sulfotransferases. In: Guengerich, F.P., ed., *Comprehensive Toxicology*, Vol. 3, *Biotransformation*, New York, Elsevier Science, pp. 365–383

Duncan, B.B., Chambless, L.E., Schmidt, M.I., Szklo, M., Folsom, A.R., Carpenter, M.A. & Crouse, J.R., III for the Atherosclerosis Risk in Communities (ARIC) Study Investigators (1995) Correlates of body fat distribution. Variation across categories of race, sex, and body mass in the atherosclerosis risk in communities study. *Ann. Epidemiol.*, **5**, 192–200

Dunn, B.P. & Curtis, J.R. (1985) Clastogenic agents in the urine of coffee drinkers and cigarette smokers. *Mutat. Res.*, **147**, 179–188

Dunn, B.P. & Stich, H.F. (1986) ^{32}P-Postlabelling analysis of aromatic DNA adducts in human oral mucosal cells. *Carcinogenesis*, **7**, 1115–1120

Dunn, B.P., Vedal, S., San, R.H.C., Kwan, W.-F., Nelems, B., Enarson, D.A. & Stich, H.F. (1991) DNA adducts in bronchial biopsies. *Int. J. Cancer*, **48**, 485–492

Dyke, G.W., Craven, J.L., Hall, R. & Garner, R.C. (1992) Smoking-related DNA adducts in human gastric cancers. *Int. J. Cancer*, **52**, 847–850

Einhaus, M., Holz, O., Meissner, R., Krause, T., Warncke, K., Held, I., Scherer, G., Tricker, A.R., Adlkofer, F. & Rüdiger, H.W. (1994) Determination of DNA single-strand breaks in lymphocytes of smokers and nonsmokers exposed to environmental tobacco smoke using the nick translation assay. *Clin. Invest.*, **72**, 930–936

Einistö, P., Nohmi, T., Watanabe, M. & Ishidate, M., Jr (1990) Sensitivity of *Salmonella typhimurium* YG1024 to urine mutagenicity caused by cigarette smoking. *Mutat. Res.*, **245**, 87–92

Ejiofor, A., Hutchison, D.C.S. & Baum, H. (1981) Inhibition of human leucocyte elastase activity by cigarette smoke. *Biosci. Rep.*, **1**, 715–720

Eke, B.C., Vural, N. & Iscan, M. (1996) Combined effects of ethanol and cigarette smoke on hepatic and pulmonary xenobiotic metabolizing enzymes in rats. *Chem.-biol. Interact.*, **102**, 155–167

Eke, B.C., Vural, N. & Iscan, M. (1997) Age dependent differential effects of cigarette smoke on hepatic and pulmonary xenobiotic metabolizing enzymes in rats. *Arch. Toxicol.*, **71**, 696–702

El Bayoumy, K., Donahue, J.M., Hecht, S.S. & Hoffmann, D. (1986) Identification and quantitative determination of aniline and toluidines in human urine. *Cancer Res.*, **46**, 6064–6067

Eliasson, M., Hägg, E., Lundblad, D., Karlsson, R. & Bucht, E. (1993) Influence of smoking and snuff use on electrolytes, adrenal and calcium regulating hormones. *Acta endocrinol.*, **128**, 35–40

Eliasson, B., Attwall, S., Taskinen, M.R. & Smith, U. (1997) Smoking cessation improves insulin sensitivity in health middle-aged men. *Eur. J. clin. Invest.*, **27**, 450–456

Ellingsen, D.G., Thomassen, Y., Aaseth, J. & Alexander, J. (1997) Cadmium and selenium in blood and urine related to smoking habits and previous exposure to mercury vapour. *J. appl. Toxicol.*, **17**, 337–343

El-Nemr, A., Al-Shawaf, T., Sabatini, L., Wilson, C., Lower, A.M. & Grudzinskas, J.G. (1998) Effect of smoking on ovarian reserve and ovarian stimulation in in-vitro fertilization and embryo transfer. *Hum. Reprod.*, **13**, 2192–2198

Endogenous Sex Hormones and Breast Cancer Collaborative Group (2002) Endogenous sex hormones and breast cancer in postmenopausal women: Reanalysis of nine prospective studies. *J. natl Cancer Inst.*, **94**, 606–616

Endoh, K. & Leung, F.W. (1994) Effects of smoking and nicotine on the gastric mucosa: A review of clinical and experimental evidence. *Gastroenterology*, **107**, 864–878

US Environmental Protection Agency (1993) *Smoking and Tobacco Control. Monograph 4. Respiratory Health Effects of Passive Smoking: Lung Cancer and Other Disorders* (NIH Publication No. 93-3605), Washington DC, US Department of Health and Human Services

Etter, J.F., Vu Duc, T. & Perneger, T.V. (2000) Saliva cotinine levels in smokers and nonsmokers. *Am. J. Epidemiol.*, **151**, 251–258

Etzel, R.A. (1990) A review of the use of saliva cotinine as a marker of tobacco smoke exposure. *Prev. Med.*, **19**, 190–197

Evans, D.A.P. (1986) Acetylation. In: Kalow, W., Goedde, H.W. & Agarwal, D.P., eds, *Ethnic Differences in Reactions to Drugs and Xenobiotics*, New York, Alan R. Liss, pp. 209–242

Everson, R.B., Randerath, E., Santella, R.M., Cefalo, R.C., Avitts, T.A. & Randerath, K. (1986) Detection of smoking-related covalent DNA adducts in human placenta. *Science*, **231**, 54–57

Everson, R.B., Randerath, E., Santella, R.M., Avitts, T.A., Weinstein, I.B. & Randerath, K. (1988) Quantitative associations between DNA damage in human placenta and maternal smoking and birth weight. *J. natl Cancer Inst.*, **80**, 567–576

Facchini, F.S., Hollenbeck, C.B., Jeppesen, J., Chen, Y.D. & Reaven, G.M. (1992) Insulin resistance and cigarette smoking. *Lancet*, **339**, 1128–1130

Fagerström, K.O., Hughes, J.R., Rasmussen, T. & Callas, P.W. (2000) Randomized trial investigating effect of a novel nicotine delivery device (Eclipse) and a nicotine oral inhaler on smoking behaviour, nicotine and carbon monoxide exposure, and motivation to quit. *Tob. Control*, **9**, 327–333

Falter, B., Kutzer, C. & Richter, E. (1994) Biomonitoring of hemoglobin adducts: Aromatic amines and tobacco-specific nitrosamines. *Clin. Invest.*, **72**, 364–371

Farmer, P.B., Neumann, H.-G. & Henschler, D. (1987) Estimation of exposure of man to substances reacting covalently with macromolecules. *Arch. Toxicol.*, **60**, 251–260

Favatier, F. & Polla, B.S. (2001). Tobacco-smoke-inducible human haem oxygenase-1 gene expression: Role of distinct transcription factors and reactive oxygen intermediates. *Biochem. J.*, **353**, 475–482

Fay, L.B., Leaf, C.D., Gremaud, E., Aeschlimann, J.-M., Steen, C., Shuker, D.E.G. & Turesky, R.J. (1997) Urinary excretion of 3-methyladenine after consumption of fish containing high levels of dimethylamine. *Carcinogenesis*, **18**, 1039–1044

Fennell, T.R., MacNeela, J.P., Morris, R.W., Watson, M., Thompson, C.L. & Bell, D.A. (2000) Hemoglobin adducts from acrylonitrile and ethylene oxide in cigarette smokers: Effects of glutathione S-transferase *T1*-null and *M1*-null genotypes. *Cancer Epidemiol. Biomarkers Prev.*, **9**, 705–712

Fernandez-Salguero, P., Hoffman, S.M., Cholerton, S., Mohrenweiser, H., Raunio, H., Rautio, A., Pelkonen, O., Huang, J.-D., Evans, W.E., Idle, J.R. & Gonzalez, F.J. (1995) A genetic poly-morphism in coumarin 7-hydroxylation: Sequence of the human *CYP2A* genes and identifica-tion of variant *CYP2A6* alleles. *Am. J. hum. Genet.*, **57**, 651–660

Ferreira, M., Jr, Buchet, J.P., Burrion, J.B., Moro, J., Cupers, L., Delavignette, J.P., Jacques, J. & Lauwerys, R. (1994) Determinants of urinary thioethers, D-glucaric acid and mutagenicity after exposure to polycyclic aromatic hydrocarbons assessed by air monitoring and measure-ment of 1-hydroxypyrene in urine: A cross-sectional study in workers of coke and graphite-electrode-producing plants. *Int. Arch. occup. environ. Health*, **65**, 329–338

Feskens, E.J.M. & Kromhout, D. (1989) Cardiovascular risk factors and the 25-year incidence of diabetes mellitus in middle-aged men. *Am. J. Epidemiol.*, **130**, 1101–1108

Fewell, J.E. & Smith, F.G. (1998) Perinatal nicotine exposure impairs ability of newborn rats to autoresuscitate from apnea during hypoxia. *J. appl. Physiol.*, **85**, 2066–2074

Fielding, S., Short, C., Davies, K., Wald, N., Bridges, B.A. & Waters, R. (1989) Studies on the abi-lity of smoke from different types of cigarettes to induce single-strand breaks in cultured human cells. *Mutat. Res.*, **214**, 147–151

Finch, G.L., Nikula, K.J., Chen, B.T., Barr, E.B., Chang, I.Y. & Hobbs, C.H. (1995) Effect of chro-nic cigarette smoke exposure on lung clearance of tracer particles inhaled by rats. *Fundam. appl. Toxicol.*, **24**, 76–85

Finch, G.L., Lundgren, D.L., Barr, E.B., Chen, B.T., Griffith, W.C., Hobbs, C.H., Hoover, M.D., Nikula, K.J. & Mauderly, J.L. (1998) Chronic cigarette smoke exposure increases the pulmo-nary retention and radiation dose of ^{239}Pu inhaled as ^{239}PuO$_2$ by F344 rats. *Health Phys.*, **75**, 597–609

Finkelstein, E.I., Nardini, M. & van der Vliet, A. (2001) Inhibition of neutrophil apoptosis by acro-lein: A mechanism of tobacco-related lung disease? *Am. J. Physiol. Lung cell. mol. Physiol.*, **281**, L732–L739

Fitzgerald, J. (2001) Cigarette smoke comparative toxicology. *Food chem. Toxicol.*, **39**, 175–176

Flamini, G., Romano, G., Curigliano, G., Chiominto, A., Capelli, G., Boninsegna, A., Signorelli, C., Ventura, L., Santella, R.M., Sgambato, A. & Cittadini, A. (1998) 4-Aminobiphenyl–DNA adducts in laryngeal tissue and smoking habits: An immunohistochemical study. *Carcino-genesis*, **19**, 353–357

Flaws, J.A., Rhodes, J.C., Langenberg, P., Hirshfield, A.N., Kjerulff, K. & Sharara, F.I. (2000) Ovarian volume and menopausal status. *Menopause*, **7**, 53–61

Flegal, K.M., Troiano, R.P., Pamuk, E.R., Kuczmarski, R.J. & Campbell, S.M. (1995) The influence of smoking cessation on the prevalence of overweight in the United States. *New Engl. J. Med.*, **333**, 1165–1170

Foiles, P.G., Akerkar, S.A., Carmella, S.G., Kagan, M., Stoner, G.D., Resau, J.H. & Hecht, S.S. (1991) Mass spectrometric analysis of tobacco-specific nitrosamine–DNA adducts in smokers and nonsmokers. *Chem. Res. Toxicol.*, **4**, 364–468

Forgacs, E., Zöchbauer-Müller, S., Oláh, E. & Minna, J.D. (2001) Molecular genetic abnormalities in the pathogenesis of human lung cancer. *Pathol. Oncol. Res.*, **7**, 6–13

Fowler, J.S., Volkow, N.D., Wang, G.J., Pappas, N., Logan, J., MacGregor, R., Alexoff, D., Shea, C., Schlyer, D., Wolf, A. P., Warner, D., Zezulkova, I. & Cilento, R. (1996a) Inhibition of monoamine oxidase B in the brains of smokers. *Nature*, **379**, 733–736

Fowler, J.S., Volkow, N.D., Wang, G.J., Pappas, N., Logan, J., Shea, C., Alexoff, D., MacGregor, R.R., Schlyer, D.J., Zezulkova, I. & Wolf, A.P. (1996b) Brain monoamine oxidase A inhibition in cigarette smokers. *Proc. natl Acad. Sci. USA*, **93**, 14065–14069

Fowler, J.S., Wang, G.J., Volkow, N.D., Franceschi, D., Logan, J., Pappas, N., Shea, C., MacGregor, R.R. & Garza, V. (1999) Smoking a single cigarette does not produce a measurable reduction in brain MAO B in nonsmokers. *Nicotine Tob. Res.*, **1**, 325–329

Fraig, M., Shreesha, U., Savici, D. & Katzenstein, A.L. (2002) Respiratory bronchiolitis: A clinicopathologic study in current smokers, ex-smokers, and never-smokers. *Am. J. Surg. Pathol.*, **26**, 647–653

Fratiglioni, L. & Wang, H.X. (2000) Smoking and Parkinson's and Alzheimer's disease: Review of the epidemiological studies. *Behav. Brain Res.*, **113**, 117–120

Fung, Y.K., Mendlik, M.G., Haven, M.C., Akhter, M.P. & Kimmel, D.B. (1998) Short-term effects of nicotine on bone and calciotropic hormones in adult female rats. *Pharmacol. Toxicol.*, **82**, 243–249

Fürstenberger, G. & Senn, H.-J. (2002) Insulin-like growth factors and cancer. *Lancet Oncol.*, **3**, 298–302

Gairola, C.G. (1987) Pulmonary aryl hydrocarbon hydroxylase activity of mice, rats and guinea pigs following long term exposure to mainstream and sidestream cigarette smoke. *Toxicology*, **45**, 177–184

Gairola, C.G., Drawdy, M.L., Block, A.E. & Daugherty, A. (2001) Sidestream cigarette smoke accelerates atherogenesis in apolipoprotein E$^{-/-}$ mice. *Atherosclerosis*, **156**, 49–55

Galdston, M., Levytska, V., Schwartz, M.S. & Magnusson, B. (1984) Ceruloplasmin. Increased serum concentration and impaired antioxidant activity in cigarette smokers, and ability to prevent suppression of elastase inhibitory capacity of alpha$_1$-proteinase inhibitor. *Am. Rev. respir. Dis.*, **129**, 258–263

Gallagher, J.E., Mumford, J., Li, X., Shank, T., Manchester, D. & Lewtas, J. (1993a) DNA adduct profiles and levels in placenta, blood and lung in relation to cigarette smoking and smoky coal emissions. In: Phillips, D.H., Castegnaro, M. & Bartsch, H., eds, *Postlabelling Methods for Detection of DNA Adducts* (IARC Scientific Publications No. 124), Lyon, IARC*Press*, pp. 283–292

Gallagher, J.E., Vine, M.F., Schramm, M.M., Lewtas, J., George, M.H., Hulka, B.S. & Everson, R.B. (1993b) ^{32}P-Postlabeling analysis of DNA adducts in human sperm cells from smokers and nonsmokers. *Cancer Epidemiol. Biomarkers Prev.*, **2**, 581–585

Gealy, R., Zhang, L., Siegfried, J.M., Luketich, J.D. & Keohavong, P. (1999) Comparison of mutations in the *p53* and *K-ras* genes in lung carcinomas from smoking and nonsmoking women. *Cancer Epidemiol. Biomarkers Prev.*, **8**, 297–302

Geisler, J., Omsjo, I.H., Helle, S.I., Ekse, D., Silsand, R. & Lonning, P.E. (1999) Plasma oestrogen fractions in postmenopausal women receiving hormone replacement therapy: Influence of route of administration and cigarette smoking. *J. Endocrinol.*, **162**, 265–270

Geneste, O., Camus, A.-M., Castegnaro, M., Petruzzelli, S., Macchiarini, P., Angeletti, C.-A., Giuntini, C. & Bartsch, H. (1991) Comparison of pulmonary DNA adduct levels, measured by ^{32}P-postlabelling and aryl hydrocarbon hydroxylase activity in lung parenchyma of smokers and ex-smokers. *Carcinogenesis*, **12**, 1301–1305

Georgiadis, P., Samoli, E., Kaila, S., Katsouyanni, K. & Kyrtopoulos, S.A. (2000) Ubiquitous presence of O[6]-methylguanine in human peripheral and cord blood DNA. *Cancer Epidemiol. Biomarkers Prev.*, **9**, 299–305

Ghittori, S., Maestri, L., Fiorentino, M.L. & Imbriani, M. (1995) Evaluation of occupational exposure to benzene by urinalysis. *Int. Arch. occup. environ. Health*, **67**, 195–200

Ghittori, S., Maestri, L., Rolandi, L., Lodola, L., Fiorentino, M.L. & Imbriani, M. (1996) The determination of trans,trans-muconic acid in urine as an indicator of occupational exposure to benzene. *Appl. occup. environ. Hyg.*, **11**, 187–191

Ghosh, R. & Ghosh, P.K. (1987) The effect of tobacco smoking on the frequency of sister chromatid exchanges in human lymphocyte chromosomes. *Cancer Genet. Cytogenet.*, **27**, 15–19

Giovannucci, E. (2001) Insulin, insulin-like growth factors and colon cancer: A review of the evidence. *J. Nutr.*, **131**, 3109S–3120S

Girre, C., Lucas, D., Hispard, E., Menez, C., Dally, S. & Menez, J.-F. (1994) Assessment of cytochrome P4502E1 induction in alcoholic patients by chlorzoxazone pharmacokinetics. *Biochem. Pharmacol.*, **47**, 1503–1508

Gocze, P.M. & Freeman, D.A. (2000) Cytotoxic effects of cigarette smoke alkaloids inhibit the progesterone production and cell growth of cultured MA-10 Leydig tumor cells. *Eur. J. Obstet. Gynecol. reprod. Biol.*, **93**, 77–83

Godden, P.M., Kass, G., Mayer, R.T. & Burke, M.D. (1987) The effects of cigarette smoke compared to 3-methylcholanthrene and phenobarbitone on alkoxyresorufin metabolism by lung and liver microsomes from rats. *Biochem. Pharmacol.*, **36**, 3393–3398

Godschalk, R.W.L., Maas, L.M., Van Zandwijk, N., van't Veer, L.J., Breedijk, A., Borm, P.J.A., Verhaert, J., Kleinjans, J.C.S. & van Schooten, F.-J. (1998) Differences in aromatic–DNA adduct levels between alveolar macrophages and subpopulations of white blood cells from smokers. *Carcinogenesis*, **19**, 819–825

Godschalk, R.W.L., Dallinga, J.W., Wikman, H., Risch, A., Kleinjans, J.C.S., Bartsch, H. & Van Schooten, F.-J. (2001) Modulation of DNA and protein adducts in smokers by genetic polymorphisms in *GSTM1*, *GSTT1*, *NAT1* and *NAT2*. *Pharmacogenetics*, **11**, 389–398

Gold, E.B., Bromberger, J., Crawford, S., Samuels, S., Greendale, G.A., Harlow, S.D. & Skurnick, J. (2001) Factors associated with age at natural menopause in a multiethnic sample of midlife women. *Am. J. Epidemiol.*, **153**, 865–874

Goldman, R., Enewold, L., Pellizzari, E., Beach, J.B., Bowman, E.D., Krishnan, S.S. & Shields, P.G. (2001) Smoking increases carcinogenic polycyclic aromatic hydrocarbons in human lung tissue. *Cancer Res.*, **61**, 6367–6371

Gontijo, Á.M.deM.C., Elias, F.N., Salvadori, D.M.F., de Oliveira, M.L.C.S., Correa, L.A., Goldberg, J., Trindade, J.C.deS. & de Camargo, J.L. (2001) Single-cell gel (comet) assay detects primary DNA damage in nonneoplastic urothelial cells of smokers and ex-smokers. *Cancer Epidemiol. Biomarkers Prev.*, **10**, 987–993

Gonzalez, F.J. & Gelboin, H.V. (1994) Role of human cytochromes P450 in the metabolic activation of chemical carcinogens and toxins. *Drug Metab. Rev.*, **26**, 165–183

Goodman-Gruen, D. & Barrett-Connor, E. (1997) Epidemiology of insulin-like growth factor-I in elderly men and women. The Rancho Bernardo Study. *Am. J. Epidemiol.*, **145**, 970–976

Gordon, S.M. (1990) Identification of exposure markers in smokers' breath. *J. Chromatogr.*, **511**, 291–302

Górecka, D. & Gorski, T. (1993) The influence of cigarette smoking on sister chromatid exchange frequencies in peripheral lymphocytes among nurses handling cytostatic drugs. *Polish J. occup. Med. environ. Health*, **6**, 143–148

Gorrod, J.W. & Schepers, G. (1999) Biotransformation of nicotine in mammalian systems. In: Gorrod, J.W. & Jacob, P., III, eds, *Analytical Determination of Nicotine and Related Compounds and their Metabolites*, New York, Elsevier, pp. 45–67

Granath, F., Westerholm, R., Peterson, A., Törnqvist, M. & Ehrenberg, L. (1994) Uptake and metabolism of ethene studied in a smoke-stop experiment. *Mutat. Res.*, **313**, 285–291

Granella, M., Priante, E., Nardini, B., Bono, R. & Clonfero, E. (1996) Excretion of mutagens, nicotine and its metabolites in urine of cigarette smokers. *Mutagenesis*, **11**, 207–211

Grimmer, G., Dettbarn, G. & Jacob, J. (1993) Biomonitoring of polycyclic aromatic hydrocarbons in highly exposed coke plant workers by measurement of urinary phenanthrene and pyrene metabolites (phenols and dihydrodiols). *Int. Arch. occup. environ. Health*, **65**, 189–199

Grimmer, G., Jacob, J., Dettbarn, G. & Naujack, K.-W. (1997) Determination of urinary metabolites of polycyclic aromatic hydrocarbons (PAH) for the risk assessment of PAH-exposed workers. *Int. Arch. occup. environ. Health*, **69**, 231–239

Grimmer, G., Dettbarn, G., Seidel, A. & Jacob, J. (2000) Detection of carcinogenic aromatic amines in the urine of nonsmokers. *Sci. total Environ.*, **247**, 81–90

Grinberg-Funes, R.A., Singh, V.N., Perera, F.P., Bell, D.A., Young, T.L., Dickey, C., Wang, L.W. & Santella, R.M. (1994) Polycyclic aromatic hydrocarbon–DNA adducts in smokers and their relationship to micronutrient levels and the glutathione-S-transferase M1 genotype. *Carcinogenesis*, **15**, 2449–2454

Grove, K.L., Sekhon, H.S., Brogan, R.S., Keller, J.A., Smith, M.S. & Spindel, E.R. (2001) Chronic maternal nicotine exposure alters neuronal systems in the arcuate nucleus that regulate feeding behavior in the newborn rhesus macaque. *J. clin. Endocrinol. Metab.*, **86**, 5420–5426

Grunberg, N.E. (1990) The inverse relationship between tobacco use and body weight. In: Kozlowski, L.T., Annis, H.M., Cappell, H.D., Glaser, F.B., Goodstadt, M.S., Israel, Y., Kalant, H., Sellers, E.M. & Vingilis, E.R., eds, *Research Advances in Alcohol and Drug Problems*, Vol. 10, New York, Plenum Press, pp. 273–315

Gu, Y., Cimino, G., Alder, H., Nakamura, T., Prasad, R., Canaani, O., Moir, D.T., Jones, C., Nowell, P.C., Croce, C.M. & Canaani, O. (1992) The (4;11)(q21;q23) chromosome translocations in acute leukemias involve the VDJ recombinase. *Proc. natl Acad. Sci. USA*, **89**, 10464–10468

Guengerich, F.P. (1997) Cytochrome P450 enzymes. In: Guengerich, F.P., ed., *Comprehensive Toxicology*, Vol. 3, *Biotransformation*, New York, Elsevier Science, pp. 37–68

Guengerich, F.P., Kim, D.-H. & Iwasaki, M. (1991) Role of human cytochrome P-450 IIE1 in the oxidation of many low molecular weight cancer suspects. *Chem. Res. Toxicol.*, **4**, 168–179

Guidotti, T.L. (1989) Critique of available studies on the toxicology of kretek smoke and its constituents by routes of entry involving the respiratory tract. *Arch. Toxicol.*, **63**, 7–12

Gündel, J. & Angerer, J. (2000) High-performance liquid chromatographic method with fluorescence detection for the determination of 3-hydroxybenzo[a]pyrene and 3- hydroxybenz[a]anthracene in the urine of polycyclic aromatic hydrocarbon-exposed workers. *J. Chromatogr.*, **B738**, 47–55

Gupta, R.C., Sopori, M.L. & Gairola, C.G. (1989) Formation of cigarette smoke-induced DNA adducts in the rat lung and nasal mucosa. *Cancer Res.*, **49**, 1916–1920

Gupta, R.C., Arif, J.M. & Gairola, C.G. (1999) Enhancement of pre-existing DNA adducts in rodents exposed to cigarette smoke. *Mutat. Res.*, **424**, 195–205

Gupta, K., Krishnaswamy, G., Karnad, A. & Peiris, A.N. (2002) Insulin: A novel factor in carcinogenesis. *Am. J. med. Sci.*, **323**, 140–145

Habib, M.P., Clements, N.C. & Garewal, H.S. (1995) Cigarette smoking and ethane exhalation in humans. *Am. J. resp. crit. Care Med.*, **151**, 1368–1372

Hackman, P., Hou, S.-M., Nyberg, F., Pershagen, G. & Lambert, B. (2000) Mutational spectra at the hypoxanthine-guanine phosphoribosyltransferase (*HPRT*) locus in T-lymphocytes of non-smoking and smoking lung cancer patients. *Mutat. Res.*, **468**, 45–61

Hageman, G.J., Stierum, R.H., van Herwijnen, M.H., van der Veer, M.S. & Kleinjans, J.C. (1998) Nicotinic acid supplementation: Effects on niacin status, cytogenetic damage, and poly(ADP-ribosylation) in lymphocytes of smokers. *Nutr. Cancer*, **32**, 113–120

Hainaut, P. & Pfeifer, G.P. (2001) Patterns of p53 G→T transversions in lung cancer reflect the primary mutagenic signature of DNA-damage by tobacco smoke. *Carcinogenesis*, **22**, 367–374

Hall, J., Brésil, H., Donato, F., Wild, C.P., Loktionova, N.A., Kazanova, O.I., Komyakov, I.P., Lemekhov, V.G., Likhachev, A.J. & Montesano, R. (1993) Alkylation and oxidative-DNA damage repair activity in blood leukocytes of smokers and nonsmokers. *Int. J. Cancer*, **54**, 728–733

Hanahan, D. & Weinberg, R.A. (2000) The hallmarks of cancer (Review). *Cell*, **100**, 57–70

Hanawalt, P.C. (2001) Controlling the efficiency of excision repair. *Mutat. Res.*, **485**, 3–13

Hankey, G.J. (1999) Smoking and risk of stroke. *J. cardiovasc. Risk*, **6**, 207–211

Hansen, C., Sørensen, L.D., Asmussen, I. & Autrup, H. (1992) Transplacental exposure to tobacco smoke in human-adduct formation in placenta and umbilical cord blood vessels. *Teratog. Carcinog. Mutag.*, **12**, 51–60

Hansen, C., Asmussen, I. & Autrup, H. (1993) Detection of carcinogen–DNA adducts in human fetal tissues by the ³²P-postlabeling procedure. *Environ. Health Perspect.*, **99**, 229–231

Hansen, Å.M., Poulsen, O.M., Sigsgaard, T. & Christensen, J.M. (1994) The validity of determination of α-naphthol in urine as a marker for exposure to polycyclic aromatic hydrocarbons. *Anal. chim. Acta*, **291**, 341–347

Hargreave, F.E. & Leigh, R. (1999) Induced sputum, eosinophilic bronchitis, and chronic obstructive pulmonary disease. *Am. J. respir. crit. Care Med.*, **160**, S53–S57

Härkönen, K., Viitanen, T., Larsen, S.B., Bonde, J.P. & Lahdetie, J. (1999) Aneuploidy in sperm and exposure to fungicides and lifestyle factors. ASCLEPIOS. A European Concerted Action on Occupational Hazards to Male Reproductive Capability. *Environ. mol. Mutag.*, **34**, 39–46

Harris, S.S., Soteriades, E., Coolidge, J.A., Mudgal, S. & Dawson-Hughes, B. (2000) Vitamin D insufficiency and hyperparathyroidism in a low income, multiracial, elderly population. *J. clin. Endocrinol. Metab.*, **85**, 4125–4130

Hasan, S.U., Simakajornboon, N., MacKinnon, Y. & Gozal, D. (2001) Prenatal cigarette smoke exposure selectively alters protein kinase C and nitric oxide synthase expression within the neonatal rat brainstem. *Neurosci. Lett.*, **301**, 135–138

Hatch, M.C., Warburton, D. & Santella, R.M. (1990) Polycyclic aromatic hydrocarbon–DNA adducts in spontaneously aborted fetal tissue. *Carcinogenesis*, **11**, 1673–1675

Haugen, A., Becher, G., Benestad, C., Vahakangas, K., Trivers, G.E., Newman, M.J. & Harris, C.C. (1986) Determination of polycyclic aromatic hydrocarbons in the urine, benzo[*a*]pyrene diol epoxide–DNA adducts in lymphocyte DNA, and antibodies to the adducts in sera from coke oven workers exposed to measured amounts of polycyclic aromatic hydrocarbons in the work atmosphere. *Cancer Res.*, **46**, 4178–4183

Hautanen, A. & Adlercreutz, H. (1993) Hyperinsulinaemia, dyslipidaemia and exaggerated adrenal androgen response to adrenocorticotropin in male smokers. *Diabetologia*, **36**, 1275–1281

Hawkins, B.T., Brown, R.C. & Davis, T.P. (2002) Smoking and ischemic stroke: A role for nicotine? *Trends pharmacol. Sci.*, **23**, 78–82

Hecht, S.S. (1998) Biochemistry, biology, and carcinogenicity of tobacco-specific *N*-nitrosamines. *Chem. Res. Toxicol.*, **11**, 559–603

Hecht, S.S. (1999) Tobacco smoke carcinogens and lung cancer. *J. natl Cancer Inst.*, **91**, 1194–1210

Hecht (2002a) Cigarette smoking and lung cancer: Chemical mechanisms and approaches to prevention. *Lancet Oncol.*, **3**, 461–469

Hecht (2002b) Human urinary carcinogen metabolites: Biomarkers for investigating tobacco and cancer. *Carcinogenesis*, **23**, 907–922

Hecht, S.S., Peterson, L.A. & Spratt, T.E. (1994) Tobacco-specific nitrosamines. In: Hemminki, K., Dipple, A., Shuker, D.E.G., Kadlubar, F.F., Segerbäck, D. & Bartsch, H., eds, *DNA Adducts: Identification and Biological Significance* (IARC Scientific Publications No. 125), Lyon, IARC*Press*, pp. 91–106

Hecht, S.S., Chung, F.-L., Richie, J.P., Jr, Akerkar, S.A., Borukhova, A., Skowronski, L. & Carmella, S.G. (1995) Effects of watercress consumption on metabolism of a tobacco-specific lung carcinogen in smokers. *Cancer Epidemiol. Biomarkers Prev.*, **4**, 877–884

Hecht, S.S., Carmella, S.G., Chen, M., Dor Koch, J.F., Miller, A.T., Murphy, S.E., Jensen, J.A., Zimmerman, C.L. & Hatsukami, D.K. (1999a) Quantitation of urinary metabolites of a tobacco-specific lung carcinogen after smoking cessation. *Cancer Res.*, **59**, 590–596

Hecht, S.S., Hatsukami, D.K., Bonilla, L.E. & Hochalter, J.B. (1999b) Quantitation of 4-oxo-4-(3-pyridyl)butanoic acid and enantiomers of 4-hydroxy-4-(3-pyridyl)butanoic acid in human urine: A substantial pathway of nicotine metabolism. *Chem. Res. Toxicol.*, **12**, 172–179

Hecht, S.S., Hochalter, J.B., Villalta, P.W. & Murphy, S.E. (2000) 2′-Hydroxylation of nicotine by cytochrome P450 2A6 and human liver microsomes: Formation of a lung carcinogen precursor. *Proc. natl Acad. Sci. USA*, **97**, 12493–12497

Hecht, S.S., Ye, M., Carmella, S.G., Fredrickson, A., Adgate, J.L., Greaves, I.A., Church, T.R., Ryan, A.D., Mongin, S.J. & Sexton, K. (2001) Metabolites of a tobacco-specific lung carcinogen in the urine of elementary school-aged children. *Cancer Epidemiol. Biomarkers Prev.*, **10**, 1109–1116

Hecht, S.S., Carmella, S.G., Ye, M., Le, K.-A., Jensen, J.A., Zimmerman, C.L. & Hatsukami, D.K. (2002) Quantitation of metabolites of 4-(methylnitrosamino)-1-(3-pyridyl)-1-butanone after cessation of smokeless tobacco use. *Cancer Res.*, **62**, 129–134

Heikkilä, P., Luotamo, M., Pyy, L. & Riihimäki, V. (1995) Urinary 1-naphthol and 1-pyrenol as indicators of exposure to coal tar products. *Int. Arch. occup. environ. Health*, **67**, 211–217

Helander, A., Löwenmo, C., Wikström, T. & Curvall, M. (1991) Inhibition of human blood aldehyde dehydrogenase activity by cigarette-smoke condensate. *Life Sci.*, **49**, 1901–1905

Hernan, M.A., Takkouche, B., Caamano-Isorna, F. & Gestal-Otero, J.J. (2002) A meta-analysis of coffee drinking, cigarette smoking, and the risk of Parkinson's disease. *Ann. Neurol.*, **52**, 276–284

Hernandez-Boussard, T.M. & Hainaut, P. (1998) A specific spectrum of *p53* mutations in lung cancer from smokers: Review of mutations compiled in the IARC *p53* database. *Environ. Health Perspect.*, **106**, 385–391

Hess, R.D. & Brandner, G. (1996) DNA damage by filtered, tar-and aerosol-free cigarette smoke in rodent cells: A novel evaluation. *Toxicol. Lett.*, **88**, 9–13

Heudorf, U. & Angerer, J. (2001) Urinary monohydroxylated phenanthrenes and hydroxypyrene — The effects of smoking habits and changes induced by smoking on monooxygenase-mediated metabolism. *Int. Arch. occup. environ. Health*, **74**, 177–183

Heusch, W.L. & Maneckjee, R. (1998) Signalling pathways involved in nicotine regulation of apoptosis of human lung cancer cells. *Carcinogenesis*, **19**, 551–556

Hirao, T., Nelson, H.H., Ashok, T.D., Wain, J.C., Mark, E.J., Christiani, D.C., Wiencke, J.K. & Kelsey, K.T. (2001) Tobacco smoke-induced DNA damage and an early age of smoking initation induce chromosome loss at 3p21 in lung cancer. *Cancer Res.*, **61**, 612–615

Hittelman, W.N. (2001) Genetic instability in epithelial tissues at risk for cancer. *Ann. N.Y. Acad. Sci.*, **952**, 1–12

Hoffmann, K., Becker, K., Friedrich, C., Helm, D., Drause, C. & Seifert, B. (2000) The German Environmental Survey 1990/1992 (GerES II): Cadmium in blood, urine and hair of adults and children. *J. Expos. Anal. environ. Epidemiol.*, **10**, 126–135

Hoffmann, D., Hoffmann, I. & El-Bayoumy, K. (2001) The less harmful cigarette: A controversial issue. A tribute to Ernst L. Wynder. *Chem. Res. Toxicol.*, **14**, 767–790

Holly, E.A., Petrakis, N.L., Friend, N.F., Sarles, D.L., Lee, R.E. & Flander, L.B. (1986) Mutagenic mucus in the cervix of smokers. *J. natl Cancer Inst.*, **76**, 983–986

Holz, O., Krause, T., Scherer, G., Schmidt-Preuss, U. & Rüdiger, H.W. (1990) ^{32}P-Postlabelling analysis of DNA adducts in monocytes of smokers and passive smokers. *Int. Arch. occup. environ. Health*, **62**, 299–303

Holz, O., Meissner, R., Einhaus, M., Koops, F., Warncke, K., Scherer, G., Adlkofer, F., Baumgartner, E. & Rüdiger, H.W. (1993) Detection of DNA single-strand breaks in lymphocytes of smokers. *Int. Arch. occup. environ. Health*, **65**, 83–88

Hou, S.M., Yang, K., Nyberg, F., Hemminki, K., Pershagen, G. & Lambert, B. (1999) *Hprt* mutant frequency and aromatic DNA adduct level in non-smoking and smoking lung cancer patients and population controls. *Carcinogenesis*, **20**, 437–444

Hou, S.M., Fält, S., Yang, K., Nyberg, F., Pershagen, G., Hemminki, K. & Lambert, B. (2001) Differential interactions between *GSTM1* and *NAT2* genotypes on aromatic DNA adduct level and *HPRT* mutant frequency in lung cancer patients and population controls. *Cancer Epidemiol. Biomarkers Prev.*, **10**, 133–140

Hou, S.M., Fält, S., Angelini, S., Yang, K., Nyberg, F., Lambert, B. & Hemminki, K. (2002) The *XPD* variant alleles are associated with increased aromatic DNA adduct level and lung cancer risk. *Carcinogenesis*, **23**, 599–603

Howard, L.A., Micu, A.L., Sellers, E.M. & Tyndale, R.F. (2001) Low doses of nicotine and ethanol induce CYP2E1 and chlorzoxazone metabolism in rat liver. *J. Pharmacol. exp. Ther.*, **299**, 542–550

Hsu, T.M., Zhang, Y.-J. & Santella, R.M. (1997) Immunoperoxidase quantitation of 4-aminobiphenyl– and polycyclic aromatic hydrocarbon–DNA adducts in exfoliated oral and urothelial cells of smokers and nonsmokers. *Cancer Epidemiol. Biomarkers Prev.*, **6**, 193–199

Huang, Y.-L., Chuang, I.-C., Pan, C.-H., Hsieh, C., Shi, T.-S. & Lin, T.-H. (2000) Determination of chromium in whole blood and urine by graphite furnace AAS [atomic absorption spectroscopy]. *Atom. Spectroscop.*, **21**, 10–16

Hughes, E.G. & Brennan, B.G. (1996) Does cigarette smoking impair natural or assisted fecundity? *Fertil. Steril.*, **66**, 679–689

Hull, M.G., North, K., Taylor, H., Farrow, A. & Ford, W.C. (2000) Delayed conception and active and passive smoking. The Avon Longitudinal Study of Pregnancy and Childhood Study Team. *Fertil. Steril.*, **74**, 725–733

Hurt, R.D., Croghan, G.A., Wolter, T.D., Croghan, I.T., Offord, K.P., Williams, G.M., Djordjevic, M.V., Richie, J.P., Jr & Jeffrey, A.M. (2000) Does smoking reduction result in reduction of biomarkers associated with harm? A pilot study using a nicotine inhaler. *Nicotine Tob. Res.*, **2**, 327–336

Husgafvel-Pursiainen, K. (1987) Sister-chromatid exchange and cell proliferation in cultured lymphocytes of passively and actively smoking restaurant personnel. *Mutat. Res.*, **190**, 211–215

Husgafvel-Pursiainen, K., Hackman, P., Ridanpää, M., Anttila, S., Karjalainen, A., Partanen, T., Taikina-Aho, O., Heikkilä, L. & Vainio, H. (1993) K-*ras* mutations in human adenocarcinoma of the lung: Association with smoking and occupational exposure to asbestos. *Int. J. Cancer*, **53**, 250–256

Hussain, S.P., Hofseth, L.J. & Harris, C.C. (2001) Tumor suppressor genes: At the crossroads of molecular carcinogenesis, molecular epidemiology and human risk assessment. *Lung Cancer*, **34** (Suppl. 2), S7–S15

Husum, B, Wulf, H.C. & Niebuhr, E. (1986) Sister chromatid exchange frequency correlates with age, sex and cigarette smoking in a 5-year material of 553 healthy adults. *Hereditas*, **105**, 17–21

IARC (1972) *IARC Monographs on the Evaluation of Carcinogenic Risk of Chemicals to Man*, Vol. 1, *Some Inorganic Substances, Chlorinated Hydrocarbons, Aromatic Amines, N-Nitroso Compounds, and Natural Products*, Lyon, IARCPress, pp. 74–79

IARC (1974) *IARC Monographs on the Evaluation of Carcinogenic Risk of Chemicals to Man*, Vol. 4, *Some Aromatic Amines, Hydrazine and Related Substances, N-Nitroso Compounds and Miscellaneous Alkylating Agents*, Lyon, IARCPress, pp. 97–111

IARC (1978a) *IARC Monographs on the Evaluation of the Carcinogenic Risk of Chemicals to Humans*, Vol. 17, *Some N-Nitroso Compounds*, Lyon, IARCPress, pp. 125–175

IARC (1978b) *IARC Monographs on the Evaluation of the Carcinogenic Risk of Chemicals to Humans*, Vol. 17, *Some N-Nitroso Compounds*, Lyon, IARCPress, pp. 303–311

IARC (1978c) *IARC Monographs on the Evaluation of the Carcinogenic Risk of Chemicals to Humans*, Vol. 17, *Some N-Nitroso Compounds*, Lyon, IARCPress, pp. 327–335

IARC (1978d) *IARC Monographs on the Evaluation of the Carcinogenic Risk of Chemicals to Humans*, Vol. 17, *Some N-Nitroso Compounds*, Lyon, IARCPress, pp. 313–326

IARC (1979) *IARC Monographs on the Evaluation of the Carcinogenic Risks of Chemicals to Humans*, Vol. 19, *Some Monomers, Plastics and Synthetic Elastomers, and Acrolein*, Lyon, IARCPress, pp. 377–438

IARC (1980) *IARC Monographs on the Evaluation of the Carcinogenic Risk of Chemicals to Humans*, Vol. 23, *Some Metals and Metallic Compounds*, Lyon, IARCPress, pp. 325–415

IARC (1982) *IARC Monographs on the Evaluation of the Carcinogenic Risk of Chemicals to Humans*, Vol. 29, *Some Industrial Chemicals and Dyestuffs*, Lyon, IARCPress, pp. 93–148

IARC (1983a) *IARC Monographs on the Evaluation of the Carcinogenic Risk of Chemicals to Humans*, Vol. 32, *Polynuclear Aromatic Compounds, Part 1, Chemical, Environmental and Experimental Data*, Lyon, IARCPress, pp. 33–91, 211–224

IARC (1983b) *IARC Monographs on the Evaluation of the Carcinogenic Risk of Chemicals to Humans*, Vol. 32, *Polynuclear Aromatic Compounds, Part 1, Chemical, Environmental and Experimental Data*, Lyon, IARCPress, pp. 419–430

IARC (1983c) *IARC Monographs on the Evaluation of the Carcinogenic Risk of Chemicals to Humans*, Vol. 32, *Polynuclear Aromatic Compounds, Part 1, Chemical, Environmental and Experimental Data*, Lyon, IARCPress, pp. 431–445

IARC (1985a) IARC *Monographs on the Evaluation of the Carcinogenic Risk of Chemicals to Humans*, Vol. 37, *Tobacco Habits Other than Smoking; Betel-Quid and Areca-Nut Chewing; and Some Related Nitrosamines*, Lyon, IARCPress, pp. 209–223

IARC (1985b) IARC *Monographs on the Evaluation of the Carcinogenic Risk of Chemicals to Humans*, Vol. 37, *Tobacco Habits Other than Smoking; Betel-Quid and Areca-Nut Chewing; and Some Related Nitrosamines*, Lyon, IARCPress, pp. 241–261

IARC (1986) *IARC Monographs on the Evaluation of the Carcinogenic Risk of Chemicals to Humans*, Vol. 38, *Tobacco Smoking*, Lyon, IARCPress

IARC (1987) *IARC Monographs on the Evaluation of Carcinogenic Risks to Humans*, Suppl. 7, *Overall Evaluations of Carcinogenicity: An Updating of* IARC Monographs *Volumes 1 to 42*, Lyon, IARCPress

IARC (1990a) *IARC Monographs on the Evaluation of Carcinogenic Risks to Humans*, Vol. 49, *Chromium, Nickel and Welding*, Lyon, IARCPress, pp. 257–445

IARC (1990b) *IARC Monographs on the Evaluation of Carcinogenic Risks to Humans*, Vol. 49, *Chromium, Nickel and Welding*, Lyon, IARCPress, pp. 49–256

IARC (1993a) *IARC Monographs on the Evaluation of Carcinogenic Risks to Humans*, Vol. 56, *Some Naturally Occurring Substances: Food Items and Constituents, Heterocyclic Aromatic Amines and Mycotoxins*, Lyon, IARCPress, pp. 229–242

IARC (1993b) *Monographs on the Carcinogenic Risk of Chemicals to Humans*, Vol. 58, *Beryllium, Cadmium, Mercury, and Exposures in the Glass Manufacturing Industry*, Lyon, IARCPress, pp. 119–237

IARC (1994a) *IARC Monographs on the Evaluation of Carcinogenic Risks to Humans*, Vol. 60, *Some Industrial Chemicals*, Lyon, IARCPress, pp. 73–159

IARC (1994b) *IARC Monographs on the Evaluation of Carcinogenic Risks to Humans*, Vol. 60, *Some Industrial Chemicals*, Lyon, IARCPress, pp. 45–71

IARC (1995a) *IARC Monographs on the Evaluation of Carcinogenic Risks to Humans*, Vol. 63, *Dry Cleaning, Some Chlorinated Solvents and Other Industrial Chemicals*, Lyon, IARCPress, pp. 337–372

IARC (1995b) *IARC Monographs on the Evaluation of Carcinogenic Risks to Humans*, Vol. 62, *Wood Dust and Formaldehyde*, Lyon, IARCPress, pp. 217–362

IARC (1999a) *IARC Monographs on the Evaluation of Carcinogenic Risks to Humans*, Vol. 71, *Re-evaluation of Some Organic Chemicals, Hydrazine and Hydrogen Peroxide (Part Three)*, Lyon, IARCPress, pp. 1037–1047

IARC (1999b) *IARC Monographs on the Evaluation of Carcinogenic Risks to Humans*, Vol. 71, *Re-evaluation of Some Organic Chemicals, Hydrazine and Hydrogen Peroxide (Part Two)*, Lyon, IARCPress, pp. 319–335

IARC (1999c) *IARC Monographs on the Evaluation of Carcinogenic Risks to Humans*, Vol. 71, *Re-evaluation of Some Organic Chemicals, Hydrazine and Hydrogen Peroxide (Part Two)*, Lyon, IARC*Press*, pp. 749–768

IARC (1999d) *IARC Monographs on the Evaluation of Carcinogenic Risks to Humans*, Vol. 71, *Re-evaluation of Some Organic Chemicals, Hydrazine and Hydrogen Peroxide (Part Two)*, Lyon, IARC*Press*, pp. 691–719

IARC (1999e) *IARC Monographs on the Evaluation of Carcinogenic Risks to Humans*, Vol. 71, *Re-evaluation of Some Organic Chemicals, Hydrazine and Hydrogen Peroxide (Part Two)*, Lyon, IARC*Press*, pp. 433–451

IARC (1999f) *IARC Monographs on the Evaluation of Carcinogenic Risks to Humans*, Vol. 71, *Re-evaluation of Some Organic Chemicals, Hydrazine and Hydrogen Peroxide (Part One)*, Lyon, IARC*Press*, pp. 109–225

IARC (1999g) *IARC Monographs on the Evaluation of Carcinogenic Risks to Humans*, Vol. 73, *Some Chemicals that Cause Tumours of the Kidney or Urinary Bladder in Rodents and Some Other Substances*, Lyon, IARC*Press*, pp. 49–58

IARC (2000) *IARC Monographs on the Evaluation of Carcinogenic Risks to Humans*, Vol. 77, *Some Industrial Chemicals*, Lyon, IARC*Press*, pp. 267–322

IARC (2002) *IARC Monographs on the Evaluation of Carcinogenic Risks to Humans*, Vol. 82, *Some Traditional Herbal Medicines, Some Mycotoxins, Naphthalene and Styrene*, Lyon, IARC*Press*, pp. 367–435

Ichiba, M., Hagmar, L., Rannug, A., Hogstedt, B., Alexandrie, A.-K., Carstensen, U. & Hemminki, K. (1994) Aromatic DNA adducts, micronuclei and genetic polymorphism for *CYP1A1* and *GST1* in chimney sweeps. *Carcinogenesis*, **15**, 1347–1352

Inoue, O., Seiji, K., Kasahara, M., Nakatsuka, H., Watanabe, T., Yin, S.-G., Li, G.-L., Cai, S.-X., Jin, C. & Ikeda, M. (1988) Determination of catechol and quinol in the urine of workers exposed to benzene. *Br. J. ind. Med.*, **45**, 487–492

Inoue, O., Seiji, K., Nakatsuka, H., Watanabe, T., Yin, S.-N., Li, G.-L., Cai, S.-X., Jin, C. & Ikeda, M. (1989) Excretion of 1,2,4-benzenetriol in the urine of workers exposed to benzene. *Br. J. ind. Med.*, **46**, 559–565

Ishizaki, M., Yamada, Y., Morikawa, Y., Noborisaka, Y., Ishida, M., Miura, K. & Nakagawa, H. (1999) The relationship between waist-to-hip ratio and occupational status and life-style factors among middle-aged male and female Japanese workers. *Occup. Med.*, **49**, 177–182

Izzotti, A., Rossi, G.A., Bagnasco, M. & De Flora, S. (1991) Benzo[*a*]pyrene diolepoxide–DNA adducts in alveolar macrophages of smokers. *Carcinogenesis*, **12**, 1281–1285

Izzotti, A., Balansky, R.M., Coscia, N., Scatolini, L., D'Agostini, F. & De Flora, S. (1992) Chemoprevention of smoke-related DNA adduct formation in rat lung and heart. *Carcinogenesis*, **13**, 2187–2190

Izzotti, A., De Flora, S., Petrilli, G.L., Gallagher, J., Rojas, M., Alexandrov, K., Bartsch, H. & Lewtas, J. (1995a) Cancer biomarkers in human atherosclerotic lesions: Detection of DNA adducts. *Cancer Epidemiol. Biomarkers Prev.*, **4**, 105–110

Izzotti, A., Balansky, R., Scatolini, L., Rovida, A. & De Flora, S. (1995b) Inhibition by N-acetylcysteine of carcinogen–DNA adducts in the tracheal epithelium of rats exposed to cigarette smoke. *Carcinogenesis*, **16**, 669–672

Izzotti, A., Balansky, R.M., Blagoeva, P.M., Mircheva, Z.I., Tulimiero, L., Cartiglia, C. & De Flora, S. (1998) DNA alterations in rat organs after chronic exposure to cigarette smoke and/or ethanol ingestion. *FASEB J.*, **12**, 753–758

Jacob, J., Grimmer, G. & Dettbarn, G. (1999) Profile of urinary phenanthrene metabolites in smokers and nonsmokers. *Biomarkers*, **4**, 319–327

Jacobson, J.S., Begg, M.D., Wang, L.W., Wang, Q., Agarwal, M., Norkus, E., Singh, V.N., Young, T.L., Yang, D. & Santella, R.M. (2000) Effects of a 6-month vitamin intervention on DNA damage in heavy smokers. *Cancer Epidemiol. Biomarkers Prev.*, **9**, 1303–1311

Jahnke, G.D., Thompson, C.L., Walker, M.P., Gallagher, J.E., Lucier, G.W. & DiAugustine, R.P. (1990) Multiple DNA adducts in lymphocytes of smokers and nonsmokers determined by ^{32}P-postlabeling analysis. *Carcinogenesis*, **11**, 205–211

Jalili, T., Murthy, G.G. & Schiestl, R.H. (1998) Cigarette smoke induces DNA deletions in the mouse embryo. *Cancer Res.*, **58**, 2633–2638

Jansen, E.H.J.M., Schenk, E., den Engelsman, G. & van de Werken, G. (1995) Use of biomarkers in exposure assessment of polycyclic aromatic hydrocarbons. *Clin. Chem.*, **41**, 1905–1906

Janssen, J.A.M.J.L., Stolk, R.P., Pols, H.A.P., Grobbee, D.E. & Lamberts, S.W.J. (1998) Serum total IGF-I, free IGF-I, and IGFBP-1 levels in an elderly population. Relation to cardiovascular risk factors and disease. *Arterioscler. Thromb. vasc. Biol.*, **18**, 277–282

Jansson, T., Curvall, M., Hedin, A. & Enzell, C.R. (1986) In vitro studies of biological effects of cigarette smoke condensate. II. Induction of sister-chromatid exchanges in human lymphocytes by weakly acidic, semivolatile contituents. *Mutat. Res.*, **169**, 129–139

Jansson, T., Curvall, M., Hedin, A. & Enzell, C.R. (1988) In vitro studies of the biological effects of cigarette smoke condensate. III. Induction of SCE by some phenolic and related constituents derived from cigarette smoke. A study of structure–activity relationships. *Mutat. Res.*, **206**, 17–24

Jansson, A., Andersson, K., Bjelke, B., Eneroth, P. & Fuxe, K. (1992) Effects of a postnatal exposure to cigarette smoke on hypothalamic catecholamine nerve terminal systems and on neuroendocrine function in the postnatal and adult male rat. Evidence for long-term modulation of anterior pituitary function. *Acta physiol. scand.*, **144**, 453–462

Jarvis, M.J., Tunstall-Pedoe, H., Feyerabend, C., Vesey, C. & Saloojee, Y. (1987) Comparison of tests used to distinguish smokers from nonsmokers. *Am. J. public Health*, **77**, 1435–1438

Jarvis, M.J., Feyerabend, C., Bryant, A., Hedges, B. & Primatesta, P. (2001) Passive smoking in the home: Plasma cotinine concentrations in non-smokers with smoking partners. *Tob. Control*, **10**, 368–374

Jensen, J. & Christiansen, C. (1988) Effects of smoking on serum lipoproteins and bone mineral content during postmenopausal hormone replacement therapy. *Am. J. Obstet. Gynecol.*, **159**, 820–825

Jensen, J., Christiansen, C. & Rodbro, P. (1985) Cigarette smoking, serum estrogens, and bone loss during hormone-replacement therapy early after menopause. *New Engl. J. Med.*, **17**, 973–975

Jensen, T.K., Henriksen, T.B., Hjollund, N.H., Scheike, T., Kolstad, H., Giwercman, A., Ernst, E., Bonde, J.P., Skakkebaek, N.E. & Olsen, J. (1998) Adult and prenatal exposures to tobacco smoke as risk indicators of fertility among 430 Danish couples. *Am. J. Epidemiol.*, **148**, 992–997

Ji, Q. & Chen, Y. (1996) *Vicia faba* root tip micronucleus test on the mutagenicity of water-soluble contents of cigarette smoke. *Mutat. Res.*, **359**, 1–6

Jick, H., Porter, J. & Morrison, A.S. (1977) Relation between smoking and age of natural menopause. Report from the Boston Collaborative Drug Surveillance Program, Boston University Medical Center. *Lancet*, **i**, 1354–1355

Jin, Y.P., Kobayashi, E., Nogawa, K., Kido, T., Suwazono, Y., Sakurada, I., Yin, K.O., Nakagawa, H. & Tsuritani, I. (1997) Lead levels in 24-h urine in Japanese adults. *Toxicol. Lett.*, **92**, 173–178

Jo, W.-K. & Pack, K.-W. (2000) Utilization of breath analysis for exposure estimates of benzene associated with active smoking. *Environ. Res.*, **A 83**, 180–187

Jones, N.J., Kadhim, M.A., Hoskins, P.L., Parry, J.M. & Waters, R. (1991) ^{32}P-Postlabelling analysis and micronuclei induction in primary Chinese hamster lung cells exposed to tobacco particulate matter. *Carcinogenesis*, **12**, 1507–1514

Jones, N.J., McGregor, A.D. & Waters, R. (1993) Detection of DNA adducts in human oral tissue: Correlation of adduct levels with tobacco smoking and differential enhancement of adducts using the butanol extraction and nuclease P1 versions of ^{32}P postlabeling. *Cancer Res.*, **53**, 1522–1528

Jongen, W.M., Hakkert, B.C. & van der Hoeven, J.C. (1985) Genotoxicity testing of cigarette-smoke condensate in the SCE and HGPRT assays with V79 Chinese hamster cells. *Food Chem. Toxicol.*, **23**, 603–607

Jongeneelen, F.J. (1994) Biological monitoring of environmental exposure to polycyclic aromatic hydrocarbons; 1-hydroxypyrene in urine of people. *Toxicol. Lett.*, **72**, 205–211

Jongeneelen, F.J. (2001) Benchmark guideline for urinary 1-hydroxypyrene as biomarker of occupational exposure to polycyclic aromatic hydrocarbons. *Ann. occup. Hyg.*, **45**, 3–13

Jongeneelen, F.J., Anzion, R.B.M., Leijdekkers, C.M., Bos, R.P. & Henderson, P.T. (1985) 1-Hydroxypyrene in human urine after exposure to coal tar and a coal tar derived product. *Int. Arch. occup. environ. Health*, **57**, 47–55

Joschko, M.A., Dreosti, I.E. & Tulsi, R.S. (1991) The teratogenic effects of nicotine in vitro in rats: A light and electron microscope study. *Neurotoxicol. Teratol.*, **13**, 307–316

Jull, B.A., Plummer, H.K., III & Schuller, H.M. (2001) Nicotinic receptor-mediated activation by the tobacco-specific nitrosamine NNK of a Raf-1/MAP kinase pathway, resulting in phosphorylation of c-myc in human small cell lung carcinoma cells and pulmonary neuroendocrine cells. *J. Cancer Res. clin. Oncol.*, **127**, 707–717

Kaaks, R., Toniolo, P., Akhmedkhanov, A., Lukanova, A., Biessy, C., Dechaud, H., Rinaldi, S., Zeleniuch-Jacquotte, A., Shore, R.E. & Riboli, E. (2000) Serum C-peptide, insulin-like growth factor (IGF)-I, IGF-binding proteins and colorectal cancer risk in women. *J. natl Cancer Inst.*, **92**, 1592–1600

Kadlubar, F.F. (1994) DNA adducts of carcinogenic aromatic amines. In: Hemminki, K., Dipple, A., Shuker, D.E.G., Kadlubar, F.F., Segerbäck, D. & Bartsch, H., eds, *DNA Adducts, Identification and Biological Significance* (IARC Scientific Publications No. 125), Lyon, IARC*Press*, pp. 199–216

Kadlubar, F.F. & Beland, F.A. (1985) Chemical properties of ultimate carcinogenic metabolites of arylamines and arylamides. In: Harvey, R.G., ed., *Polycyclic Hydrocarbons and Carcinogenesis* (ACS Symposium Series 283), Washington DC, American Chemical Society, pp. 341–370

Kado, N.Y., Langley, D. & Eisenstadt, E. (1983) A simple modification of the *Salmonella*, liquid incubation assay. *Mutat. Res.*, **121**, 25–32

Kado, N.Y., Manson, C., Eisenstadt, E. & Hsieh, D.P. (1985) The kinetics of mutagen excretion in the urine of cigarette smokers. *Mutat. Res.*, **157**, 227–233

Kadohama, N., Shintani, K. & Osawa, Y. (1993) Tobacco alkaloid derivatives as inhibitors of breast cancer aromatase. *Cancer Lett.*, **75**, 175–182

Kaklamani, V.G., Linos, A., Kaklamani, E., Markaki, I. & Mantzoros, C. (1999) Age, sex, and smoking are predictors of circulating insulin-like growth factor 1 and insulin-like growth factor-binding protein 3. *J. clin. Oncol.*, **17**, 813–817

Kalra, R., Singh, S.P., Savage, S.M., Finch, G.L. & Sopori, M.L. (2000) Effects of cigarette smoke on immune response: Chronic exposure to cigarette smoke impairs antigen-mediated signaling in T cells and depletes IP3-sensitive Ca²⁺ stores. *J. Pharmacol. exp. Ther.*, **293**, 166–171

Kanaoka, T., Miyakawa, M. & Yoshida, O. (1990) [Study on influence of cigarette smoking on the mutagenicity of urine. 1. Influence of cigarette smoking on the mutagenicity of urine in health smokers and bladder cancer patients.] *Acta. urol. jpn.*, **36**, 385–393 (in Japanese)

Kang, M.K. & Park, N.H. (2001) Conversion of normal to malignant phenotype: Telomere shortening, telomerase activation, and genomic instability during immortalization of human oral keratinocytes. *Crit. Rev. oral Biol. Med.*, **12**, 38–54

Kao-Shan, C.-S., Fine, R.L., Whang-Peng, J., Lee, E.C. & Chabner, B.A. (1987) Increased fragile sites and sister chromatid exchanges in bone marrow and peripheral blood of young cigarette smokers. *Cancer Res.*, **47**, 6278–6282

Karube, T., Odagiri, Y., Takemoto, K. & Watanabe, S. (1989) Analyses of transplacentally induced sister chromatid exchanges and micronuclei in mouse fetal liver cells following maternal exposure to cigarette smoke. *Cancer Res.*, **49**, 3550–3552

Kasai, H., Iwamoto-Tanaka, N., Miyamoto, T., Kawanami, K., Kawanami, S., Kido, R. & Ikeda, M. (2001) Life style and urinary 8-hydroxydeoxyguanosine, a marker of oxidative DNA damage: Effects of exercise, working conditions, meat intake, body mass index, and smoking. *Jpn J. Cancer Res.*, **92**, 9–15

Kato, I., Tominaga, S. & Suzuki, T. (1988) Factors related to late menopause and early menarche as risk factors for breast cancer. *Jpn. J. Cancer Res.*, **79**, 165–172

Kato, S., Bowman, E.D., Harrington, A.M., Blomeke, B. & Shields, P.G. (1995) Human lung carcinogen–DNA adduct levels mediated by genetic polymorphisms *in vivo*. *J. natl Cancer Inst.*, **87**, 902–907

Kato, I., Toniolo, P., Akhmedkhanov, A., Koenig, K.L., Shore, R. & Zeleniuch-Jacquotte, A. (1998) Prospective study of factors influencing the onset of natural menopause. *J. clin. Epidemiol.*, **51**, 1271–1276

Kaufman, D.W., Slone, D., Rosenberg, L., Miettinen, O.S. & Shapiro, S. (1980) Cigarette smoking and age at natural menopause. *Am. J. public Health*, **70**, 420–422

Kaur, J., Srivastava, A. & Ralhan, R. (1998) Prognostic significance of p53 protein overexpression in betel- and tobacco-related oral oncogenesis. *Int. J. Cancer*, **79**, 370–375

Kawakami, N., Takatsuka, N., Shimizu, H. & Ishibashi, H. (1997) Effects of smoking on the incidence of non-insulin-dependent diabetes mellitus. Replication and extension in a Japanese cohort of male employees. *Am. J. Epidemiol.*, **145**, 103–109

Kelsey, K.T., Wiencke, J.K., Little, F.F., Baker, E.L., Jr & Little, J.B. (1988) Effects of cigarette smoking and solvent exposure on sister chromatid exchange frequency in painters. *Environ. mol. Mutag.*, **11**, 389–399

Kharitonov, S.A., Robbins, R.A., Yates, D., Keatings, V. & Barnes, P.J. (1995) Acute and chronic effects of cigarette smoking on exhaled nitric oxide. *Am. J. respir. crit. Care Med.*, **152**, 609–612

Kidd, L.C., Stillwell, W.G., Yu, M.C., Wishnok, J.S., Skipper, P.L., Ross, R.K., Henderson, B.E. & Tannenbaum, S.R. (1999) Urinary excretion of 2-amino-1-methyl-6-phenylimidazo[4,5-*b*]-pyridine (PhIP) in white, African-American, and Asian-American men in Los Angeles County. *Cancer Epidemiol. Biomarkers Prev.*, **8**, 439–445

Kim, S.Y., Chung, J.H., Kang, K.W., Joe, C.O. & Park, K.H. (1992) Relationship between activities of cytochrome P-450 monooxygenases in human placental microsomes and binding of benzo(a)pyrene metabolites to calf thymus DNA. *Drug chem. Toxicol.*, **15**, 313–327

Kim, H., Kim, Y.-D., Lee, H., Kawamoto, T., Yang, M. & Katoh, T. (1999) Assay of 2-naphthol in human urine by high-performance liquid chromatography. *J. Chromatogr.*, **B734**, 211–217

Kim, D.-H., Nelson, H.H., Wiencke, J.K., Christiani, D.C., Wain, J.C., Mark, E.J. & Kelsey, K.T. (2001) Promoter methylation of DAP-kinase: Association with advanced stage in non-small cell lung cancer. *Oncogene*, **20**, 1765–1770

Kim, H., Cho, S.-H., Kang, J.-W., Kim, Y.-D., Nan, H.-M., Lee, C.-H., Lee, H. & Kawamoto, T. (2001) Urinary 1-hydroxypyrene and 2-naphthol concentrations in male Koreans. *Int. Arch. occup. environ. Health*, **74**, 59–62

King, M.M., Hollingsworth, A., Cuzick, J. & Garner, R.C. (1994) The detection of adducts in human cervix tissue DNA using ^{32}P-postlabelling: A study of the relationship with smoking history and oral contraceptive use. *Carcinogenesis*, **15**, 1097–1100

Kitagawa, K., Kunugita, N., Katoh, T., Yang, M. & Kawamoto, T. (1999) The significance of the homozygous *CYP2A6* deletion on nicotine metabolism: A new genotyping method of *CYP2A6* using a single PCR–RFLP. *Biochem. biophys. Res. Commun.*, **262**, 146–151

Kivistö, H., Pekari, K., Peltonen, K., Svinhufvud, J., Veidebaum, T., Sorsa, M. & Aitio, A. (1997) Biological monitoring of exposure to benzene in the production of benzene and in a cokery. *Sci. total Environ.*, **199**, 49–63

Kiyosawa, H., Suko, M., Okudaira, H., Murata, K., Miyamoto, T., Chung, M.-H., Kasai, H. & Nishimura, S. (1990) Cigarette smoking induces formation of 8-hydroxydeoxyguanosine, one of the oxidative DNA damages in human peripheral leukocytes. *Free Radic. Res. Commun.*, **11**, 23–27

Klesges, R.C., Meyers, A.W., Klesges, L.M. & La Vasque, M.E. (1989) Smoking, body weight, and their effects on smoking behavior: A comprehensive review of the literature. *Psychol. Bull.*, **106**, 204–230

Kopplin, A., Eberle-Adamkiewicz, G., Glüsenkamp, K.-H., Nehls, P. & Kirstein, U. (1995) Urinary excretion of 3-methyladenine and 3-ethyladenine after controlled exposure to tobacco smoke. *Carcinogenesis*, **16**, 2637–2641

Kriebel, D., Henry, J., Gold, J.C., Bronsdson, A. & Commoner, B. (1985) The mutagenicity of cigarette smokers' urine. *J. environ. Pathol. Toxicol. Oncol.*, **6**, 157–169

Kriek, E., Rojas, M., Alexandrov, K. & Bartsch, H. (1998) Polycyclic aromatic hydrocarbon–DNA adducts in humans: Relevance as biomarkers for exposure and cancer risk. *Mutat. Res.*, **400**, 215–231

Krokan, H., Grafstrom, R.C., Sundqvist, K., Esterbauer, H. & Harris, C.C. (1985) Cytotoxicity, thiol depletion and inhibition of O^6-methylguanine–DNA methyltransferase by various aldehydes in cultured human bronchial fibroblasts. *Carcinogenesis*, **6**, 1755–1759

Kuenemann-Migeot, C., Callais, F., Momas, I. & Festy, B. (1996) Urinary promutagens of smokers: Comparison of concentration methods and relation to cigarette consumption. *Mutat. Res.*, **368**, 141–147

Kulkarni, J.R., Sarkar, S. & Bhide, S.V. (1987) Mutagenicity of extracts of brown and black masheri, pyrolysed products of tobacco using short-term tests. *Mutagenesis*, **2**, 263–266

Kulp, K.S., Knize, M.G., Malfatti, M.A., Salmon, C.P. & Felton, J.S. (2000) Identification of urine metabolites of 2-amino-1-methyl-6- phenylimidazo[4,5-*b*]pyridine following consumption of a single cooked chicken meal in humans. *Carcinogenesis*, **21**, 2065–2072

Kwon, J.T., Nakajima, M., Chai, S., Yom, Y.K., Kim, H.K., Yamazaki, H., Sohn, D.R., Yamamoto, T., Kuroiwa, Y. & Yokoi, T. (2001) Nicotine metabolism and CYP2A6 allele frequencies in Koreans. *Pharmacogenetics*, **11**, 317–323

Lafi, A. & Parry, J.M. (1988) Cytogenetic activities of tobacco particulate matter (TPM) derived from a low to middle tar British cigarette. *Mutat. Res.*, **201**, 365–374

Lähdetie, J., Engström, K., Husgafvel-Pursiainen, K., Nylund, L., Vainio, H. & Sorsa, J. (1993) Maternal smoking induced cotinine levels and genotoxicity in second trimester amniotic fluid. *Mutat. Res.*, **300**, 37–43

Landin-Wilhelmsen, K., Wilhelmsen, L., Lappas, G., Rosen, T., Lindstedt, G., Lundberg, P.A. & Bengtsson, B.A. (1994) Serum insulin-like growth factor I in a random population sample of men and women: Relation to age, sex, smoking habits, coffee consumption and physical activity, blood pressure and concentrations of plasma lipids, fibrinogen, parathyroid hormone and osteocalcin. *Clin. Endocrinol.*, **4**, 351–357

Larramendy, M.L. & Knuutila, S. (1991) Increased frequency of micronuclei in B and T8 lymphocytes from smokers. *Mutat. Res.*, **259**, 189–195

LaRue, H., Allard, P., Simoneau, M., Normand, C., Pfister, C., Moore, L., Meyer, F., Têtu, B. & Fradet, Y. (2000) P53 point mutations in initial superficial bladder cancer occur only in tumors from current or recent cigarette smokers. *Carcinogenesis*, **21**, 101–106

Lauwerys, R.R., Buchet, J.P. & Andrien, F. (1994) Muconic acid in urine: A reliable indicator of occupational exposure to benzene. *Am. J. ind. Med.*, **25**, 297–300

LaVoie, E.J., Adams, J.D., Reinhardt, J., Rivenson, A. & Hoffmann, D. (1986) Toxicity studies on clove cigarette smoke and constituents of clove: Determination of the LD_{50} of eugenol by intratracheal instillation in rats and hamsters. *Arch. Toxicol.*, **59**, 78–81

Law, M.R. & Hackshaw, A.K. (1997) A meta-analysis of cigarette smoking, bone mineral density and risk of hip fracture: Recognition of a major effect. *Br. med. J.*, **315**, 841–846

Law, M.R., Cheng, R., Hackshaw, A.K., Allaway, S. & Hale, A.K. (1997) Cigarette smoking, sex hormones and bone density in women. *Eur. J. Epidemiol.*, **13**, 553–558

Lazutka, J.R., Dedonyte, V. & Krapavickaite, D. (1994) Sister-chromatid exchanges and their distribution in human lymphocytes in relation to age, sex and smoking. *Mutat. Res.*, **306**, 173–180

Leanderson, P. (1993) Cigarette smoke-induced DNA damage in cultured human lung cells. *Ann. N.Y. Acad. Sci.*, **686**, 249–259, 259–261

Leanderson, P. & Tagesson, C. (1990) Cigarette smoke-induced DNA-damage: Role of hydroquinone and catechol in the formation of the oxidative DNA–adduct, 8-hydroxydeoxyguanosine. *Chem.-biol. Interact.*, **75**, 71–81

Leanderson, P. & Tagesson, C. (1994) Cigarette tar promotes neutrophil-induced DNA damage in cultured lung cells. *Environ. Res.*, **64**, 103–111

Lechner, J.F., Neft, R.E., Gilliland, F.D., Crowell, R.E. & Belinsky, S.A. (1997) Molecular identification of individuals at high risk for lung cancer. *Radiat. oncol. Inves.*, **5**, 103–105

Lee, C.K., Brown, B.G., Rice, W.Y., Jr & Doolittle, D.J. (1989) Role of oxygen free radicals in the induction of sister chromatid exchanges by cigarette smoke. *Environ. mol. Mutag.*, **13**, 54–59

Lee, C.K., Brown, B.G., Reed, E.A., Lowe, G.D., McKarns, S.C., Fulp, C.W., Coggins, C.R., Ayres, P.H. & Doolittle, D.J. (1990a) Analysis of cytogenetic effects in bone-marrow cells of rats subchronically exposed to smoke from cigarettes which burn or only heat tobacco. *Mutat. Res.*, **240**, 251–257

Lee, C.K., Doolittle, D.J., Burger, G.T. & Hayes, A.W. (1990b) Comparative genotoxicity testing of mainstream whole smoke from cigarettes which burn or heat tobacco. *Mutat. Res.*, **242**, 37–45

Lee, C.K., Brown, B.G., Reed, B.A., Rahn, C.A., Coggins, C.R., Doolittle, D.J. & Hayes, A.W. (1992) Fourteen-day inhalation study in rats, using aged and diluted sidestream smoke from a reference cigarette. *Fundam. appl. Toxicol.*, **19**, 141–146

Lee, B.L., New, A.L., Kok, P.W., Ong, H.Y., Shi, C.Y. & Ong, C.N. (1993) Urinary *trans,trans-*muconic acid determined by liquid chromatography: Application in biological monitoring of benzene exposure. *Clin. Chem.*, **39**, 1788–1792

Lee, C.K., Brown, B.G., Reed, E.A., Coggins, C.R., Doolittle, D.J. & Hayes, A.W. (1993) Ninety-day inhalation study in rats, using aged and diluted sidestream smoke from a reference cigarette: DNA adducts and alveolar macrophage cytogenetics. *Fundam. appl. Toxicol.*, **20**, 393–401

Le Houezec, J. & Benowitz, N.L. (1991) Basic and clinical psychopharmacology of nicotine. *Clin. Chest. Med.*, **12**, 681–699

Le Houezec, J., Martin, C., Cohen, C. & Molimard, R. (1989) Failure of behavioral dependence induction and oral nicotine biovailability in rats. *Physiol. Behav.*, **45**, 103–108

Lemasters, G.K., Livingston, G.K., Lockey, J.E., Olsen, D.M., Shukla, R., New, G., Selevan, S.G. & Yiin, J.H. (1997) Genotoxic changes after low-level solvent and fuel exposure on aircraft maintenance personnel. *Mutagenesis*, **12**, 237–243

Levin, J.O. (1995) First international workshop on hydroxypyrene as a biomarker for PAH exposure in man — Summary and conclusions. *Sci. total Environ.*, **163**, 165–168

Leyden, D.E., Leitner, E. & Siegmund, B. (1999) Determination of nicotine in pharmaceutical products and dietary sources. In: Gorrod, J.W. & Jacob, P., III, eds, *Analytical Determination of Nicotine and Related Compounds and Their Metabolites*, New York, Elsevier

Li, D., Wang, M., Dhingra, K. & Hittelman, W.N. (1996) Aromatic DNA adducts in adjacent tissues of breast cancer patients: Clues to breast cancer etiology. *Cancer Res.*, **56**, 287–293

Li, H., Krieger, R.I. & Li, Q.X. (2000) Improved HPLC method for analysis of 1-hydroxypyrene in human urine specimens of cigarette smokers. *Sci. total Environ.*, **257**, 147–153

Li, L., Ruan, Y., Chen, Y., Chu, Y. & Xu, X. (2002) [The role of transforming growth factor-beta(1) in smoking-induced chronic bronchitis and emphysema in hamsters.] *Zhonghua Jie He He Hu Xi Za Zhi*, **25**, 284–286 (in Chinese)

Linert, W., Bridge, M.H., Huber, M., Bjugstad, K.B., Grossman, S. & Arendash, G.W. (1999) In-vitro and in-vivo studies investigating possible antioxidant actions of nicotine: Relevance to Parkinson's and Alzheimer's diseases. *Biochim. biophys. Acta*, **1454**, 143–152

Lipkin, M. & Newmark, H.L. (1999) Vitamin D, calcium and prevention of breast cancer: A review. *J. Am. Coll. Nutr.*, **18** (Suppl. 5), 392–397

Lippman, S.M., Peters, E.J., Wargovich, M.J., Stadnyk, A.N., Dixon, D.O., Dekmezian, R.H., Loewy, J.W., Morice, R.C., Cunningham, J.E. & Hong, W.K. (1990) Broncial micronuclei as a marker of an early stage of carcinogenesis in the human tracheobronchial epithelium. *Int. J. Cancer*, **45**, 811–815

Littlefield, L.G. & Joiner, E.E. (1986) Analysis of chromosome aberrations in lymphocytes of long-term heavy smokers. *Mutat. Res.*, **170**, 145–150

Liu, X., Lu, J. & Liu, S. (1999) Synergistic induction of hydroxyl radical-induced DNA single-strand breaks by chromium (VI) compound and cigarette smoke solution. *Mutat. Res.*, **440**, 109–117

Liu, Y., Egyhazi, S., Hansson, J., Bhide, S.V., Kulkarni, P.S. & Grafström, R.C. (1997) O^6-Methyl-guanine–DNA methyltransferase activity in human buccal mucosal tissue and cell cultures. Complex mixtures related to habitual use of tobacco and betel quid inhibit the activity *in vitro*. *Carcinogenesis*, **18**, 1889–1895

Lodovici, M., Akpan, V., Giovannini, L., Migliani, F. & Dolara, P. (1998) Benzo[*a*]pyrene diol-epoxide DNA adducts and levels of polycyclic aromatic hydrocarbons in autoptic samples from human lungs. *Chem.-biol. Interact.*, **116**, 199–212

Loechler, E.L., Green, C.L. & Essigmann, J.M. (1984) In-vivo mutagenesis by O^6-methylguanine built into a unique site in a viral genome. *Proc. natl Acad. Sci. USA*, **81**, 6271–6275

Loennechen, J.P., Beisvag, V., Arbo, I., Waldum, H.L., Sandvik, A.K., Knardahl, S. & Ellingsen, O. (1999) Chronic carbon monoxide exposure in vivo induces myocardial endothelin-1 expression and hypertrophy in rat. *Pharmacol. Toxicol.*, **85**, 192–197

Loft, S. & Poulsen, H.E. (1998) Estimation of oxidative DNA damage in man from urinary excretion of repair products. *Acta biochim. polon.*, **45**, 133–144

Loft, S., Vistisen, K., Ewertz, M., Tjonneland, A., Overvad, K. & Poulsen, H.E. (1992) Oxidative DNA damage estimated by 8-hydroxydeoxyguanosine excretion in humans: Influence of smoking, gender and body mass index. *Carcinogenesis*, **13**, 2241–2247

Longcope, C. & Johnston, C.C., Jr (1988) Androgen and estrogen dynamics in pre- and postmeno-pausal women: A comparison between smokers and nonsmokers. *J. clin. Endocrinol. Metab.*, **67**, 379–383

Lucero, J., Harlow, B.L., Barbieri, R.L., Sluss, P. & Cramer, D.W. (2001) Early follicular phase hormone levels in relation to patterns of alcohol, tobacco, and coffee use. *Fertil. Steril.*, **76**, 723–729

Lukanova, A., Toniolo, P., Akhmedkhanov, A., Hunt, K., Rinaldi, S., Zeleniuch-Jacquotte, A., Haley, N.J., Riboli, E., Stattin, P., Lundin, E. & Kaaks, R. (2001) A cross-sectional study of IGF-1 determinants in women. *Eur. J. Cancer Prev.*, **10**, 443–452

Luoto, R., Kaprio, J. & Uutela, A. (1994) Age at natural menopause and sociodemographic status in Finland. *Am. J. Epidemiol.*, **139**, 64–76

Ma, L., Chow, J.Y. & Cho, C.H. (1998) Effects of cigarette smoking on gastric ulcer formation and healing: Possible mechanisms of action. *J. clin. Gastroenterol.*, **27** (Suppl. 1), S80–S86

Ma, J., Pollak, M.N., Giovannucci, E., Chan, J.M., Tao, Y., Hennekens, C.H. & Stampfer, M.J. (1999) Prospective study of colorectal cancer risk in men and plasma levels of insulin-like growth factor (IGF)-I and IGF-binding protein-3. *J. natl Cancer Inst.*, **91**, 620–625

van Maanen, J.M.S., Welle, I.J., Hageman, G., Dallinga, J.W., Mertens, P.L.J.M. & Kleinjans, J.C.S. (1996) Nitrate contamination of drinking water: Relationship with *HPRT* variant frequency in lymphocyte DNA and urinary excretion of *N*-nitrosamines. *Environ. Health Perspect.*, **104**, 522–528

Mackenzie, P.I., Miners, J.O. & McKinnon, R.A. (2000) Polymorphisms in UDP glucuronosyltransferase genes: Functional consequences and clinical relevance. *Clin. Chem. Lab. Med.*, **38**, 889–892

Maclure, M., Katz, R.B.-A., Bryant, M.S., Skipper, P.L. & Tannenbaum, S.R. (1989) Elevated blood levels of carcinogens in passive smokers. *Am. J. public Health*, **79**, 1381–1384

Maclure, M., Bryant, M.S., Skipper, P.L. & Tannenbaum, S.R. (1990) Decline of the hemoglobin adduct of 4-aminobiphenyl during withdrawal from smoking. *Cancer Res.*, **50**, 181–184

Maestrelli, P., Saetta, M., Mapp, C.E. & Fabbri, L.M. (2001) Remodeling in response to infection and injury. Airway inflammation and hypersecretion of mucus in smoking subjects with chronic obstructive pulmonary disease. *Am. J. respir. crit. Care Med.*, **164**, S76–S80

Maggio, R., Riva, M., Vaglini, F., Fornai, F., Molteni, R., Armogida, M., Racagni, G. & Corsini, G.U. (1998) Nicotine prevents experimental parkinsonism in rodents and induces striatal increase of neurotrophic factors. *J. Neurochem.*, **71**, 2439–2446

Mahimkar, M.B. & Bhisey, R.A. (1995) Occupational exposure to bidi tobacco increases chromosomal aberrations in tobacco processors. *Mutat. Res.*, **334**, 139–144

Malaveille, C., Vineis, P., Estève, J., Ohshima, H., Brun, G., Hautefeuille, A., Gallet, P., Ronco, G., Terracini, B. & Bartsch, H. (1989) Levels of mutagens in the urine of smokers of black and blond tobacco correlate with their risk of bladder cancer. *Carcinogenesis*, **10**, 577–586

Malin, D.H. (2001) Nicotine dependence. Studies with a laboratory model. *Pharmacol. Biochem. Behav.*, **70**, 551–559

Manchester, D.K. & Jacoby, E.H. (1981) Sensitivity of human placental monooxygenase activity to maternal smoking. *Clin. Pharmacol. Ther.*, **30**, 687–692

Manchester, D.K., Weston, A., Choi, J.-S., Trivers, G.E., Fennessey, P.V., Quintana, E., Farmer, P.B., Mann, D.L. & Harris, C.C. (1988) Detection of benzo[*a*]pyrene diol epoxide–DNA adducts in human placenta. *Proc. natl Acad. Sci. USA*, **85**, 9243–9247

Manchester, D.K., Wilson, V.L., Hsu, I.-C., Choi, J.S., Parker, N.B., Mann, D.L., Weston, A. & Harris, C.C. (1990) Synchronous fluorescence spectroscopic, immunoaffinity chromatographic and ^{32}P-postlabeling analysis of human placental DNA known to contain benzo[*a*]pyrene diol epoxide adducts. *Carcinogenesis*, **11**, 553–559

Manchester, D.K., Bowman, E.D., Parker, N.B., Caporaso, N.E. & Weston, A. (1992) Determinants of polycyclic aromatic hydrocarbon–DNA adducts in human placenta. *Cancer Res.*, **52**, 1499–1503

Mancini, R., Romano, G., Sgambato, A., Flamini, G., Giovagnoli, M.R., Boninsegna, A., Carraro, C., Vecchione, A. & Cittadini, A. (1999) Polycyclic aromatic hydrocarbon–DNA adducts in cervical smears of smokers and nonsmokers. *Gynecol. Oncol.*, **75**, 68–71

Manson, J.E., Ajani, U.A., Liu, S., Nathan, D.M. & Hennekens, C.H. (2000) A prospective study of cigarette smoking and the incidence of diabetes mellitus among US male physicians. *Am. J. Med.*, **109**, 538–542

Manson, J.M., Sammel, M.D., Freeman, E.W. & Grisso, J.A. (2001) Racial differences in sex hormone levels in women approaching the transition to menopause. *Fertil. Steril.*, **75**, 297–304

Mao, L., Lee, J.S., Kurie, J.M., Fan, Y.H., Lippman, S.M., Lee, J.J., Ro, J.Y., Broxson, A., Yu, R., Morice, R.C., Kemp, B.L., Khuri, F.R., Walsh, G.L., Hittelman, W.N. & Hong, W.K. (1997)

Clonal genetic alterations in the lungs of current and former smokers. *J. natl. Cancer Inst.*, **89**, 834–836

March, T.H., Barr, E.B., Finch, G.L., Hahn, F.F., Hobbs, C.H., Menache, M.G. & Nikula, K.J. (1999) Cigarette smoke exposure produces more evidence of emphysema in B6C3F1 mice than in F344 rats. *Toxicol. Sci.*, **51**, 289–290

Marchetti, A., Pelligrini, S., Sozzi, G., Bertacca, G., Gaeta, P., Buttitta, F., Carnicelli, V., Griseri, P., Chella, A., Angeletti, C.A., Pierotti, M. & Bevilacqua, G. (1998) Genetic analysis of lung tumours of non-smoking subjects: p53 Gene mutations are constantly associated with loss of heterozygosity at the FHIT locus. *Br. J. Cancer*, **78**, 73–78

Martinez, M.E. & Willett, W.C. (1998) Calcium, vitamin D, and colorectal cancer: A review of the epidemiologic evidence. *Cancer Epidemiol. Biomarkers Prev.*, **7**, 163–168

Marubio, L.M. & Changeux, J.-P. (2000) Nicotinic acetylcholine receptor knockout mice as animal models for studying receptor function. *Eur. J. Pharmacol.*, **393**, 113–121

Mascher, D.G., Mascher, H.J., Scherer, G. & Schmid, E.R. (2001) High-performance liquid chromatographic–tandem mass spectrometric determination of 3-hydroxypropylmercapturic acid in human urine. *J. Chromatogr.*, **B750**, 163–169

Massey, E., Aufderheide, M., Koch, W., Lodding, H., Pohlmann, G., Windt, H., Jarck, P. & Knebel, J.W. (1998) Micronucleus induction in V79 cells after direct exposure to whole cigarette smoke. *Mutagenesis*, **13**, 145–149

Matikainen, T., Perez, G.I., Jurisicova, A., Pru, J.K., Schlezinger, J.J., Ryu, H.-Y., Laine, J., Sakai, T., Korsmeyer, S.J., Capser, R.F., Sherr, D.H. & Tilly, J.L. (2001) Aromatic hydrocarbon receptor-driven *Bax* gene expression is required for premature ovarian failure caused by biohazardous environmental chemicals. *Nat. Genet.*, **28**, 355–360

Matsukura, N., Willey, J., Miyashita, M., Taffe, B., Hoffmann, D., Waldren, C., Puck, T.T. & Harris, C.C. (1991) Detection of direct mutagenicity of cigarette smoke condensate in mammalian cells. *Carcinogenesis*, **12**, 685–689

Mattison, D.R. (1982) The effects of smoking on fertility from gametogenesis to implantation. *Environ. Res.*, **28**, 410–433

Mattison, D.R. & Thorgeirsson, S.S. (1978) Smoking and industrial pollution, and their effects on menopause and ovarian cancer. *Lancet*, **i**, 187–188

Matullo, G., Palli, D., Peluso, M., Guarrera, S., Carturan, S., Celentano, E., Krogh, V., Munnia, A., Tumino, R., Polidoro, S., Piazza, A. & Vineis, P. (2001) *XRCC1*, *XRCC3*, *XPD* gene polymorphisms, smoking and ^{32}P–DNA adducts in a sample of healthy subjects. *Carcinogenesis*, **22**, 1437–1445

Mauderly, J.L., Chen, B.T., Hahn, F.F., Lundgren, D.L., Cuddihy, R.G., Namenyi, J. & Rebar, A.H. (1989) The effect of chronic cigarette smoke inhalation on the long-term pulmonary clearance of inhaled particles in the rat. In: Wehner, A.P., ed., *Biological Interaction of Inhaled Mineral Fibers and Cigarette Smoke*, Columbus, OH, Battelle Press, pp. 223–239

McFadden, D., Wright, J.L., Wiggs, B. & Churg, A. (1986) Smoking inhibits asbestos clearance. *Am. Rev. respir. Dis.*, **133**, 372–374

McKinlay, S.M., Bifano, N.L. & McKinlay, J.B. (1985) Smoking and age at menopause in women. *Ann. intern. Med.*, **103**, 350–356

Meger, M., Meger-Kossien, I., Dietrich, M., Tricker, A.R., Scherer, G. & Adlkofer, F. (1996) Metabolites of 4-(*N*-methylnitrosamino)-1-(3-pyridyl)-1-butanone in urine of smokers. *Eur. J. Cancer Prev.*, **5** (Suppl. 1), 121–124

Meger, M., Meger-Kossien, I., Riedel, K. & Scherer, G. (2000) Biomonitoring of environmental tobacco smoke (ETS)-related exposure to 4-(methylnitrosamino)-1-(3-pyridyl)-1-butanone (NNK). *Biomarkers*, **5**, 33–45

Melikian, A.A., Prahalad, A.K. & Hoffmann, D. (1993) Urinary trans,trans-muconic acid as an indicator of exposure to benzene in cigarette smokers. *Cancer Epidemiol. Biomarkers Prev.*, **2**, 47–51

Melikian, A.A., Prahalad, A.K. & Secker-Walker, R.H. (1994) Comparison of the levels of the urinary benzene metabolite trans,trans-muconic acid in smokers and nonsmokers, and the effects of pregnancy. *Cancer Epidemiol. Biomarkers Prev.*, **3**, 239–244

Melikian, A.A., Sun, P., Pierpont, C., Coleman, S. & Hecht, S.S. (1997) Gas chromatographic–mass spectrometric determination of benzo[a]pyrene and chrysene diol epoxide globin adducts in humans. *Cancer Epidemiol. Biomarkers Prev.*, **6**, 833–839

Melikian, A.A., Sun, P., Prokopczyk, B., El-Bayoumy, K., Hoffmann, D., Wang, X. & Waggoner, S. (1999) Identification of benzo[a]pyrene metabolites in cervical mucus and DNA adducts in cervical tissues in humans by gas chromatography–mass spectrometry. *Cancer Lett.*, **146**, 127–134

Mellstrom, D., Johansson, C., Johnell, O., Lindstedt, G., Lundberg, P.A., Obrant, K., Schoon, I.M., Toss, G. & Ytterberg, B.O. (1993) Osteoporosis, metabolic aberrations, and increased risk for vertebral fractures after partial gastrectomy. *Calcif. Tissue int.*, **53**, 370–377

Memisoglu, A. & Samson, L. (2000) Base excision repair in yeast and mammals. *Mutat. Res.*, **451**, 39–51

Merchant, C., Tang, M.X., Albert, S., Manly, J., Stern, Y. & Mayeux, R. (1999) The influence of smoking on the risk of Alzheimer's disease. *Neurology*, **52**, 1408–1412

Merlo, F., Andreassen, Å., Weston, A., Pan, C.-F., Haugen, A., Valerio, F., Reggiardo, G., Fontana, V., Garte, S., Puntoni, R. & Abbondandolo, A. (1998) Urinary excretion of 1-hydroxypyrene as a marker for exposure to urban air levels of polycyclic aromatic hydrocarbons. *Cancer Epidemiol. Biomarkers Prev.*, **7**, 147–155

Meschia, M., Pansini, F., Modena, A.B., de Aloysio, D., Gambacciani, M., Parazzini, F., Campagnoli, C., Maiocchi, G. & Peruzzi, E. (2000) Determinants of age at menopause in Italy: Results from a large cross-sectional study. ICARUS Study Group. Italian Climacteric Research Group Study. *Maturitas*, **34**, 119–125

Messina, E.S., Tyndale, R.F. & Sellers, E.M. (1997) A major role for CYP2A6 in nicotine C-oxidation by human liver microsomes. *J. Pharmacol. exp Ther.*, **282**, 1608–1614

Michnovicz, J.J., Hershcopf, R.J., Naganuma, H., Bradlow, H.L. & Fishman, J. (1986) Increased 2-hydroxylation of estradiol as a possible mechanism for the anti-estrogenic effect of cigarette smoking. *New Engl. J. Med.*, **315**, 1305–1309

Michnovicz, J.J., Naganuma, H., Hershcopf, R.J., Bradlow, H.L. & Fishman, J. (1988) Increased urinary catechol estrogen excretion in female smokers. *Steroids*, **52**, 69–83

Midgette, A.S. & Baron, J.A. (1990) Cigarette smoking and the risk of natural menopause. *Epidemiology*, **1**, 474–480

Minoia, C., Apostoli, P., Maranelli, G., Baldi, C., Pozzoli, L. & Capodaglio, E. (1988) Urinary chromium levels in subjects living in two north Italy regions. *Sci. total Environ.*, **71**, 527–531

Miyaura, S., Eguchi, H. & Johnston, J.M. (1992) Effect of a cigarette smoke extract on the metabolism of the proinflammatory autacoid, platelet-activating factor. *Circ. Res.*, **70**, 341–347

Modan, M., Meytes, D., Rozeman, P., Yosef, S.B., Sehayek, E., Yosef, N.B., Lusky, A. & Halkin, H. (1988) Significance of high HbA1 levels in normal glucose tolerance. *Diabetes Care*, **11**, 422–428

Mohtashamipur, E., Norpoth, K. & Straeter, H. (1987) Clastogenic effect of passive smoking on bone marrow polychromatic erythrocytes of NMRI mice. *Toxicol. Lett.*, **35**, 153–156

Mohtashamipur, E., Steinforth, T. & Norpoth, K. (1988) Comparative bone marrow clastogenicity of cigarette sidestream, mainstream and recombined smoke condensates in mice. *Mutagenesis*, **3**, 419–422

Molarius, A., Seidell, J.C., Kuulasmaa, K., Dobsen, A.J. & Sans, S. (1997) Smoking and relative body weight: An international perspective from the WHO MONICA Project. *J. Epidemiol. Community Health*, **51**, 252–260

Mollerup, S., Ryberg, D., Hewer, A., Phillips, D.H. & Haugen, A. (1999) Sex differences in lung *CYP1A1* expression and DNA adduct levels among lung cancer patients. *Cancer Res.*, **59**, 3317–3320

Mooney, L.A., Santella, R.M., Covey, L., Jeffrey, A.M., Bigbee, W., Randall, M.C., Cooper, T.B., Ottman, R., Tsai, W.Y., Wazneh, L., Glassman, A.H., Young, T.-L. & Perera, F.P. (1995) Decline of DNA damage and other biomarkers in peripheral blood following smoking cessation. *Cancer Epidemiol. Biomarkers Prev.*, **4**, 627–634

Mooney, L.A., Bell, D.A., Santella, R.M., Van Bennekum, A.M., Ottman, R., Paik, M., Blaner, W.S., Lucier, G.W., Covey, L., Young, T.L., Cooper, T.B., Glassman, A.H. & Perera, F.P. (1997) Contribution of genetic and nutritional factors to DNA damage in heavy smokers. *Carcinogenesis*, **18**, 503–509

Moorman, A.V., Roman, E., Cartwright, R.A. & Morgan, G.J. (2002) Smoking and the risk of acute myeloid leukaemia in cytogenetic subgroups. *Br. J. Cancer*, **86**, 60–62

Morabia, A., Bernstein, M.S., Curtin, F. & Berode, M. (2001) Validation of self-reported smoking status by simultaneous measurement of carbon monoxide and salivary thiocyanate. *Prev. Med.*, **32**, 82–88

Mori, Y., Iimura, K., Furukawa, F., Nishikawa, A., Takahashi, M. & Konishi, Y. (1995) Effect of cigarette smoke on the mutagenic activation of various carcinogens in hamster. *Mutat. Res.*, **346**, 1–8

Morimoto, T., Nakaya, K., Sugitani, A., Yamada, F. & Imai, J. (1977) Studies on the influence of environmental pollution with heavy metals on human health. IV. Nickel and chromium contents in human urine. *Gifu-Ken Eisei Kenkyusho Ho*, **22**, 13–17

Morin, R.S., Tulis, J.J. & Claxton, L.D. (1987) The effect of solvent and extraction methods on the bacterial mutagenicity of sidestream cigarette smoke. *Toxicol. Lett.*, **38**, 279–290

Mostafa, M.H., Helmi, S., Badawi, A.F., Tricker, A.R., Spiegelhalder, B. & Preussmann, R. (1994) Nitrate, nitrite and volatile *N*-nitroso compounds in the urine of *Schistosoma haematobium* and *Schistosoma mansoni* infected patients. *Carcinogenesis*, **15**, 619–625

Motykiewicz, G., Malusecka, E., Michalska, J., Kalinowska, E., Wloch, J., Butkiewicz, D., Mazurek, A., Lange, D., Perera, F.P. & Santella, R.M. (2001) Immunoperoxidase detection of polycyclic aromatic hydrocarbon–DNA adducts in breast tissue sections. *Cancer Detect. Prev.*, **25**, 328–335

Moxham, J. (2000) Nicotine addiction. *Br. med. J.*, **320**, 391–392

Müller, M., Krämer, A., Angerer, J. & Hallier, E. (1998) Ethylene oxide–protein adduct formation in humans: Influence of glutathione-*S*-transferase polymorphisms. *Int. Arch. occup. environ. Health,* **71**, 499–502

Mumford, J.L., Li, X., Hu, F., Lu, X.B. & Chuang, J.C. (1995) Human exposure and dosimetry of polycyclic aromatic hydrocarbons in urine from Xuan Wei, China with high lung cancer mortality associated with exposure to unvented coal smoke. *Carcinogenesis,* **16**, 3031–3036

Muranaka, H., Higashi, E., Itani, S. & Shimizu, Y. (1988) Evaluation of nicotine, cotinine, thiocyanate, carboxyhemoglobin, and expired carbon monoxide as biochemical tobacco smoke uptake parameters. *Int. Arch. occup. environ. Health,* **60**, 37–41

Mure, K., Hayatsu, H., Takeuchi, T., Takeshita, T. & Morimoto, K. (1997) Heavy cigarette smokers show higher mutagenicity in urine. *Mutat. Res.,* **373**, 107–111

Murthy, M.K., Bhargava, M.K. & Augustus, M. (1997) Sister chromatid exchange studies in oral cancer patients. *Indian J. Cancer,* **34**, 49–58

Mustonen, R. & Hemminki, K. (1992) 7-Methylguanine levels in DNA of smokers' and nonsmokers' total white blood cells, granulocytes and lymphocytes. *Carcinogenesis,* **13**, 1951–1955

Mustonen, R., Schoket, B. & Hemminki, K. (1993) Smoking-related DNA adducts: ^{32}P-Postlabeling analysis of 7-methylguanine in human bronchial and lymphocyte DNA. *Carcinogenesis,* **14**, 151–154

Myers, S.R., Spinnato, J.A., Pinorini-Godly, M.T., Cook, C., Boles, B. & Rodgers, G.C. (1996) Characterization of 4-aminobiphenyl–hemoglobin adducts in maternal and fetal blood samples. *J. Toxicol. environ. Health,* **47**, 553–566

Nagaya, T. & Toriumi, H. (1985) Effects of smoking on spontaneous and induced sister chromatid exchanges in lymphocytes. *Toxicol. Lett.,* **25**, 293–296

Nakajima, M., Yamamoto, T., Nunoya, K.-I., Yokoi, T., Nagashima, K., Inoue, K., Funae, Y., Shimada, N., Kamataki, T. & Kuroiwa, Y. (1996) Role of human cytochrome P4502A6 in *C*-oxidation of nicotine. *Drug Metab. Dispos.,* **24,** 1212–1217

Nakajima, M., Yamagishi, S.-I., Yamamoto, H., Yamamoto, T., Kuroiwa, Y. & Yokoi, T. (2000) Deficient cotinine formation from nicotine is attributed to the whole deletion of the *CYP2A6* gene in humans. *Clin. Pharmacol. Ther.,* **67**, 57–69

Nakajima, M., Kwon, J.-T., Tanaka, N., Zenta, T., Yamamoto, Y., Yamamoto, H., Yamazaki, H., Yamamoto, T., Kuroiwa, Y. & Yokoi, T. (2001) Relationship between interindividual differences in nicotine metabolism and *CYP2A6* genetic polymorphism in humans. *Clin. Pharmacol. Ther.,* **69**, 72–78

Nakayama, T., Kaneko, M., Kodama, M. & Nagata, C. (1985) Cigarette smoke induces DNA single-strand breaks in human cells. *Nature,* **314**, 462–464

Nan, H.-M., Kim, H., Lim, H.-S., Choi, J.K., Kawamoto, T., Kang, J.-W., Lee, C.-H., Kim, Y.-D. & Kwon, E.H. (2001) Effects of occupation, lifestyle and genetic polymorphisms of CYP1A1, CYP2E1, GSTM1 and GSTT1 on urinary 1-hydroxypyrene and 2-naphthol concentrations. *Carcinogenesis,* **22**, 787–793

Nath, R.G., Ocando, J.E., Guttenplan, J.B. & Chung, F.L. (1998) 1,N^2-Propanodeoxyguanosine adducts: Potential new biomarkers of smoking-induced DNA damage in human oral tissue. *Cancer Res.,* **58**, 581–584

National Research Council (1986) *Environmental Tobacco Smoke. Measuring Exposures and Assessing Health Effects*, Washington DC, National Academy Press

Need, A.G., Kemp, A., Giles, N., Morris, H.A., Horowitz, M. & Nordin, B.E. (2002) Relationships between intestinal calcium absorption, serum vitamin D metabolites and smoking in post-menopausal women. *Osteoporos. int.*, **13**, 83–88

Nersessian, A.K. & Arutyunyan, R.M. (1994) The comparative clastogenic activity of mainstream tobacco smoke from cigarettes widely consumed in Armenia. *Mutat. Res.*, **321**, 89–92

Nerurkar, P.V., Okinaka, L., Aoki, C., Seifried, A., Lum-Jones, A., Wilkens, L.R. & Le Marchand, L. (2000) *CYP1A1*, *GSTM1*, and *GSTP1* genetic polymorphisms and urinary 1-hydroxypyrene excretion in non-occupationally exposed individuals. *Cancer Epidemiol. Biomarkers Prev.*, **9**, 1119–1122

Newman, M.G., Lindsay, M.K. & Graves, W. (2001) Cigarette smoking and pre-eclampsia: Their association and effects on clinical outcomes. *J. matern. fetal Med.*, **10**, 166–170

Nguyen, H., Finkelstein, E., Reznick, A., Cross, C. & van der Vliet, A. (2001). Cigarette smoke impairs neutrophil respiratory burst activation by aldehyde-induced thiol modifications. *Toxicology*, **160**, 207–217

Nilsson, P.M., Lind, L., Pollare, T., Berne, C. & Lithell, H.O. (1995) Increased level of hemoglobin A1c, but not impaired insulin sensitivity, found in hypertensive and normotensive smokers. *Metabolism*, **44**, 557–561

Nishio, E. & Watanabe, Y. (1997) Cigarette smoke extract inhibits plasma paraoxonase activity by modification of the enzyme's free thiols. *Biochem. biophys. Res. Commun.*, **236**, 289–293

Norbury, C.J. & Hickson, I.D. (2001) Cellular responses to DNA damage. *Ann. Rev. Pharmacol. Toxicol.*, **41**, 367–401

Nordic Study Group on the Health Risk of Chromosome Damage (1990) A Nordic data base on somatic chromosome damage in humans. *Mutat. Res.*, **241**, 325–337

Nunoya, K., Yokoi, T., Takahashi, Y., Kimura, K., Kinoshita, M. & Kamataki, T. (1999) Homologous unequal cross-over within the human *CYP2A* gene cluster as a mechanism for the deletion of the entire *CYP2A6* gene associated with the poor metabolizer phenotype. *J. Biochem. (Tokyo)*, **126**, 402–407

Nylander, G. & Berg, K. (1991) Mutagenicity study of urine from smoking and non-smoking road tanker drivers. *Int. Arch. occup. environ. Health*, **63**, 229–232

Obe, G., ed. (1984) *Mutations in Man*, Berlin, Springer

Ogushi, F., Hubbard, R.C., Vogelmeier, C., Fells, G.A. & Crystal, R.G. (1991) Risk factors for emphysema. Cigarette smoking is associated with a reduction in the association rate constant of lung α_1-antitrypsin for neutrophil elastase. *J. clin. Invest.*, **87**, 1060–1065

O'Hara, P., Connett, J.E., Lee, W.W., Nides, M., Murray, R. & Wise, R. (1998) Early and late weight gain following smoking cessation in the Lung Health Study. *Am. J. Epidemiol.*, **148**, 821–830

Ohshima, H. & Bartsch, H. (1981) Quantitative estimation of endogenous nitrosation in humans by monitoring *N*-nitrosoproline excreted in the urine. *Cancer Res.*, **41**, 3658–3662

Okonofua, F.E., Lawal, A. & Bamgbose, J.K. (1990) Features of menopause and menopausal age in Nigerian women. *Int. J. Gynecol. Obstet.*, **31**, 341–345

Ong, T.-M., Stewart, J., Wen, Y.-F. & Whong, W.-Z. (1987) Application of SOS *umu*-test for the detection of genotoxic volatile chemicals and air pollutants. *Environ. Mutag.*, **9**, 171–176

Ong, C.N., Lee, B.L., Shi, C.Y., Ong, H.Y. & Lee, H.P. (1994) Elevated levels of benzene-related compounds in the urine of cigarette smokers. *Int. J. Cancer*, **59**, 177–180

Ong, C.N., Kok, P.W., Lee, B.L., Shi, C.Y., Ong, H.Y., Chia, K.S., Lee, C.S. & Luo, X.W. (1995) Evaluation of biomarkers for occupational exposure to benzene. *Occup. environ. Med.*, **52**, 528–533

Ong, C.N., Kok, P.W., Ong, H.Y., Shi, C.Y., Lee, B.L., Phoon, W.H. & Tan, K.T. (1996) Biomarkers of exposure to low concentrations of benzene: A field assessment. *Occup. environ. Med.*, **53**, 328–333

Ortego-Centeno, N., Muñoz-Torres, M., Hernandez-Quero, J., Jurado-Duce, A. & de la Higuera Torres-Puchol, J. (1994) Bone mineral density, sex steroids, and mineral metabolism in premenopausal smokers. *Calcif. Tissue int.*, **55**, 403–407

Oscarson, M., Gullstén, H., Rautio, A., Bernal, M.L., Sinues, B., Dahl, M.-L., Stengård, J.H., Pelkonen, O., Raunio, H. & Ingelman-Sundberg, M. (1998) Genotyping of human cytochrome P450 2A6 (CYP2A6), a nicotine *C*-oxidase. *FEBS Lett.*, **438**, 201–205

Oscarson, M., McLellan, R.A., Gullstén, H., Agúndez, J.A., Benítez, J., Rautio, A., Raunio, H., Pelkonen, O. & Ingelman-Sundberg, M. (1999) Identification and characterisation of novel polymorphisms in the *CYP2A* locus: Implications for nicotine metabolism. *FEBS Lett.*, **460**, 321–327

Osterman-Golkar, S.M., MacNeela, J.P., Turner, M.J., Walker, V.E., Swenberg, J.A., Sumner, S.J., Youtsey, N. & Fennell, T.R. (1994) Monitoring exposure to acrylonitrile using adducts with *N*-terminal valine in hemoglobin. *Carcinogenesis*, **15**, 2701–2707

Pachinger, A., Begutter, H., Ultsch, I. & Klus, H. (1993) Determination of 4-(methylnitrosamino)-4-(3-pyridyl)-butyric acid in tobacco, tobacco smoke and the urine of rats and smokers. *J. Chromatogr.*, **620**, 55–60

Parazzini, F., Negri, E. & La Vecchia, C. (1992) Reproductive and general lifestyle determinants of age at menopause. *Maturitas*, **15**, 141–149

Parsons, W.D., Carmella, S.G., Akerkar, S., Bonilla, L.E. & Hecht, S.S. (1998) A metabolite of the tobacco-specific lung carcinogen 4-(methylnitrosamino)-1-(3-pyridyl)-1-butanone (NNK) in the urine of hospital workers exposed to environmental tobacco smoke. *Cancer Epidemiol. Biomarkers Prev.*, **7**, 257–260

Paschal, D.C., Burt, V., Caudill, S.P., Gunter, E.W., Pirkle, J.L., Sampson, E.J., Miller, D.T. & Jackson, R.J. (2000) Exposure of the US population aged 6 years and older to cadmium: 1988–1994. *Arch. environ. Contam. Toxicol.*, **38**, 377–383

Pasquini, R., Scassellati Sforzolini, G., Savino, A., Angeli, G. & Monarca, S. (1987) Enzyme induction in rat lung and liver by condensates and fractions from main-stream and side-stream cigarette smoke. *Environ. Res.*, **44**, 302–311

Pastorelli, R., Guanci, M., Cerri, A., Negri, E., La Vecchia, C., Fumagalli, F., Mezzetti, M., Cappelli, R., Panigalli, T., Fanelli, R. & Airoldi, L. (1998) Impact of inherited polymorphisms in glutathione *S*-transferase M1, microsomal epoxide hydrolase, cytochrome P450 enzymes on DNA, and blood protein adducts of benzo(*a*)pyrene-diolepoxide. *Cancer Epidemiol. Biomarkers Prev.*, **7**, 703–709

Pastorelli, R., Guanci, M., Restano, J., Berri, A., Micoli, G., Minoia, C., Alcini, D., Carrer, P., Negri, E., La Vecchia, C., Fanelli, R. & Airoldi, L. (1999) Seasonal effect on airborne pyrene, urinary 1-hydroxypyrene, and benzo(a)pyrene diol epoxide–hemoglobin adducts in the general population. *Cancer Epidemiol. Biomarkers Prev.*, **8**, 561–565

Pavanello, S., Favretto, D., Brugnone, F., Mastrangelo, G., Dal Pra, G. & Clonfero, E. (1999). HPLC/fluorescence determination of *anti*-BPDE–DNA adducts in mononuclear white blood cells from PAH-exposed humans. *Carcinogenesis*, **20**, 431–435

Paz-y-Miño, C., Pérez, J.C., Dávalos, V., Sánchez, M.E. & Leone, P.E. (2001) Telomeric associations in cigarette smokers exposed to low levels of X-rays. *Mutat. Res.*, **490**, 77–80

Pegg, A.E. (2000) Repair of O^6-alkylguanine by alkyltransferases. *Mutat. Res.*, **462**, 83–100

Peluso, M., Amasio, E., Bonassi, S., Munnia, A., Altrupa, F. & Parodi, S. (1997) Detection of DNA adducts in human nasal mucosa tissue by ^{32}P-postlabeling analysis. *Carcinogenesis*, **18**, 339–344

Peluso, M., Airoldi, L., Magagnotti, C., Fiorini, L., Munnia, A., Hautefeuille, A., Malaveille, C. & Vineis, P. (2000) White blood cell DNA adducts and fruit and vegetable consumption in bladder cancer. *Carcinogenesis*, **21**, 183–187

Perera, F.P., Santella, R.M., Brenner, D., Poirier, M.C., Munshi, A.A., Fischman, H.K. & Van Ryzin, J. (1987) DNA adducts, protein adducts, and sister chromatid exchange in cigarette smokers and nonsmokers. *J. natl Cancer Inst.*, **79**, 449–456

Perera, F., Mayer, J., Jaretzki, A., Hearne, S., Brenner, D., Young, T.L., Fischman, H.K., Grimes, M., Grantham, S., Tang, M.X., Tsai, W.-Y. & Santella, R.M. (1989) Comparison of DNA adducts and sister chromatid exchange in lung cancer cases and controls. *Cancer Res.*, **49**, 4446–4451

Perera, F.P., Estabrook, A., Hewer, A., Channing, K., Rundle, A., Mooney, L.A., Whyatt, R. & Phillips, D.H. (1995) Carcinogen–DNA adducts in human breast tissue. *Cancer Epidemiol. Biomarkers Prev.*, **4**, 233–238

Pérez-Stable, E.J., Herrera, B., Jacob, P., III & Benowitz, N.L. (1998) Nicotine metabolism and intake in black and white smokers. *J. Am. med. Assoc.*, **280**, 152–156

Perkins, K.A. (1993) Weight gain following smoking cessation. *J. consult. clin. Psychol.*, **61**, 768–777

Persson, M.G., Zetterström, O., Agrenius, V., Ihre, E. & Gustafsson, L.E. (1994) Single-breath nitric oxide measurements in asthmatic patients and smokers. *Lancet*, **343**, 146–147

Petruzzelli, S., Franchi, M., Gronchi, L., Janni, A., Oesch, F., Pacifici, G.M. & Giuntini, C. (1992) Cigarette smoke inhibits cytosolic but not microsomal epoxide hydrolase of human lung. *Hum. exp. Toxicol.*, **11**, 99–103

Petruzzelli, S., Tavanti, L.M., Celi, A. & Giuntini, C. (1996) Detection of N^7-methyldeoxyguanosine adducts in human pulmonary alveolar cells. *Am. J. respir. Cell mol. Biol.*, **15**, 216–223

Petruzzelli, S., Celi, A., Pulerà, N., Baliva, F., Viegi, G., Carrozzi, L., Ciacchini, G., Bottai, M., Di Pede, F., Paoletti, P. & Giuntini, C. (1998) Serum antibodies to benzo(*a*)pyrene diol epoxide–DNA adducts in the general population: Effects of air pollution, tobacco smoking, and family history of lung diseases. *Cancer Res.*, **58**, 4122–4126

Pezzagno, G., Maestri, L. & Fiorentino, M.L. (1999) trans,trans-Muconic acid, a biological indicator to low levels of environmental benzene: Some aspects of its specificity. *Am. J. ind. Med.*, **35**, 511–518

Phillips, D.H. (1996) DNA adducts in human tissues: Biomarkers of exposure to carcinogens in tobacco smoke. *Environ. Health Perspect.*, **104** (Suppl 3), 453–458

Phillips, D.H. (1997) Detection of DNA modifications by the ^{32}P-postlabelling assay. *Mutat. Res.*, **378**, 1–12

Phillips, D.H. & Farmer, P.B. (1995) Protein and DNA adducts as biomarkers of exposure to environmental mutagens. In: Phillips, D.H. & Venitt, S., eds, *Environmental Mutagenesis*, Oxford, Bioscience, pp. 367–395

Phillips, D.H. & Hewer, A. (1993) DNA adducts in human urinary bladder and other tissues. *Environ. Health Perspect.*, **99**, 45–49

Phillips, D.H. & Ni She, M. (1993) Smoking-related DNA adducts in human cervical biopsies. In: Phillips, D.H., Castegnaro, M. & Bartsch, H., eds, *Postlabelling Methods for Detection of DNA Adducts* (IARC Scientific Publications No. 124), Lyon, IARC*Press*, pp. 327–330

Phillips, D. H. & Ni She, M. (1994) DNA adducts in cervical tissue of smokers and nonsmokers. *Mutat. Res.*, **313**, 277–284

Phillips, D.H., Hewer, A., Martin, C.N., Garner, R.C. & King, M.M. (1988) Correlation of DNA adduct levels in human lung with cigarette smoking. *Nature*, **336**, 790–792

Phillips, D.H., Schoket, B., Hewer, A., Bailey, E., Kostic, S. & Vincze, I. (1990a) Influence of cigarette smoking on the levels of DNA adducts in human bronchial epithelium and white blood cells. *Int. J. Cancer*, **46**, 569–575

Phillips, D.H., Hewer, A., Malcolm, A.D., Ward, P. & Coleman, D.V. (1990b) Smoking and DNA damage in cervical cells (Letter to the Editor). *Lancet*, **335**, 417

Pianezza, M.L., Sellers, E.M. & Tyndale, R.F. (1998) Nicotine metabolism defect reduces smoking. *Nature*, **393**, 750

Picciotto, M.R., Caldarone, B.J., King, S.L. & Zachariou, V. (2000) Nicotinic receptors in the brain: Links between molecular biology and behavior. *Neuropsychopharmacology*, **22**, 451–465

Pickworth, W.B., Moolchan, E.T., Berlin, I. & Murty, R. (2002) Sensory and physiologic effects of menthol and nonmenthol cigarettes with different nicotine delivery. *Pharmacol. Biochem. Behav.*, **71**, 55–61

Pietilä, K. & Ahtee, L. (2000) Chronic nicotine administration in the drinking water affects the striatal dopamine in mice. *Pharmacol. Biochem. Behav.*, **66**, 95–103

Pignatelli, B., Li, C.-Q., Boffetta, P., Chen, Q., Ahrens, W., Nyberg, F., Mukera, A., Bruske-Holfeld, I., Fortes, C., Constantinescu, V., Ischiropoulos, H. & Oshima, H. (2001) Nitrated and oxidized plasma proteins in smokers and lung cancer patients. *Cancer Res.*, **61**, 778–784

Piipari, R., Savela, K., Nurminen, T., Hukkanen, J., Raunio, H., Hakkola, J., Mantyla, T., Beaune, P., Edwards, R.J., Boobis, A.R. & Anttila, S. (2000) Expression of CYP1A1, CYP1B1 and CYP3A, and polycyclic aromatic hydrocarbon–DNA adduct formation in bronchoalveolar macrophages of smokers and nonsmokers. *Int. J. Cancer*, **86**, 610–616

Pilger, A., Germadnik, D., Riedel, K., Meger-Kossien, I., Scherer, G. & Rüdiger, H.W. (2001) Longitudinal study of urinary 8-hydroxy-2'-deoxyguanosine excretion in healthy adults. *Free Radic. Res.*, **35**, 273–280

Piperakis, S.M., Visvardis, E.-E., Sagnou, M. & Tassiou, A.M. (1998) Effects of smoking and aging on oxidative DNA damage of human lymphocytes. *Carcinogenesis*, **19**, 695–698

Pirkle, J.L., Flegal, K.M., Bernert, J.T., Brody, D.J., Etzel, R.A. & Maurer, K.R. (1996) Exposure of the US population to environmental tobacco smoke: The Third National Health and Nutrition Examination Survey, 1988 to 1991. *J. Am. med. Assoc.*, **275**, 1233–1240

Pluth, J.M., Ramsey, M.J. & Tucker, J.D. (2000) Role of maternal exposures and newborn genotypes on newborn chromosome aberration frequencies. *Mutat. Res.*, **465**, 101–111

Podlutsky, A., Hou, S.-M., Nyberg, F., Pershagen, G. & Lambert, B. (1999) Influence of smoking and donor age on the spectrum of in vivo mutation at the *HPRT*-locus in T lymphocytes of healthy adults. *Mutat. Res.*, **431**, 325–339

Poirier, M.C., Santella, R.M. & Weston, A. (2000) Carcinogen macromolecular adducts and their measurement. *Carcinogenesis*, **21**, 353–359

Polek, T.C. & Weigel, N.L. (2002) Vitamin D and prostate cancer. *J. Androl.*, **23**, 9–17

Poli, P., Buschini, A., Spaggiari, A., Rizzoli, V., Carlo-Stella, C. & Rossi, C. (1999) DNA damage by tobacco smoke and some antiblastic drugs evaluated using the Comet assay. *Toxicol. Lett.*, **108**, 267–276

Popp, W., Schell, C., Kraus, R., Vahrenholz, C., Wolf, R., Radtke, J., Bierwirth, K. & Norpoth, K. (1993) DNA strand breakage and DNA adducts in lymphocytes of oral cancer patients. *Carcinogenesis*, **14**, 2251–2256

Potts, R.J., Newbury, C.J., Smith, G., Notarianni, L.J. & Jefferies, T.M. (1999) Sperm chromatin damage associated with male smoking. *Mutat. Res.*, **423**, 103–111

Pourcelot, S., Faure, H., Firoozi, F., Ducros, V., Tripier, M., Hee, J., Cadet, J. & Favier, A. (1999) Urinary 8-oxo-7,8-dihydro-2′-deoxyguanosine and 5-(hydroxymethyl)uracil in smokers. *Free Radic. Res.*, **30**, 173–180

Pressl, S., Edwards, A. & Stephan, G. (1999) The influence of age, sex and smoking habits on the background level of FISH-detected translocations. *Mutat. Res.*, **442**, 89–95

Preussmann, R. & Stewart, B.W. (1984) *N*-Nitroso carcinogens. In: Searle, C.E., ed., *Chemical Carcinogens*, Vol. 2, 2nd Ed. (ACS Monograph 182), Washington DC, American Chemical Society, pp. 643–828

Prévost, V. & Shuker, D.E. (1996) Cigarette smoking and urinary 3-alkyladenine excretion in man. *Chem. Res. Toxicol.*, **9**, 439–444

Prévost, V., Shuker, D.E.G., Friesen, M.D., Eberle, G., Rajewsky, M.F. & Bartsch, H. (1993) Immunoaffinity purification and gas chromatography–mass spectrometric quantification of 3-alkyladenines in urine: Metabolism studies and basal excretion levels in man. *Carcinogenesis*, **14**, 199–204

Priemé, H., Loft, S., Kharlund, M., Grønbæk, K., Tønnesen, P. & Poulsen, H.E. (1998) Effect of smoking cessation on oxidative DNA modification estimated by 8-oxo-7,8-dihydro-2′-deoxyguanosine excretion. *Carcinogenesis*, **19**, 347–351

Probst-Hensch, N.M., Bell, D.A., Watson, M.A., Skipper, P.L., Tannenbaum, S.R., Chan, K.K., Ross, R.K. & Yu, M.C. (2000) *N*-Acetyltransferase 2 phenotype but not *NAT1*10* genotype affects aminobiphenyl–hemoglobin adduct levels. *Cancer Epidemiol. Biomarkers Prev.*, **9**, 619–623

Probst-Hensch, N.M., Yuan, J.M., Stanczyk, F.Z., Gao, Y.T., Ross, R.K. & Yu, M.C. (2001) IGF-1, IGF-2 and IGFBP-3 in prediagnostic serum: Association with colorectal cancer in a cohort of Chinese men in Shanghai. *Br. J. Cancer*, **85**, 1695–1699

Prokopczyk, B., Cox, J.E., Hoffmann, D. & Waggoner, S.E. (1997) Identification of tobacco-specific carcinogen in the cervical mucus of smokers and nonsmokers. *J. natl Cancer Inst.*, **89**, 868–873

Prokopczyk, B., Trushin, N., Leszczynska, J., Waggoner, S.E. & El-Bayoumy, K. (2001) Human cervical tissue metabolizes the tobacco-specific nitrosamine, 4-(methylnitrosamino)-1-(3-pyridyl)-1-butanone, via α-hydroxylation and carbonyl reduction pathways. *Carcinogenesis*, **22**, 107–114

Prokopczyk, B., Hoffmann, D., Bologna, M., Cunningham, A.J,. Trushin, N., Akerkar, S., Boyiri, T., Amin, S., Desai, D., Colosimo, S., Pittman, B., Leder, G., Ramadani, M., Henne-Bruns, D., Beger, H.G. & El-Bayoumy, K. (2002) Identification of tobacco-derived compounds in human pancreatic juice. *Chem. Res. Toxicol.*, **15**, 677–685

Pryor, W.A. (1997) Cigarette smoke radicals and the role of free radicals in chemical carcinogenicity. *Environ. Health Perspect.*, **105** (Suppl. 4), 875–882

Pulera, N., Petruzzelli, S., Celi, A., Puntoni, R., Fornai, E., Sawe, U., Paoletti, P. & Giuntini, C. (1997) Presence and persistence of serum anti-benzo[a]pyrene diolepoxide–DNA adduct antibodies in smokers: Effects of smoking reduction and cessation. *Int. J. Cancer*, **70**, 145–149

Putnam, K.P., Bombick, D.W., Avalos, J.T. & Doolittle, D.J. (1999) Comparison of the cytotoxic and mutagenic potential of liquid smoke food flavourings, cigarette smoke condensate and wood smoke condensate. *Food chem. Toxicol.*, **37**, 1113–1118

Putzrath, R.M., Langley, D. & Eisenstadt, E. (1981) Analysis of mutagenic activity in cigarette smokers' urine by high performance liquid chromatography. *Mutat. Res.*, **85**, 97–108

Qu, Q., Melikian, A.A., Li, G., Shore, R., Chen, L., Cohen, B., Yin, S., Kagan, M.R., Li, H., Meng, M., Jin, X., Winnik, W., Li, Y., Mu, R. & Li, K. (2000) Validation of biomarkers in humans exposed to benzene: Urine metabolites. *Am. J. ind. Med.*, **37**, 522–531

Rahn, C.A., Howard, G., Riccio, E. & Doolittle, D.J. (1991) Correlations between urinary nicotine or cotinine and urinary mutagenicity in smokers on controlled diets. *Environ. mol. Mutag.*, **17**, 244–252

Rajah, T. & Ahuja, Y.R. (1995) In vivo genotoxic effects of smoking and occupational lead exposure in printing press workers. *Toxicol. Lett.*, **76**, 71–75

Ramsey, M.J., Moore, D.H., II, Briner, J.F., Lee, D.A., Olsen, L.A., Senft, J.R. & Tucker, J.D. (1995) The effects of age and lifestyle factors on the accumulation of cytogenetic damage as measured by chromosome painting. *Mutat. Res.*, **338**, 95–106

Randerath, E., Avitts, T.A., Reddy, M.V., Miller, R.H., Everson, R.B. & Randerath, K. (1986) Comparative ^{32}P-analysis of cigarette smoke-induced DNA damage in human tissues and mouse skin. *Cancer Res.*, **46**, 5869–5877

Randerath, E., Miller, R.H., Mittal, D., Avitts, T.A., Dunsford, H.A. & Randerath, K. (1989) Covalent DNA damage in tissues of cigarette smokers as determined by ^{32}P-postlabeling assay. *J. natl Cancer Inst.*, **81**, 341–347

Rao, Y., Hoffmann, E., Zia, M., Bodin, L., Zeman, M., Sellers, E.M. & Tyndale, R.F. (2000) Duplications and defects in the *CYP2A6* gene: Identification, genotyping, and in vivo effects on smoking. *Mol. Pharmacol.*, **58**, 747–755

Rapuri, P.B., Gallagher, J.C., Balhorn, K.E. & Ryschon, K.L. (2000) Smoking and bone metabolism in elderly women. *Bone*, **27**, 429–436

Rasky, E., Stronegger, W.J. & Freidi, W. (1996) The relationship between body weight and patterns of smoking in women and men. *Int. J. Epidemiol.*, **25**, 1208–1212

Rauscher, D., Bader, M. & Angerer, J. (1994) The t,t-muconic acid excretion of the general population caused by environmental benzene exposures. In: *Proceedings of the 1st International Congress on Environmental Medicine, February 23–26, Duisburg*

Read, G.A. & Thornton, R.E. (1985) Preliminary studies of urinary hydroxyproline levels in rodents and in smokers. *Tokai J. exp. clin. Med.*, **10**, 445–450

Reidy, J.A., Annest, J.L., Chen. A.T.L. & Welty, T.K. (1988) Increased sister chromatid exchange associated with smoking and coffee consumption. *Environ. mol. Mutag.*, **12**, 311–318

Renner, T., Fechner, T. & Scherer, G. (2000) Fast quantification of the urinary marker of oxidative stress 8-hydroxy-2'-deoxyguanosine using solid-phase extraction and high-performance liquid chromatography with triple-stage quadrupole mass detection. *J. Chromatogr.*, **B738**, 311–317

Richie, J.P., Jr, Carmella, S.G., Muscat, J.E., Scott, D.G., Akerkar, S.A. & Hecht, S.S. (1997) Differences in the urinary metabolites of the tobacco-specific lung carcinogen 4-(methylnitrosamino)-1-(3-pyridyl)-1-butanone in black and white smokers. *Cancer Epidemiol. Biomarkers Prev.*, **6**, 783–790

Riffelmann, M., Müller, G., Schmieding, W., Popp, W. & Norpoth, K. (1995) Biomonitoring of urinary aromatic amines and arylamine hemoglobin adducts in exposed workers and nonexposed control persons. *Int. Arch. occup. environ. Health*, **68**, 36–43

Rimm, E.B., Manson, J.E., Stampfer, M.J., Colditz, G.A., Willett, W.C., Rosner, B., Hennekens, C.H. & Speizer, F.E. (1993) Cigarette smoking and the risk of diabetes in women. *Am. J. public Health*, **83**, 211–214

Rimm, E.B., Chan, J., Stampfer, M.J., Colditz, G.A. & Willett, W.C. (1995) Prospective study of cigarette smoking, alcohol use, and the risk of diabetes in men. *Br. med. J.*, **310**, 555–559

Rioux, N. & Castonguay, A. (2000) The induction of cyclooxygenase-1 by a tobacco carcinogen in U937 human macrophages is correlated to the activation of NF-κB. *Carcinogenesis*, **21**, 1745–1751

Rithidech, K., Chen, B.T., Mauderly, J.L., Whorton, E.B., Jr & Brooks, A.L. (1989) Cytogenetic effects of cigarette smoke on pulmonary alveolar macrophages of the rat. *Environ. mol. Mutag.*, **14**, 27–33

Robbins, W.A., Vine, M.F., Truong, K.Y. & Everson, R.B. (1997) Use of fluoresence in situ hybridization (FISH) to assess effects of smoking, caffeine, and alcohol on aneuploidy load in sperm of healthy men. *Environ. mol. Mutag.*, **30**, 175–183

Robertson, A.S., Burge, P.S. & Cockrill, B.L. (1987) A study of serum thiocyanate concentrations in office workers as a means of validation of smoking histories and assessing passive exposure to cigarette smoke. *Br. J. ind. Med.*, **44**, 351–354

Robinson, D.R., Goodall, K., Albertini, R.J., O'Neill, J.P., Finette, B., Sala-Trepat, M., Moustacchi, E., Tates, A.D., Beare, D.M., Green, M.H.L. & Cole, J. (1994) An analysis of in vivo *hprt* mutant frequency in circulating T-lymphocytes in the normal human population: A comparison of four datasets. *Mutat. Res.*, **313**, 227–247

Rodin, S.N. & Rodin, A.S. (2000) Human lung cancer and p53: The interplay between mutagenesis and selection. *Proc. natl Acad. Sci. USA*, **97**, 12244–12249

Roemer, E., Tewes, F.J., Meisgen, T.J., Veltel, D.J. & Carmines, E.L. (2002) Evaluation of the potential effects of ingredients added to cigarettes. Part 3: In vitro genotoxicity and cytotoxicity. *Food chem. Toxicol.*, **40**, 105–111

Roggi, C., Minoia, C., Sciarra, G.F., Apostoli, P., Maccarini, L., Magnaghi, S., Cenni, A., Fonte, A., Nidasio, G.F. & Micoli, G. (1997) Urinary 1-hydroxypyrene as a marker of exposure to pyrene: An epidemiological survey on a general population group. *Sci. total Environ.*, **199**, 247–254

Rojas, M., Alexandrov, K., Van Schooten, F.-J., Hillebrand, M., Kriek, E. & Bartsch, H. (1994) Validation of a new fluorometric assay for benzo[*a*]pyrene diolepoxide–DNA adducts in human white blood cells: Comparisons with ^{32}P-postlabeling and ELISA. *Carcinogenesis*, **15**, 557–560

Rojas, M., Alexandrov, K., Auburtin, G., Wastiaux-Denamur, A., Mayer, L., Mahieu, B., Sebastien, P. & Bartsch, H. (1995) Anti-benzo[*a*]pyrene diolepoxide–DNA adduct levels in peripheral mononuclear cells from coke oven workers and the enhancing effect of smoking. *Carcinogenesis*, **16**, 1373–1376

Rojas, E., Valverde, M., Sordo, M. & Ostrosky-Wegman, P. (1996) DNA damage in exfoliated buccal cells of smokers assessed by the single cell gel electrophoresis assay. *Mutat. Res.*, **370**, 115–120

Rojas, M., Alexandrov, K., Cascorbi, I., Brockmöller, J., Likhachev, A., Pozharisski, K., Bouvier, G., Auburtin, G., Mayer, L., Kopp-Schneider, A., Roots, I. & Bartsch, H. (1998) High benzo-[*a*]pyrene diol-epoxide DNA adduct levels in lung and blood cells from individuals with combined *CYP1A1 MspI/MspI-GSTM1*0/*0* genotypes. *Pharmacogenetics*, **8**, 109–118

Rojas, M., Cascorbi, I., Alexandrov, K., Kriek, E., Auburtin, G., Mayer, L., Kopp-Schneider, A., Roots, I. & Bartsch, H. (2000) Modulation of benzo[*a*]pyrene diolepoxide–DNA adduct levels in human white blood cells by *CYP1A1*, *GSTM1* and *GSTT1* polymorphism. *Carcinogenesis*, **21**, 35–41

Romano, G., Mancini, R., Fedele, P., Curigliano, G., Flamini, G., Giovagnoli, M.R., Malara, N., Boninsegna, A., Vecchione, A., Santella, R.M. & Cittadini, A. (1997) Immunohistochemical analysis of 4-aminobiphenyl–DNA adducts in oral mucosal cells of smokers and nonsmokers. *Anticancer Res.*, **17**, 2827–2830

Romano, G., Sgambato, A., Boninsegna, A., Flamini, G., Curigliano, G., Yang, Q., La Gioia, V., Signorelli, C., Ferro, A., Capelli, G., Santella, R.M. & Cittadini, A. (1999a) Evaluation of polycyclic aromatic hydrocarbon–DNA adducts in exfoliated oral cells by an immunohistochemical assay. *Cancer Epidemiol. Biomarkers Prev.*, **8**, 91–96

Romano, G., Garagnani, L., Boninsegna, A., Ferrari, P., Flamini, G., De Gaetani, C., Sgambato, A., Giovanni, F., Curigliano, G., Ferretti, G., Cittadini, A. & Trentini, G. (1999b) Analysis of 4-ABP–DNA adducts and p53 alterations in urinary bladder carcinoma. *Anticancer Res.*, **19**, 4571–4576

Romert, L., Jansson, T., Curvall, M. & Jenssen, D. (1994) Screening for agents inhibiting the mutagenicity of extracts and constituents of tobacco products. *Mutat. Res.*, **322**, 97–110

Ronco, G., Vineis, P., Bryant, M.S., Skipper, P.L. & Tannenbaum, S.R. (1990) Haemoglobin adducts formed by aromatic amines in smokers: Sources of inter-individual variability. *Br. J. Cancer*, **61**, 534–537

Rose, J.E., Behm, F.M., Ramsey, C. & Ritchie, J.C., Jr (2001) Platelet monoamine oxidase, smoking cessation, and tobacco withdrawal symptoms. *Nicotine Tob. Res.*, **3**, 383–390

Ross, G.W. & Petrovitch, H. (2001) Current evidence for neuroprotective effects of nicotine and caffeine against Parkinson's disease. *Drugs Aging*, **18**, 797–806

Routledge, M.N., Garner, R.C., Jenkins, D. & Cuzick, J. (1992) ^{32}P-Postlabelling analysis of DNA from human tissues. *Mutat. Res.*, **282**, 139–145

Rowland, R.E. & Harding, K.M. (1999) Increased sister chromatid exchange in the peripheral blood lymphocytes of young women who smoke cigarettes. *Hereditas*, **131**, 143–146

Rubes, J., Lowe, X., Moore, D., Perreault, S., Slott, V., Evenson, D., Selevan, S.G. & Wyrobek, A.J. (1998) Smoking cigarettes is associated with increased sperm disomy in teenage men. *Fertil. Steril.*, **70**, 715–723

Rubin, D.T. & Hanauer, S.B. (2000) Smoking and inflammatory bowel disease. *Eur. J. Gastroenterol. Hepatol.*, **12**, 855–862

Ruiz, E., Osorio, E. & Ortega, E. (1992) Androgenic status in cyclic and postmenopausal women: A comparison between smokers and nonsmokers. *Biochem. int.*, **27**, 841–845

Rundle, A., Tang, D., Hibshoosh, H., Estabrook, A., Schnabel, F., Cao, W., Grumet, S. & Perera, F.P. (2000) The relationship between genetic damage from polycyclic aromatic hydrocarbons in breast tissue and breast cancer. *Carcinogenesis*, **21**, 1281–1289

Ruppert, T., Scherer, G., Tricker, A.R., Rauscher, D. & Adlkofer, F. (1995) Determination of urinary *trans, trans*-muconic acid by gas chromatography–mass spectrometry. *J. Chromatogr.*, **B666**, 71–76

Ruppert, T., Scherer, G., Tricker, A.R. & Adlkofer, F. (1997) *trans, trans*-Muconic acid as a biomarker of non-occupational environmental exposure to benzene. *Int. Arch. occup. environ. Health*, **69**, 247–251

Russell, M.A.H., Jarvis, M.J., Feyerabend, C. & Saloojee, Y. (1986) Reduction of tar, nicotine and carbon monoxide intake in low tar smokers. *J. Epidemiol. Community Health*, **40**, 80–85

Rutten, A.A. & Wilmer, J.W. (1986) Effect of cigarette-smoke condensate and norharman on the induction of SCEs by direct and indirect mutagens in CHO cells. *Mutat. Res.*, **172**, 61–67

Ryberg, D., Hewer, A., Phillips, D.H. & Haugen, A. (1994) Different susceptibility to smoking-induced DNA damage among male and female lung cancer patients. *Cancer Res.*, **54**, 5801–5803

Ryberg, D., Skaug, V., Hewer, A., Phillips, D.H., Harries, L.W., Wolf, C.R., Øgreid, D., Ulvik, A., Vu, P. & Haugen, A. (1997) Genotypes of glutathione transferase M1 and P1 and their significance for lung DNA adduct levels and cancer risk. *Carcinogenesis*, **18**, 1285–1289

Safe, S. & McDougal, A. (2002) Mechanism of action and development of selective aryl hydrocarbon receptor modulators for treatment of hormone-dependent cancers (Review). *Int. J. Oncol.*, **20**, 1123–1128

Safe, S., Wang, F., Porter, W., Duan, R. & McDougal, A. (1998) Ah receptor agonists as endocrine disruptors: Antiestrogenic activity and mechanisms. *Toxicol. Lett.*, **102–103**, 343–347

Safe, S.H., Pallaroni, L., Yoon, K., Gaido, K., Ross, S., Saville, B. & McDonnell, D. (2001) Toxicology of environmental estrogens. *Reprod. Fertil. Dev.*, **13**, 307–315

Salomaa, S., Tuominen, J. & Skytta, E. (1988) Genotoxicity and PAC analysis of particulate and vapour phases of environmental tobacco smoke. *Mutat. Res.*, **204**, 173–183

Sanchez-Cespedes, M., Ahrendt, S.A., Piantadosi, S., Rosell, R., Monzo, M., Wu, L., Westra, W.H., Yang, S.C., Jen, J. & Sidransky, D. (2001) Chromosomal alterations in lung adenocarcinoma from smokers and nonsmokers. *Cancer Res.*, **61**, 1309–1313

Sandler, D.P., Shore, D.L., Anderson, J.R., Davey, F.R., Arthur, D., Mayer, R.J., Silver, R.T., Weiss, R.B., Moore, J.O., Schiffer, C.A., Wurster-Hill, D.H., McIntyre, O.R. & Bloomfield, C.D. (1993) Cigarette smoking and risk of acute leukemia: Associations with morphology and cytogenetic abnormalities in bone marrow. *J. natl. Cancer Inst.*, **85**, 1994–2003

Santella, R.M., Grinberg-Funes, R.A., Young, T.L., Dickey, C., Singh, V.N., Wang, L.W. & Perera, F.P. (1992) Cigarette smoking related polycyclic aromatic hydrocarbon–DNA adducts in peripheral mononuclear cells. *Carcinogenesis*, **13**, 2041–2045

Santella, R.M., Gammon, M.D., Zhang, Y.J., Motykiewicz, G., Young, T.L., Hayes, S.C., Terry, M.B., Schoenberg, J.B., Brinton, L.A., Bose, S., Teitelbaum, S.L. & Hibshoosh, H. (2000) Immunohistochemical analysis of polycyclic aromatic hydrocarbon–DNA adducts in breast tumor tissue. *Cancer Lett.*, **154**, 143–149

Sanyal, M.K., Li, Y.L. & Belanger, K. (1994) Metabolism of polynuclear aromatic hydrocarbon in human term placenta influenced by cigarette smoke exposure. *Reprod. Toxicol.*, **8**, 411–418

Sardas, S., Walker, D., Akyol, D. & Karakaya, A.E. (1995) Assessment of smoking-induced DNA damage in lymphocytes of smoking mothers of newborn infants using the alkaline single-cell gel electrophoresis technique. *Mutat. Res.*, **335**, 213–217

Sargeant, L.A., Khaw, K.T., Bingham, S., Day, N.E., Luben, R.N., Oakes, S., Welch, A. & Wareham, N.J. (2001) Cigarette smoking and glycaemia: The EPIC-Norfolk Study. European prospective investigation into cancer. *Int. J. Epidemiol.*, **30**, 547–554

Sarto, F., Faccioli, M.C., Cominato, I. & Levis, A.G. (1985) Aging and smoking increase the frequency of sister-chromatid exchanges (SCE) in man. *Mutat. Res.*, **144**, 183–187

Sarto, F., Mustari, L., Mazzotti, D., Tomanin, R. & Levis, A.G. (1987) Variations of SCE frequencies in peripheral lymphocytes of ex-smokers. *Mutat. Res.*, **192**, 157–162

Sastry, B.V.R. (1991) Placental toxicology: Tobacco smoke, abused drugs, multiple chemical interactions, and placental function. *Reprod. Fertil. Dev.*, **3**, 355–372

Savela, K. & Hemminki, K. (1991) DNA adducts in lymphocytes and granulocytes of smokers and nonsmokers detected by the ^{32}P-postlabelling assay. *Carcinogenesis*, **12**, 503–508

Schaller, K.H. & Zober, A. (1982) [Renal excretion of toxicologically relevant metals in occupationally non-exposed individuals.] *Ärztl. Lab.*, **28**, 209–214 (in German)

Schell, C., Popp, W., Kraus, R., Vahrenholz, C. & Norpoth, K. (1995) ^{32}P-Postlabeling analysis of DNA adducts in different populations. *Toxicol. Lett.*, **77**, 299–307

Scherer, G., Conze, C., von Meyerinck, L., Sorsa, M. & Adlkover, F. (1990) Importance of exposure to gaseous and particulate phase components of tobacco smoke in active and passive smokers. *Int. Arch. occup. environ. Health*, **62**, 459–466

Scherer, G., Doolittle, D.J., Ruppert, T., Meger-Kossien, I., Riedel, K., Tricker, A.R. & Adlkofer, F. (1996) Urinary mutagenicity and thioethers in nonsmokers: Role of environmental tobacco smoke (ETS) and diet. *Mutat. Res.*, **368**, 195–204

Scherer, G., Renner, T. & Meger, M. (1998) Analysis and evaluation of *trans,trans*-muconic acid as a biomarker for benzene exposure. *J. Chromatogr.*, **B717**, 179–199

Scherer, G., Frank, S., Riedel, K., Meger-Kossien, I. & Renner, T. (2000) Biomonitoring of exposure to polycyclic aromatic hydrocarbons of nonoccupationally exposed persons. *Cancer Epidemiol. Biomarkers Prev.*, **9**, 373–380

Scherer, G., Urban, M. & Meger, M. (2001a) Biological monitoring of the tobacco smoke-related exposure to alkylating agents (Abstract No. 802). *Proc. Am. Assoc. Cancer Res.*, **42**, 149–150

Scherer, G., Meger, M., Meger-Kossien, I. & Pachinger, A. (2001b) Biological monitoring of the tobacco-smoke related exposure to benzene (Abstract No. 803). *Proc. Am. Assoc. Cancer Res.*, **42**, 150

Schilling, J., Holzer, P., Guggenbach, M., Gyurech, D., Marathia, K. & Geroulanos, S. (1994) Reduced endogenous nitric oxide in the exhaled air of smokers and hypertensives. *Eur. respir. J.*, **7**, 467–471

Schneider, M., Diemer, K., Engelhart, K., Zankl, H., Trommer, W.E. & Biesalski, H.K. (2001) Protective effects of vitamins C and E on the number of micronuclei in lymphocytes in smokers and their role in ascorbate free radical formation in plasma. *Free Radic. Res.*, **34**, 209–219

Schoket, B., Kostic, S. & Vincze, I. (1993) Determination of smoking-related DNA adducts in lung-cancer and non-cancer patients. In: Phillips, D.H., Castegnaro, M. & Bartsch, H., eds, *Postlabelling Methods for Detection of DNA Adducts* (IARC Scientific Publications No. 124), Lyon, IARC*Press*, pp. 315–319

Schoket, B., Phillips, D.H., Kostic, S. & Vincze, I. (1998) Smoking-associated bulky DNA adducts in bronchial tissue related to *CYP1A1 MspI* and *GSTM1* genotypes in lung patients. *Carcinogenesis*, **19**, 841–846

Schoket, B., Papp, G., Lévay, K., Mracková, G., Kadlubar, F.F. & Vincze, I. (2001) Impact of metabolic genotypes on levels of biomarkers of genotoxic exposure. *Mutat. Res.*, **482**, 57–69

Schreiber, G., Fong, K.M., Peterson, B., Johnson, B.E., O'Briant, K.C. & Bepler, G. (1997) Smoking, gender, and survival association with allele loss for the LOH11B lung cancer region on chromosome 11. *Cancer Epidemiol. Biomarkers Prev.*, **6**, 315–319

Schwartz, G.G. & Hulka, B.S. (1990) Is vitamin D deficiency a risk factor to prostate cancer? (Hypothesis). *Anticancer Res.*, **10**, 1307–1311

Seagrave, J. (2000) Oxidative mechanisms in tobacco smoke-induced emphysema. *J. Toxicol. environ. Health*, **A61**, 69–78

Seidman, D.S., Paz, I., Merlet-Aharoni, I., Vremen, H., Stevenson, D.K. & Gale, R. (1999) Non-invasive validation of tobacco smoke exposure in late pregnancy using end-tidal carbon monoxide measurements. *J. Perinatol.*, **19**, 358–361

Sekido, Y., Fong, K.M. & Minna, J.D. (1998) Progress in understanding the molecular pathogenesis of human lung cancer. *Biochim. biophys. Acta*, **1378**, F21–F59

Seller, M.J. & Bnait, K.S. (1995) Effects of tobacco smoke inhalation on the developing mouse embryo and fetus. *Reprod. Toxicol.*, **9**, 449–459

Sellers, E.M., Kaplan, H.L. & Tyndale, R.F. (2000) *Inhibition of Cytochrome P450 2A6 Increases Nicotine's Oral Bioavailability and Decreases Smoking*, Toronto, University of Toronto, Departments of Pharmacology, Medicine, and Psychiatry and the Centre for Research in Women's Health

Selman, M., Montano, M., Ramos, C., Vanda, B., Becerril, C., Delgado, J., Sansores, R., Barrios, R. & Pardo, A. (1996) Tobacco smoke-induced lung emphysema in guinea pigs is associated with increased interstitial collagenase. *Am. J. Physiol.*, **271**, 734–743

Senthilmohan, S.T., McEwan, M.J., Wilson, P.F., Milligan, D.B. & Freeman, C.G. (2001) Real time analysis of breath volatiles using SIFT-MS in cigarette smoking. *Redox Rep.*, **6**, 185–187

Seree, E.M., Villard, P.H., Re, J.L., De Meo, M., Lacarelle, B., Attolini, L., Dumenil, G., Catalin, J., Durand, A. & Barra, Y. (1996) High inducibility of mouse renal CYP2E1 gene by tobacco smoke and its possible effect on DNA single strand breaks. *Biochem. biophys. Res. Commun.*, **219**, 429–434

Seto, H., Ohkubo, T., Kanoh, T., Koike, M., Nakamura, K. & Kawahara, Y. (1993) Determination of polycyclic aromatic hydrocarbons in the lung. *Arch. environ. Contam. Toxicol.*, **24**, 498–503

Sharara, F.I., Beatse, S.N., Leonardi, M.R., Navot, D. & Scott, R.T., Jr (1994) Cigarette smoking accelerates the development of diminished ovarian reserve as evidenced by the clomiphene citrate challenge test. *Fertil. Steril.*, **62**, 257–262

Sherman, M.P., Aeberhard, E.E., Wong, V.Z., Simmons, M.S., Roth, M.D. & Tashkin, D.P. (1995) Effects of smoking marijuana, tobacco or cocaine alone or in combination on DNA damage in human alveolar macrophages. *Life Sci.*, **56**, 2201–2207

Shen, H.-M., Chia, S.-E., Ni, Z.-Y., New, A.-L., Lee, B.-L. & Ong, C.-N. (1997) Detection of oxidative DNA damage in human sperm and the association with cigarette smoking. *Reprod. Toxicol.*, **11**, 675–680

Shen, H.M., Chia, S.E. & Ong, C.N. (1999) Evaluation of oxidative DNA damage in human sperm and its association with male infertility. *J. Androl.*, **20**, 718–723

Shi, Q., Ko, E., Barclay, L., Hoang, T., Rademaker, A. & Martin, R. (2001) Cigarette smoking and aneuploidy in human sperm. *Mol. Reprod. Dev.*, **59**, 417–421

Shinozaki, R., Inoue, S., Choi, K.S. & Tatsuno, T. (1999) Association of benzo[*a*]pyrene-diol-epoxide–deoxyribonucleic acid (BPDE–DNA) adduct level with aging in male smokers and nonsmokers. *Arch. environ. Health*, **54**, 79–85

Shuker, D.E.G. & Bartsch, H. (1994) DNA adducts of nitrosamines. In: Hemminki, K., Dipple, A., Shuker, D.E.G., Kadlubar, F.F., Segerbäck, D. & Bartsch, H., eds, *DNA Adducts: Identification and Biological Significance* (IARC Scientific Publications No. 125), Lyon, IARC*Press*, pp. 73–89

Shuker, D.E.G., Friesen, M.D., Garren, L. & Prévost, V. (1991) A rapid gas chromatography–mass spectrometry method for the determination of urinary 3-methyladenine: Application in human subjects. In: O'Neill, I.K., Chen, J. & Bartsch, H., eds, *Relevance to Human Cancer of N-Nitroso Compounds, Tobacco Smoke and Mycotoxins* (IARC Scientific Publications No. 105), Lyon, IARC*Press*, pp. 102–106

Simon, D., Senan, C., Garnier, P., Saint-Paul, M. & Papoz, L. (1989) Epidemiological features of glycated haemoglobin A1c-distribution in a healthy population. The Telecom Study. *Diabetologia*, **32**, 864–869

Simon, P., Lafontaine, M., Delsaut, P., Morele, Y. & Nicot, T. (2000) Trace determination of urinary 3-hydroxybenzo[*a*]pyrene by automated column-switching high-performance liquid chromatography. *J. Chromatogr.*, **B748**, 337–348

Simons, A.M., Phillips, D.H. & Coleman, D.V. (1993) Damage to DNA in cervical epithelium related to smoking tobacco. *Br. med. J.*, **306**, 1444–1448

Simons, A.M., Mugica van Herckenrode, C., Rodriguez, J.A., Maitland, N., Anderson, M., Phillips, D.H. & Coleman, D.V. (1995) Demonstration of smoking-related DNA damage in cervical epithelium and correlation with human papillomavirus type 16, using exfoliated cervical cells. *Br. J. Cancer*, **71**, 246–249

Simpson, C.D., Wu, M.-T., Christiani, D.C., Santella, R.M., Carmella, S.G. & Hecht, S.S. (2000) Determination of *r*-7,*t*-8,9,*c*-10-tetrahydroxy-7,8,9,10-tetrahydrobenzo[*a*]pyrene in human urine by gas chromatography negative ion chemical ionization mass spectrometry. *Chem. Res. Toxicol.*, **13**, 271–280

Singer, B. & Grunberger, D. (1983) *Molecular Biology of Mutagens and Carcinogens*, New York, Plenum Press

Sinués, B., Izquierdo, M. & Viguera, J.P. (1990) Chromosome aberrations and urinary thioethers in smokers. *Mutat. Res.*, **240**, 289–293

Sithisarankul, P., Vineis, P., Kang, D., Rothman, N., Caporaso, N. & Strickland, P. (1997) The association of 1-hydroxypyrene-glucuronide in human urine with cigarette smoking and broiled or roasted meat consumption. *Biomarkers*, **2**, 217–221

van Sittert, N.J., Boogaard, P.J. & Beulink, G.D.J. (1993) Application of the urinary *S*-phenylmercapturic acid test as a biomarker for low levels of exposure to benzene in industry. *Br. J. ind. Med.*, **50**, 460–469

Skipper, P.L., Peng, X., Soohoo, C.K. & Tannenbaum, S.R. (1994) Protein adducts as biomarkers of human carcinogen exposure. *Drug Metab. Rev.*, **26**, 111–124

Slattery, M.L., Curtin, K., Anderson, K., Ma, K.-N., Ballard, L., Edwards, S., Schaffer, D., Potter, J., Leppert, M. & Samowitz, W.S. (2000) Associations between cigarette smoking, lifestyle factors, and microsatellite instability in colon tumors. *J. natl Cancer Inst.*, **92**, 1831–1836

Slebos, R.J., Hruban, R.H., Dalesio, O., Mooi, W.J., Offerhaus, G.J. & Rodenhuis, S. (1991) Relationship between K-ras oncogene activation and smoking in adenocarcinoma of the human lung. *J. natl Cancer Inst.*, **83**, 1024–1027

Slotkin, T.A., Saleh, J.L., McCook, E.C. & Seidler, F.J. (1997) Impaired cardiac function during postnatal hypoxia in rats exposed to nicotine prenatally: Implications for perinatal morbidity and mortality, and for sudden infant death syndrome. *Teratology*, **55**, 177–184

Smith, C.J. & Fischer, T.H. (2001) Particulate and vapor phase constituents of cigarette mainstream smoke and risk of myocardial infarction. *Atherosclerosis*, **158**, 257–267

Smith, C.J. & Hansch, C. (2000) The relative toxicity of compounds in mainstream cigarette smoke condensate. *Food chem. Toxicol.*, **38**, 637–646

Smith, C.J., McKarns, S.C., Davis, R.A., Livingston, S.D., Bombick, B.R., Avalos, J.T., Morgan, W.T. & Doolittle, D.J. (1996) Human urine mutagenicity study comparing cigarettes which burn or primarily heat tobacco. *Mutat. Res.*, **361**, 1–9

Smith, L.E., Denissenko, M.F., Bennett, W.P., Li, H., Amin, S., Tang, M.-S. & Pfeifer, G.P. (2000) Targeting of lung cancer mutational hotspots by polycyclic aromatic hydrocarbons. *J. natl Cancer Inst.*, **92**, 803–811

Smith, C.J., Perfetti, T.A., Bombick, D.W., Rodgman, A. & Doolittle, D.J. (2001) Response to 'cigarette smoke comparative toxicology'. *Food chem. Toxicol.*, **39**, 177–180

Sopori, M.L., Cherian, S., Chilukuri, R. & Shopp, G.M. (1989) Cigarette smoke causes inhibition of the immune response to intratracheally administered antigens. *Toxicol. appl. Pharmacol.*, **97**, 489–499

Sowers, M., Beebe, J., McConnell, D., Randolph, J. & Jannausch, M. (2001) Testosterone concentrations in women aged 25–50 years: Associations with lifestyle, body composition, and ovarian status. *Am. J. Epidemiol.*, **153**, 256–264

Sozzi, G., Sard, L., De Gregorio, L., Marchetti, A., Musso, K., Buttitta, F., Tornielli, S., Pellegrini, S., Veronese, M.L., Manenti, G., Incarbone, M., Chella, A., Angeletti, C.A., Pastorino, U., Huebner, K., Bevilaqua, G., Pilotti, S., Croce, C.M. & Pierotti, M.A. (1997) Association between cigarette smoking and *FHIT* gene alterations in lung cancer. *Cancer Res.*, **57**, 2121–2123

Spencer, J.P., Jenner, A., Chimel, K., Aruoma, O.I., Cross, C.E., Wu, R. & Halliwell, B. (1995) DNA damage in human respiratory tract epithelial cells: Damage by gas phase cigarette smoke apparently involves attack by reactive nitrogen species in addition to oxygen radicals. *FEBS Lett.*, **375**, 179–182

Spitz, M.R., Fueger, J.J., Halabi, S., Schantz, S.P., Sample, D. & Hsu, T.C. (1993) Mutagen sensitivity in upper aerodigestive tract cancer: A case–control analysis. *Cancer Epidemiol. Biomarkers Prev.*, **2**, 329–333

Spruck, C.H., III, Rideout, W.M., III, Olumi, A.F., Ohneseit, P.F., Yang, A.S., Tsai, Y.C., Nichols, P.W., Horn, T., Hermann, G.G., Steven, K., Ross, R.K., Yu, M.C. & Jones, P.A. (1993) Distinct pattern of p53 mutations in bladder cancer: Relationship to tobacco usage. *Cancer Res.*, **53**, 1162–1166

Steele, R.H., Payne, V.M., Fulp, C.W., Rees, D.C., Lee, C.K. & Doolittle, D.J. (1995) A comparison of the mutagenicity of mainstream cigarette smoke condensates from a representative sample of the US cigarette market with a Kentucky reference cigarette (K1R4F). *Mutat. Res.*, **342**, 179–190

Stenstrand, K. (1985) Effects of ionizing radiation on chromosome aberrations, sister chromatid exchanges and micronuclei in lymphocytes of smokers and nonsmokers. *Hereditas*, **102**, 71–76

Stillwell, W.G., Glogowski, J., Xu, H.-X., Wishnok, J.S., Zavala, D., Montes, G., Correa, P. & Tannenbaum, S.R. (1991) Urinary excretion of nitrate, *N*-nitrosoproline, 3-methyladenine, and 7-methylguanine in a Colombian population at high risk for stomach cancer. *Cancer Res.*, **51**, 190–194

Stoichev, I.I., Todorov, D.K. & Christova, L.T. (1993) Dominant-lethal mutations and micronucleus induction in male BALB/c, BDF1 and H mice by tobacco smoke. *Mutat. Res.*, **319**, 285–292

Stommel, P., Müller, G., Stücker, W., Verkoyen, C., Schöbel, S. & Norpoth, K. (1989) Determination of *S*-phenylmercapturic acid in the urine — An improvement in the biological monitoring of benzene exposure. *Carcinogenesis*, **10**, 279–282

Stone, J.G., Jones, N.J., McGregor, A.D. & Waters, R. (1995) Development of a human biomonitoring assay using buccal mucosa: Comparison of smoking-related DNA adducts in mucosa *versus* biopsies. *Cancer Res.*, **55**, 1267–1270

Stratton, K., Shetty, P., Wallace, R. & Bondurant, S. (2001) *Clearing the Smoke: Assessing the Science Base for Tobacco Harm Reduction*, Washington DC, National Academy Press

Strickland, P.T., Routledge, M.N. & Dipple, A. (1993) Methodologies for measuring carcinogen adducts in humans. *Cancer Epidemiol. Biomarkers Prev.*, **2**, 607–619

Strom, S.S., Wu, X., Sigurdon, A.J., Hsu, T.C., Fueger, J.J., Lopez, J., Tee, P.G. & Spitz, M.R. (1995) Lung cancer, smoking patterns, and mutagen sensitivity in Mexican-Americans. *J. natl Cancer Inst. Monogr.*, **18**, 29–33

Swislocki, A.L., Tsuzuki, A., Tait, M., Khuu, D. & Fann, K. (1997) Smokeless nicotine administration is associated with hypertension but not with a deterioration in glucose tolerance in rats. *Metabolism*, **46**, 1008–1012

Syrop, C.H., Willhoite, A. & Van Voorhis, B.J. (1995) Ovarian volume: A novel outcome predictor for assisted reproduction. *Fertil. Steril.*, **64**, 1167–1171

Szaniszló, J. & Ungváry, G. (2001) Polycyclic aromatic hydrocarbon exposure and burden of outdoor workers in Budapest. *J. Toxicol. environ. Health*, **A62**, 297–306

Szostak-Wegierek, D., Bjorntorp, P., Marin, P., Lindstedt, G. & Andersson, B. (1996) Influence of smoking on hormone secretion in obese and lean female smokers. *Obes. Res.*, **4**, 321–328

Szyfter, K., Hemminki, K., Szyfter, W., Szmeja, Z., Banaszewski, J. & Yang, K. (1994) Aromatic DNA adducts in larynx biopsies and leukocytes. *Carcinogenesis*, **15**, 2195–2199

Szyfter, K., Hemminki, K., Szyfter, W., Szmeja, Z., Banaszewski, J. & Pabiszczak, M. (1996) Tobacco smoke-associated *N*7-alkylguanine in DNA of larynx tissue and leucocytes. *Carcinogenesis*, **17**, 501–506

Taioli, E., Garbers, S., Bradlow, H.L., Carmella, S.G., Akerkar, S. & Hecht, S.S. (1997) Effects of indole-3-carbinol on the metabolism of 4-(methylnitrosamino)-1-(3-pyridyl)-1-butanone in smokers. *Cancer Epidemiol. Biomarkers Prev.*, **6**, 517–522

Takubo, Y., Guerassimov, A., Ghezzo, H., Triantafillopoulos, A., Bates, J.H., Hoidal, J.R. & Cosio, M.G. (2002) Alpha1-antitrypsin determines the pattern of emphysema and function in tobacco smoke-exposed mice: Parallels with human disease. *Am. J. respir. crit. Care Med.*, **15**, 166

Talaska, G., Al-Juburi, A.Z.S.S. & Kadlubar, F.F. (1991a) Smoking related carcinogen–DNA adducts in biopsy samples of human urinary bladder: Identification of *N*-(deoxyguanosin-8-yl)-4-aminobiphenyl as a major adduct. *Proc. natl Acad. Sci. USA*, **88**, 5350–5354

Talaska, G., Schamer, M., Skipper, P., Tannenbaum, S., Caporaso, N., Unruh, L., Kadlubar, F.F., Bartsch, H., Malaveille, C. & Vineis, P. (1991b) Detection of carcinogen–DNA adducts in exfoliated urothelial cells of cigarette smokers: Association with smoking, hemoglobin adducts, and urinary mutagenicity. *Cancer Epidemiol. Biomarkers Prev.*, **1**, 61–66

Talaska, G., Schamer, M., Casetta, G., Tizzani, A. & Vineis, P. (1994) Carcinogen–DNA adducts in bladder biopsies and urothelial cells: A risk assessment exercise. *Cancer Lett.*, **84**, 93–97

Tang, D., Santella, R.M., Blackwood, A.M., Young, T.-L., Mayer, J., Jaretzki, A., Grantham, S., Tsai, W.-Y. & Perera, F.P. (1995) A molecular epidemiological case-control study of lung cancer. *Cancer Epidemiol. Biomarkers Prev.*, **4**, 341–346

Tang, D., Phillips, D.H., Stampfer, M., Mooney, L.A., Hsu, Y., Cho, S., Tsai, W.-Y., Ma, J., Cole, K.J., Shé, M.N. & Perera, F.P. (2001) Association between carcinogen–DNA adducts in white blood cells and lung cancer risk in the Physicians Health Study. *Cancer Res.*, **61**, 6708–6712

Tavares, R., Ramos, P., Palminha, J., Bispo, M.A., Paz, I., Bras, A., Rueff, J., Farmer, P.B. & Bailey, E. (1994) Transplacental exposure to genotoxins. Evaluation in haemoglobin of hydroxyethylvaline adduct levels in smoking and non-smoking mothers and their newborns. *Carcinogenesis*, **15**, 1271–1274

Tavares, R., Borba, H., Monteiro, M., Proenca, M.J., Lynce, N., Rueff, J., Bailey, E., Sweetman, G.M.A., Lawrence, R.M. & Farmer, P.B. (1996) Monitoring of exposure to acrylonitrile by determination of N-(2-cyanoethyl)valine at the N-terminal position of haemoglobin. *Carcinogenesis*, **17**, 2655–2660

Tawn, E.J. & Whitehouse, C.A. (2001) Frequencies of chromosome aberrations in a control population determined by G banding. *Mutat. Res.*, **490**, 171–177

Thomas, E.J., Edridge, W., Weddell, A., McGill, A. & McGarrigle, H.H. (1993) The impact of cigarette smoking on the plasma concentrations of gonadotrophins, ovarian steroids and androgens and upon the metabolism of oestrogens in the human female. *Hum. Reprod.*, **8**, 1187–1193

Thompson, C.L., McCoy, Z., Lambert, J.M., Andries, M.J. & Lucier, G.W. (1989) Relationships among benzo(*a*)pyrene metabolism, benzo(*a*)pyrene-diol-epoxide:DNA adduct formation, and sister chromatid exchanges in human lymphocytes from smokers and nonsmokers. *Cancer Res.*, **49**, 6503–6511

Tokiwa, H., Sera, N., Horikawa, K., Nakanishi, Y. & Shigematu, N. (1993) The presence of mutagens/carcinogens in the excised lung and analysis of lung cancer induction. *Carcinogenesis*, **14**, 1933–1938

Tolcos, M., Mallard, C., McGregor, H., Walker, D. & Rees, S. (2000) Exposure to prenatal carbon monoxide and postnatal hyperthermia: Short and long-term effects on neurochemicals and neuroglia in the developing brain. *Exp. Neurol.*, **162**, 235–246

Tomingas, R., Pott, F. & Dehnen, W. (1976) Polycyclic aromatic hydrocarbons in human bronchial carcinoma. *Cancer Lett.*, **1**, 189–195

Toniolo, P., Bruning, P.F., Akhmedkhanov, A., Bonfrer, J.M., Koenig, K.L., Lukanova, A., Shore, R.E. & Zeleniuch-Jacquotte, A. (2000) Serum insulin-like growth factor-I and breast cancer. *Int. J. Cancer*, **88**, 828–832

Torgerson, D.J., Avenell, A., Russell, I.T. & Reid, D.M. (1994) Factors associated with onset of menopause in women aged 45–49. *Maturitas*, **19**, 83–92

Törnqvist, M., Osterman-Golkar, S., Kautiainen, A., Jensen, S., Farmer, P.B. & Ehrenberg, L. (1986) Tissue doses of ethylene oxide in cigarette smokers determined from adduct levels in hemoglobin. *Carcinogenesis*, **7**, 1519–1521

Törnqvist, M., Svartengren, M. & Ericsson, C.H. (1992) Methylations in hemoglobin from mono-zygotic twins discordant for cigarette smoking: Hereditary and tobacco-related factors. *Chem.-biol. Interact.*, **82**, 91–98

Trauth, J.A., McCook, E.C., Seidler, F.J. & Slotkin, T.A. (2000) Modeling adolescent nicotine exposure: Effects on cholinergic systems in rat brain regions. *Brain Res.*, **873**, 18–25

Tricker, A.R. (1997) *N*-Nitroso compounds and man: Sources of exposure, endogenous formation and occurrence in body fluids. *Eur. J. Cancer Prev.*, **6**, 226–268

Tricker, A.R., Scherer, G., Conze, C., Adlkofer, F., Pachinger, A. & Klus, H. (1993) Evaluation of 4-(*N*-methylnitrosamino)-4-(3-pyridyl)butyric acid as a potential monitor of endogenous nitrosation of nicotine and its metabolites. *Carcinogenesis*, **14**, 1409–1414

Trivedi, A.H., Dave, B.J. & Adhvaryu, S.G. (1990) Assessment of genotoxicity of nicotine employ-ing in vitro mammalian test system. *Cancer Lett.*, **54**, 89–94

Trivedi, A.H., Dave, B.J. & Adhvaryu, S.S. (1993) Genotoxic effects of nicotine in combination with arecoline on CHO cells. *Cancer Lett.*, **74**, 105–110

Trivedi, A.H., Roy, S.K., Jaju, R.J., Patel, R.K., Adhvaryu, S.G. & Balar, D.B. (1995) Urine of tobacco/areca nut chewers causes genomic damage in Chinese hamster ovary cells. *Carcino-genesis*, **16**, 205–208

Trummer, H., Habermann, H., Haas, J. & Pummer, K. (2002) The impact of cigarette smoking on human semen parameters and hormones. *Hum. Reprod.*, **17**, 1554–1559

Trushin, N. & Hecht, S.S. (1999) Stereoselective metabolism of nicotine and tobacco-specific *N*-nitrosamines to 4-hydroxy-4-(3-pyridyl)butanoic acid in rats. *Chem. Res. Toxicol.*, **12**, 164–171

Tseng, J.E., Kemp, B.L., Khuri, F.R., Kurie, J.M., Lee, J.S., Zhou, X., Liu, D., Hong, W.K. & Mao, L. (1999) Loss of Fhit is frequent in stage I non-small cell lung cancer and in the lungs of chronic smokers. *Cancer Res.*, **59**, 4798–4803

Tsuda, M. & Kurashima, Y. (1991) Tobacco smoking, chewing, and snuff dipping: Factors contri-buting to the endogenous formation of N-nitroso compounds. *Crit. Rev. Toxicol.*, **21**, 243–253

Tsutsumi, M., Lasker, J.M., Takahashi, T. & Lieber, C.S. (1993) In vivo induction of hepatic P450E1 by ethanol: Role of increased enzyme synthesis. *Arch. Biochem. Biophys.*, **304**, 209–218

Tunstall-Pedoe, H., Woodward, M. & Brown, C.A. (1991) The drinking, passive smoking, smoking deception and serum cotinine in the Scottish Hearth Health Study. *J. clin. Epidemiol.*, **44**, 1411–1414

Tuomisto, J., Kolonen, S., Sorsa, M. & Einistö, P. (1986) No difference between urinary muta-genicity in smokers of low-tar and medium-tar cigarettes: A double-blind cross-over study. *Arch. Toxicol.*, **Suppl. 9**, 115–119

Ulrik, C.S. & Lange, P. (2001) Cigarette smoking and asthma. *Monaldi Arch. Chest Dis.*, **56**, 349–353

Upadhyaya, P., Kenney, P.M.J., Hochalter, J.B., Wang, M. & Hecht, S.S. (1999) Tumorigenicity and metabolism of 4-(methylnitrosamino)-1-(3-pyridyl)-1-butanol enantiomers and meta-bolites in the A/J mouse. *Carcinogenesis*, **20**, 1577–1582

Upadhyaya, P., McIntee, E.J. & Hecht, S.S. (2001) Preparation of pyridine-*N*-glucuronides of tobacco-specific nitrosamines. *Chem. Res. Toxicol.*, **14**, 555–561

US Department of Health and Human Services (DHHS) (1983) *The Health Consequences of Smoking. Cardiovascular Disease. A Report of the Surgeon General* (DHHS Publ. No. (CDC) 84-50204), Washington DC, US Government Printing Office

US Department of Health and Human Services (DHHS) (1984) *The Health Consequences of Smoking. Chronic Obstructive Disease. A Report of the Surgeon General* (DHHS Publ. No. (PHS) 84-50205), Washington DC, US Government Printing Office

US Department of Health and Human Services (DHHS) (1986) *The Health Consequences of Involuntary Smoking. A Report of the Surgeon General* (US DHHS Pub. No. (PHS) 87-8398), Washington DC, Public Health Service, Office of the Assistant Secretary for health, Office of Smoking and Health

US Department of Health and Human Services (DHHS) (1988) *The Health Consequences of Smoking: Nicotine Addiction. A Report of the Surgeon General* (DHHS Publ. No. (CDC) 88-8406), Washington DC, US Government Printing Office

US Department of Health and Human Services (DHHS) (1989) *Reducing the Health Consequences of Smoking: 25 Years of Progress. A Report of the Surgeon General* (DHHS Publ. No. (CDC) 89-8411), Washington DC, US Government Printing Office

US Department of Health and Human Services (DHHS) (2001) *Women and Smoking. A Report of the Surgeon General*, Rockville, MD [available at http://www.cdc.gov/tobacco/sgr/sgr_for-women/index]

Van Rooij, J.G.M., Veeger, M.M.S., Bodelier-Bade, M.M., Scheepers, P.T.J. & Jongeneelen, F.J. (1994) Smoking and dietary intake of polycyclic aromatic hydrocarbons as sources of inter-individual variability in the baseline excretion of 1- hydroxypyrene in urine. *Int. Arch. occup. environ. Health*, **66**, 55–65

Van Schooten, F.J., Hillebrand, M.J.X., van Leeuwen, F.E., Lutgerink, J.T., van Zandwijk, N., Jansen, H.M. & Kriek, E. (1990a) Polycyclic aromatic hydrocarbon–DNA adducts in lung tissue from lung cancer patients. *Carcinogenesis*, **11**, 1677–1681

Van Schooten, F.J., van Leeuwen, F.E., Hillebrand, M.J.X., de Rijke, M.E., Hart, A.A.M., van Veen, H.G., Oosterink, S. & Kriek, E. (1990b) Determination of benzo[*a*]pyrene diol epoxide–DNA adducts in white blood cell DNA from coke-oven workers: The impact of smoking. *J. natl Cancer Inst.*, **82**, 927–933

Van Schooten, F.J., Hillebrand, M.J., van Leeuwen, F.E., Van Zandwijk, N., Jansen, H.M., den Engelse, L. & Kriek, E. (1992) Polycyclic aromatic hydrocarbon–DNA adducts in white blood cells from lung cancer patients: No correlation with adduct levels in lung. *Carcinogenesis*, **13**, 987–993

Van Schooten, F.J., Godschalk, R.W., Breedijk, A., Maas, L.M., Kriek, E., Sakai, H., Wigbout, G., Baas, P., Van't Veer, L. & Van Zandwijk, N. (1997) ^{32}P-Postlabelling of aromatic DNA adducts in white blood cells and alveolar macrophages of smokers: Saturation at high exposures. *Mutat. Res.*, **378**, 65–75

Van Schooten, F.J., Hirvonen, A., Maas, L.M., De Mol, B.A., Kleinjans, J.C.S., Bell, D.A. & Durrer, J.D. (1998) Putative susceptibility markers of coronary artery disease: Association between *VDR* genotype, smoking, and aromatic DNA adduct levels in human right atrial tissue. *FASEB J.*, **12**, 1409–1417

Van Schooten, F.J., Nia, A.B., De Flora, S., D'Agostini, F., Izzotti, A., Camoirano, A., Balm, A.J., Dallinga, J.W., Bast, A., Haenen, G.R., Van't Veer, L., Baas, P., Sakai, H. & Van Zandwijk, N. (2002) Effects of oral administration of *N*-acetyl-L-cysteine: A multi-biomarker study in smokers. *Cancer Epidemiol. Biomarkers Prev.*, **11**, 167–175

Vaught, J.B., Gurtoo, H.L., Parker, N.B., LeBoeuf, R. & Doctor, G. (1979) Effect of smoking on benzo(a)pyrene metabolism by human placental microsomes. *Cancer Res.*, **39**, 3177–3183

Velasco, E., Malacara, J.M., Cervantes, F., de Leon, J.D., Davalos, G. & Castillo, J. (1990) Gonadotropins and prolactin serum levels during the perimenopausal period: Correlation with diverse factors. *Fertil. Steril.*, **53**, 56–60

Veltel, D. & Hoheneder, A. (1996) Characterization of cigarette smoke-induced micronuclei *in vitro*. *Exp. Toxicol. Pathol.*, **48**, 548–550

Venier, P., Clonfero, E., Cottica, D., Gava, C., Zordan, M., Pozzoli, L. & Levis, A.G. (1985) Mutagenic activity and polycyclic aromatic hydrocarbon levels in urine of workers exposed to coal tar pitch volatiles in an anode plant. *Carcinogenesis*, **6**, 749–752

Verkasalo, P.K., Thomas, H.V., Appleby, P.N., Davey, G.K. & Key, T.J. (2001) Circulating levels of sex hormones and their relation to risk factors for breast cancer: A cross-sectional study in 1092 pre- and postmenopausal women (United Kingdom). *Cancer Causes Control*, **12**, 47–59

Villablanca, A.C., McDonald, J.M. & Rutledge, J.C. (2000) Smoking and cardiovascular disease. *Clin. Chest Med.*, **21**, 159–172

Villard, P.H., Seree, E., Lacarelle, B., Therene-Fenoglio, M.C., Barra, Y., Attolini, L., Bruguerole, B., Durand, A. & Catalin, J. (1994) Effect of cigarette smoke on hepatic and pulmonary cytochromes P450 in mouse: Evidence for CYP2E1 induction in lung. *Biochem. biophys. Res. Commun.*, **202**, 1731–1737

Villard, P.H., Herber, R., Seree, E.M., Attolini, L., Magdalou, J. & Lacarelle, B. (1998a) Effect of cigarette smoke on UDP-glucuronosyltransferase activity and cytochrome P450 content in liver, lung and kidney microsomes in mice. *Pharmacol. Toxicol.*, **82**, 74–79

Villard, P.H., Seree, E.M., Re, J.L., De Meo, M., Barra, Y., Attolini, L., Dumenil, G., Catalin, J., Durand, A. & Lacarelle, B. (1998b) Effects of tobacco smoke on the gene expression of the *Cyp1a*, *Cyp2b*, *Cyp2e*, and *Cyp3a* subfamilies in mouse liver and lung: Relation to single strand breaks of DNA. *Toxicol. appl. Pharmacol.*, **148**, 195–204

Vine, M.F. (1996) Smoking and male reproduction: A review. *Int. J. Androl.*, **19**, 323–337

Vine, M.F., Margolin, B.H., Morrison, H.I. & Hulka, B.S. (1994) Cigarette smoking and sperm density: A meta-analysis. *Fertil. Steril.*, **61**, 35–43

Vineis, P., Estève, J. & Terracini, B. (1984) Bladder cancer and smoking in males: Types of cigarettes, age at start, effect of stopping and interaction with occupation. *Int. J. Cancer*, **34**, 165–170

Vineis, P., Caporaso, N., Tannenbaum, S.R., Skipper, P.L., Glogowski, J., Bartsch, H., Coda, M., Talaska, G. & Kadlubar, F. (1990) Acetylation phenotype, carcinogen–hemoglobin adducts, and cigarette smoking. *Cancer Res.*, **50**, 3002–3004

Vineis, P., Talaska, G., Malaveille, C., Bartsch, H., Martone, T., Sithisarankul, P. & Strickland, P. (1996) DNA adducts in urothelial cells: Relationship with biomarkers of exposure to arylamines and polycyclic aromatic hydrocarbons from tobacco smoke. *Int. J. Cancer*, **65**, 314–316

Vineis, P., d'Errico, A., Malats, N. & Boffetta, P. (1999) Overall evaluation and research perspectives. In: Ryder, W., ed., *Metabolic Polymorphisms and Susceptibility in Cancer* (IARC Scientific Publications No. 148), Lyon, IARCPress, pp. 403–408

Voncken, P., Rustemeier, K. & Schepers, G. (1990) Identification of *cis*-3′-hydroxycotinine as a urinary nicotine metabolite. *Xenobiotica*, **20**, 1353–1356

Vulimiri, S.V., Wu, X., Baer-Dubowska, W., de Andrade, M., Detry, M., Spitz, M.R. & DiGiovanni, J. (2000) Analysis of aromatic DNA adducts and 7,8-dihydro-8-oxo-2′-deoxyguanosine in lymphocyte DNA from a case–control study of lung cancer involving minority populations. *Mol. Carcinog.*, **27**, 34–46

Wagenknecht, L.E., Manolio, T.A., Sidney, S., Burke, G.L. & Haley, N.J. (1993) Environmental tobacco smoke exposure as determined by cotinine in black and white young adults: The CARDIA study. *Environ. Res.*, **63**, 39–46

Wallace, L.A. & Pellizzari, E.D. (1986) Personal air exposures and breath concentrations of benzene and other volatile hydrocarbons for smokers and nonsmokers. *Toxicol. Lett.*, **35**, 113–116

Wallace, L.A., Pellizzari, E.D., Hartwell, T.D., Perritt, R. & Ziegenfus, R. (1987) Exposures to benzene and volatile compounds from active and passive smoking. *Arch. environ.* Health, **42**, 272–279

Wang, M., Dhingra, K., Hittelman, W.N., Liehr, J.G., de Andrade, M. & Li, D. (1996) Lipid peroxidation-induced putative malondialdehyde–DNA adducts in human breast tissues. *Cancer Epidemiol. Biomarkers Prev.*, **5**, 705–710

Wang, Y., Ichiba, M., Oishi, H., Iyadomi, M., Shono, N. & Tomokuni, K. (1997) Relationship between plasma concentrations of β-carotene and α-tocopherol and life-style factors and levels of DNA adducts in lymphocytes. *Nutr. Cancer*, **27**, 69–73

Wang, M., Abbruzzese, J.L., Friess, H., Hittelman, W.N., Evans, D.B., Abbruzzese, M.C., Chiao, P. & Li, D. (1998) DNA adducts in human pancreatic tissues and their potential role in carcinogenesis. *Cancer Res.*, **58**, 38–41

Wang, L.-E., Bondy, M.L., de Andrade, M., Strom, S.S., Wang, X., Sigurdson, A., Spitz, M.R. & Wei, Q. (2000) Gender difference in smoking effect on chromosome sensitivity to gamma radiation in a health population. *Radiat. Res.*, **154**, 20–27

Wang, Q., Fan, J., Wang, H. & Liu, S. (2000) DNA damage and activation of *c-ras* in human embryo lung cells exposed to chrysotile and cigarette smoking solution. *J. environ. Pathol. Toxicol. Oncol.*, **19**, 13–19

Wang, H., Liu, X., Umino, T., Skold, C.M., Zhu, Y., Kohyama, T., Spurzem, J.R., Romberger, D.J. & Rennard, S.I. (2001) Cigarette smoke inhibits human bronchial epithelial cell repair processes. *Am. J. respir. Cell mol. Biol.*, **25**, 772–779

Wardlaw, S.A., Nikula, K.J., Kracko, D.A., Finch, G.L., Thornton-Manning, J.R. & Dahl, A.R. (1998) Effect of cigarette smoke on CYP1A1, CYP1A2 and CYP2B1/2 of nasal mucosae in F344 rats. *Carcinogenesis*, **19**, 655–662

Wehner, A.P., Olson, R.J. & Busch, R.H. (1976) Increased life span and decreased weight in hamsters exposed to cigarette smoke. *Arch. environ. Health*, **31**, 146–153

Wei, Q., Cheng, L., Amos, C.I., Wang, L.-E., Guo, Z., Hong, W.K. & Spitz, M.R. (2000) Repair of tobacco carcinogen-induced DNA adducts and lung cancer risk: A molecular epidemiologic study. *J. natl Cancer Inst.*, **92**, 1764–1772

Weitberg, A.B. & Corvese, D. (1993) Oxygen radicals potentiate the genetic toxicity of tobacco-specific nitrosamines. *Clin. Genet.*, **43**, 88–91

Westhoff, C., Murphy, P. & Heller, D. (2000) Predictors of ovarian follicle number. *Fertil. Steril.*, **74**, 624–628

Westman, E.C., Levin, E.D. & Rose, J.E. (1995) Nicotine as a therapeutic drug. *N.C. med. J.*, **56**, 48–51

Weston, A. (1993) Physical methods for the detection of carcinogen–DNA adducts in humans. *Mutat. Res.*, **288**, 19–29

Weston, A. & Bowman, E.D. (1991) Fluorescence detection of benzo[*a*]pyrene–DNA adducts in human lung. *Carcinogenesis*, **12**, 1445–1449

Weston, A., Rowe, M.L., Manchester, D.K., Farmer, P.B., Mann, D.L. & Harris, C.C. (1989a) Fluorescence and mass spectral evidence for the formation of benzo[*a*]pyrene *anti*-diol-epoxide–DNA and –hemoglobin adducts in humans. *Carcinogenesis*, **10**, 251–257

Weston, A., Manchester, D.K., Poirier, M.C., Choi, J.S., Trivers, G.E., Mann, D.L. & Harris, C.C. (1989b) Derivative fluorescence spectral analysis of polycyclic aromatic hydrocarbon–DNA adducts in human placenta. *Chem. Res. Toxicol.*, **2**, 104–108

Weston, A., Caporaso, N.E., Taghizadeh, K., Hoover, R.N., Tannenbaum, S.R., Skipper, P.L., Resau, J.H., Trump, B.F. & Harris, C.C. (1991) Measurement of 4-aminobiphenyl–hemoglobin adducts in lung cancer cases and controls. *Cancer Res.*, **51**, 5219–5223

Westra, W.H., Slebos, R.J.C., Offerhaus, G.J.A., Goodman, S.N., Evers, S.G., Kensler, T.W., Askin, F.B., Rodenhuis, S. & Hruban, R.H. (1993) K-*ras* oncogene activation in lung adenocarcinomas from former smokers. *Cancer*, **72**, 432–438

White, J.L., Conner, B.T., Perfetti, T.A., Bombick, B.R., Avalos, J.T., Fowler, K.W., Smith, C.J. & Doolittle, D.J. (2001) Effect of pyrolysis temperature on the mutagenicity of tobacco smoke condensate. *Food chem. Toxicol.*, **39**, 499–505

WHO (1992) *Cadmium* (Environmental Health Criteria No. 134), Geneva, International Programme on Chemical Safety

Whyatt, R.M., Bell, D.A., Jedrychowski, W., Santella, R.M., Garte, S.J., Cosma, G., Manchester, D.K., Young, T.L., Cooper, T.B., Ottman, R. & Perera, F.P. (1998) Polycyclic aromatic hydrocarbon–DNA adducts in human placenta and modulation by CYP1A1 induction and genotype. *Carcinogenesis*, **19**, 1389–1392

Whyatt, R.M., Jedrychowski, W., Hemminki, K., Santella, R.M., Tsai, W.Y., Yang, K. & Perera, F.P. (2001) Biomarkers of polycyclic aromatic hydrocarbon–DNA damage and cigarette smoke exposures in paired maternal and newborn blood samples as a measure of differential susceptibility. *Cancer Epidemiol. Biomarkers Prev.*, **10**, 581–588

Wiencke, J.K., Kelsey, K.T., Varkonyi, A., Semey, K., Wain, J.C., Mark, E. & Christiani, D.C. (1995) Correlation of DNA adducts in blood mononuclear cells with tobacco carcinogen-induced damage in human lung. *Cancer Res.*, **55**, 4910–4914

Wiencke, J.K., Thurston, S.W., Kelsey, K.T., Varkonyi, A., Wain, J.C., Mark, E.J. & Christiani, D.C. (1999) Early age at smoking initiation and tobacco carcinogen DNA damage in the lung. *J. natl Cancer Inst.*, **91**, 614–619

Wild, C.P. & Pisani, P. (1998) Carcinogen DNA and protein adducts as biomarkers of human exposure in environmental cancer epidemiology. *Cancer Detect. Prev.*, **22**, 273–283

Wilkins, J.N., Carlson, H.E., Van Vunakis, H., Hill, M.A., Gritz, E. & Jarvik, M.E. (1982) Nicotine from cigarette smoking increases circulating levels of cortisol, growth hormone, and prolactin in male chronic smokers. *Psychopharmacology*, **78**, 305–308

Willett, W., Stampfer, M.J., Bain, C., Lipnick, R., Speizer, F.E., Rosner, B., Cramer, D. & Hennekens, C.H. (1983) Cigarette smoking, relative weight, and menopause. *Am. J. Epidemiol.*, **117**, 651–658

Willey, J.C., Grafstrom, R.C., Moser, C.E., Jr, Ozanne, C., Sundqvist, K. & Harris, C.C. (1987) Biochemical and morphological effects of cigarette smoke condensate and its fractions on normal human bronchial epithelial cells *in vitro*. *Cancer Res.*, **47**, 2045–2049

Williams, K. & Lewtas, J. (1985) Metabolic activation of organic extracts from diesel, coke oven, roofing tar, and cigarette smoke emissions in the Ames assay. *Environ. Mutag.*, **7**, 489–500

Williams, R.W., Watts, R., Inmon, J., Pasley, T. & Claxton, L. (1990) Stability of the mutagenicity in stored cigarette smokers' urine and extract. *Environ. mol. Mutag.*, **16**, 246–249

Williamson, D.F., Madans, J., Anda, R.F., Kleinman, J.C., Giovino, G.A. & Byers, T. (1991) Smoking cessation and severity of weight gain in a national cohort. *New Engl. J. Med.*, **324**, 739–745

Windham, G.C., Von Behren, J., Waller, K. & Fenster, L. (1999) Exposure to environmental and mainstream tobacco smoke and risk of spontaneous abortion. *Am. J. Epidemiol.*, **149**, 243–247

Winternitz, W.W. & Quillen, D. (1977) Acute hormonal response to cigarette smoking. *J. clin. Pharmacol.*, **17**, 389–397

Wistuba, I.I., Lam, S., Behrens, C., Virmani, A.K., Fong, K.M., LeRiche, J., Samet, J.M., Srivastava, S., Minna, J.D. & Gazdar, A.F. (1997) Molecular damage in the bronchial epithelium of current and former smokers. *J. natl Cancer Inst.*, **89**, 1366–1373

Wistuba, I.I., Gazdar, A.F. & Minna, J.D. (2001) Molecular genetics of small cell lung carcinoma. *Semin. Oncol.*, **28** (Suppl. 4), 3–13

Wong, W.Y., Thomas, C.M., Merkus, H.M., Zielhuis, G.A., Doesburg, W.H. & Steegers-Theunissen, R.P. (2000) Cigarette smoking and the risk of male factor subfertility: Minor association between cotinine in seminal plasma and semen morphology. *Fertil. Steril.*, **74**, 930–935

Woodward, M. & Tunstall-Pedoe, H. (1992) Do smokers of lower tar cigarettes consume lower amounts of smoke components? Results from the Scottish Heart Health Study. *Br. J. Addict.*, **87**, 921–928

Wright, J.L., Dai, J., Zay, K., Price, K., Gilks, C.B. & Churg, A. (1999) Effects of cigarette smoke on nitric oxide synthase expression in the rat lung. *Lab. Invest.*, **79**, 975–983

Wu, X., Lippman, S.M., Lee, J.J., Zhu, Y., Wei, Q.V., Thomas, M., Hong, W.K. & Spitz, M.R. (2002) Chromosome instability in lymphocytes: A potential indicator of predisposition to oral premalignant lesions. *Cancer Res.*, **62**, 2813–1818

Wulf, H.C., Kromann, N., Kousgaard, N., Hansen, J.C., Niebuhr, E. & Albøge, K. (1986) Sister chromatid exchange (SCE) in Greenlandic Eskimos. Dose–response relationship between SCE and seal diet, smoking, and blood cadmium and mercury concentrations. *Sci. total Environ.*, **48**, 81–94

Wurzel, H., Yeh, C.E., Gairola, C.C. & Chow, C.K. (1995) Oxidative damage and antioxidant status in the lungs and bronchoalveolar lavage fluid of rats exposed chronically to cigarette smoke. *J. Biochem. Toxicol.*, **10**, 11–17

Xu, C., Rao, Y.S., Xu, B., Hoffmann, E., Jones, J., Sellers, E.M. & Tyndale, R.F. (2002) An *in vivo* pilot study characterizing the new *CYP2A6*7, *8*, and **10* alleles. *Biochem. biophys. Res. Commun.*, **290**, 318–324

Yadav, J.S. & Thakur, S. (2000a) Cytogenetic damage in bidi smokers. *Nicotine Tob. Res.*, **2**, 97–103

Yadav, J.S. & Thakur, S. (2000b) Genetic risk assessment in hookah smokers. *Cytobios*, **101**, 101–113

Yamasaki, E., & Ames, B.N. (1977) Concentration of mutagens from urine by adsorption with the nonpolar resin XAD-2: Cigarette smokers have mutagenic urine. *Proc. natl Acad. Sci. USA*, **74**, 3555–3559

Yamazaki, H., Inoue, K., Hashimoto, M. & Shimada, T. (1999) Roles of CYP2A6 and CYP2B6 in nicotine *C*-oxidation by human liver microsomes. *Arch. Toxicol.*, **73**, 65–70

Yang, X., Nakao, Y., Pater, M.M., Tang, S.-C. & Pater, A. (1997) Expression of cellular genes in HPV16-immortalized and cigarette smoke condensate-transformed human endocervical cells. *J. cell. Biochem.*, **66**, 309–321

Yang, Q., Hergenhahn, M., Weninger, A. & Bartsch, H. (1999) Cigarette smoke induces direct DNA damage in the human B-lymphoid cell line Raji. *Carcinogenesis*, **20**, 1769–1775

Yang, M., Koga, M., Katoh, T. & Kawamoto, T. (1999) A study for the proper application of urinary naphthols, new biomarkers for airborne polycyclic aromatic hydrocarbons. *Arch. environ. Contam. Toxicol.*, **36**, 99–108

Yang, M., Kunugita, N., Kitagawa, K., Kang, S.-H., Coles, B., Kadlubar, F.F., Katoh, T., Matsuno, K. & Kawamoto, T. (2001) Individual differences in urinary cotinine levels in Japanese smokers: Relation to genetic polymorphism of drug-metabolizing enzymes. *Cancer Epidemiol. Biomarkers Prev.*, **10**, 589–593

Yates, D.H., Breen, H. & Thomas, P.S. (2001) Passive smoke inhalation decreases exhaled nitric oxide in normal subjects. *Am. J. respir. crit. Care Med.*, **164**, 1043–1046

Yeowell-O'Connell, K., Rothman, N., Waidyanatha, S., Smith, M.T., Hayes, R.B., Li, G., Bechtold, W.E., Dosemeci, M., Zhang, L., Yin, S. & Rappaport, S.M. (2001) Protein adducts of 1,4-benzoquinone and benzene oxide among smokers and nonsmokers exposed to benzene in China. *Cancer Epidemiol. Biomarkers Prev.*, **10**, 831–838

Yokoi, T. & Kamataki, T. (1998) Genetic polymorphism of drug metabolizing enzymes: New mutations in *CYP2D6* and *CYP2A6* genes in Japanese. *Pharm. Res.*, **15**, 517–524

Yong, V.W. & Perry, T.L. (1986) Monoamine oxidase B, smoking, and Parkinson's disease. *J. neurol. Sci.*, **72**, 265–272

Yoshie, Y. & Ohshima, H. (1997) Synergistic induction of DNA strand breakage by cigarette tar and nitric oxide. *Carcinogenesis*, **18**, 1359–1363

Yu, H. & Rohan, T. (2000) Role of the insulin-like growth factor family in cancer development and progression. *J. natl Cancer Inst.*, **92**, 1472–1489

Yu, M.C., Skipper, P.L., Taghizadeh, K., Tannenbaum, S.R., Chan, K.K., Henderson, B.E. & Ross, R.K. (1994) Acetylator phenotype, aminobiphenyl–hemoglobin adduct levels, and bladder cancer risk in white, black, and Asian men in Los Angeles, California. *J. natl Cancer Inst.*, **86**, 712–716

Yu, H., Spitz, M.R., Mistry, J., Gu, J., Hong, W.K. & Wu, X. (1999) Plasma levels of insulin-like growth factor-I and lung cancer risk: A case–control analysis. *J. natl Cancer Inst.*, **91**, 151–156

Zavaroni, I., Bonini, L., Gasparini, P., Dall'Aglio, E., Passeri, M. & Reaven, G.M. (1994) Cigarette smokers are relatively glucose intolerant, hyperinsulinemic and dyslipidemic. *Am. J. Cardiol.*, **73**, 904–905

Zavos, P.M., Correa, J.R., Antypas, S., Zarmakoupis-Zavos, P.N. & Zarmakoupis, C.N. (1998) Effects of seminal plasma from cigarette smokers on sperm viability and longevity. *Fertil. Steril.*, **69**, 425–429

van Zeeland, A.A., de Groot, A.J., Hall, J. & Donato, F. (1999) 8-Hydroxydeoxyguanosine in DNA from leukocytes of healthy adults: Relationship with cigarette smoking, environmental tobacco smoke, alcohol and coffee consumption. *Mutat. Res.*, **439**, 249–257

Zeleniuch-Jacquotte, A., Bruning, P.F., Bonfrer, J.M., Koenig, K.L., Shore, R.E., Kim, M.Y., Pasternack, B.S. & Toniolo, P. (1997) Relation of serum levels of testosterone and dehydroepiandrosterone sulfate to risk of breast cancer in postmenopausal women. *Am. J. Epidemiol.*, **145**, 1030–1038

Zeman, M.V., Hiraki, L. & Sellers, E.M. (2002) Gender differences in tobacco smoking: Higher relative exposure to smoke than nicotine in women. *J. Women Health Gender-based Med.*, **11**, 147–153

Zenzes, M.T. (2000) Smoking and reproduction: Gene damage to human gametes and embryos. *Hum. Reprod. Update 2000*, **6**, 122–131

Zenzes, M.T., Wang, P. & Casper, R.F. (1995) Cigarette smoking may affect meiotic maturation of human oocytes. *Hum. Reprod.*, **10**, 3213–3217

Zenzes, M.T., Puy, L.A. & Bielecki, R. (1998) Immunodetection of benzo[*a*]pyrene adducts in ovarian cells of women exposed to cigarette smoke. *Mol. hum. Reprod.*, **4**, 159–165

Zenzes, M.T., Bielecki, R. & Reed, T.E. (1999a) Detection of benzo(*a*)pyrene diol epoxide–DNA adducts in sperm of men exposed to cigarette smoke. *Fertil. Steril.*, **72**, 330–335

Zenzes, M.T., Puy, L.A., Bielecki, R. & Reed, T.E. (1999b) Detection of benzo[*a*]pyrene diol epoxide–DNA adducts in embryos from smoking couples: Evidence for transmission by spermatozoa. *Mol. hum. Reprod.*, **5**, 125–131

Zevin, S. & Benowitz, N.L. (1999) Drug interactions with tobacco smoking. An update. *Clin. Pharmacokinet.*, **36**, 425–438

Zhang, Y.J., Hsu, T.M. & Santella, R.M. (1995) Immunoperoxidase detection of polycyclic aromatic hydrocarbon–DNA adducts in oral mucosa cells of smokers and nonsmokers. *Cancer Epidemiol. Biomarkers Prev.*, **4**, 133–138

Zhang, Z.-F., Shu, X.-M., Cordon-Cardo, C., Orlow, I., Lu, M.-L., Millon, T.V., Cao, P.-Q., Connolly-Jenks, C., Dalbagni, G., Lianes, P., Lacombe, L., Reuter, V.E. & Scher, H. (1997) Cigarette smoking and chromosome 9 alterations in bladder cancer. *Cancer Epidemiol. Biomarkers Prev.*, **6**, 321–326

Zhang, Y.J., Weksler, B.B., Wang, L., Schwartz, J. & Santella, R.M. (1998) Immunohistochemical detection of polycyclic aromatic hydrocarbon–DNA damage in human blood vessels of smokers and nonsmokers. *Atherosclerosis*, **140**, 325–331

Zhang, Y.J., Chen, S.-Y., Hsu, T.M. & Santella, R.M. (2002) Immunohistochemical detection of malondialdehyde–DNA adducts in human oral mucosa cells. *Carcinogenesis*, **23**, 207–211

Zhao, C., Georgellis, A., Flato, S., Palmberg, L., Thunberg, E. & Hemminki, K. (1997) DNA adducts in human nasal mucosa and white blood cells from smokers and nonsmokers. *Carcinogenesis*, **18**, 2205–2208

5. Summary of Data Reported and Evaluation

5.1   Exposure data

Smoking of tobacco is practised worldwide by over one thousand million people. However, while smoking prevalence has declined in many developed countries, it remains high in others and is increasing among women and in developing countries. Between one-fifth and two-thirds of men in most populations smoke. Women's smoking rates vary more widely but rarely equal male rates.

Tobacco is most commonly smoked as cigarettes, both manufactured — which are a highly sophisticated nicotine-delivery system — and hand-rolled. Pipes, cigars, bidis and other products are used to a lesser extent or predominantly in particular regions. Cigarettes are made from fine-cut tobaccos which are wrapped in paper or a maize leaf. Cigars consist of cut tobacco filler formed in a binder leaf and with a wrapper leaf rolled spirally around the bunch. Bidis contain shredded tobacco wrapped in non-tobacco leaves, usually dried *temburni* leaves.

The chemical composition of tobacco smoke, although influenced by the specific manner in which individuals smoke, is primarily determined by the type of tobacco. It is also influenced by the design of the smoking device or product and, for cigarettes, by the presence or absence of filters, and by other factors including ventilation, paper porosity and types of additives. As a result, concentrations of individual chemicals in smoke vary. Analysis of the ways in which people smoke modern cigarettes shows that actual doses of nicotine, carcinogens and toxins depend on the intensity and method of smoking and have little relation to stated tar yields. The total volume of smoke drawn from cigarettes as a result of specific smoking patterns is the principal determinant of dose to the smoker. All presently available tobacco products that are smoked deliver substantial amounts of established carcinogens to their users.

The yields of tar, nicotine and carbon monoxide from cigarettes, as measured by standard machine-smoking tests, have fallen over recent decades in cigarettes sold in most parts of the world, but have remained higher in some countries. The tar and nicotine yields as currently measured are misleading and have only little value in the assessment of human exposure to carcinogens.

The regulation of smoking and smoke yields varies widely around the world in scope and degree of enforcement. Certain regulatory actions, such as taxes and workplace smoking bans, are effective in reducing smoking rates and protecting nonsmokers.

5.2   Human carcinogenicity data

In the previous 1986 *IARC Monograph* on tobacco smoking, cancers of the lung, oral cavity, pharynx, larynx, oesophagus (squamous-cell carcinoma), pancreas, urinary bladder and renal pelvis were identified as caused by cigarette smoking. Many more studies published since this earlier monograph support these causal links. In addition, there is now sufficient evidence for a causal association between cigarette smoking and cancers of the nasal cavities and nasal sinuses, oesophagus (adenocarcinoma), stomach, liver, kidney (renal-cell carcinoma), uterine cervix and myeloid leukaemia.

In cancer sites that were causally linked to cigarette smoking in the previous *IARC Monograph* on tobacco smoking, the observed relative risks ranged generally from approximately 3 for pancreatic cancer to more than 20 for lung cancer. For those cancer sites that were now also linked to cigarette smoking in this monograph, generally two- to threefold increased risks were observed.

Cigarettes

Lung

Lung cancer is the most common cause of death from cancer in the world. The total number of cases is now estimated to be 1.2 million annually and is still increasing. The major cause of lung cancer is tobacco smoking, primarily of cigarettes. In populations with prolonged cigarette use, the proportion of lung cancer cases attributable to cigarette smoking has reached 90%.

The duration of smoking is the strongest determinant of lung cancer in smokers. Hence, the earlier the age of starting and the longer the continuation of smoking in adult-hood, the greater the risk. Risk of lung cancer also increases in proportion to the numbers of cigarettes smoked.

Tobacco smoking increases the risk of all histological types of lung cancer including squamous-cell carcinoma, small-cell carcinoma, adenocarcinoma (including bronchiolar/-alveolar carcinoma) and large-cell carcinoma. The association between adenocarcinoma of the lung and smoking has become stronger over time. The carcinogenic effects of ciga-rette smoking appear similar in both women and men.

Stopping smoking at any age avoids the further increase in risk of lung cancer incurred by continued smoking. The younger the age at cessation, the greater the benefit.

Urinary tract

Tobacco smoking is a major cause of transitional-cell carcinomas of the bladder, ureter and renal pelvis. Risk increases with the duration of smoking and number of ciga-rettes smoked. As for lung cancer, stopping smoking at any age avoids the further increase in risk incurred by continued smoking.

Evidence from several cohort and case–control studies published since the previous *IARC Monograph* on tobacco smoking has indicated that renal-cell carcinoma is asso-ciated with tobacco smoking in both men and women. The association is not explained by confounding. A dose–response relationship with the number of cigarettes smoked has been noted in most studies, and a few also noted a reduction in risk after cessation.

Oral cavity

Tobacco smoking, including cigarette smoking, is causally associated with cancer of the oral cavity (including lip and tongue) in both men and women. Since the previous *IARC Monograph* on tobacco smoking, evidence from many more studies has accumulated that further confirms this association. Use of smokeless tobacco and/or alcohol in combination with tobacco smoking greatly increases the risk of oral cancer. Risk increases substantially with duration of smoking and number of cigarettes smoked. Risk among former smokers is consistently lower than among current smokers and there is a trend of decreasing risk with increasing number of years since quitting.

Nasal cavity and paranasal sinuses

An increased risk of sinonasal cancer among cigarette smokers has been reported in all nine case–control studies for which results are available. Of seven studies that have analysed dose–response relationships, a positive trend was found in five and was suggested in the other two. In all the five studies that have analysed squamous-cell carcinoma and adenocarcinoma separately, the relative risk was clearly increased for squamous-cell carcinoma.

Nasopharynx

An increased risk for nasopharyngeal cancer among cigarette smokers was reported in one cohort study and nine case–control studies. Increased relative risks were reported in both high- and low-risk geographical regions for nasopharyngeal cancer. A dose–response relationship was detected with either duration or amount of smoking. A reduction in risk after quitting was also detected. The potential confounding effect of infection with Epstein–Barr virus was not controlled for in these studies; however, such an effect was not considered to be plausible. No important role was shown for other potential confounders.

Oropharynx and hypopharynx

Oropharyngeal and hypopharyngeal cancer are causally associated with cigarette smoking. The risk increased with increased duration of smoking and daily cigarette consumption and decreased with increasing time since quitting.

Oesophagus

Tobacco smoking is causally associated with cancer of the oesophagus, particularly squamous-cell carcinoma. Tobacco smoking is also causally associated with adenocarcinoma of the oesophagus. In most of the epidemiological studies, the risk for all types of oesophageal cancer increased with numbers of cigarettes smoked daily and duration of smoking. However, risk for oesophageal cancer remains elevated many years after cessation of smoking.

Tobacco and alcohol in combination with tobacco smoking greatly increase the risk for squamous-cell carcinoma of the oesophagus. In India, use of smokeless tobacco in combination with smoking also greatly increases the risk.

Larynx

Laryngeal cancer is causally associated with cigarette smoking. The risk increases substantially with duration and number of cigarettes smoked. Use of alcohol in combination with tobacco smoking greatly increases the risk for laryngeal cancer. A few studies also reported that relative risks for cancer of the larynx increased with decreasing age at start of smoking. The relative risk decreased with increasing time since quitting smoking.

Pancreas

Cancer of the pancreas is causally associated with cigarette smoking. The risk increases with duration of smoking and number of cigarettes smoked daily. The risk remains elevated after allowing for potential confounding factors such as alcohol consumption. The relative risk decreased with increasing time since quitting smoking.

Stomach

The data available in 1986 did not permit the earlier IARC Working Group to conclude that the association between tobacco smoking and stomach cancer was causal. Since that time, further studies have shown a consistent association of cancer of the stomach with cigarette smoking in both men and women in many cohort and case–control studies conducted in various parts of the world. Confounding by other factors (e.g. alcohol consumption, *Helicobacter pylori* infection and dietary factors) can be reasonably ruled out. Risk increases with duration of smoking and number of cigarettes smoked, and decreases with increasing duration of successful quitting. In studies that had adequate numbers, the relative risks for men and women were similar.

Liver

In the previous *IARC Monograph* on tobacco smoking, a causal relationship between liver cancer and smoking could not be established, chiefly due to possible confounding from alcohol intake and hepatitis B and hepatitis C virus infections. Many cohort studies and case–control studies have provided additional information on smoking and liver cancer since then. Most of the cohort studies and the largest case–control studies (most notably those that included community controls) showed a moderate association between tobacco smoking and risk of liver cancer. In many studies, the risk for liver cancer increased with the duration of smoking or the number of cigarettes smoked daily. Former smokers who had stopped smoking for more than 10 years showed a decline in liver cancer risk. Confounding from alcohol can be ruled out, at least in the best case–control studies, by means of careful adjustment for drinking habits. An association with smoking has also been demonstrated among non-drinkers. Many studies, most notably from Asia, have shown no attenuation of the association between smoking and liver cancer after adjustment/stratification for markers of hepatitis B/hepatitis C virus infection. There is now sufficient evidence to judge the association between tobacco smoking and liver cancer as causal.

Cervix

An association of invasive cervical squamous-cell carcinoma with smoking has been observed in the large number of studies reviewed. The most recent studies have controlled for infection with human papillomavirus, a known cause of cervical cancer. The effect of smoking was not diminished by the adjustment for human papillomavirus infection, or analysis restricted to cases and controls both positive for human papillomavirus (as ascertained by human papillomavirus DNA or human papillomavirus serological methods). There is now sufficient evidence to establish a causal association of squamous-cell cervical carcinoma with smoking. In the small number of studies available for adeno- and adeno-squamous-cell carcinoma, no consistent association was observed.

Leukaemia

Myeloid leukaemia in adults was observed to be causally related to smoking. Risk increased with amount of tobacco smoked in a substantial number of adequate studies. No clear evidence of any risk was seen for lymphoid leukaemia/lymphoma.

Support for a causal relationship of smoking with myeloid leukaemia is provided by the finding of known leukaemogens in tobacco smoke, one of which (benzene) is present in sufficient amounts to account for up to half of the estimated excess of acute myeloid leukaemia.

Colorectal cancer

There is some evidence from prospective cohort studies and case–control studies that the risk of colorectal cancer is increased among tobacco smokers. However, it is not possible to conclude that the association between tobacco smoking and colorectal cancer is causal. Inadequate adjustment for various potential confounders could account for some of the small increase in risk that appears to be associated with smoking.

Female breast

Most epidemiological studies have found no association with active smoking, after controlling for established risk factors (e.g. age at time of first birth, parity, family history of breast cancer and alcohol). The large multicentre pooled analysis of the association of smoking with breast cancer in non-drinkers confirms the lack of an increased risk of breast cancer associated with smoking.

Endometrium

Cigarette smoking is not associated with an increased risk for endometrial cancer.

An inverse relationship of cigarette smoking with endometrial cancer is observed consistently in most case–control and cohort studies, after adjustment for major confounders. This pattern is stronger in post-menopausal women.

Prostate

No clear evidence of any risk for prostate cancer is seen in case–control studies or in studies of incident cases in cohort studies. The small excess observed in some analytical mortality studies can reasonably be explained by bias in the attribution of the underlying cause of death.

Other

There is inconsistent and/or sparse evidence for association between cigarette smoking and other cancer sites that were considered by the Working Group.

Cigars and pipes

Cigar and/or pipe smoking is strongly related to cancers of the oral cavity, oropharynx, hypopharynx, larynx and oesophagus, the magnitude of risk being similar to that from cigarette smoking. These risks increase with the amount of cigar and/or pipe smoking and with the combination of alcohol and tobacco consumption. Cigar and/or pipe smoking is causally associated with cancer of the lung and there is evidence that cigar and/or pipe smoking are also causally associated with cancers of the pancreas, stomach and urinary bladder.

Bidi

Bidi smoking is the most common form of tobacco smoking in India and is also prevalent in other south-Asian countries and an emerging problem in the USA. Bidi smoke was considered as carcinogenic in the earlier *IARC Monograph* on tobacco smoking, and later studies have provided further evidence of causality. Case–control studies demonstrated a strong association at various sites: oral cavity (including subsites), pharynx, larynx, oesophagus, lung and stomach. Almost all studies show significant trends with duration of bidi smoking and number of bidis smoked.

Synergy

For public health purposes, synergy should be characterized as a positive departure from additivity. The epidemiological literature often inadequately describes combined effects of smoking with co-exposures to other carcinogenic agents and in many studies power is limited for characterizing combined effects. The issue of synergistic effects can be appropriately addressed by epidemiological studies that show stratified analysis and have sufficient power. The studies reviewed found evidence of synergy between smoking and several occupational causes of lung cancer (arsenic, asbestos and radon), and between smoking and alcohol consumption for cancers of the oral cavity, pharynx, larynx and oesophagus and between smoking and human papillomavirus infection for cancer of the cervix. Data were inadequate to evaluate the evidence for synergy between smoking and other known causes of cancer (e.g. hepatitis B and alcohol for liver cancer).

5.3 Animal carcinogenicity data

Cigarette smoke has been tested for carcinogenicity by inhalation studies in rodents, rabbits and dogs. The model systems for animal exposure to tobacco smoke do not fully simulate human exposure to tobacco smoke, and the tumours that develop in animals are not completely representative of human cancer. Nevertheless, the animal data provide valuable insights regarding the carcinogenic potential of tobacco smoke.

The most compelling evidence for a positive carcinogenic effect of tobacco smoke in animals is the reproducible increase observed in several studies in the occurrence of laryngeal carcinomas in hamsters exposed to whole tobacco smoke or to its particulate phase. In four of five studies in rats, exposure to whole smoke led to modest increases in the occurrence of malignant and/or benign lung tumours. Similarly, in four of eight studies in mice of varying susceptibility to lung tumour development, exposure to whole smoke led to a modest increase in the frequency of lung adenomas. An increased incidence of lung 'tumours' has also been reported in dogs exposed to tobacco smoke, but it is uncertain whether the histopathological features of the lesions are consistent with malignancy. In hamsters exposed to both cigarette smoke and chemical carcinogens (N-nitrosodiethylamine and 7,12-dimethylbenz[a]anthracene), the tumour response in the respiratory tract was higher than in hamsters exposed to either agent alone. The same is true in rats exposed simultaneously to cigarette smoke and radionuclides (radon progeny and plutonium oxide).

Cigarette smoke condensate both initiates and promotes tumour development in animals. It reproducibly induces both benign and malignant skin tumours in mice following topical application. Similarly, it produces skin tumours in rabbits following topical application. Topical application to the oral mucosa also produced an increased incidence of lung tumours and lymphomas in mice. In rats, cigarette smoke condensate produced lung tumours after intrapulmonary injection. In initiation/promotion assays in mouse skin, a single topical application of cigarette smoke condensate followed by application of croton oil was sufficient to initiate both benign and malignant skin tumours. Smoke condensates of Indian bidi administered to mice by gavage were found to induce tumours in a number of organs. Collectively, these data provide evidence of the carcinogenic effect of mainstream tobacco smoke in experimental animals.

5.4 Other relevant data

Causal associations have been clearly established between active smoking and adverse reproductive outcomes and numerous non-neoplastic diseases, including chronic obstructive pulmonary disease and cardiovascular diseases.

Tobacco smoking is addictive, and nicotine has been established as the major addictive constituent of tobacco products. Measurement of the nicotine metabolite, cotinine, in human blood, urine or saliva provides a specific and sensitive test for exposure to tobacco smoke and can be used to distinguish active and passive smokers from nonsmokers.

Active smoking raises the concentrations of carbon monoxide, benzene and volatile organic compounds in exhaled air. The concentrations of urinary metabolites of some important tobacco smoke carcinogens and related compounds are consistently higher in smokers than in nonsmokers. These include metabolites of benzene, a known carcinogen in humans, as well as metabolites of several carcinogens that cause lung tumours in rodents. Covalent binding to blood proteins by carcinogens present in tobacco smoke has been demonstrated to occur at significantly higher levels in smokers than in nonsmokers. The adducts are derived from various compounds including aromatic amines (e.g. 4-aminobiphenyl), polycyclic aromatic hydrocarbons (e.g. benzo[a]pyrene), tobacco-specific nitrosamines (e.g. 4-(methylnitrosamino)-1-(3-pyridyl)-1-butanone), benzene, acrylamide and acrylonitrile.

Smoking-related DNA adducts have been detected by a variety of analytical methods in the respiratory tract, urinary bladder, cervix and other tissues. In many studies the levels of carcinogen–DNA adducts have been shown to be higher in tissues of smokers than in tissues of nonsmokers. Some but not all studies have demonstrated elevated levels of these adducts in the peripheral blood and in full-term placenta. Smoking-related adducts have also been detected in cardiovascular tissues. Collectively, the available biomarker data provide convincing evidence that carcinogen uptake, activation and binding to cellular macromolecules, including DNA, are higher in smokers than in nonsmokers.

The exposure of experimental animals, primarily rodents, to mainstream tobacco smoke results in a number of biological effects that include (i) increases or decreases in the activities of phase I and phase II enzymes involved in carcinogen metabolism, (ii) increases in the activation of antioxidant enzymes, (iii) increased expression of nitric oxide synthase and of various protein kinases and collagenase, (iv) the formation of tobacco smoke-related DNA adducts in several tissues and (v) reduced clearance of particulate material from the lung.

Smoking is known to have inhibitory or inducing effects on the activities of many enzymes in human tissues. These include xenobiotic metabolizing enzymes, which affect drug and carcinogen metabolism. Numerous studies have reported effects on enzymes in cells treated in culture with tobacco smoke or tobacco smoke condensates.

In humans, smoking produces gene mutations and chromosomal abnormalities. Urine from smokers is mutagenic. Relative to nonsmokers, lung tumours of smokers contain higher frequencies of TP53 and KRAS mutations, and the spectrum of mutations has unique features. Most of the genetic effects seen in smokers are also observed in cultured cells or in experimental animals exposed to tobacco smoke or smoke condensate. Tobacco smoke is genotoxic in humans and in experimental animals.

5.5   Evaluation

There is *sufficient evidence* in humans that tobacco smoking causes cancer of the lung, oral cavity, naso-, oro- and hypopharynx, nasal cavity and paranasal sinuses, larynx, oesophagus, stomach, pancreas, liver, kidney (body and pelvis), ureter, urinary bladder, uterine cervix and bone marrow (myeloid leukaemia).

There is *evidence suggesting lack of carcinogenicity* of tobacco smoking in humans for cancers of the female breast and endometrium.

There is *sufficient evidence* in experimental animals for the carcinogenicity of tobacco smoke and tobacco smoke condensates.

Overall evaluation

Tobacco smoking and tobacco smoke *are carcinogenic to humans (Group 1)*.

INVOLUNTARY SMOKING

1.   Composition, Exposure and Regulations

1.1   Composition

1.1.1   *Secondhand smoke*

During smoking of cigarettes, cigars, pipes and other tobacco products, in addition to the mainstream smoke drawn and inhaled by smokers, a stream of smoke is released between puffs into the air from the burning cone. Once released, this stream (also known as the sidestream smoke) is mixed with exhaled mainstream smoke as well as the air in an indoor environment to form the secondhand smoke to which both smokers and nonsmokers are exposed. A small additional contribution to the smoke issues from the tip of the cigarette and through the cigarette paper during puffing and through the paper and from the mouth end of the cigarette between puffs (IARC, 1986; NRC, 1986; US EPA, 1992). Thus, secondhand tobacco smoke is composed of aged exhaled mainstream smoke and diluted sidestream smoke.

Secondhand tobacco smoke contains a variable proportion of exhaled mainstream smoke ranging from 1 to 43% (Baker & Proctor, 1990). Because of its rapid dilution and dispersion into the indoor environment, secondhand tobacco smoke acquires different physicochemical properties to those of mainstream smoke and sidestream smoke and the concentrations of the individual constituents are decreased. The principal physical change is a decrease in the proportion of smoke constituents found in the particulate phase as opposed to the vapour phase of the smoke. The median particle size of secondhand tobacco smoke is subsequently smaller than that of the particles of mainstream smoke. The principal chemical change is in the composition (i.e. in the relative quantities of the individual constituents present); this is caused by differences in the ways in which individual constituents respond to ventilation and to contact with indoor surfaces. There is some indication that chemical transformation of reactive species also occurs.

The effects of exposure to secondhand tobacco smoke, or involuntary (passive) smoking, cannot be estimated from any individual constituents. Secondhand tobacco smoke is actually a complex mixture, containing many compounds for which concentrations can vary with time and environmental conditions. Cigarette smoking is the main source for involuntary exposure because it is by far the most prevalent form of tobacco smoking although specific patterns may differ between countries. Emissions of sidestream smoke in indoor environments with low ventilation rates can result in concentrations of toxic and carcinogenic agents above those generally encountered in ambient air in urban areas (IARC, 1986; Jenkins *et al.*, 2000).

Studies on the complex composition of secondhand tobacco smoke in 'real world' conditions have been limited partly because of the presence of additional sources of secondhand smoke constituents. Therefore compositional and physical studies of second-hand tobacco smoke have often been performed in environmental chambers (also known as a 'controlled experimental atmosphere'). The disadvantage of the controlled experi-mental atmosphere is that it does not reflect real life situations. The studies of the chemical composition of secondhand tobacco smoke, either in a controlled experimental atmosphere or in the field, have been limited. This is mainly because there are still no standardized criteria for the development of experimental atmospheres that represent secondhand tobacco smoke (Jenkins *et al.*, 2000).

Respirable suspended particles (only those particles that are small enough to reach the lower airways of the human lung) can exist in many forms in indoor air: those resulting from secondhand tobacco smoke are present in the form of liquid or waxy droplets. They are smaller than the particles in mainstream smoke. The mass median diameter of mainstream smoke particles averages 0.35–0.40 μm. Gravimetric determination indicates that the respirable suspended particles of secondhand tobacco smoke in typically encoun-tered environments may comprise one-third of the respirable suspended particles in indoor air. However, in some environments, this fraction may be as much as two-thirds (Jenkins *et al.*, 2000).

Respirable suspended particle concentrations of 4091 μg/m^3 were measured in an experimental room in which 120 cigarettes were smoked during 9 hours in 1 day for the evaluation of exposure to benzene and other toxic compounds (Adlkofer *et al.*, 1990).

Worldwide in indoor environments where people smoke, the mean levels of respirable suspended particles ranged from 24 to 1947 μg/m^3. Background levels of respirable sus-pended particles depend on many factors including local vehicular traffic patterns, quality of ventilation systems and the presence of other sources (e.g. cooking and wood-burning stoves). Comparisons between smoking and nonsmoking locations revealed up to threefold higher concentrations of respirable suspended particles in smoking areas. The US EPA-proposed maximal level for fine particles in outdoor ambient air (65 μg/m^3 parti-culate matter, that is 2.5 μm or smaller in size, for 24 h) is frequently exceeded in indoor situations where people are smoking (Jenkins *et al.*, 2000).

Besides respirable suspended particles and nicotine (see Section 1.2), carbon monoxide (CO) has been the most extensively studied constituent of secondhand tobacco smoke. The contemporary commercial cigarettes in the USA deliver approximately 15 mg CO in mainstream smoke and an additional 50 mg in sidestream smoke (Jenkins *et al.*, 2000). In an indoor environment, CO concentrations are rapidly diluted. The measured mean concentrations reported for CO in offices, other workplaces, functions and public gatherings, transportation, restaurants and cafeterias, bars and taverns where people smoke ranged from 0.2 to 33 ppm. The American Society of Heating, Refrigerating and

Air-Conditioning Engineers (ASHRAE) standard for CO concentration in indoor air is 9 ppm (Jenkins *et al.*, 2000).

The mean levels of nitric oxide (NO) in indoor areas were reported from not detected to 500 ppb and those of nitrogen dioxide (NO_2) from not detected to 76 ppb (Jenkins *et al.*, 2000).

There are a number of studies that have addressed the composition of secondhand tobacco smoke beyond the 'common' constituents such as nicotine, CO and respirable suspended particles. A few of these are shown in Table 1.1 (Eatough *et al.*, 1989; Löfroth *et al.* 1989; Higgins *et al.*, 1990; Löfroth, 1993; Martin *et al.*, 1997). The focus of these studies was primarily on vapour-phase constituents. Vapour phase represents the bulk of the mass of secondhand tobacco smoke whereas the respirable suspended particle-related constituents are present at very low concentrations that are very difficult to quantify. For example, if the levels of respirable suspended particles are in the range of 20 to 1000 $\mu g/m^3$, constituents of the particulate phase present at concentrations of 1–100 ppm in the particles themselves will be present at airborne concentrations from 20 pg/m^3 to 100 ng/m^3. These are very low concentrations for detection by any sampling and analysis method (Jenkins *et al.*, 2000).

As can be seen from the data in Table 1.1, the field studies show considerable variation in the measured levels of constituents of secondhand tobacco smoke. Similar concentrations of benzene and isoprene to those shown in Table 1.1 were reported in a smoke-filled bar (from 26 to 36 $\mu g/m^3$ and 80–106 $\mu g/m^3$, respectively), although the nicotine levels were much lower (22 $\mu g/m^3$). The concentration of 1,3-butadiene measured in the smoke-filled bar was from 2.7 to 4.5 $\mu g/m^3$ (Brunnemann *et al.*, 1990). In a field study of 25 homes of smokers, Heavner *et al.* (1995) estimated that the median fraction of benzene contributed by secondhand tobacco smoke was 13% (ranging from 0 to 63%).

In a study of six homes of smokers, secondhand tobacco smoke was found to make a substantial contribution to the concentrations of 1,3-butadiene (Kim *et al.*, 2001).

The levels of carbonyl compounds measured in an experimental room under extremely high concentrations of secondhand tobacco smoke (Adlkofer *et al.*, 1990) were: formaldehyde, 49 $\mu g/m^3$; acetaldehyde, 1390 $\mu g/m^3$ and propionaldehyde, 120 $\mu g/m^3$. The concentrations of other constituents of secondhand tobacco smoke were: nicotine, 71 $\mu g/m^3$; benzene, 206 $\mu g/m^3$; benzo[*a*]pyrene, 26.7 ng/m^3; pyrene, 25 ng/m^3 and chrysene, 70.5 ng/m^3.

Benzo[*a*]pyrene was also detected in natural environments containing secondhand tobacco smoke, with concentrations ranging from not detected to 3.6 ng/m^3 (or up to 3.35 ng/m^3 when the background concentration was subtracted) (Jenkins *et al.*, 2000). Trace levels of some other polycyclic aromatic hydrocarbons (PAHs; such as naphthalene, chrysene, anthracene, phenanthrene and benzofluoranthenes) were also reported. The vapour-phase 2- to 3-ring PAHs predominate quantitatively over the higher-ring system PAHs.

Table 1.1. Concentrations (in µg/m³) of selected constituents of secondhand tobacco smoke in some experimental and real-life situations[a]

Constituent	18-m³ chamber: mean for 50 best-selling US cigarettes (Martin et al., 1997)	Living quarters (Löfroth, 1993)	Tavern (Löfroth et al., 1989)	Discothèque (Eatough et al., 1989)	Home (Higgins et al., 1990)
Respirable suspended particles	1440	240–480	420	801[b]	–
Nicotine	90.8	8–87	71	120	51.8
CO (ppm)	5.09	–	4.8	22.1	–
Benzene	30	–	27	–	17.6
Formaldehyde	143	–	104	–	–
1,3-Butadiene	40	–	19	–	–
Acetaldehyde	268	–	204	–	–
Isoprene	657	50–200	150	–	83.3
Styrene	10	–	–	–	7.3
Catechol	1.24	–	–	–	–
3-Ethenyl pyridine	37.1	–	–	18.2	–
Ethylbenzene	8.5	–	–	–	8.0
Pyridine	23.8	–	–	–	6.5
Toluene	54.5	–	–	17.6	51.2
Limonene	29.1	–	–	–	22.0

Modified from Jenkins et al. (2000)
–, not reported
[a] These are not typical average concentrations, but represent the higher end of the exposure scale.
[b] Fine particles (< 2 µm size)

The levels of *N*-nitrosodimethylamine (NDMA) measured in the field (e.g. in workrooms, conference rooms, restaurants and bars where people smoked) ranged from less than 10 ng/m^3 to 240 ng/m^3 (Jenkins *et al.*, 2000). In unventilated offices in which 11–18 cigarettes were smoked during a 2-h period, up to 8.6 ng/m^3 *N*-nitrosodiethylamine (NDEA) and up to 13 ng/m^3 *N*-nitrosopyrrolidine (NPYR) were measured.

The *N'*-nitrosonornicotine (NNN) concentrations measured in a poorly ventilated office where heavy smoking of cigarettes, cigars and pipes took place ranged from not detected to 6 ng/m^3 and those of 4-(methylnitrosamino)-1-(3-pyridyl)-1-butanone (NNK) from not detected to 13.5 ng/m^3 (Klus *et al.*, 1992). The upper levels reported by Klus *et al.* (1992) and by Adlkofer *et al.* (1990) for the 'heavily smoked rooms' (11 cigarettes smoked in 2 h in a 84 m^2 office) were somewhat lower than those measured by Brunnemann *et al.* (1992): NNN concentrations ranged from not detected to 22.8 ng/m^3 and NNK concentrations between 1.4 and 29.3 ng/m^3, measured inside bars, restaurants, trains, and a car, an office and a smoker's home (Brunnemann *et al.*, 1992).

The effects of cigar smoking on indoor levels of CO, respirable suspended particles and particle-bound PAH particles were investigated in an office where several brands of cigar were machine smoked, in a residence where two cigars were smoked by a person and at cigar social events where up to 18 cigars were smoked at a time. The average concentrations of CO at cigar social events were comparable with, or larger than, those measured on a main road during rush-hour traffic. A mass balance model developed for predicting secondhand tobacco smoke was used in this study to obtain CO, respirable suspended particle and PAH emission. These factors show that cigars can be a stronger source of CO than cigarettes. In contrast, cigars may have lower emissions of respirable suspended particles and PAHs per gram of tobacco consumed than cigarettes, but the greater size and longer smoking time of a single cigar results in greater total respirable suspended particle and PAH emission than from a single cigarette (Klepeis *et al.*, 1999). Nelson *et al.* (1997) tested six brands of cigar and the yields of respirable suspended particles averaged 52 mg/cigar. Yields of CO, nitric oxide (NO) and nitrogen dioxide (NO$_2$) averaged 32, 10.5 and 2.1 mg/cigar, respectively, and that of volatile organic compounds (VOC) (analysed with gas chromatograph-flame ionization detection (FID)) was estimated to be 340 mg/cigar (propane equivalent). Ratios of secondhand tobacco smoke respirable suspended particles to the surrogate standards for the particulate markers ultraviolet particulate matter (UVPM) and fluorescent particulate matter (FPM) were 6.5 and 27.8, respectively. Another particulate marker, solanesol, made up 2.1% of the particles from cigars. For the two gas-phase markers, the ratio of 3-ethenyl pyridine to other gasphase species was more consistent than ratios involving nicotine.

The comparative analysis of the composition of secondhand tobacco smoke from Eclipse (a cigarette that primarily heats tobacco rather than burning it) and from four commercial cigarettes with a wide range of Federal Trade Commission (FTC) yields is shown in Table 1.2 (Bombick *et al.*, 1998). Eclipse contributed similar amounts of CO to secondhand tobacco smoke to those contributed by burning-tobacco cigarettes but contributed 86–90% less respirable suspended particles. Commercial cigarettes, however,

Table 1.2. Mean concentrations (in μg/m³) of selected components of secondhand smoke of four commercial cigarette brands and Eclipse[a] measured in a chamber with a controlled experimental atmosphere

Constituent	Full-flavour brand	Full-flavour light	100-mm brand	Ultra-light	Eclipse
Respirable suspended particles	1458	1345	1706	1184	181
Nicotine	54	63	58	51	4.3
CO (ppm)	6.5	6.2	7.9	6.6	5.2
3-Ethenylpyridine	25	28	28	34	0.56
Acetaldehyde	313	301	384	312	46
Phenol	17.4	16.7	20.0	16.8	4
NO_x (ppb)	241	233	268	250	24
Total hydrocarbons[b]	2.6	2.6	3.0	2.8	0.47

From Bombick *et al.* (1998)
[a] A cigarette that primarily heats (rather than burns) tobacco
[b] Analysed with gas chromatograph–flame ionizing detector (ppm)

contributed a similar amount of constituents to secondhand tobacco smoke, regardless of their ranking on the FTC scale.

1.1.2 *Exhaled mainstream smoke*

Baker and Proctor (1990) estimated that exhaled mainstream smoke contributes 3–11% of CO, 15–43% of particles and 1–9% of nicotine to secondhand tobacco smoke. Non-inhaling smokers can contribute larger amounts. There is little information on how much exhaled mainstream smoke contributes to the overall composition of secondhand tobacco smoke except that the contribution to the particulate phase is more significant than that to the vapour phase (see monograph on tobacco smoke/Section 4 — breath compounds).

1.1.3 *Sidestream smoke*

The composition of cigarette sidestream smoke is similar to that of mainstream smoke. However, the relative quantities of many of the individual constituents of side-stream smoke are different from those found in mainstream smoke. Also, the absolute quantities of most of the constituents released in sidestream smoke differ from those delivered in mainstream smoke (Jenkins *et al.*, 2000).

Like mainstream cigarette smoke, sidestream smoke contains many compounds that are emitted as gases and particles. The distinction between particle and vapour-phase constituents is appropriate for those constituents that are non-volatile (e.g. high-molecular-weight organic compounds and most metals) and those that are clearly gases (e.g. CO). Constituents with appreciable vapour pressure (i.e. most of the constituents of tobacco smoke) can be found in both the particulate phase and the vapour phase of cigarette smoke. The term 'semivolatiles' has been used to describe such constituents. The degree to which these compounds are distributed between the particle and vapour phases is determined by their volatility (and stability) and the characteristics of their environment. These constituents are distributed preferentially in the particulate phase in highly concentrated smokes, such as those inhaled by smokers, and preferentially in the particle and vapour phases in highly diluted smokes, such as those encountered by involuntary smokers. The phase distribution and the ultimate fate of any given constituent released into the ambient environment is likely to differ depending upon ambient conditions and upon the chemical or physical properties of that constituent.

The manner in which cigarettes are smoked greatly influences their mainstream delivery and sidestream emissions. For the different machine-smoking protocols referred to in this monograph, see Table 1.9 in the monograph on tobacco smoke. Particulate matter that is released in mainstream smoke during active smoking enters the respiratory tract largely intact, whereas the particulate matter in sidestream smoke is available for inhalation only after dilution in ambient air and after the physical and chemical changes that occurred during that dilution. However, conventional analysis of sidestream smoke provides only information on the quantities of individual smoke constituents released into the air. Moreover, the methods for analysis of sidestream smoke are not as well defined as those for mainstream smoke (Jenkins *et al.*, 2000).

As they leave the cigarette, sidestream smoke particles are initially slightly smaller than mainstream smoke particles (geometric mean diameter, 0.1 µm versus 0.18 µm; Guerin *et al.*, 1987). The natural dissipation rates of sidestream smoke particles dispersed in an experimental chamber were studied from the standpoint of a static atmosphere and were expressed as half-lives of residence in the air. The half-lives for particles with diameters less than 0.3 µm, 0.3–0.5 µm and 0.5–1 µm were found to be 25.5, 12.8 and 4.9 h, respectively. Total particulate matter decreased by half over 6.2 h (Vu Duc & Huynh, 1987). However in real-life situations the ageing of sidestream smoke over several minutes may lead to an increase in particle size of secondhand tobacco smoke due to the coagulation of particles and the removal of smaller particles that attach to surfaces in the environment. Sidestream smoke is produced at generally lower temperatures and with a very different oxygen flux to that of mainstream smoke.

The ratio of sidestream smoke to mainstream smoke is customarily used to express the distribution of individual constituents between the two smoke matrices. The distribution of specific components is dependent on their mechanism of formation. Higher ratios of sidestream smoke to mainstream smoke between cigarettes or smoking conditions generally reflect a lower mainstream smoke delivery with no significant change in sidestream smoke delivery. Under similar smoking conditions, filter-tipped cigarettes will have lower mainstream smoke yields than their untipped analogues. Sidestream smoke yields will not vary greatly, because they reflect the weight of tobacco burned during smouldering. In general, more tobacco is burned during smouldering than during puffing (Guerin *et al.*, 1987).

Adams *et al.* (1987) reported that sidestream smoke contains more alkaline and neutral compounds than mainstream smoke (the pH of the sidestream smoke of cigarettes with a wide range of FTC yields averaged 7.5 [7.2–7.7], whereas the pH of mainstream smoke averaged 6.1 [6.0–6.3]). The differences are due to temperature during burning and mechanisms of chemical transfer (release) from unburned tobacco.

Many constituents of sidestream smoke belong to chemical classes known to be geno-toxic and carcinogenic. These include the IARC group 1 carcinogens benzene, cadmium, 2-aminonaphthalene, nickel, chromium, arsenic and 4-aminobiphenyl; the IARC group 2A carcinogens formaldehyde, 1,3-butadiene and benzo[*a*]pyrene; and the IARC group 2B carcinogens acetaldehyde, isoprene, catechol, acrylonitrile, styrene, NNK, NNN and lead among others.

Adams *et al.* (1987) determined the levels of selected toxic and carcinogenic agents in the mainstream and sidestream smoke of four different types of US commercial ciga-rette brands — untipped and filter-tipped — with a wide range of FTC yields. In this study, smoke was generated by a machine using the standard FTC method. The concen-trations of all agents except NNN were higher in the sidestream than in the mainstream smoke of both untipped and filter-tipped brands. The tar yields in sidestream smoke ranged from 14 to 24 mg per cigarette (similar to the range reported by Ramsey *et al.*, 1990) and were, on average, 5.3 times higher than those in mainstream smoke. The highest sidestream smoke/mainstream smoke ratio for tar was calculated for ultra low-yield cigarettes (ratio, 15.7) and the lowest for untipped cigarettes (ratio, 1.12). The mainstream smoke yields are strongly affected by variables that only slightly affect side-stream smoke yields (Guerin *et al.*, 1987). The ratios of sidestream smoke to mainstream smoke for nicotine, CO and NNK for the ultra low-yield brand were 21.1, 14.9 and 22.3, respectively. The highest emissions of nicotine, NNK and NNN were measured in the sidestream smoke of untipped cigarettes (4.62 mg, 1444 ng and 857 ng, respectively). In mainstream smoke, these values were 2.04 mg, 425 ng and 1007 ng, respectively. The levels of volatile *N*-nitrosamines in sidestream smoke greatly exceeded those measured in mainstream smoke (e.g. 735 ng versus 31.1 ng NDMA per untipped cigarette and 685 ng versus 4.1 ng NDMA for ventilated filter-tipped cigarettes; average ratio, 95). The average ratio of sidestream smoke to mainstream smoke for the carcinogen NPYR was 10. The authors concluded that the availability of cigarettes with greatly reduced amounts of carcinogens in mainstream smoke had little bearing on the emissions of carcinogens in sidestream smoke.

Chortyk and Schlotzhauer (1989) compared the emissions of various smoke compo-nents for 19 low-yield brands of filter-tipped cigarettes with those measured for a refe-rence high-yield untipped brand. It was found that low-yield cigarettes produced large quantities of tar in sidestream smoke, about equal to that of the high-yield cigarette. On an equal weight basis, the low-tar cigarettes emitted more of these hazardous compounds into sidestream and secondhand smoke than did the high-tar cigarette.

The yields of various constituents of sidestream smoke of 15 Canadian cigarette brands measured using the FTC machine-smoking protocol with the exception that cigarettes were smoked to a butt length of 30 mm, ranged as follows: tar, from 15.8 to 29.3 mg per cigarette in non-ventilated brands and from 24.2 mg to 36.0 mg in ventilated brands; nicotine, from 2.7 mg to 4.6 mg in non-ventilated brands and 3.0 mg to 6.1 mg in ventilated brands, and CO, from 40.5 mg to 67.3 mg in non-ventilated brands and 46.5 mg to 63.1 mg in ventilated brands. Yields in sidestream smoke were much higher than those in mainstream smoke for all brands tested. The average ratios for sidestream smoke to mainstream smoke were 3.5, 6.6 and 6.8 for tar, nicotine and CO, respectively. The highest yields from sidestream smoke were obtained from the brands with the lowest mainstream smoke yields (Rickert et al., 1984). The concentrations of carbon monoxide in the sidestream smoke in the Canadian cigarettes were higher than those reported for four different types of American blend cigarettes smoked according to the FTC protocol (Adams et al., 1987). Differences in the tobacco blend may be one explanation for this discrepancy and Canadian cigarettes are made predominantly from flue-cured tobacco.

The average yields of total particulate matter and nicotine in sidestream smoke generated by the machine-smoking of two cigarette brands that are popular among smokers in India (one filter-tipped and one untipped) were 16.51 and 0.9 mg per cigarette, respectively (Pakhale & Maru, 1998). In the sidestream smoke from bidis, these concentrations were 5.5 mg total particulate matter and 0.25 mg nicotine. The sidestream smoke released from chuttas contained 19.8 mg total particulate matter and 2.07 mg nicotine per unit. In all Indian products, the emissions of total particulate matter were much higher in mainstream smoke than in sidestream smoke, which is demonstrated clearly by the ratio of sidestream smoke to mainstream smoke which ranged from 0.13 to 0.49 (see also the monograph on tobacco smoke, Section 1.2.7). This is a modified, more intensive smoking standard (two puffs per minute instead of one) used because of the poor burning properties of the tobacco in Indian products.

In the 1999 Massachusetts Benchmark Study (Borgerding et al., 2000), a subset of 12 brands was analysed for the chemical composition of the sidestream smoke that was generated by machine-smoking using the 'more intense' Massachusetts method. The data obtained are summarized in Table 1.3. The concentrations of the constituents of the sidestream smoke determined in this study differed significantly from those obtained using the standard FTC method that had been reported by Adams et al. (1987): the yields of CO, ammonia and benzo[a]pyrene were higher, those of tar and catechol were of the same order of magnitude and those of NNN and NNK were significantly lower. NNN and NNK levels were even lower than those measured in the mainstream smoke generated by the same intense machine-smoking method. The values obtained by the Massachusetts Study for some gaseous compounds such as 1,3-butadiene, acrolein, isoprene, benzene and toluene were also far below those obtained by machine-smoking using the FTC method (Brunnemann et al., 1990; Table 1.4). For the 12 commercial cigarette brands tested by the Massachusetts puffing parameters, the highest median sidestream smoke/mainstream smoke ratios in the Massachusetts study were obtained for ammonia (ratio, 147),

Table 1.3. Average values of 44 smoke constituents in the sidestream smoke of 12 commercial cigarette brands assayed in the 1999 Massachusetts Benchmark Study using Massachusetts smoking parameters

Constituent	Unit	Range	SS/MS ratio[a]
Ammonia	mg/cig.	4.0–6.6	147
1-Aminonaphthalene	ng/cig.	165.8–273.9	7.10
2-Aminonaphthalene	ng/cig.	113.5–171.6	8.83
3-Aminobiphenyl	ng/cig.	28.0–42.2	10.83
4-Aminobiphenyl	ng/cig.	20.8–31.8	5.41
Benzo[a]pyrene	ng/cig.	51.8–94.5	3.22
Formaldehyde	µg/cig.	540.4–967.5	14.78
Acetaldehyde	µg/cig.	1683.7–2586.8	1.31
Acetone	µg/cig.	811.3–1204.8	1.52
Acrolein	µg/cig.	342.1–522.7	2.53
Propionaldehyde	µg/cig.	151.8–267.6	1.06
Crotonaldehyde	µg/cig.	62.2–121.8	1.95
Methyl ethyl ketone	µg/cig.	184.5–332.6	1.49
Butyraldehyde	µg/cig.	138.0–244.9	2.68
Hydrogen cyanide	mg/cig.	0.19–0.35	0.77
Mercury	ng/cig.	5.2–13.7	1.09
Nickel	ng/cig.	ND–NQ	
Chromium	ng/cig.	ND–ND	
Cadmium	ng/cig.	122–265	1.47
Arsenic	ng/cig.	3.5–26.5	1.51
Selenium	ng/cig.	ND–ND	
Lead	ng/cig.	2.7–6.6	0.09
Nitric oxide	mg/cig.	1.0–1.6	2.79
Carbon monoxide	mg/cig.	31.5–54.1	1.87
'Tar'	mg/cig.	10.5–34.4	0.91
Nicotine	mg/cig.	1.9–5.3	2.31
Pyridine	µg/cig.	195.7–320.7	16.08
Quinoline	µg/cig.	9.0–20.5	12.09
Phenol	µg/cig.	121.3–323.8	9.01
Catechol	µg/cig.	64.5–107.0	0.85
Hydroquinone	µg/cig.	49.8–134.1	0.94
Resorcinol	µg/cig.	ND–5.1	
meta-Cresol + para-Cresol[b]	µg/cig.	40.9–113.2	4.36
ortho-Cresol	µg/cig.	12.4–45.9	4.15[c]
NNN	ng/cig.	69.8–115.2	0.43
NNK	ng/cig.	50.7–95.7	0.40
NAT	ng/cig.	38.4–73.4	0.26
NAB	ng/cig.	11.9–17.8	0.55
1,3-Butadiene	µg/cig.	81.3–134.7	1.30

Table 1.3 (contd)

Constituent	Unit	Range	SS/MS ratio[a]
Isoprene	μg/cig.	743.2–1162.8	1.33
Acrylonitrile	μg/cig.	24.1–43.9	1.27
Benzene	μg/cig.	70.7–134.3	1.07
Toluene	μg/cig.	134.9–238.6	1.27
Styrene	μg/cig.	23.2–46.1	2.60

From Borgerding *et al.* (2000)

SS, sidestream smoke; MS, mainstream smoke; NNN, *N*′-nitrosonornicotine; NNK, 4-(*N*-nitrosomethylamino)-1-(3-pyridyl)-1-butanone; NAT, *N*′-nitroso-anatabine; NAB, *N*′-nitrosoanabasine; ND, not detected; limit of detection for chromium, 8 ng/cigarette; for selenium, 5 ng/cigarette; for resorcinol, 0.6 μg/cigarette; for nickel, 6.8 ng/cigarette; NQ, not quantifiable; limit of quantification for nickel, 10 ng/cigarette

[a] Median value for the sidestream/mainstream smoke ratios for the 12 commercial cigarette brands

[b] Reported together

Table 1.4. Concentrations of selected gas-phase compounds in sidestream smoke of commercial cigarettes

Compound	Federal Trade Commission method (Adams *et al.*, 1987; Brunnemann *et al.*, 1990)	1999 Massachusetts Benchmark Study (Borgerding *et al.*, 2000)
NNN (ng/cig.)	185–857	70–115
NNK (ng/cig.)	386–1444	51–96
1,3-Butadiene (μg/cig.)	205–250[a]	81–135
Acrolein (μg/cig.)	723–1000	342–523
Isoprene (μg/cig.)	4380–6450	743–1163
Benzene (μg/cig.)	345–529	71–134
Toluene (μg/cig.)	758–1060	135–239

NNN, *N*′-nitrosonornicotine; NNK, 4-(*N*-nitrosomethylamino)-1-(3-pyridyl)-1-butanone)

[a] 400 μg 1,3-butadiene measured in the sidestream smoke collected after emission into an environmental chamber (Löfroth, 1989)

Table 1.5. Yields of IARC carcinogens in regular-sized Canadian cigarettes. Comparison of International Organization for Standardization (ISO)[a] and Health Canada (HC)[b] machine-smoking parameters[c]

Compound	ISO smoking parameters						
	Regular (full flavour)	Light	Extra light	Ultra light	ISO/ISO regular/ light	ISO/ISO regular/ extra light	ISO/ISO regular/ ultra light
IARC Group 1 carcinogens							
Benzene (µg/cig.)	222.0	250.0	260.0	296.0*	0.9	0.9	0.8*
Cadmium (ng/cig.)	438.0	484.0	502.0*	627.0*	0.9	0.9*	0.7*
2-Aminonapththalene (ng/cig.)	157.0	147.0	175.0	186.0	1.1	0.9	0.8
Nickel (ng/cig.)	34.3	45.1	74.4*	73.0*	0.8	0.5*	0.5*
Chromium (ng/cig.)	61.0	62.0	121*	82.9*	1.0	0.5*	0.7*
Arsenic (ng/cig.)	ND	NQ	ND	ND			
4-Aminobiphenyl (ng/cig.)	22.1	19.5	21.0	21.2	1.1	1.1	1.0
IARC Group 2A carcinogens							
Formaldehyde (µg/cig.)	378.0	326.0	414.0	431.0	1.2	0.9	0.9
1,3-Butadiene (µg/cig.)	196.0	185.0	264.0	299.0	1.1	0.7	0.7
Benzo[a]pyrene (ng/cig.)	48.8	98.3	92.2	113.0	0.5	0.5	0.4
IARC Group 2B carcinogens							
Acetaldehyde (µg/cig.)	1416.0	1454.0	1449.0	1492.0	1.0	1.0	0.9
Isoprene (µg/cig.)	1043.0	1164.0	1060.0	1172.0	0.9	1.0	0.9
Catechol (µg/cig.)	130.0	117.0	149.0	148.0	1.1	0.9	0.9
Acrylonitrile (µg/cig.)	78.6	85.6	74.1	81.8	0.9	1.1	1.0
Styrene (µg/cig.)	74.0	84.7	87.5	108.0*	0.9	0.8	0.7*
NNK (ng/cig.)	95.2	153.4	38.3	34.7	0.6	2.5	2.7
NNN (ng/cig.)	23.3	53.9	43.7	45.2	0.4	0.5	0.5
Lead (ng/cig.)	54.8	39.4	22.3	18.5	1.4	2.5	3.0

Source: Government of British Columbia (2003)

NNN, N'-nitrosonornicotine; NNK, 4-(N-nitrosomethylamino)-1-(3-pyridyl)-1-butanone; ND, not detectable; NQ, not quantifiable
[a] ISO smoking parameters: 35 mL puff in 2 sec, interval 60 sec, ventilation holes not blocked
[b] HC: Health Canada smoking parameters: 56 mL puff in 2 sec, interval 26 sec, ventilation holes fully blocked
[c] Reporting period: year 1999
* Changed according to personal communication with B. Beech, Health Canada

3-aminobiphenyl (ratio, 10.8), formaldehyde (ratio, 14.8), pyridine (ratio, 16.1) and quinoline (ratio, 12.1).

Often, conflicting results concerning the phase distribution of individual constituents and poor agreement between laboratories for quantitation of sidestream emissions are attributed to different methods used for smoke generation and collection.

Table 1.5 shows the yields of IARC carcinogens in sidestream smoke generated under standard International Organization for Standardization (ISO) and the more intense Health Canada methods, of four popular regular-size Canadian cigarette brands.

On the basis of their mainstream smoke tar yields as measured by the ISO/FTC machine-smoking method, the four cigarette brands may be classified as 'full flavour', 'light', 'extra light' and 'ultra light'. British Columbia has established the Tobacco Testing and Disclosure Regulation and became the first jurisdiction in the world to require Canadian tobacco manufacturers to disclose on a brand-by-brand basis the contents of cigarettes and tobacco and the levels of potentially toxic chemicals in tobacco smoke.

Table 1.5. (contd)

HC smoking parameters

Regular (full flavour)	Light	Extra light	Ultra light	HC/HC regular/ light	HC/HC regular/ extra light	HC/HC regular/ ultra light	HC/ISO Regular	HC/ISO Light	HC/ISO Extra light	HC/ISO Ultra light
98.1	140.0	141.0	158.0	0.7	0.7	0.6	0.4	0.6	0.5	0.5*
256.0	276.0	282.0	355.0	0.9	0.9	0.7	0.6	0.6	0.5*	0.5*
113.0	71.1	112.0	102.0	1.6	1.0	1.1	0.7	0.5	0.6	0.5
17.6	49.3	35.5	34.8	0.4	0.5	0.5	0.5	1.1	0.5*	0.5*
47.1	57.2	54.6	69.4	0.8	0.9	0.7	0.8	0.9	0.5*	0.8*
ND	ND	ND	ND							
16.3	12.5	17.2	15.1	1.3	0.9	1.1	0.7	0.6	0.8	0.7
311.0	208.0	256.0	327.0	1.5	1.2	1.0	0.8	0.6	0.6	0.8
120.0	109.0	168.0	175.0	1.1	0.7	0.7	0.6	0.6	0.6	0.6
31.9	39.5	41.2	44.0	0.8	0.8	0.7	0.7	0.4	0.4	0.4
1174.0	969.0	1079.0	1277.0	1.2	1.1	0.9	0.8	0.7	0.7	0.9
525.0	818.0	763.0	858.0	0.6	0.7	0.6	0.5	0.7	0.7	0.7
104.0	82.0	96.1	109.0	1.3	1.1	1.0	0.8	0.7	0.6	0.7
41.1	50.1	47.6	51.9	0.8	0.9	0.8	0.5	0.6	0.6	0.6
38.7	61.6	50.8	55.6	0.6	0.8	0.7	0.5	0.7	0.6	0.5*
69.8	116.5	65.6	89.9	0.6	1.1	0.8	0.7	0.8	1.7	2.6
19.3	37.8	24.3	30.1	0.5	0.8	0.6	0.8	0.7	0.6	0.7
40.0	30.1	27.0	24.3	1.3	1.5	1.6	0.7	0.8	1.2	1.3

Among the 44 smoke components reported by the manufacturers on a yearly basis, there are seven IARC group 1 carcinogens (benzene, cadmium, 2-aminonaphthalene, nickel, chromium, arsenic and 4-aminobiphenyl), three IARC group 2A carcinogens (formaldehyde, 1,3-butadiene and benzo[a]pyrene) and eight IARC group 2B carcinogens (acetaldehyde, isoprene, catechol, acrylonitrile, styrene, NNK, NNN and lead).

Of the seven IARC group 1 carcinogens, arsenic yields in sidestream smoke were below the detection limits of both the ISO and Health Canada smoking methods. In general, yields of the six other IARC group 1 carcinogens in sidestream smoke were higher when measured by the ISO than by the Health Canada smoking method. The ISO and Health Canada methods gave similar yields for nickel and chromium in the 'light' cigarette and for chromium in the 'ultra light' cigarette.

For most IARC group 2A and 2B carcinogens, the yields in sidestream smoke measured by the Health Canada method were 40–80% of corresponding yields measured by the ISO method. Exceptionally, for NNK and lead the yields measured by the Health Canada method were higher than the yields measured by the ISO method, but only for the 'extra light' and 'ultra light' brands. The yields of NNK measured by the Health Canada method were up to 2.6-fold higher than the yields measured by the ISO method (Government of British Columbia, 2003).

Table 1.5 also allows comparisons of sidestream smoke yields between the brands. There is no significant difference between the total sidestream smoke yields of IARC group 1 carcinogens of 'full flavour' and 'light', extra light and ultra light cigarettes when measured by either the ISO or Health Canada methods.

The data in Tables 1.3 and 1.5 suggest that during more intense smoking (as employed by the Massachusetts and Health Canada methods: i.e. larger puffs, shorter interval between puffs and partial or complete blockage of ventilation holes), smaller quantities of tobacco are burned during the smouldering of the cigarette, thus affecting the emissions of toxins in sidestream smoke. Therefore, the real-life contribution of sidestream smoke to the overall concentrations of selected components of secondhand tobacco smoke may have been overestimated in the past because most smokers draw smoke from their cigarettes with an intensity more similar to that of the Massachusetts or Health Canada methods than the FTC machine-smoking method (Djordjevic et al., 2000). This concept needs to be investigated more thoroughly, especially in view of the finding that an increase in puff volume from 17.5 mL to 50 mL and in filter ventilation from 0 to 83% failed to reduce the levels of tar, CO and nicotine in the sidestream smoke, whereas the yields in mainstream smoke and subsequently the ratios of sidestream smoke to mainstream smoke changed significantly (Guerin et al., 1987).

In addition to the constituents listed in Table 1.3, some further constituents have been quantified in sidestream smoke since the publication of the 1986 *IARC Monograph*. These are NDMA (up to 735 ng per cigarette), *N*-nitrosopiperidine (NPIP, 19.8 ng) and NPYR (up to 234 ng) (Adams et al., 1987); and volatile hydrocarbons, e.g. ethene up to 1200 µg, propene up to 1300 µg, butenes up to 900 µg and pentenes up to 2100 µg. The sidestream smoke emissions of various unsaturated gaseous hydrocarbons were 3–30 times those reported for the mainstream smoke emissions. These compounds constitute a potential health risk as they are metabolized *in vivo* to reactive genotoxic epoxides (Löfroth et al., 1987; Löfroth, 1989). High-molecular-weight *n*-alkanes (C_{27} [66–86.5 µg per cigarette], C_{29} [28–39 µg per cigarette] C_{31} [148–197 µg per cigarette], C_{33} [43.5–62 µg per cigarette]) were also quantified in the sidestream smoke of commercial cigarettes (Ramsey et al., 1990).

The co-mutagenic beta-carbolines, norharman and harman, were quantified in the sidestream smoke condensates of some Japanese cigarette brands. The concentrations per cigarette were 4.1–9.0 µg for norharman and 2.1–3.0 µg for harman (Totsuka et al., 1999).

1.2   Exposure

Exposure to secondhand smoke can take place in any of the environments where people spend time. A useful conceptual framework for considering exposure to secondhand smoke is offered by the microenvironmental model that describes personal exposure to secondhand smoke as the weighted sum of the concentrations of secondhand smoke in the microenvironments where time is spent and the weights supplied by the time spent in each (Jaakkola & Jaakkola, 1997). A microenvironment is a space, e.g. a room in a dwelling or an office area, with a relatively uniform concentration of secondhand smoke during the time that is spent in that particular microenvironment. For research purposes and for considering health risks, personal exposure is the most relevant measure for evaluating and projecting risk (Samet & Yang, 2001).

Within the framework of the microenvironmental model, there are several useful indicators of exposure to secondhand smoke, ranging from surrogate indicators to direct measurements of exposure and of biomarkers that reflect dose (Table 1.6). One useful surrogate, and the only indicator available for many countries, is the prevalence rate of smoking among men and women. It provides at least a measure of likelihood of exposure. For the countries of Asia, for example, where smoking rates among men are very high and those among women are low, the prevalence data for men imply that most women are exposed to tobacco smoke at home (Samet & Yang, 2001).

The components of secondhand smoke include a number of irritating and odiferous gaseous components, such as aldehydes. Nonsmokers typically identify the odour of secondhand smoke as annoying, and the odour detection thresholds determined for secondhand smoke is at concentrations that are three or more orders of magnitude lower

Table 1.6. Indicators of exposure to secondhand tobacco smoke

Measure	Indicator
Surrogate measures	Prevalence of smoking in men and women
Indirect measures	Report of secondhand tobacco smoke exposure in the home and in the workplace

	Smoking in the household
	   Number of smokers
	   Smoking by parent(s)
	   Number of cigarettes smoked

	Smoking in the workplace
	   Presence of secondhand tobacco smoke
	   Number of smokers

Direct measures	Concentration of secondhand tobacco smoke components
	   Nicotine
	   Respirable particles
	   Other markers

	Biomarker concentrations
	   Cotinine
	   Carboxyhaemoglobin

From Samet & Yang (2001)

than the secondhand smoke concentrations measured in field settings and correspond to a fresh air dilution volume > 19 000 m³ per cigarette (Junker *et al.*, 2001).

The indirect measures listed in Table 1.6 are generally obtained by questionnaires. These measures include self-reported exposure and descriptions of the source of second-hand smoke (e.g. smoking), in relevant microenvironments, most often the home and workplace. Self-reported exposure to secondhand smoke is a useful indicator of being exposed, although questionnaire-based reports of intensity of exposure are of uncertain validity. Questionnaires have been used to ascertain the prevalence of passive smoking; some of these have included questions directly related to the WHO definition of passive smoking: i.e. exposure for at least 15 minutes per day on more than 1 day per week (Samet & Yang, 2001).

Questionnaires have been used widely for research purposes to characterize smoking (the source of secondhand smoke) in the home and work environments. A simple mass-balance model gives the concentration of secondhand smoke as reflecting the rate of its generation, i.e., the number of smokers and of cigarettes smoked, the volume of the space into which the smoke is released, and the rate of smoke removal by either air exchange or air cleaning (Ott, 1999). Information on smoking can be collected readily by adults within the household (the source term), although reports of numbers of cigarettes smoked in the home are probably less valid than exposure predicted using the mass balance model. For workplace environments, smoking can be reported by co-workers, although the com-plexity of some workplace environments may preclude the determination of the numbers of smokers in the work area or the numbers of cigarettes smoked. The other determinants of secondhand smoke concentration, namely, room volume and air exchange are not readily determined by questionnaire and are assessed only for specific research purposes (Samet & Yang, 2001).

The direct measures of exposure to secondhand smoke include measurement of the concentrations of components of secondhand smoke in the air and of the levels of second-hand smoke biomarker in biological specimens. Using the microenvironmental model, researchers can estimate exposure to secondhand smoke by measuring the concentration of secondhand smoke in the home, workplace, or other environments and then combining the data on concentrations with information on the time spent in the microenvironments where exposure took place. For example, to estimate exposure to secondhand smoke in the home, the concentration of a marker in the air, e.g. nicotine, would be measured and the time spent in the home would be assessed, possibly using a time–activity diary in which information on all locations where time is spent is collected (Samet & Yang, 2001).

Because cigarette smoke is a complex mixture, exposure assessment depends on the choice of a suitable marker compound that is found in both mainstream smoke and secondhand tobacco smoke. No compound has a consistent ratio with all other com-ponents. Therefore, the choice of marker can affect the estimate of exposure.

The selection of a particular secondhand smoke component for monitoring is largely based on technological feasibility. Air can be sampled either actively, using a pump that passes air through a filter or a sorbent, or passively, using a badge that operates on the principle of diffusion. A number of secondhand smoke components have been proposed as potential indicators; these include small particles in the respirable size range and the gases, nicotine, which is present in the vapour phase in secondhand smoke, and carbon monoxide. Other proposed indicators include more specific measures of particles and other gaseous components (Guerin et al., 1992; Jenkins & Counts, 1999). The most widely studied components have been respirable particles, which are sampled actively with a pump and filter, and nicotine, which can be collected using either active or passive sampling methods. The respirable particles in indoor air have sources other than active smoking and are nonspecific indicators of secondhand smoke; nicotine in air, by contrast, is highly specific because smoking is its only source (Jenkins et al., 2000). Nicotine concentration can be measured readily using a passive filter badge, which is sufficiently small to be worn by a child or an adult or to be placed in a room (Hammond, 1999).

Biomarkers of exposure are compounds that can be measured in biological materials such as blood, urine or saliva. Cotinine, a metabolite of nicotine, is a highly specific indicator of exposure to secondhand smoke in nonsmokers (Benowitz, 1999). Some foods contain small amounts of nicotine, but for most persons cotinine level offers a highly specific and sensitive indicator of exposure to secondhand smoke (Benowitz, 1999). In nonsmokers, the half-life of cotinine is about 20 h; it therefore provides a measure of exposure to secondhand smoke over several days. It is an integrative measure that reflects exposure to secondhand smoke in all environments where time has been spent. Cotinine can be readily measured in blood, urine and even saliva with either radioimmunoassay or chromatography. New methods for analysis extend the sensitivity to extremely low levels (Benowitz, 1996; Benowitz, 1999). Alternatives to nicotine as a tobacco-specific marker substance are few. One such compound is 3-ethenylpyridine (also called 3-vinyl pyridine); it is a pyrolisis product of nicotine degradation during smoking present almost exclusively in the vapour phase of tobacco smoke. It has been employed to a small extent for measuring the concentrations of secondhand tobacco smoke in air (Heavner et al., 1995; Hodgson et al., 1996; Scherer et al., 2000; Vainiotalo et al., 2001), and a correlation between nicotine and 3-ethenylpyridine has been reported in some studies (Jenkins et al., 1996; Moschandreas & Vuilleumier, 1999; Hyvärinen et al., 2000). 3-Ethenylpyridine, solanesol and ultraviolet-absorbing particulate matter as markers of secondhand smoke have been suggested as being potentially better correlated with other constituents of secondhand smoke than nicotine and respirable particles (Hodgson et al., 1996; Jenkins et al., 1996). There are however many fewer data available on measurements using other tobacco-specific marker compounds than those based on air nicotine.

1.2.1 *Measurements of nicotine and particulate matter in indoor air*

The report of the US Environmental Protection Agency (US EPA, 1992) summarizes over 25 separate studies that reported concentrations of nicotine in air measured in more than 100 different indoor microenvironments. Hammond (1999) also reported an extensive survey of the concentrations of nicotine in air. Based on the large numbers of measurements made in various indoor environments in the USA between 1957 and 1991, the average concentrations of nicotine in air showed about 100-fold variation, i.e. from 0.3–30 µg/m³ (US EPA, 1992). The average concentrations in homes with one or more smokers typically ranged from 2 to 10 µg/m³, with the highest averages being up to 14 µg/m³. Data from the mid 1970s until 1991 indicate that the nicotine concentrations in offices were similar to those measured in homes, with a large overlap in the range of air concentrations for the two types of environment. The maximum levels of nicotine, however, were considerably higher in offices than in domestic environments (US EPA, 1992; California EPA, 1997). In studies using controlled and field conditions, the concentrations of nicotine in air were found to increase as a function of the number of smokers present and the number of cigarettes consumed (US EPA, 1992).

Jenkins et al. (1996) studied exposure to secondhand tobacco smoke in 16 cities in the USA by sampling personal breathing zone air from about 100 nonsmokers in each city. The demographics of the study subjects were comparable with the population of the USA in general, although more women than men participated in the study. The mean 24-h time-weighted average concentration of nicotine was 3.27 µg/m³ for those exposed to secondhand tobacco smoke both at work and away from work, 1.41 µg/m³ for those only exposed away from work and 0.69 µg/m³ for those who were exposed only at work. The mean 24-h time-weighted average concentration of nicotine in air measured by personal monitoring, for those who were not exposed to secondhand tobacco smoke was 0.05 µg/m³ (Jenkins et al., 1996).

Personal exposure to particulate matter associated with secondhand tobacco smoke was determined using the set of specific markers such as respirable suspended particles, fluorescent particulate matter and solanesol-particulate matter. The ranges of mean concentrations of these particles for workers exposed to secondhand smoke in 11 countries were: respirable suspended particles, from 24 to 112 µg/m³; fluorescent particulate matter, from 5.7 to 57 µg/m³; and solanesol-particulate matter, from 3.6 to 64 µg/m³ (Jenkins et al., 2000). By measuring the levels of solanesol-particulate matter and nicotine, the exposure to secondhand tobacco smoke of office workers living and working with smokers was determined to be higher in winter than in summer (median 24-h time-weighted average concentrations, 25 µg versus 2.4 µg solanesol-particulate matter and 1.3 µg versus 0.26 µg nicotine, respectively) (Phillips & Bentley, 2001).

1.2.2   Population-based measurements of exposure

Most population-based estimates of exposure to secondhand tobacco smoke have been obtained from self-reports. When measuring exposure to secondhand smoke in indoor areas, nicotine or respirable suspended particles can be measured in air sampled using personal monitors. In a few studies, biomarkers such as cotinine have been measured in physiological fluids.

(a)   *Adults*

Some studies suggest that exposure to secondhand tobacco smoke is related to occupation and socioeconomic status, and that higher exposure is more common among adults employed in blue-collar jobs, service occupations and poorly paid jobs and among the less well educated (Gerlach *et al.*, 1997; Curtin *et al.*, 1998; Whitlock *et al.*, 1998). Exposure to secondhand tobacco smoke may also be higher among racial and ethnic minority groups in areas of the USA, although it is unclear if this is due to different socioeconomic status (Gerlach *et al.*, 1997).

Relatively few data are available on the prevalence of nonsmokers' exposure to secondhand tobacco smoke on a population basis, using biomarkers. Survey data from a study in the USA in 1988–91 showed that 37% of adult non-tobacco users lived in a home with at least one smoker or reported exposure to secondhand tobacco smoke at work, whereas serum cotinine levels indicated more widespread exposure to nicotine. Of all the non-tobacco users surveyed including children, 88% had detectable serum cotinine levels, indicating widespread exposure to secondhand tobacco smoke in residents of the USA (Pirkle *et al.*, 1996). Data were recently published on the serum cotinine levels measured in 2263 nonsmokers in 12 locations across the USA (Figure 1.1) (CDC, 2001). As reported previously (Pirkle *et al.*, 1996), exposure to secondhand tobacco smoke tended to be higher among men than among women. Among racial/ethnic groups, blacks had the highest cotinine levels. People younger than 20 years of age had higher cotinine levels than those aged 20 years and older.

Table 1.7 summarizes the data obtained from a number of recent population-based studies that used questionnaires to characterize exposure. Some of these studies were national in scope, e.g. the national samples in Australia, China and the USA, whereas others were from single states or specific localities. Several of the studies incorporated cotinine as a biomarker. Unfortunately, few data are available from developing countries (Samet & Yang, 2001). In a case–control study of lung cancer and exposure to secondhand smoke in 12 centres from seven European countries, 1542 control subjects up to 74 years of age were interviewed between 1988 and 1994 about their exposure to secondhand smoke. Exposure of adults to secondhand smoke from a spouse who smoked was reported by 45% of the subjects (including 2% who were exposed to smoke from cigars or pipes only); an additional 8% were not exposed to spousal smoke, but reported exposure to secondhand smoke produced by cohabitants other than spouses. Exposure to secondhand smoke in the workplace was reported by 71% of men and 46% of women. Combined exposure to secondhand smoke both from the spouse and at the workplace was reported by 78%. Exposure to secondhand smoke in vehicles was reported by 20% and exposure in public indoor settings such as restaurants was reported by 29% (Boffetta *et al.*, 1998). Recent data from Finland illustrate trends in self-reported exposure to secondhand tobacco smoke at work and at home over a 15-year period. In 1985, 25% of employed nonsmoking men and 15% of employed nonsmoking women were exposed to

Figure 1.1. 75th percentile of serum cotinine concentrations for the US nonsmoking population aged 3 years and older, National Health and Nutrition Examination Survey, 1999

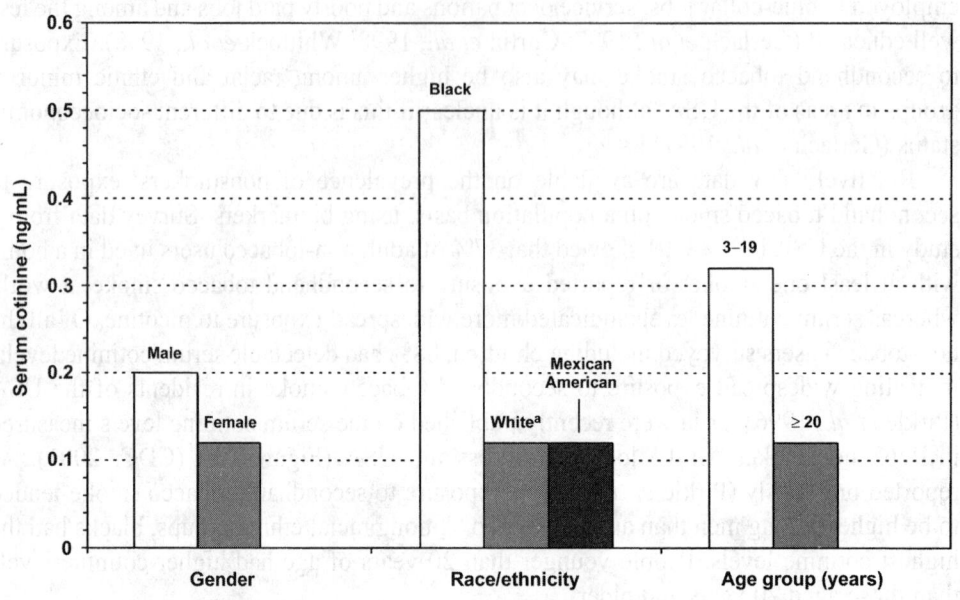

From CDC (2001)
[a] Includes other racial/ethnic groups

secondhand tobacco smoke at work. In contrast, the figures for exposure to secondhand smoke in 2000 were 8% of men and 4% of women (Jousilahti & Helakorpi, 2002).

In a 1993 review of existing studies, Siegel (1993) noted wide variation in the concentrations of secondhand tobacco smoke by location when measured by weighted mean levels of nicotine in the ambient air of offices (4.1 μg/m³), restaurants (6.5 μg/m³), bars (19.7 μg/m³) and dwellings with at least one smoker (4.3 μg/m³).

The recently published study in the USA of the median serum cotinine concentration measured in nonsmokers aged 3 years and older found a 75% decrease over the period 1991–99 (CDC, 2001), suggesting positive effects of policies for cleaner indoor air.

(b)   Children

Because the home is a predominant location for smoking, children are exposed to tobacco smoke as they go about their daily lives, i.e. while eating, playing and even sleeping. The exposure at home may be added to exposure at school and in vehicles. Consequently, in many countries, children cannot avoid inhaling tobacco smoke (Samet & Yang, 2001).

Table 1.7. Prevalence of exposure to secondhand tobacco smoke — population-based studies

Reference	Study design and population	Results
Europe		
Somerville *et al.* (1988)	Cross-sectional study; 4337 children aged 5–11 years in England and 766 in Scotland, from the 1982 National Health Interview Survey on Child Health in the United Kingdom	Prevalence = 42% in England and 60% in Scotland
Dijkstra *et al.* (1990)	Cohort study; nonsmoking children aged 6–12 years over a 2-year period, in the Netherlands	Prevalence = 66%
Jaakkola *et al.* (1994)	Population-based cross-sectional study; random sample of 1003 children aged 1–6 years in Espoo, Finland	25.2% reported exposure to secondhand tobacco smoke at home; 74.8% of children did not, assessed by parent-completed questionnaire.
Brenner *et al.* (1997)	Cross-sectional study; survey of 974 predominantly blue-collar employees of a south German metal company	> 60% of nonsmoking blue collar workers reported being exposed to secondhand smoke at work; 52% of nonsmoking white collar workers exposed if smoking allowed in immediate work area, and 18% if smoking not allowed
Boffetta *et al.* (1998)	Case–control study of lung cancer and exposure to secondhand tobacco smoke in 12 centres from seven European countries, 1542 control subjects up to 74 years of age were interviewed between 1988 and 1994 about exposure to secondhand tobacco smoke	Prevalence during childhood was 66%. Prevalence in adulthood (spousal smoke) was 45% (including 2% with exposure to cigar or pipe smoke only). In addition, 8% who were not exposed to spousal smoke were exposed to secondhand tobacco smoke produced by cohabitants other than spouse. Prevalence in the workplace was 71% among men and 46% among women. Combined prevalence from the spouse and at the workplace was 78%. Prevalence of exposure to secondhand tobacco smoke in vehicles was 20% and in public indoor settings such as restaurants, it was 29%.

Table 1.7 (contd)

Reference	Study design and population	Results
Lund et al. (1998)	Children born in 1992; descriptive study of exposure to secondhand tobacco smoke at home in 3547 households in Denmark, Finland, Iceland, Norway and Sweden in 1995–96	Prevalence of weekly exposure was 47% in Denmark, 7% in Finland, 46% in Iceland, 32% in Norway and 15% in Sweden.
Jousilahti & Helakorpi (2002)	A cohort of 58 721 men and women aged 15 to 64 years was followed-up by annual questionnaires on exposure to secondhand smoke at work and at home between 1985 and 2000 in Finland.	In the middle of the 1980s, about a quarter of employed nonsmoking men and 15% of nonsmoking women were exposed for at least 1 hour daily to environmental tobacco smoke at work. In 2000, the proportions were 7.9% and 4.4%, respectively. Exposure to environmental tobacco smoke at home also decreased slightly. In 2000, 14.3% of the nonsmoking men and 13% of the nonsmoking women aged 15 to 64 years were exposed to secondhand smoke either at work or at home.
America		
Coultas et al. (1987)	Cross-sectional study; 2029 Hispanic children and adults in New Mexico (1360 nonsmokers and ex-smokers also had salivary cotinine measured)	Prevalence = 39% ≥ 18 years; 48%, 13–17 years; 45%, 6–12 years, and 54% < 5 years. Mean salivary cotinine concentrations = 0 to 6 ng/mL; 35% of members of nonsmoking households had detectable levels of cotinine.
Greenberg et al. (1989)	Questionnaire-based cross-sectional study; mothers of 433 infants from a representative population of healthy neonates from 1986–87 in North Carolina	55% lived in a household with at least one smoker; 42% of infants had been exposed during the week preceding data collection; cotinine was detected in 60% of urine samples (median = 121 ng/mg creatinine).
Chilmonczyk et al. (1990)	Cross-sectional study; 518 infants aged 6–8 weeks receiving well-child care in the offices of private physicians in greater Portland, Maine	91% of infants living in households where only the mother smoked (43 households) had urinary cotinine levels ≥ 10 μg/L; 8% of infants living in households where no smoking was reported (305 households) had urinary cotinine levels ≥ 10 μg/L.

Table 1.7 (contd)

Reference	Study design and population	Results
Overpeck & Moss (1991)	Cross-sectional study; sample of 5356 children ≤ 5 years of age from the National Health Interview Survey in 1988	Approximately 50% of all US children ≤ 5 years of age exposed to prenatal maternal smoking and/or secondhand smoke from household members after birth; 28% were exposed both prenatally and postnatally, 21% only after birth and 1.2% only prenatally.
Borland et al. (1992)	Cross-sectional study; sample of 7301 nonsmokers from the larger study of Burns & Pierce (1992)	31.3% of nonsmoking workers reported exposure at work ≥ 1 time in the preceding 2 weeks; 35.8% males vs 22.9% females; 41.9% < 25 years vs 26.4% for older workers; 43.1% with < 12 years of education vs 18.6% with ≥ 16 years of college education
Burns & Pierce (1992)	Cross-sectional study; head of household in 32 135 homes in California, contacted by stratified random-digit dialling from June 1990 to July 1991	32.2% of children aged 5–11 years and 36.5% of adolescents aged 12–17 years were exposed at home.
Jenkins et al. (1992)	Cross-sectional study; telephone interviews with 1579 English-speaking adults and 183 adolescents (12–17 years of age) from October 1987 to September 1988 in California	46% of nonsmokers were exposed during the day: 43% of adult nonsmokers and 64% of adolescent nonsmokers. Exposure most frequently occurred at home, in restaurants or in cars. The average duration of exposure was longest in workplaces.
Jenkins et al. (1992); Lum (1994)	Cross-sectional study; same population as described above and additional 1200 children aged ≤ 11 years (< 8 years old with a parent or guardian) from April 1989 to February 1990 in California	Prevalence of exposure among smokers and nonsmokers = 61% for adults and 70% for adolescents during the day; 35% to 45% of children, infants, and preschoolers were reported to be exposed to secondhand smoke; average duration = 3.5 h.
Pierce et al. (1994)	Cross-sectional study; using the California Adult Tobacco Surveys in 1990, 1992 and 1993 with 8224 to 30 716 adults 18 years and older and 1789 to 5531 teenagers 12–17 years of age interviewed	15.1% smoked prior to pregnancy and of these, 37.5% quit after the pregnancy (between 1988 and 1992, 9.4% of women smoked during pregnancy).

Table 1.7 (contd)

Reference	Study design and population	Results
Pletsch (1994)	Cross-sectional study; 4256 Hispanic women aged 12–49 years who participated in the Hispanic Health and Nutrition Examination Survey (HHANES) from 1982 to 1984	Age-specific household exposure for nonsmokers was 31%–62% for Mexican-Americans, 22%–59% for Puerto Ricans and 40%–53% for Cuban-Americans; 59% of Puerto Rican and 62% of Cuban-American adolescents had high levels of exposure.
Thompson et al. (1995)	Cross-sectional study; 20 801 US employees from 114 work sites	52.4% of respondents reported being exposed to secondhand tobacco smoke at work
Kurtz et al. (1996)	Questionnaire-based cross-sectional survey; sample of 675 African-American students enrolled in grades 5–12 in an urban public school district in Detroit, Michigan	Smoking rates were higher among students with parents who smoked; 48% reported paternal smoking; 46% reported maternal smoking.
Mannino et al. (1996)	17 448 children aged 1–10 years from 1991 US National Health Interview Survey	41% of children with lower socioeconomic status experienced daily exposure at home; 21% of children with higher socioeconomic status experienced daily exposure at home.
Pirkle et al. (1996)	Cross-sectional study; 9744 adults aged 17 years or older from the NHANES III Study, 1988–91	Prevalence for males was 43.5% and for females, 32.9%; 87.9% had detectable serum cotinine levels.
Stamatakis et al. (2002)	Cross-sectional study of ethnically diverse non-smoking women, aged 40 years and older, across the United States ($n = 2326$)	Exposure to secondhand tobacco smoke at home was associated with being American Indian/Alaska Native (aOR, 1.5; 95% CI, 1.0–2.6). Compared with college graduates, exposure to secondhand tobacco smoke at work was higher among women with some high school education (aOR, 2.8; 95% CI, 1.5–5.3) and high school graduates (aOR, 3.1; 95% CI, 1.9–5.1) and substantially higher for women who worked where smoking was allowed in some (aOR, 15.1; 95% CI, 10.2–22.4) or all (aOR, 44.8; 95% CI, 19.6–102.4) work areas.

Table 1.7 (contd)

Reference	Study design and population	Results
Asia		
Lam *et al.* (1998)	Questionnaire-based cross-sectional study; sample of 6304 students aged 12–15 years, from 172 classes of 61 schools in Hong Kong	53.1% were living in a household with at least one smoker; 35.2% had only one smoker; 9.5% had two and 2.5% had three or more smokers in the household; 38% of fathers and 3.5% of mothers smoked.
Yang *et al.* (1999)	Cross-sectional study; 120 298 records (63 793 males and 56 020 females) of persons aged 15–69 years from the 1996 National Prevalence Survey of Smoking in China	Of the nonsmoking respondents, 53.5% reported passive exposure to smoke. Over 60% of female nonsmokers between ages 25 and 50 years were passively exposed to tobacco smoke; 71% of participants reported exposure to smoke at home, 32% in public places and 25% in their workplace.
Africa		
Steyn *et al.* (1997)	Questionnaire-based cross-sectional study; 394 pregnant women attending antenatal services in Johannesburg, Cape Town, Port Elizabeth and Durban in urban South Africa, 1992	Most women who smoked stopped or reduced tobacco use during their pregnancy; 70% lived with at least one smoker in the house.
Australia and New Zealand		
Sherrill *et al.* (1992)	Cohort study; 634 children aged 9–15 years; New Zealand	Overall prevalence = 40%
Lister & Jorm (1998)	Cross-sectional study; data from the Australian Bureau of Statistics 1989–90 National Health Survey of parents and their children (*n* = 4281) aged 0–4 years; Australia	45% of children lived in households with ≥ 1 current smoker; 29% had a mother who smoked.

Modified from Samet & Yang (2001)

aOR, adjusted odds ratio for sociodemographic characteristics (race, age, education, location and having children in the home), health risk behaviours, and the type of smoking policy in the workplace

Data on the exposure of children to secondhand tobacco smoke are limited. In perhaps the most comprehensive cross-sectional study to date, researchers examined exposure to secondhand tobacco smoke in 17 448 children aged 1–10 years in the USA. Exposure varied considerably according to socioeconomic status: 41% of children of lower socioeconomic status experienced daily exposure to secondhand tobacco smoke in their home, whereas only 21% of children of higher socioeconomic status were exposed daily. Exposure to secondhand tobacco smoke did not vary by race, family size, gender or season (Mannino *et al.*, 1996). In a multicentre study conducted in 1988–94 in seven European countries, exposure to secondhand smoke in childhood was reported by 66% of respondents (Boffetta *et al.*, 1998). Parent-reported exposure to secondhand tobacco smoke among children varied widely across the countries of Denmark, Finland, Iceland, Norway and Sweden (Lund *et al.*, 1998). For example, Finnish parents were more likely than all other Nordic parents to protect their children from secondhand tobacco smoke. Exposure was highest in Denmark and Iceland, where children were exposed in almost half of all households and in nine of ten households with daily smokers. The lack of common metrics for measuring exposure to secondhand tobacco smoke in children is a significant challenge when comparing data between countries.

1.3   Regulations

1.3.1   *Policy options*

There are a range of options available for the regulation of secondhand tobacco smoke. Of these options, the least effective is designating smoking areas that have no separate ventilation. This option provides only minimal protection to nonsmokers; studies have shown that substantial exposure to secondhand tobacco smoke occurs in workplaces where there are smoking areas without separate ventilation (Repace, 1994). A more effective option is the use of separately ventilated smoking lounges; this protects non-smokers but is costly and may elevate lung cancer risk in smokers (Siegel *et al.*, 1995). Separately ventilated smoking lounges also endanger workers (e.g. waiting staff) who must enter these areas as part of their job. Finally, the most effective alternative is a totally smoke-free workplace (Brownson *et al.*, 2002).

1.3.2   *Prevalence of regulations*

In 1985, only about 38% of workers in the USA were employed by firms that had policies restricting smoking (Farrelly *et al.*, 1999). Since that time, smoking restrictions have become increasingly common. According to the 1999 National Worksite Health Promotion Survey, 79% of workplaces with 50 or more employees had formal smoking policies that prohibited smoking or allowed it only in separately ventilated areas (US Department of Health and Human Services, 2000). Data showed that, from 1995–96, 64% of indoor workers in the USA were covered by a total ban on smoking in the workplace.

The proportion of workers in the USA who work in a smoke-free workplace varies considerably by state — from 84% in Maryland and Utah to 40% in Nevada (Burns et al., 2000). There are few systematic data available on the enforcement of existing policies to restrict smoking in the workplace, although existing studies suggest that compliance is likely to be high (Stillman et al., 1990; Wakefield et al., 1996). National data from the USA also suggest that despite some protective laws, workers in blue-collar and service occupations remain much more likely to be exposed to secondhand tobacco smoke in the workplace than other categories of workers (Gerlach et al., 1997). In the USA, hospitals are the only sector that has voluntarily implemented a nationwide smoking ban. This ban was announced in November 1991 and full implementation was required by December 31, 1993. Two years after implementation, the policy was found to have been successful with 96% of hospitals complying with the smoking ban standard (Longo et al., 1995; Brownson et al., 2002).

A recent overview of the legislation restricting smoking at work in different countries has been provided by the American Cancer Society (Corrao et al., 2000) (Table 1.8). Despite using a wide range of already published sources together with Internet searches, no information could be found for many countries. Thus, absence of an entry in this Table does not imply certainty that no legislation exists in a particular country. Conversely, the existence of a law banning or restricting smoking implies nothing about its enforcement. In general, it appears that voluntary restrictions under control of the employer are more common in developing countries than in developed countries (Brownson et al., 2002). A country that relies on voluntary action to ban or restrict smoking may have quite high rates of worker protection. For example, although Australia banned smoking in all federal government workplaces in 1988, it has been left to individual employers to determine their own policies. Yet, in 1999, 71% of indoor workers in the state of Victoria reported a total ban on smoking at their workplace, 21% reported some restrictions on smoking and 8% reported unrestricted smoking (Letcher & Borland, 2000). As in other countries, employees in small Australian workplaces are less likely to report protection, as are workers in particular types of employment (Wakefield et al., 1996; McMaugh & Rissell, 2000). In a survey of indoor workers, 38% of those employed in a restaurant or hotel, 15% of warehouse/store workers and 17% of those working in a workshop or factory reported unrestricted smoking where they worked, compared with only 3% of workers in open-plan offices (Letcher & Borland, 2000). In the United Kingdom, workplace restrictions are also voluntary. In 1997, 40% of the workforce was estimated to be working in a totally smoke-free environment (Freeth, 1998). A survey of 1500 workplaces in Scotland found that 79% of them had designated nonsmoking areas, but only 22% had banned smoking completely (ASH, 2001). Despite the limitations of the data presented in Table 1.9, it is apparent that most countries have some laws that restrict smoking. However, it is very likely that there is considerable need for improvement in protection of workers from secondhand tobacco smoke in almost all countries (Brownson et al., 2002).

A few researchers have begun to examine the prevalence of smoking restrictions in the home because such restrictions are likely to have beneficial effects on the health of

Table 1.8. Variations in workplace smoking policies in selected countries

Country	Type of policy[a]				Comments
	B	R	V	X	
Africa					
Benin	x				Certain workplaces only
Botswana	x				Areas accessible to public, common areas
Mali	x				Public service offices
Nigeria	x				Offices
South Africa	x				Designated smoking areas
Uganda				x	
Tanzania				x	
Zambia	x				
Americas					
Argentina			x		
Barbados				x	
Belize				x	Some private workplaces
Brazil				x	
Canada	x				
Chile	x				Areas accessible to public
Costa Rica	x				
Cuba				x	
Dominican Republic	x				Offices
Ecuador	x				Working areas
El Salvador			x		
Grenada				x	
Guatemala	x				Areas accessible to the public
Honduras	x				
Mexico	x				Working areas
Panama	x				Areas accessible to public
Peru	x				
Trinidad and Tobago				x	
United States				x	State and local levels
Venezuela			x		
Eastern Mediterranean					
Cyprus	x				Private and public
Egypt	x				Enclosed public places
Iran	x				Areas accessible to public
Iraq			x		Administrative measures
Kuwait				x	
Lebanon				x	Upon request by nonsmokers
Morocco	x				Public administration and service offices
Sudan	x				Areas accessible to public
Syria	x				

Table 1.8 (contd)

Country	Type of policy[a]				Comments
	B	R	V	X	
Tunisia			x		
Europe					
Austria	x				Unless appropriate ventilation exists
Belarus		x			
Belgium	x		x		Areas accessible to public and other areas
Bosnia & Herzegovina		x			
Bulgaria	x				Unless nonsmokers give written permission for smoking
Croatia	x				
Czech Republic	x				During work hours when nonsmokers are present
Denmark	x				Voluntary restrictions in private workplaces
Estonia	x				Labour environments
Finland	x				Designated smoking areas
France	x				Except individual offices
Germany			x		
Greece		x			
Hungary	x				Areas accessible to public
Iceland	x				Areas accessible to public
Ireland	x				Areas accessible to public
Israel	x				Except in designated areas
Krygyzstan			x		
Latvia		x			
Lithuania	x				Enclosed areas
Netherlands		x			Public and private
Norway	x				With 2 or more employees
Poland	x				
Portugal		x			
Moldova	x				
Romania			x		
Russia	x				
San Marino	x				
Slovakia		x			
Slovenia		x			
Spain		x			
Sweden		x			
Switzerland		x			
Turkey	x				With 5 or more employees
Ukraine	x				
United Kingdom			x		

Table 1.8 (contd)

Country	Type of policy[a]				Comments
	B	R	V	X	
South-East Asia					
Bangladesh				x	
India		x			
Nepal		x			
Sri Lanka				x	Administrative measures
Thailand	x				
Western Pacific					
Australia				x	
Cambodia	x				Partial ban
China	x				Administrative measures
Cook Islands			x		
Fiji				x	
Japan				x	Guideline, set by Ministry of Labour
Kiribati				x	
Lao People's Democratic Republic				x	
Malaysia	x				Areas accessible to the public
Micronesia			x		
Mongolia	x				Designated smoking areas
New Zealand	x				Common work areas and public areas
Niue				x	
Philippines	x				
Republic of Korea		x			
Samoa				x	
Solomon Islands			x		
Tokelau			x		
Tonga				x	

Brownson *et al.* (2002); adapted from Corrao *et al.* (2000); number of additional countries for which no information is available: Africa = 38; Americas = 15; Eastern Mediterranean = 13; Europe = 15; South-East Asia = 5; Western Pacific = 11.

[a] B, smoking is prohibited in workplaces according to national legislation and/or regulations; facilities with a designated smoking area are included in this category if nonsmoking areas must always remain uncontaminated by smoke; R, smoking is restricted, but not prohibited, in workplaces according to national legislation and/or regulations; V, employers voluntarily prohibit or restrict smoking in areas under their management; X, different state and county laws apply.

Table 1.9. Summary of selected studies on the effects of workplace smoking bans and restrictions on exposure to secondhand tobacco smoke

Reference/location	Industry/setting	Sample size	Outcome(s) studied/size of effect[a]
Millar (1988)/ Ontario, Canada	Department of Health and Welfare	4200 (12 locations)	Change in mean respirable suspended particulates = -6 µg/m^3 to -22 µg/m^3 (depending on the storey of the building)
Becker *et al.* (1989)/ Maryland, USA	Children's hospital	951 (9 locations)	Change in average nicotine vapour concentrations = -12.53 µg/m^3 to $+0.08$ µg/m^3 (depending on the location)
Biener *et al.* (1989)/ Rhode Island, USA	Hospital	535	Percentage of workers 'bothered' by secondhand smoke in various workplace locations: offices = -20%; lounges = -20%
Gottlieb *et al.* (1990)/Texas, USA	Government agency	1158	Percentage of workers 'never bothered' by secondhand smoke = $+38.8\%$
Mullooly *et al.* (1990)/Oregon, USA	Health maintenance organization	13 736 1985: pre-ban 764 post-ban 1027 1986: pre-ban 1352 post-ban 1219	Presence of smoke in workplace = -21% (1985 sites); -35% (1986 sites)
Stillman *et al.* (1990)/Maryland, USA	Medical centre	8742 (7 locations)	Change in average 7-day nicotine vapour concentrations = -7.71 µg/m^3 to -0.72 µg/m^3 (depending on the location)
Borland *et al.* (1992)/ California, USA	Indoor workers in California	7301	Percentage of employees exposed to secondhand smoke at work = -42.1% between no policy and smoke-free policy
Broder *et al.* (1993)/ Toronto, Canada	Public sector workplaces	179 (3 buildings; 8–12 samples per floor)	Change in the mean measurements (for several secondhand smoke components) Volatile organic compounds = -0.7 mg/m^3
Patten *et al.* (1995)/California, USA	Statewide workers	8580 (at baseline survey)	Percentage of employees exposed to secondhand smoke at work = -56.3% difference between work area ban and no ban

Table 1.9 (contd)

Reference/location	Industry/setting	Sample size	Outcome(s) studied/size of effect[a]
Etter *et al.* (1999)/ Geneva, Switzerland	University	2908	Exposure to secondhand smoke (score 0–100; 'not at all' (0) to 'very much' (100)) = –4% (follow-up compared to baseline)

Brownson *et al.* (2002); modified from Hopkins *et al.* (2001)
[a] Values noted are absolute differences from baseline.

children. In 1997, a population-based, cross-sectional telephone survey was conducted using random-digit-dialling asking 6199 adult Oregonians to provide baseline data on tobacco use in Oregon. Seventy per cent of the households were composed of nonsmokers only, and 85% of those had a full ban on smoking inside the home. Of the households containing one or more smokers, 38% had a full household ban on smoking. Fifty per cent of households with at least a smoker and a child present did not have a full ban on indoor smoking (Pizacani *et al.*, 2003). Face-to-face interviews were conducted with 380 rural, low-income Native American and white parents of children aged 1–6 years in Oklahoma. The prevalence of complete smoking bans was 49% in Native American homes and 43% in white homes. Bans on smoking in cars were less common, with 35% of Native American and 40% of white caregivers reporting complete bans (Kegler & Malcoe, 2002). In Victoria, Australia, the percentage of respondents who reported discouraging visitors from smoking in the home rose from 27% in 1989 to 53% in 1997 (Borland *et al.*, 1999), and not smoking in the presence of children rose from 14% in 1989 to 33% in 1996. Similarly, attitudes toward smoking in the home have changed in Ontario, Canada. The percentage of respondents favouring not smoking in homes where there were children increased from 51% in 1992 to 70% in 1996 (Ashley *et al.*, 1998).

Only minimal regulation applies to constituents of cigarettes and tobacco smoke. This covers only the content of tar, nicotine and carbon monoxide (cf. Section 1.4(*e*) of the monograph on tobacco smoke).

1.3.3   *Effectiveness of regulations*

Evaluations of the effects and effectiveness of workplace smoking policies have used a wide variety of study designs and measurements of exposure to secondhand tobacco smoke and tobacco use behaviours. Most of the published studies are simple assessments conducted before and after adoption of a workplace policy, although more recent (and more complex) investigations have employed cross-sectional surveys of workers in workplaces operating different policies. Few studies have evaluated or controlled for potential bias and confounding of the observed differences or changes in exposure to secondhand smoke or in tobacco use behaviours (Brownson *et al.*, 2002).

The effectiveness of workplace smoking policies has been measured by differences or changes in perceived air quality in the workplace following a ban or restriction, and by differences or changes in active measurements of nicotine vapour concentrations, metabolites, or levels of particles. Overall, workplace smoking policies have been highly effective in reducing the exposure of nonsmokers to secondhand tobacco smoke. The 'best evidence subset' comprised ten studies, including cross-sectional surveys, before-and-after comparisons, different settings or locations (offices, public sector workplaces, medical centres, workplaces community-wide) and different outcome measurements (Table 1.9) (Briss *et al.*, 2000; Hopkins *et al.*, 2001). In nine of ten studies, workplace smoking policies had a significant impact on exposure to secondhand tobacco smoke. In assessments conducted between 4 and 18 months after implementation of the policy, the median relative percentage difference in self-reported exposure to secondhand tobacco smoke was –60%, range +4% to –97%. Workplaces with smoking bans tended to show greater reduction in exposure to secondhand tobacco smoke than did workplaces with smoking restrictions (Hopkins *et al.*, 2001; Brownson *et al.*, 2002).

Hammond (1999) summarized the existing literature on average indoor nicotine concentrations when various workplace smoking policies were enacted. In workplaces with policies that had banned smoking, nicotine concentrations were generally decreased to less than 1 $\mu g/m^3$. The mean concentrations of nicotine in workplaces that allowed smoking ranged from 2 to 6 $\mu g/m^3$ in offices, 3 to 8 $\mu g/m^3$ in restaurants and from 1 to 6 $\mu g/m^3$ in the workplaces of blue-collar workers. By comparison, studies of nicotine concentrations that included at least 10 homes of smokers and that were sampled for 14 h to 1 week found average nicotine concentrations of between 1 and 6 $\mu g/m^3$.

References

Adams, J.D., O'Mara-Adams, K.J. & Hoffmann, D. (1987) Toxic and carcinogenic agents in undiluted mainstream smoke and sidestream smoke of different types of cigarettes. *Carcinogenesis*, **8**, 729–731

Adlkofer, F., Scherer, G., Conze, C., Angerer, J. & Lehnert, G. (1990) Significance of exposure to benzene and other toxic compounds through environmental tobacco smoke. *J. Cancer Res. clin. Oncol.*, **116**, 591–598

ASH (Action on Smoking and Health) (2001) Smoking in the workplace. ASH, National Asthma Campaign and Trade Union Congress. WHO-Europe Partnership Project, Copenhagen [http://www.ash.org.uk/html/workplace/html/workplace.html]

Ashley, M.J., Cohen, J., Ferrence, R., Bull, S., Bondy, S., Poland, B. & Pederson, L. (1998) Smoking in the home: Changing attitudes and current practices. *Am. J. public Health*, **88**, 797–800

Baker, R.R. & Proctor, C.J. (1990) The origins and properties of environmental tobacco smoke. *Environ. int.*, **16**, 231–245

Becker, D.M., Conner, H.F., Waranch, H.R., Stillman, F., Pennington, L., Lees, P.S. & Oski, F. (1989) The impact of a total ban on smoking in the Johns Hopkins Children's Center. *J. Am. med. Assoc*, **262**, 799–802

Benowitz, N.L. (1996) Cotinine as a biomarker of environmental tobacco smoke exposure. *Epidemiol. Rev.*, **18**, 188–204

Benowitz, N.L. (1999) Biomarkers of environmental tobacco smoke exposure. *Environ. Health Perspect.*, **107** (Suppl. 2), 349–355

Biener, L., Abrams, D.B., Follick, M.J. & Dean, L. (1989) A comparative evaluation of a restrictive smoking policy in a general hospital. *Am. J. public Health*, **79**, 192–195

Boffetta, P., Agudo, A., Ahrens, W., Benhamou, E., Benhamou, S., Darby, S.C., Ferro, G., Fortes, C., Gonzalez, C.A., Jöckel, K.H., Krauss, M., Kreienbrock, L., Kreuzer, M., Mendes, A., Merletti, F., Nyberg, F., Pershagen, G., Pohlabeln, H., Riboli, E., Schmid, G., Simonato, L., Trédaniel, J., Whitley, E., Wichmann, H.E., Winck, C., Zambon, P. & Saracci, R. (1998) Multicenter case–control study of exposure to environmental tobacco smoke and lung cancer in Europe. *J. natl Cancer Inst.*, **90**, 1440–1450

Bombick, B.R., Avalos, J.T., Nelson, P.R., Conrad, F.W. & Doolittle, D.J. (1998) Comparative studies of the mutagenicity of environmental tobacco smoke from cigarettes that burn or primarily heat tobacco. *Environ. Mol. Mutag.*, **31**, 169–175

Borgerding, M.F., Bodnar, J.A. & Wingate, D.E. (2000) *The 1999 Massachusetts Benchmark Study. Final Report. A Research Study Conducted after Consultation with the Massachusetts Department of Public Health*, Department of Health, Massachusetts

Borland, R., Pierce, J.P., Burns, D.M., Gilpin, E., Johnson, M. & Bal, D. (1992) Protection from environmental tobacco smoke in California. The case for a smoke-free workplace. *J. Am. med. Assoc.*, **268**, 749–752

Borland, R., Mullins, R., Trotter, L. & White, V. (1999) Trends in environmental tobacco smoke restrictions in the home in Victoria, Australia. *Tob. Control*, **8**, 266–271

Brenner, H., Born, J., Novak, P. & Wanek, V. (1997) Smoking behavior and attitude toward smoking regulations and passive smoking in the workplace. A study among 974 employees in the German metal industry. *Prev. Med.*, **26**, 138–143

Briss, P.A., Zaza, S., Pappaioanou, M., Fielding, J., Wright-De Aguero, L., Truman, B.I., Hopkins, D.P., Mullen, P.D., Thompson, R.S., Woolf, S.H., Carande-Kulis, V.G., Anderson, L., Hinman, A.R., McQueen, D.V., Teutsch, S.M., Harris, J.R. & The Task Force on Community Preventive Services (2000) Developing an evidence-based Guide to Community Preventive Services — Methods. *Am. J. prev. Med.*, **18**, 35–43

Broder, I., Pilger, C. & Corey, P. (1993) Environment and well-being before and following smoking ban in office buildings. *Can. J. public Health*, **84**, 254–258

Brownson, R.C., Hopkins, D.P. & Wakefield, M.A. (2002) Effects of smoking restrictions in the workplace. *Ann. Rev. public Health*, **23**, 333–348

Brunnemann, K.D., Kagan, M.R., Cox, J.E. & Hoffmann, D. (1990) Analysis of 1,3-butadiene and other selected gas-phase components in cigarette mainstream and sidestream smoke by gas chromatography–mass selective detection. *Carcinogenesis*, **11**, 1863–1868

Brunnemann, K.D., Cox, J.E. & Hoffmann, D. (1992) Analysis of tobacco-specific N-nitrosamines in indoor air. *Carcinogenesis*, **13**, 2415–2418

Burns, D. & Pierce, J.P. (1992) *Tobacco Use in California 1990–1991*, Sacramento, CA, California Department of Health Services

Burns, D.M., Shanks, T.G., Major, J.M., Gower, K.B. & Shopland, D.R. (2000) Restrictions on smoking in the workplace. In: *Population Based Smoking Cessation, Proceedings of a Conference on what Works to Influence Cessation in the General Population. Smoking and Tobacco*

Control Monograph No. 12, Bethesda, MD, US Department of Health and Human Services, National Institutes of Health, National Cancer Institute (NIH Pub. No. 00-4892), pp. 99–128

CDC (Centers for Disease Control and Prevention) (2001) *National Report on Human Exposure to Environmental Chemicals*, Atlanta, GA

California EPA (California Environmental Protection Agency) (1997) *Health Effects of Exposure to Environmental Tobacco Smoke, Final Report,* California Environmental Protection Agency, Office of Environmental Health Hazard Assessment

Chilmonczyk, B.A., Knight, G.J., Palomaki, G.E., Pulkkinen, A.J., Williams, J. & Haddow, J.E. (1990) Environmental tobacco smoke exposure during infancy. *Am. J. Public Health*, **80**, 1205–1208

Chortyk, O.T. & Schlotzhauer, W.W. (1989) The contribution of low-tar cigarettes to environmental tobacco smoke. *J. anal. Toxicol.*, **13**, 129–134

Corrao, M.A., Guindon, G.E., Sharma, N. & Shokoohi, D.F., eds (2000) *Tobacco Control Country Profiles*, Atlanta, GA, American Cancer Society [http://www.cancer.org/eprise/main/docroot/res/content/res_6_4x_other_publications]

Coultas, D.B., Howard, C.A., Peake, G.T., Skipper, B.J. & Samet, J.M. (1987) Salivary cotinine levels and involuntary tobacco smoke exposure in children and adults in New Mexico. *Am. Rev. Respir. Dis.*, **136**, 305–309

Curtin, F., Morabia, A. & Bernstein, M. (1998) Lifetime exposure to environmental tobacco smoke among urban women: Differences by socioeconomic class. *Am. J. Epidemiol.*, **148**, 1040–1047

Dijkstra, L., Houthuijs, D., Brunekreef, B., Akkerman, I. & Boleij, J.S. (1990) Respiratory health effects of the indoor environment in a population of Dutch children. *Am. Rev. Respir. Dis.*, **142**, 1172–1178

Djordjevic, M.V., Stellman, S.D. & Zang, E. (2000) Doses of nicotine and lung carcinogens delivered to cigarette smokers. *J. natl Cancer Inst.*, **92**, 106–111

Eatough, D.J., Benner, C.L., Tang, H., Landon, V., Richards, G., Caka, F.M., Crawford, J., Lewis, E.A., Hansen, L.D. & Eatough, N.L. (1989) The chemical composition of environmental tobacco smoke. III. Identification of conservative tracers of environmental tobacco smoke. *Environ. int.*, **15**, 19–28

Etter, J.-F., Ronchi, A. & Perneger, T.V. (1999) Short-term impact of a university based smoke free campaign. *J. Epidemiol. Community Health*, **53**, 710–715

Farrelly, M.C., Evans, W.N. & Sfekas, A.E. (1999) The impact of workplace smoking bans: Results from a national survey. *Tob. Control*, **8**, 272–277

Freeth, S. (1998) *Smoking-related Behaviour and Attitudes, 1997. A Report on Research using the Omnibus Survey produced on behalf of the Department of Health*, London, Office for National Statistics, p. 13

Gerlach, K.K., Shopland, D.R., Hartman, A.M., Gibson, J.T. & Pechacek, T.F. (1997) Workplace smoking policies in the United States: Results from a national survey of more than 100 000 workers. *Tob. Control*, **6**, 199–206

Gottlieb, N.H., Eriksen, M.P., Lovato, C.Y., Weinstein, R.P. & Green, L.W. (1990) Impact of a restrictive work site smoking policy on smoking behavior, attitudes, and norms. *J. occup. Med.*, **32**, 16–23

Government of British Columbia (2003) What is in cigarettes? Mainstream smoke and sidestream smoke chemical constituents by cigarette brand. [http://www.healthplanning.gov.bc.ca/ttdr/index.html Accessed 07.03.2003]

Greenberg, R.A., Bauman, K.E., Glover, L.H., Strecher, V.J., Kleinbaum, D.G., Haley, N.J., Stedman, H.C., Fowler, M.G. & Loda, F.A. (1989) Ecology of passive smoking by young infants. *J. Pediatr.*, **114**, 774–780

Guerin, M.R., Higgins, C.E. & Jenkins, R.A. (1987) Measuring environmental emissions from tobacco combustion: Sidestream cigarette smoke literature review. *Atmos. Environ.*, **21**, 291–297

Guerin M.R., Jenkins, R.A. & Tomkins, B.A., eds (1992) *The Chemistry of Environmental Tobacco Smoke: Composition and Measurement*. Center for Indoor Air Research, Chelsea, MI, Lewis Publishers

Hammond, S.K. (1999) Exposure of U.S. workers to environmental tobacco smoke. *Environ. Health Perspect.*, **107** (Suppl. 2), 329–340

Heavner, D.L., Morgan, W.T. & Ogden, M.W. (1995) Determination of volatile organic compounds and ETS apportionment in 49 homes. *Environ. int.*, **21**, 3–21

Higgins, C.E., Thompson, C.V., Ilgner, L.H., Jenkins, R.A. & Guerin, M.R. (1990) *Determination of Vapor Phase Hydrocarbons and Nitrogen-containing Constituents in Environmental Tobacco Smoke. Internal Progress Report*, Analytical Chemistry Division, Oak Ridge National Laboratory, Oak Ridge, TN 37831-6120

Hodgson, A.T., Daisey, J.M., Mahanama, K.R.R., Brinke, T. & Alevantis, L.E. (1996) Use of volatile tracers to determine the contribution of environmental tobacco smoke to concentrations of volatile organic compounds in smoking environments. *Environ. Int.*, **22**, 295–307

Hopkins, D.P., Briss, P.A., Ricard, C.J., Husten, C.G., Carande-Kulis, V.G., Fielding, J.E., Alao, M.O., McKenna, J.W., Sharp, D.J., Harris, J.R., Woollery, T.A., Harris, K.W. & The Task Force on Community Preventive Services (2001) Reviews of evidence regarding interventions to reduce tobacco use and exposure to environmental tobacco smoke. *Am. J. prev. Med.*, **20**, 16–66

Hyvärinen, M.J., Rothberg, M., Kähkönen, E., Mielo, T. & Reijula, K. (2000) Nicotine and 3-ethenylpyridine concentrations as markers for environmental tobacco smoke in restaurants. *Indoor Air*, **10**, 121–125

IARC (1986) *IARC Monographs on the Evaluation of the Carcinogenic Risk of Chemicals to Humans*, Vol. 38, *Tobacco Smoking*, Lyon, IARCPress

IARC (1999) *IARC Monographs on the Evaluation of Carcinogenic Risks to Humans*, Vol. 71, *Re-evaluation of Some Organic Chemicals, Hydrazine and Hydrogen Peroxide*, Lyon, IARCPress

Jaakkola, M.S. & Jaakkola, J.J.K. (1997) Assessment of exposure to environmental tobacco smoke. *Eur. Respir. J.*, **10**, 2384–2397

Jaakkola, N., Ruotsalainen, R. & Jaakkola, J.J.K. (1994) What are the determinants of children's exposure to environmental tobacco smoke at home? *Scand. J. Soc. Med.*, **22**, 107–112

Jenkins, R.A. & Counts, R.W. (1999) Occupational exposure to environmental tobacco smoke: Results of two personal exposure studies. *Environ. Health Perspect.*, **107** (Suppl. 2), 341–348

Jenkins, P.L., Phillips, T.J., Mulberg, E.J. & Hui, S.P. (1992) Activity patterns of Californians: Use of and proximity to indoor pollutant sources. *Atmos. Environ.*, **26A**, 2141–2148

Jenkins, R.A., Palausky, A., Counts, R.W., Bayne, C.K., Dindal, A.B. & Guerin, M.R. (1996) Exposure to environmental tobacco smoke in sixteen cities in the United States as determined by personal breathing zone air sampling. *J. Expo. anal. environ. Epidemiol.*, **6**, 473–502

Jenkins, R.A., Guerin, M.R. & Tomkins, B.A. (2000) Properties and measure of environmental tobacco smoke. In: *The Chemistry of Environmental Tobacco Smoke. Composition and Measurement*, 2nd Ed., Boca Raton, FL, Lewis Publishers, CRC Press

Jousilahti, P. & Helakorpi, S. (2002) Prevalence of exposure to environmental tobacco smoke at work and at home — 15-year trends in Finland. *Scand. J. Work Environ. Health*, **28** (Suppl. 2), 16–20

Junker, M.H., Danuser, B., Monn, C. & Koller, T. (2001) Acute sensory responses of nonsmokers at very low environmental tobacco smoke concentrations in controlled laboratory settings. *Environ. Health Perspect.*, **109**, 1045–1052

Kegler, M.C. & Malcoe, L.H. (2002) Smoking restrictions in the home and car among rural Native American and white families with young children. *Prev. Med*, **35**, 334–342

Kim, Y.M., Harrad, S. & Harrison, R.M. (2001) Concentrations and sources of VOCs in urban domestic and public microenvironments. *Environ. Sci. Technol.*, **35**, 997–1004

Klepeis, N.E., Ott, W.R. & Repace, J.L. (1999) The effect of cigar smoking on indoor levels of carbon monoxide and particles. *J. exp. anal. environ. Epidemiol.*, **9**, 622–635

Klus, H., Begutter, H., Scherer, G., Tricker, A.R. & Adlkofer, F. (1992) Tobacco-specific and volatile N-nitrosamines in environmental tobacco smoke of offices. *Indoor Environ.*, **1**, 348–350

Kurtz, M.E., Kurtz, J.C., Johnson, S.M. & Beverly, E.E. (1996) Exposure to environmental tobacco smoke — Perceptions of African American children and adolescents. *Prev. Med.*, **25**, 286–292

Lam, T.H., Chung, S.F., Betson, C.L., Wong, C.M. & Hedley, A.J. (1998) Respiratory symptoms due to active and passive smoking in junior secondary school students in Hong Kong. *Int. J. Epidemiol.*, **27**, 41–48

Letcher, T. & Borland, R. (2000) Smoking bans in Victorian workplaces: 1999 update. In: Trotter, L. & Letcher, T., eds, *Quit Evaluation Studies*, Vol. 10, pp. 49–57, Centre for Behavioural Research on Cancer [http://www.quit.org.au/quit/qe10/10home.html], Melbourne, Australia. Victorian Smoking and Health Program, The Anti-Cancer Council of Victoria

Lister, S.M. & Jorm, L.R. (1998) Parental smoking and respiratory illnesses in Australian children aged 0–4 years: ABS 1989–1990 National Health Survey results. *Australian and New Zealand J. Public Health*, **22**, 781–786

Löfroth, G. (1989) Environmental tobacco smoke: Overview of chemical composition and geno-toxic components. *Mutat. Res.*, **222**, 73–80

Löfroth, G. (1993) Environmental tobacco smoke. Multicomponent analysis and room to room distribution in homes. *Tob. Control*, **2**, 222–225

Löfroth, G., Burton, R., Goldstein, G., Forehand, L., Hammond, K., Mumford, J., Seila, R. & Lewtas, J. (1987) Genotoxic emission factors for sidestream cigarette smoke components (Abstract). *Environ. Mutag.*, **9** (Suppl. 8), 61

Löfroth, G., Burton, R.M., Forehand, L., Hammond, S.K., Seila, R.L., Zweidinger, R.B. & Lewtas, J. (1989) Characterization of environmental tobacco smoke. *Environ. Sci. Technol.*, **23**, 610–614

Longo, D.R., Brownson, R.C. & Kruse, R.L. (1995) Smoking bans in US hospitals. Results of a national survey. *J. Am. med. Assoc.*, **274**, 488–491

Lum, S. (1994) Duration and location of ETS exposure for the California population. Memorandum from S. Lum, Indoor Exposure Assessment Section, Research Division, California Air Resources Board, to L. Haroun, Reproductive and Cancer Hazard Assessment Section, Office of Environmental Health Hazard Assessment, 3 February (cited according to Samet and Yang, 2001)

Lund, K.E., Skrondal, A., Vertio, H. & Helgason, A.R. (1998) Children's residential exposure to environmental tobacco smoke varies greatly between the Nordic countries. *Scand. J. soc. Med.*, **26**, 115–120

Mannino, D.M., Siegel, M., Husten, C., Rose, D. & Etzel, R. (1996) Environmental tobacco smoke exposure and health effects in children: Results from the 1991 National Health Interview Survey. *Tob. Control*, **5**, 13–18

Martin, P., Heavner, D.L., Nelson, P.R., Maiolo, K.C., Risner, C.H., Simmons, P.S., Morgan, W.T. & Ogden, M.W. (1997) Environmental tobacco smoke (ETS): A market cigarette study. *Environ. int.*, **23**, 75–90

McMaugh, K. & Rissell, C. (2000) Smoking restrictions in small businesses of inner West Sydney: A management perspective. *J. occup. Health Saf.-Aust. NZ*, **16**, 37–45

Millar, W.J. (1988) Evaluation of the impact of smoking restrictions in a government work setting. *Can. J. public Health*, **79**, 379–382

Moschandreas, D.J. & Vuilleumier, K.L. (1999) ETS levels in hospitality environments satisfying ASHRAE standard 62-1989: 'Ventilation for acceptable indoor air quality'. *Atmos. Env.*, **33**, 4327–4340

Mullooly, J.P., Schuman, K.L., Stevens, V.J., Glasgow, R.E. & Vogt, T.M. (1990) Smoking behavior and attitudes of employees of a large HMO before and after a work site ban on cigarette smoking. *Public Health Rep.*, **105**, 623–628

Nelson, P.R., Kelly, S.P. & Conrad, F.W. (1997) Generation of environmental tobacco smoke by cigars (Abstract No. 46). In: *Proceedings of the 51st Tobacco Chemist's Research Conference, Winston-Salem, NC, September 14–17, 1997*

NRC (National Research Council) (1986) *Environmental Tobacco Smoke. Measuring Exposures and Assessing Health Effects*, Washington DC, National Academy Press

Ott, W.R. (1999) Mathematical models for predicting indoor air quality from smoking activity. *Environ. Health Perspect.*, **107** (Suppl. 2), 375–381

Overpeck, M.D. & Moss, A.J. (1991) Children's exposure to environmental cigarette smoke before and after birth. Health of our nation's children, United States, 1988. *Adv. Data*, **202**, 1–11

Pakhale, S.S. & Maru, G.B. (1998) Distribution of major and minor alkaloids in tobacco, mainstream and sidestream smoke of popular Indian smoking products. *Food Chem. Toxicol.*, **36**, 1131–1138

Patten, C.A., Pierce, J.P., Cavin, S.W., Berry, C.C. & Kaplan, R.M. (1995) Progress in protecting non-smokers from environmental tobacco smoke in California workplaces. *Tob. Control*, **4**, 139–144

Phillips, K. & Bentley, M.C. (2001) Seasonal assessment of environmental tobacco smoke and respirable suspended particle exposures for nonsmokers in Bremen using personal monitoring. *Environ. int.*, **27**, 69–85

Pierce, J.P., Evans, N., Farkas, S.J., Cavin, S.W., Berry, C., Kramer, M., Kealey, S., Rosbrook, B., Choi, W. & Kaplan, R.M. (1994) *Tobacco Use in California: An Evaluation of the Tobacco Control Program, 1989–1993*. La Jolla, CA. Cancer Prevention and Control, University of California, San Diego

Pirkle, J., Flegal, K., Bernert, J., Brody, D., Etzel, R. & Maurer, K. (1996) Exposure of the US population to environmental tobacco smoke. The Third National Health and Nutrition Examination Survey,1988 to 1991. *J. Am. med. Assoc.*, **275**, 1233–1240

Pizacani, B.A., Martin, D.P., Stark, M.J., Koepsell, T.D., Thompson, B. & Diehr, P. (2003) Household smoking bans: Which households have them and do they work? *Prev. Med.*, **36**, 99–107

Pletsch, P.K. (1994) Environmental tobacco smoke exposure among Hispanic women of reproductive age. *Public Health Nursing*, **11**, 229–235

Ramsey, R.S., Moneyhun, J.H. & Jenkins, R.A. (1990) Generation, sampling and chromatographic analysis of particulate matter in dilute sidestream tobacco smoke. *Anal. chem. Acta*, **236**, 213–220

Repace, J.L. (1994) Risk management of passive smoking at work and at home. *Saint Louis University Public Law Review*, **13**, 763–785

Rickert, W.S., Robinson, J.C. & Collishaw, N. (1984) Yields of tar, nicotine, and carbon monoxide in the sidestream smoke from 15 brands of Canadian cigarettes. *Am. J. public Health*, **74**, 228–231

Samet, J. & Yang, G. (2001) Passive smoking, women and children. In: Samet, J. & Yoon, S.-Y., eds, *Women and the Tobacco Epidemic, Challenges for the 21st Century* (WHO/NMH/TF1/01.1), Geneva, World Health Organization

Scherer, G., Frank, S., Riedel, K., Meger-Kossien, I. & Renner, T. (2000) Biomonitoring of exposure to polycyclic aromatic hydrocarbons of nonoccupationally exposed persons. *Cancer Epidemiol. Biomarkers Prev.*, **9**, 373–380

Sherrill, D.L., Martinez, F.D., Lebowitz, M.D., Holdaway, M.D., Flannery, E.M., Herbison, G.P., Stanton, W.R., Silva, P.A. & Sears, M.R. (1992) Longitudinal effects of passive smoking on pulmonary function in New Zealand children. *Am. Rev. Respir. Dis.*, **145**, 1136–1141

Siegel, M. (1993) Involuntary smoking in the restaurant workplace. A review of employee exposure and health effects. *J. Am. med. Assoc.*, **270**, 490–493

Siegel, M., Husten, C., Merritt, R.K., Giovino, G.A. & Eriksen, M.P. (1995) Effects of separately ventilated smoking lounges on the health of smokers: Is this an appropriate public health policy ? *Tob. Control*, **4**, 22–29

Somerville, S.M., Rona, R.J. & Chinn, S. (1988) Passive smoking and respiratory conditions in primary school children. *J. Epidemiol. Community Health*, **42**, 105–110

Stamatakis, K.A., Brownson, R.C. & Luke, D.A. (2002) Risk factors for exposure to environmental tobacco smoke among ethnically diverse women in the United States. *J. Women's Health Gend. Based Med.*, **11**, 45–51

Steyn, K., Yach, D., Stander, I. & Fourie, J.M. (1997) Smoking in urban pregnant women in South Africa. *S. Afr. Med. J.*, **87**, 460–463

Stillman, F.A., Becker, D.M., Swank, R.T., Hantula, D., Moses, H., Glantz, S. & Waranch, H.R. (1990) Ending smoking at the Johns Hopkins Medical Institutions. An evaluation of smoking prevalence and indoor air pollution. *J. Am. med. Assoc.*, **264**, 1565–1569

Thompson, B., Emmons, K., Abrams, D., Ockene, J.K. & Feng, Z. (1995) ETS exposure in the workplace. Perceptions and reactions by employees in 114 work sites. Working Well Research Group [corrected]. *J. Occup. environ. Med.*, **37**, 1086–1092

Totsuka, Y., Ushiyama, H., Ishihara, J., Sinha, R., Goto, S., Sugimura, T. & Wakabayashi, K. (1999) Quantification of the co-mutagenic beta-carbolines, norharman and harman, in cigarette smoke condensates and cooked foods. *Cancer Lett.*, **143**, 139–143

US Department of Health and Human Services (2000) *National Worksite Health Promotion Survey*. Available at: http://www.cdc.gov/nchs/data/hp2000/safety/sumtable.pdf (accessed 24 January 2003), Washington DC, Office of Disease Prevention and Health Promotion

US EPA (US Environmental Protection Agency) (1992) *Respiratory Health Effects of Passive Smoking: Lung Cancer and Other Disorders* (EPA/600/6-90/006F), Washington DC, United States Environmental Protection Agency

Vainiotalo, S., Vaaranrinta, R., Tornaeus, J., Aremo, N., Hase, T. & Peltonen, K. (2001) Passive monitoring method for 3-ethenylpyridine: A marker for environmental tobacco smoke. *Environ. Sci. Technol.*, **35**, 1818–1822

Vu Duc, T. & Huynh, C.K. (1987) Deposition rates of sidestream tobacco smoke particles in an experimental chamber. *Toxicol. Lett.*, **35**, 59–65

Wakefield, M., Roberts, L. & Owen, N. (1996) Trends in prevalence and acceptance of workplace smoking bans among indoor workers in South Australia. *Tob. Control*, **5**, 205–208

Whitlock, G., MacMahon, S., Vander Hoorn, S., Davis, P., Jackson, R. & Norton, R. (1998) Association of environmental tobacco smoke exposure with socioeconomic status in a population of 7725 New Zealanders. *Tob. Control*, **7**, 276–280

Yang, G., Fan, L., Tan, J., Qi, G., Zhang, Y., Samet, J.M., Taylor, C.E., Becker, K. & Xu, J. (1999) Smoking in China. Findings of the 1996 National Prevalence Survey. *JAMA*, **282**, 1247–1253

2. Studies of Cancer in Humans

2.1 Lung cancer

The section summarizes the results of the relevant cohort studies and case–control studies of the association between lung cancer and exposure to secondhand smoke. They are ordered by source of exposure, i.e. secondhand smoke from partners at home, at the workplace, during childhood and from other sources. For each type of study, the results are presented first without differentiation according to the levels of exposure and then the exposure–response relationship is described.

The most commonly used measure of exposure to secondhand smoke has been from the spouse. This is because it is well defined and has been validated using cotinine studies of never-smokers who do or do not live with smokers. Spousal exposure is also a marker of exposure to tobacco smoke in general because people who live with smokers tend to mix with smokers outside the home. Other measures of exposure, at the workplace or during childhood, are not so well validated. It is more difficult to quantify exposure at the workplace than spousal exposure; the extent of exposure may vary considerably between different working environments (exposure from the spouse is clearly defined and fairly consistent); people are more likely to change jobs than to remarry or divorce and, in studies based on people who have died from lung cancer, it may be more difficult for the next of kin or other respondent to know whether or not the subject had been exposed to secondhand smoke at work. Exposure during childhood has not been validated and, in studies of exposure to secondhand smoke, the relative risk for lung cancer associated with exposure during childhood should be stratified according to spousal exposure. Few studies have done this, and, even when they have, the number of lung cancer cases has been too small to enable robust conclusions to be drawn.

2.1.1 *Cohort studies*

There have been eight cohort studies of nonsmokers who were followed for several years to determine the risk for lung cancer (these are described in Table 2.1). Six of these studies (Garfinkel, 1981; Hirayama, 1984; Butler, 1988; Cardenas *et al.*, 1997; Jee *et al.*, 1999; Nishino *et al.*, 2001) reported the risk of lung cancer associated with exposure to secondhand smoke from the spouse. All six studies found that the risk for nonsmoking women with partners who smoked was higher than that for those whose partner did not

Table 2.1. Cohort studies of secondhand smoke and lung cancer

Reference (country, years of study)	Cohort sample	Cohort eligibility; follow-up	Source of exposure	Incidence/death; covariates adjusted for; comments
Garfinkel (1981) (USA, 1960–72)	176 739 married nonsmoking women	ACS Study: friends, neighbours and relatives of American Cancer Society volunteers; deaths reported by volunteers; death certificates obtained from state health departments; 93% follow-up Veterans Study: questionnaire mailed to veterans holding a US Government life insurance; 85% response; death certificates supplied to the Veterans' Administration or through field work at health departments	Active smoking by current spouse	Deaths 1) Crude death rates; 2) analysis with women matched by age, race, highest educational status of husband or wife, residence and occupational exposure of husband
Hirayama (1984) (Japan, 1965–81)	91 540 married nonsmoking women	95% of the census population in the study area in 29 health centre districts; follow-up consisted of special annual census and special death registry system.	Active smoking by current spouse	Deaths SMRs
Butler (1988) (USA, 1974–82)	Spouse pairs: 9378 subjects; AHSMOG cohort: 6467 subjects (66% overlap)	Non-Hispanic white Adventists; spouse pairs with a non-smoking wife; AHSMOG cohort enrolled for air pollution study; deaths ascertained by linkage to California death certificate file, national death index and notification of death by church clerks; cases ascertained with hospital history forms and review of hospital and tumour registry records; 99% histologically confirmed	Spouse pair cohort: active smoking by current spouse; AHSMOG cohort: exposure at work	Cases/deaths Adjusted for age
DeWaard et al. (1995) (the Netherlands, 1977–91)	23 cases and 191 controls	Nested case–control study among women enrolled in breast cancer screening projects (DOM project, enrolment 1975–77, aged 50–64 years and Lutine Study, enrolment 1982–83, aged 40–49 years)	Exposure assessed by measurement of urinary cotinine levels in declared nonsmokers	Cases/deaths Cotinine excretion adjusted for creatinine resulted in higher odds ratios.

Table 2.1 (contd)

Reference (country, years of study)	Cohort sample	Cohort eligibility; follow-up	Source of exposure	Incidence/death; covariates adjusted for; comments
Cardenas et al. (1997) (USA, 1982–89)	288 776 (96 542 men, 192 234 women) nonsmoking subjects	Friends, neighbours and relatives of American Cancer Society volunteers in all 50 States; aged > 30 years; death monitored by volunteers and through national death index; cause of death classified according to ICD-9.	Active smoking by current spouse; self-reported exposure at home, at work or in other areas	Deaths Adjusted for age, race, education, blue-collar employment, asbestos exposure, consumption of vegetables, citrus fruits and fat, history of chronic lung disease
Jee et al. (1999) (Republic of Korea, 1992–97)	157 436 married nonsmoking women	Both spouses had to have completed the Korean Medical Insurance Corporation medical examination; aged > 40 years; cases ascertained from diagnosis on discharge summary	Active smoking by current husband	Cases Univariate analysis; multivariate analysis adjusted for age of husband and wife, socioeconomic status, residence, husband's vegetable consumption and occupation
Speizer et al. (1999) (USA, 1976–92)	121 700 women, US registered nurses in 1976; unknown subcohort of nonsmokers	Female nurses aged 30–55 years, Nurses' Health Study; deaths ascertained by family members, postal service or through national death index; cases confirmed by pathology reports	Information on exposure to second-hand smoke during childhood and adulthood ascertained in 1982	Cases Adjusted for age
Nishino et al. (2001) (Japan, 1984–92)	31 345 (13 992 men, 17 353 women) non-smokers	Residents of six primary school sectors in a city and the whole area of two towns in north-eastern Honshu, aged > 40 years; cases ascertained by linkage to the prefectural cancer registry; cancer sites coded according to ICD-9	Any smoker in the household	Cases 1) Crude relative risk; 2) stratification by smoking status of husband and other household members; 3) multivariate relative risk adjusted for age, study area, alcohol intake, green and yellow vegetable intake, fruit intake, meat intake and past history of lung disease

SMR, standardized mortality ratio

smoke (see Table 2.2). In both cohort studies that reported on the effect in nonsmoking men whose wives smoked, the relative risk was increased (Hirayama 1984; Cardenas *et al.*, 1997). The two other cohort studies, which were based on general exposure to secondhand smoke (deWaard *et al.*, 1995; Speizer *et al.*, 1999), obtained similar results.

Table 2.2. Epidemiological studies[a] of the risk for lung cancer in lifelong non-smokers whose spouses smoked relative to the risk in those whose spouses did not smoke[b]

Reference (country)	No. of cases of lung cancer	Crude relative risk (95% CI)	Adjusted relative risk (95% CI)[c]
Women			
Case–control studies (n = 40)			
Chan & Fung (1982) (Hong Kong, SAR)	84	0.8 [0.4–1.3]	NR[d]
Correa *et al.* (1983) (USA)	22	2.1 [0.8–5.3]	NR
Trichopoulos *et al.* (1983) (Greece)	62	2.1 [1.2–3.8]	NR
Buffler *et al.* (1984) (USA)	41	0.8 [0.3–1.9]	0.8 (0.3–1.8)
Kabat & Wynder (1984) (USA)	24	0.8 [0.3–2.5]	NR
Lam (1985) (Hong Kong, SAR)	60	2.0 [1.1–3.7][e]	NR
Garfinkel *et al.* (1985) (USA)	134	1.2 [0.8–1.9]	1.2 (0.9–1.6)
Wu *et al.* (1985) (USA)	29	NR	1.2 (0.5–3.3)
Akiba *et al.* (1986) (Japan)	94	1.5 [0.9–2.6]	1.5 [0.8–2.8][f]
Lee *et al.* (1986) (United Kingdom)	32	1.0 [0.4–2.6]	1.0 (0.4–2.7)
Brownson *et al.* (1987) (USA)[g]	19	1.5 (0.4–6.0)	
Gao *et al.* (1987) (China)	246	1.2 (0.8–1.7)	1.3 (1.0–1.8)
Humble *et al.* (1987) (USA)	20	2.3 [0.8–6.8]	2.2 (0.7–6.6)
Koo *et al.* (1987) (Hong Kong, SAR)	86	1.6 [0.9–2.7]	1.6 (0.9–3.1)
Lam *et al.* (1987) (Hong Kong, SAR)	199	1.7 [1.2–2.4]	NR
Pershagen *et al.* (1987) (Sweden)	70	1.0 [0.6–1.7]	1.2 (0.7–2.1)
Geng *et al.* (1988) (China)	54	2.2 [1.1–4.3]	NR
Inoue & Hirayama (1988) (Japan)	22	2.6 (0.7–8.8)[h]	NR
Shimizu *et al.* (1988) (Japan)	90	1.1 [0.6–1.8]	1.1 (NR)
Choi *et al.* (1989) (Republic of Korea)	75	1.6 (0.9–2.9)	1.6 (NR)
Kalandidi *et al.* (1990) (Greece)	90	1.6 [0.9–2.9]	2.1 (1.1–4.1)
Sobue (1990) (Japan)	144	1.1 [0.7–1.5]	1.1 (0.8–1.6)
Wu-Williams *et al.* (1990) (China)	417	0.8 [0.6–1.0]	0.7 (0.6–0.9)
Liu & Chapman (1991)[i] (China)	54	0.7 [0.3–1.7]	0.8 (0.3–2.0)
Brownson *et al.* (1992) (USA)	431	1.0 [0.8–1.2]	1.0 (0.8–1.2)
Stockwell *et al.* (1992) (USA)	210	NR	1.6 (0.8–3.0)
Du *et al.* (1993) (China)	75	1.2 (0.7–2.1)	NR
Liu *et al.* (1993) (China)	38	1.7 (0.7–3.8)	NR
Fontham *et al.* (1994) (USA)	651	1.3 (1.0–1.5)	1.3 (1.0–1.6)
Kabat *et al.* (1995) (USA)	67	1.1 [0.6–2.0]	1.1 (0.6–1.9)
Sun *et al.* (1996) (China)	230	NR	1.2 (0.8–1.7)

Table 2.2 (contd)

Reference (country)	No. of cases of lung cancer	Crude relative risk (95% CI)	Adjusted relative risk (95% CI)[c]
Wang et al. (1996) (China)	135	1.1 [0.7–1.8]	NR
Boffetta et al. (1998) (Europe)	508	1.0 [0.8–1.3]	1.1 (0.9–1.4)
Shen et al. (1998) (China)	70	[1.5 (0.7–3.3)]	1.6 (0.7–3.9)
Zaridze et al. (1998) (Russia)	189	1.6 [1.1–2.3]	1.5 (1.1–2.2)
Rapiti et al. (1999) (India)	41	1.0 [0.4–2.4]	1.2 (0.5–2.9)
Zhong et al. (1999) (China)	407	1.2 [0.8–1.6]	1.1 (0.8–1.5)
Kreuzer et al. (2000)[j] (Germany)	100	0.9 [0.6–1.4]	0.8 (0.5–1.3)
Lee et al. (2000)[k] (Taiwan, China)	268	1.7 [1.3–2.4]	1.8 (1.3–2.5)
Johnson et al. (2001) (Canada)	71	NR	1.2 (0.6–4.0)
Cohort studies (n = 6)			
Garfinkel (1981) (USA)	153	NR	1.2 [0.9–1.4]
Hirayama (1984) (Japan)	200	NR	1.5 [1.0–2.1][l]
Butler (1988) (USA)	8	NR	2.0 (0.5–8.6)
Cardenas et al. (1997) (USA)	150	NR	1.2 (0.8–1.6)
Jee et al. (1999) (Republic of Korea)	63	NR	1.9 (1.0–3.5)
Nishino et al. (2001) (Japan)	24	NR	1.9 (0.8–4.4)
Men			
Case–control studies (n = 9)			
Correa et al. (1983) (USA)	8	2.0 [0.2–11.8][m]	NR
Buffler et al. (1984) (USA)	11	0.5 (0.1–2.2)[m]	0.5 (0.2–1.7)
Kabat & Wynder (1984) (USA)	12	1.0 [0.2–6.7][m]	NR
Akiba et al. (1986) (Japan)	19	2.1 (0.5–8.6)	1.8 (0.5–7.0)[f]
Lee et al. (1986) (United Kingdom)	15	1.3 (0.3–5.4)[m]	1.3 (0.4–4.4)
Choi et al. (1989) (Republic of Korea)	13	2.7 (0.5–15.2)[m]	2.7 (NR)
Kabat et al. (1995) (USA)	39	1.6 [0.7–3.9]	1.6 (0.7–3.8)
Boffetta et al. (1998) (Europe)	141	1.3 [0.8–2.2]	NR
Kreuzer et al. (2000)[j] (Germany)	23	0.4 (0.1–3.0)	NR
Cohort studies (n = 2)			
Hirayama (1984) (Japan)	64	NR	2.3 [1.1–4.8]
Cardenas et al. (1997) (USA	97	NR	1.1 (0.6–1.8)

CI, confidence interval

[a] Only the most recent publication is used for studies that have been updated from previously published reports. Also, studies based on subjects who are included in a larger series are not listed here.

[b] In addition, there are four studies that gave results for men and women combined: Hole et al. (1989) (7 cases), relative risk, 2.1 (95% CI, 0.5–12.8); Janerich et al. (1990) (188 cases), relative risk, 0.9 (95% CI, 0.6–1.6) for analysis based on subjects interviewed directly and 0.4 (0.2–1.0) for analysis based on interviews with surrogate respondents; Schwartz et al. (1996) (257 cases), relative risk, 1.1 (95% CI, 0.8–1.6); Boffetta et al. (1999a) (69 cases), relative risk 1.22 (95% CI, 0.7–2.1).

[c] Adjusted for at least age (other factors included dietary habits, education and social class)

Table 2.2 (contd)

---

[d] Not reported or estimatable from the reported results

[e] Results for adenocarcinoma only

[f] The original report presented 90% confidence intervals that were converted to 95% confidence intervals for this table.

[g] The raw data came from the US Environmental Protection Agency (1992).

[h] Results reported in the US Environmental Protection Agency report (1992), which also noted that the results reported in this article (odds ratio, 2.3) were erroneous

[i] One of the 202 controls was a smoker, but this would have a negligible effect on the result, so this study was included.

[j] Results from analysis excluding cases and controls already included in the study by Boffetta et al. (1998) [personal communication M. Kreuzer]

[k] Crude results are for comparisons between women married to smokers and those married to non-smokers. The adjusted result was obtained by pooling the odds ratio corresponding to women married to smokers who smoked in their presence with the odds ratio corresponding to women married to smokers who did not smoke in their presence.

[l] Authors reported a 90% confidence interval that was adjusted to a 95% confidence interval for this table. It should also be noted that this result was for a comparison of women whose husbands smoked 1–19 cigarettes/day with women whose husbands were nonsmokers, and did not include the highest exposure group (≥ 20 cigarettes/day).

[m] Fisher's exact 95% confidence intervals were estimated.

Exposure–response relationships

The analysis of exposure–response relationships provides critical evidence for or against a causal relationship between exposure to secondhand smoke and the development of lung cancer.

In the study by Garfinkel (1981), the relative risk did not increase with increasing exposure levels.

In the study by Hirayama (1984), the relative risks for women were 1.4, 1.4, 1.6 and 1.9 when their husbands were ex-smokers, and when they smoked 1–14, 15–19 or ≥ 20 cigarettes/day, respectively (*p* value for trend test, 0.002). Similarly the relative risk for nonsmoking men increased with exposure level: it was 2.1 when the wives smoked 1–19 cigarettes/day and 2.3 when they smoked ≥ 20 cigarettes/day (*p* value for trend test, 0.02).

The study by Cardenas et al. (1997) also found a significant exposure–response relationship. When the husbands smoked 1–19, 20–39 and ≥ 40 cigarettes/day, the relative risks for women exposed to secondhand smoke were 1.1, 1.2 and 1.9 respectively (*p* value for trend test, 0.03). There was no evidence of an association between risk and the length of time the couples had been married. A similar analysis for nonsmoking men exposed to secondhand smoke would not be robust because the number of cases was too small. The particular strengths of this study were the near complete data on cause of death (97%), direct questioning of both partners about their smoking habits, and the taking into account of numerous potential confounders such as previous lung disease, occupational exposure to asbestos, dietary habits and education.

Taken together, the three large cohort studies demonstrate an increased incidence of deaths from lung cancer associated with exposure to secondhand smoke from the spouse. The increase in deaths from lung cancer in the study by Hirayama (1984) is significant, and this study and that by Cardenas *et al.* (1997) also reported a significant exposure–response relationship.

2.1.2 Case–control studies

Many case–control studies have been undertaken in several countries (mostly China and the USA) (described in Table 2.3). In these studies lung cancer cases were ascertained and matched with controls (usually for age and other factors). The controls were selected from either the general population or the hospital in which the patients with lung cancer were diagnosed. Details of the smoking habits of the partners of both cases and controls were obtained either by interview or questionnaire. In some instances the next of kin provided the relevant information. These studies were based on various measures of exposure to secondhand smoke, including exposure from the partner, at the workplace, during childhood or exposure from other sources. The following section describes only large, relevant studies in which all cases and controls were interviewed in person and no information from the next of kin was used to reconstruct exposure.

(a) Description of studies

The study of Lam *et al.* (1987) included 199 cases and 335 controls from Hong Kong, Special Administrative Region of China. The study is characterized by good data on exposure (from various sources) to secondhand smoke, valid classification of the smoking habits of the husband and a consideration of potential confounders (including education, place of birth, duration of residence and marital status).

The study from China by Gao *et al.* (1987) included 246 cases and 375 controls. The cases were identified using a system built upon the Shanghai Cancer Registry. The analyses were controlled for age and education.

The study of Wu-Williams *et al.* (1990), also from China, included 417 cases and 602 controls. A limitation of this study is that it was not able to control for important indoor sources of exposure to potential lung carcinogens such as those produced during burning of coal and frying in oil.

The study of Brownson *et al.* (1992) in the USA included 431 cases and 1166 controls. It is characterized by good documentation of data on exposure in the home and the workplace, and took into account potential confounders (age, sex and socioeconomic status).

In the study of Fontham *et al.* (1994) in the USA, 651 cases and 1253 controls were interviewed. Possible misclassification of smokers and potential confounding by age, occupational exposure to known carcinogens, eating habits, familial history of lung cancer and education were taken into account. The smoking status was verified by means of cotinine determination to minimize the misclassification of smokers as nonsmokers.

Table 2.3. Main study design characteristics of case–control studies on exposure to secondhand smoke and lung cancer

Reference (country, years of study)	No. of non-smoking cases and controls	Eligibility criteria and comments	Covariates adjusted for	Source of exposure data
Chan & Fung (1982) (Hong Kong, SAR, 1976–77)	Women: 84 cases, 139 controls	Histologically confirmed cases of bronchial cancer were identified in five hospitals in Hong Kong. Controls were identified from patients in the orthopaedic ward at the same hospitals and were selected from the 'same general age group' as the cases.	None	Patients were interviewed using a questionnaire that included a question on exposure to passive smoke at home.
Correa et al. (1983) (USA, not reported)	Men: 8 cases, 178 controls Women: 22 cases, 133 controls	Cases of primary lung cancer identified from admission and pathology records at 29 hospitals. Patients with bronchioalveolar cancer were excluded. Controls were randomly selected from patients attending the same hospital and matched for race, sex and age. Patients with smoking-related diseases were excluded from the controls.	None	Study subjects were interviewed with a questionnaire including questions on history of exposure from smoking spouses and parental smoking.
Trichopoulos et al. (1983) (Greece, 1978–82)	Men and women: 77 cases, 225 controls	Cases of lung cancer other than adenocarcinoma of the terminal bronchi were identified from three hospitals in Athens. Controls were drawn from an orthopaedic hospital in the same area as the cases. The cases and controls had 'similar demographic and socioeconomic profiles'.	None	Physicians interviewed subjects concerning smoking habits of their spouses.
Buffler et al. (1984) (USA, 1976–80)	Men: 11 cases, 90 controls Women: 41 cases, 196 controls	Patients aged 30–79 years with histologically confirmed lung cancer were identified from hospital and state records in six counties in Texas. Population-based and deceased controls were selected from state and federal records that were matched to cases on age, race, sex, region of residence and vital status.	Age, race, sex, region of residence and vital status	Questionnaires were administered to study subjects or next of kin, which included questions on household members who smoked regularly.
Kabat & Wynder (1984) (USA, 1971–80)	Men: 25 cases, 25 controls Women: 53 cases, 53 controls	Cases of primary cancer of the lung were selected from hospitals. One control was matched to each case on age, sex, race, hospital and date of interview. Controls were selected from other hospitalized patients who had diseases that were not tobacco related.	None	Study subjects were interviewed in hospital using a standardized questionnaire that included questions on spousal and workplace exposure.

Table 2.3 (contd)

Reference (country, years of study)	No. of non-smoking cases and controls	Eligibility criteria and comments	Covariates adjusted for	Source of exposure data
Lam (1985) (Hong Kong, SAR, 1981–84)	Women: 60 cases, 144 controls	Cases of primary lung cancer were identified from a hospital in Hong Kong. Controls were selected from patients in the orthopaedic wards of the same hospital and were reported to be comparable in age and social class to the cases. Sufficient numbers of cases were available to permit a meaningful analysis only for adenocarcinoma.	Although age and social class appear to have been matched for, they were not controlled for in the analysis.	Exposure assessment used interviews of study subjects or next of kin, which included questions on exposure to secondhand smoke from parents, spouse or other family members.
Garfinkel et al. (1985) (USA, 1971–81)	Women: 134 cases, 402 controls	Cases and controls were identified from three hospitals in New Jersey and one in Ohio. Controls were colon and rectum cancers matched to the cases on age and hospital. Both cases and controls were histologically confirmed.	Age and hospital in all analyses. Logistic regression also controlled for socioeconomic status and year of diagnosis	Study subjects or next of kin were interviewed using a questionnaire designed to elicit information on exposure to secondhand smoke from the spouse or other household member(s).
Wu et al. (1985) (USA, 1981–82)	Women: 29 patients with adenocarcinomas and 62 controls; 2 with squamous-cell carcinomas and 30 controls[a]	Cases diagnosed by microscopy were identified from a population-based tumour registry in Los Angeles County. Cases were white residents, under 76 years of age who had no prior history of cancer (except melanoma). Neighbourhood controls met the same criteria and were matched to cases on date of birth.	Age. Active smoking was included in analyses that were not restricted to nonsmokers.	A structured telephone questionnaire was used to elicit information on exposure to secondhand smoke from spouse or other household members, and during childhood from household members.

Table 2.3 (contd)

Reference (country, years of study)	No. of non-smoking cases and controls	Eligibility criteria and comments	Covariates adjusted for	Source of exposure data
Akiba *et al.* (1986) (Japan, 1971–80)	Women: 94 cases, 270 controls Men: 19 cases, 241 controls	Cases and controls were identified from a cohort of atomic bomb survivors in Hiroshima and Nagasaki. Cases were identified from tumour, mortality and other medical registries. Controls were matched to cases by birth, sex, city of residence, vital status and whether they participated in an annual medical programme. For deceased cases, the corresponding controls were required to have died from a disease other than cancer or chronic respiratory diseases, and were matched to cases on year of death.	Age, sex, city, and year of death	Subjects or next of kin were interviewed using a structured questionnaire to elicit information on exposure to secondhand smoke from a spouse or parent.
Lee *et al.* (1986) (United Kingdom, 1979–82)	Women: 32 cases, 66 controls Men: 15 cases, 30 controls	Cases and controls were nonsmokers identified from several hospitals in England. Controls were patients who did not have lung cancer, chronic bronchitis, ischaemic heart disease or stroke. Two controls for each case were selected and matched on sex, age, marital status, and as far as possible, hospital.	Age, sex, hospital and marital status	The patients and their spouses were interviewed to obtain a history of spousal smoking.
Schwartz (1996) (USA, 1984–87)	Men and women: 401 cases, 398 controls	Cases between the ages of 40 and 84 years were identified in Detroit from an Occupational Cancer Incidence Surveillance Study (OCISS) in conjunction with the Metropolitan Detroit Cancer Surveillance System. Population-based controls were randomly selected from the controls who took part in the OCISS study. Controls were frequency-matched to cases on age, sex, race and county of residence.	Age, sex and race	Telephone interviews were conducted with cases (17%) or controls (78%) or their proxies. The questionnaire included information on exposure to secondhand smoke at work or at home.

Table 2.3 (contd)

Reference (country, years of study)	No. of non-smoking cases and controls	Eligibility criteria and comments	Covariates adjusted for	Source of exposure data
Brownson et al. (1987) (USA, 1979–82)	Women: 19 cases, 47 controls Men: 4 cases, 19 controls	Cases of adenocarcinoma and controls were identified from the Colorado Central Cancer Registry. All cases were confirmed by microscopy. Controls were patients with colon and bone marrow cancer and were group-matched to cases on age and sex. Cases and controls were required to have resided for a minimum of 6 months in the Denver metropolitan area prior to diagnosis.	Age, sex and socioeconomic status	Cases and controls or next of kin were interviewed and information collected on the smoking status of the spouse and the number of hours per day exposed to secondhand smoke.
Gao et al. (1987) (China, 1984–86)	Women: 246 cases, 375 controls	Cases of lung cancer were identified among female residents of Shanghai aged 35–69 from a system built upon the Shanghai Cancer Registry. Female controls were randomly selected from the Shanghai area and approximately frequency-matched on age.	Age and education	Cases and controls were interviewed to obtain information on exposure in childhood and adulthood.
Geng et al. (1988) (China, not stated)	Women: 54 cases, 93 controls	Cases were identified among females who had lived for more than 10 years in Tianjin, China. Controls were matched to the cases on sex, race, age and marital status. The precise source of the cases or controls is not stated.	None[b]	The methods used to collect information on exposure to secondhand smoke are not described.
Humble et al. (1987) (USA, 1980–82)	Men: 8 cases, 130 controls Women: 20 cases, 162 controls	Cases were identified from the New Mexican Tumor Registry. An initial series was selected between 1980 and 1982 that included all individuals less than 50 years of age, Hispanics aged over 50 years, and a random sample of male (40%) and female (50%) non-Hispanics over 50 years.	Ethnicity and age	Interviews of study subjects (48% cases) or their next of kin (52% cases) were conducted to collect information on spousal smoking habits.
Koo et al. (1987) (Hong Kong, SAR, 1981–83)	Women: 86 cases, 136 controls	Cases were identified as part of a larger study on female lung cancer in Hong Kong from the wards and outpatient departments of eight hospitals. An equal number of 'healthy' controls were selected and matched to cases on age, district and socioeconomic status (housing type).	Age, district and housing type, formal schooling and number of live births	Cases and controls were interviewed to elicit information on exposure to secondhand smoke from spouses and other relatives at home.

Table 2.3 (contd)

Reference (country, years of study)	No. of non-smoking cases and controls	Eligibility criteria and comments	Covariates adjusted for	Source of exposure data
Lam et al. (1987) (Hong Kong SAR, 1983–86)	Women: 199 cases, 35 controls	Pathologically confirmed cases of lung cancer were identified from eight hospitals. Controls were matched to the cases on age and drawn from the same neighbourhood as the corresponding case.	None	Study subjects were interviewed using a questionnaire that included questions concerning the husband's smoking habits.
Pershagen et al. (1987) (Sweden, 1963–80)	Women: 70 cases[c]	Cases and controls were selected from two cohort studies in Sweden. The first was a sample of men and women aged 15–65 years in the 1960 National Census who were mailed a questionnaire on smoking habits in 1963. The second was from a study of Swedish twins born between 1886 and 1925. Lung cancer cases were identified until 1980 by links with the Swedish Cancer Registry and the National Register on Causes of Death. Two control series were selected at random from the cohort. One was based on matching controls to cases based on year of birth, and the other on vital status at the end of follow-up as well as year of birth.	Age and vital status	A questionnaire was mailed in 1984 to each study subject, or if they were dead, to their next of kin (excluding the husband). The questionnaire included questions on exposure to secondhand smoke from husbands and parents.
Inoue & Hirayama (1988) (Japan, 1972–83)	Women: 22 cases[d], 62 controls	Cases and controls are from Kamakure and Miura, Japan. The methods used to identify the cases and controls were not clearly stated. Controls were individuals with cerebrovascular disease who were matched to the cases on age, year of death and district.	Age, year of death and district	Interviews were conducted using 'standard questionnaires'.
Shimizu et al. (1988) (Japan, 1982–85)	Women: 90 cases, 163 controls	Cases of primary lung cancer were identified from 4 hospitals in Nagoya, Japan. Controls were patients from adjacent wards with diseases other than lung cancer who were matched to the cases on age and date of admission.	Age, hospital and date of admission	Participants answered a questionnaire on the first or second day of admission that included questions on exposure to secondhand smoke from the spouse and other family members, and at the workplace.

Table 2.3 (contd)

Reference (country, years of study)	No. of non-smoking cases and controls	Eligibility criteria and comments	Covariates adjusted for	Source of exposure data
Choi et al. (1989) (Republic of Korea, 1985–88)	Women: 75 cases, 144 controls	375 patients with lung cancer admitted to Korean Cancer Centre Hospital with histopathologically confirmed diagnosis. Two controls were selected per case matched by age (± 5 years), gender, admission date and area (urban/rural); patients with smoking-related diseases were excluded.	Unmatched analysis of subgroup of non-smoking study subjects	A questionnaire was administered face-to-face including questions on smoking.
Janerich et al. (1990) (USA, 1982–85)	Men and women: 191 cases, 191 controls	Cases were identified from 125 diagnostic or treatment facilities covering 23 counties in New York State, and from the New York State cancer registry. Cases were between 20 and 80 years of age, and had to have been resident of one of the 23 counties. Controls were identified from records of the New York Department of Motor Vehicles, and matched to the cases on age, county of residence and smoking history (i.e. nonsmokers).	Age and county of residence	Face-to-face interviews were conducted with cases or controls or their next of kin. When a next-of-kin interview was required, the next of kin of the matching controls were also interviewed. The questionnaire included questions on exposure to smoke from the spouse, at the workplace and during childhood.
Kalandidi et al. (1990) (Greece, 1987–89)	Women: 90 cases, 120 controls	Cases with a 'definite' diagnosis of lung cancer were identified from 7 hospitals in the greater Athens area. Controls were women hospitalized in the orthopaedic department of the same or a nearby hospital, and were randomly selected from those who entered within a week of a corresponding case. Controls had to be 35 years or older.	Age, years of schooling, interviewer and total energy consumption	A questionnaire was administered face-to-face to the cases and controls that included questions on exposure to secondhand smoke from the spouse, other household members and at the workplace.

Table 2.3 (contd)

Reference (country, years of study)	No. of non-smoking cases and controls	Eligibility criteria and comments	Covariates adjusted for	Source of exposure data
Sobue (1990) (Japan, 1986–88)	Women: 144 cases, 731 controls	Cases of lung cancer and controls aged 40–79 years were identified from eight hospitals in Osaka, Japan. Controls were individuals with diseases other than lung cancer.	Age and education	A self-administered questionnaire was given to cases and controls at the time of admission which included questions on exposure to secondhand smoke.
Wu-Williams et al. (1990) (China, 1985–87)	Women: 417 cases, 602 controls	Patients under the age of 70 years with primary lung cancers were identified in the cancer registries of Shenyang and Harbin, China and of major hospitals serving these areas. Controls were randomly selected from the populations of Shenyang and Harbin, and were frequency-matched to the cases by age.	Age, education and centre	Cases and controls were interviewed using a questionnaire that included questions concerning exposure to secondhand smoke from the spouse and other co-habitants, and at the workplace.
Liu et al. (1991) (China, 1985–86)	Men and women: 4 cases, 19 controls	Cases of lung cancer were identified from hospitals and clinics in Xuanwei. Controls were matched to the cases on age, sex and village of residence.	Age, sex, village of residence and cooking history	Cases and controls were personally interviewed using a questionnaire that included a question on exposure to second-hand smoke at home (primarily from the spouse)
Brownson et al. (1992) (USA, 1986–91)	Women: 431 cases, 1166 controls	Cases of primary lung cancer among white females were identified from the Missouri cancer registry; 76% of the cases were histologically verified. Controls were selected for women under 65 years from the state driver's license files, and for women 65 years or over from the Health Care Finance Administration's roster of Medicare recipients. Controls were frequency-matched to cases on age.	Age, previous lung disease and dietary β-carotene and fat	Telephone interviews were conducted that included questions concerning exposure to secondhand smoke during childhood and adulthood.

Table 2.3 (contd)

Reference (country, years of study)	No. of non-smoking cases and controls	Eligibility criteria and comments	Covariates adjusted for	Source of exposure data
Stockwell et al. (1992) (USA, 1987–91)	Women: 210 cases, 301 controls	Cases of histologically confirmed primary lung cancer were identified from hospital tumour registries, and a state-wide cancer registry in 28 counties in central Florida. Population-based controls were selected using random digit dialling.	Age, race and education	Interviews of patients or next of kin were conducted in person, by telephone or occasionally by post. The questionnaire included questions on exposure to secondhand smoke at home, at work or in social settings.
Du et al. (1993) (China, 1985–86)	**1985 analysis** Men and women: 120 cases, 120 controls with non-respiratory disease, 120 controls with non-respiratory cancer **1986 analysis** Women: 75 cases, 128 non-cancer patients as controls plus 126 controls with tumours other than of the lung	Cases in this study were apparently identified from deaths reported to the local police stations in Guanghzo. Two separate analyses are presented (1) for nonsmokers in 1985 and (2) for female nonsmokers in 1986. Two control groups were selected for each analysis, but it is not clear how these controls were selected. The control groups for the first analysis consisted of (1) non-respiratory system diseases and (2) non-respiratory cancers. The control groups for the second analysis consisted of (1) non-tumour disease and (2) tumours other than of the lung. In the first analysis, controls were matched to cases on sex and age, and were matched on residence in both analyses.	First analysis sex, age and residence Second analysis did not adjust for covariates.	A questionnaire was used by trained personnel to obtain information from family members; it included questions on spousal smoking habits.

Table 2.3 (contd)

Reference (country, years of study)	No. of non-smoking cases and controls	Eligibility criteria and comments	Covariates adjusted for	Source of exposure data
Liu et al. (1993) (China, 1983–84)	Women: 38 cases, 69 controls	Cases of primary lung cancer were identified from eight major hospitals covering most of Guangzhou. Controls were selected from inpatients at six of these hospitals and patients with chronic obstructive lung diseases, pulmonary tuberculosis, cancers and coronary heart disease were excluded. Controls were matched to cases on age, sex, residential district and date of diagnosis or admission to hospital.	Age, sex, residential area, calendar time, education and occupation	Interviews were carried out in the homes of the subjects using a questionnaire that included questions on spousal smoking habits.
Fontham et al. (1994) (USA, 1986–90)	Women: 651 cases, 1253 controls	Cases of primary lung cancer confirmed by microscopy were identified between 1986 and 1988 among residents of Atlanta, and Houston; and between 1989 and 1990 among residents of New Orleans, Los Angeles and San Francisco. Population-based controls were chosen using random digit dialling and random sampling from the Health Care Financing Administration's files. Controls were frequency-matched to cases on race, study centre and age. Cases and controls were required to be between 20 and 79 years of age, to speak English, Spanish or Chinese, and to have no prior history of cancer.	Age, race, study centre, education, family history of cancer, occupational and dietary factors	In-person interviews were conducted with cases and controls or with next of kin. The questionnaire included questions on exposure to secondhand smoke during adulthood (from spouse and at work), and during childhood (from parents or other household members). Urine cotinine measurements were made and used to eliminate individuals who may have been smokers.
Kabat et al. (1995) (USA, 1983–90)	Women: 69 cases, 187 controls Men: 100 cases, 117 controls	Histologically confirmed cases were identified in hospitals in New York City, Chicago, Detroit and Philadelphia. Controls were patients admitted to the same hospitals with diseases thought to be unrelated to tobacco smoke. Cases were matched to controls on age, sex, race, hospital and date of interview.	Age, sex, race, education and type of hospital (cancer centre versus other)	In-person interviews were conducted that included questions on exposure to secondhand smoke in childhood and adulthood (at home and in the workplace)

Table 2.3 (contd)

Reference (country, years of study)	No. of non-smoking cases and controls	Eligibility criteria and comments	Covariates adjusted for	Source of exposure data
de Waard et al. (1995) (the Netherlands, 1989, 1991, 1992)	Women: 23 cases, 305 controls	Cases and controls were identified from two cohorts of women screened for breast cancer in Utrecht. The first cohort included women aged 50–64 years who were screened in 1975 and 1977, and re-examined 1 year later. The second cohort included women aged 40–49 years who were screened between 1982 and 1983. Lung cancer cases were identified from mortality and cancer incidence registries. Cancer cases and controls were identified for the first cohort in 1989, 1991 and 1992, whereas cases and controls for the second cohort were identified only in 1992. Four controls were selected for each case identified in 1989 and 1991, and two controls per case in 1992 from the cohort files. Controls were matched to cases on 'about the same age and day of urine collection' for the 1989 cases, and it is unclear whether this matching criterion was also applied to cases and controls from the other years.	Possibly age and calendar time, but it is not clear if these were matched for in all cases or adjusted for in the analyses.	Urinary cotinine concentrations measured in samples collected during the screenings. Non-smokers were defined as subjects with creatinine adjusted cotinine levels of < 9.2 ng/mg creatinine
Sun et al. (1996) (China, not reported)	Women: 230 cases, 230 controls	This was a population based case–control study in Harbin. Only an abstract was available, and the source of the cases and controls was not described in it.	Age and education	In-person interviews of cases and controls included questions on exposure to secondhand smoke during childhood, adolescence and adulthood.
Wang et al. (1996) (China, 1992–94)	Women: 135 cases, 135 controls	Cases of primary lung cancer who were between 35 and 69 years of age were identified in 18 hospitals in Shenyang. Controls were randomly selected from the urban population in Shenyang, and matched to cases on age.	Cases and controls were matched for age, but it is unclear whether an unmatched analysis was performed.	Cases and controls were interviewed face-to-face using a questionnaire that included questions on exposure to secondhand smoke in childhood and adulthood.

Table 2.3 (contd)

Reference (country, years of study)	No. of non-smoking cases and controls	Eligibility criteria and comments	Covariates adjusted for	Source of exposure data
Boffetta *et al.* (1998) (Europe, 1988–94)	Men: 141 cases, 531 controls Women: 508 cases, 1011 controls	Cases and controls were ≤ 74 years of age and had smoked < 400 cigarettes in their lifetimes. Cases were identified from 12 centres in seven European countries and 96.5% were confirmed by microscopy. Controls were hospital-based in some centres and community-based in others. Hospital-based controls were chosen to exclude those with other diseases related to smoking. Community-based controls were drawn from population registries. Controls were matched to cases on age and sex using individual matching in some centres and frequency matching in others. Questionnaire response rates ranged from 53 to > 95% except for 3 centres who had response rates < 50% among controls.	Sex, age and centre	Questionnaire on exposure to secondhand smoke from spouse, during childhood, in the workplace and from other sources was developed based on a previous study of urine cotinine levels and exposure to secondhand smoke including smoke from cigarillos, cigars and pipes as well as cigarettes.
Jöckel *et al.* (1998b) (Germany, 1988–93)	Men and women: 71 cases, 236 controls	Cases and controls were also a part of the study by Boffetta *et al.* (1998). Nonsmokers were identified from a larger case–control study from Bremen, Frankfurt and the surrounding areas. Controls were population based and matched to the cases on sex, age and region.	Sex, age, region, exposure to asbestos, social class, and intake of vegetables and fruits	Compatible with questionnaire used in study by Boffetta 1998. Individuals who had never smoked regularly for more than 6 months were classified as 'never-smokers', and were combined with workers exposed to low levels of secondhand smoke (<75th percentile) to form the referent group.

Table 2.3 (contd)

Reference (country, years of study)	No. of non-smoking cases and controls	Eligibility criteria and comments	Covariates adjusted for	Source of exposure data
Shen et al. (1998) (China, 1993)	Women: 70 cases, 70 controls	Cases of primary lung cancer (adenocarcinoma) living ≥ 20 years in Nanjing; healthy controls came from the same neighbourhood, 1:1 matched by sex and age (± 5 years); response rate was 100%.	Chronic lung disease, cooking conditions, family history of lung cancer	Standardized questionnaire administered by trained staff covered exposure to secondhand smoke for the 20 years preceding diagnosis: no. of cigarettes smoked/day, no. of years of exposure to secondhand smoke.
Zaridze et al. (1998) (Russia, not reported)	Women: 189 cases, 358 controls	Histologically confirmed cases of primary lung cancer were identified in two cancer treatment hospitals in Moscow. Controls were female oncology patients from the same hospitals who did not have lung or upper respiratory cancers. Cases and controls were required to be nonsmokers who lived in Moscow.	Age and education	In-person interviews were conducted within 2–3 days of hospital admission; they included questions on exposure to secondhand smoke in adulthood and childhood.
Boffetta et al. (1999a) (Europe, 1988–94)	Women: 208 cases, 361 controls	Same as Boffetta et al. (1998) except that results are stratified by type of exposure to secondhand smoke (cigarettes or cigars, cigarillos and pipes)	Age and centre	Same as Boffetta et al. (1998)
Boffetta et al. (1999b) (Europe, 1994–96)	Men: 4 cases, 41 controls Women: 66 cases, 137 controls	Histologically confirmed lung adenocarcinomas were identified from 9 centres in 7 countries from a larger study designed to assess the role of biomarkers of susceptibility in lung cancer among nonsmokers. Controls were selected from nonsmokers in the source populations or in hospital patients. Controls were frequency-matched to cases on age and gender.	Age, gender, and centre. Some models also included urban residence, education and occupational exposure.	Exposure to secondhand smoke was assessed using the same questionnaire as in Boffetta et al. (1998).

Table 2.3 (contd)

Reference (country, years of study)	No. of non-smoking cases and controls	Eligibility criteria and comments	Covariates adjusted for	Source of exposure data
Rapiti et al. (1999) (India, 1991–92)	Men: 17 cases, 56 controls Women: 41 cases, 67 controls	Histologically or cytologically confirmed cases of primary lung cancer were identified in a hospital in Chandigarh, Northern India. Two controls were selected for each case. One control was a patient at the same hospital who was not hospitalized for more than a month and did not have a disease related to active or passive smoking, alcohol or diet. The other control was a visitor of the patient. No matching of cases and controls was performed.	Sex, age, religion and residence	Interviews of subjects were conducted that included questions on exposure to secondhand smoke from the spouse, at the workplace and during childhood.
Zhong et al. (1999) (China, 1992–94)	Women: 504 cases, 601 controls	Cases of primary lung cancer aged 35–69 years were identified from the Shanghai cancer registry. Controls were randomly selected from a Shanghai residential registry and frequency-matched to the age distribution of female lung cancer patients in Shanghai in 1987–89.	Age, income, vitamin C intake, kitchen smokiness, family history of lung cancer, and potentially high risk occupations, and respondent status	Personal interviews with study subjects or their next of kin (2.3% for controls, and 20.2% for cases). The interview included questions on exposure to secondhand smoke from the spouse, at the workplace and during childhood.
Brennan et al. (2000) (Europe, 1994–96)	Subset of cases and controls from centres included in Boffetta et al. (1998) for whom dietary information was available	Same as Boffetta et al. (1998), but analyses were restricted to centres that had information on subjects' consumption of fruit, lettuce, tomato, carrot, cheese, carotenoids, β-carotene or retinol. Analyses were stratified by high and low consumption of these dietary variables, and high and low exposure to secondhand smoke.	Age, gender and centre	Same as Boffetta et al. (1998). High exposure to secondhand smoke was defined as being in the upper quartile from combined spousal and workplace exposures.

Table 2.3 (contd)

Reference (country, years of study)	No. of non-smoking cases and controls	Eligibility criteria and comments	Covariates adjusted for	Source of exposure data
Kreuzer et al. (2000) (Germany, 1990–96)	Men and women: 292 cases, 1338 controls	An extension of the German part of the European multicentre study (Boffetta et al., 1998). The cases and controls were a subset of nonsmokers from a larger study of radon exposure in Germany. Cases were identified from 15 hospitals in the study area and were restricted to those who were < 75 years of age; resident in the study area; had lived for > 25 years in Germany; interviewed within 3 months of diagnosis, and not too ill. Controls satisfying the first three criteria listed above were identified from mandatory registries or by modified random digit dialling and were frequency-matched to the cases on sex, age and region. The response rate in the cases was 76%, but that of the controls was only 41%.	Age, region, gender; some models included occupational exposure, exposure to radon, diet, family history of cancer, previous non-malignant respiratory disease and social class.	Same as Boffetta et al. (1998)
Lee et al. (2000) (China (Province of Taiwan), 1992–98)	Women: 268 cases, 445 controls	Histologically verified cases were identified from Kaohsiung Medical University Hospital in Taiwan. Controls were patients with conditions unrelated to tobacco smoking who were selected within 3 weeks of the case admission from the same hospital, and matched on age.	Age, date of hospital admission, residential area, education, occupation, tuberculosis, cooking fuels and presence of a fume extractor	Interviews were conducted using a structured questionnaire designed to elicit information on exposure to secondhand smoke.

Table 2.3 (contd)

Reference (country, years of study)	No. of non-smoking cases and controls	Eligibility criteria and comments	Covariates adjusted for	Source of exposure data
Wang et al. (2000) (China, 1994–98)	Men: 33 cases, 1214 controls Women: 200 cases, 407 controls	Cases of lung cancer who were aged 30–75 years and residents of Pingliang or Qingyang prefectures were identified from hospitals and clinics in these and neighbouring regions. Controls were randomly selected from 1990 census lists for the 2 prefectures and frequency matched to cases on age, sex and prefecture.	Age, sex and prefecture	In person interviews were conducted with cases and controls or with their next of kin when necessary. The questionnaire included questions on exposure to secondhand smoke during adulthood, childhood and in the workplace.
Johnson et al. (2001) (Canada, 1994–97)	Women: 71 cases, 761 controls	Cases of histologically confirmed primary lung cancer were identified from a national cancer surveillance system that covers 8 of Canada's 10 provinces. In five provinces controls were identified from health insurance plans, in one from property assessment databases, and in two using random digit dialling. Controls were frequency-matched to the expected distribution of cancer cases by age and province.	Age, province, education and fruit and vegetable consumption	Mailed questionnaires were completed by cases and controls except in one province where next of kin completed them. The questionnaires included questions on exposure to secondhand smoke at work, at home and during childhood.
Kreuzer et al. (2001) (Germany, 1990–96)	Men: 58 cases, 803 controls	Same as Kreuzer et al. (2000) except that analyses were restricted to men.	Same as Kreuzer et al. (2000)	Same as Boffetta et al. (1998). Results only presented for low and high exposure to secondhand smoke where high was defined as having greater than the 75th percentile of cumulative duration of exposure weighted by a subjective index of intensity.

Table 2.3 (contd)

Reference (country, years of study)	No. of non-smoking cases and controls	Eligibility criteria and comments	Covariates adjusted for	Source of exposure data
Kreuzer et al. (2002) (Germany, 1990–96)	Women: 234 cases, 535 controls	Same as Kreuzer et al. (2000) except that analyses were restricted to women	Same as Kreuzer et al. (2000)	Same as Boffetta et al. (1998). Results only presented for high and medium exposure to secondhand smoke versus low or non-exposed. High was defined as having greater than the 90th percentile of cumulative duration of exposure, and low was defined as having less than the 75th percentile.

[a] This study presented results separately for patients with adenocarcinoma and for patients with squamous-cell carcinoma. However, the numbers for the squamous-cell carcinomas were too few to present meaningful results for secondhand smoke in nonsmokers.

[b] Although this study did match cases to controls on several potential confounders, an unmatched analysis was published.

[c] The study had a total of 184 controls in each of the control groups. However, it is unclear how many controls were used in the analysis of exposure to secondhand smoke because several cases (and presumably their matched controls) were dropped from these analyses.

[d] Information on spousal smoking habits was available for only some of the cases and controls. The actual number of cases and controls included in the analysis was not reported, but was smaller than the given numbers.

The study from China by Sun *et al.* (1996) included 230 cases and 230 controls. The study controlled for age and education, but not for burning of coal and frying in oil.

The study of Lee *et al.* (2000) from China (Province of Taiwan) included 268 cases and 445 controls and was an extension of the study of Ko *et al.* (1997). Detailed information on exposure to secondhand smoke was collected, and nonsmoking status was verified by household members. Potential confounding by age, education, occupation, cooking fuels and other factors was allowed for.

The participants in a European multicentre study included 650 cases and 1542 controls from 12 centres in seven countries. Potential confounders such as occupational exposure, socioeconomic status and intake of fruits and vegetables were taken into account. The main publication was by Boffetta *et al.* (1998), but additional analyses were made of effects of secondhand smoke from cigars, cigarillos and pipes (Boffetta *et al.*, 1999b) and of exposure to secondhand smoke and diet (Brennan *et al.*, 2000). In addition, the data from some centres on specific aspects have been published separately and in some cases with additional data (Germany: Jöckel *et al.*, 1998a,b; Kreuzer *et al.*, 2000, 2001, 2002; Sweden: Nyberg *et al.*, 1998).

The study of Zaridze *et al.* (1998) from Russia included 189 cases and 358 controls. Information on exposure to secondhand smoke in the family and from colleagues at work was obtained, and potential confounders (age and education) were considered.

(b)   *Exposure to secondhand smoke from the partner*

Table 2.2 shows the relative risk for lung cancer associated with exposure to second-hand smoke from the spouse. Taking the crude relative risks, or the adjusted estimates when the crude ones are not available (in any event, the crude and adjusted estimates are similar) 25 of the 40 case–control studies of nonsmoking women showed an increased risk; the results of seven of the 25 studies were statistically significant (Trichopolous *et al.*, 1983; Lam, 1985; Lam *et al.*, 1987; Geng *et al.*, 1988; Fontham *et al.*, 1994; Zaridze *et al.*, 1998; Lee *et al.*, 2000). In studies of nonsmoking men, five of the nine studies showed an increased risk, although none were statistically significant.

Exposure–response relationships

Several studies reported the risk of lung cancer associated with increasing levels of exposure, in particular, the number of cigarettes smoked by the spouse per day, the number of years of living with a smoker and pack–years; these studies are listed in Table 2.4. Because most of these studies were relatively small, they would not have had sufficient statistical power to find an exposure–response relationship. Eight studies found a statistically significant trend (p value < 0.05) between lung cancer risk and the number of cigarettes smoked by the spouse (Trichopolous *et al.*, 1983; Hirayama, 1984; Garfinkel *et al.*, 1985; Lam *et al.*, 1987; Geng *et al.*, 1988; Inoue & Hirayama, 1988; Liu *et al.*, 1993; Cardenas *et al.*, 1997) and one other found an almost statistically significant trend (Akiba *et al.*, 1986; $p = 0.06$). Six studies found a statistically significant trend (p value < 0.05) for lung cancer risk and the number of years of marriage to a smoker (Gao *et al.*,

Table 2.4. Relative risk of lung cancer in lifelong nonsmoking women comparing those with the highest exposure to secondhand smoke from a smoking partner to women with nonsmoking partners (the relative risks are ranked in ascending order for each type of exposure)

Reference	Exposure level	Relative risk[a] (95% CI)	
	No. of cigarettes smoked per day by the spouse		
Garfinkel (1981)	≥ 20	1.1	(0.8–1.6)
Kabat et al. (1995)	> 10	1.1	(0.5–2.3)
Humble et al. (1987)	≥ 21	1.2	(0.3–5.2)
Koo et al. (1987)	≥ 21	1.2	(0.5–3.0)
Boffetta et al. (1998)	> 18.1	1.3	(0.8–2.2)
Wang et al. (1996)	≥ 20	1.4	(0.8–2.6)
Zhong et al. (1999)	> 20	1.4	(0.7–2.6)
Jee et al. (1999)	≥ 20	1.5	(0.7–3.3)
Du et al. (1993)	> 20	1.6[b]	(0.8–3.2)
Kalandidi et al. (1990)	≥ 41	1.6	(0.5–4.6)
Hirayama (1984)[c,d]	≥ 20	1.7	(1.1–2.7)
Cardenas et al. (1997)	≥ 40	1.9	(1.0–3.6)
Trichopoulos et al. (1983)	≥ 31	1.9	(0.7–5.0)
Akiba et al. (1986)[d]	≥ 30	2.1	(1.7–2.6)
Garfinkel et al. (1985)	≥ 20	2.1	(1.1–4.0)
Lam et al. (1987)	≥ 21	2.1	(1.1–4.0)
Geng et al. (1988)	≥ 20	2.8	(1.9–4.1)
Liu et al. (1993)	≥ 20	2.9	(1.2–7.3)
Pershagen et al. (1987)	≥ 16[e]	3.2	(1.0–9.5)
Inoue & Hirayama (1988)	≥ 20	3.4	(1.2–9.7)
	No. of years of marriage to a smoker		
Buffler et al. (1984)	≥ 33	0.9	(0.4–2.3)
Sun et al. (1996)	≥ 35	0.9	(0.5–1.7)
Boffetta et al. (1998)	≥ 43	1.0	(0.7–1.7)
Cardenas et al. (1997)	≥ 30	1.1	(0.6–2.1)
Wang et al. (1996)	≥ 41	1.1	(0.4–3.1)
Zhong et al. (1999)	≥ 36	1.1	(0.7–1.8)
Du et al. (1993)	≥ 30	1.2	(0.6–2.3)
Fontham et al. (1994)	≥ 31	1.2	(0.9–1.7)
Akiba et al. (1986)[d]	≥ 40	1.3	(0.6–2.8)
Zaridze et al. (1998)	> 15	1.4	(1.0–2.1)
Gao et al. (1987)	≥ 40	1.7	(1.0–2.9)
Kalandidi et al. (1990)	≥ 40	1.9	(0.8–4.3)
Wu et al. (1985)	≥ 31[f]	2.0	NA[g]
Humble et al. (1987)	≥ 27	2.1	(0.7–6.9)

Table 2.4 (contd)

Reference	Exposure level	Relative risk[a] (95% CI)	
Choi *et al.* (1989)	≥ 41	2.3	(1.0–5.6)
Stockwell *et al.* (1992)	≥ 40	2.4	(1.1–5.3)
Jee *et al.* (1999)	≥ 30	3.1	(1.4–6.6)
Geng *et al.* (1988)	≥ 40	3.3	(2.1–5.2)
No. of pack–years of exposure[h]			
Rapiti *et al.* (1999)	> 128	0.4	(0.1–1.8)
Kreuzer *et al.* (2000)[i]	> 23	0.8	(0.2–3.1)
Brownson *et al.* (1992)	≥ 40	1.3	(1.0–1.7)
Boffetta *et al.* (1998)	≥ 23	1.5	(1.0–2.4)
Cardenas *et al.* (1997)	≥ 36	1.5	(0.8–2.6)
Fontham *et al.* (1994)	≥ 80	1.8	(1.0–3.3)
Lee *et al.* (2000)	> 40	3.3	(1.7–6.2)
Correa *et al.* (1983)	≥ 41	3.5	[1.2–10.2][j]

[a] Rate ratios for cohort studies (Garfinkel (1981), Hirayama (1984), Cardenas (1997) & Jee (1999)); odds ratios for case–control studies (all the other studies); adjusted relative risk, where not available crude relative risk

[b] Results are from an analysis using non-tumour controls. The paper also presents results using controls with tumours of sites other than lung (odds ratio, 1.4; 95% CI, 0.7–2.5).

[c] The results are from Table 2 of Hirayama (1984), which were adjusted by the wife's age.

[d] The report presented 90% CIs; 95% CIs were estimated for this table.

[e] For ≥ 30 years of marriage

[f] Years of exposure for adults (from partner and at workplace)

[g] Not available or estimatable from data presented in the paper

[h] Pack–years = number of packs of cigarettes smoked daily by the partner × years of smoking

[i] Some of the cases and controls reported on in Kreuzer *et al.* (2000) were part of another study included in this table (Boffetta *et al.*, 1998). The results given here for the study by Kreuzer are based on those cases and controls that were not part of the study by Boffetta (personal communication M. Kreuzer).

[j] Confidence intervals in brackets were not given in the original report and were estimated for this table using an approximate method.

1987; Geng *et al.*, 1988; Stockwell *et al.*, 1992; Fontham *et al.*, 1994; Cardenas *et al.*, 1997; Jee *et al.*, 1999) and the results of two others were almost significant (Kalandidi *et al.*, 1990; Zaridze *et al.*, 1998; *p* value = 0.07 in both).

Table 2.4 shows the increase in risk in nonsmoking women who have the highest level of exposure according to each measure. All 20 of the studies that reported on the number of cigarettes smoked showed an increased risk in the highest exposure group, and seven of the studies reported a doubling of risk or more. Similarly, of the 18 studies that looked at the number of years of marriage to a smoker, all but three showed an increased risk in the highest exposure group; six reported a relative risk of at least 2.0.

In summary, there is evidence of an exposure–response relationship, thus providing further support for a causal relationship between the development of lung cancer and exposure to secondhand smoke from partners.

(c)   Exposure to secondhand smoke at the workplace

In total, 23 studies have been published on exposure to secondhand smoke at the workplace (Table 2.5). The results from these studies are mixed with some showing a positive association and others not. Only one study reported a statistically significant association between exposure to secondhand smoke at the workplace and risk for lung cancer (Reynolds et al., 1996). Many of the studies assessed only recent workplace exposure to secondhand smoke; this is likely to result in a serious misclassification of exposure because past exposure is more likely to be etiologically relevant.

Exposure–response relationships

Two studies found no statistically significant exposure–response relationship (Kalandidi et al., 1990; Kabat et al., 1995).

In the study by Reynolds et al. (1996) in the USA, the risk for lung cancer in women who were exposed to secondhand smoke at work was significantly increased to 1.6 (95% CI, 1.2–2.0). For women who had been exposed to secondhand smoke for 1–15, 16–30 or > 30 years, the relative risk for developing lung cancer increased significantly ($p < 0.001$) with the length of the exposure period: 1.5 (95% CI, 1.1–1.9), 1.6 (95% CI, 1.1–2.2) and 2.1 (95% CI, 1.4–3.2), respectively.

In the European multicentre study (Boffetta et al. 1998), the relative risk for lung cancer after exposure to secondhand smoke at work was 1.2 (95% CI, 0.9–1.5). No exposure–response relationship was seen when the data were analysed according to duration of exposure but a significant trend was observed after analysis of weighted exposure, which is most likely a better index of exposure than duration. A significant relative risk of 2.1 (95% CI, 1.3–3.2) was observed in the group with the highest weighted exposure.

Two studies from Germany which are included in part in Boffetta et al. (1998) also showed an increased risk in the highest exposure group of 1.9 (95% CI, 1.1–3.6) and 2.5 (women only, 95% CI, 1.1–5.7) (Jöckel et al., 1998b; Kreuzer et al., 2000).

The study of Rapiti et al. (1999) reported increasing relative risks with increasing duration of exposure, but the trend did not reach statistical significance.

In the study of Zhong et al. (1999), women ever exposed to secondhand smoke at work showed an odds ratio of 1.7 (95% CI, 1.3–2.3). There was a statistically significant ($p < 0.001$) increase in risk associated with the number of hours of exposure per day at work with odds ratios of 1.0 (95% CI, 0.6–1.7), 1.6 (95% CI, 1.0–2.5) and 2.9 (95% CI, 1.8–4.7) for 1–2, 3–4 and > 4 h per day. When the number of co-workers who smoked was considered there was again a statistically significant trend ($p < 0.001$) with odds ratios of 1.0 (95% CI, 0.6–1.6), 1.7 (95% CI, 1.1–2.8) and 3.0 (95% CI, 1.8–4.9) for 1–2,

Table 2.5. The relative risk for lung cancer in nonsmokers exposed to secondhand smoke at the workplace compared with nonsmokers who were not

Reference	Sex of subjects	No. of cases of lung cancer	Relative risk for lung cancer (95% CI) if exposed at the workplace	
			Crude analysis	Adjusted analysis
Kabat et al. (1984)	Men	25	3.3 [1.0–10.6]	NR
	Women	53	0.7 [0.3–1.5]	NR
Koo et al. (1984)	Women	88	1.2 [0.5–3.0]	NR
Garfinkel et al. (1985)	Women	76	NR	0.9 (0.7–1.2)[a]
Wu et al. (1985)	Women	29	NR	1.3 (0.5–3.3)[b]
Lee et al. (1986)	Men	10	1.6 [0.4–6.6]	NR
	Women	15	0.6 [0.2–2.3]	NR
Butler (1988)	Men	6	NR	1.0 [0.2–5.4]
	Women	7	NR	0.98 [0.2–5.4]
Shimizu et al. (1988)	Women	90	1.2 [0.6–2.6][c]	NR
Kalandidi et al. (1990)	Women	89	1.4 [0.8–2.5]	NR
Wu-Williams et al. (1990)	Women	415	1.2 [1.0–1.6]	1.2 (0.9–1.6)
Kabat et al. (1995)	Men	41	NR	1.0 (0.5–2.1)
	Women	58	NR	1.2 (0.6–2.1)
Reynolds et al. (1996)	Women	528	1.4 [1.1–1.7]	1.6 (1.2–2.0)
Schwartz et al. (1996)	Men + women	257	NR	1.5 (1.0–2.2)
Sun et al. (1996)	Women	230	NR	1.4 (0.9–2.0)
Wang et al. (1996)	Women	135	0.9 (0.5–1.8)	NR
Boffetta et al. (1998)	Men + women	650	1.1 [0.9–1.3]	1.2 (0.9–1.5)
	Men	141	1.2 [0.8–1.8]	NR
	Women	509	1.3 [1.0–1.6]	1.2 (0.9–1.5)
Zaridze et al. (1998)	Women	189	1.0 [0.7–1.6]	0.9 (0.6–1.4)
Boffetta et al. (1999a)	Men + women	70	1.2 (0.7–2.1)	1.0 (0.5–1.8)
Rapiti et al. (1999)	Men + women	58	NR	1.1 (0.3–4.1)[d]
Zhong et al. (1999)	Women	504	1.4 [1.0–1.8]	1.7 (1.3–2.3)
Kreuzer et al. (2000)[e]	Men + women	123	0.7 [0.5–1.0]	1.1 (0.7–1.7)
	Men	23	0.5 [0.2–1.3]	NR
	Women	100	1.1 [0.7–1.7]	1.4 (0.8–2.2)
Lee et al. (2000)	Women	268	1.2 [0.7–1.9]	0.9 [0.5–1.7]
Wang et al. (2000)	Men + women	233	NR	1.6 (0.7–3.3)
Johnson et al. (2001)	Women	71	1.2 [0.7–2.0]	NR

NR, not reported

[a] Results shown are for exposure over the preceding 25 years

[b] Results are for adenocarcinoma. There were too few cases in this study to permit an analysis for squamous-cell carcinoma or other histological types.

[c] The 95% CI was not reported. It was estimated using the average standard error taken from Kalandidi et al. (1990) and Nyberg et al. (1998), because all three studies included similar numbers of cases of lung cancer.

[d] The reported result was 1.1 (95% CI, 0.9–1.6); the authors reported the correct estimates in Wells et al. (1998).

[e] Some of the cases and controls in the study by Kreuzer et al. (2000) were also part of another study included in this table (Boffetta et al., 1998). The results given here are based on those cases and controls that were not part of the study by Boffetta et al. [personal communication M. Kreuzer].

3–4 and > 4 co-workers who smoked, whereas there was no increase in relative risk with increasing numbers of years of exposure to secondhand smoke. Risk estimates were not affected when analyses were restricted to personal interviews excluding proxy interviews.

In summary, the studies in which exposure–response relationships were analysed generally revealed an increase in the relative risk for lung cancer associated with exposure to secondhand smoke at work and statistically significant increases in relative risk in those groups with the highest level of exposure. The associations are stronger in studies with better assessment of exposure and other aspects of study design.

(d)   Exposure during childhood

The studies on exposure to secondhand smoke during childhood are summarized in Table 2.6. The results of these studies have been somewhat contradictory. Out of 23 studies, only three studies of exposure from the mother reported a significantly increased relative risk (Brownson et al., 1992; Sun et al., 1996; Rapiti et al., 1999) and two studies reported a significant increase in relative risk related to exposure from the father or either parent (Sun et al., 1996; Rapiti et al., 1999). One study found a significant inverse association with exposure from the father or either parent (Boffetta et al., 1998).

Exposure–response relationships

The study of Wang et al. (2000) observed a significant trend ($p < 0.01$) with increasing pack–years of childhood exposure to secondhand smoke with odds ratios for men and women combined of 1.0, 1.4 (95% CI, 1.0–2.1), 1.8 (95% CI, 1.0–3.3) and 3.0 (95% CI, 1.0–8.9) for < 1, 1–9, 10–19 and ≥ 20 pack–years. In contrast, the study of Boffetta et al. (1998) suggested a negative trend for cumulative exposure, which was statitistically significant for all subjects combined ($p = 0.02$).

In summary, there is no clear indication that lung cancer risk in later life is associated with exposure to secondhand smoke in childhood. However, an important problem in interpreting these studies is the very poor quality of the assessment of exposure that occurred 50 or more years in the past.

(e)   Exposure from other sources

Few studies have addressed exposure to secondhand smoke from other sources. Kreuzer et al. (2000) reported a significantly increased relative risk of 2.6 (95% CI, 1.3–5.4) for exposure in vehicles in the highest category of weighted duration of exposure.

Other studies have either not addressed these other sources of exposure or have considered them only as part of a cumulative exposure from all sources.

In summary, insufficient data are available to evaluate the risk from exposure to secondhand smoke from other sources.

Table 2.6. The relative risk[a] for lung cancer in nonsmokers exposed to second-hand smoke during childhood compared with that in nonsmokers who were not

Reference	Sex of subjects	No. of cases of lung cancer	Relative risk (95% CI) for lung cancer according to exposure during childhood		
			Mother	Father	Either parent
Garfinkel et al. (1985)	Women	134	NR	NR	0.9 (0.7–1.1)
Wu et al. (1985)	Women	29	NR	NR	0.6 (0.2–1.7)
Koo et al. (1987)	Women	88	NR	NR	0.6 [0.2–1.8]
Pershagen et al. (1987)	Women	47	NR	NR	1.0 (0.4–2.3)
Shimizu et al. (1988)	Women	90	4.0 [1.0–15.7][b]	1.1 [0.6–2.0][b]	NR
Svensson et al. (1989)	Women	34	3.1 [0.7–14.0]	0.9 [0.4–1.9]	NR
Janerich et al. (1990)	Men + women	191	NR	NR	1.3 [0.9–2.0]
Sobue (1990)	Women	144	1.4 [0.8–2.5]	0.8 [0.5–1.2]	NR
Wu-Williams et al. (1990)	Women	417	0.9 (0.7–1.1)	1.1 (0.8–1.4)	NR
Brownson et al. (1992)	Women	431	NR	NR	0.6 [0.5–0.8]
Stockwell et al. (1992)	Women	210	1.6 (0.6–4.3)	1.2 (0.6–2.3)	NR
Fontham et al. (1994)	Women	651	0.9 (0.7–1.2)	0.9 (0.7–1.0)	NR
Kabat et al. (1995)	Men	40	NR	NR	0.9 (0.4–1.9)
	Women	69	NR	NR	1.6 (0.95–2.8)
Sun et al. (1996)	Women	230	2.1 (1.3–3.3)	2.4 (1.6–3.5)	2.3 (1.6–3.4)
Wang et al. (1996)	Women	135	NR	NR	0.9 (0.6–1.5)
Zaridze et al. (1998)	Women	189	NR	1.0 [0.7–1.4]	NR
Boffetta et al. (1998)	Men + women	641	0.9 (0.6–1.5)	0.8 (0.6–0.9)	0.8 [0.6–0.9]
	Men	140	NR	NR	0.7 [0.5–1.1]
	Women	501	NR	NR	0.7 [0.6–0.9]

Table 2.6 (contd)

Reference	Sex of subjects	No. of cases of lung cancer	Relative risk (95% CI) for lung cancer according to exposure during childhood		
			Mother	Father	Either parent
Boffetta et al. (1999a)	Men + women	67	0.3 (0.1–1.1)	0.6 (0.3–1.0)	0.5 (0.3–0.9)
Rapiti et al. (1999)	Men + women	58	5.7 [1.3–25.6]	4.5 [2.3–8.8]	3.6 [1.8–6.9]
	Men	17	–[c]	0.2 [0.0–1.7]	0.2 [0.0–1.5]
	Women	41	7.7 [1.6–37.2]	12.6 [4.9–32.7]	8.7 [3.6–21.2]
Zhong et al. (1999)	Women	504	NR	NR	1.0 [0.8–1.3]
Kreuzer et al. (2000)[d]	Men + women	123	NR	NR	1.0 [0.7–1.5]
	Men	23	NR	NR	0.97 [0.4–2.3]
	Women	100	NR	NR	0.9 [0.5–1.4]
Lee et al. (2000)[e]	Women	268	1.5 [0.6–3.9]	1.2 [0.9–1.6]	NR
Wang et al. (2000)	Men + women	228	NR	NR	1.4 [1.0–2.0]
	Men	32	NR	NR	1.7 [0.8–3.9]
	Women	196	NR	NR	1.3 [0.9–1.9]
Johnson et al. (2001)	Women	71	NR	NR	1.3 [0.8–2.2]

NR, not reported

[a] The crude results are given in the table and where these were not available, the adjusted ones are given.

[b] Only the p value was reported (p < 0.05 mother; p > 0.05 father); the standard error used to estimate the 95% CI was taken to be the same as in Nyberg et al. (1998) because both studies have a similar number of cases.

[c] There were no exposed cases and controls, and thus the odds ratio is undefined.

[d] Results from an analysis that excluded cases and controls that were included in Boffetta et al. (1998)

[e] The adjusted results are for children whose parents smoked in their presence whereas the crude results are for having a parent who was a smoker which is consistent with the definition used in the other studies.

(f)   Bias and confounding

There are two sources of bias (misclassification bias and bias resulting from exposure to secondhand smoke in the reference group) and several potential confounders (e.g. dietary confounding) that can result in the relative risk being overestimated or underestimated in the studies of the association between lung cancer and exposure to secondhand smoke described above.

(i)   *Misclassification bias*

Misclassification bias occurs when some of the subjects recorded as never-smokers who are included in the studies are in fact current or former smokers who have mis-reported their smoking status. Their true smoking status makes these subjects more likely to develop lung cancer and because smokers tend to live with smokers, this bias will over-estimate the true risk for lung cancer from exposure to secondhand smoke from the spouse. There has been much discussion in the literature on this bias, and it is the main factor proposed as partly or fully explaining the increased risk for lung cancer observed in epidemiological studies. The bias has four determinants:

- *The prevalence of smoking in a particular population.* This can be obtained directly from some of the studies or from national statistics.
- *The aggregation ratio (the extent to which a smoker is more likely to live with another smoker rather than a nonsmoker).* It is generally accepted to be between 2 and 4 (Wald et al., 1986; US Environmental Protection Agency, 1992; Lee, 1992; Hackshaw et al., 1997).
- *The relative risk for lung cancer in current and former smokers misclassified as never-smokers.* Some meta-analyses have assumed that the risk for lung cancer in misclassified smokers is the same as that in all reported smokers (US Environ-mental Protection Agency, 1992; Lee, 1992, 1998). However, misclassified current smokers tend to be light smokers and misclassified former smokers have usually given up smoking many years before the study, so the risk in both groups will be less than the average risk in all current or former smokers. The overall relative risk for lung cancer in misclassified ever smokers has been estimated to be about 3 (Hackshaw et al., 1997).
- *The percentage of current and former smokers misclassified as never-smokers.* The percentage of misclassified current smokers can be estimated by comparing self-reported smoking status with serum, urine or salivary cotinine levels; current smokers who report themselves to be never-smokers would tend to have high concentrations (for example, a urinary cotinine concentration > 50 ng/mg creati-nine). Wells et al. (1998) combined the results of 13 studies, seven of which were used in the US Environmental Protection Agency (1992) report, and concluded that the rates of misclassification of smokers are low; 1.6% of Caucasian women who were current smokers reported themselves as never-smokers. The estimate was higher, though still low, for women from a minority background (4.9%). Similar conclusions had been drawn from a review of six studies on cotinine and nicotine (two of which were included in the review by Wells et al., 1998) in which it was estimated that 3.1% of ever smokers were current smokers who reported themselves as never-smokers (Hackshaw et al., 1997). Two of the case–control studies on secondhand smoke and risk of lung cancer in female never-smokers (Table 2.2) measured urinary cotinine in the subjects and compared this with their reported smoking status. The percentage of reported never-smoking women with urinary cotinine concentrations > 50 ng/mg creatinine was 3.5% in the study by

Riboli *et al.* (1995) (included in Boffetta *et al.*, 1998 in Table 2.2) and 3.1% of patients with lung cancer and 5.0% of controls in the study by Fontham *et al.* (1994).

    (ii)   *Bias resulting from exposure to secondhand smoke in the reference group*

Studies of the risk for lung cancer and exposure to secondhand smoke have defined the reference group as never-smoking women with husbands who are nonsmokers. However, these women, although not exposed at home, may be exposed to secondhand smoke outside the home. This bias will tend to underestimate the true relative risk.

    (iii)   *Dietary confounding*

Several potential confounders have been proposed that may partly or fully explain the increased risk of lung cancer associated with exposure to secondhand smoke from the spouse. None of these potential confounders have been established as having a causal link with lung cancer. For example, dietary confounding (perhaps the main potential confounder) may arise because (i) nonsmokers who live with smokers tend to have similar diets, (ii) the diets of smokers tend to be poorer than those of nonsmokers (i.e. lower consumption of fruits and vegetables) and (iii) people who consume less fruits and vegetables may be more likely to develop lung cancer. Several of the observational studies listed in Table 2.2 had attempted to adjust for consumption of fruits and vegetables or other dietary factors (Dalager *et al.*, 1986 [used data from Correa *et al.* (1983) and Buffler *et al.* (1984) in Table 2.2]; Hirayama, 1989 [used data from Hirayama (1984)]; Kalandidi *et al.*, 1990; Alavanja *et al.*, 1993 [used data from Brownson *et al.* (1992)]; Fontham *et al.*, 1994; Mayne *et al.*, 1994 [used data from Janerich *et al.* (1990)]; Cardenas *et al.*, 1997; Boffetta *et al.*, 1998; Zhong *et al.*, 1999; Brennan *et al.*, 2000; Johnson *et al.*, 2001); they showed that the effect of dietary confounding was negligible.

2.1.3   *Meta-analyses of observational studies of exposure to secondhand smoke and lung cancer in adults*

    (a)   *Introduction*

Since the publication of the first epidemiological studies that reported directly on the association between exposure to secondhand smoke and the risk of lung cancer in nonsmokers (Garfinkel, 1981; Hirayama, 1981), there have been several other cohort studies and case–control studies. Most of these studies were based on a relatively small number of lung cancer cases and did not, therefore, have enough power to show a statistically significant association on their own. Meta-analyses have therefore been performed with the aim of pooling the available data and thus providing a more precise estimate of the risk. A meta-analysis is a formal statistical technique used to combine the estimates of relative risk across studies into a single estimate. Originally developed for clinical trials, it has also been applied to observational studies (see Peto, 1992, for a brief discussion of some aspects of meta-analyses of case–control and cohort studies on cancer). In spite of some concerns over the application of meta-analysis to studies of secondhand smoke and lung cancer, it is an appropriate approach for interpreting the published data collectively.

(b)   Published meta-analyses

This section presents the results of selected published reports.

(i)   Exposure to secondhand smoke from the spouse

Table 2.7 shows the main results of published meta-analyses on the risk for lung cancer in never-smokers associated with exposure to secondhand smoke from the spouse, including an indication of whether any adjustment was made for bias and confounding. All the pooled estimates show an increased risk (relative risks of 1.1–1.6), despite using different combinations of studies and methodology.

Some meta-analyses adjusted for the misclassification of ever-smokers as never-smokers (which will tend to overestimate risk). For example, in the analysis by Hackshaw et al. (1997) the relative risk was reduced from 1.24 to 1.18 after allowing for misclassification bias in 37 studies of nonsmoking women. In the analysis by Lee et al. (2001), which was based on 47 studies and used a different methodology, after allowing for misclassification bias the relative risk was reduced from 1.23 to 1.17. The effect is small.

Few meta-analyses have adjusted for background exposure to secondhand smoke from sources other than the spouse in the reference group (which will tend to underestimate risk). Hackshaw et al. (1997) reported that the effect of such an adjustment was to increase the observed relative risk from 1.24 to 1.42.

Few reviews have attempted to adjust for diet as a potential confounder. Hackshaw et al. (1997) used pooled data from nine studies of the risk of lung cancer associated with fruit and vegetable consumption in nonsmokers and pooled data from three studies on the difference in diet between nonsmokers who did and did not live with a smoker; the relative risk for lung cancer due to exposure to secondhand smoke from the spouse was reduced from 1.24 (as observed) to 1.21 after adjusting for fruit and vegetable consumption. A similarly small effect was reported by Lee et al. (2001), after adjusting for consumption of dietary fat and education as well as consumption of fruits and vegetables, and using different methodology and a larger set of studies (for the risk of lung cancer associated with each confounder: 17 studies on consumption of fruits and vegetables, seven on dietary fat and 12 on education; for the difference between nonsmokers who do and do not live with a smoker: nine studies on consumption of fruits and vegetables, seven on dietary fat and nine on education). The relative risk for lung cancer when the husband smoked 10 cigarettes/day was reduced from 1.10 (observed) to 1.09, after allowing for these three confounders (Lee et al., 2001). In both analyses the effect of allowing for confounding was small.

Table 2.7. Summary results of selected published meta-analyses of the risk for lung cancer in never-smokers exposed to secondhand smoke from the spouse

Reference	No. of studies	Sex of subjects	Pooled relative risk (95% CI)	Pooled estimate adjusted for			Adjusted pooled relative risk
				Misclassification bias	Exposure to secondhand smoke other than from the spouse	Dietary confounding	
National Research Council (1986)	13	Men and women	1.34 (1.18–1.53)	Yes	Yes	No	1.42
	13	Women	1.32 (1.16–1.53)	No	No	No	
Wald et al. (1986)	13	Men and women	1.35 (1.19–1.54)	Yes	Yes	No	1.53
Fleiss & Gross (1991)	9 (USA only)	Women	1.12 (0.95–1.30)	No	No	No	
Lee (1992)	28	Men and women	1.20 (1.09–1.31)	No	No	No	
	28	Women	1.18 (1.07–1.30)	No	No	No	
	11	Men	1.39 (0.97–1.99)	No	No	No	
Tweedie & Mengersen (1992)	26	Women	1.17 (1.06–1.28)	Yes	Yes	No	1.08
US Environmental Protection Agency (1992)	11 (USA only)	Women	1.19 (1.04–1.35)	Yes	Yes	No	1.59
Hackshaw (1998)	37	Women	1.24 (1.13–1.36)	Yes	Yes	Yes	1.26
	9	Men	1.34 (0.97–1.84)	No	No	No	
Zhong et al. (2000)	40	Women	1.20 (1.12–1.29)	No	No	No	
Lee et al. (2001)	47	Women	1.23 (1.12–1.36)	Yes	No	No	1.17
Boffetta et al. (2002)	45	Women	1.25 (1.14–1.38)	No	No	No	
	9	Men	1.25 (0.95–1.65)			No	

Generally, the overestimation due to misclassification bias and potential confounding seems to be balanced by the underestimation due to exposure to secondhand smoke in the reference group (Hackshaw et al., 1997).

(ii)   Exposure at the workplace

Interest in the risk of lung cancer associated with exposure to secondhand smoke at work has increased over the years and several meta-analyses have been published. These are listed in Table 2.8; some report no association, for example, Lee (1992) and Levois and Layard (1994), whereas others do report an association (Biggerstaff et al., 1994; Wells, 1998; Zhong et al., 2000). However, the results of some of the studies may be unreliable because they used levels of exposure reported by next of kin (who may not know the true exposure status of the case or control), and because some studies evaluated only recent exposure to secondhand smoke in the workplace. Wells et al. (1998) excluded studies that documented only recent exposure and also studies that (i) included more than 50% surrogate responses for cases, (ii) had only minimal exposure, (iii) included exposure to other respiratory carcinogens, (iv) included subjects who had smoked, and (v) did not report appropriate data to allow the confidence intervals to be checked. Based on these criteria, Wells et al. (1998) identified the following studies for inclusion in their meta-analysis: Wu et al. (1985), Shimizu et al. (1988), Kalandidi et al. (1990), Kabat et al. (1995) and Reynolds et al. (1996); the pooled risk estimate was 1.4 (1.2–1.7). Overall, there seems to be an increased risk of lung cancer in subjects exposed to secondhand smoke at the workplace.

Table 2.8. Summary of results from published meta-analyses of exposure to secondhand smoke and lung cancer in never-smokers exposed at the workplace

Reference	No. of studies included	Sex	Pooled relative risk (95% CI)
Lee (1992)	9	Men and women	0.98 (0.84–1.08)
Biggerstaff et al. (1994)	8	Women	1.12 (0.93–1.34)
Levois & Layard (1994)	14	Men and women	1.01 (0.92–1.11)
Chappell & Gratt (1996)	8	Men and women	0.99 (0.91–1.08)
Wells et al. (1998)	5[a]	Men and women	1.39 (1.15–1.68)
Zhong et al. (2000)	14	Men and women	1.16 (1.05–1.28)

[a] Restricted to studies that were based on self-reported exposure

(iii)   Exposure during childhood

There have been few meta-analyses on the risk of lung cancer in adulthood following exposure to secondhand smoke during childhood; the results of three of these meta-analyses are given in Table 2.9. None suggested an association, although no stratification

Table 2.9. Results from published meta-analyses of exposure to second-hand smoke and lung cancer in adult never-smokers exposed during childhood

Reference	No. of studies included	Sex	Pooled relative risk (95% CI)
Lee *et al.* (1992)	10	Men and women	0.98 (0.86–1.12)
Boffetta *et al.* (2000)	11	Men and women	
		Men and women	0.91 (0.80–1.05)
		From father	0.83 (0.72–0.95)
		From mother	0.99 (0.78–1.26)
Zhong *et al.* (2000)	18	Men and women	0.91 (0.83–1.00)

according to gender or exposure from the mother or father was carried out. Overall, published meta-analyses have found no evidence for an increased risk for lung cancer associated with childhood exposure to secondhand smoke.

(iv)   *Statistical methods and other considerations*

Pooling relative risks

Different methods of combining relative risk estimates from individual studies have generally tended to give similar results. For example, in 37 studies of the risk for lung cancer of never-smoking women exposed or unexposed to secondhand smoke from the spouse, the relative risks (95% CI) using the fixed or random effects model were 1.21 (1.12–1.30) and 1.24 (1.13–1.36), respectively (Hackshaw *et al.*, 1997) (the random effects model allows for heterogeneity between the risk estimates).

More complex approaches, such as Bayesian analysis, also do not yield materially different results. The difference between the pooled estimates obtained using a Bayesian model and those obtained using a simpler random effects model was small. Tweedie *et al.* (1996) pooled 40 studies of male or female never-smokers exposed to secondhand smoke from the spouse, the pooled relative risk for lung cancer was 1.20 (95% CI, 1.07–1.34) using the random effects model and 1.22 (95% CI, 1.08–1.37) using a Bayesian model (Tweedie *et al.*, 1996).

Pooling results relating to exposure–response relationships

Several studies on the effects of exposure to secondhand smoke in never-smokers have reported the relative risk for lung cancer according to the number of cigarettes smoked by the spouse or the number of years that the nonsmoker has lived with a spouse who smokes. A few researchers, using various combinations of studies and methodology, have attempted to pool the results of epidemiological studies of exposure–response in never-smoking women. For an increase of 10 cigarettes per day smoked by the husband, the excess relative risk for lung cancer compared with never-smoking husbands was estimated to be 23% (95% CI, 14–32) by Hackshaw et al. (1997), 17% (95% CI, 12–22) by Brown (1999) and 10% (95% CI, 5–15) by Lee et al. (2000). The excess relative risk that resulted from living for 10 years with a husband who smokes compared with one who does not was estimated to be 11% (95% CI, 4–17) by Hackshaw et al. (1997) and 7% (95% CI, 4–11) by Lee et al. (2000). The estimates are reasonably consistent between different reports and all found a statistically significant increase in risk associated with increasing exposure.

Heterogeneity between the estimates of relative risk

Performing a meta-analysis when there are statistically significant differences between the estimates of relative risk may yield an incorrect pooled estimate. If heterogeneity exists, an attempt should be made to explain it. If it can be explained by a single factor (or factors), then estimates should be stratified according to that factor. The authors of several reviews of the association between exposure to secondhand smoke and lung cancer have allowed for the existence of heterogeneity between geographical regions or found evidence of it and therefore stratified the relative risk estimates according to region (for example, US Environmental Protection Agency, 1992; Lee, 1998). Lee (1998) assessed heterogeneity related to several factors including geographical region, study publication date, study type and study size and concluded that there were statistically significant differences between the relative risk estimates by almost all factors. However, this was shown to be due to a single large discrepant study that unduly influenced the assessment of heterogeneity; this may be a problem especially when there are relatively few studies in the meta-analysis. In the meta-analysis by Hackshaw et al. (1997), the test for heterogeneity based on 37 studies on nonsmoking women was almost significant ($p = 0.10$), although when one study was excluded the p value became 0.46. The discrepant study, from China, was large (417 cases of lung cancer) and reported an almost statistically significant *reduction* in the risk of lung cancer associated with exposure to secondhand smoke from the spouse (relative risk, 0.8; 95% CI, 0.6–1.0), making its results inconsistent with those of the other studies. When this study was excluded, no evidence of heterogeneity was found for several factors (Hackshaw et al., 1997; Hackshaw, 1998; Zhong et al., 2000).

Publication bias

In meta-analyses of studies of the relationship between secondhand smoke and lung cancer there is a possibility of publication bias if studies with positive results (those that show an increased risk of lung cancer) are more likely to be published than studies with negative ones (those that show a decreased risk or no difference in risk). The pooled estimate of risk would then be biased upwards. Simple methods to ascertain whether much publication bias exists suggest that there is little evidence of this, for example funnel plots (Lubin, 1999) or estimating the number of negative unpublished studies that would be required to explain the increased risk observed from epidemiological studies — about 300 (Hackshaw et al., 1997; Lee, 1998); it is implausible that there would be so many unpublished negative studies. Copas and Shi (2000) used a complex method to adjust the observed relative risk for lung cancer (reported in Hackshaw *et al.*, 1997) for publication bias; the pooled estimate was reduced from 1.24 to 1.15, but Copas and Shi assumed that 40% of all studies are unpublished. Even with such an extreme assumption, the adjusted estimate is consistent with the reported relative risk adjusted for bias and confounding (1.26; 95% CI, 1.06–1.47). The problem with assessing publication bias is that it is difficult to determine empirically how many studies are unpublished (Bero *et al.*, 1994).

(c) Updated meta-analyses

Several individual studies on secondhand smoke and the risk of lung cancer in non-smokers have been published since one of the last detailed meta-analyses on the subject (Hackshaw *et al.*, 1997). This section presents updated meta-analyses using currently available results. The selection of studies to be included is as described by Hackshaw *et al.* (1997), and the method of pooling the relative risk estimates is that described by Dersimonian and Laird (1986), which allows for any heterogeneity between the estimates. Some case–control studies reported only crude estimates of relative risk, some reported only adjusted estimates (adjusted for various factors such as age and diet) and others reported both crude and adjusted estimates. Consideration therefore needed to be given to which should be used in the meta-analyses. Pooled estimates were obtained based on the crude relative risks and, where these were not available, the adjusted relative risks. This reduces the effect of those studies that adjusted for factors that are not established confounders. The pooled estimate was also obtained based on the adjusted relative risks, and where these were not available, the crude relative risks to show that the two approaches yielded similar results.

Table 2.10 shows the results of the updated meta-analyses according to type of exposure to secondhand smoke and gender of the subject (for the estimates from the individual studies, see Tables 2.2, 2.5 and 2.6).

(i) Exposure from the spouse

Among nonsmoking women who lived with a spouse who smoked, the risk of lung cancer was increased by 24% (relative risk, 1.24; 95% CI, 1.14–1.3; Table 2.10). This estimate was based on the crude estimates of relative risk found in the studies and, where these were not available, the adjusted estimates. Use of the adjusted estimates and, where these were not available, the crude estimates yielded a similar relative risk of 1.27 (95% CI, 1.15–1.41). The studies came from several countries, and the test for heterogeneity between the relative risk estimates across all 46 studies just misses statistical significance (*p* value = 0.08). However, if the discrepant study from China by Wu-Williams *et al.* (1990) that reported an almost statistically significant decrease in risk due to exposure to secondhand smoke is excluded, the pooled relative risk is not materially changed (1.25; 95% CI, 1.17–1.33), but the test for heterogeneity yields a *p* value of 0.34. Among nonsmoking men who lived with a smoker, the risk of lung cancer was increased by 37%. The risk estimates for both nonsmoking men and women are statistically significant.

Table 2.10. Summary of the updated meta-analyses of the relative risk for lung cancer in never-smokers exposed to specified sources of secondhand smoke

Source of exposure	No. of studies (total no. of lung cancer cases)	Sex of subject	Pooled relative risk (95% CI)[a]	p value	Evidence of significant heterogeneity between the studies
Spouse	46 (6257)	Women	1.24 (1.14–1.34)	< 0.001	No, $p = 0.08$[b]
	11 (442)	Men	1.37 (1.02–1.83)	0.03	No, $p = 0.80$
Workplace	19 (3588)	Women	1.19 (1.09–1.30)	< 0.001	No, $p = 0.87$
	6 (246)	Men	1.12 (0.80–1.56)	0.51	No, $p = 0.38$
	7 (1582)	Women and men combined	1.03 (0.86–1.23)	0.74	No, $p = 0.10$
Childhood					
Mother	9 (2085)	Women	1.50 (1.04–2.14)	0.03	Yes, $p = 0.004$
Father	10 (2274)	Women	1.25 (0.94–1.68)	0.13	Yes, $p < 0.001$
Either parent	14 (2576)	Women	1.11 (0.87–1.42)	0.41	Yes, $p < 0.001$
Either parent	5 (252)	Men	0.86 (0.62–1.20)	0.38	No, $p = 0.35$
Either parent	6 (1306)	Women and men combined	1.14 (0.77–1.70)	0.51	Yes, $p < 0.001$

[a] Based on the crude relative risks from the individual reports and where these were not available, the adjusted estimates

[b] When the study by Wu-Williams et al. (1990) from China is excluded (it reported an almost statistically significant decrease in risk for lung cancer associated with exposure to secondhand smoke), the pooled relative risk is similar 1.25 (1.17–1.33), but the test for heterogeneity yields a p value of 0.34.

(ii)   *Exposure at the workplace*

The increase in risk for lung cancer in nonsmoking women is about 20% (relative risk, 1.19; 95% CI, 1.09–1.30; Table 2.10). If the pooled estimate was based on the adjusted relative risks reported in the studies and, where these were not available, the crude estimates, the result was similar (relative risk, 1.21; 95% CI, 1.09–1.35). There was also an increase in risk in men (12%) though this result was not statistically significant (probably because of the smaller number of studies and fewer cases of lung cancer in the meta-analysis). There was no evidence of heterogeneity between the individual risk estimates.

(iii)   *Exposure during childhood*

There is a statistically significant increase in risk among women exposed to second-hand smoke from the mother during childhood (50% increase in risk, but the confidence interval is wide, 4–114%). There is a lower, and non-significant increase in risk for exposure to secondhand smoke from the father (25%). However, there is significant heterogeneity between the estimates of relative risk. The results on exposure during childhood are less clear than those on exposure from the spouse or at the workplace.

Overall, the evidence from the meta-analyses is clear; adult nonsmokers exposed to secondhand smoke have a higher risk for lung cancer. Although the precise quantitative estimate of risk may vary between different measures of exposure, it is consistently raised. The data on exposure to secondhand smoke from the spouse also show that risk increases with increasing exposure. The evidence for an association between lung cancer and childhood exposure to secondhand smoke is less consistent than that for exposure in adulthood.

2.2   Breast cancer

Five prospective cohort studies (Hirayama, 1984; Jee *et al.*, 1999; Wartenberg *et al.*, 2000; Nishino *et al.*, 2001; Egan *et al.*, 2002) and 12 reports of 10 case–control studies (Sandler *et al.*, 1985a,b; Smith *et al.*, 1994; Morabia *et al.*, 1996; Millikan *et al.*, 1998; Lash & Aschengrau, 1999; Delfino *et al.*, 2000; Johnson *et al.*, 2000; Marcus *et al.*, 2000; Morabia *et al.*, 2000; Chang-Claude *et al.*, 2002; Kropp & Chang-Claude, 2002) have examined the role of secondhand smoke in breast cancer. The cohort studies are summarized in Table 2.11 and the reports from the case–control studies are summarized in Table 2.12.

2.2.1   *Cohort studies*

The first cohort study that suggested a possible association of exposure to secondhand smoke with breast cancer was reported by Hirayama in 1984. Specific details of how risk estimates for breast cancer were calculated were provided by Wells (1991). A total of 115 deaths from breast cancer were identified after 15 years of follow-up (1966–81) of over

Table 2.11. Cohort studies of breast cancer and involuntary exposure to tobacco smoke

Reference	Country	Sample	Source of information on exposure	Duration and completeness of follow-up	Relative risk (95% CI)
Hirayama (1984)	Japan	115 breast cancer deaths among 91 540 nonsmoking married women	In-person interview (baseline)	15 years of follow-up. Completeness not reported	*Husband ever smoked* 1.26 (0.8–2.0)
Jee et al. (1999)	Republic of Korea	138 breast cancer cases among 157 436 non-smoking married women	Self-administered questionnaire: husband's active smoking in 1992 and 1994; wife's involuntary smoking in 1993	3.5 years of follow-up of breast cancer cases. Completeness not reported	*Husband's smoking status* Former smoker 1.2 (0.8–1.8) Current smoker 1.3 (0.9–1.8) Current smoker for 1.7 (1.0–2.8) > 30 years
Wartenberg et al. (2000)	USA	669 breast cancer deaths among 146 488 never-smoking single-marriage women	Postal questionnaire to both husband and wife	12 years of follow-up. 98% completeness	*Husband's smoking status* Former smoker 1.0 (0.8–1.2) Current smoker (baseline) 1.0 (0.8–1.2) *Years husband smoked* 1–10 0.9 (0.6–1.3) 11–20 0.7 (0.5–1.0) 21–30 1.0 (0.7–1.3) ≥31 1.1 (0.8–1.3) *p* trend = 0.9

Table 2.11 (contd)

Reference	Country	Sample	Source of information on exposure	Duration and completeness of follow-up	Relative risk (95% CI)
Nishino et al. (2001)	Japan	67 incident cases of breast cancer among 9675 never-smoking women aged ≥ 40	Self-administered questionnaires	9 years of follow-up. Completeness not reported	*Husband smoked* 0.6 (0.3–1.1) *Other household member smoked* 0.8 (0.4–1.5)
Egan et al. (2002)	USA	1359 breast cancer cases among 35 193 never-smoking women	Postal questionnaire	14 years of follow-up of invasive breast cancer. 96% completeness	*Parental smoking* Mother only 1.0 (0.7–1.4) Father only 1.1 (1.0–1.3) Both parents 0.9 (0.8–1.1) *Current exposure to secondhand smoke* Occasional 1.2 (1.0–1.4) Regular at home or at work 1.0 (0.8–1.2) Regular at home and at work 0.9 (0.7–1.2)

Table 2.12. Case–control studies of breast cancer and involuntary exposure to tobacco smoke

Reference	Country	Sample	Source of information on exposure	Duration and completeness of follow-up	Relative risk (95% CI)	
Sandler et al. (1985a)	USA	29 nonsmoking incident cases; 223 nonsmoking controls	Postal questionnaire	22 months; cases diagnosed in women aged 15–59 years. 70% case response rate; 57% control response rate	Maternal smoking	0.9
					Paternal smoking	0.9
Sandler et al. (1985b)	USA	32 nonsmoking incident cases; 247 nonsmoking controls	Postal questionnaire	22 months; cases diagnosed in women aged 15–59 years. 70% case response rate; 75% response rate for telephone controls; 60% response rate for friend controls	Husband's smoking	2.0 (0.9–4.3)
Smith et al. (1994)	United Kingdom	94 nonsmoking incident cases; 99 nonsmoking controls	In-person interview with postal questionnaire on exposure to secondhand smoke	3 years; cases diagnosed in women aged < 36 years. 72% case response rate; 89% control response rate. Data on exposure to secondhand smoke available on 65% of matched pairs	*Childhood exposure in cigarette–years*	
					1–200	1.2 (0.5–2.9)
					> 200	1.1 (0.5–2.7)
					Adult exposure	
					From partner in cigarette–years	
					≥ 1	1.6 (0.8–3.1)
					From other household smokers (years)	
					1–5	1.5 (0.7–3.2)
					≥ 6	1.1 (0.5–2.8)
					At work (years)	
					1–5	1.7 (0.7–3.8)
					≥ 6	1.4 (0.6–3.1)
					Period of exposure	
					Child only	1.3 (0.2–10.8)
					Adult only	3.1 (0.7–13.3)
					Both	2.6 (0.7–9.4)

Table 2.12 (contd)

Reference	Country	Sample	Source of information on exposure	Duration and completeness of follow-up	Relative risk (95% CI)
Morabia *et al.* (1996)	Switzerland	126 never-smoking incident cases; 620 never-smoking controls	In-person interview	22 months for cases diagnosed in women < 75 years of age. 71% case response rate; 70% control response rate	Ever exposed to second-hand smoke *(Hours/day) × year* 1–50 3.1 (1.5–6.2) > 50 3.2 (1.6–6.3) Ever exposed to second-hand smoke from spouse *From spouse (hours/day) × year* 1–50 3.1 (1.3–7.5) > 50 3.2 (1.5–6.5)
Millikan *et al.* (1998)	USA	248 never-smoking incident cases; 253 never-smoking controls	In-person interview plus 30-mL blood sample	3.5 years for cases diagnosed in women 20–74 years of age. 77% case response rate; 68% control response rate; 98% of study subjects provided blood samples	*Exposed to secondhand smoke after age 18 years* All-nonsmokers 1.3 (0.9–1.9) Premenopausal 1.5 (0.8–2.8) NAT1*10 1.7 (0.7–4.3) NAT1non*10 1.3 (0.5–3.2) NAT2rapid 2.3 (0.9–6.2) NAT2slow 1.2 (0.5–2.8) Postmenopausal 1.2 (0.7–2.2) NAT1*10 1.2 (0.6–2.6) NAT1non*10 1.3 (0.5–3.6) NAT2rapid 0.8 (0.4–1.8) NATslow 1.9 (0.7–5.2)

The relative-risk value for "Ever exposed to second-hand smoke" (Morabia *et al.*) is 3.2 (1.7–5.9).

Table 2.12 (contd)

Reference	Country	Sample	Source of information on exposure	Duration and completeness of follow-up	Relative risk (95% CI)	
Lash & Aschengrau (1999)	USA	120 never-smoking cases, 406 never-smoking controls	Proxy interview; 33% of cases and 45% of controls	3 years for cases diagnosed in women. 79% case response rate; 75% control response rate	Passive smoking	2.0 (1.1–3.7)
					By years of exposure to secondhand smoke	
					≤ 20	3.2 (1.5–7.1)
					> 20	2.1 (1.0–4.1)
Delfino et al. (2000)	USA	64 never-smoking cases; 149 never-smoking controls (benign breast disease)	Self-administered questionnaire	Cases diagnosed in women 40 years of age and above (duration not reported). 82% case response rate; 85% control response rate	Any exposure to second-hand smoke	1.3 (0.7–2.5)
					High versus low exposure to secondhand smoke	1.5 (0.8–2.9)
					Premenopausal cases	2.7 (0.9–8.0)
					Postmenopausal cases	1.0 (0.5–2.3)
Johnson et al. (2000)	Canada	378 premenopausal and 700 postmenopausal never-smoking cases; 369 pre- and 845 postmenopausal never-smoking controls	Postal questionnaire	≥ 3 years for cases diagnosed in women 20–74 years of age. 72% case response rate; 64% control response rate	*Premenopausal*	
					Any exposure to second-hand smoke	2.3 (1.2–4.6)
					Childhood exposure only	1.6 (0.6–4.4)
					Adult exposure only	2.6 (1.1–6.0)
					Exposure during childhood and adulthood	2.6 (1.2–5.5)
					Postmenopausal	
					Any exposure to second-hand smoke	1.2 (0.8–1.8)
					Childhood exposure only	0.9 (0.4–2.0)
					Adult exposure only	1.1 (0.6–1.8)
					Exposure during childhood and adulthood	1.3 (0.8–2.0)

Table 2.12 (contd)

Reference	Country	Sample	Source of information on exposure	Duration and completeness of follow-up	Relative risk (95% CI)
Marcus et al. (2000)	USA	445 never-smoking cases; 423 never-smoking controls	In-person interview	3.5 years for cases diagnosed in women 20–74 years of age. 77% case response rate; 68% control response rate	Never-smokers exposed to secondhand smoke before age 18 years 0.8 (0.6–1.1)
Morabia et al. (2000)	Switzerland	84 never-smoking cases; 99 never-smoking controls	In-person interview and buccal swab	1 year for incident cases diagnosed in women <75 years of age. 71% case response rate; 70% control response rate in original study; 83% response rate in substudy	Any exposure to secondhand smoke 3.1 (1.5–6.0) *NAT2 acetylation genotype* Slow 1.9 (0.7–4.6) Fast 5.9 (2.0–17.4)
Chang-Claude et al. (2002)	Germany	174 never-smoking cases; 365 never-smoking controls	Self-administered questionnaire and for passive smoking questions by telephone interview	4 years for cases; passive smoking response rates: ~46% of total eligible and 48% of eligible controls	*Ever exposed by NAT2 acetylator status* Rapid 2.0 (1.0–4.1) Slow 1.2 (0.7–2.0)
Kropp & Chang-Claude (2002)	Germany	197 never-smoking cases; 459 never-smoking controls	Self-administered questionnaire and for passive smoking questions by telephone interview	4 years for cases; passive smoking response rates: ~46% of total eligible and 48% of eligible controls	*Exposure to secondhand smoke* As a child only 1.1 (0.6–2.3) As an adult only 1.9 (1.2–3.0) Both 1.6 (1.0–2.6) *Lifetime in (hours/day) ×years* 1–50 1.4 (0.9–2.3) ≥ 51 1.8 (1.2–2.9) $p = 0.009$

91 000 married nonsmoking Japanese women. Women whose husbands had ever smoked had a small non-significantly increased risk of breast cancer (relative risk, 1.26; 95% CI, 0.8–2.0). [The Working Group noted this was a first prospective report with a number of limitations. For example, it reported mortality rather than incidence; there was limited assessment of risk specific to breast cancer (spouse only); there was no adjustment for potential confounders; exposure was assessed at only one time-point.]

In a study in the Republic of Korea, Jee et al. (1999) also found small non-significantly increased risks of breast cancer associated with husbands' smoking status: for former smokers the relative risk was 1.2 (95% CI, 0.8–1.8) and for current smokers the relative risk was 1.3 (95% CI, 0.9–1.8). Relative risks were adjusted for age of husbands and wives, socioeconomic status, residence, vegetable consumption and occupation of the husband. These findings were based on 138 incident and prevalent breast cancer cases in 3.5 years of follow-up (July 1994–December 1997) of a cohort of 157 436 nonsmoking Korean women. A higher risk, of borderline significance, was observed for women married to current smokers who had smoked for more than 30 years (relative risk, 1.7; 95% CI, 1.0–2.8). [The Working Group noted that this study had several limitations, i.e. prevalent cases were not excluded; limited adjustment was made for potential confounders, and the adjustment did not include reproductive or hormonal factors; assessment of exposure included only secondhand smoke from the spouse.]

Wartenberg et al. (2000) reported findings from the large American Cancer Society Cancer Prevention Study II cohort based on 12 years of follow-up (1982–94) of never-smoking women who had been married once. A total of 669 deaths from breast cancer were included and risk estimates were adjusted for year of age at baseline, race, number of years of education, history of breast cancer in mother or sister, personal history of breast cysts, age at first live birth, age at menopause, number of spontaneous abortions, use of oral contraceptives, use of estrogen replacement therapy, body mass index, alcohol intake, fat consumption, vegetable consumption, occupation and occupation of spouse. No increased risks were found for women married to current smokers (relative risk, 1.0; 95% CI, 0.8–1.2) or former smokers (relative risk, 1.0; 95% CI, 0.8–1.2) when compared with never-smokers married to nonsmoking husbands. No association was found by type of tobacco. No trend in risk was observed by years, packs per day or pack–years of spousal smoking. No significant associations were noted between breast cancer and all exposures at home (relative risk, 1.1; 95% CI, 0.9–1.3), at work (relative risk, 0.8; 95% CI; 0.6–1.0), or in other places (relative risk, 0.9; 95% CI, 0.7–1.2). When reported exposures from all sources were combined and examined according to daily hours of exposure using no exposure from any source as referent (0 hour), no trend was observed. [The Working Group considered that the strengths of this study included the large number of cases, the excellent follow-up, the thorough statistical adjustment for potential confounders and that the spouse directly reported his own tobacco use. The limitations include the use of mortality rather than incidence as the outcome and that the assessment of spousal smoking was made at only one time-point.]

A smaller cohort study that included 9675 Japanese female never-smokers over the age of 40 years accrued 67 incident cases over a 9-year follow-up period (1984–92) (Nishino *et al.*, 2001). Relative risks were adjusted for age, study area, alcohol consumption, intake of green and yellow vegetables, intake of fruit, age at first birth, number of live births, age at menarche and body mass index. The age-adjusted relative risk for breast cancer was 0.6 (95% CI, 0.3–1.0) among women whose husbands smoked when compared to that in women married to nonsmokers. The age-adjusted risk associated with living in a household with other smokers was also below unity (relative risk, 0.4; 95% CI, 0.2–0.8) when compared with women living in households where there were no smokers. Further adjustment of these relative risks for the potential confounders listed above did not appreciably change the risk estimates, but the relative risks were no longer statistically significant after full adjustment: exposure from spouse, 0.6 (95% CI, 0.3–1.1), and other household members, 0.8 (95% CI, 0.4–1.5). [The Working Group considered that the strengths of this study include adjustment for some reproductive or hormonal and dietary factors; its limitations include the very small sample size, lack of information on marital status at baseline and inclusion of unmarried women at high risk of breast cancer as unexposed which may have reduced point estimates of relative risk.]

The Nurses' Health Study in the USA has provided the largest number of prospectively accrued breast cancer cases in never-smoking women (Egan *et al.*, 2002). After 14 years of follow-up (1982–96), 1359 cases of invasive breast cancer were diagnosed among 35 193 never-smokers. Exposure to secondhand smoke was assessed as exposure during childhood as well as during adult life at home, at work and in other settings. Relative risks were adjusted for many variables including age, parity, age at first birth, menopausal status, age at menopause, change in weight (i.e. weight at age 18 years compared to the most recent reported weight), age at menarche, history of benign breast disease, family history of breast cancer, post-menopausal hormone treatment, alcohol intake and carotenoid intake. No statistically significant associations were found for exposure between breast cancer and exposure to secondhand smoke in adult life or in childhood, and most relative risks were near unity. No trends were apparent either for number of years lived with a smoker as an adult (*p* for trend = 0.87) or for a categorized index of adult exposures (*p* for trend = 0.97). Women who reported the highest levels of exposure to secondhand smoke during adulthood had a rate of breast cancer similar to that of women who reported no current exposure to secondhand smoke (relative risk, 1.0; 95% CI, 0.8–1.3). The findings were similar for pre- and postmenopausal women. [The Working Group noted that this study's main strength is that it is the largest and most methodologically rigorous prospective study to date. Other strengths were that exposure assessments were updated over time, incident cases rather than mortality were studied and comprehensive adjustment was made for potential confounders.]

2.2.2   *Case–control studies*

The first two reports (Sandler *et al.*, 1985a,b) on involuntary smoking and breast cancer were based on a case–control study conducted in North Carolina, USA. Cases were selected from a single hospital tumour registry and included patients diagnosed between 1 July 1979 and 31 March 1981, who were between the ages of 15 and 59 years at the time of diagnosis. Approximately 60% of the controls were friends or acquaintances identified by cases and the remaining 40% were selected by systematic telephone sampling. The two control groups were combined after separate analyses of the two groups indicated similar results. The risk for breast cancer in nonsmoking women was not associated with exposure to secondhand smoke during childhood from either mother (relative risk, 0.9) or father (relative risk, 0.9) (Sandler *et al.*, 1985a). Exposure to secondhand smoke in non-smoking women based on husband's smoking was associated with a two-fold, non-significant increase in risk (relative risk, 2.0; 95% CI, 0.9–4.3) (Sandler *et al.*, 1985b). Risk estimates of childhood exposure were adjusted for age and education, and risk esti-mates of exposure during adulthood were adjusted for age, race and education. Both reports included only a few lifetime nonsmokers with breast cancer (29 and 32 cases, respectively). [The Working Group noted that the limitations of this study include small sample size, lack of adjustment for reproductive factors and the potentially inappropriate control group (i.e. friends and neighbours of cases supplemented with controls selected by random digit dialling.]

Smith *et al.* (1994) investigated the relationship between exposure to secondhand smoke and risk for breast cancer in a sample of nonsmokers including 94 incident cases and 99 controls drawn from a larger study of breast cancer diagnosed in young women below the age of 36 years between 1982 and 1985. This study was conducted in the United Kingdom and information on exposure to secondhand smoke was collected by postal questionnaire in a sample of participants from the main study. Controls were selected randomly from the list of the case's general practitioner and matched to the case on age. Risk estimates were adjusted for age, residence, age at menarche, family history of breast cancer, history of biopsy for benign breast disease, oral contraceptive use and history of breastfeeding. Although most of the risk estimates exceeded unity as shown in Table 2.12, none were statistically significant and there was no evidence of a positive trend in risk associated with increasing exposure. When total lifetime exposure as measured in ciga-rette–years was considered, elevations in risk were found for all levels above zero (referent). However, the trend was not statistically significant. No effect of active smoking was found in this study. [The Working Group considered this study to have limited gene-ralizability (cases < 36 years of age) and noted that no exposure–response relationship was observed despite comparatively high point estimates of risk.]

A population-based case–control study conducted in Switzerland by Morabia *et al.* (1996) was designed specifically to evaluate the role of exposure to secondhand smoke in risk of breast cancer. It included 126 cases and 620 controls who were lifetime never-smokers. Never-smokers were defined as having smoked fewer than 100 cigarettes in a lifetime. Eligible cases were women less than 75 years of age who had been diagnosed with invasive breast cancer between 1 January 1992 and 31 October 1993. Population controls were selected from the official registers of residents of Geneva and were 30–74 years of age. This study included a detailed assessment of exposure to secondhand smoke and risk estimates were adjusted for the following potential confounders: age, education, body mass index, age at menarche, age at first live birth, oral contraceptive use, breast cancer in mother or sister, history of breast biopsy, alcohol intake and saturated fat intake. The referent unexposed group in this study included women who were never regularly exposed (< 1 (h/day) $\times$ years) to either active or passive smoking (28/244 cases and 241/1032 controls). Estimates of relative risk associated with any exposure to secondhand smoke, duration of exposure to secondhand smoke, exposure to spousal secondhand smoke only and duration of spousal smoking were all approximately three and were statistically significant; however, risk estimates stratified by duration (1–50 or > 50 (h/day) $\times$ years) were virtually identical and there was no suggestion of an exposure–response relationship. [The Working Group considered that the strengths of the study were its comprehensive assessment of exposure, being population-based and the large number of potential confounders included in the analysis. Concerns included the following: magnitude of the association between cancer and passive smoking is the same as that for active smoking in same study, no exposure–response relationship was found for secondhand smoke and the very restrictive reference category used may have biased the results.]

Morabia *et al.* (2000) next conducted a sub-study from the above-mentioned case–control study. It was designed to evaluate the role of *N*-acetyltransferase 2 (NAT2) in the relationship between breast cancer and active and passive smoking. Cases believed to be alive and living in Geneva in 1996–97 were re-contacted, as were a subset of controls, and asked to provide a buccal swab for DNA extraction and NAT2 genotyping for subsequent classification as slow or fast acetylators. This sub-study included 84 cases who were never-smokers and 99 controls who were never-smokers. As in the parent study, a three-fold increase in risk of breast cancer was associated with any reported exposure to secondhand smoke (relative risk, 3.1; 95% CI, 1.5–6.0). The association between exposure to secondhand smoke and breast cancer appeared to be modified by acetylation status; breast cancer risk was higher in persons with the fast acetylation genotype (relative risk, 5.9; 95% CI, 2.0–17.4) than in slow acetylators (relative risk, 1.9; 95% CI, 0.7–4.6). [The Working Group's comments on the parent study also applied to this sub-study.]

Millikan *et al.* (1998) conducted a population-based case–control study in North Carolina, USA, that also examined the effect of *N*-acetylation genotypes (NAT1 and NAT2), exposure to secondhand smoke and breast cancer risk. Cases included women between 20 and 74 years of age who were diagnosed with invasive primary breast cancer between May 1993 and December 1996. Controls less than 65 years of age were selected from files of the North Carolina Division of Motor Vehicles and those from 65 to 74 years of age from the United States Health Care Financing Administration (HCFA) files. All African–American cases and a sample of white cases were selected. This report was based on cases and controls who provided a blood sample. Cases and controls were broadly frequency-matched on race (African–American and white) and age (age less than 50 years and 50 years and above). Relative risk estimates were adjusted for age, race, age at menarche, age at first full-term pregnancy, parity, family history of breast cancer, breast biopsies showing benign tumours and alcohol consumption. Statistically non-significant increases in risk were associated with exposure to secondhand smoke after the age of 18 years in never-smokers (relative risk, 1.3; 95% CI, 0.9–1.9). The point estimates for premenopausal (relative risk, 1.5; 95% CI, 0.8–2.8) and postmenopausal women (relative risk, 1.2; 95% CI, 0.7–2.2) were not substantially different. Stratification by menopausal status and NAT1 and NAT2 genotypes resulted in statistically non-significant relative risks for all subgroups. The point estimates for exposure to secondhand smoke after the age of 18 years were highest for pre-menopausal never-smoking women for NAT1*10 (relative risk, 1.7; 95% CI, 0.7–4.3) and NAT2rapid (relative risk, 2.3; 95% CI, 0.9–6.2).

Marcus et al. (2000) included additional cases from this North Carolina study without the requirement for a blood sample and addressed the issue of exposure to secondhand smoke before the age of 18 years. Exposure to secondhand smoke at home during childhood showed no statistically significant association with risk of breast cancer in this study (relative risk, 0.8; 95% CI, 0.6–1.1). [The Working Group considered that the strengths of this study included the large number of never-smoking cases and controls; the multiethnic study population (although no ethnicity-specific risk estimates for exposure to secondhand smoke were reported and that the study investigated possible high-risk subgroups.]

Lash and Aschengrau (1999) reported the findings of a case–control study conducted in five towns in Massachusetts, USA. The incident cases of breast cancer were diagnosed from 1983–1986. Population controls from these towns for living cases under 65 years of age were selected using random-digit dialling and for women 65 years and older from the US Health Care Financing Administration (HCFA) files. Because deceased cases were also eligible for this study, deceased controls were selected from Massachusetts Department of Vital Statistics and Research. A total of 120 cases and 406 controls were never-smokers. About one-third of the interviews relating to cases and 45% of the interviews relating to controls were with proxy respondents. Age, parity, history of breast cancer other than index diagnosis, family history of breast cancer, history of benign breast disease, and history of radiation therapy were adjusted for in the analyses. A twofold increase in risk (relative risk, 2.0; 95% CI, 1.1–3.7) was associated with any exposure to secondhand smoke; however, increasing duration was not associated with increasing risk. The relative risk estimates for exposure to secondhand smoke and for active smoking also determined in this study were similar. [The Working Group noted that the limitations of the study were that the original study was not designed to evaluate exposure to secondhand smoke; it was unclear whether controls from the parent study which included three types of cancer cases were matched to breast cancer cases in this substudy, and that this substudy included a large number of proxy respondents.]

Findings from a small clinic-based case–control study, conducted in Orange County, California, USA, were reported by Delfino et al. (2000). Three breast cancer centres were included in the study. Subjects diagnosed with a suspicious breast mass detected either clinically or radiographically who were over the age of 39 years were considered to be eligible. Information on exposure was obtained from a self-administered questionnaire completed prior to biopsy in order to minimize recall bias and interviewer bias. Among women who were never-smokers, 64 were subsequently found to have malignant tumours and comprised the case series, and 149 never-smokers with benign breast disease were classified as controls. Risk estimates for exposure to secondhand smoke in the home were adjusted for age, menopausal status, age at menarche, age at first full-term pregnancy, total months of pregnancy, lactation history, education, race/ethnicity, body mass index and family history of breast cancer. NAT2 genotype was also determined, but was not associated with risk for breast cancer in this study. No statistically significant association was found between exposure to secondhand smoke and breast cancer risk in these never-smokers (relative risk, 1.3; 95% CI, 0.7–2.5) for any exposure to secondhand smoke in the home. [The Working Group considered that the strengths of this study included the fact that exposure data were collected prior to determination of case–control status. Its limitations were that it was a small study and that information on exposure to secondhand smoke was limited to exposure in the household.]

A large Canadian study (Johnson *et al.*, 2000) identified population-based incident cases of breast cancer aged 25–74 years at diagnosis from the National Enhanced Cancer Surveillance System beginning in April 1994 in some provinces (later in others) and continuing until July 1997. The study included 378 premenopausal and 700 postmeno-pausal never-smoking cases and 369 pre- and 845 postmenopausal population-based never-smoking controls. Exposure to secondhand smoke in the household during child-hood and adult life as well as in the workplace were assessed. Relative risk estimates were adjusted for age, province, education, body mass index, alcohol use, physical activity, age at menarche, age at the end of first pregnancy lasting 5 months or longer, number of live births, months of breastfeeding and height. There was no evidence of an association between breast cancer and exposure to secondhand smoke during childhood or adulthood in postmenopausal women (relative risk estimates ranged from 0.9 to 1.3, none were statistically significant). However, premenopausal women had significantly elevated risks for breast cancer associated with any exposure to secondhand smoke (relative risk, 2.3; 95% CI, 1.2–4.6), exposure to secondhand smoke during adulthood (relative risk, 2.6; 95% CI, 1.1–6.0), and exposure to secondhand smoke during both childhood and adult-hood (relative risk, 2.6; 95% CI, 1.2–5.5). There was evidence of a strong dose–response relationship in premenopausal women associated with duration of residential and occupa-tional exposure (*p* for trend = 0.0007). [The Working Group noted that the risk associated with passive smoking was similar in magnitude to that in former active smokers (relative risk, 2.6) and was higher than that for current active smokers (relative risk, 1.9) in the same study. The limitations of the study were that information was missing on a large number of cases and controls who were excluded from this study and information on exposure to secondhand smoke was available for only 59% of never-smokers.]

Two recent reports from a case–control study of breast cancer in German women aged 50 years and younger have used as the referent for assessing the risks of both active and involuntary smoking those women who have experienced no active and no passive exposure to tobacco smoke (lifetime non-exposed: < 1 (h/day) × year) (Kropp & Chang-Claude, 2002; Chang-Claude et al., 2002). The study included 706 cases (response rate, 70.1%) and 1381 controls (response rate, 61.2%). Data were initially collected by self-administered questionnaires for active smoking, and later, living cases and controls were re-contacted for information on involuntary exposure to tobacco smoke. Of the original participants, approximately 66% of the cases and 79% of the controls completed this part of the study. Risk estimates were adjusted for daily alcohol intake, total number of months of breastfeeding, education, first-degree family history of breast cancer, menopausal status and body mass index. For active smoking, a relative risk of 1.1 (95% CI, 0.6–2.0) was recorded, whereas never-smokers exposed to involuntary smoking had a statistically increased risk of about 60% (Kropp & Chang-Claude, 2002). In a subgroup analysis of 422 cases and 887 controls, the effect of NAT2 on the association between tobacco and breast cancer was considered (Chang-Claude et al., 2002). When compared to women who had never been exposed to any tobacco smoke, no association with active smoking was seen in rapid acetylators and a modest statistically non-significant increase in risk was observed in slow acetylators. In contrast, passive smoking was associated with a statistically non-significant risk that was higher in rapid than in slow acetylators (relative risk, 2.0; 95% CI, 1.0–4.1; and 1.2; 95% CI, 0.7–2.0, respectively). [The Working Group noted that this study has included many subgroup analyses, had reported incongruent findings related to active and involuntary smoking in the same study AND had obtained passive smoking data for only about 50% of study subjects. However, the strength of this study was the inclusion of a referent group of subjects who had not been exposed to any tobacco smoke during their lifetimes by self-report.]

2.3   Childhood cancers

Many studies have evaluated the association of cancer risk in childhood with exposure to parental smoking since this issue was considered previously in the IARC Monograph Volume 38 (IARC, 1986). These associations will be evaluated below for all cancers combined and separately, for brain tumours, leukaemias and lymphomas, and other childhood cancers.

Few studies distinguish times of exposure to tobacco smoke from parents, i.e. whether the exposure was preconception, in utero or postnatal. Exposure may have occurred in all three periods even when a study reports on only one, or exposure may also be reported as 'ever'. Involuntary smoking during each of these time periods tends to be correlated, in particular exposure to secondhand smoke from the father because father's smoking habits are less likely to change.

2.3.1 *All sites combined*

Four cohort studies (Neutel & Buck, 1971; Golding *et al.*, 1990; Pershagen *et al.*, 1992; Klebanoff *et al.*, 1996) and ten case–control studies (Buckley *et al.*, 1986; McKinney *et al.*, 1986; Stjernfeldt *et al.*, 1986; Forsberg & Kallen, 1990; John *et al.*, 1991; Golding *et al.*, 1992; Sorahan *et al.*, 1995; Ji *et al.*, 1997; Sorahan *et al.*, 1997a,b) (Table 2.13) have examined the role of involuntary exposure to tobacco smoke in risk for childhood cancers in general.

All four cohort studies specifically reported on the risk associated with cancer related to mothers' smoking during pregnancy. Neutel and Buck (1971) identified 97 deaths from childhood cancer in a cohort of 89 302 births from Ontario (Canada), and England and Wales followed from 7 to 10 years. Children with a mother who had smoked during pregnancy had a relative risk of 1.3 (95% CI, 0.8–2.2). No exposure–response relationship was apparent. [The Working Group noted several limitations of this study: no control for potential confounders; completeness of follow-up unknown, and limited assessment of exposure to secondhand smoke.]

Golding *et al.* (1990) followed a cohort of 16 193 births for 10 years (1970–80) and a total of 33 cancers were diagnosed. After adjustment for social class, exposure to X-rays during pregnancy, term delivery, administration of pethidine in labour and of drugs during infancy, a statistically significant increase in risk was found for children whose mothers smoked five or more cigarettes per day during the index pregnancy (relative risk, 2.5; 95% CI, 1.2–5.1). [The Working Group noted that the strength of this study was that the effect of exposure to secondhand smoke was independent of other risk factors found in this study. Its limitations were that the completeness of follow-up was unknown and that there was limited assessment of exposure to secondhand smoke.]

Pershagen *et al.* (1992), in Sweden, followed a large cohort of 497 051 births. In 5 years of follow-up, a total of 327 cancers that could be linked to data on maternal smoking were diagnosed. Relative risks were adjusted for year and county of birth, birth order and maternal age. No association was found for any maternal smoking during pregnancy (relative risk, 1.0; 95% CI, 0.8–1.3) and no exposure–response relationship was seen for number of cigarettes smoked during pregnancy (< 10 cigarettes per day, relative risk, 1.0; ≥ 10 cigarettes per day, relative risk, 0.9). No cancer at any of the sites evaluated individually was associated with maternal smoking. [The Working Group noted that the strengths of this study were that it was the largest cohort study, some statistical adjustment of risk estimates had been made and there was a high rate of follow-up. Its limitation was that there had been limited assessment of exposure to secondhand smoke.]

The most recent prospective study to evaluate the association between maternal smoking during pregnancy and childhood cancer is the US Collaborative Perinatal Project that included 54 795 children born from 1959–66 who were followed until the age of seven or eight years (Klebanoff *et al.*, 1996). The hazard ratio for cancer in children whose mother smoked during pregnancy compared to those whose mother did not was 0.7 (95% CI, 0.4–1.2). Adjustment of the hazard ratio for maternal race, age, education,

Table 2.13. Childhood cancers, all sites combined, and involuntary exposure to parental smoking

Reference (country)	Sample	Source of information on exposure	Duration (from birth) and completeness of follow-up	Exposure	Relative risk (95% CI)
Cohort studies					
Neutel & Buck (1971) (Canada, United Kingdom)	72 952 births in Ontario; 16 350 births in England and Wales	Interview	7–10 years in Ontario; 7 years in England and Wales; completeness not reported	Maternal smoking during pregnancy	1.3 (0.8–2.2)
Golding et al. (1990) (United Kingdom)	16 193 births, 33 cases	Cancer registry, medical record	10 years diagnosis of children ≤ 10 years of age; completeness not reported	Maternal smoking ≥ 5 cigarettes/day during pregnancy	2.5 (1.2–5.1)
Pershagen et al. (1992) (Sweden)	497 051 births, 327 cases	Cancer registry	5 years follow-up; 327 of 422 cancers linked to births with smoking data; 99% complete follow-up	Maternal smoking during pregnancy *Cigarettes/day* < 10 ≥ 10	1.0 (0.8–1.3) 1.0 (0.8–1.4) 0.9 (0.6–1.3)
Klebanoff et al. (1996) (USA)	54 795 births, 51 cases		7–8 years follow-up of cancers diagnosed in children ≤ 8 years old; completeness of follow-up not reported	Maternal smoking during pregnancy *Incidence rate* Smoker Nonsmoker *Hazard ratio*	0.9 per 1000 4 per 1000 p < 0.15 0.7 (0.4–1.2)

Table 2.13 (contd)

Reference (country)	Sample	Source of information on exposure	Duration (from birth) and completeness of follow-up	Exposure	Relative risk (95% CI)
Case–control studies					
Buckley *et al.* (1986) (USA, Canada)	1814 cases, 720 controls	In-person interview	3 years diagnosis in children (age not reported); 100% response rate	Maternal smoking during pregnancy *Cigarettes/day* <10 ≥10	1.3 (0.9–1.9) 1.0 (0.8–1.2)
McKinney *et al.* (1986) (United Kingdom)	555 cases, 1110 controls	Not reported	Duration and response rate not reported; children <15 years of age	Maternal smoking during pregnancy *Cigarettes/day* 1–10 ≥11	1.1 (0.9–1.5) 0.8 (0.7–1.1)
Stjernfeldt *et al.* (1986) (Sweden)	305 cases, 340 controls	Physician-distributed questionnaire	3 years diagnosis of children <17 years old; >95% response rate	Maternal smoking during pregnancy *Cigarettes/day* 1–9 ≥10	1.1 1.6, $p < 0.01$
Forsberg & Kallen (1990) (Sweden)	69 cases, 139 controls	Medical record	2 years diagnosis of children <10 years of age; response rate not reported	Any maternal smoking	1.1 (0.6–2.0)
John *et al.* (1991) (USA)	223 cases, 196 controls	Telephone interview	7 years diagnosis of children <15 years of age; 71% case response rate; 63% control response rate	Any maternal smoking in first trimester Paternal smoking in year prior to birth	1.3 (0.7–2.1) 1.2 (0.8–2.1)

Table 2.13 (contd)

Reference (country)	Sample	Source of information on exposure	Duration (from birth) and completeness of follow-up	Exposure	Relative risk (95% CI)
Golding et al. (1992) (United Kingdom)	195 cases, 558 controls	Medical record	20 years diagnosis of children (age not reported); response rate not reported	Maternal smoking in pregnancy	2.0 (1.3–3.2)
Sorahan et al. (1995) (United Kingdom)	1641 cases, 1641 controls	In-person interview	Deaths 1977–81 in children < 16 years of age; 61% case response rate; control response rate not reported	Maternal prenatal smoking *Cigarettes/day* 1–9 10–19 20–29 30–39 ≥ 40	1.0 (0.7–1.3) 1.2 (1.0–1.4) 1.0 (0.8–1.2) 0.9 (0.6–1.5) 1.6 (0.9–3.0)
				Paternal prenatal smoking *Cigarettes/day* 1–9 10–19 20–29 30–39 ≥ 40	1.2 (0.8–1.8) 1.2 (1.0–1.6) 1.3 (1.1–1.5) 1.4 (1.0–1.8) 1.5 (1.1–2.0)
Sorahan et al. (1997a) (United Kingdom)	1549 cases, 1549 controls	In-person interview	Deaths 1953–55 in children < 16 years of age; 88% case response rate; 94% control response rate	Maternal smoking *Cigarettes/day* 1–9 10–20 > 20	1.0 (0.8–1.2) 1.2 (1.0–1.5) 1.2 (0.7–2.3) *p* for trend = 0.09

Table 2.13 (contd)

Reference (country)	Sample	Source of information on exposure	Duration (from birth) and completeness of follow-up	Exposure	Relative risk (95% CI)
Sorahan et al. (1997a) (contd)				Paternal smoking *Cigarettes/day* 1–9 10–20 > 20	1.0 (0.8–1.3) 1.3 (1.1–1.6) 1.4 (1.1–1.9) *p* for trend < 0.001
Sorahan et al. (1997b) (United Kingdom)	2587 cases, 2587 controls	In-person interview	Deaths 1971–76 in children < 16 years of age; 63% case response rate; control response rate not reported	Maternal smoking only Paternal smoking only Both parents smoking	1.0 (0.8–1.1) 1.3 (1.1–1.5) 1.3 (1.3–2.4)
Ji et al. (1997) (China)	642 cases, 642 controls	In-person interview	10 years diagnosis of children < 15 years of age; 83% case response rate; 100% control response rate	Paternal smoking *Cigarettes/day* < 10 10–14 ≥ 15 Paternal smoking (years) < 10 10–14 ≥ 15	1.5 (1.1–2.3) 1.1 (0.8–1.6) 1.5 (1.0–2.3) 1.2 (0.7–1.8) 1.1 (0.8–1.7) 1.7 (1.2–2.5) *p* for trend = 0.007

socioeconomic status, height and pre-pregnancy weight as well as previous pregnancies, exposure to diagnostic radiation during pregnancy, feeding of infant in hospital, sex of infant and date of delivery had only a minimal effect on the point estimates, all of which remained in the range of 0.6. [The Working Group noted that the limitations of this study were that the completeness of follow-up was unknown, but the estimates of expected incidence suggest that few cases were missed, and that assessment of exposure to secondhand smoke was limited.]

Buckley *et al.* (1986) conducted a case–control analysis using data from the US/ Canada Children's Cancer Study Group. These investigators compared smoking by mothers and fathers of 1814 childhood cancer cases with that of parents of 720 controls selected at random from approximately the same geographical regions as cases. Smoking in the periods before and during pregnancy was assessed. No association was found between maternal smoking during pregnancy (< 10 cigarettes per day, relative risk, 1.3; 95% CI, 0.9–1.9; ≥ 10 cigarettes per day, relative risk, 1.0; 95% CI, 0.8–1.2) and no association with paternal smoking was found [relative risk not reported]. Adjustment for potential confounders such as year of birth, age of mother, illnesses during pregnancy and socioeconomic factors, did not alter findings. [The Working Group noted that the strength of this study was the large sample size and its limitations were that the report lacked details of the study and the control group was not well described.]

In a case–control study based on the Inter-Regional Epidemiological Study of Childhood Cancer in the United Kingdom, 555 cases of cancer in children < 15 years of age and 1110 controls matched for age and sex were compared for exposure to maternal smoking during pregnancy (McKinney *et al.*, 1986). There was no evidence of an association between maternal smoking and risk for childhood cancer (1–10 cigarettes per day, relative risk, 1.1; 95% CI, 0.9–1.5; > 11 cigarettes per day, relative risk, 0.8; 95% CI, 0.7–1.1). [The Working Group noted that the strength of this study was the large sample size. The limitations were that the report provided few study details; other than matching for age and sex there was no adjustment for potential confounders, and there was limited assessment of exposure to secondhand smoke.] This dataset was recently re-evaluated (Sorahan *et al.*, 2001). Microfilmed interview records of all study subjects were reviewed and information on parental cigarette smoking habits was re-abstracted. There was a statistically significant positive trend (*p* = 0.02) associated with daily paternal cigarette consumption before pregnancy for all cancers combined when cases were compared with controls selected from General Practitioners' (GPs') lists (*n* = 555), but no significant association was observed when cases were compared with hospital controls (*n* = 555). The opposite was seen for maternal smoking before pregnancy: an inverse trend (*p* < 0.001) was noted between daily cigarette consumption when cases were compared with hospital controls, but not when compared with GP controls. Risk estimates were adjusted for socioeconomic status, ethnicity, parental age at child's birth and other parent's smoking. [The Working Group noted that the two sets of controls produced very different results that are not easily explained.]

Stjernfeldt *et al.* (1986) reported the findings of a nationwide case–control study in Sweden that included 305 cases of cancer in children ≤ 16 years of age and 340 children with insulin-dependent diabetes mellitus who served as controls. Estimates of relative risk were adjusted for year of child's birth and maternal age, illness during pregnancy, occupation and place of residence. A 50% ($p < 0.01$) increase in risk for cancer was associated with in-utero exposure to maternal smoking. [The Working Group noted that the strengths of the study included the good response rate and the attempt to control for response bias by using children with diabetes mellitus as controls; its limitation was that the appropriateness of the control group was unknown.]

A case–control study from Sweden by Forsberg and Kallen (1990) found no association between childhood cancers and maternal smoking (relative risk, 1.1; 95% CI, 0.6–2.0) based on 69 cases and 139 controls for whom maternal smoking status was known. [The Working Group noted that the limitations of this study included the small sample size, uncertainty as to whether original case–control matching also applied to the substudy sample and the limited assessment of exposure.]

John *et al.* (1991) evaluated both maternal and paternal prenatal smoking histories in relation to risk for childhood cancer. The study included 223 incident cases < 15 years of age diagnosed from 1976 to 1983 in Denver, CO, USA. Controls were selected using random digit dialling and were matched to cases on age, sex and telephone exchange, and 196 controls were included in the analysis. Mothers' and fathers' smoking was highly correlated. Of the 109 children exposed to mother's smoking during the first trimester, 81% were also exposed to father's tobacco smoking while an additional 105 children were exposed to father's smoking alone. Mother's smoking during the first trimester was associated with a modest statistically nonsignificant increase in risk for childhood cancer after adjustment for father's education (relative risk, 1.3; 95% CI, 0.7–2.1). Children whose mothers did not smoke who were exposed to father's smoking also had a modest, statistically non-significant increase in risk (relative risk, 1.2; 95% CI, 0.8–2.1). [The Working Group noted that this study included a more detailed assessment of exposure to secondhand smoke than did earlier studies.]

Golding *et al.* (1992) conducted a case–control study in the United Kingdom to assess the association of childhood cancer with administration of intramuscular vitamin K and pethidine during labour. Data on mothers' smoking during pregnancy as a potential confounder were collected. A twofold increase in risk (relative risk, 2.0; 95% CI, 1.3–3.2) adjusted for year of delivery was found. [The Working Group noted that this study was not designed to investigate exposure to secondhand smoke, that only maternal smoking during pregnancy was recorded and that there was only minimal control for potential confounders.]

Three reports from the Oxford Survey of Childhood Cancer (OSCC) provided data from large case–control studies of childhood cancer deaths during different time periods: 1977–81 (Sorahan *et al.*, 1995), 1953–55 (Sorahan *et al.*, 1997a) and 1971–76 (Sorahan *et al.*, 1997b). The first report in 1995 included 1641 cases and an equal number of controls. There was no association with prenatal maternal cigarette smoking; however, paternal smoking was associated with a statistically significant positive trend (p for trend = 0.003). When cigarette use by one or both parents was adjusted for social class, maternal age at birth and use of alcohol, the relative risk was 1.4 (95% CI, 1.1–1.7) for father's use of cigarettes and 1.4 (95% CI, 1.1–1.7) for cigarette use by both parents, whereas cigarette use by mother was not statistically significantly associated with an increased risk (relative risk, 1.2; 95% CI, 1.0–1.6). A total of 1549 deaths from childhood cancer between 1953 and 1955 and 1549 matched healthy controls were used to further investigate the earlier findings from the OSCC (Sorahan *et al.*, 1997a). After adjustment for smoking by the spouse, social class, age of father, age of mother, birth order, and exposure to obstetric radiography, no statistically significant dose–response trend was found to be associated with maternal smoking, but maternal smoking only was associated with a 30% increased risk for childhood cancer (relative risk, 1.3; 95% CI, 1.1–1.5). At the highest level of paternal smoking (> 20 cigarettes per day), a clear trend was noted (p for trend < 0.001) with a relative risk of 1.4 (95% CI, 1.1–1.9); paternal smoking only was also associated with increased risk (relative risk, 1.7; 95% CI, 1.3–2.2). The third report (Sorahan *et al.*, 1997b) which examined deaths from 1971 to 1976 provided very similar results to those in the first two reports, i.e. no clear association with childhood cancer was evident for maternal smoking and there was a statistically significant positive trend for paternal smoking. [The Working Group noted the very large sample sizes, the consistent findings over time, the adjustment for potential confounders and the assessment of exposure from mothers and fathers with data for trends.]

A large case–control study in China by Ji *et al.* (1997) also examined paternal smoking and risk for cancer in children (< 15 years of age) of nonsmoking mothers. Relative risks were adjusted for birth weight, income, paternal age, education and alcohol drinking. For all sites combined, the relative risk for 'ever smoking' by the father was 1.3 (95% CI, 1.0–1.7). Statistically significant trends were found for duration of paternal smoking (p for trend = 0.007) and pack–years (p for trend = 0.01), but not age of starting smoking (p for trend = 0.28) or cigarettes per day (p for trend = 0.07). [The Working Group noted the large sample size, the minimization of exposure misclassification by including only children of nonsmoking mothers, the adjustment for potential confounders and the extensive exposure assessment for fathers.]

Boffetta *et al.* (2000) conducted a meta-analysis of childhood cancers associated with passive exposure to smoke based on the random effects model. The relative risk estimate for maternal smoking during pregnancy for all cancers combined included all cohort studies and eight of the ten case–control studies listed in Table 2.13 (Sorahan *et al.* 1997b; Ji *et al.* 1997; were not included). The results suggest a small increase in risk for all cancers for maternal smoking during pregnancy (relative risk, 1.1; 95% CI, 1.0–1.2), but not for specific cancer sites. Results on exposure before and after pregnancy were too sparse for any conclusion to be drawn. Studies of exposure to paternal tobacco smoke and risk for all cancers combined are fewer than those addressing maternal smoking and no relative risk was reported in this meta-analysis.

2.3.2   *Brain and central nervous system*

Table 2.14 lists one cohort study (Pershagen *et al.* 1992) and 15 case–control studies (Gold *et al.*, 1979; Preston-Martin *et al.*, 1982; Stjernfeldt *et al.*, 1986; Howe *et al.*, 1989; Kuijten *et al.*, 1990; Gold *et al.*, 1993; Bunin *et al.*, 1994; Cordier *et al.*, 1994; Filippini *et al.*, 1994; McCredie *et al.*, 1994; Norman *et al.*, 1996; Ji *et al.*, 1997; Sorahan *et al.*, 1997a,b; Filippini *et al.*, 2000) that have examined parental smoking and risk for brain tumours or for all tumours of the central nervous system combined.

Only the cohort study of Pershagen *et al.* (1992) (see section 2.3.1) has published a relative risk for tumours of the central nervous system. No association was found between maternal smoking in pregnancy and risk for tumours of the central nervous system.

The first case–control study to examine risk for brain tumour and maternal smoking was reported by Gold *et al.* (1979). This study was conducted in the USA and included 84 children with brain tumours and two control groups. One control group comprised 78 children with other malignancies matched on sex, race, date and age at diagnosis, and the other, 73 children selected from the state birth certificate file and matched on sex, date of birth and race. Risk associated with maternal smoking before and during pregnancy was associated with large non-statistically significant risks for childhood brain tumour that were based on a small sample size.

Preston-Martin *et al.* (1982) reported the findings from a larger case–control study in the USA designed to evaluate the risk for brain tumour associated with childhood exposure to *N*-nitroso compounds, including those from tobacco smoke. No increased risk was associated with maternal smoking, but a relative risk of 1.5 ($p = 0.03$) was found for children of mothers living with a smoker during pregnancy. The small Swedish case–control study by Stjernfeldt *et al.* (1986) (see section 2.3.1) found no increased risk for tumours of the central nervous system associated with maternal smoking in pregnancy.

An exploratory case–control study of brain tumours in Canadian children diagnosed in Ontario between 1977 and 1983 included 74 cases and 138 age- and sex-matched controls. The study found neither maternal nor paternal smoking during pregnancy to be statistically significantly associated with risk for brain tumours (Howe *et al.*, 1989). Similarly, a population-based case–control study in the USA of childhood astrocytomas that included 163 case–control pairs found no increased risk associated with any smoking by either mother or father (Kuijten *et al.*, 1990).

A large population-based case–control study in the USA of childhood brain tumours examined smoking by both parents in some detail. The study included exposure assessments for the preconception period as well as the pre- and postnatal period (year of birth of child) and dose–response estimates (Gold *et al.*, 1993). There was no statistically significant association between risk for brain tumours and any indicator of parental smoking. [The Working Group noted that this was a well-conducted study designed to examine parental smoking in detail, and having sufficient statistical power.]

Bunin *et al.* (1994) studied the two most common types of brain tumour, astrocytoma and primitive neuroectodermal tumour, in children less than six years of age. Controls,

Table 2.14. Tumours of the brain and central nervous system and involuntary exposure to parental smoking

Reference (country)	Sample	Source of information on exposure	Duration (from birth) and completeness of follow-up	Exposure	Results Relative risk (95% CI)
Cohort study					
Pershagen et al. (1992) (Sweden)	497 051 births, 81 CNS tumours	Cancer registry	Up to 5 years follow-up; 99% complete	Maternal smoking during pregnancy *Cigarettes/day* <10, ≥10	0.9 (0.5–1.6), 1.1 (0.6–2.1)
Case–control studies					
Gold et al. (1979) (USA)	84 brain tumours, 73 population controls, 78 cancer controls	In-person interview	10 years diagnosis of children <20 years old; 66% case response rate; 20% population control response rate; 44% cancer control response rate	Maternal smoking during pregnancy With population controls With cancer controls	5.0, $p < 0.22$ ∞
Preston-Martin et al. (1982) (USA)	209 brain tumours, 209 controls	Telephone interview	5 years diagnosis of cases <25 years old; 66% case response rate; 78% control response rate	Maternal smoking during pregnancy Mother living with a smoker	1.1 (one-sided $p = 0.42$) 1.5 (one sided $p = 0.03$)
Stjernfeldt et al. (1986) (Sweden)	43 brain and CNS tumours, 332 controls	Physician-distributed questionnaire	3 years diagnosis in children <17 years old; > 95% response rate	Maternal smoking during pregnancy *Cigarettes/day* 1–9, ≥10	1.0 0.9

Table 2.14 (contd)

Reference (country)	Sample	Source of information on exposure	Duration (from birth) and completeness of follow-up	Exposure	Results Relative risk (95% CI)	
Howe et al. (1989) (Canada)	74 brain tumours, 138 controls	In-person interview	6 years diagnosis of children <20 years of age; 60% case response rate; 86% control response rate	Any smoking	Mother 1.4 (0.7–3.0)	Father 1.1 (0.6–2.1)
Kuijten et al. (1990) (USA)	163 astrocytomas, 163 controls	In-person interview	6 years diagnosis of children <15 years of age; 80% case response rate; 73% control response rate	Any smoking	Mother 1.0 (0.6–1.7)	Father 0.8 (0.5–1.3)
Gold et al. (1993) (USA)	361 brain tumours, 1083 controls	In-person interview	4 years diagnosis of children <18 years of age; 85% case response rate; 85% control response rate	Any smoking	Mother 0.9 (0.7–1.2)	Father 1.1 (0.8–1.4)
				During year of birth (packs/day)		
				< 1	0.8 (0.6–1.3)	0.7 (0.4–1.2)
				≥ 1	1.0 (0.7–1.4)	1.1 (0.8–1.5)
				Two years before birth (packs/day)		
				< 1	0.8 (0.5–1.1)	0.9 (0.5–1.5)
				≥ 1	1.0 (0.7–1.4)	1.2 (0.9–1.6)

Table 2.14 (contd)

Reference (country)	Sample	Source of information on exposure	Duration (from birth) and completeness of follow-up	Exposure	Results Relative risk (95% CI)	
					Mother	Father
Bunin et al. (1994) (USA)	155 astrocytic gliomas, 166 primitive neuroectodermal tumours and 155 and 166 controls, respectively	Telephone interview	3 years diagnosis of children < 6 years of age; 65% case response rate; 83% control response rate	**Astrocytic glioma** Ever smoked Smoked during pregnancy **Primitive neuro-ectodermal tumour** Ever smoked Smoked during pregnancy	1.1 (0.7–1.8) 1.0 (0.6–1.7) 0.9 (0.6–1.5) 1.0 (0.6–1.7)	1.1 (0.7–1.8) 1.0 (0.6–1.7) 0.9 (0.6–1.5) 1.0 (0.6–1.7)
Cordier et al. (1994) (France)	75 brain tumours, 113 controls	In-person interview	2 years diagnosis of children < 15 years of age; 69% case response rate; 72% control response rate	Any smoking by mother	1.6 (0.7–3.5)	

Filippini et al. (1994) (Italy)	91 brain tumours, 321 controls	In-person interview	3 years diagnosis of children < 15 years of age; 88% case response rate; 75% control response rate	Maternal smoking during pregnancy
				Maternal smoking
				  1–10 cigarettes/day
				  > 10 cigarettes/day
				Paternal smoking before pregnancy
					1.7 (0.8–3.8)
					
					2.0 (1.0–4.0)
					1.6 (0.5–4.8)
					1.3 (0.8–2.4)	

McCredie et al. (1994) (Australia)	82 brain tumours, 164 controls	In-person interview	4 years diagnosis of children < 15 years of age; 85% case response rate; 60% control response rate	Questions related to sources of exposure to N-nitroso compounds including tobacco smoke	No association	

Table 2.14 (contd)

Reference (country)	Sample	Source of information on exposure	Duration (from birth) and completeness of follow-up	Exposure	Results Relative risk (95% CI)	
					Mother	Father
Norman et al. (1996) (USA)	540 brain tumours, 801 controls	In-person and telephone interviews	6 years diagnosis of children < 15 years of age; 71% case response rate; 74% control response rate	Any smoking	1.0 (0.7–1.3)	1.2 (0.9–1.5)
Ji et al. (1997) (China)	107 brain tumours, 107 controls	In-person interview	10 years diagnosis of children < 15 years of age; 83% case response rate; 100% control response rate	Paternal smoking *Cigarettes/day*		
				1–9	1.5 (0.5–4.5)	
				10–14	1.6 (0.6–4.7)	
				≥ 15	2.1 (0.6–8.1)	
				Duration of exposure (years)		
				< 10	0.8 (0.2–3.8)	
				10–14	1.3 (0.4–4.1)	
				≥ 15	3.4 (0.9–12.5)	
Sorahan et al. (1997a) (United Kingdom)	229 CNS tumours, 229 controls	In-person interview	Deaths 1953–55 in children < 16 years of age; 88% case response rate; 94% control response rate	Parental smoking	1.0 (0.8–1.4)	1.2 (1.0–1.5)
Sorahan et al. (1997b) (United Kingdom)	410 CNS tumours, 410 controls	In-person interview	Deaths 1971–76 in children < 16 years of age; 63% case response rate; control response rate not reported	Parental smoking	1.1 (1.0–1.2)	1.0 (0.9–1.1)

Table 2.14 (contd)

Reference (country)	Sample	Source of information on exposure	Duration (from birth) and completeness of follow-up	Exposure	Results Relative risk (95% CI)
Filippini et al. (2000) (Italy)	244 CNS tumours, 502 controls	Telephone interview	5 years diagnosis of children < 16 years old; 85% case response rate; 88% control response rate	*Maternal smoking* Before pregnancy Before she knew she was pregnant *Maternal exposure to secondhand smoke* During early pregnancy During late pregnancy	1.2 (0.9–1.7) 1.5 (1.0–2.3) 1.8 (1.2–2.6) 1.7 (1.2–2.5)

CNS, central nervous system

selected by random-digit dialling, were matched to cases on race, year of birth, and telephone area code and prefix. Estimates of relative risk for astrocytoma were adjusted for income level, but primitive neuroectodermal tumour estimates were unadjusted. No association was found between either of these types of tumour and maternal active (ever and/or during pregnancy) or passive smoking (during pregnancy) or paternal smoking (ever and/or during pregnancy).

A non-statistically significant increase in risk for brain tumours (relative risk, 1.6; 95% CI, 0.7–3.5) associated with any smoking by the mother was found in a small case–control study in France (Cordier *et al.* 1994). Filippini *et al.* (1994) in Italy assessed the risk associated with active and passive smoking by mothers during pregnancy in a case–control study with 91 cases. Active smoking by the mother during pregnancy was associated with a relative risk of 1.7 (95% CI, 0.8–3.8); no dose–response relationship was observed. Relative risks were adjusted for education level. Among nonsmoking mothers, the relative risks for light and heavy exposure to secondhand smoke were 1.7 (95% CI, 0.8–3.6) and 2.2 (95% CI, 1.1–4.5; *p* trend = 0.02). McCredie *et al.* (1994) conducted another small, population-based case–control study of brain tumours in Australia. Two controls were matched to each case by age and sex. No association was found with exposure to tobacco smoke from another member of the household, but no risk estimates were provided. [The Working Group noted that the limitations of these studies were that they lacked statistical power; there was limited adjustment for potential confounders and limited assessment of exposure.]

The findings from a large, population-based case–control study of brain tumours in children < 15 years of age diagnosed from 1984 to 1991 provided no support for an association between brain tumour risk and maternal or paternal smoking before pregnancy or maternal smoking during pregnancy (Norman *et al.* 1996). Risk estimates were at or below unity and there was no evidence of a relationship between risk for brain tumours and amount or timing of exposure. [The Working Group noted that the strengths of this study were that it was large and included a relatively detailed assessment of exposure.]

Three studies discussed previously (Ji *et al.* 1997; Sorahan *et al.* 1997a,b) found no increased risk for brain tumours associated with father's smoking (Ji *et al.*, 1997) or of tumours of the central nervous system associated with maternal or paternal smoking (Sorahan *et al.*, 1997a,b; 2001).

Filippini *et al.* (2000) in northern Italy, conducted a population-based case–control study of childhood tumours of the central nervous system with cases diagnosed from 1988 to 1993. Cases from their previous study (Filippini *et al.*, 1994) were excluded. Active smoking by parents before pregnancy was not associated with increased risk. Active smoking by mothers in early pregnancy was associated with a small increase in risk (relative risk, 1.5; 95% CI, 1.0–2.3). An increase in risk was also associated with passive smoking by nonsmoking mothers in early pregnancy (relative risk, 1.8; 95% CI, 1.2–2.6) and late pregnancy (relative risk, 1.7; 95% CI, 1.2–2.5).

The results of the meta-analysis by Boffetta *et al.* (2000) indicated no significant increase in risk for tumours of the central nervous system associated with maternal smoking during pregnancy (relative risk, 1.0; 95% CI, 0.9–1.2), but exposure to paternal smoking suggested an increased risk for brain tumours (relative risk, 1.1; 95% CI, 1.1–1.4). [The Working Group noted that this meta-analysis included two studies of neuroblastoma and one study of retinoblastoma with tumours of the central nervous system.]

2.3.3   Leukaemias and lymphomas

The only cohort study to report specifically on lymphatic and haematopoietic cancers (Pershagen et al., 1992) and 16 case–control studies with data on one or more of these types of malignancy are included in Table 2.15 (Manning & Carroll, 1957; Stewart et al., 1958; Van Steensel-Moll et al., 1985; Buckley et al., 1986; McKinney et al., 1986; Stjernfeldt et al., 1986; Magnani et al., 1990; John et al., 1991; Roman et al., 1993; Severson et al., 1993; Shu et al., 1996; Ji et al., 1997; Sorahan et al., 1997a,b; Brondum et al., 1999; Infante-Rivard et al., 2000).

A total of 129 lymphatic and haematopoietic cancers were diagnosed during 5 years of follow-up in the Swedish cohort (Pershagen et al., 1992). No association was observed between the development of these cancers and smoking during pregnancy or any amount of smoking by the mother.

Manning and Carroll (1957) found no difference in the proportion of mothers of children with leukaemia who smoked 10 or more cigarettes per day at the time of interview when compared to control mothers (39% versus 38%) and a somewhat lower proportion of mothers of children with lymphoma (31%) who smoked at that level. A second early study (Stewart et al., 1958) reported a very small but statistically significant increase in risk for death from leukaemia among children of mothers who had ever smoked (relative risk, 1.1; $p < 0.04$). [The Working Group noted that neither study was designed specifically to study the effects of involuntary smoking; only unadjusted proportions were reported.]

Van Steensel-Moll et al. (1985) found no association between maternal smoking in the year before pregnancy and risk for acute lymphocytic leukaemia in a study in the Netherlands designed to assess maternal fertility problems and this risk. [The Working Group noted that the strength of this study was the large number of cases. Its limitations are the limited assessment of exposure and the questionable time period.] The case–control study in Sweden by Stjernfeldt et al. (1986) included 157 cases of acute lympho-blastic leukaemia, 16 cases of non-Hodgkin lymphoma and 15 cases of Hodgkin disease. A statistically significant positive trend (p trend < 0.01) was found for number of cigarettes smoked per day by the mother during pregnancy and risk for acute lymphoblastic leukaemia. No statistically significant association with smoking was observed for either non-Hodgkin lymphoma or Hodgkin disease based on a very small number of cases.

McKinney et al. (1986) found no association between maternal smoking during pregnancy and risk for childhood leukaemia or lymphoma. Buckley et al. (1986) also failed to find an association between maternal smoking during pregnancy in their large

Table 2.15. Childhood leukaemias and lymphomas and involuntary exposure to parental smoking

Reference (country)	Sample	Source of information on exposure	Duration (from birth) and completeness of follow-up	Exposure	Results Relative risk (95% CI)
Cohort study					
Pershagen et al. (1992) (Sweden)	497 051 births, 129 lymphatic and haematopoietic cancers	Cancer registry	5 years follow-up; 327 of 422 cancers linked to births with smoking data.	Maternal smoking during pregnancy *Cigarettes/day* <10 ≥10	1.0 (0.7–1.5) 1.2 (0.8–1.9) 0.8 (0.4–1.5)
Case–control studies					
Manning & Carroll (1957) (USA)	188 leukaemias, 42 lymphomas, 50 hospital controls	Interview	3 years diagnosis of children <15 years of age	Proportion of mothers smoking ≥ 10 cigarettes/day at time of interview	Leukaemia 39% Lymphoma 31% Controls 38%
Stewart et al. (1958) (United Kingdom)	677 leukaemias, 739 other cancers, 1416 living controls	In-person interview	3 years diagnosis of children <15 years of age	Mother ever smoked	1.1 ($p < 0.04$)
Van Steensel-Moll et al. (1985) (the Netherlands)	519 ALL, 507 controls	Postal questionnaire	7 years diagnosis of children <15 years of age; 90% case response rate; 69% control response rate	Maternal smoking during year before pregnancy	1.0 (0.8–1.3)
Stjernfeldt et al. (1986) (Sweden)	157 ALL, 16 NHL, 15 HD, 340 controls	Physician-delivered questionnaire	3 years diagnosis of children <17 years of age; 95% response rate for both cases and controls	*Maternal smoking during pregnancy* 1–9 cigarettes/day ≥ 10 cigarettes/day	ALL NHL HD 1.3 2.0 1.1 2.1 2.1 0.3
McKinney et al. (1986) (United Kingdom)	171 leukaemias, 74 lymphomas, 2 controls/case	Not reported	Response rate not reported	*Maternal smoking during pregnancy* 1–10 cigarettes/day >10 cigarettes/day	Leukaemia Lymphoma 1.0 (0.6–1.7) 1.9 (0.9–4.0) 0.6 (0.4–1.0) 1.0 (0.5–2.1)
Buckley et al. (1986) (USA, Canada)	742 ALL, 169 NHL, 720 controls	Questionnaire	3 years diagnosis of cancer in children (age not given). Response rate not reported	*Maternal smoking during pregnancy* 1–9 cigarettes/day ≥10 cigarettes/day	ALL NHL 1.0 (0.6–1.0) 0.8 (0.3–1.8) 0.9 (0.7–1.1) 1.0 (0.7–1.4)

Table 2.15 (contd)

Reference (country)	Sample	Source of information on exposure	Duration (from birth) and completeness of follow-up	Exposure	Results Relative risk (95% CI)
Magnani et al. (1990) (Italy)	142 ALL, 22 other leukaemias (non-ALL), 19 NHL, 307 controls	In-person interview	10 years diagnosis in cases <15 years of age. Response rate not reported	Maternal smoking up to child's birth Paternal smoking	ALL Non-ALL NHL 0.7 (0.5–1.1) 2.0 (0.8–4.8) 1.7 (0.7–4.5) 0.9 (0.6–1.5) 0.9 (0.3–2.1) 6.7 (1.0–43.4)
John et al. (1991) (USA)	73 leukaemias, 26 lymphomas, 196 controls	Telephone interview	7 years diagnosis in children <15 years of age; 71% case response rate; 63% control response rate	*Maternal smoking* 3 months before conception First trimester All 3 trimesters	ALL Non-ALL Lymphoma 2.1 (1.0–4.3) 0.8 (0.2–2.7) 1.9 (0.7–5.2) 2.3 (1.1–5.0) 1.1 (0.3–4.0) 2.5 (0.9–7.0) 2.5 (1.2–5.4) 0.6 (0.1–3.0) 2.7 (1.0–7.6)
Severson et al. (1993) (USA, Canada)	187 acute myeloid leukaemias, 187 controls	Telephone interview	4 years diagnosis in children <18 years of age; 78% case response rate; 79% control response rate	*Maternal smoking* During pregnancy Current smoker Ever smoker	 1.2 (0.8–1.9) 0.9 (0.6–1.4) 1.3 (0.9–2.1)
Roman et al. (1993) (United Kingdom)	54 leukaemias and NHL, 324 controls	Interview, birth certificates, occupational and medical records	17 years diagnosis in cases <5 years of age; 76% case response rate; 95% control response rate	*Smoking during pregnancy* From obstetric records From interview	 0.9 (0.3–2.5) 0.5 (0.2–1.2)
Shu et al. (1996) (USA, Canada, Australia)	302 leukaemias, 558 controls	Telephone interview	5 years diagnosis of children ≤18 months of age; 79% case response rate; 75% control response rate	Smoking during pregnancy *Cigarettes/day* 1–10 11–20 > 20	Mother Father 1.2 (0.9–1.8) 0.7 (0.4–1.0) 0.6 (0.4–1.1) 0.6 (0.2–1.8) p for trend = 0.03
Ji et al. (1997) (China)	166 acute leukaemias, 87 lymphomas, 166 and 87 controls, respectively	In-person interview	10 years diagnosis of children <15 years of age; 83% case response rate; 100% control response rate	Paternal smoking before conception *Cigarettes/day* < 10 10–14 ≥ 15	Acute leukaemia Lymphoma 1.6 (0.7–3.9) 3.4 (0.8–14.0) 0.9 (0.4–1.5) 1.1 (0.3–4.8) 1.9 (0.8–4.6) 3.8 (0.9–16.5) p for trend = 0.27 p for trend = 0.09

Table 2.15 (contd)

Reference (country)	Sample	Source of information on exposure	Duration (from birth) and completeness of follow-up	Exposure	Results Relative risk (95% CI)	
Ji et al. (1997) (contd)				*Pack-years*		
				≤ 5	0.9 (0.4–2.2)	2.8 (0.6–12.8)
				> 5–< 10	1.1 (0.5–2.6)	1.3 (0.3–5.5)
				≥ 10	1.9 (0.8–4.6)	5.7 (1.3–26.0)
					p for trend = 0.06	*p* for trend = 0.03
Sorahan et al. (1997a) (United Kingdom)	367 ALL, 115 myeloid leukaemias, 27 monocytic leukaemias, 216 other, unspecified leukaemias, 125 lymphomas, equal numbers of controls	In-person interview	2 years diagnosis of children < 16 years old; 88% case response rate; 60% control response rate	Parental smoking	Mother	Father
				Leukaemias		
				ALL	1.2 (1.0–1.5)	1.1 (0.9–1.3)
				Myeloid	1.2 (0.9–1.7)	1.0 (0.7–1.3)
				Monocytic	1.2 (0.6–2.5)	1.1 (0.6–2.0)
				Other	1.2 (0.9–1.6)	1.1 (0.9–1.4)
				Lymphomas	0.8 (0.6–1.1)	1.4 (1.0–1.8)
Sorahan et al. (1997b) (United Kingdom)	573 ALL, 190 myeloid leukaemias, 25 monocytic leukaemias, 47 other unspecified leukaemias, 165 lymphomas, equal numbers of controls	In-person interview	5 years diagnosis in children < 16 years of age; 57% case response rate; 52% control response rate	Parental smoking	Mother	Father
				Leukaemias		
				ALL	1.0 (0.9–1.1)	1.1 (1.0–1.2)
				Myeloid	1.0 (0.8–1.2)	1.3 (1.1–1.5)
				Monocytic	0.7 (0.4–1.2)	0.8 (0.6–1.3)
				Other	0.9 (0.7–1.2)	1.0 (0.8–1.3)
				Lymphomas	1.1 (0.9–1.2)	1.1 (0.9–1.2)
Brondum et al. (1999) (USA)	1842 ALL, 1987 controls, 517 AML, 612 controls	Telephone interview	3.5 years diagnosis of acute leukaemia < 5–18 years of age. Case response rates: 92% ALL, 83% AML; control response rates: 76.5% ALL controls, 79.4% AML controls	Father ever smoked Mother ever smoked	ALL 1.0 (0.9–1.2) 1.0 (0.9–1.2)	AML 0.9 (0.7–1.2) 1.0 (0.7–1.2)

Table 2.15 (contd)

Reference (country)	Sample	Source of information on exposure	Duration (from birth) and completeness of follow-up	Exposure	Results Relative risk (95% CI)		
Infante-Rivard *et al.* (2000)	491 ALL, 491 controls	Telephone interview	13 years diagnosis of ALL in children < 10 yrs of age. 96.3% case response rate; 83.8% control response rate	Parental smoking during childhood	Mother	Father	
				Cigarettes/day			
				1–20	1.0 (0.7–1.4)	1.0 (0.7–1.4)	
				> 20	1.0 (0.6–1.3)	1.0 (0.7–1.3)	
					1st trimester	2nd trimester	3rd trimester
				Maternal smoking			
				Cigarettes/day			
				1–20	1.1 (0.8–1.6)	1.2 (0.8–1.6)	1.2 (0.8–1.6)
				> 20	1.0 (0.7–1.6)	1.2 (0.7–1.9)	1.2 (0.8–2.0)
	158 cases, 491 controls (case–case substudy)			*At > 20 cigarettes/day*			
				CYP1A1*2A allele	Moderate risk increases		
				CYP1A1*2B allele	Reduced risk		
				CYP1A1*4 allele	Lower increases associated with father's smoking; mother's smoking risks higher in 3rd trimester		

ALL, acute lymphocytic leukaemia; NHL, non-Hodgkin lymphoma; HD, Hodgkin disease; AML, acute myeloblastic leukaemia study that included 742 cases of acute lymphocytic leukaemia and 169 cases of non-Hodgkin lymphoma.

Magnani *et al.* (1990) found no association between acute lymphocytic leukaemia, other leukaemias or non-Hodgkin lymphoma during childhood and the mother's smoking up to the time of the child's birth. The father's history of smoking was associated with a risk for non-Hodgkin lymphoma (relative risk, 6.7; 95% CI, 1.0–43.4), but not for acute lymphocytic leukaemia or other leukaemias. This Italian hospital-based case–control study included 142 cases of acute lymphocytic leukaemia, but only a small number of non-Hodgkin lymphoma ($n = 19$) and other types of leukaemia ($n = 22$). Risk estimates were adjusted for socioeconomic status only.

The case–control study in the USA reported by John *et al.* (1991) included 73 cases of leukaemia and 26 cases of lymphoma. Statistically significant increases in risk were associated with maternal smoking 3 months before conception for acute lymphocytic leukaemia; with smoking during the first trimester for acute lymphocytic leukaemia; and during all three trimesters for acute lymphocytic leukaemia (relative risk, 2.5; 95% CI, 1.2–5.4) and lymphoma (relative risk, 2.7; 95% CI, 1.0–7.6).

A US–Canadian case–control study of acute myeloid leukaemia found no association between risk for acute myeloid leukaemia and maternal smoking before, during or after pregnancy (Severson *et al.* 1993). No association was observed with smoking by the father, but this was not quantified. [The Working Group noted the reasonably detailed exposure assessment, but although relative risks were adjusted for potential confounders, the factors were not named.]

A small case–control study of leukaemia and non-Hodgkin lymphoma in the United Kingdom examined maternal smoking based on obstetric notes and by interview (Roman *et al.*, 1993). Both relative risks were below unity. [The Working Group noted that very little information was provided, that no adjustment was made for confounders, and the small size of the sample.]

Shu *et al.* (1996) found that maternal smoking during pregnancy was negatively associated with risk for leukaemia (all leukaemias, acute lymphocytic leukaemia or acute myeloblastic leukaemia) in infants. Paternal smoking one month prior to pregnancy was related to an elevated risk for acute lymphocytic leukaemia (relative risk, 1.6; 95% CI, 1.0–2.4), but not acute myeloblastic leukaemia and smoking by the father during pregnancy did not lead to a statistically significant increase in risk for any type of leukaemia. [The Working Group noted that the strengths of this study included the relatively detailed exposure from mothers' and fathers' smoking, and the adjustment for some potential confounders (sex, parental age, education and alcohol consumption by the mother during pregnancy).]

The case–control study of paternal smoking and childhood cancer in China reported by Ji *et al.* (1997) included 166 cases of acute leukaemia and 87 of lymphoma. No statistically significant association with paternal smoking was found for leukaemia, although a borderline positive trend was found for the father's number of pack–years of smoking (trend, $p = 0.06$). The father's smoking was associated with a fourfold increase in risk for lymphoma (relative risk, 4.0; 95% CI, 1.3–12.5) and statistically significant positive dose–response trends for lymphoma were observed for number of years smoked pre-conception and pack–year history, but not for number of cigarettes smoked per day.

Sorahan *et al.* (1997a) reported a modest association between risk for acute lymphocytic leukaemia and maternal smoking (relative risk, 1.2; 95% CI, 1.0–1.5), but no increased risk was found for myeloid, monocytic or other types of leukaemia or lymphoma. This study found no relationship between paternal smoking and any type of leukaemia, but the risk estimate for lymphoma was 1.4 (95% CI, 1.0–1.8). No increased risks associated with parental smoking were found when cases and controls from a later time period, 1971–76, were examined (Sorahan *et al.* 1997b).

A large case–control study in the USA of parental cigarette smoking and risk for acute leukaemia collected detailed information on exposure to smoke from the mothers and fathers of 1842 children with acute lymphocytic leukaemia and 517 with acute myelo-blastic leukaemia and controls matched on age, race, and telephone area code/exchange (Brondum *et al.*, 1999). There was no association between risk for acute lymphocytic leukaemia and ever smoking by the father (relative risk, 1.0; 95% CI, 0.9–1.2) or mother (relative risk, 1.0; 95% CI, 0.9–1.2); similarly, no associations were observed between acute myeloblastic leukaemia and ever smoking by the father (relative risk, 0.9; 95% CI, 0.7–1.2) or the mother (relative risk, 1.0; 95% CI, 0.7–1.2). Parental smoking during or around the time of the index pregnancy was not related to risk, nor were the number of cigarettes smoked, years of smoking or pack–years. Risk estimates were adjusted for household income, mother's race and education and father's race and education. [The Working Group noted the good statistical power and the detailed histories of both parents and also that some adjustment has been made for potential confounders.]

A case–control study in Canada of acute lymphocytic leukaemia assessed the role of parental smoking and *CYP1A1* genetic polymorphisms (Infante-Rivard *et al.*, 2000). There was no statistically significant association between parents' smoking and leukaemia overall. However, a substudy that included 158 of the 491 cases suggested that the effect of parental smoking may be modified by variant alleles in the *CYP1A1*. *CYP1A1*2B* tended to decrease risks and *CYP1A1*2A* and *CYP1A1*4* increased the risks associated with smoking in the second and third trimesters. [The Working Group noted that this was the first study to look at the interaction between parental smoking, *CYP1A1* and leukaemia.]

Sorahan *et al.* (2001) (see Section 2.3.1) found a statistically non-significant positive association between risk for acute lymphocytic leukaemia and daily cigarette consump-tion by fathers before pregnancy and a statistically non-significant inverse association between risk for acute lymphocytic leukaemia and daily smoking by mothers before pregnancy.

The results of the meta-analysis for maternal smoking during pregnancy indicated that there were no statistically significant associations for all lymphatic and haematopoietic neoplasms (relative risk, 1.0; 95% CI, 0.9–1.2), for non-Hodgkin lymphoma or total lym-phomas (relative risk, 1.1; 95% CI, 0.9–1.5) or for all leukaemias, acute leukaemia or acute lymphocytic leukaemia (relative risk, 1.1; 95% CI, 0.8–1.3) (Boffetta *et al.*, 2000). The authors found evidence of publication bias for the data available on lymphomas ($p = 0.04$). Published studies with a small number of cases reported positive associations between exposure to tobacco smoke and childhood leukaemia, whereas larger studies showed no association. This suggests that small studies that had found no association or a negative association failed to be published. The meta-analysis for paternal smoking indicated no statistically significant association with acute lymphocytic leukaemia, but a twofold increase in risk for non-Hodgkin lymphoma (relative risk, 2.1; 95% CI, 1.1–4.0).

2.3.4   *Other childhood cancers*

Several other types of childhood cancer have been studied in relation to parental smoking in epidemiological investigations.

The cohort study by Pershagen *et al.* (1992) reported no statistically significant associations between mother's smoking during pregnancy and kidney cancer (30 cases; relative risk, 0.6; 95% CI, 0.2–1.5), eye tumours (28 cases; relative risk, 1.4; 95% CI, 0.6–2.8), endocrine tumours (13 cases; relative risk, 1.9; 95% CI, 0.6–6.0) or tumours of the connective tissue and muscle (15 cases; relative risk, 1.2; 95% CI, 0.4–3.6).

Magnani *et al.* (1989) conducted a hospital-based case–control study of soft-tissue sarcomas in Italy during 1983–84. The cases included 36 children with rhabdomyo-sarcoma and 16 cases of other soft-tissue sarcomas who were compared with 326 controls from the same hospitals. No associations were found between soft-tissue sarcoma or rhabdomyosarcoma and either mother's or father's smoking (all point estimates of relative risks were below unity). Smoking during several time periods, before, during and after birth was then looked at separately and the results were the same as for any smoking by the parents. [The Working Group noted that this was a small study, but that the exposure assessment included different time periods.]

Two studies in the USA (Holly *et al.*, 1992; Winn *et al.*, 1992) examined risk factors for Ewing's sarcoma. In their population-based study, Holly *et al.* (1992) looked at 43 cases and 193 controls selected by random digit dialling and matched to cases by sex and age. This tumour was not associated with smoking by the mother during pregnancy (relative risk, 1.1; 95% CI, 0.5–2.4) or by the father (relative risk, 0.9; 95% CI, 0.4–1.9). Risk estimates were adjusted for agricultural occupation of the father, poison or overdose of medication, area of residence, year of child's birth and income. [The Working Group noted that this was a small study that had made a detailed assessment of many factors, but less for parental smoking.] Winn *et al.* (1992) reported the findings of a larger case–control study that included 208 cases throughout the USA and two control groups with equal numbers of controls (sibling controls and regional controls). When cases were compared to regional controls, no significant risk estimates were found for smoking by either parent; however, parents were more likely to have smoked during pregnancy with the child with Ewing's sarcoma than during the pregnancy with the unaffected sibling; if only the mother smoked, the relative risk was 1.5 (95% CI, 0.3–9.0); if only the father smoked, the relative risk was 3.1 (95% CI, 0.7–14.0); if both parents smoked, the relative risk was 7.3 (95% CI, 1.3–41.6).

Two case–control studies in the USA evaluated prenatal drug consumption by the mother and risk for neuroblastoma (Kramer et al., 1987; Schwartzbaum, 1992). The first study was population-based and included 104 cases diagnosed from 1970 to 1979, a first group of 104 controls matched on date of birth, race and the first five digits of case's telephone number and a second group of controls comprising siblings of the index case. No significant increase in risk was associated with maternal smoking during pregnancy when cases were compared to either control group. The second study compared 101 newly diagnosed cases of neuroblastoma and 690 controls diagnosed with other types of childhood cancer at St Jude Children's Research Hospital. Cigarette smoking by the mother during pregnancy was found to increase the risk for neuroblastoma (relative risk, 1.9; 95% CI, 1.1–3.2). [The Working Group noted the questionable appropriateness of the control group in the study by Schwartzbaum and the limited exposure assessments in both studies.]

Olshan et al. (1993) reported findings from the National Wilms Tumour Study, a case–control study from a national collaborative clinical trial group in the USA. The study was conducted using interviews with 200 cases and 233 matched controls identified by random-digit dialling. No association was found for mother's smoking during pregnancy and risk for Wilms tumour (relative risk for smoking ten or more cigarettes per day, 0.7; 95% CI, 0.4–1.3).

2.4   Other cancers

2.4.1   All cancer sites combined

Hirayama (1984) reported a statistically significant association (p for trend < 0.001) between husband's smoking and cancer mortality in wives for all sites combined in the Japanese cohort (relative risk for former smoker: 1–19 cigarettes per day, 1.1; 95% CI, 1.0–1.2; relative risk for ≥ 20 cigarettes per day, 1.2; 95% CI, 1.1–1.4).

Sandler et al. (1985b), in their study previously described in detail (Section 2.2.2), found an increased risk of all cancers combined among nonsmokers passively exposed to cigarette smoke in adulthood (relative risk, 2.1; 95% CI, 1.4–3.0). Risk did not differ according to race (white or non-white), but was statistically significant only among women aged 30–49 years.

Miller (1990) reported the findings from a case–control study in the USA of cancer deaths among nonsmoking women in which next-of-kins were interviewed by telephone. Data on 906 nonsmoking wives were included in this report. The cases were women who had died of any type of cancer and the controls were nonsmoking wives who had died of cardiovascular, respiratory, kidney and other non-cancer diseases, excluding trauma. A nonsmoker was defined as a person who had smoked fewer than 20 packs of cigarettes during her lifetime. The percentage of deaths from cancer among non-exposed, non-employed wives was 2.2%; for exposed, non-employed wives, 18.9%, and for employed wives, 34.3% (*p* < 0.001). [The Working Group noted that the study used a questionable comparison group and a non-standard definition of a nonsmoker.]

2.4.2   *Cervical cancer*

Three Asian cohort studies described in Section 2.1 also reported on involuntary smoking and risk for cancer of the cervix. Risk for cervical cancer associated with involuntary exposure to smoking in nonsmokers was examined in a Japanese cohort study that found no significant increase in risk associated with husbands' smoking (Hirayama, 1984). A second cohort study also considered exposure to husbands' smoking and risk for cervical cancer in nonsmoking Korean women (Jee *et al.*, 1999). The relative risk based on 203 cases of cervical cancer in nonsmokers was 0.9 (95% CI, 0.6–1.3) for women married to former and 0.9 (95% CI, 0.6–1.2) for women married to current smokers when compared with women married to nonsmokers. The cohort study by Nishino *et al.* (2001) included 11 incident cases of cervical cancer. Again, no association with husband's smoking status was observed (relative risk, 1.1; 95% CI, 0.3–4.5). [The Working Group noted that these cohort studies consistently indicated no association between exposure to secondhand smoke and cervical cancer.]

The case–control study from the USA reported by Sandler *et al.* (1985b; see Section 2.2.2) found an increased risk of cervical cancer associated with spousal smoking (relative risk, 2.1; 95% CI, 1.2–3.9). A second case–control study in the USA was conducted from 1984 to 1987 in Utah where a large percentage of the population are members of the Church of Jesus Christ of the Latter-day Saints which proscribes tobacco smoking (Slattery *et al.*, 1989). The cases were population-based and controls were selected by random-digit dialling and matched to cases on age and county of residence. The response rates for cases and controls were 66% and 76%, respectively. Nonsmokers involuntarily exposed for 3 hours or more per day to secondhand smoke were found to have an increased risk for cervical cancer (relative risk, 3.4; 95% CI, 1.2–9.5). Self-characterized exposure to 'a lot' of secondhand smoke was also associated with increased risk (in-home relative risk, 2.9; 95% CI, 1.1–7.9; outside the home relative risk, 1.6; 95% CI, 0.6–4.5). [The Working Group noted that a statistically non-significant increase in risk was also observed in active smokers exposed to smoking by others.]

Coker *et al.* (1992) examined the risk of exposure to secondhand smoke in a case–control study of cervical intraepithelial neoplasma (CIN) of grades II (*n* = 40) and III (*n* = 63) in the USA. No statistically significant association was found between exposure to secondhand smoke and CIN II/III in nonsmokers, after adjustment for age, race, education, number of partners, contraceptive use, history of sexually transmitted disease and history of Pap smear. Another case–control study conducted in the USA compared 582 women with abnormal Pap smears (class 2–4) with 1866 controls with normal cytology (Scholes *et al.*, 1999). Nonsmokers exposed to secondhand smoke from spouses, partners or other household members were found to have a borderline increase in risk for abnormal cervical cytology compared to nonsmokers who were not exposed to these sources of secondhand smoke (relative risk, 1.4; 95% CI, 1.0–2.0). Risk estimates were adjusted for age, age at first sexual intercourse, and number of sexual partners during lifetime.

2.4.3   Gastrointestinal cancers

The incidence of colorectal cancer in relation to passive exposure to smoke, which was defined as having lived with a person who smoked, was examined in a 12-year prospective cohort study in Washington County, MD, USA (Sandler et al., 1988). A statistically significant reduction in risk for colorectal cancer was observed for nonsmoking women who were involuntarily exposed to smoking (relative risk, 0.7; 95% CI, 0.6–1.0), but an increased risk for this cancer was found for nonsmoking men exposed to secondhand smoke in the household (relative risk, 3.0; 95% CI, 1.8–5.0).

In a Swedish population-based case–control study, Gerhardsson de Verdier et al. (1992) found an increased risk for colon cancer in women (relative risk, 1.8; 95% CI, 1.2–2.8) and rectal cancer in men (relative risk, 1.9; 95% CI, 1.0–3.6) in association with passive smoking after adjustment for numerous potential confounders. [The Working Group noted that it is unclear whether the analysis was restricted to never-smokers.]

A large Canadian case–control study of 1171 patients newly diagnosed with histologically confirmed stomach cancer and 2207 population controls evaluated the risk associated with active and passive smoking (Mao et al., 2002). Response rates of approximately 65% were obtained for both cases and controls. The analysis of passive smoking was conducted in male never-smokers (132 cases, 343 controls). Questionnaires were mailed to respondents and provided information on lifetime exposure to secondhand smoke through residential and occupational histories and also looked at source, intensity, and duration of exposure. Risk estimates for passive smoking were adjusted for 10-year age group, province of residence, education, social class, total consumption of meat and total consumption of vegetables, fruits and juices. A positive trend ($p = 0.03$) in risk for cancer of the gastric cardia was associated with lifetime exposure to secondhand smoke (sum of years of residential plus occupational exposure) in male never-smokers. At the highest level of exposure (≥ 43 years), the relative risk was 5.8 (95% CI, 1.2–27.5). No increased risks or trends were associated with risk for distal gastric cancer. Risks assessed by subsite (cardia and distal), were similar for active and passive smoking.

2.4.4   Nasopharyngeal and nasal sinus cavity cancer

The relationship between involuntary exposure of nonsmokers to secondhand smoke and risk for these rare cancers of the upper respiratory tract has been examined in one cohort study (Hirayama, 1984) and four case–controls studies (Fukuda & Shibata, 1990; Zheng et al., 1993; Cheng et al., 1999; Yuan et al., 2000). A positive association was found in most of these studies.

Hirayama (1984) found an increased risk of nasal sinus cancer in women (histology not noted) associated with increasing numbers of cigarettes smoked by husbands of non-smoking women. When compared with nonsmoking women married to nonsmokers, wives whose husbands smoked had a relative risk of 1.7 (95% CI, 0.7–4.2) for 1–14 cigarettes per day, 2.0 (95% CI, 0.6–6.3) for 15–19 cigarettes per day and 2.55 (95% CI, 1.0–6.3) for ≥ 20 cigarettes per day (p for trend = 0.03).

Fukuda and Shibata (1990) reported the results of the first Japanese case–control study based on 169 cases of squamous-cell carcinoma of the maxillary sinus and 338 controls matched on sex, age and residence in Hokkaido, Japan. Among nonsmoking women, a relative risk of 5.4 ($p < 0.05$) was associated with exposure in the household to secondhand smoke from one or more smokers. Active smoking was associated with an increased risk for squamous-cell carcinoma in men in the same study.

Zheng *et al.* (1993) used data from the 1986 US National Mortality Followback Survey to assess risk for cancer of the nasal cavity and sinuses in relation to exposure to secondhand smoke in white men. A total of 147 deaths from cancer of the nasal cavity and sinuses were compared to 449 controls who had died from one of a variety of causes (excluding any causes strongly linked to alcohol and/or tobacco use). Data were obtained from postal questionnaires completed by next-of-kins. Among nonsmokers, patients with nasal cancer were more likely to have a spouse who smoked cigarettes (relative risk, 3.0; 95% CI, 1.0–8.9) after adjustment for age and alcohol use. When the analysis of cases was restricted to those with cancer of the maxillary sinus, the risk was somewhat higher (relative risk, 4.8; 95% CI, 0.9–24.7). The risks reported for active and for involuntary smoking were of similar magnitude in this study.

Neither involuntary exposure to tobacco smoke during childhood nor exposure during adult life were positively associated with an increased risk for nasopharyngeal cancer in a study in China (Province of Taiwan) (Cheng *et al.*, 1999). Although histological type was not specified, all cases were histologically confirmed. Among never-smokers, the risk estimates for cumulative exposure to passive smoking (pack–person–years) in childhood declined as exposure increased (p for trend = 0.05); a similar but non-significant inverse relationship was found for exposure during adulthood. Significant elevations in risk of nasopharyngeal cancer were observed for active smokers in this study. [The Working Group noted that the exposure assessment was relatively detailed and that the estimates of relative risk were adjusted for age, sex, education and family history of nasopharyngeal cancer.]

A large population-based case–control study conducted in Shanghai, China, included 935 cases of nasopharyngeal carcinoma and 1032 population controls randomly selected from a population-registry and frequency-matched by sex and 5-year age group (Yuan *et al.*, 2000). All cases were histologically confirmed, but the cell type was not specified. The study subjects were interviewed face to face, and the response rates were 84% for cases and 99% for controls. In female never-smokers, a consistent increase in risk related to exposure to secondhand smoke during childhood was noted. If the mother smoked, the relative risk was 3.4 (95% CI, 1.4–8.1); if the father smoked, the relative risk was 3.0

(95% CI, 1.4–6.2); if another household member smoked, the relative risk was 2.7 (95% CI, 1.1–6.9), and if any household member smoked, the relative risk was 3.0 (95% CI, 1.4–6.2). Risks associated with exposure to secondhand smoke during adult-hood in women were also statistically significantly increased. For male never-smokers, the associations were weaker and were not statistically significant for exposure during childhood and adulthood. Gender-specific risk estimates were adjusted for age, level of education, consumption of preserved foods, oranges and tangerines, exposure to rapeseed oil, exposure to burning coal during cooking, occupational exposure to chemical fumes, history of chronic ear and nose conditions and family history of nasopharyngeal cancer. [The Working Group noted that this was a large, well-conducted study that included a detailed exposure assessment and adjustment for numerous potential confounders.]

2.4.5   *Tumours of the brain and central nervous system*

A population-based case–control study of patients with incident primary brain tumours diagnosed from 1987 through 1990 in Adelaide, Australia, was reported by Ryan *et al.* (1992). Controls were selected from the Australian electoral rolls which cover 95% of the population. Response rates of 90% and 63% were obtained for cases and controls, respectively. The study included 110 histologically confirmed cases of glioma, 60 menin-gioma cases and 417 controls. An increased risk of meningioma was associated with invo-luntary exposure to tobacco from the spouse, particularly among women (relative risk, 2.7; 95% CI, 1.2–6.1). No statistically significant association was found between active smoking and either glioma or meningioma in this study.

References

Akiba, S., Kato, H. & Blot, W.J. (1986) Passive smoking and lung cancer among Japanese women. *Cancer Res.*, **46**, 4804–4807

Alavanja, M.C.R., Brown, C.C., Swanson, C., Brownson, R.C. (1993) Saturated fat intake and lung cancer risk among non-smoking women in Missouri. *J. nat. Cancer Inst.*, **85**, 6–16

Bennett, W.P., Alavanja, M.C.R., Blomeke, B., Vähäkangas, K.H., Castren, K., Welsh, J.A., Bowman, E.D., Khan, M.A., Flieder, D.B. & Harris, C.C. (1999) Environmental tobacco smoke, genetic susceptibility, and risk of lung cancer in never-smoking women. *J. natl Cancer Inst.*, **91**, 2009–2014

Berlin, J.A., Longnecker, M.P. & Greenland, S. (1993) Meta-analysis of epidemiologic dose-response data. *Epidemiology*, **4**, 218–228

Bero, L.A., Glantz, S.A. & Rennie D. (1994) Publication bias and public health policy on environ-mental tobacco smoke. *J. Am. med. Assoc.*, **272**, 133–136

Biggerstaff, B.J., Tweedie, R.L. & Mengersen, K.L. (1994) Passive smoking in the workplace: Classical and Bayesian meta-analysis. *Int. Arch. occup. environ. Health*, **66**, 269–277

Boffetta, P. (2002) Involuntary smoking and lung cancer. *Scand. J. Work Environ. Health*, **28** (Suppl. 2), 30–40

Boffetta, P., Agudo, A., Ahrens, W., Benhamou, E., Benhamou, S., Darby, S.C., Ferro, G., Fortes, C., Gonzales, C.A., Jöckel, K.-H., Krauss, M., Kreienbrock, L., Kreuzer, M., Mendes, A., Merletti, F., Nyberg, F., Pershagen, G., Pohlabeln, H., Riboli, E., Schmid, G., Simonato, L., Tredaniel, J., Whitley, E., Wichmann, H.-E., Winck, C., Zambon, P. & Saracci, R. (1998) Multicenter case–control study of exposure to environmental tobacco smoke and lung cancer. *J. natl Cancer Inst.*, **90**, 1440–1450

Boffetta, P., Ahrens, W., Nyberg, F., Mukeria, A., Brüske-Hohlfeld, I., Fortes, C., Constantinescu, V., Simonato, L., Batura-Gabryel, H., Lea, S., Gaborieau, V. & Benhamou, S. (1999a) Exposure to environmental tobacco smoke and risk of adenocarcinoma of the lung. *Int. J. Cancer*, **83**, 635–639

Boffetta, P., Nyberg, F., Agudo, A., Benhamou, E., Joeckel, K.H., Kreuzer, M., Merletti, F., Pershagen, G., Pohlabeln, H., Simonato, L., Wichmann, H.E. & Saracci, R. (1999b) Risk of lung cancer from exposure to environmental tobacco smoke from cigars, cigarillos and pipes. *Int. J. Cancer*, **83**, 805–806

Boffetta, P., Tredaniel, J. & Greco, A. (2000) Risk of childhood cancer and adult lung cancer after childhood exposure to passive smoke: A meta-analysis. *Environ. Health Perspect.*, **108**, 73–82

Brennan, P., Butler, J., Agudo, A., Benhamou, S., Darby, S., Fortes, C., Joeckel, K.H., Kreuzer, M., Nyberg, F., Pohlabeln, H., Saracci, R., Wichmann, H.E. & Boffetta, P. (2000) Joint effect of diet and environmental tobacco smoke on risk of lung cancer among nonsmokers. *J. natl Cancer Inst.*, **92**, 426–427

Brondum, J., Shu, X.-O., Steinbuch, M., Severson, R.K., Potter, J.D. & Robison, L.L. (1999) Parental cigarette smoking and the risk of acute leukemia in children. *Cancer*, **85**, 1380–1388

Brown, K.G. (1999) Lung cancer and environmental tobacco smoke: Occupational risk to non-smokers. *Environ. Health Perspect.*, **107** (Suppl. 6), 885–890

Brownson, R.C., Reif, J.S., Keefe, T.J., Ferguson, S.W. & Pritzl, J.A. (1987) Risk factors for adenocarcinoma of the lung. *Am. J. Epidemiol.*, **125**, 25–34

Brownson, R.C., Alavanja, M.C., Hock, E.T. & Loy, T.S. (1992) Passive smoking and lung cancer in nonsmoking women. *Am. J. public Health*, **82**, 1525–1530

Buckley, J.D., Hobbie, W.L., Ruccione, K., Sather, H.N., Woods, W.G. & Hammond, G.D. (1986) Maternal smoking during pregnancy and risk of childhood cancer [Letter]. *Lancet*, **ii**, 519–520

Buffler, P.A., Pickle, L.W., Mason, T.J. & Contant, C. (1984) The causes of lung cancer in Texas. In: Mizell, M. & Corres, P., eds, *Lung Cancer: Causes and Prevention*, New York, Verlag Chemie International, pp. 83–99

Bunin, G.R., Buckley, J.D., Boesel, C.P., Rorke, L.B. & Meadows, A.T. (1994) Risk factors for astrocytic glioma and primitive neuroectodermal tumor of the brain in young children: A report from the Children's Cancer Group. *Cancer Epidemiol. Biomarkers Prev.*, **3**, 197–204

Butler, T.L. (1988) *The Relationship of Passive Smoking to Various Health Outcomes Among Seventh-day Adventists in California*, Los Angeles, University of California, Doctoral thesis

Cardenas, V.M., Thun, M.J., Austin, H., Lally, C.A., Clark, W.S., Greenberg, S. & Heath, C.W., Jr (1997) Environmental tobacco smoke and lung cancer mortality in the American Cancer Society's cancer prevention study II. *Cancer Causes Control*, **8**, 57–64

Chan, W.C. & Fung, S.C. (1982) Lung cancer in non-smokers in Hong Kong. In: Grundmann, E., ed., *Cancer Epidemiology* (Cancer Campaign 6), Stuttgart, Gustav Fischer Verlag, pp. 199–202

Chang-Claude, J., Krupp, S., Jager, B., Bartsch, H. & Risch, A. (2002) Differential effect of NAT2 on the association between active and passive smoke exposure and breast cancer risk. *Cancer Epidemiol. Biomarkers Prev.*, **8**, 698–704

Chappell, W.R. & Gratt, L.B. (1996) A graphical method for pooling epidemiological studies. *Am. J. public Health*, **88**, 1011–1012

Cheng, Y.-J., Hildesheim, A., Hsu, M.-M., Chen, I.-H., Brinton, L.A., Levine, P.H., Chen, C.-J. & Yang, C.-S. (1999) Cigarette smoking, alcohol consumption and risk of nasopharyngeal carcinoma in Taiwan. *Cancer Causes Control*, **10**, 201–207

Choi, S.-Y., Lee, K.-H. & Lee, T.-O. (1989) A case–control study on risk factors in lung cancer. *Korean J. Epidemiol.*, **11**, 66–80

Coker, A.L., Rosenberg, A.J., McCann, M.F. & Hulka, B.S. (1992) Active and passive cigarette smoke exposure and cervical intraepithelial neoplasia. *Cancer Epidemiol. Biomarkers Prev.*, **1**, 349–356

Copas, J.B. & Shi, J.Q. (2000) Reanalysis of epidemiological evidence on lung cancer and passive smoking. *Br. med. J.*, **320**, 417–418

Cordier, S., Iglesias, M.-J., LeGoaster, C., Guyot, M.-M., Mandereau, L. & Hemon, D. (1994) Incidence and risk factors for childhood brain tumors in the Ile de France. *Int. J. Cancer*, **59**, 776–782

Correa, P., Pickle, L.W., Fontham, E., Lin, Y. & Haenszel, W. (1983) Passive smoking and lung cancer. *Lancet*, **ii**, 595–597

Dalager, N.A., Pickle, L.W., Mason, T.J., Correa, P., Fontham, E.T.H., Stemhagen, A., Buffler, P.A., Ziegler, R.G. & Fraumeni, J.F., Jr (1986) The relation of passive smoking to lung cancer. *Cancer Res.*, **46**, 4808–4811

Delfino, R.J., Smith, C., West, J.G., Lin, H.J., White, E., Liao, S.-Y., Gim, J.S.Y., Ma, H.L., Butler, J. & Anton-Culver, H. (2000) Breast cancer, passive and active cigarette smoking and *N*-acetyltransferase 2 genotype. *Pharmacogenetics*, **10**, 461–469

Dersimonian, R. & Laird, N. (1986) Meta-analysis in clinical trials. *Controlled clin. Trials*, 177–188

Du, Y.X., Cha, Q., Chen, Y.Z. & Wu, J.M. (1993) Exposure to environmental tobacco smoke and female lung cancer in Guangzhou, China. *Proc. Indoor Air*, **1**, 511–516

Egan, K.M., Stampfer, M.J., Hunter, D., Hankinson, S., Rosner, B.A., Holmes, M., Willett, W.C. & Colditz, G.A. (2002) Active and passive smoking in breast cancer: Prospective results from the Nurses' Health Study. *Epidemiology*, **13**, 138–145

Filippini, G., Farinotti, M., Lovicu, G., Maisonneuve, P. & Boyle, P. (1994) Mothers' active and passive smoking during pregnancy and risk of brain tumors in children. *Int. J. Cancer*, **57**, 769–774

Filippini, G., Farinotti, M. & Ferrarini, M. (2000) Active and passive smoking during pregnancy and risk of central nervous system tumours in children. *Paediatr. perinatal Epidemiol.*, **14**, 78–84

Fleiss, J.L. & Gross, A.J. (1991) Meta-analysis in epidemiology, with special reference to studies of the association between exposure to environmental tobacco smoke and lung cancer: A critique. *J. clin. Epidemiol.*, **44**, 127–139

Fontham, E.T.H., Correa, P., Wu-Williams, A.H., Reynolds, P., Greenberg, R.S., Buffler, P.A., Chen, V.W., Boyd, P., Alterman, T., Austin, D.F., Liff, J. & Greenberg, S.D. (1991) Lung cancer in nonsmoking women: A multicenter case–control study. *Cancer Epidemiol. Biomarkers Prev.*, **1**, 35–43

Fontham, E.T.H., Correa, P., Reynolds, P., Wu-Williams, A., Buffler, P.A., Greenberg, R.S., Chen, V.W., Alterman, T., Boyd, P., Austin, D.F. & Liff, J. (1994) Environmental tobacco smoke and lung cancer in nonsmoking women. A multicenter study. *J. Am. med. Assoc.*, **271**, 1752–1759

Forsberg, J.-G. & Kallen, B. (1990) Pregnancy and delivery characteristics of women whose infants develop child cancer. *APMIS*, **98**, 37–42

Fukuda, K. & Shibata, A. (1990) Exposure–response relationships between woodworking, smoking or passive smoking and squamous cell neoplasms of the maxillary sinus. *Cancer Causes Control*, **1**, 165–168

Gao, Y.-T., Blot, W.J., Zheng, W., Ershow, A.G., Hsu, C.W., Levin, L.I., Zhang, R. & Fraumeni, J.F., Jr (1987) Lung cancer among Chinese women. *Int. J. Cancer*, **40**, 604–609

Garfinkel, L. (1981) Time trends in lung cancer mortality among nonsmokers and a note on passive smoking. *J. natl Cancer Inst.*, **66**, 1061–1066

Garfinkel, L., Auerbach, O. & Joubert, L. (1985) Involuntary smoking and lung cancer: A case–control study. *J. natl Cancer Inst.*, **75**, 463–469

Geng, G.Y., Liang, Z.H., Zhang, A.Y. & Wu, G.L. (1988) On the relationship between smoking and female lung cancer. In: Aoki, M., Hisamichi, S. & Tominaga, S., eds, *Smoking and Health*, Amsterdam, Elsevier, pp. 483–486

Gerhardsson de Verdier, M., Plato, N., Steineck, G. & Peters, J.M. (1992) Occupational exposures and cancer of the colon and rectum. *Am. J. ind. Med.*, **22**, 291–303

Gold, E., Gordis, L., Tonascia, J. & Szklo, M. (1979) Risk factors for brain tumors in children. *Am. J. Epidemiol*, **109**, 309–319

Gold, E.B., Leviton, A., Lopez, R., Gilles, F.H., Hedley-Whyte, E.T., Kolonel, L.N., Lyon, J.L., Swanson, G.M., Weiss, N.S., West, D., Aschenbrener, C. & Austin, D.F. (1993) Parental smoking and risk of childhood brain tumors. *Am. J. Epidemiol.*, **137**, 620–628

Golding, J., Paterson, M. & Kinlen, L.J. (1990) Factors associated with childhood cancer in a national cohort study. *Br. J. Cancer*, **62**, 3034–3038

Golding, J., Greenwood, R., Birmingham, K. & Mott, M. (1992) Childhood cancer, intramuscular vitamin K, and pethidine given during labor. *Br. med. J.*, **305**, 341–346

Hackshaw, A.K. (1998) Lung cancer and passive smoking. *Stat. Meth. med. Res.*, **7**, 119–136

Hackshaw, A.K., Law, M.R. & Wald, N.J. (1997) The accumulated evidence on lung cancer and environmental tobacco smoke. *Br. med. J.*, **315**, 980–988

Hackshaw, A.K., Law, M.R. & Wald, N.J. (2000) Increased risk is not disputed. *Br. med. J.*, **321**, 1221–1222

Heller, W.-D., Scherer, G., Sennewald, E. & Adlkofer, F. (1998) Misclassification of smoking in a follow-up population study in southern Germany. *Clin. Epidemiol.*, **51**, 211–218

Hirayama, T. (1981) Nonsmoking wives of heavy smokers have a higher risk of lung cancer: A study from Japan. *Br. med. J.*, **282**, 183–185

Hirayama, T. (1984) Cancer mortality in nonsmoking women with smoking husbands based on a large-scale cohort study in Japan. *Prev. Med.*, **13**, 680–690

Hirayama, T. (1989) Dietary habits are of limited importance in influencing the lung cancer risk among Japanese females who never smoked. In: Bieva, C.J., Courtois, Y. & Govaerts, M., eds, *Present and Future Indoor Air Quality. Proceedings of the Brussels Conference*, Amsterdam, Elsevier Science

Hole, D.J., Gills, C.R., Chopra, C. & Hawthorne, V.M. (1989) Passive smoking and cardiorespiratory health in a general population in the west of Scotland. *Br. med. J.*, **299**, 423–427

Holly, E.A., Aston, D.A., Ahn, D.K. & Kristiansen, J.J. (1992) Ewing's bone sarcoma, paternal occupational exposure, and other factors. *Am. J. Epidemiol.*, **135**, 122–129

Howe, G.R., Burch, J.D., Chiarelli, A.M., Risch, H. & Choi, B.C.K. (1989) An exploratory case–control study of brain tumors in children. *Cancer Res.*, **49**, 4349–4352

Humble, C.G., Samet, J.M. & Pathak, D.R. (1987) Marriage to a smoker and lung cancer risk. *Am. J. public Health*, **77**, 598–602

IARC (1986) *IARC Monographs on the Evaluation of the Carcinogenic Risk of Chemicals to Humans*, Vol. 38, *Tobacco Smoking*, Lyon, IARCPress

Infante-Rivard, C., Krajinovic, M., Labuda, D. & Sinnett, D. (2000) Parental smoking, *CYP1A1* genetic polymorphisms and childhood leukemia (Quebec, Canada). *Cancer Causes Control*, **11**, 547–553

Inoue, R. & Hirayama, T. (1988) Passive smoking and lung cancer in women. In: Aoki, M., Hisamichi, S. & Tominaga, S., eds, *Smoking and Health*, Amsterdam, Elsevier, pp. 283–285

Janerich, D.T., Thompson, W.D., Varela, L.R., Greenwald, P., Chorost, S., Tucci, C., Zaman, M.B., Melamed, M., Kiely, M. & McKneally, M.F. (1990) Lung cancer and exposure to tobacco smoke in the household. *New Engl. J. Med.*, **323**, 632–636

Jee, S.H., Ohrr, H. & Kim, I.-S. (1999) Effects of husbands' smoking on the incidence of lung cancer in Korean women. *Int. J. Epidemiol.*, **28**, 824–828

Ji, B.T., Shu, X.O., Linet, M.S., Zheng, W., Wacholder, S., Gao, Y.T., Ying, D.M. & Jin, F. (1997) Paternal cigarette smoking and the risk of childhood cancer among offspring of nonsmoking mothers. *J. natl Cancer Inst.*, **89**, 238–244

Jöckel, K.-H., Krauss, M., Pohlabeln, H., Ahrens, W., Kreuzer, M., Kreienbrock, L., Möhner, M. & Wichmann, H.E. (1998a) Lungenkrebsrisiko durch berufliche Exposition – Passivrauchen. In: Wichmann, H.E., Jöckel, K.-H. & Robra, B.P., eds, *Fortschritte in der Epidemiologie, Lungenkrebsrisiko durch berufliche Exposition*, Landsberg, Ecomed, pp. 227–236

Jöckel, K.-H., Pohlabeln, H., Ahrens, W. & Krauss, M. (1998b) Environmental tobacco smoke and lung cancer. *Epidemiology*, **9**, 672–675

John, E., Savitz, D.A. & Sandler, D.P. (1991) Prenatal exposure to parents smoking and childhood cancer. *Am. J. Epidemiol.*, **133**, 123–132

Johnson, K.C., Hu, J., Mao, Y. & The Canadian Cancer Registries Epidemiology Research Group. (2000) Passive and active smoking and breast cancer risk in Canada, 1994–97. *Cancer Causes Control*, **11**, 211–221

Johnson, K.C., Hu, J., Mao, Y. & Canadian Cancer Registries Epidemiology Research Group (2001) Lifetime residential and workplace exposure to environmental tobacco smoke and lung cancer in never-smoking women, Canada 1994–1997. *Int. J. Cancer*, **93**, 902–906

Kabat, G.C. (1990) Epidemiologic studies of the relationship between passive smoking and lung cancer. In: *Proceedings of the 1990 Annual Winter Meeting of the Toxicology Forum*, Washington DC

Kabat, G.C. & Wynder, E.L. (1984) Lung cancer in nonsmokers. *Cancer*, **53**, 1214–1221

Kabat, G.C., Stellman, S.D. & Wynder, E.L. (1995) Relation between exposure to environmental tobacco smoke and lung cancer in lifetime nonsmokers. *Am. J. Epidemiol.*, **142**, 141–148

Kalandidi, A., Trichopoulos, D., Hatzakis, A., Tzannes, S. & Saracci, R. (1987) Passive smoking and chronic obstructive lung disease. *Lancet*, **ii**, 1325–1326

Kalandidi, A., Katsouyanni, K., Voropoulou, N., Bastas, G., Saracci, R. & Trichopoulos, D. (1990) Passive smoking and diet in the etiology of lung cancer among non-smokers. *Cancer Causes Control*, **1**, 15–21

Katada, H., Mikami, R., Konishi, M., Koyama, Y. & Narita, N. (1988) Effect of passive smoking in lung cancer development in women in the Nara region. *Gan No Rinsho*, **34**, 21–27

Keil, U., Stieber, J., Filipiak, B., Löwel, H. & Wichmann, H.E. (1998) On misclassification of smoking (Letter to the Editor). *J. clin. Epidemiol.*, **52**, 91–93

Klebanoff, M.A., Clemens, J.D. & Read, J.S. (1996) Maternal smoking during pregnancy and childhood cancer. *Am. J. Epidemiol.*, **144**, 1028–1033

Ko, Y.-C., Lee, C.-H., Chen, M.-J., Huang, C.-C., Chang, W.-Y., Lin, H.-J., Wang, H.-Z. & Chang, P.-Y. (1997) Risk factors for primary lung cancer among non-smoking women in Taiwan. *Int. J. Epidemiol.*, **26**, 24–31

Koo, L.C., Ho, J.H.-C. & Saw, D. (1983) Active and passive smoking among female lung cancer patients in Hong Kong. *J. exp. clin. Cancer Res.*, **4**, 367–375

Koo, L.C., Ho, J.H.-C. & Saw, D. (1984) Is passive smoking an added risk factor for lung cancer in Chinese women? *J. exp. clin. Cancer Res.*, **3**, 277–283

Koo, L.C., Ho, J.H., Saw, D. & Ho, C.Y. (1987) Measurements of passive smoking and estimates of lung cancer risk among non-smoking Chinese females. *Int. J. Cancer*, **39**, 162–169

Koo, L.C., Ho, J.H.-C. & Rylander, R. (1988) Life-history correlates of environmental tobacco smoke: A study on nonsmoking Hong Kong Chinese wives with smoking versus nonsmoking husbands. *Soc. Sci. Med.*, **26**, 751–760

Kramer, S., Ward, E., Meadows, A.T. & Malone, K.E. (1987) Medical and drug risk factors associated with neuroblastoma: A case–control study. *J. natl Cancer Inst.*, **78**, 797–804

Kreuzer, M., Krauss, M., Kreienbrock, L., Jockel, K.-H. & Wichmann, H.-E. (2000) Environmental tobacco smoke and lung cancer: A case–control study in Germany. *Am. J. Epidemiol.*, **151**, 241–250

Kreuzer, M., Gerken, M., Kreienbrock, L., Wellmann, J., Wichmann, H.E. (2001) Lung cancer in lifetime nonsmoking men – results of a case–control study in Germany. *Br. J. Cancer*, **84**, 134–140

Kreuzer, M., Heinrich, J., Kreienbrock, L., Rosario, A.S., Gerken, M. & Wichmann, H.E. (2002) Risk factors for lung cancer among nonsmoking women. *Int. J. Cancer*, **100**, 706–713

Kropp, S. & Chang-Claude, J. (2002) Active and passive smoking and risk of breast cancer by age 50 years among German women. *Am. J. Epidemiol.*, **156**, 616–626

Kuijten, R.R., Bunin, G.R., Nass, C.C. & Meadows, A.T. (1990) Gestational and familial risk factors for childhood astrocytoma: Results of a case–control study. *Cancer Res.*, **50**, 2608–2612

Lam, W.K. (1985) *A Clinical and Epidemiological Study of Carcinoma of the Lung in Hong Kong*, Hong Kong, University of Hong Kong, Doctoral thesis

Lam, T.H., Kung, I.T., Wong, C.M., Lam, W.K., Kleevens, J.W., Saw, D., Hsu, C., Seneviratne, S., Lam, S.Y. & Lo, K.K. (1987) Smoking, passive smoking and histological types in lung cancer in Hong Kong Chinese women. *Br. J. Cancer*, **56**, 673–678

Lash, T.L. & Aschengrau, A. (1999) Active and passive cigarette smoking and the occurrence of breast cancer. *Am. J. Epidemiol.*, **149**, 5–12

Lee, P.N. (1987a) Lung cancer and passive smoking: Association of an artifact due to misclassification of smoking habits? *Toxicol. Lett.*, **35**, 157–162

Lee, P.N. (1987b) Passive smoking and lung cancer association: A result of bias? *Hum. Toxicol.*, **6**, 517–524

Lee, P.N. (1988) *Misclassification of Smoking Habits and Passive Smoking*, Berlin, Springer Verlag

Lee, P.N. (1991a) *Correcting Meta-analyses of the Association of Lung Cancer in Females with Spouse (or Household) Exposure for Bias due to Misclassification of Active Smoking Status* (Report submitted to US Environmental Protection Agency, dated 29 November 1991)

Lee, P.N. (1991b) An estimate of adult mortality in the United States from passive smoking. *Environ. int.*, **17**, 379–381

Lee, P.N. (1992) *Environmental Tobacco Smoke and Mortality*, Basel, Karger

Lee, P.N. (1998) Difficulties in assessing the relationship between passive smoking and lung cancer. *Stat. Meth. med. Res.*, **7**, 137–163

Lee, P.N., Chamberlain, J. & Alderson, M.R. (1986) Relationship of passive smoking to risk of lung cancer and other smoking-associated diseases. *Br. J. Cancer*, **54**, 97–105

Lee, C.H., Ko, Y.C., Goggins, W., Huang, J.J., Huang, M.S., Kao, E.L. & Wang, H.Z. (2000) Lifetime environmental exposure to tobacco smoke and primary lung cancer of non-smoking Taiwanese women. *Int. J. Epidemiol.*, **29**, 224–231

Lee, P.N., Forey, B. & Fry, J.S. (2001) Revisiting the association between environmental tobacco smoke and exposure to lung cancer risk. III. Adjustment for the biasing effect of misclassification of smoking habits. *Indoor Built Environ.*, **10**, 384–398

Levois, M.E. & Layard, M.W. (1994) Inconsistency between workplace and spousal studies of environmental tobacco smoke and lung cancer. *Regul. Toxic. Pharmacol.*, **19**, 309–316

Liu, Z., He, X. & Chapman, R.S. (1991) Smoking and other risk factors for lung cancer in Xuanwei, China. *Int. J. Epidemiol.*, **20**, 26–31

Liu, Q., Sasco, A.J., Riboli, E. & Hu, M.X. (1993) Indoor air pollution and lung cancer in Ghuangzhou, People's Republic of China. *Am. J. Epidemiol.*, **137**, 145–154

Lubin, J.H. (1999) Estimating lung cancer risk with exposure to environmental tobacco smoke. *Environ. Health Perspect.*, **107** (Suppl. 6), 879–883

McCredie, M., Maisonneuve, P. & Boyle, P. (1994) Perinatal and early postnatal risk factors for malignant brain tumours in New South Wales children. *Int. J. Cancer*, **56**, 11–15

McKinney, P.A., Stiller, C.A. (for the IRESCC group) (1986). Maternal smoking during pregnancy and the risk of childhood cancer [Letter]. *Lancet*, **ii**, 519

Magnani, C., Pastore, G., Luzzatto, L., Carli, M., Lubrano, P. & Terracini, B. (1989) Risk factors for soft tissue sarcomas in childhood: A case–control study. *Tumori*, **75**, 396–400

Magnani, C., Pastore, G., Luzzatto, L. & Terracini, B. (1990) Parental occupation and other environmental factors in the etiology of leukemias and non-Hodgkin's lymphomas in childhood: A case–control study. *Tumori*, **76**, 413–419

Manning, M.D. & Carroll, B.E. (1957) Some epidemiological aspects of leukemia in children. *J. natl Cancer Inst.*, **19**, 1087–1094

Mao, Y., Hu, J., Semenciw, R., White, K., and the Canadian Cancer Registries Epidemiology Research Group (2002) Active and passive smoking and the risk of stomach cancer, by subsite, in Canada. *Eur. J. Cancer Prev.*, **11**, 27–38

Marcus, P.M., Newman, B., Millikan, R.C., Moorman, P.G., Baird, D.D. & Qaqish, B. (2000) The associations of adolescent cigarette smoking, alcoholic beverage consumption, environmental tobacco smoke, and ionizing radiation with subsequent breast cancer risk (United States). *Cancer Causes Control*, **11**, 271–278

Mayne, S.T., Janerich, D.T., Greenwald, P., Chorost, S., Tucci, C., Zaman, M.B., Melamed, M.R., Kiely, M. & McKneally, M.F. (1994) Dietary beta carotene and lung cancer risk in US non-smokers. *J. natl Cancer Inst.*, **86**, 33–38

Miller, G.H. (1990) The impact of passive smoking: Cancer deaths among nonsmoking women. *Cancer Detect. Prev.*, **14**, 497–503

Millikan, R.C., Pittman, G.S., Newman, B., Tse, C.-K.J., Selmin, O., Rockhill, B., Savitz, D., Moorman, P.G. & Bell, D.A. (1998) Cigarette smoking, *N*-acetyltransferases 1 and 2, and breast cancer risk. *Cancer Epidemiol. Biomarkers Prev.*, **7**, 371–378

Morabia, A., Bernstein, M., Heritier, S. & Khatchatrian, N. (1996) Relation of breast cancer with passive and active exposure to tobacco smoke. *Am. J. Epidemiol.*, **143**, 918–928

Morabia, A., Bernstein, M.S., Bouchardy, I., Kurtz, J. & Morris, M.A. (2000) Breast cancer and active and passive smoking: The role of the *N*-acetyltransferase 2 genotype. *Am. J. Epidemiol.*, **152**, 226–232

National Research Council (1986) *Environmental Tobacco Smoke: Measuring Exposures and Assessing Health Effects*, Washington DC, National Academy Press

Neutel, C.I. & Buck, C. (1971) Effect of smoking during pregnancy on the risk of cancer in children. *J. natl Cancer Inst.*, **47**, 59–63

Nishino, Y., Tsubono, Y., Tsuji, I., Komatsu, S., Kanemura, S., Nakatsuka, H., Fukao, A., Satoh, H. & Hisamichi, S. (2001) Passive smoking at home and cancer risk: A population-based prospective study in Japanese nonsmoking women. *Cancer Causes Control*, **12**, 797–802

Norman, M.A., Holly, E.A., Ahn, D.K., Preston-Martin, S., Mueller, B.A. & Bracci, P.M. (1996) Prenatal exposure to tobacco smoke and childhood brain tumors: Results from the United States West Coast Childhood Brain Tumor Study. *Cancer Epidemiol. Biomarkers Prev.*, **5**, 127–133

Nyberg, F., Isaksson, I., Harris, J.R. & Pershagen, G. (1997) Misclassification of smoking status and lung cancer risk from environmental tobacco smoke in never-smokers. *Epidemiology*, **8**, 304–309

Nyberg, F., Agrenius, V., Svartengren, K., Svensson, C. & Pershagen, G. (1998) Environmental tobacco smoke and lung cancer in nonsmokers: Does time since exposure play a role? *Epidemiology*, **9**, 301–308

Olshan, A.F., Breslow, N.E., Falletta, J.M., Grufferman, S., Pendergrass, T., Robison, L.L., Waskerwitz, M., Woods, W.G., Vietti, T.J. & Hammond, G.D. (1993) Risk factors for Wilms tumor: Report from the National Wilms Tumor Study. *Cancer*, **72**, 938–944

Pershagen, G., Hrubec, Z. & Svensson, C. (1987) Passive smoking and lung cancer in Swedish women. *Am. J. Epidemiol.*, **125**, 17–24

Pershagen, G., Ericson, A. & Otterblad-Olausson, P. (1992) Maternal smoking in pregnancy: Does it increase the risk of childhood cancer? *Int. J. Epidemiol.*, **21**, 1–5

Peto, J. (1992) Meta-analysis of epidemiological studies of carcinogenesis. In: Vainio, H., Magee, P.N., McGregor, D.B. & McMichael, A.J., eds, *Mechanisms of Carcinogenesis in Risk Identification* (IARC Scientific Publications No. 116), Lyon, IARC*Press*, pp. 571–577

Preston-Martin, S., Yu, M.C., Benton, B. & Henderson, B.E. (1982) N-nitroso compounds and childhood brain tumors: A case–control study. *Cancer Res.*, **42**, 5240–5245

Rapiti, E., Jindal, S.K., Gupta, D. & Boffetta, P. (1999) Passive smoking and lung cancer in Chandigarh, India. *Lung Cancer*, **23**, 183–189

Reynolds, P., Von Behren, J., Fontham, E.T.H., Wu, A., Buffler, P. & Greenberg, R. (1996) Occupational exposure to environmental tobacco smoke [Letter]. *J. Am. med. Assoc.*, **275**, 441–442

Riboli, E., Haley, N.J., Tredaniel, J., Saracci, R., Preston-Martin, S. & Trichopolous, D. (1995) Misclassification of smoking status among women in relation to exposure to environmental tobacco smoke. *Eur. respir. J.*, **8**, 285–290

Roman, E., Watson, A., Beral, V., Buckle, S., Bull, D., Baker, K., Ryder, H. & Barton, C. (1993) Case–control study of leukaemia and non-Hodgkin's lymphoma among children aged 0–4 years living in West Berkshire and North Hampshire health districts. *Br. med. J.*, **306**, 615–621

Ryan, P., Lee, M.W., North, J.B. & McMichael, A.J. (1992) Risk factors for tumors of the brain and meninges: Results from the Adelaide Adult Brain Tumor study. *Int. J. Cancer*, **51**, 20–27

Sandler, D.P., Everson, R.B., Wilcox, A.J. & Browder, J.P. (1985a) Cancer risk in adulthood from early life exposure to parents' smoking. *Am. J. public Health*, **75**, 487–492

Sandler, D.P., Everson, R.B. & Wilcox, A.J. (1985b). Passive smoking in adulthood and cancer risk. *Am. J. Epidemiol.*, **121**, 37–48

Sandler, R.S., Sandler, D.P., Comstock, G.W., Helsing, K.J. & Shore, D.L. (1988) Cigarette smoking and the risk of colorectal cancer in women. *J. natl Cancer Inst.*, **80**, 1329–1333

Scholes, D., McBride, C., Grothaus, L., Curry, S., Albright, J. & Ludman, E. (1999) The association between cigarette smoking and low-grade cervical abnormalities in reproductive-age women. *Cancer Causes Control*, **10**, 339–344

Schwartz, A.G., Yang, P. & Swanson, G.M. (1996) Familial risk of lung cancer among nonsmokers and their relatives. *Am. J. Epidemiol.*, **144**, 554–562

Schwartzbaum, J.A. (1992) Influence of the mother's prenatal drug consumption on risk of neuroblastoma in the child. *Am. J. Epidemiol.*, **135**, 1358–1367

Severson, R.K., Buckley, J.D., Woods, W.G., Benjamin, D. & Robison, L.L. (1993) Cigarette smoking and alcohol consumption by parents of children with acute myeloid leukemia: An analysis within morphological subgroups—a report from the Childrens Cancer Group. *Cancer Epidemiol. Biomarkers Prev.*, **2**, 433–439

Shen, X.B., Wang, G.X. & Zhou, B.S. (1998) Relation of environmental tobacco smoke and pulmonary adenocarcinoma in non-smoking women: A case–control study in Nanjing. *Oncol. Rep.*, **5**, 1221–1223

Shimizu, H., Morishita, M., Mizuno, K., Masuda, T., Ogura, Y., Santo, M., Nishimura, M., Kunishima, K., Karasawa, K., Nishiwaki, K., Yamamoto, M., Hisamichi, S. & Tominaga, S. (1988) A case–control study of lung cancer in non-smoking women. *Tohoku J. exp. Med.*, **154**, 389–397

Shu, X.-O., Ross, J.A., Pendergrass, T.W., Reaman, G.H., Lampkin, B. & Robison, L.L. (1996) Parental alcohol consumption, cigarette smoking, and risk of infant leukemia: A Childrens Cancer Group study. *J. natl Cancer Inst.*, **88**, 24–31

Slattery, M.L., Robison, L.M., Schuman, K.L., French, T.K., Abbott, T.M., Overall, J.C., Jr & Gardner, J.W. (1989) Cigarette smoking and exposure to passive smoke are risk factors for cervical cancer. *J. Am. med. Assoc.*, **262**, 1593–1598

Smith, S.J., Deacon, J.M., Chilvers, C.E.D. & members of the UK National Case–Control Study Group. (1994) Alcohol, smoking, passive smoking and caffeine in relation to breast cancer risk in young women. *Br. J. Cancer*, **70**, 113–119

Sobue, T. (1990) Association of indoor air pollution and lifestyle with lung cancer in Osaka, Japan. *Int. J. Epidemiol.*, **19** (Suppl. 1), S62–S66

Sorahan, T., Lancashire, R., Prior, P., Peck, I. & Stewart, A. (1995) Childhood cancer and prenatal use of alcohol and tobacco. *Ann. Epidemiol.*, **5**, 354–359

Sorahan, T., Lancashire, R.J., Hulten, M.A., Peck, I. & Stewart, A.M. (1997a) Childhood cancer and parental use of tobacco: Deaths from 1953 to 1955. *Br. J. Cancer*, **75**, 134–138

Sorahan, T., Prior, P., Lancashire, R.J., Faux, S.P., Hulten, M.A., Peck, I.M. & Stewart, A.M. (1997b) Childhood cancer and parental use of tobacco: Deaths from 1971 to 1976. *Br. J. Cancer*, **76**, 1525–1531

Sorahan, T., McKinney, P.A., Mann, J.R., Lancashire, R.J., Stiller, C.A., Birch, J.M., Dodd, H.E. and Cartwright, R.A. (2001) Childhood cancer and parental use of tobacco: Findings from the inter-regional epidemiological study of childhood cancer (IRESCC) *Br. J. Cancer*, **84**, 141–148

Speizer, F.E., Colditz, G.A., Hunter, D.J., Rosner, B. & Hennekens, C. (1999) Prospective study of smoking, antioxidant intake, and lung cancer in middle-aged women (USA). *Cancer Causes Control*, **10**, 475–482

Stewart, A., Webb, J. & Hewitt, D. (1958) A survey of childhood malignancies. *Br. med. J.*, **5086**, 1495–1508

Stjernfeldt, M., Berglund, K., Lindsten, J. & Ludvigsson, J. (1986) Maternal smoking during pregnancy and risk of childhood cancer. *Lancet*, **i**, 1350–1352

Stockwell, H.G., Goldman, A.L., Lyman, G.H., Noss, C.I., Armstrong, A.W., Pinkham, P.A., Candelora, E.C. & Brusa, M.R. (1992) Environmental tobacco smoke and lung cancer risk in nonsmoking women. *J. natl Cancer Inst.*, **84**, 1417–1422

Sun, X.-W., Dai, X.-D., Lin, C.-Y., Shi, Y.-B., Ma, Y.-Y. & Li, W. (1996) Passive smoking and lung cancer among nonsmoking women in Harbin, China. International symposium on lifestyle factors and human lung cancer, China 1994. *Lung Cancer*, **14**, 237

Svensson, C., Pershagen, G. & Klominek, J. (1988) *Smoking and Passive Smoking in Relation to Lung Cancer in Women*, Stockholm, National Institute of Environmental Medicine

Svensson, C., Pershagen, G. & Klominek, J. (1989) Smoking and passive smoking in relation to lung cancer in women. *Acta oncol.*, **28**, 623–629

Trichopoulos, D. (1988) Passive smoking and lung cancer. *Scand. J. soc. Med.*, **16**, 75–79

Trichopoulos, D., Kalandidi, A., Sparros, L. & MacMahon, B. (1981) Lung cancer and passive smoking. *Int. J. Cancer*, **27**, 1–4

Trichopoulos, D., Kalandidi, A. & Sparros, L. (1983) Lung cancer and passive smoking: Conclusion of Greek study. *Lancet*, **ii**, 677–678

Tweedie, R.L. & Mengersen, K.L. (1992) Lung cancer and passive smoking: Reconciling the biochemical and epidemiological approaches. *Br. J. Cancer*, **66**, 700–705

Tweedie, R.L., Scott, D.J., Biggerstaff, B.J. & Mengersen, K.L. (1996) Bayesian meta-analysis, with application to studies of ETS and lung cancer. *Lung Cancer*, **14** (Suppl. 1), S171–S194

US Environmental Protection Agency (1992) *Respiratory Health Effects of Passive Smoking: Lung Cancer and Other Disorders (No. EPA/600/6-90/006F)*, Washington DC, Office of Research and Development, Office of Health and Environmental Assessment

Van Steensel-Moll, H.A., Valkenburg, H.A., Vandenbroucke, J.P. & Van Zanen, G.E. (1985) Are maternal fertility problems related to childhood leukaemia? *Int. J. Epidemiol.*, **14**, 555–559

de Waard, F., Kemmeren, J.M., van Ginkel, L.A. & Stolker, A.A. (1995) Urinary cotinine and lung cancer risk in a female cohort. *Br. J. Cancer*, **72**, 784–787

Wald, N.J., Nanchahal, K., Thompson, S.G. & Cuckle, H.S. (1986) Does breathing other people's tobacco smoke cause lung cancer? *Br. med. J.*, **293**, 1217–1222

Wang, L., Lubin, J.H., Zhang, S.R., Metayer, C., Xia, Y., Brenner, A., Shang, B., Wang, Z. & Kleinerman, R.A. (2000) Lung cancer and environmental tobacco smoke in a non-industrial area of China. *Int. J. Cancer*, **88**, 139–145

Wang, T.-J., Zhou, B.-S. & Shi, J.-P. (1996) Lung cancer in nonsmoking Chinese women: A case-control study. International symposium on lifestyle factors and human lung cancer, China 1994. *Lung Cancer*, **14**, 93–98

Wartenberg, D., Calle, E.E., Thun, M.J., Heath, C.W., Jr, Lally, C. & Woodruff, T. (2000) Passive smoking exposure and female breast cancer. *J. natl Cancer Inst.*, **92**, 1666–1673

Wells, A.J. (1991) Breast cancer, cigarette smoking, and passive smoking [Letter]. *Am. J. Epidemiol.*, **133**, 208–210

Wells, A.J. (1998) Lung cancer from passive smoking at work. *Am. J. public Health*, **88**, 1025–1029

Wells, A.J., English, P.B., Posner, S.F., Wagenknecht, L.E. & Perez-Stable, E.J. (1998) Misclassification rates for current smokers misclassified as nonsmokers. *Am. J. public Health*, **88**, 1053–1059

Whitehead, J. & Whitehead, A. (1991) A general parametric approach to the meta-analysis of randomised clinical trials. *Stat. Med.*, **10**, 1665–1677

Winn, D.M., Li, F.P., Robison, L.L., Mulvihill, J.J., Daigle, A.E. & Fraumeni, J.F., Jr (1992) A case–control study of the etiology of Ewing's sarcoma. *Cancer Epidemiol. Biomarkers Prev.*, **1**, 525–532

Wu, A.H., Henderson, B.E., Pike, M.C. & Yu, M.C. (1985) Smoking and other risk factors for lung cancer in women. *J. natl Cancer Inst.*, **74**, 747–751

Wu-Williams, A.H., Dai, X.D., Blot, W., Xu, Z.Y., Sun, X.W., Xiao, H.P., Stone, B.J., Yu, S.F., Feng, Y.P., Ershow, A.G., Sun, J., Fraumeni, J.F., Jr & Henderson, B.E. (1990) Lung cancer among women in north-east China. *Br. J. Cancer*, **62**, 982–987

Yuan, J.-M., Wang, X.-L., Xiang, Y.-B., Gao, Y.-T., Ross, R.K. & Yu, M.C. (2000) Non-dietary risk factors for nasopharyngeal carcinoma in Shanghai, China. *Int. J. Cancer*, **85**, 364–369

Zaridze, D.G., Zemlianaia, G.M. & Aitakov, Z.N. (1995) [Contribution of out- and indoor air pollution to the etiology of lung cancer.] *Vestn. Ross. Akad. Med. Nauk*, **4**, 6–10 (in Russian)

Zaridze, D., Maximovitch, D., Zemlyana, G., Aitakov, Z.N. & Boffetta, P. (1998) Exposure to environmental tobacco smoke and risk of lung cancer in non-smoking women from Moscow, Russia. *Int. J. Cancer*, **75**, 335–338

Zheng, W., McLaughlin, J.K., Chow, W.-H., Co Chien, H.T. & Blot, W.J. (1993) Risk factors for cancers of the nasal cavity and paranasal sinuses among white men in the United States. *Am. J. Epidemiol.*, **138**, 965–972

Zhong, L., Goldberg, M.S., Gao, Y.-T. & Jin, F. (1999) A case–control study of lung cancer and environmental tobacco smoke among non-smoking women living in Shanghai, China. *Cancer Causes Control*, **10**, 607–616

Zhong, L., Goldberg, M.S., Parent, M.-E. & Hanley, J.A. (2000) Exposure to environmental tobacco smoke and the risk of lung cancer: A meta-analysis. *Lung Cancer*, **27**, 3–18

3. Studies of Cancer in Experimental Animals

3.1   Inhalation exposure: simulated environmental tobacco smoke

Since the previous *IARC Monograph* on tobacco smoking (IARC, 1986), studies that include exposure to sidestream cigarette smoke or to simulated environmental tobacco smoke from cigarettes have been conducted. For experimental purposes, many of the studies employed a mixture of 89% sidestream and 11% mainstream tobacco smoke prepared by smoking machines from standard reference cigarettes, referred to in the published literature and in this section as simulated environmental tobacco smoke (Teague *et al.*, 1994). Although this experimental exposure system was designed to mimic human exposure, it provides an exposure pattern that differs from that encountered by humans exposed to secondhand smoke. No studies were available on sidestream smoke or simulated environmental smoke from other tobacco products.

The mice used in the studies described below were of the specially inbred strain A/J and outbred strain Swiss, both of which are highly susceptible to lung tumour development (Shimkin & Stoner, 1975). Both strains carry the pulmonary adenoma susceptibility-1 genetic locus (*Pas1*), a locus affecting genetic predisposition to lung tumours in mice (Manenti *et al.*, 1997). Strain A/J mice carry the *Eco*RI-generated 0.55 Kb DNA fragment of the K-*ras* oncogene which is associated with high susceptibility to lung tumour development (Malkinson, 1992). Both strains are highly susceptible to chemical induction of peripheral lung tumours that originate primarily from type II pneumocytes. It should be noted that type II pneumocytes are precursors for a relatively small fraction (~5–10%) of human adenocarcinomas (i.e. bronchiolo-alveolar carcinomas). Most adenocarcinoma cells are derived from bronchiolar cells and not from type II pneumocytes.

Mouse

Male strain A/J mice (6–8 weeks old) were exposed in chambers to sidestream smoke generated from Kentucky 1R4F reference cigarettes. Mice were exposed for 6 h/day, 5 days/week at chamber concentrations of 4 mg/m^3 total suspended respirable particulate matter. The experiment was terminated after 6 months. The fraction of animals bearing lung tumours was the same in those exposed to smoke (33%; 12/36) as in those exposed to filtered air (33%; 12/36). The average number of tumours per lung (0.42 tumours/smoke-exposed mouse; 0.39 tumours/control mouse) was also similar (Witschi *et al.*,

1995). [The Working Group noted the low concentration of tobacco smoke used and the short duration of the study.]

　　Male strain A/J mice (6–8 weeks old) were exposed to simulated environmental tobacco smoke that consisted of a mixture of 89% sidestream and 11% mainstream smoke from Kentucky 1R4F reference cigarettes, at a chamber concentration of 87 mg/m³ total suspended particulate matter. Mice were exposed in 0.44 m³ stainless steel inhalation chambers for 6 h/day, 5 days/week for 5 months and then killed for assessment of lung tumour incidence and multiplicity (see Table 3.1). The incidence of lung tumours in mice exposed to simulated environmental tobacco smoke (25%; 6/24) was not significantly different from that in controls (8.3%; 2/24). There was no significant difference between lung tumour multiplicities (total number of lung tumours per total number of animals) in exposed and control animals (0.3 ± 0.1 and 0.1 ± 0.1 tumour/mouse, respectively [mean ± SE]). A second group of mice exposed for 5 months to simulated environmental tobacco smoke was allowed to recover for a further 4 months in filtered air before being killed for analysis of lung tumour incidence and multiplicity. Tumour incidence was significantly greater in mice exposed to smoke (83.3%; 20/24) than in controls kept in air (37.5%; 9/24; $p < 0.05$, Fisher's

Table 3.1. Lung tumours in strain A/J mice exposed to filtered and unfiltered simulated environmental tobacco smoke

Exposure conditions	Parameter	Filtered air controls	Animals exposed to ETS
5 months in simulated ETS (87 mg TSP/m³), 6 h/day, 5 days/week	Tumour incidence[a] Tumour multiplicity[b]	8.3% (2/24) 0.1 ± 0.1	25.0% (6/24) 0.3 ± 0.1
5 months in simulated ETS (87 mg TSP/m³), 6 h/day, 5 days/week, then 4 months recovery in air	Tumour incidence Tumour multiplicity	37.5% (9/24) 0.5 ± 0.2	83.3% (20/24)[c] 1.4 ± 0.2[d]
5 months in unfiltered simulated ETS (78.5 mg TSP/m³) and 4 months recovery in air	Tumour incidence Tumour multiplicity	41.6% (10/24) 0.5 ± 0.1	57.7% (15/26) 1.3 ± 0.3[d]
5 months in filtered simulated ETS (0.1 mg TSP/m³) and 4 months recovery in air	Tumour incidence Tumour multiplicity	37.5% (9/24) 0.5 ± 0.1	66.7% (16/24) 1.2 ± 0.3[d]
5 months in filtered simulated ETS (0.1 mg TSP/m³)	Tumour incidence Tumour multiplicity	20% (4/20) 0.3 ± 0.1	50% (12/24) 0.7 ± 0.2

Modified from Witschi et al. (1997a,b)

ETS, simulated environmental tobacco smoke; TSP, total suspended particulate matter

[a] Percentage of animals with lung tumours (incidence)

[b] Total number of lung tumours/total number of mice in the group (mean ± SE)

[c] $p < 0.05$, Fisher's exact test

[d] $p < 0.05$, Welch's alternate t-test

exact test) and tumour multiplicities were significantly higher in the group exposed to smoke (1.4 ± 0.2 versus 0.5 ± 0.2, $p < 0.05$, Welch's alternate t-test). More than 80% of all tumours were adenomas and the remainder were adenocarcinomas (Witschi et al., 1997a).

Female strain A/J mice (10 weeks old) were exposed to unfiltered (one group of 26 animals) or high efficiency particulate air (HEPA)-filtered simulated environmental tobacco smoke (two groups of 24 animals) which consisted of a mixture of 89% side-stream and 11% mainstream smoke from Kentucky 1R4F reference cigarettes. The concentration of total suspended particulates was 78.5 mg/m^3 in the unfiltered smoke exposure chamber and 0.1 mg/m^3 in the filtered smoke chamber (see Table 3.1). In addition, three groups of 24 control animals were exposed to filtered air. Lung tumour incidence and multiplicity in animals exposed to filtered smoke for 6 h/day, 5 days/week, and killed after 5 months were not significantly greater than those in controls kept in filtered air. Mice exposed as above to filtered tobacco smoke and then allowed to recover in air for 4 months had a lung tumour incidence of 16/24 (67%) and an average lung tumour multiplicity of 1.2 ± 0.3, compared with an incidence of 9/24 (37.5%) and a lung tumour multiplicity of 0.5 ± 0.1 in control mice breathing filtered air. Lung tumour multiplicity was significantly higher in mice exposed to filtered smoke than in controls ($p < 0.05$). Mice exposed to unfiltered smoke had a lung tumour incidence of 15/26 (57.5%) and a lung tumour multiplicity of 1.3 ± 0.3, whereas controls kept in filtered air had a tumour incidence of 10/24 (41.6%) and a lung tumour multiplicity of 0.5 ± 0.1 (multiplicity greater in treated mice, $p < 0.05$ than in controls kept in filtered air, Welch's alternate t-test). The authors concluded that the gas phase of simulated environmental tobacco smoke is as carcinogenic as unfiltered environmental tobacco smoke (Witschi et al., 1997b).

In a study of the effects of the experimental chemopreventive agents, phenethyl iso-thiocyanate and N-acetylcysteine, on the occurrence of lung tumours, male and female strain A/J mice (6–8 weeks old) were exposed to simulated environmental tobacco smoke that consisted of a mixture of 89% sidestream and 11% mainstream smoke from Kentucky 1R4F reference cigarettes. Mice were exposed for 6 h/day, 5 days/week for 5 months in 0.4 m^3 stainless steel inhalation chambers in which the concentration of total airborne suspended particulates was 82.5 mg/m^3. Controls were placed, within their cages, into chambers of the same size as the inhalation chambers. At the conclusion of the exposure period, the mice were transferred to a conventional animal holding facility. Nine months after the beginning of the experiment, the animals were killed and the lungs prepared for tumour analysis and histopathological examination. Lung tumour multiplicity, but not incidence, was increased in mice exposed to simulated environmental tobacco smoke. Lung tumours occurred in 20/29 (69%) of the controls with a multiplicity of 0.9 ± 0.2, and in 24/33 (73%) of the mice exposed to smoke with a multiplicity of 1.3 ± 0.2 (mean $\pm$ SEM, $p < 0.05$ by two-way ANOVA) (Witschi et al., 1998).

As part of a study on chemoprevention of tobacco smoke-induced lung tumours by dietary supplements of *myo*-inositol/dexamethasone, male strain A/J mice (8–10 weeks old) were exposed for 5 months to a mixture of 89% sidestream and 11% mainstream cigarette smoke. The animals were placed, within their cages, in stainless steel inhalation chambers ventilated with tobacco smoke or filtered air (controls). Exposure to simulated environmental tobacco smoke took place for 6 h/day, 5 days/week. Exposure during the first 2 weeks was to an average of 71 mg total suspended particles/m³; this was followed by exposure for 3 weeks to 86 mg/m³ and finally to an average of 132 mg/m³ for the remainder of the exposure period. After 5 months, all mice were removed from the inhalation chambers and transferred to a conventional animal holding facility with controlled temperature and humidity. Mice were killed 9 months after the beginning of the experiment. The incidence of lung tumours in control mice was 15/30 (50%) and the lung tumour multiplicity was 0.6 ± 0.1; the incidence of tumours in mice exposed to simulated environmental tobacco smoke was 30/35 (86%) and the multiplicity was 2.1 ± 0.3. The difference in lung tumour multiplicity between exposed and control mice was statistically significant ($p < 0.05$) (Witschi et al., 1999).

As part of a study on chemoprevention of lung tumours induced by exposure to tobacco smoke, male strain A/J mice (10 weeks old) were exposed in stainless steel inhalation chambers for 6 h/day, 5 days/week to a mixture of 89% sidestream cigarette smoke and 11% mainstream smoke prepared from Kentucky 1R4F reference cigarettes. The total suspended particulate concentration was 137 mg/m³. Inhalation exposure took place for 5 months and was followed by a recovery period of 4 months in filtered air in a conventional animal facility. Control mice were kept in chambers of the same size as the inhalation chambers, but ventilated with filtered air, for the first 5 months of the study. Mice were killed 9 months after the beginning of exposure. In the first of two studies, the lung tumour incidence in control mice was 35/54 (65%) and lung tumour multiplicity was 1.0 ± 0.1. In mice exposed to smoke, the tumour incidence was 25/28 (89%; i.e. significantly different from controls, $p < 0.05$, Fisher's exact test) and tumour multiplicity was 2.4 ± 0.3 (i.e. significantly different from controls, $p < 0.01$ by parametric or non-parametric ANOVA). In the second experiment, conducted under the same conditions of exposure, lung tumour incidence in control mice was 18/30 mice and the incidence in mice exposed to smoke was 38/38 ($p < 0.01$, Fisher's exact test). Lung tumour multiplicity was 0.9 ± 0.2 in control mice and 2.8 ± 0.2 in animals exposed to smoke ($p < 0.01$, ANOVA) (Witschi et al., 2000).

In a third study conducted using the same experimental design, strain A/J mice [sex not specified] were exposed continuously to simulated environmental tobacco smoke for 9 months. There was no statistically significant increase in lung tumour incidence (85% [23/27] versus 63% [53/84]) or lung tumour multiplicity (1.5 ± 0.2 versus 1.0 ± 0.1) (Witschi, 2000).

Female strain A/J mice (4 weeks of age) were exposed to simulated environmental tobacco smoke (89% sidestream and 11% mainstream smoke) from Kentucky 2R1 reference cigarettes. Exposure continued for 5 months for 6 h/day, 5 days/week. The concentration of total suspended particulates was 120 mg/m³ air. Control mice were kept in chambers ventilated with filtered air. Mice were then kept for a 4-month recovery period in filtered air, after which they were killed and lungs tumours were counted. The lung tumour incidence in mice exposed to smoke was 15/20 (75%); the incidence in sham-exposed controls was 5/20 (25%; $p < 0.01$). Lung tumour multiplicity in mice exposed to smoke was 1.05 ± 0.17 and that in control mice was 0.25 ± 0.10 ($p < 0.01$). In a third group of mice exposed to simulated environmental tobacco smoke under the same conditions for 9 months and killed immediately at the end of the exposure period, the lung tumour incidence (6/20; 30%) and multiplicity (0.4 ± 0.15) were not significantly different from the tumour incidence and multiplicity in control mice. In a fourth group of mice exposed to simulated tobacco smoke under the same conditions for 2 months, followed by a recovery period of 7 months, lung tumour incidence (8/20; 40%) and multiplicity (0.50 ± 0.15) were also not significantly greater than in control mice. These data are in agreement with the results of Witschi et al. (1997a,b, 1998 and 1999) which indicate that strain A/J mice require a 4-month recovery period following a smoke exposure for 5 months to demonstrate a positive carcinogenic effect of environmental tobacco smoke (D'Agostini et al., 2001).

Witschi et al. (2002) exposed male Swiss albino mice to simulated environmental tobacco smoke for 5 months, followed by 4 months of recovery in air. The lung tumour incidence was 1/26 (4%) in sham-exposed mice and 6/31 (20%) in mice exposed to simulated environmental tobacco smoke, with a fivefold increase ($p = 0.075$). Lung tumour multiplicity was 0.04 ± 0.04 in sham-exposed mice and 0.35 ± 0.14 in mice exposed to environmental tobacco smoke ($p < 0.05$). When BALB/c mice were exposed to simulated environmental tobacco smoke under identical conditions, the incidence of lung tumours was increased (33%, 9/27 versus 20%, 6/30), but the multiplicity was not (0.4 versus 0.2).

As part of a series of pilot experiments on chemoprevention of cancer induced by environmental tobacco smoke, De Flora et al. (2003) reported studies of the effects of environmental tobacco smoke in Swiss albino mice. However, these studies were published in a review, and the reporting of study details was incomplete.

Groups of gestating female Swiss albino mice were exposed for 20 days to simulated environmental tobacco smoke. The exposure conditions were similar to those described by D'Agostini et al. (2001). The exposure of gestating mice to environmental tobacco smoke decreased the body weights of dams during the 3 months following delivery [details not given]. Similarly, in the female progeny of dams exposed to smoke, the body weight 10 days after birth was slightly, but significantly lower than that of female progeny from sham-exposed dams [details not given]. Dams exposed to tobacco smoke during gestation had significantly higher yields of lung tumours than sham-exposed dams. The lung tumour incidence at 8.5 months of age was increased from 1/22 (4.5%) in sham-exposed dams to 4/14 (28.6%) in dams exposed to tobacco smoke. The lung tumour multiplicity at 8.5 months of age was increased from 0.05 ± 0.5 in sham-exposed dams to 0.36 ± 0.17 (mean $\pm$ SE; $p < 0.05$) in dams exposed to tobacco smoke. The progeny of sham-exposed dams and dams exposed to environmental tobacco smoke, kept either 8.5 or 15 months after birth in filtered air, had identical yields of lung tumours. The incidence of lung tumours in the progeny at 8.5 months was 10% (1/10) and the lung tumour multiplicity was 0.1 ± 0.1. At 15 months, the lung tumour incidence in the progeny was 20% (2/10) and the lung tumour multiplicity was 0.3 ± 0.21 (De Flora et al., 2003).

In a second experiment (see Table 3.2), De Flora *et al.* (2003) investigated the effects of gestation and length of the exposure period on lung tumours induced by environmental tobacco smoke in Swiss mice. The exposure to environmental tobacco smoke during gestation (for 20 days) increased the tumour incidence from 4.4% (1/23) in sham-exposed dams to 23.8% (10/42; $p < 0.05$) in dams exposed to smoke. The lung tumour multiplicity in sham-exposed dams (0.09 ± 0.09) was significantly lower than that in the mice exposed to smoke (0.38 ± 0.13; $p < 0.05$). A similar trend was seen in non-gestating Swiss albino mice exposed for an equivalent period (20 days), but the increases in tumour incidence and lung tumour multiplicity were not significant. When non-gestating mice were exposed to environmental tobacco smoke for 5 months, followed by 4 months of recovery in filtered air, there was an increase in lung tumour incidence from 9.1% (2/22) in sham-exposed mice to 42.9% (9/21; $p < 0.01$) in mice exposed to tobacco smoke and in lung tumour multiplicity from 0.14 to 0.57 ($p < 0.01$) in sham-exposed compared to smoke-exposed mice. The increases were more pronounced if the animals were exposed to environmental tobacco smoke for 9 consecutive months.

In summary, when strain A/J mice of either sex are exposed to sufficiently high concentrations of simulated environmental tobacco smoke for a period of 5 months and are then kept in filtered air for a further 4 months, lung tumour multiplicities are consistently and significantly higher in mice exposed to tobacco smoke than in concomitant controls.

Table 3.2. Lung tumour yield in female Swiss albino mice, either gestating or non-gestating, exposed to simulated environmental tobacco smoke for varying time periods

Exposure to simulated ETS (time)	Gestating	Percentage of animals with lung tumour (incidence)	Lung tumour multiplicity[a]
0[b]	–	9.1% (2/22)	0.14 ± 0.10
0[b]	+	4.4% (1/23)	0.09 ± 0.09
20 days[c]	–	20.9% (9/43)	0.28 ± 0.09
20 days[c]	+	23.8% (10/42)[e]	0.38 ± 0.13[e]
5 months[d]	–	42.9% (9/21)[f]	0.57 ± 0.16[f]
9 months	–	50.0% (11/22)[f]	0.68 ± 0.17[f]

From De Flora *et al.* (2003)

ETS, environmental tobacco smoke

[a] Total number of lung tumours/total number of mice in the group (mean ± SE)

[b] Sham-exposed mice kept in filtered air for 9 months

[c] Exposed to ETS throughout gestation, or for an equivalent period in non-gestating mice, followed by 8 months and 10 days of recovery in filtered air

[d] Followed by 4 months of recovery in filtered air

[e] $p < 0.05$

[f] $p < 0.01$, compared with the corresponding sham-exposed mice, assessed by χ^2 analysis (incidence data) or Student's *t* test for unpaired data (multiplicity data)

In one experiment, filtered simulated environmental tobacco smoke induced lung tumours as effectively as whole simulated environmental tobacco smoke. At the higher levels of exposure, the incidences of lung tumour were also significantly higher in mice exposed to simulated environmental tobacco smoke than in controls. Similarly, the exposure of Swiss mice to environmental tobacco smoke for 5 months followed by a 4-month recovery period resulted in a significant increase in lung tumour response. In contrast to the findings in A/J mice, however, treatment of Swiss mice with environmental tobacco smoke for 9 consecutive months also resulted in a significant increase in the lung tumour response. Moreover, the short-term exposure of Swiss mice to environmental tobacco smoke led to an increased occurrence of lung tumours after 9 months.

3.2   Administration of condensates of sidestream smoke

3.2.1   *Mouse*

The comparative carcinogenicity of cigarette sidestream and mainstream smoke condensates was tested on the skin of female NMRI mice. Commercial brand German blond tobacco cigarettes were smoked to a defined butt length on a smoking machine using a puff duration of 2 s/min. Sidestream and mainstream smoke condensates were collected separately, dissolved in acetone, and administered on the shaved skin of the animal's lower back. Mice received half a dose twice a week for 3 months to give total weekly doses of 5, 10 and 15 mg. The animals were kept until natural death. No cutaneous or subcutaneous tumours developed in any of three control groups (42, 44 and 43 mice). In animals given mainstream smoke condensate, there were four malignant and three benign tumours in seven of 177 treated mice: two mammary adenocarcinomas, one haemangiosarcoma and one schwannoma in 58 mice that received the 5-mg dose; no tumours in any of the 61 mice that received the 10-mg dose, and three squamous-cell papillomas of the skin in 58 mice that received the 15-mg weekly dose. In the mice given sidestream smoke condensate, there were 16 malignant and 14 benign tumours in 30 of 182 treated mice: one mammary adenocarcinoma, three squamous-cell carcinomas and one squamous-cell papilloma of the skin in 60 mice that received the 5-mg dose; two mammary adenocarcinomas, one squamous-cell carcinoma and two squamous-cell papillomas of the skin in 61 mice that received the 10-mg dose; and two mammary adeno-carcinomas, one mixed mammary tumour, six squamous-cell carcinomas and 11 squamous-cell papillomas in 61 mice that received the 15-mg dose. The overall carcinogenic effect of sidestream smoke condensate was significantly higher than that of mainstream smoke condensate ($p < 0.001$) (Mohtashamipur *et al.*, 1990).

3.2.2   *Rat*

The carcinogenicity of sidestream cigarette smoke condensate was studied by collecting particles and semivolatiles from commercial German cigarettes smoked on a smoking machine and implanting the condensed material in a mixture of trioctanoin and beeswax into the lungs of female Osborne-Mendel rats at a dose corresponding to the products of a single cigarette. The fraction containing PAHs with four and more rings (dose, 1.06 mg/rat) induced five lung carcinomas in 35 treated rats. A sixfold higher dose (6.4 mg/rat) induced two lung carcinomas in five treated rats. The combined fractions containing no PAHs and PAHs of two and three rings (16 mg/rat) caused one lung carcinoma in 35 treated rats, and the semivolatiles (11.8 mg/rat) gave rise to no carcinoma in 35 treated rats (Grimmer *et al.*, 1988).

3.3   Observational studies of cancer in companion animals

Many species of animals are kept as pets, or companion animals, and these animals commonly share the environments of their owners. In consequence they are also exposed to toxic agents that may be present in the shared environment. The use of epidemiological methods to investigate environmental carcinogens through analysis of the occurrence of tumours in companion animals has been reviewed by Bukowski and Wartenberg (1997). Such data have been used in previous *IARC Monographs*, notably in the evaluation of carcinogenic risks associated with surgical implants and other foreign bodies (IARC, 1999).

3.3.1   *Case reports*

Case reports of lung cancer in the household pets of smokers are useful for generating hypotheses, but usually contain insufficient details to allow useful analysis (Cummins, 1994).

3.3.2   *Case–control studies*

(*a*)   *Dog*

Lung: A case–control study was conducted using 51 pet dogs with confirmed primary lung cancer from two veterinary teaching hospitals in the USA during 1985–87. Dogs with cancers at sites other than the lung (i.e. breast, soft connective tissues, skin, gastrointestinal tract, thyroid, bone, lymphoid and others) and not suspected of being related to cigarette smoking were chosen as controls ($n = 83$). Types of exposure to secondhand smoke that were assessed for both case and control dogs included the number of smokers who resided in the household, the number of packs of cigarettes smoked per day by the heaviest smoker and the time per day spent by the dog inside the home. Age, sex, body size and skull shape were included in a stratified analysis. A weak, statistically non-significant association was found between exposure to secondhand tobacco smoke and the risk of canine lung cancer. The crude odds ratio for exposure to environmental tobacco smoke was 1.5 (95% CI, 0.7–3.0). After adjustment for age, sex, skull shape, time spent indoors, and hospital of origin, the odds ratio rose slightly to 1.6 (95% CI, 0.7–3.7). The risk estimate for dogs aged 10 years or less was 2.7 (95% CI, 1.0–7.2); that for older dogs was 0.8 (95% CI, 0.3–2.2). A suggestion that skull shape exerted a modifying effect on risk for lung cancer was noted: the odds ratio was non-significantly increased in dogs of breeds with short (brachycephalic) and medium length (mesocephalic) noses (odds ratio, 2.4; 95% CI, 0.7–7.8), but not in dogs with long noses. It was noted that primary canine lung cancer is rare (approximately 4 cases per 100 000 hospitalizations) (Reif *et al.*, 1992).

Nasal cavity and paranasal sinuses: Sinonasal cancer is estimated to be tenfold more prevalent in dogs than lung cancer (Bukowski *et al.*, 1998).

A case–control study of nasal cancer in pet dogs treated at the veterinary teaching hospital at Colorado State University, USA, included 103 dogs with cancer of the nasal cavity and paranasal sinuses. Dogs with cancers at other sites (chiefly lymphoma, melanoma, haemangiosarcoma, and breast, bone and oral cavity) served as controls. The controls were similar to cases with respect to age, sex, breed and time spent outdoors. Telephone interviews were conducted with the owners of the pets to obtain data on exposure to environmental tobacco smoke. These data included the number of smokers in the household, the number of packs of cigarettes smoked per day at home by each smoker, the number of years that each person had smoked during the dog's lifetime and the time spent by the dog inside the home. The crude odds ratio for the presence of a smoker in the home and risk of nasal cancer was 1.1 (95% CI, 0.7–1.8). After stratification by anatomical features, the risk appeared to be restricted to long-nosed (dolichocephalic) dogs (odds ratio, 2.0; 95% CI, 1.0–4.1) (Reif *et al.*, 1998).

A case–control study was conducted to investigate the environmental causes of sinonasal cancers among pet dogs. Data on indoor environmental exposure including the presence of smokers in the household were collected for 129 dogs with histologically confirmed sinonasal cancer diagnosed during 1989–93 at the University of Pennsylvania School of Veterinary Medicine, USA. These were compared with 176 control dogs diagnosed with primary stomach, bowel, omental or liver cancers during the same period. Long-nosed dogs were significantly more likely to present with sinonasal cancer than dogs with short or medium-length noses (odds ratio, 3.2; 95% CI, 1.1–10). Elevated odds ratios were reported for dogs living in households that used coal fires or kerosene heaters for indoor heating (2.7; 95% CI, 1.4–5.4) and in which household chemicals were stored in the living area (5.5; 95% CI, 1.2–29). There was no excess risk associated with smokers living in the home (odds ratio, 0.70; 95% CI, 0.41–1.2) (Bukowski *et al.*, 1998).

Urinary bladder: A case–control study of household dogs was conducted to determine whether exposure to sidestream cigarette smoke, chemicals in the home, use of topical insecticides or obesity are associated with the occurrence of bladder cancer in canines. Information was obtained by interviewing the owners of 59 dogs with transitional cell carcinoma of the urinary bladder, diagnosed histologically at the University of Pennsylvania School of Veterinary Medicine, USA, between January 1982 and June 1985. Dogs matched on age and size of breed (*n* = 71) with other chronic diseases or neoplasms, excluding diseases of the urinary tract, served as controls. The risk of bladder cancer was correlated with use of topical insecticide and was enhanced in overweight dogs. The risk of bladder cancer was not found to be related to exposure to household chemicals or to sidestream cigarette smoke at the levels of 1–3000 lifetime pack–years (odds ratio, 1.3; 95% CI, 0.5–3.1) or > 3000 lifetime pack–years (odds ratio, 0.8; 95% CI, 0.3–2.0) (Glickman *et al.*, 1989). [The Working Group noted that the exposure is most likely expressed as lifetime number of packs.]

(b)   Cat

Malignant lymphoma

A case–control study of domestic cats was conducted to determine whether exposure to household environmental tobacco smoke is associated with the occurrence of feline malignant lymphoma. Information on the level of smoking in the household two years prior to diagnosis was obtained from questionnaires sent to the owners of 80 cats with malignant lymphoma diagnosed during 1993–2000 at the Foster Small Animal Hospital, MA, USA. These cases were compared with 114 control cats diagnosed with renal disease during the same period. The relative risk of malignant lymphoma for cats exposed to any household tobacco smoke was 2.4 (95% CI, 1.2–4.5). The risk increased with both duration and level of exposure, with evidence of a linear trend. Cats exposed to tobacco smoke for five or more years had a relative risk of 3.2 (95% CI, 1.5–6.9; *p* for trend = 0.003) when compared with cats in nonsmoking households (Bertone *et al.*, 2002).

References

Bertone, E.R., Snyder, L.A. & Moore, A.S. (2002) Environmental tobacco smoke and risk of malignant lymphoma in pet cats. *Am. J. Epidemiol.*, **156**, 268–273

Bukowski, J.A. & Wartenberg, D. (1997) An alternative approach for investigating the carcinogenicity of indoor air pollution: Pets as sentinels of environmental cancer risk. *Environ. Health Perspect.*, **105**, 1312–1319

Bukowski, J.A., Wartenberg, D. & Goldschmidt, M. (1998) Environmental causes for sinonasal cancers in pet dogs, and their usefulness as sentinels of indoor cancer risk. *J. Toxicol. environ. Health*, **A54**, 579–591

Cummins, D. (1994) Pets and passive smoking [Letter to the editor]. *Br. med. J.*, **309**, 960

D'Agostini, F., Balansky, R.M., Bennicelli, C., Lubet, R.A., Kelloff, G.J. & De Flora, S. (2001) Pilot studies evaluating the lung tumor yield in cigarette smoke-exposed mice. *Int. J. Oncol.*, **18**, 607–615

De Flora, S., D'Agostini, F., Balansky, R., Camoirano, A., Bennicelli, C., Bagnasco, M. Cartiglia, C., Tampa, E., Longobardi, M.G., Lubet, R.A. & Izzotti, A. (2003) Modulation of cigarette smoke-related end-points in mutagenesis and carcinogenesis. *Mutat. Res.*, **523–524**, 237–252

Glickman, L.T., Schofer, F.S., McKee, L.J., Reif, J.S. & Goldschmidt, M.H. (1989) Epidemiologic study of insecticide exposures, obesity, and risk of bladder cancer in household dogs. *J. Toxicol. environ. Health*, **28**, 407–414

Grimmer, G., Brune, H., Dettbarn, G., Naujack, K.-W., Mohr, U. & Wenzel-Hartung, R. (1988) Contribution of polycyclic aromatic compounds to the carcinogenicity of sidestream smoke of cigarettes evaluated by implantation into the lungs of rats. *Cancer Lett.*, **43**, 173–177

IARC (1986) *IARC Monographs on the Evaluation of the Carcinogenic Risk of Chemicals to Humans*, Vol. 38, *Tobacco smoking*, Lyon, IARC*Press*

IARC (1999) *IARC Monographs on the Evaluation of Carcinogenic Risks to Humans*, Vol. 74, *Surgical Implants and other Foreign Bodies*, Lyon, IARC*Press*, pp. 173–177

Malkinson, A.M. (1992) Primary lung tumors in mice: An experimentally manipulable model of human adenocarcinoma. *Cancer Res.*, **52** (Suppl.), 2670S–2676S

Manenti, G., Gariboldi, M., Fiorino, A., Zanesi, N., Pierotti, M.A. & Dragani, T.A. (1997) Genetic mapping of lung cancer modifier loci specifically affecting tumor initiation and progression. *Cancer Res.*, **57**, 4164–4166

Mohtashamipur, E., Mohtashamipur, A., Germann, P.-G., Ernst, H., Norpoth, K. & Mohr, U. (1990) Comparative carcinogenicity of cigarette mainstream and sidestream smoke condensates on the mouse skin. *J. Cancer Res. clin. Oncol.*, **116**, 604–608

Reif, J.S., Dunn, K., Ogilvie, G.K. & Harris, C.K. (1992) Passive smoking and canine lung cancer risk. *Am. J. Epidemiol.*, **135**, 234–239

Reif, J.S., Bruns, C. & Lower, K.S. (1998) Cancer of the nasal cavity and paranasal sinuses and exposure to environmental tobacco smoke in pet dogs. *Am. J. Epidemiol.*, **147**, 488–492

Shimkin, M.B. & Stoner, G.D. (1975) Lung tumours in mice: Application to carcinogenesis bioassay. *Adv. Cancer Res.*, **21**, 1–58

Teague, S.V., Pinkerton, K.E., Goldsmith, M., Gebremichael, A., Chang, S., Jenkins, R.A. & Moneyhun, J.H. (1994) Sidestream cigarette smoke generation and exposure system for environmental tobacco smoke studies. *Inhal. Toxicol.*, **6**, 79–93

Witschi, H. (2000) Successful and not so successful chemoprevention of tobacco smoke-induced lung tumors. *Exp. Lung Res.*, **26**, 743–755

Witschi, H., Oreffo, V.I.C. & Pinkerton, K.E. (1995) Six-month exposure of strain A/J mice to cigarette sidestream smoke: Cell kinetics and lung tumor data. *Fundam. appl. Toxicol.*, **26**, 32–40

Witschi, H., Espiritu, I., Peake, J.L., Wu, K, Maronpot, R.R. & Pinkerton, K.E. (1997a) The carcinogenicity of environmental tobacco smoke. *Carcinogenesis*, **18**, 575–586

Witschi, H., Espiritu, I., Maronpot, R.R., Pinkerton, K.E. & Jones, A.D. (1997b) The carcinogenic potential of the gas phase of environmental tobacco smoke. *Carcinogenesis*, **18**, 2035–2042

Witschi, H., Espiritu, I., Yu, M. & Willits, N.H. (1998) The effects of phenethyl isothiocyanate, *N*-acetylcysteine and green tea on tobacco smoke-induced lung tumors in strain A/J mice. *Carcinogenesis*, **19**, 1789–1794

Witschi, H., Espiritu, I. & Uyeminami, D. (1999) Chemoprevention of tobacco smoke-induced lung tumors in A/J strain mice with dietary *myo*-inositol and dexamethasone. *Carcinogenesis*, **20**, 1375–1378

Witschi, H., Uyeminami, D., Moran, D. & Espiritu, I. (2000) Chemoprevention of tobacco-smoke lung carcinogenesis in mice after cessation of smoke exposure. *Carcinogenesis*, **21**, 977–982

Witschi, H., Espiritu, I., Dance, S.T. & Miller, M.S. (2002) A mouse lung tumor model of tobacco smoke carcinogenesis. *Toxicol. Sci.*, **68**, 322–330

4. Other Data Relevant to an Evaluation of Carcinogenicity and its Mechanisms

The Working Group attempted to provide comprehensive coverage of the published literature on other data relevant to the evaluation of the carcinogenic hazards of second-hand smoke (since 1985), in some cases referring to recent reviews.

4.1 Absorption, distribution, metabolism and excretion

For a description of the absorption, distribution, metabolism and excretion of components of tobacco smoke, the reader is referred to the monograph on tobacco smoke.

4.1.1 *Humans*

(*a*) *Enzyme activities and metabolism*

In a study of human placental monooxygenase activity, as measured by in-vitro oxidation of 7-ethoxyresorufin, O-deethylase activity was significantly inhibited ($p < 0.05$) by 7,8-benzoflavone with placental microsomes from women passively exposed to cigarette smoke, but not with those from women who had not been exposed (Manchester & Jacoby, 1981).

A pharmacokinetic study reported a significantly faster clearance of theophylline in a group of seven nonsmokers exposed to secondhand tobacco smoke, as determined by questionnaire data and cotinine levels, than in a matched group of non-exposed individuals, as determined by clearance rate, terminal elimination half-time and mean residence time ($T_{1/2} = 6.93$ h versus 8.69 h, $p < 0.05$) (Matsunga *et al.*, 1989). Conversely, no changes in theophylline clearance rate were observed in five male subjects who were heavily exposed to secondhand tobacco smoke for 3 h/day on 5 consecutive days under controlled conditions (Casto *et al.*, 1990).

(*b*) *Tobacco smoke carcinogen biomarkers*

(i) *Urinary compounds*

The use of urinary compounds as biomarkers of carcinogen uptake from environmental tobacco smoke was reviewed by Scherer and Richter (1997).

4-(Methylnitrosamino)-1-(3-pyridyl)-1-butanol (NNAL) and its glucuronides (NNAL-Gluc) are metabolites of the tobacco-specific lung carcinogen 4-(methylnitrosamino)-1-(3-pyridyl)-1-butanone (NNK). The use of the assay for NNAL and NNAL-Gluc in urine for investigations of exposure to secondhand tobacco smoke offers several advantages. Firstly, it has the sensitivity required to measure relatively low concentrations (typically about 0.05 pmol/mL urine). Secondly, because NNK is a tobacco-specific compound, the detection of NNAL and NNAL-Gluc in urine specifically signals exposure to tobacco smoke. All studies reported to date have found significantly higher concentrations of NNAL plus NNAL-Gluc, or NNAL-Gluc alone, in the urine of nonsmokers exposed to secondhand tobacco smoke than in the urine of unexposed controls, and a good correlation between urinary levels of cotinine and NNAL plus NNAL-Gluc (Table 4.1). In one study, the uptake of NNK was more than six times higher in women who lived with smokers than in women who lived with nonsmokers (Anderson *et al.*, 2001). In another investigation, widespread uptake of NNK was demonstrated in a group of economically disadvantaged school-children heavily exposed to tobacco smoke at home (Hecht *et al.*, 2001). Correlations have been consistently observed between levels of urinary cotinine and NNAL + NNAL-Gluc in people exposed to secondhand tobacco smoke (Hecht, 2002). Because NNAL is a meta-bolite of the lung carcinogen NNK, these data imply that there is elevated carcinogen uptake in subjects with raised concentrations of urinary cotinine.

Mixed results have been obtained in studies on the relationship between *tt*-muconic acid, a metabolite of benzene, and exposure to secondhand tobacco smoke. Some studies have shown significantly increased concentrations in people exposed to secondhand tobacco smoke (Yu & Weisel, 1996; Taniguchi *et al.*, 1999; Carrer *et al.*, 2000) whereas others found no effect (Scherer *et al.*, 1995; Weaver *et al.*, 1996; Ruppert *et al.*, 1997; Scherer *et al.*, 1999), the levels being primarily dependent on whether the subject's home is in the city or the suburbs and on dietary intake of sorbic acid rather than on exposure to secondhand tobacco smoke. The levels of 1-hydroxypyrene and hydroxyphenanthrenes in urine are generally not increased by exposure to secondhand tobacco smoke (Hoepfner *et al.*, 1987; Scherer *et al.*, 1992; Scherer *et al.*, 2000), although significant increases have been reported under some high exposure conditions (Van Rooij *et al.*, 1994; Siwinska *et al.*, 1999).

The concentrations of aromatic amines (Grimmer *et al.*, 2000) and 8-hydroxy-2'-deoxyguanosine (8-OHdG) (Pilger *et al.*, 2001) in urine were also unaffected by exposure to secondhand tobacco smoke. The concentration of urinary 5-(hydroxymethyl)uracil was significantly elevated in nonsmokers exposed to high levels of secondhand tobacco smoke, in a dose-dependent manner (Bianchini *et al.*, 1998). Exposure to secondhand tobacco smoke did not affect urinary concentrations of 3-ethyladenine (Kopplin *et al.*, 1995). Elevated concentrations of thioethers, in particular of 3-hydroxypropylmercapturic acid, were observed under controlled, high exposure conditions (Scherer *et al.*, 1990, 1992), but not in a field study (Scherer *et al.*, 1996).

Lackmann *et al.* (1999) first reported the presence of NNAL and NNAL-Gluc in the urine of newborns of women who smoked (Table 4.1). The available data indicate that

Table 4.1. Urinary NNAL and its glucuronides (NNAL-Gluc): biomarkers of NNK uptake in studies of involuntary exposure to tobacco smoke

Study group	Main conclusions[a]	Reference
Exposure of adults to secondhand smoke		
5 men exposed to second-hand smoke	Significantly increased levels of NNAL + NNAL-Gluc after exposure in a chamber: 127 ± 74 pmol/day (approx. 0.16 ± 74 pmol/mL urine)	Hecht *et al.* (1993)
5 men, 4 women exposed to secondhand smoke 5 unexposed controls	Significantly increased levels of NNAL-Gluc in exposed workers compared to unexposed controls: 0.059 ± 0.028 pmol/mL urine	Parsons *et al.* (1998)
29 nonsmokers (13 women)	NNAL + NNAL-Gluc levels correlated with nicotine levels from personal samplers. NNAL, 20.3 ± 21.8 pmol/day; NNAL-Gluc, 22.9 ± 28.6 pmol/day in exposed nonsmokers	Meger *et al.* (2000)
45 nonsmoking women, 23 exposed to secondhand smoke in the home, 22 non-exposed	NNAL + NNAL-Gluc significantly higher in exposed women: 0.050 ± 0.068 pmol/mL urine	Anderson *et al.* (2001)
204 nonsmoking elementary school-aged children	34% with total cotinine ≥ 5 ng/mL; 52/54 of these samples had detectable NNAL or NNAL-Gluc, 93-fold range. NNAL + NNAL-Gluc, 0.056 ± 0.076 pmol/mL urine	Hecht *et al.* (2001)
In-utero exposure to mother's smoking		
31 newborns of mothers who smoked; 17 newborns of mothers who did not smoke	NNAL-Gluc detected in 71%, NNAL in 13% of urine samples of newborns of smokers; neither detected in urine of newborns of nonsmokers ($p < 0.001$); NNAL + NNAL-Gluc in urine of newborns of smoking mothers, 0.13 ± 0.15 pmol/mL urine	Lackmann *et al.* (1999)
21 smokers and 30 non-smokers	NNAL detected in amniotic fluid of 52.4% of smokers and 6.7% of nonsmokers ($p = 0.0006$). NNAL concentration in amniotic fluid of smokers, 0.025 ± 0.029 pmol/mL	Milunsky *et al.* (2000)
12 smokers and 10 nonsmokers	NNAL and NNAL-Gluc not detected in follicular fluid	Matthews *et al.* (2002)

[a] Values represent mean $\pm$ SD.

NNAL, 4-(methylnitrosamino)-1-(3-pyridyl)-1-butanol; NNK, 4-(methylnitrosamino)-1-(3-pyridyl)-1-butanone

NNK, a transplacental carcinogen, is taken up by the fetus and metabolized to NNAL and NNAL-Gluc by fetal enzymes (Lackmann *et al.*, 1999). Consistent with these results, NNAL was detected in the amniotic fluid of pregnant smokers (Milunksy *et al.*, 2000). However, neither NNAL nor NNAL-Gluc could be detected in follicular fluid (Matthews *et al.*, 2002).

Urinary excretion of 8-OHdG by newborn babies ($n = 12$) whose mothers were exposed to secondhand tobacco smoke was significantly higher ($p = 0.047$) than that of babies whose mothers were not exposed ($n = 8$). In both groups, the concentration of 8-OHdG excreted was also significantly higher for babies whose mothers had the *GSTM1* null genotype (Hong *et al.*, 2001).

(ii)   *Protein adducts*

To determine whether involuntary smoking increased the levels of aromatic amine-haemoglobin adducts, a group of 14 volunteers who reported negligible exposure to secondhand tobacco smoke was compared with a group of 15 nonsmokers who reported exposure to at least one pack of cigarettes per day smoked by others, and one of 15 non-smokers with unknown levels of exposure to secondhand tobacco smoke. No measurable quantities of cotinine were detected in the blood of members of any of the three groups (see Section 4.1.1.(d) for measurement of cotinine). A further group of 13 nonsmokers, including six bartenders who were heavily exposed to secondhand tobacco smoke, had measurable levels of cotinine in their blood. Background levels of adducts from 4-amino-biphenyl (ABP) and 3-aminobiphenyl were detected in all subjects, but higher levels were found in subjects with detectable cotinine levels ($p = 0.05$ and 0.027, respectively) (Maclure *et al.*, 1989). In another study, the levels of 4-ABP-haemoglobin adducts in 15 nonsmokers who reported being exposed to secondhand tobacco smoke were not signifi-cantly higher than those in 35 nonsmokers who were not exposed to secondhand tobacco smoke (87.9 ± 19 [SE] pg/g haemoglobin and 69.5 ± 7 pg/g, respectively). Only four out of 15 of those subjects who reported exposure to secondhand tobacco smoke and four out of 35 of those who reported no exposure had measurable levels of urinary cotinine (Bartsch *et al.*, 1990). The level of exposure of 40 nonsmoking women to secondhand tobacco smoke was determined by questionnaire, use of a diary and a personal air monitor and was stratified by average nicotine concentration. There was a significant correlation between the concentration of 4-ABP–haemoglobin and exposure category ($p = 0.009$) (Hammond *et al.*, 1993).

Exposure of pre-school children to secondhand tobacco smoke from their mothers was investigated by measuring plasma cotinine levels and PAH–albumin adducts in peri-pheral blood, the latter detected by ELISA. The study involved 87 mother–child pairs; 31 mothers smoked and 56 did not. Not only did the mothers who smoked have higher levels of adducts (see monograph on tobacco smoke), but the levels in their children were also significantly higher ($p < 0.05$). There was also a significant correlation between adduct levels in the mothers and in their children ($p = 0.014$) (Crawford *et al.*, 1994). In a sub-sequent study, PAH–albumin and 4-ABP–haemoglobin adducts were also found to be significantly higher in children whose mothers smoked or who lived with other smokers ($p < 0.05$) (Tang *et al.*, 1999). In a study in children from three different-sized cities, levels of 4-ABP adducts and other aromatic amines correlated with the size of the city. Exposure to secondhand tobacco smoke was associated with a non-significant increase in levels of 4-ABP adducts and a significant decrease in adducts of *ortho-* and *m*-toluidine ($p < 0.05$) (Richter *et al.*, 2001).

In a study of 69 adults, 27 were smokers, and 19 of the 42 nonsmokers were classified as passive smokers as determined by self-report and cotinine levels. The levels of benzo-[*a*]pyrene adducts with albumin and haemoglobin were similar for nonsmokers and passive smokers (Scherer *et al.*, 2000).

The levels of *N*-hydroxyethylvaline in haemoglobin were reported to be similar in nonsmokers who did not live or work with a smoker ($n = 74$) and in those who did ($n = 28$). Cotinine levels in passive smokers were not higher than in nonsmokers (Bono *et al.*, 1999).

There was a significantly higher level ($p = 0.02$) of nitrated proteins in blood plasma of nonsmokers who were exposed to secondhand tobacco smoke ($n = 30$) than in non-smokers who were unexposed ($n = 23$) (Pignatelli *et al.*, 2001).

Measurements of maternal–fetal exchange of 4-ABP in pregnant women who smoked ($n = 14$) and in nonsmoking ($n = 38$) pregnant women (see monograph on tobacco smoke) showed consistently lower levels of haemoglobin adducts in cord blood than in maternal blood, with an average maternal to fetal ratio of 2. A significant correlation was found between maternal and fetal levels for all subjects ($p < 0.001$) and for smokers only ($p = 0.002$), but not for nonsmokers only ($p = 0.06$) (Coghlin *et al.* 1991). Another study also found that adduct levels were lower in fetal blood than in maternal blood and were correlated with the smoking status of the mothers (subjects included 74 smokers and 74 nonsmokers) (Myers *et al.*, 1996). Another study of 73 nonsmoking pregnant women whose cotinine:creatinine ratios correlated with self-reported exposure to secondhand tobacco smoke, found no association with levels of haemoglobin adducts formed by any of nine aromatic amines (Branner *et al.*, 1998).

Blood samples from smoking and nonsmoking mothers and cord blood from their newborns were analysed for *N*-hydroxyethylvaline in haemoglobin. The average adduct concentration in newborns of mothers who smoked ($n = 13$; 147 ± 68 [mean $\pm$ SD] pmol/g) was significantly higher ($p < 0.01$) than in those from mothers who were nonsmokers ($n = 10$; 42 ± 18 pmol/g). There was also a significant correlation ($p < 0.01$) between adduct levels in the newborns and in their mothers (Tavares *et al.*, 1994). The same samples showed a strong correlation between the concentration of *N*-(2-cyanoethyl)valine (CEVal) adducts in the mothers who smoked and in their newborns ($p < 0.001$). The adduct levels in the babies were also strongly correlated with the numbers of cigarettes smoked per day by their mothers ($p = 0.009$). The levels of CEVal in babies of mothers who did not smoke were below the limit of detection of the assay (1 pmol/g) (Tavares *et al.*, 1996).

(iii)   DNA adducts

Although many studies have investigated the levels of DNA adducts or other measures of DNA damage in the tissues of smokers, ex-smokers and nonsmokers (see monograph on tobacco smoke), relatively few studies have investigated the use of these biomarkers to monitor the exposure of nonsmokers to secondhand tobacco smoke, probably because they may not distinguish the effects of exposure to secondhand tobacco smoke from those of exposure to other sources of environmental carcinogens.

In a study in which declining DNA adduct levels in the white blood cells of smokers enrolled in a smoking cessation programme were measured by ELISA, the levels of PAH–DNA adducts both at baseline and 10 weeks after cessation were significantly associated with number of hours of exposure to secondhand tobacco smoke at home ($p = 0.009$ and $p = 0.02$, respectively) and were also higher if the subject lived with another smoker ($p = 0.02$). However, there was no observable influence of exposure to secondhand tobacco smoke at the workplace (Mooney et al., 1995).

Using the prevalence of serum antibodies to benzo[a]pyrene diol epoxide (BPDE)–DNA adducts as a biomarker of exposure to environmental PAHs in an Italian population, no association between the percentage of subjects with DNA adducts and passive smoking was found (Petruzzelli et al., 1998). In a study in which significant differences were observed between the levels of BPDE–DNA adducts in the peripheral lymphocytes of smokers ($n = 40$) and nonsmokers ($n = 35$), as determined by a flow cytometric method using BPDE–DNA antibodies, the mean value for nonsmokers with no or low exposure to secondhand tobacco smoke ($n = 17$) was marginally *higher* than that of exposed nonsmokers ($n = 18$), but the difference was not statistically significant (Shinozaki et al., 1999). Using antibodies to BPDE–DNA adducts, immunohistochemical staining of ovarian granulosa-lutein cells from women undergoing in-vitro fertilization showed a strong correlation between smoking status and adduct levels in nonsmokers ($n = 11$), passive smokers ($n = 7$) and active smokers ($n = 14$); all pairwise comparisons were highly significant ($p < 0.0001$) (Zenzes et al., 1998).

Oxidative damage caused by exposure to secondhand tobacco smoke was assessed by measuring the concentration of 8-OHdG in the blood of 74 nonsmokers. The levels were, on average, 63% higher in the subjects exposed to secondhand tobacco smoke in the workplace ($n = 27$) than in the unexposed group ($n = 29$) and this difference was statistically significant ($p < 0.05$) (Howard et al., 1998a). However, in another study, the levels of 8-OHdG in leukocytes were significantly *lower* in smokers than in nonsmokers (see monograph on tobacco smoke) and no association was observed with exposure to secondhand tobacco smoke (van Zeeland et al., 1999).

Five nonsmokers were exposed to secondhand tobacco smoke under controlled conditions (exposure to gas phase only for 8 h, followed by exposure to whole secondhand tobacco smoke for 8 h, 40 h later). When their monocyte DNA was analysed by ^{32}P-post-labelling, no changes in the adduct patterns were seen after either exposure period, when compared with the samples obtained before exposure (Holz et al., 1990). In a study of biomarkers of exposure to air pollution in three Greek populations, one urban, one rural and one on a university campus, ^{32}P-postlabelling analysis of lymphocyte DNA revealed the presence of DNA adducts that significantly ($p < 0.001$) paralleled the level of exposure to secondhand tobacco smoke, as determined by self-report, plasma cotinine concentrations and profiles of personal exposure to PAHs that were characteristic of secondhand tobacco smoke, rather than other environmental sources (Georgiadis et al., 2001).

DNA adducts of PAHs were detected by ELISA in 6/14 placentas and in 5/12 matched fetal lung samples from spontaneous abortions. None of the samples were from women who reported smoking during pregnancy, suggesting that the adducts are due to some other source of hydrocarbon exposure (Hatch et al., 1990). In another study using ELISA, BPDE–DNA adducts were detected in 13/15 placental samples from smokers and 3/10 from nonsmokers. There was a strong correlation between concentrations of both adducts and urinary cotinine for both placental DNA and umbilical cord DNA, the former tissue having the higher adduct levels (transfer coefficient = 0.37–0.74) (Arnould et al., 1997). When placental DNA was analysed both for bulky DNA adducts by ^{32}P-postlabelling and for 8-OHdG by electrochemical detection, neither method showed a difference between 11 smokers, ten nonsmokers and nine nonsmokers exposed to passive smoking (Daube et al., 1997). Using ^{32}P-postlabelling with nuclease P1 digestion, DNA adducts were detected in placental and umbilical cord DNA regardless of the smoking status of the mothers and were significantly higher in maternal tissue than in fetal tissue (maternal/fetal ratio = 2.0). When considered separately, tissues showed only marginally increased adduct levels in smokers, but total DNA adduct levels in all tissues combined were significantly higher in smokers ($n = 8$) than in nonsmokers ($n = 11$) (Hansen et al., 1992, 1993).

(c) Other biomarkers

(i) Breath compounds

Carbon monoxide

Carbon monoxide (CO) in expired air has been reported to be an indirect measure of passive smoking both in adults and children. Given its very short half-life, CO concentration must be measured shortly after exposure.

After a 9-h period of exposure to secondhand tobacco smoke at the workplace, 100 nonsmoking waiters exhaled on average 5.0 ppm CO (the pre-exposure CO concentration was 2.0 ppm) compared to a concentration of 2.5 ppm CO exhaled by 100 medical students who spent the day in a nonsmoking environment ($p < 0.001$; Laranjeira et al., 2000). A study in Japan found that mean concentrations of exhaled CO in passive smokers were also significantly higher ($p < 0.001$) than those of nonsmokers who were not exposed to secondhand tobacco smoke (Taniguchi et al., 1999).

The concentrations of exhaled CO were also measured in 235 healthy and 54 asthmatic children (Ece et al., 2000). Regardless of the parents' smoking habits, CO concentrations were higher in asthmatic than in healthy children (1.32 ppm versus 0.86 ppm; $p = 0.028$). Significant relationships were found between the number of cigarettes smoked in the house and concentrations of exhaled CO in both healthy ($p = 0.003$) and asthmatic children ($p = 0.01$).

Both women exposed to secondhand smoke during pregnancy and their newborns exhaled higher concentrations of CO than non-exposed women (1.95 ppm versus 1.33 ppm and 2.51 versus 1.74 ppm, respectively) (Seidman et al., 1999).

Nitric oxide

Fifteen nonsmoking subjects were exposed to secondhand tobacco smoke or asked to smoke for 60 min in a ventilated chamber. Within 15 min of exposure, the concentrations of exhaled nitric oxide (NO) had fallen by 23.6% or 30.3%, respectively, and remained low during the entire time of exposure (Yates et al., 2001). Similarly, newborns exposed prenatally to cigarette smoke ($n = 7$) exhaled significantly less NO than non-exposed ($n = 13$) newborns (Hall et al., 2002).

Benzene

The concentrations of exhaled benzene in children exposed to secondhand tobacco smoke were not significantly related to the smoking status of the household members, but depended primarily on the location of the home (Scherer et al., 1999). Passive smokers not exposed at home, but exposed for more than 50% of their time at work had significantly higher levels of benzene, ethylbenzene, *meta*-xylene + *para*-xylene and *ortho*-xylene in their breath than did non-exposed nonsmokers (Wallace et al., 1987) .

(ii)   *Blood compounds*

Carboxyhaemoglobin

Measurements of the concentration of carboxyhaemaglobin in subjects exposed to secondhand tobacco smoke and in subjects who were not, are consistent with measurements of CO in the environment (Russell et al., 1973; Hugod et al., 1978; Jarvis et al., 1983). However, carboxyhaemoglobin measurements may be largely confounded by endogenous formation and environmental factors, and are thus not a reliable means for monitoring passive smoking (Scherer & Richter, 1997).

Thiocyanate

It is not possible to distinguish between nonsmokers who are exposed to secondhand smoke and those who are not by measuring serum thiocyanate concentrations (Robertson et al., 1987; Scherer & Richter, 1997).

(iii)   *Particles*

Experimental deposition of particulate matter with a diameter of < 1 μm from secondhand tobacco smoke within the human respiratory tract was evaluated in 15 nonsmokers and three regular smokers (Morawska et al., 1999). On average, smokers had a higher rate of deposition than nonsmokers ($65.3 \pm 24.1\%$ versus $56.0 \pm 15.9\%$ for nose breathing and $66.1 \pm 17.6\%$ versus $48.7 \pm 11.6\%$ for mouth breathing). The large variations observed between individuals indicate that deposition of environmental tobacco smoke is governed by an individual's airway anatomy and breathing patterns.

(d)   Nicotine and its metabolites as biomarkers

Many of the biological markers other than nicotine or cotinine that are used as indicators of exposure and uptake in smokers (e.g. carboxyhaemoglobin and thiocyanate; see monograph on tobacco smoke) are not suitable for accurate measurement of exposure to secondhand tobacco smoke because of potential confounding exposure from diet and environment (US National Research Council, 1986; US Environmental Protection Agency, 1992; California Environmental Protection Agency, 1997; Benowitz, 1999).

In addition to nicotine from use of tobacco products, pharmaceutical products for nicotine replacement therapy or exposure from secondhand tobacco smoke, small quantities of nicotine may enter the body from dietary sources, mainly from consumption of tea and some solanaceous plants such as aubergine, potato peel and tomato (Castro & Monji, 1986; Sheen, 1988; Davis et al., 1991; Domino et al., 1993; reviewed in Leyden et al., 1999). The contribution from dietary sources has, however, been estimated to be minimal and is generally thought not to influence the concentrations of nicotine or cotinine in body fluids significantly enough to affect their use as a biomarker for exposure to secondhand tobacco smoke (Tunstall-Pedoe et al., 1991; Henningfield, 1993; Benowitz, 1996), although there has been some disagreement on the subject (Davis et al., 1991). It has been calculated that even very high consumption of these nicotine-containing products would equal, at most, about 10% of the amount of nicotine generally taken up by nonsmokers exposed to secondhand tobacco smoke (Jarvis, 1994; Repace, 1994; Pirkle et al., 1996).

Measurements of nicotine and/or cotinine in body fluids of smokers have demonstrated that nicotine and cotinine are biomarkers of high sensitivity (96–97%) and specificity (99–100%) of exposure to tobacco smoke (Jarvis et al., 1987; see monograph on tobacco smoke). Owing to its longer half-life, cotinine measured in the blood, saliva or urine of nonsmokers is presently the most widely used biomarker for assessment of exposure to secondhand tobacco smoke (IARC, 1986; US National Research Council, 1986; US Environmental Protection Agency, 1992).

(i)   Adults

Numerous studies have investigated the dependence of concentrations of cotinine in the serum, saliva and urine on exposure to secondhand tobacco smoke (concentration and duration of exposure) in experimental conditions as well as in nonsmokers exposed to secondhand tobacco smoke, as reviewed in the reports of IARC (1986), US National Research Council (1986), the US DHHS (1986), the US Environmental Protection Agency (1992) and the California Environmental Protection Agency (1997). Studies involving several thousands of subjects have demonstrated that cotinine concentrations measured in the blood, saliva or urine of nonsmokers exposed to secondhand tobacco smoke at home or at work are significantly higher than the concentrations in non-exposed nonsmokers (Coultas *et al.*, 1987; Cummings *et al.*, 1990; Riboli *et al.*, 1990; Tunstall-Pedoe *et al.*, 1991; Pirkle *et al.*, 1996; Wagenknecht *et al.*, 1993; Fontham *et al.*, 1994; Jarvis *et al.*, 2001). In nonsmokers exposed to secondhand tobacco smoke, cotinine levels are typically 0.6–2% of those detected in smokers (Hackshaw *et al.*, 1997; Jarvis *et al.*, 1987, 2001; Etzel *et al.*, 1990; Benowitz, 1999; Etter, 2000), and they correlate well with self-reported exposure (Jarvis *et al.*, 1985; Haley *et al.*, 1989; Coultas *et al.*, 1987; Cummings *et al.*, 1990; Riboli *et al.*, 1990; Jarvis *et al.*, 1991, 2001, and also discussed in the reviews of the US Environmental Protection Agency (1992) and the California Environmental Protection Agency (1997)).

Cut-points have been introduced in these studies to distinguish occasional smokers from nonsmokers exposed to secondhand smoke. The cut-off values used in the various studies are typically in the range of 10–30 ng/mL for salivary cotinine, 10–15 ng/mL for cotinine in serum, 20–40 ng/mL for cotinine in plasma, and 50–90 ng/mL for cotinine in urine (reviewed in Etzel, 1990; Pérez-Stable *et al.*, 1992; California Environmental Protection Agency, 1997), but higher values may sometimes be applied (Riboli *et al.*, 1995).

The relationships between exposure to secondhand tobacco smoke and cotinine concentrations in body fluids have been investigated. Cummings and co-workers (1990) found a clear association between concentrations of urinary cotinine and the number of reported exposures to secondhand tobacco smoke in the 4 days before sampling in 663 nonsmokers. Another study that investigated almost 200 nonsmokers who were exposed to secondhand tobacco smoke at home or at work showed that concentrations of urinary cotinine increased with increasing duration of exposure (Thompson *et al.*, 1990). Every additional 10-h period of exposure was found to result in an increase in urinary cotinine of 44% (95% CI, 23–67%; $p < 0.001$).

In a large multicentre, multinationality study conducted among 1300 nonsmoking women, a clear linear increase in mean concentrations of urinary cotinine was observed from the group of women not exposed to secondhand smoke either at work or at home (mean, 2.7 ng/mg creatinine) to those exposed both at work and at home (mean, 10.0 ng/mg creatinine) (Riboli *et al.*, 1990). Cotinine concentrations have been demonstrated to be dependent both on the duration of exposure and the number of cigarettes smoked by others. When the number of cigarettes was corrected for duration of exposure and room volume, it was estimated that a similar increase in concentration of cotinine (5 ng/mg) is predicted with 7.2 cigarettes smoked at home versus 17.9 cigarettes smoked at the workplace. Based on the measured cotinine concentrations, the number of cigarettes smoked by the spouse was found to be the best estimate for domestic exposure, and duration of exposure provided the best estimate for occupational exposure (Riboli *et al.*, 1990).

Cotinine concentrations associated with occupational exposure to secondhand tobacco smoke vary somewhat more than those related to domestic exposure. This is because occupational exposure is subject to larger variations in several variables including the number of smokers present, ventilation conditions and variation in physical workload of the nonsmokers. Studies of flight attendants and workers in restaurants, bars, casinos and other similar public settings have found that these occupations lead to greater expo-sure to secondhand tobacco smoke than that of the average population, with cotinine con-centrations generally reflecting those of tobacco smoke concentrations measured in the workplace (Mattson *et al.*, 1989; Jarvis *et al.*, 1992; Siegel, 1993; Dimich-Ward *et al.*, 1997; Trout *et al.*, 1998; Maskarinec *et al.*, 2000). One study showed that in addition to exposure in the workplace, exposure of bartenders to secondhand smoke at home further elevated their cotinine concentrations (Maskarinec *et al.*, 2000). Jarvis *et al.* (1992) reported a median salivary cotinine concentration of 7.95 ng/mL and a maximum concen-tration of 31.3 ng/mL among 42 nonsmoking staff working in a bar. Thus, under certain circumstances of exposure, peak values detected in people exposed to secondhand tobacco smoke may exceed the cut-points used to distinguish smokers from nonsmokers in many studies (Pérez-Stable *et al.*, 1992; California Environmental Protection Agency, 1997).

(ii)   *Children*

The reports of the US Environmental Protection Agency (1992) and the California Environmental Protection Agency (1997) summarize studies that have reported increased concentrations of cotinine in children exposed to secondhand tobacco smoke at home. Many more recent studies have also found a significant correlation between cotinine con-centrations in children and the amount of smoking by the parent(s) (Jarvis *et al.*, 1985; reviewed in Hovell *et al.*, 2000a). A cross-sectional survey of secondary-school children conducted in 1998 found that salivary cotinine concentrations were correlated with parental smoking, but that the concentrations had halved since the late 1980s (Jarvis *et al.*, 2000). Counselling, during 3 months, of non-employed mothers who smoked and who had children under school age significantly reduced the children's urine cotinine concen-tration at 12 months (Hovell *et al.*, 2000b).

(iii)   *Newborns*

Higher concentrations of cotinine were found in amniotic fluid than in maternal urine in both smokers and nonsmokers (Jordanov, 1990). Studies of isolated perfused human placental cotyledon indicated that less than 1% of nicotine is metabolized to cotinine by the placenta. Rather, after rapid transfer across the placenta, nicotine is metabolized to cotinine by fetal tissues (Pastrakuljic *et al.*, 1998; Sastry *et al.*, 1998). The elimination kinetics of nicotine, cotinine, trans-3'-hydroxycotinine and their conjugates in the urine of newborns were first reported by Dempsey *et al.* (2000). The results indicated that the half-life of nicotine in newborns was 3–4 times longer than that in adults, whereas the half-life of cotinine was essentially the same in newborns as in adults. The data indicate that new-borns are capable of metabolizing nicotine to cotinine and of conjugating nicotine, coti-nine and 3'-OH cotinine. However, it is not known what percentage of cotinine is formed by the fetus and what percentage is acquired transplacentally, and which P450 isozymes are involved in fetal metabolism of nicotine (Dempsey *et al.*, 2000).

Etzel *et al.* (1985) used a radio-immunoassay to detect cotinine in the 1-day urine of infants born to self-identified smokers and nonsmokers. The median concentration of urinary cotinine for newborns of smokers was 1233 ng/mg creatinine as opposed to 14.5 ng/mg for newborns whose mothers were nonsmokers.

A study of 31 mothers and their newborns was conducted in Bulgaria (Jordanov, 1990). Analysis of 1-day urine by a direct colorimetric method found a mean urinary cotinine concentration of 13 ± 3 µmol/L for the newborns of nonsmokers not exposed to tobacco smoke, 18 ± 4 µmol/L for the newborns of passive smokers and 44 ± 18 µmol/L for the newborns of active smokers who smoked an average of 15 cigarettes per day; all differences were statistically significant. First-day urine of newborns was analysed in a large study of 429 mothers in Barcelona, Spain (Pichini *et al.*, 2000). Concentrations of urinary cotinine higher than the cut-off value of 50 ng/mL were measured in 17% of samples from newborns of nonsmoking mothers exposed to secondhand smoke, versus 2% for nonsmoking mothers who were not exposed to secondhand smoke. The concentrations of cotinine in the urine and cord serum of newborns of nonsmoking women with a calculated daily exposure to nicotine of more than 4 mg were significantly higher than the levels in newborns of nonsmoking mothers who were not exposed (30.9 versus 6.2 ng/mL; $p < 0.05$), after adjustment for creatinine, maternal age and sex. Daily intake of nicotine for active smokers was stratified into ≤ 3.6 mg nicotine per day, 3.6–9 mg per day, and > 9 mg per day. Urinary and cord serum cotinine concentrations were 515 ng/mL for newborns of mothers with intermediate daily nicotine intake and 568 ng/mL for the newborns of mothers with high daily nicotine intake and were statistically different ($p < 0.05$) from the concentrations in newborns of mothers with a low daily nicotine intake (161 ng/mL).

Nicotine has recently been demonstrated to occur in newborn urine. Lackmann *et al.* (1999) used gas chromatography–mass spectrometry with selective ion monitoring to detect nicotine in first voided urine samples in newborns of mothers who smoked an average of 12.4 cigarettes per day. The average concentration of nicotine in 18/31 (58%) samples was 0.63 nmol/mL. Nicotine was not detected in the urine of 17 newborns of women who did not smoke ($p < 0.001$). In the same study, cotinine was detected in 28/31 (90%) of the urine samples from newborns of mothers who were smokers, at a mean concentration of 0.87 nmol/mL. The newborns of women who were nonsmokers had a mean urine cotinine concentration of 0.049 nmol/mL. The difference was statistically significant ($p < 0.001$). Similarly, using high-performance liquid chromatography, Köhler *et al.* (2001) were able to detect nicotine and cotinine in the urine of newborns of active smokers (mean ± SD, 374 ± 765 nmol/L for nicotine and 500 ± 572 nmol/L for cotinine), but not in the urine of the newborns of nonsmokers, whether or not they were exposed to secondhand tobacco smoke ($p < 0.05$ and $p < 0.001$ for nicotine and cotinine, respectively). They also observed a strong correlation between the nicotine and cotinine concentrations in the mothers and in their newborns.

(iv)   *Alternative nicotine-related measures of exposure*

The analysis of nicotine in hair has been suggested as an alternative and non-invasive measure of exposure to tobacco smoke, particularly in children. This method may allow past exposure to be measured over a longer time period than is possible using measurements of nicotine in blood, saliva or urine. Several studies have shown a strong correlation between nicotine levels in hair and self-reported exposure to tobacco smoke or exposure in experimental chambers (Zahlsen *et al.*, 1996; Nafstad *et al.*, 1997; Dimich-Ward *et al.*, 1997; Al-Delaimy *et al.*, 2000). In fact, this has been proposed to be a more precise indicator of exposure to secondhand tobacco smoke than concentrations of urinary cotinine (Al-Delaimy *et al.*, 2002).

The concentrations in the urine of minor nicotine-related tobacco alkaloids not present in nicotine medications, such as anabasine or anatabine, have been proposed as indicators of exposure to tobacco smoke in individuals undergoing nicotine replacement therapy (Jacob *et al.*, 1999).

In summary, cotinine and its parent compound nicotine have a very high specificity and sensitivity for exposure to secondhand tobacco smoke, and, as such, cotinine is presently the best suited biomarker for assessing exposure to secondhand smoke and its uptake and metabolism in adults, children and newborns.

4.1.2   *Experimental systems*

The studies in which experimental animals were exposed to sidestream smoke alone or to simulated environmental tobacco smoke are reviewed below (see Section 3.1 for definitions).

In most studies the amount of smoke administered to the animals was monitored by measuring its total particulate matter (TPM), carbon monoxide (CO) and/or nicotine content. Internal dose measurements include those of carboxyhaemoglobin (COHb) adducts and/or cotinine in blood or urine.

(a)   *Effects of tobacco smoke on enzyme activities*

Studies in animals on the effects of sidestream smoke on enzyme concentrations have evaluated changes in phase I and phase II enzymes in liver, lung and trachea (Table 4.2). A few studies have looked at changes in enzyme activities in brain and heart.

(i)   *Phase I enzymes*

The ability of sidestream smoke to induce hepatic P450 activity was investigated in male Wistar rats (Kawamoto *et al.*, 1993). Animals were exposed for 8 h/day to the smoke from 1, 3 or 5 cigarettes/h for 5 days (6–500 ppm CO). Total cytochrome P450 and nicotinamide-adenine dinucleotide phosphate (reduced form; NADPH) cytochrome c reductase activities were not affected, but cytochrome b_5 was increased 1.6-fold and aryl hydrocarbon hydroxylase (AHH) activity was significantly decreased in the highest exposure

Table 4.2. Effect of sidestream or simulated environmental tobacco smoke on enzyme concentration or activity

Species	Strain/sex	Exposure conditions (mg/m³ TPM)	Enzyme affected	Effect (tissue)	Reference
Rat	S-D/M	n.g.	Ornithine decarboxylase	+ (trachea); 0 (lung)	Olson (1985)
			S-Adenosyl-methionine decarboxylase	– (trachea, lung)	
Mouse	C57BL/M	n.g.	Aryl hydrocarbon hydroxylase	+ (lung)	Gairola (1987)
Rat	S-D/M		Aryl hydrocarbon hydroxylase	+ (lung)	
Guinea-pig	Hartley/M		Aryl hydrocarbon hydroxylase	0 (lung)	
Mouse	C57BL/F	5.21 mg/kg bw	Aryl hydrocarbon hydroxylase	+ (lung)	Gairola et al. (1993)
	DBA/F	7.05 mg/kg bw	Aryl hydrocarbon hydroxylase	0 (lung)	
Rat	Wistar/M	6–500 ppm CO	Total P450s	0 (liver)	Kawamoto et al. (1993)
			P450 1A1, 1A2, 2B1	+ (liver)	
			NADPH cytochrome C reductase	0 (liver)	
			Cytochrome b5	+ (liver)	
			Aryl hydrocarbon hydroxylase	– (liver)	Ji et al. (1994)
	S-D/M	1	P450 1A1	+ (lung)	
			NADPH reductase	+ (lung)	
			P450 2B	0 (lung)	
Rat	S-D/M	1	P450 1A1	0 (trachea, liver); + (lung)	Gebremichael et al. (1995)
			P450 2B1	0 (lung, liver)	
			P450s	– (liver)	Sindhu et al. (1995)
Ferret	European/M&F	38; 381	P450 reductase	– (liver)	
			7-Ethoxycoumarin O-deethylase	– (liver)	
			P450 1A	– (liver)	
Rat	European/F		Cytochrome b5	– (liver)	
			Cytochrome b5 reductase	– (liver)	

Table 4.2 (contd)

Species	Strain/sex	Exposure conditions (mg/m³ TPM)	Enzyme affected	Effect (tissue)	Reference
Mouse	C57BL/6N/M DBA/2N/M	1	P450 1A1 P450 1A1	+ (lung) 0 (lung)	Gebremichael et al. (1996)
Mouse	AJ/M	87.3	P450 1A1 P450 2B1, 2E1	+ (trachea, lung) 0 (lung)	Witschi et al. (1997a)
Rat	Wistar/M	n.g.	P450s	0 (liver)	Kurata et al. (1998)
Rat	Sprague-Dawley/n.g.	73–93	Aryl hydrocarbon hydroxylase Glutathione-S-transferase	+ (lung) + (lung)	Izzotti et al. (1999)
Rat	Wistar/M	n.g.	Protein kinase C	+ (lung)	Maehira et al. (1999)
Rat	Wistar/M	10	Inducible nitric oxide synthase*	+ (alveolar macrophages)	Morimoto et al. (1999)
Rat	Sprague-Dawley/ M&F	1	P450 1A1 P450 1B1, 2B1 NADPH reductase	+ (lung) 0 (lung) 0 (lung)	Lee et al. (2000)
Rat	Sprague-Dawley/F	1	Adenylyl cyclase	+ (brain, heart)	Slotkin et al. (2001)
Rat	Wistar/M	90	P450 1A1	+ (lung)	Nadadur et al. (2002)

TPM, total particulate matter; M, male; F, female; bw, body weight; +, significant increase; 0, unchanged; –, significant decrease; n.g., not given
* With mineral fibre treatment

group. Although total cytochrome P450s did not change, P450 1A1, P450 1A2, and P450 2B1 were elevated by the high exposure regimen.

The effect of sidestream smoke on bronchiolar epithelial cell expression of P450 1A1 was studied in postnatal male Sprague-Dawley rats that were exposed to aged and diluted sidestream smoke (1 mg/m³ TPM; 6 ppm CO; 350 µg/m³ nicotine) for 6 h/day, 5 days/ week from birth until 7, 14, 21, 50 or 100 days of age. Exposure to sidestream smoke significantly increased the expression of P450 1A1 in Clara cells of the proximal and distal airways and in alveolar Type II cells in the lung parenchyma at all times, with a maximal expression occurring at 50 days of age. NADPH reductase was increased in bronchiolar epithelial cells at 21 and 50 days, but not at 7 or 100 days. Cytochrome P450 2B expression was not affected by sidestream smoke in any airway epithelial cells during this study (Ji et al., 1994).

Sindhu et al. (1995) studied hepatic cytochrome P450s after the exposure of ferrets to simulated environmental tobacco smoke. Six-week old male and female European ferrets were exposed to simulated environmental tobacco smoke (38 mg/m³ TPM (low-dose) and 381 mg/m³ TPM (high-dose)) for 2 h/day, 5 days/week for 8 weeks. In both male and female animals, there was a significant decrease in P450 content, and in P450 reductase and 7-ethoxycoumarin O-deethylase activities after exposure to both high and low concentrations. Immunoblot analysis revealed a decrease in P450 1A in exposed animals compared with controls. In addition, cytochrome b_5 content and the activity of its reductase were decreased in females.

The expression of P450 1A1 and 2B1 was evaluated in newborn male rats which were exposed to aged and diluted sidestream smoke for 6 h/day, 5 days/week (1 mg/m³ TPM). Sidestream smoke induced pulmonary P450 1A1 activity as early as day 7 after birth, whereas it was not detected in controls. Pulmonary P450 1A1 activity remained significantly (3- to 4-fold) elevated until 100 days, whereas pulmonary P450 2B1 activity did not change at any age. Hepatic P450 1A1 and P450 2B1 were generally unchanged following exposure to sidestream smoke, except that P450 2B1 activity was decreased by 30% at 100 days. The effects of short-term exposure were studied in 47-day-old rats exposed for 6 h/day for 4 days, to either filtered or unfiltered sidestream smoke (0.03 and 1 mg/m³ TPM, respectively). Whole, but not filtered, sidestream smoke increased pulmonary P450 1A1 more than threefold; P450 2B1 was unchanged by either type of exposure (Gebremichael et al., 1995).

The role of the Ah receptor in response to exposure to sidestream smoke was evaluated (Gebremichael et al., 1996). Male C57BL/6N and DBA/2N mice were exposed for 6 h/day for 4 days to aged and diluted sidestream smoke (1 mg/m³ TPM; 3.4 ppm CO; 703 µg/m³ nicotine). Sidestream smoke induced ethoxyresorufin-O-dealkylase activity in the lungs of C57BL/6N mice, but had no effect in mice of the DBA/2N strain, which has a reduced AhR functionality.

The induction of pulmonary tumours and P450 1A1 after exposure to simulated environmental tobacco smoke was examined in male A/J mice (Witschi et al., 1997a). Mice, 12 weeks of age, were exposed to simulated environmental tobacco smoke (87.3 mg/m³

TPM) for 6 h/day, 5 days/week for 5 months. The expression of P450 1A1 was significantly increased in airway epithelium and lung parenchyma of the smoke-exposed mice
after 5 months of exposure; however, after a 4-month recovery period, no expression of
P450 1A1 could be detected. P450 2B1 and 2E1 were not affected by exposure to tobacco
smoke. No enhanced expression of P450 1A1 was detected in lung tumours. Filtered
smoke containing 0.1 mg/m^3 TPM did not induce P450 1A1 expression in female A/J
mice under the same conditions (Witschi *et al.*, 1997b).

The effect of sidestream smoke on the expression of pulmonary cytochrome P450
mRNAs in rats has been examined following in-utero and postnatal exposure (Lee *et al.*,
2000). Gestating Sprague-Dawley rats were exposed to aged and diluted sidestream
smoke (1 mg/m^3 TPM; 7.3 ppm CO; 250 µg/m^3 nicotine) beginning on gestational day 5.
None of the P450 isozymes analysed were increased in fetal lungs when evaluated at 17,
19 or 21 days of gestation. In contrast, postnatal exposure to sidestream smoke induced
P450 1A1 expression as early as 1 day after birth. No induction of P450 1B1, 2B1 or
NADPH cytochrome P450 reductase was observed following continuous in-utero and
postnatal exposure to sidestream smoke.

Total liver content of P450 remained unchanged in male Wistar rats following exposure to sidestream smoke for 2 h/day for 25 days [no information on TPM or other
measurements of smoke concentration was given] (Kurata *et al.*, 1998).

Spontaneously hypertensive (SH) rats exhibit heritable risk factors similar to those
found in patients with chronic obstructive pulmonary disease, and are more susceptible to
lung injury and inflammation, to oxidative stress resulting from exposure to combustion
by-products and to induction of pulmonary diseases in general. Nadadur *et al.* (2002) used
this model to examine the differential gene expression following exposure to sidestream
smoke. Male SH rats were exposed to sidestream smoke (90 mg/m^3 TPM) for 6 h/day on
2 consecutive days. Total RNAs were isolated from lungs on the third day and cDNA was
examined by gene-expression array filters containing 588 genes. Exposure to sidestream
smoke resulted in a differential expression of 16 genes, including P450 1A1.

The effect of sidestream smoke on AHH activity was investigated in different species
and strains. Male C57BL mice, Sprague-Dawley rats and Hartley guinea-pigs [ages not
stated] were exposed to sidestream smoke once or twice daily, on 7 days/week for 16
weeks. AHH levels were significantly increased in mice and rats (3.7-fold and 2.7-fold,
respectively), but remained unchanged in guinea-pigs (Gairola, 1987). In a later study by
Gairola *et al.* (1993), female C57BL and DBA mice, 8–9 weeks old, were exposed to sidestream smoke daily [duration of exposure not stated] for 65–70 weeks (average TPM
intake, 5.21 and 7.05 mg/kg body weight, respectively). Exposure to sidestream smoke
induced pulmonary AHH activity two- to threefold in C57BL mice, but no effect was
found in DBA mice. In a later study, male Sprague-Dawley rats were exposed to
simulated environmental tobacco smoke (a mixture of 89% sidestream smoke and 11%
mainstream smoke) for 6 h/day, 5 days/week for up to 5 weeks (73–93 mg/m^3 TPM; 350
ppm CO). Exposure to simulated environmental tobacco smoke resulted in a significant
induction of AHH activity in lung microsomal fractions, which increased over the first 4

weeks of exposure; however, within 1 week after termination of the exposure, AHH activity decreased to the same levels as those measured in sham-treated rats (Izzotti *et al.*, 1999).

(ii)   *Phase II enzymes*

Male Sprague-Dawley rats were exposed to simulated environmental tobacco smoke for 6 h/day, 5 days/week for up to 5 weeks (73–93 mg/m^3 TPM; 350 ppm CO) (Izzotti *et al.*, 1999). This exposure resulted in the concentrations of GSH in lung post-mito-chondrial (S12) fractions undergoing a progressive and consistent decrease, which became significant after 4 weeks. After 5 weeks, GSH levels in exposed animals were 67% of the levels in controls. The activity of glutathione-*S*-transferase (GST) in lung cyto-solic fractions from exposed animals increased steadily and became significantly elevated after 5 weeks.

(iii)   *Other enzymatic alterations*

The effect of chronic exposure to sidestream smoke on ornithine decarboxylase and *S*-adenosyl-methionine decarboxylase activity was determined in the rat trachea and lung. Male Sprague-Dawley rats were exposed for 10 min daily, 7 days/week, for 4 or 8 weeks to 25% sidestream smoke, or for 20 weeks to either 50%, 25% or 10% sidestream smoke (Olson, 1985). Ornithine decarboxylase activity in the lung was elevated in the group exposed for 8 weeks, but not in the group exposed for 20 weeks at any dose. Ornithine decarboxylase in the trachea was significantly elevated by all concentrations of sidestream smoke at all times. None of the treated rats showed any significant increase in *S*-adenosyl-methionine decarboxylase activity at any concentration or duration of exposure.

In 8-week-old male Wistar rats exposed to sidestream smoke [concentration not reported] for 1-h periods, twice daily, for 8, 12 or 20 weeks, protein kinase C activity in lung was increased by 120% at 8 weeks, and by 86% and 81% at 12 and 20 weeks, res-pectively (Maehira *et al.*, 1999).

The synergistic effects of sidestream smoke and mineral fibres were investigated by Morimoto *et al.* (1999). Ten-week-old male Wistar rats were first given an intratracheal instillation of chrysotile or ceramic fibres and subsequently exposed to sidestream smoke for 4 h/day, 5 days/week for 4 weeks (10 mg/m^3 TPM; 79 ppm CO). Control groups included animals exposed to saline only, chrysotile only, ceramic fibres only and side-stream smoke only. Both exposure to mineral fibres and/or to sidestream smoke increased the number of cells recovered from bronchoalveolar lavage; alveolar macrophages accounted for > 95% of the total cells. Levels of IL-1α mRNA were significantly increased ($p < 0.05$) in all exposed groups (i.e. those exposed to sidestream smoke, mineral fibres, and sidestream smoke plus mineral fibres) in alveolar macrophages, but not in lung (when compared to saline-treated controls). Increased expression of IL-6 mRNA was only seen in the lung when sidestream smoke was combined with chrysotile, but neither exposure alone was sufficient to induce expression of IL-6 mRNA. No such increase was observed in alveolar macrophages. Similarly, inducible nitric oxide synthase (iNOS) was not increased in the alveolar macrophages of rats treated with mineral fibres or sidestream smoke alone, but was significantly increased in animals that received combination treatments ($p < 0.01$). iNOS was not induced in the lungs by any treatment.

To mimic fetal and childhood exposure to secondhand smoke, gestating Sprague-Dawley rats were exposed to mainstream smoke (29 mg/m³ TPM; 93 ppm CO; 4.6 mg/m³ nicotine) for 6 h/day, 7 days/week, from gestational day 5 to day 20. One or two days after parturition, dams and pups were exposed to sidestream smoke (1 mg/m³ TPM; 5.6 ppm CO; 117 μg/m³ nicotine) until postnatal day 21. Animals were exposed either prenatally or postnatally or both. Adenylyl cyclase (AC) activity was evaluated under four different conditions in brain and heart tissues: basal AC, after isoproterenol or forskolin stimulation, and after forskolin stimulation followed by carbachol inhibition. In the brain, both prenatal and postnatal exposure were effective in upregulating AC when measured by forskolin response, but not when measured by the other methods. In the heart, AC activity as measured by all methods was significantly elevated after prenatal exposure, postnatal exposure, or both. The authors concluded that postnatal exposure to sidestream smoke elicited changes similar to, or more severe than, those observed during prenatal exposure from maternal smoking (see also Section 4.3.2(iii)) (Slotkin et al., 2001).

Male SH rats were exposed to sidestream smoke (90 mg/m³ TPM) for 6 h/day for 2 days (Nadadur et al., 2002; see Section 4.1.2(a)(i) for details). A two- to threefold increase was observed in expression of macrophage inflammatory protein-2, suggesting the potential for lung inflammation. Over-expression of matrix metalloproteinase-7 was also observed; this may play a role in cell migration and invasion.

(b)   Tobacco smoke carcinogen biomarkers

Animal studies on the formation of carcinogen biomarkers following exposure to sidestream smoke have evaluated protein and DNA adducts, including those in lung and liver. These studies are summarized in Table 4.3; only the main studies are described in detail in the text.

(i)   Urinary compounds

Urine samples from male and female Fischer 344 rats exposed to sidestream smoke for 15 min four times/day for 5 days elicited DNA adducts in a plasmid assay in vitro (Takenawa et al., 1994).

(ii)   DNA adducts

Lee et al. (1992, 1993) evaluated the formation of DNA adducts in various tissues following 14-day and 90-day periods of exposure to sidestream smoke. In these studies, 7-week-old male Sprague-Dawley rats were exposed to aged and diluted sidestream smoke for 6 h/day for 14 or 90 days at target exposure concentrations of 0, 0.1, 1.0 and 10 mg/m³ TPM. DNA adducts were observed only in the lung and heart of animals that received the highest dose. Adducts in lung were observed after 7 and 14 days and were

Table 4.3. Effects of sidestream or simulated environmental tobacco smoke on DNA adducts and other biomarkers

Species	Strain/sex	Biomarker	Effect (tissue)	Reference
		DNA adducts		
Rat	S-D/*	Smoke-related (14-day exposure)	+ (lung, heart/high dose) – (lung, heart/low dose)	Lee *et al.* (1992)
Rat	S-D/M	Smoke-related (90-day exposure)	+ (lung, heart, larynx) – (liver, bladder)	Lee *et al.* (1993)
Mouse	Parkes/M	Smoke-related	+++ (skin, lung, bladder) ++ (heart, kidney)	Carmichael *et al.* (1993)
Mouse	C7BL/F DBA/F	Smoke-enhanced	+ (lung); – (liver) + (lung); – (liver)	Gairola *et al.* (1993)
Rat	F344/M&F	Smoke-related	+ (bladder, kidney) – (testis)	Takenawa *et al.* (1994)
Mouse	BALB/c/F BALB/c/F	Smoke-related 8-Hydroxy-2′-deoxyguanosine	+ (lung, liver, heart) + (lung, liver, heart)	Howard *et al.* (1998b)
Rat	S-D/M	Smoke-related 8-Hydroxy-2′-deoxyguanosine	+ (lung, heart, bladder, trachea, bronchi) 0 (liver), ± (testes) + (lung)	Izzotti *et al.* (1999)
Rat	Wistar/M	8-Hydroxy-2′-deoxyguanosine	+ (lung)	Maehira *et al.* (1999)
	S-D/F	Smoke-related	+++ (lung), ++ (trachea, heart) + (bladder)	Arif *et al.* (2000)
Rat	S-D/M	Smoke-related 8-Hydroxy-2′-deoxyguanosine	+ (lung, trachea, heart) + (lung)	Izzotti *et al.* (2001)
Mouse	SKH-1	Smoke-related 8-Hydroxy-2′-deoxyguanosine	+ (skin), ++ (lung) + (lung)	De Flora *et al.* (2003)

Table 4.3 (contd)

Species	Strain/sex	Biomarker	Effect (tissue)	Reference
		Other biomarkers and metabolites		
Ferret	EUR/M&F	(+)-*Anti*-BaP 7,8-dihydrodiol-9,10-epoxide	– (liver) (female only)	Sindhu *et al.* (1995)
		- glutathione	0 (liver)	
		- glucuronide	0 (liver)	
		- sulfate	– (liver)	
		total BaP	0 (liver)	
		(-)-7R *trans*-BaP-7,8-dihydrodiol-9,10-epoxide		
Rat	Wistar/M	L-Ascorbic acid	+ (urine, plasma, tissues)	Kurata *et al.* (1998)
Rat	n.g./n.g.	Cotinine	+ (urine)	Oddoze *et al.* (1998)
Rat	S-D/M	8-Iso-prostaglandin-$F_{2\alpha}$	+ (urine)	Visioli *et al.* (2000)
Rat	S-D/M	BaP-7,8-diol-9,10-epoxide haemoglobin	+ (blood)	Izzotti *et al.* (2001)

M, male; F, female; S-D, Sprague-Dawley; +, significant increase; 0, unchanged; –, significant decrease; n.g., not given
* Sex not stated, but likely to be males (see Lee *et al.*, 1993)

still present after 14 days of recovery. Adducts in heart tissue were first seen after 14 days and persisted through the 14-day recovery period. Neither liver nor larynx exhibited expo-sure-related adducts at any time period or any dose. In the 90-day study, animals were killed at 28 and 90 days, and after a 90-day recovery period. After 28 and 90 days, a signi-ficant elevation in adducts in lung, heart and larynx was seen only in the animals exposed to 10 mg/m³ TPM, and liver and bladder were unaffected by exposure at any time or any dose. After a 90-day recovery period, adduct levels in all organs in which there had been a response to exposure decreased, but were still elevated compared to the levels in controls [no statistical test performed]. These data establish a no-observed-effect-level of at least 1.0 mg/m³ TPM for DNA adducts.

Sidestream smoke condensate was applied topically on mouse skin and DNA adducts formed from the condensate in several organs were quantified by ³²P-postlabelling techniques. When compared with unexposed controls, sidestream smoke condensate was found to induce approximately five- to sevenfold higher levels of adducts in skin, lung and bladder and two- to threefold higher levels in heart and kidney (Carmichael et al., 1993).

Long-term studies of exposure of female C57BL and DBA mice to sidestream smoke were conducted by Gairola et al. (1993). DNA adducts were assayed in lung and liver after 65–70 consecutive weeks of exposure (average TPM intake, 5.21 and 7.05 mg/kg body weight, respectively). Sidestream smoke enhanced DNA adducts in lung in both strains of mice; the increase was about 16-fold in C57BL mice and 8-fold in DBA mice (the difference between the two strains was not statistically significant. Adduct maps showed no qualitative difference between strains, or between treated and control mice. No increase in adduct levels was observed in the liver.

Male and female Fischer 344 rats were exposed to sidestream smoke for 15 min four times/day for 5 days (Takenawa et al., 1994). [No monitoring of exposure was reported.] A significant increase in DNA adducts in bladder and kidney was seen in exposed animals when compared to control samples, but not in testicular tissues; this suggests that the DNA adducts were formed in the tissues along the urinary tract.

Adult female BALB/c mice were exposed to a regimen of 30-min exposures to sidestream smoke followed by a 90-min recovery, for three consecutive cycles. The level of 8-OHdG adducts was increased by exposure to sidestream smoke in heart, lung and liver (about 1.6-fold) and remained elevated in lung and heart after the recovery period [limited statistical analysis was performed] (Howard et al., 1998b).

In a study to evaluate the inhibitory effect of indole-3-carbinol on cigarette smoke-related formation of DNA adducts in target organs, Arif et al. (2000) found that whole-body exposure of female Sprague-Dawley rats to sidestream smoke (6 h/day, 7 days/week for 4 weeks; 27 mg/m³ TPM) induced smoke-related adducts in all tissues examined, including (in descending order) lung, heart, trachea and bladder. The adducts were quali-tatively similar in all organs, but were present in different proportions.

Male Sprague-Dawley rats were exposed to simulated environmental tobacco smoke for 6 h/day, 5 days/week for up to 5 weeks (73–93 mg/m³ TPM; 350 ppm CO) (Izzotti et al., 1999, 2001). The exposure continued for 1, 2, 3, 4 or 5 weeks and rats were killed

16 h after the last exposure. Samples of heart, lung, liver, testes, bladder, bronchial alveolar macrophages and tracheal epithelium were analysed for adducts. Examination of the autoradiograph patterns revealed the existence of four major and two minor spots in tracheal epithelium, three major spots in macrophages, and one major and one minor spot in lung, heart and bladder. All organs showed a time-related increase in adducts during the first 4 weeks, and the trachea and macrophages continued to accumulate adducts through the fifth week. When animals were allowed 1 week of recovery after 4 weeks of exposure, levels of adducts decreased significantly in all tissues except heart, but remained significantly higher than in control animals. There was a slight but significant increase in 8-OHdG adducts in lung of animals exposed to smoke for 4 weeks when compared with sham-treated rats (Izzotti *et al.*, 2001).

In a preliminary experiment reported by De Flora *et al.* (2003), SKH-1 hairless mice were exposed to simulated environmental tobacco smoke for 28 days [exposure concentrations not given]. Whole-body exposure resulted in bulky DNA and 8-OHdG-adducts in the skin and lungs of treated animals. A potential synergistic effect was noted between exposure to simulated environmental tobacco smoke and exposure to sunlight-simulating lamps with respect to the induction of bulky DNA adducts in the lung.

(c)   *Other biomarkers and metabolites*

The results of animal studies that have reported changes in metabolites and carboxyhaemoglobin levels in various tissues are summarized below and in Table 4.3.

(i)   *Blood compounds*

Serum concentrations of carboxyhaemoglobin, together with nicotine and/or cotinine, are commonly used as biomarkers of exposure in experimental models as they are strongly correlated with the estimated total particulate matter (von Meyerink *et al.*, 1989; Coggins *et al.*, 1992, 1993; Zhu *et al.*, 1994; Sun *et al.*, 2001).

(ii)   *Particles*

A comparison of the deposition of environmental tobacco smoke particles in human and rat tracheobronchial tree and pulmonary region was performed by Oberdörster and Pott (1986). Their calculations showed that the relative deposition of particles (mass median aerodynamic diameter of 0.2 μm) was about the same in the tracheobronchial tree of rats and humans, and was less in the pulmonary region in rats than in humans. However, the rate of deposition in the transitional region of the lung was about twice as high in rats as in humans. These data should be taken into consideration when using the results of experiments in rats to predict the results of human exposure.

(iii)   *Urinary compounds including cotinine*

L-Ascorbic acid is a potential scavenger of free radicals under normal conditions and following most carcinogenic insults, including the free radicals contained in and generated by cigarette smoke. To evaluate the effect of sidestream smoke on the metabolism and excretion of L-ascorbic acid, Kurata *et al.* (1998) exposed 7-week-old male Wistar rats to the sidestream smoke generated by two cigarettes every 30 min, four times/day, for 25 days [concentrations of TPM, CO and nicotine not stated]. The excretion of L-ascorbic acid into urine increased steadily with duration of exposure to sidestream smoke, and became significantly higher than in controls after day 12. At 25 days, L-ascorbic acid in liver, adrenal glands, lungs and kidneys in exposed animals was higher than in controls.

The exposure of rats to sidestream smoke produces a smoke-related oxidative stress, resulting in lipid peroxidation, that can be monitored by the urinary excretion of F_2 iso-prostanes (e.g. 8-*iso*-prostaglandin $F_{2\alpha}$), produced from arachidonic acid by free radical-catalysed mechanisms. Visioli *et al.* (2000) evaluated the antioxidant effect of olive oil on the excretion of 8-*iso*-prostaglandin $F_{2\alpha}$. Male Sprague-Dawley rats were exposed to side-stream smoke for 20 min/day for 4 days (2600 ppm CO). The excretion of 8-*iso*-prosta-glandin $F_{2\alpha}$ increased from 237 to 319 pg/mg creatinine after 2 days of exposure, an increase of 44%. After four exposures, the excretion of 8-*iso*-prostaglandin $F_{2\alpha}$ was 55% higher than in control rats. Treatment with olive oil reduced the excretion to pre-exposure levels and to a 34% increase over pre-exposure levels, after 2 and 4 days of exposure, respectively.

Oddoze *et al.* (1998) developed a rapid and sensitive assay for measuring urinary metabolites in human nonsmokers and rats. In rats exposed to sidestream smoke for 4 days [strain and sex of rats and conditions of exposure not stated], 24-h urine samples were collected before the exposure began and after the last exposure. No cotinine was found in sham-exposed samples, but the amount of cotinine in the urine of exposed rats ($n = 5$) ranged from 525 to 675 ng/mL and one sample had a cotinine concentration of 1587 ng/mL.

4.2   Toxic effects

Exposure to secondhand tobacco smoke is a cause of cardiovascular and respiratory disease. The studies reviewed here add to the knowledge of the adverse effects of expo-sure to secondhand tobacco smoke on the health of adult humans.

4.2.1   *Humans*

(a)   *Nicotine addiction*

No data on nicotine addiction resulting from involuntary exposure to tobacco smoke were available to the Working Group.

(b)   *Cardiovascular system*

A causal association between active smoking and coronary heart disease (CHD) is well established (US Department of Health and Human Services, 1983, 1990). Since 1984, some 20 studies have examined the association between exposure to secondhand tobacco smoke and risk of CHD in nonsmokers. The available literature was first reviewed in 1986 in a report from the US National Research Council (US National

Research Council, 1986) and a report of the Surgeon General (US DHHS, 1986). Both reviews concluded that an association between exposure to secondhand tobacco smoke and CHD was biologically plausible, but that the epidemiological evidence was inconclusive. Since then, numerous reviews and reports have become available (Wells, 1988; Wu-Williams & Samet, 1990; Glantz & Parmley, 1991; Steenland, 1992; Wells, 1994; Glantz & Parmley, 1995; Kritz *et al.*, 1995; Law *et al.*, 1997; Wells, 1998; He *et al.*, 1999; Thun *et al.*, 1999; US National Cancer Institute, 1999). Nine of these reviews included a meta-analysis to calculate a pooled relative risk for CHD in relation to exposure to secondhand tobacco smoke (Wells, 1988; Glantz & Parmley, 1991; Wells, 1994 ; Glantz & Parmley, 1995; Kritz *et al.*, 1995; Law *et al.*, 1997; Wells, 1998; He *et al.*, 1999; Thun *et al.*, 1999).

(i)   *Epidemiological studies*

The results of three recent meta-analyses (Law *et al.*, 1997; He *et al.*, 1999; Thun *et al.*, 1999) are summarized in Tables 4.4 and 4.5.

Law *et al.* (1997) carried out five sets of meta-analyses using published data (Table 4.4). In the first analysis, which included 19 studies of exposure to secondhand tobacco smoke and ischaemic heart disease (IHD), it was estimated that never-smokers living with a smoker have a 30% increased risk of IHD. In the second analysis, which included five large cohorts of men, it was estimated that the risk for CHD in nonsmokers living with a smoker was similar to the excess risk from smoking one cigarette per day. The third analysis, which included three cohorts, estimated that almost all the excess risk reversed after cessation of smoking; the residual excess risk was 6%. The fourth analysis was conducted on 18 studies to estimate the potential effect of confounding attributable to differences in diet between passive smokers and nonsmokers. People exposed to secondhand smoke were more likely than nonsmokers not exposed to tobacco smoke to consume diets with few vegetables and fruits and were less likely to take antioxidant vitamin supplements. However, clinical trials have indicated that taking β-carotene and vitamin E supplements does not reduce the risk for CHD in persons with no history of myocardial infarction (Alpha-Tocopherol β Carotene Cancer Prevention Study Group, 1994; Hennekens *et al.*, 1996). It was estimated that nonsmokers living with smokers eat a diet that gives them a 6% increased risk for IHD. The relative risk of exposure to secondhand smoke for ischaemic heart disease adjusted for diet was 1.2 (95% CI, 1.1–1.3). In the fifth analysis, which was based on eight studies, the increase in risk for IHD attributable to secondhand tobacco smoke-related platelet aggregation was estimated. It was concluded that the increase in experimentally produced platelet aggregation caused by exposure to secondhand tobacco smoke would be expected to have acute effects increasing the risk for IHD by 34%.

In the meta-analysis conducted by He *et al.* (1999), passive smoking was consistently associated with an increased relative risk for CHD. This association was observed in cohort studies, in case–control studies, in men, in women and in those exposed to

Table 4.4. Relative risk for coronary (or ischaemic) heart disease (and/or death from coronary heart disease) in never-smokers exposed to secondhand tobacco smoke in meta-analyses

Focus of meta-analysis	Relative risk (95% CI)	Exposure to tobacco smoke	Number of studies included and references
Secondhand tobacco smoke and IHD	1.30 (1.22–1.38; $p < 0.001$)	Never-smokers living with a smoker	Meta-analysis of 19 studies (Garland et al., 1985; Lee et al., 1986; Svendsen et al., 1987; He, 1989; Hole et al., 1989; Sandler et al., 1989; Hirayama, 1990; Humble et al., 1990; Dobson et al., 1991; Lee, 1992; La Vecchia et al., 1993; He et al., 1994; Layard, 1995; LeVois & Layard, 1995; Muscat & Wynder, 1995; Tunstall-Pedoe et al., 1995; Steenland et al., 1996; Kawachi et al., 1997; Ciruzzi et al., 1998)
Smoking at low doses and IHD	1.39 (1.18–1.64) 1.78 (1.31–2.44)	Active smoking of 1 cig/day Active smoking of 20 cig/day	Five large cohorts of men (660 IHD events) (Hammond & Horn, 1958; Doll & Hill, 1964; 1966; Hammond, 1966; Kahn, 1966; Hammond & Garfinkel, 1969; Pooling Project Research Group, 1978)
Smoking cessation and reversibility of excess risk of IHD	1.06 (1.02–1.10)	Former smokers (smoking cessation)	Meta-analysis of 3 studies (Hammond & Garfinkel, 1969; Rogot & Murray, 1980; Doll & Peto, 1976)
Dietary differences between nonsmokers living with a smoker and nonsmokers living with a nonsmoker and IHD	1.06	Diet of nonsmokers living with a smoker	Meta-analysis of 18 studies (Keith & Driskell, 1980; Fehily et al., 1984; Stryker et al., 1988; Sidney et al., 1989; Larkin et al., 1990; Subar et al., 1990; Cade & Margetts, 1991; Le Marchand et al., 1991; Nuttens et al., 1992; Bolton-Smith et al., 1993; Margetts & Jackson, 1993; Midgette et al., 1993; Tribble et al., 1993; Järvinen et al., 1994; McPhillips et al., 1994; Thornton et al., 1994; Emmons et al., 1995; Zondervan et al., 1996)
Secondhand tobacco smoke-related platelet aggregation and risk of IHD	1.34 (1.19–1.50)	Platelets experimentally exposed to second-hand tobacco smoke	Meta-analysis of 8 studies (cohort of 2398 men) (Davis & Davis, 1981; Davis et al., 1982; Schmidt & Rasmussen, 1984; Davis et al., 1985a,b, 1986; 1989; Blache et al., 1992)

CI, confidence interval; IHD, ischaemic heart disease; cig, cigarettes

Table 4.5. Relative risk for coronary heart disease (and/or death from coronary heart disease) in never-smokers exposed to secondhand tobacco smoke in meta-analyses

Meta-analyses	Number of studies analysed	Number of cases of CHD	Relative risk (95% CI)	References
He et al. (1999)	10 cohort studies, 8 case–control studies	6813	1.25 (1.17–1.32) in all studies 1.21 (1.14–1.30) in cohort studies 1.51 (1.26–1.81) in case–control studies 1.22 (1.10–1.35) in men 1.24 (1.15–1.34) in women 1.17 (1.11–1.24) at home 1.11 (1.00–1.23) at work 1.26 (1.16–1.38) pooled adjusted relative risk[a] *Intensity of exposure to secondhand smoke* 1–19 cig/day, 1.23 (1.13–1.34) ≥ 20 cig/day, 1.31 (1.21–1.42) (p for linear trend = 0.006) *Duration of exposure to secondhand smoke* 1–9 years, 1.18 (0.98–1.42) 10–19 years, 1.31 (1.11–1.55) ≥ 20 years, 1.29 (1.16–1.43) (p for linear trend = 0.01)	Cohort studies: Hirayama (1984); Garland et al. (1985); Svendsen et al. (1987); Butler (1988); Hole et al. (1989); Sandler et al. (1989); Hirayama (1990); Humble et al. (1990); Steenland et al. (1996); Kawachi et al. (1997) Case–control studies: Lee et al. (1986); He (1989); Jackson (1989); Dobson et al. (1991); La Vecchia et al. (1993); He et al. (1994); Muscat & Wynder (1995); Ciruzzi et al. (1998)
Thun et al. (1999)	9 cohort studies, 8 case–control studies	7345	1.25 (1.17–1.33) in all studies 1.23 (1.15–1.31) in cohort studies 1.47 (1.19–1.81) in case–control studies 1.24 (1.15–1.32) in men 1.23 (1.15–1.32) in women 1.22 (1.13–1.30) in USA 1.41 (1.21–1.65) in other countries 1.22 (1.14–1.30) for fatal CHD 1.32 (1.04–1.67) for non-CHD	Cohort studies: Hirayama (1984); Garland et al. (1985); Svendsen et al. (1987); Butler (1988); Hole et al. (1989); Sandler et al. (1989); Hirayama (1990); Humble et al. (1990); Steenland et al. (1996); Kawachi et al. (1997) Case–control studies: Lee et al. (1986); He (1989); Jackson (1989); Dobson et al. (1991); La Vecchia et al. (1993); He et al. (1994); Muscat & Wynder (1995); Lam & He (1997); Ciruzzi et al. (1998)

CHD, coronary heart disease; IHD, ischaemic heart disease; CI, confidence interval; cig, cigarettes
[a] Analysis confined to 10 studies that adjusted for age, sex, blood pressure, body weight and serum cholesterol

smoking at home or in the workplace. Positive dose–response relationships for intensity and duration of exposure were observed (Table 4.5).

Thun *et al.* (1999) found that never-smokers married to smokers had an increased relative risk for fatal or non-fatal coronary events when compared with never-smokers married to nonsmokers. The increase in relative risk was similar in men and women, in cohort and case–control studies, in the USA and other countries and in studies of fatal and non-fatal coronary events (Table 4.5).

(ii)   *Other human data*

Several mechanisms may increase the risk of CHD in nonsmokers exposed to second-hand tobacco smoke (US DHHS, 1990; Wells, 1994; He *et al.*, 1999). The acute effects of passive smoking include alterations in heart rate (Pope *et al.*, 2001), blood pressure, concentrations of carboxyhaemoglobin and carbon monoxide in the blood, in the blood's ability to use oxygen in the formation of adenosine triphosphate (ATP), and reduced exercise capability in people breathing secondhand smoke (Glantz & Parmley, 1995). An increase in the ratio of serum total cholesterol to high-density lipoprotein cholesterol (HDL-C), a decrease in the serum level of HDL-C (Feldman *et al.*, 1991), an increase in platelet aggregation (Davis *et al.*, 1989) and endothelial cell dysfunction (Otsuka *et al.*, 2001) have also been described. Exposure to secondhand tobacco smoke may also contribute to atherosclerosis by priming and sensitizing neutrophils, resulting in their activation and subsequent oxidant-mediated tissue damage (Anderson *et al.*, 1991).

(c)   *Respiratory system*

The relationship between exposure to secondhand tobacco smoke and a variety of non-malignant respiratory health endpoints has been examined extensively in epidemiological and experimental studies. When this topic was first raised in the 1972 Report of the Surgeon General (US DHHS, 1972), the handful of studies that had addressed this issue had provided only limited information.

Since then, several reviews of the literature on secondhand tobacco smoke have addressed some aspects of the effects of secondhand tobacco smoke on the risk for non-neoplastic respiratory diseases in adults (Weiss *et al.*, 1983; US DHHS, 1984, 1986; US National Research Council, 1986; Crawford, 1988; Eriksen *et al.*, 1988; Spitzer *et al.*, 1990; Trédaniel *et al.*, 1994; Jinot & Bayard, 1996; California Environmental Protection Agency, 1997; Coultas, 1998; Weiss *et al.*, 1999; US National Academy of Sciences, 2000).

A variety of adverse respiratory health outcomes in children have been causally linked to exposure to secondhand tobacco smoke or there is suggestive evidence of a causal association (see Table 4.6). For a detailed discussion of the relevant studies, the reader is referred to the recent reviews of the California Environmental Protection Agency (1997) and the US National Academy of Sciences (2000).

In adults, irritation of the eyes and nasal irritation have been causally associated with exposure to secondhand tobacco smoke and other annoyance has been described in

Table 4.6. Respiratory effects associated with exposure to secondhand tobacco smoke in children

Effects causally associated with exposure to secondhand tobacco smoke	Effects for which there is suggestive evidence of a causal association with exposure to secondhand tobacco smoke
Acute infections of the lower respiratory tract (e.g. bronchitis and pneumonia) Induction and exacerbation of asthma Chronic respiratory symptoms Middle-ear infections	Exacerbation of cystic fibrosis Decreased pulmonary function

Modified from California Environmental Protection Agency (1997)

several studies (US DHHS, 1999). For decreased pulmonary function, especially in combination with other exposures (e.g. prior exposure to occupational irritants) and for exacerbation of asthma, there is suggestive evidence of a causal association (California Environmental Protection Agency, 1997; US National Academy of Sciences, 2000). Some of the studies on exposure to secondhand tobacco smoke and respiratory health effects are briefly summarized below; for more comprehensive details, the reader is referred to some recent reviews (California Environmental Protection Agency, 1999; US National Academy of Sciences, 2000).

(i) Acute effects of sensory irritation and annoyance

The determination of the acute effects of secondhand tobacco smoke is difficult, because the observed reactions, although immediate, are largely subjective (Speer, 1968). A review of the irritation and annoyance attributable to exposure to secondhand tobacco smoke was published by the California Environmental Protection Agency (1997). The chemical constituents of secondhand tobacco smoke thought to be responsible for sensory irritation include organic acids (acetic acid and propionic acid), aldehydes (formaldehyde and acrolein), nicotine, ammonia, pyridine, toluene, sulfur dioxide and nitrogen oxides, among others (Ayer & Yeager, 1982; Triebig et al., 1984; US DHHS, 1986).

Nonsmokers seem to react significantly more than smokers (Weber, 1984a). The most common effect is tissue irritation, especially of the eyes (Speer, 1968; Basu et al., 1978; Shephard et al., 1979a; Bascom et al., 1991; White et al., 1991), but also of the nose, throat and airways (Bascom et al., 1991; Willes et al., 1992, 1998). The complaints are especially marked among aircraft passengers (US National Institute for Occupational Safety and Health, 1971; US National Academy of Sciences, 1986; Mattson et al., 1989).

Weber and co-workers (Weber et al., 1976; Weber, 1984b; Weber & Grosjean, 1987) and Muramatsu et al. (1983) conducted experiments in which volunteers were exposed to progressively increasing concentrations of secondhand tobacco smoke; as duration and intensity of exposure increased, subjects began to report subjective eye irritation, and blink rate also increased.

Lebowitz *et al.* (1992) found an increased prevalence of acute respiratory symptoms as levels of indoor secondhand tobacco smoke increased, especially in the households of subjects with lower socioeconomic status.

(ii)   *Chronic respiratory symptoms*

In an early study, 25% of 10 320 nonsmoking office workers reported exacerbation of pre-existing pulmonary conditions when working with a smoker (Barad, 1979).

Other studies have shown no association (or a weak and statistically non-significant association) between the frequency of major respiratory symptoms and exposure to secondhand tobacco smoke from family members or spouse (Lebowitz & Burrows, 1976; Schilling *et al.*, 1977; Comstock *et al.*, 1981; Kauffmann *et al.*, 1983; Gillis *et al.*, 1984; Hole *et al.*, 1989; Kauffmann *et al.*, 1989).

Since 1990, however, several investigations have demonstrated a significant increase in risk for many respiratory symptoms (including cough, phlegm, breathlessness, wheeze, chest illness and dyspnoea) in subjects exposed to secondhand smoke at home and/or at work (Schwartz & Zeger, 1990; White *et al.*, 1991; Ng *et al.*, 1993; Leuenberger *et al.*, 1994; Janson *et al.*, 2001).

(iii)   *Lung function testing*

A number of studies have been published that have examined the effects of second-hand tobacco smoke on pulmonary function in adults. These investigations were often initiated within the framework of research projects not primarily concerned with secondhand tobacco smoke; as a result, certain limitations apply regarding the validity of some of the findings, because of the low sensitivity and low power of these studies.

Acute exposure

Many studies have shown that exposure of nonsmoking adults to secondhand tobacco smoke is associated with a decrease in maximum expiratory flow at 25% (MEF25), FVC, FEV_1 and FEF25–75 and a decrease in dynamic lung volume (Pimm *et al.*, 1978; Shephard *et al.*, 1979a,b,c; Bascom *et al.*, 1991; Smith *et al.*, 2001).

Chronic exposure

A number of studies failed to detect any association between exposure to secondhand tobacco smoke and ventilatory parameters of lung function (Schilling *et al.*, 1977; Comstock *et al.*, 1981; Jones *et al.*, 1983; Lebowitz, 1984a,b; Kentner *et al.*, 1984; Laurent *et al.*, 1992; Jaakkola *et al.*, 1995; Frette *et al.*, 1996).

Other investigators have reported an association between exposure to secondhand tobacco smoke and pulmonary function determined using different test parameters. In numerous studies, FEV_1 and/or FVC were reported to be significantly decreased (Brunekreef *et al.*, 1985; Svendsen *et al.*, 1987; Hole *et al.*, 1989; Kauffmann *et al.*, 1989; Masjedi *et al.*, 1990; Xu & Li, 1995; Carey *et al.*, 1999; Chen *et al.*, 2001). Other studies reported a significant decrease in the ventilatory parameters FEF25–75, PEF or FEF75–85 (Kauffmann & Perdrizet, 1981; Kauffmann *et al.*, 1983; Salem *et al.*, 1984; Masi *et al.*,

1988; White & Froeb, 1980; Masjedi *et al.*, 1990; Lebowitz *et al.*, 1992). Decreases in MEF50 and/or MEF75 were reported to occur only in nonsmoking men exposed at home (Masi *et al.*, 1988) or nonsmoking women exposed at home (Brunekreef *et al.*, 1985).

(iv) *Chronic obstructive pulmonary disease*

Few studies have examined the possible association between exposure to secondhand tobacco smoke and development of chronic obstructive pulmonary disease (COPD). With the exception of two studies that reported a negative association (Hirayama, 1981; Lee *et al.*, 1986), most of them found an increased risk for COPD including emphysema and bronchitis, airways obstructive disease (AOD) and obstructive respiratory disease associated with exposure to secondhand smoke (Euler *et al.*, 1987; Kalandidi *et al.*, 1987; Sandler *et al.*, 1989; Kalandidi *et al.*, 1990; Robbins *et al.*, 1993; Dayal *et al.*, 1994).

(v) *Asthma*

Many patients regard secondhand tobacco smoke as a major factor in the exacerbation of asthma (Cockcroft, 1988).

Symptoms and lung function. Many studies have shown that patients with allergies and/or asthma experienced more nasal symptoms, headache, cough, wheezing, sore throat, hoarseness (Speer, 1968), eye irritation (Weber & Fisher, 1980), aggravation of the asthma (Dales *et al.*, 1992) and restrictions in activity (Ostro *et al.*, 1994) in response to secondhand smoke. Other studies have reported a statistically significant association between the new onset of asthma, asthma ever diagnosed by a physician or current asthma and exposure to secondhand tobacco smoke at the workplace (Greer *et al.*, 1993), in the home environment and among young adults exposed to parental smoking (Hu *et al.*, 1997; Thorn *et al.*, 2001).

Two studies have found no statistically significant change in dynamic lung volume of asthmatic subjects exposed for 1 or 2 h to tobacco smoke (Shephard *et al.*, 1979b; Wiedeman *et al.*, 1986), whereas other studies have reported a statistically significant decrease in FEV_1, FVC and FEF25–75 in asthmatic subjects exposed to smoke in a chamber study (Dahms *et al.*, 1981), to secondhand tobacco smoke from the spouse and/or other close contacts (Jindal *et al.*, 1994) or in the workplace, particularly in asthmatic women (Künzli *et al.*, 2000).

Chamber studies. Chamber studies have been used to investigate potential relationships between controlled exposure to secondhand smoke and lung function and airway reactivity in asthmatic subjects. The principal advantage of this methodology over epidemiological studies is that the exposure to secondhand tobacco smoke can, in theory, be measured precisely.

Most of the studies of exposure to secondhand tobacco smoke in inhalation chambers reported slight-to-moderate transient effects on lung function in at least some of the study subjects. In several studies, some participants experienced decreases in lung function of more than 20% and a marked increase in bronchial reactivity to inhaled histamine or methacholine. These changes in lung function are considered clinically significant, particularly when they occur in conjunction with lower respiratory symptoms such as chest tightness, dyspnoea and cough (Dahms *et al.*, 1981; Knight & Breslin, 1985; Stankus *et al.*, 1988; Menon *et al.*, 1991, 1992; Nowak *et al.*, 1997). However, these results were not confirmed by Magnussen and colleagues (Jörres & Magnussen, 1992; Magnussen *et al.*, 1992) who exposed adults with mild and moderate asthma to secondhand tobacco smoke for a short period (1 h) and then conducted a bronchoprovocation test with methacholine.

Suggestion can induce an attack of asthma (Spector *et al.*, 1976). Most of the above-mentioned studies were unable to exclude the possibility that the changes reported in asthmatic subjects were emotionally related to cigarette smoke which might result in psychological suggestion being the cause of the observed symptoms, such as changes in lung function and others (Witorsch, 1992). Urch *et al.* (1988) argued that, if physiological responses were dominant, changes in pulmonary function should show a dose–response relationship to secondhand tobacco smoke, whereas, if psychological reactions were dominant, correlations between functional changes and specific measures of suggestibility would be expected. Sixteen nonsmoking asthmatic subjects were exposed to high or low concentrations of secondhand tobacco smoke or to ambient air for 65 min. Cigarette smoke was generated by a machine located outside the exposure chamber, but visible to the subjects; during sham-exposure, the smoke from the cigarettes was diverted from the study chamber. Subjects with asthma showed significant dose–response relationships for MEF50 at 5 min, and for FVC and FEV_1 at 30 min of exposure; these results support a physiological rather than psychological explanation of the findings. In the study by Danuser *et al.* (1993), the subjects wore noseclips and were exposed to secondhand tobacco smoke administered by a mouthpiece, thus blinding them to the differences in the concentrations of secondhand tobacco smoke delivered. In these conditions subjective airway symptoms were weak, but most of the symptomatic responses of the subjects with airway hyperresponsiveness appeared to be dose-related.

4.2.2   *Experimental systems*

Studies in which experimental animals were exposed to sidestream smoke alone or to simulated environmental tobacco smoke were reviewed, and the results of studies on adult animals are summarized in Tables 4.7 and 4.8 (see also Witschi *et al.*, 1997c) (see Section 3.1 for definitions).

(*a*)   *Exposure of adult animals*

(i)   *Effects on the respiratory tract*

Rats and hamsters were exposed to sidestream smoke (4 mg/m³ TPM; 25–30 ppm CO) for 10 h/day, 5 days/week for 90 days. Hyperplasia and metaplasia in the epithelium of the dorsal nasal turbinates were the only changes seen in the rats. The changes partially receded after 30 days and had completely reversed 60 days after exposure. No signs of toxicity were observed in the hamster respiratory tract (Von Meyerinck *et al.*, 1989).

Table 4.7. Toxicity of sidestream or simulated environmental tobacco smoke on respiratory tract in adult animals

Species	Strain/sex	Exposure concentration (mg/m³ TPM)	Exposure duration; conditions	Effects	Reference
Rat	F344/CrlBr/M+F	4	90 days; 10 h/d; 5 d/wk	Hyperplasia/metaplasia of the dorsal nasal epithelium	von Meyerinck et al. (1989)
Hamster	Syrian golden/M+F			No effect	
Rat	SD/M+F	0.1; 1; 10	14 d; 6 h/d	Slight-to-mild hyperplasia and inflammation in rostral nasal cavity at high dose only	Coggins et al. (1992)
Rat	SD/M	0.1; 1; 10	4 d; 28 d; 90 d; 6 h/d; 5 d/wk	Slight-to-mild hyperplasia and inflammation in rostral nasal cavity at high dose only	Coggins et al. (1993)
Rat	SD/F	1	3 h; 4 d	No effect	Joad et al. (1993)
Mouse	A/J/M	1	3 d; 5 d; 6 h/day	Increased cell proliferation in airways	Rajini & Witschi (1994)
Mouse	C57BL/6/M		5 d	No effect	
Hamster	Syrian golden/M	1	1 wk; 6 h/d; 7 d/wk	Increased cell proliferation in respiratory epithelium of nasal septum; increase after 1-week recovery period in terminal bronchioles	Witschi & Rajini (1994)
Rat	Wistar/M+F	35 ppm CO	3 mths; 90 min/d; 5 d/wk	Emphysema in lungs	Escolar et al. (1995)
Mouse	A/J/M	83.5	20 wks; 6 h/d; 5 d/wk	Increased cell proliferation in airways during the first 2 wks. No changes in lung parameters (volume and cell number)	Witschi et al. (1997a)

TPM, total particulate matter; M, male; F, female; h, hour; d, day; wk, week; mths, months; SD, Sprague-Dawley

Table 4.8. Toxicity of sidestream or simulated environmental tobacco smoke on cardiovascular system in adult animals

Species	Strain/sex	Exposure concentration (mg/m^3 TPM)	Exposure duration; conditions	Effects	Reference
Cockerel	–	8	16 wks; 6 h/d; 5 d/wk	Increase in size of arteriosclerotic plaques, but not in number or distribution	Penn & Snyder (1993)
Rabbit	New Zealand/M	4 or 33	10 wks; 6 h/d; 5 d/wk	Dose-dependent increase in formation of arteriosclerotic plaques in cholesterol-fed animals	Zhu et al. (1993)
Cockerel	–	2.5	16 wks; 6 h/d; 5 d/wk	Increase in size of arteriosclerotic plaques, but not in number or distribution	Penn et al. (1994)
Rat	SD/not given	60	3 d; 3 wks; 6 wks; 6 h/d; 7 d/wk	Time-dependent increase in infarct size	Zhu et al. (1994)
Mouse	Apolipoprotein E$^{-/-}$/F	25	7, 10, 14 wks; 6 h/d; 5 d/wk	Increased percentage of atherosclerotic lesions in aortic intimal surface	Gairola et al. (2001)
Rabbit	New Zealand White/M	24	10 wk; 6 h/d; 5 d/wk	Increased percentage of surface lipid lesions in aorta and pulmonary artery	Sun et al. (2001)

TPM, total particulate matter; h, hour; d, day; wk, week; M, male; F, female; SD, Sprague-Dawley

Rats were exposed, nose-only, for 6 h/day for 4, 14, 28 or 90 days to sidestream smoke at concentrations of 0.1, 1 or 10 mg/m^3 TPM. The only pathological response observed was slight to mild epithelial hyperplasia and chronic active inflammation in the most rostral part of the nasal cavity, in the group exposed to the high dose (10 mg/m^3 TPM). No time-dependent increase in the severity of the lesions was observed. After a 14-day recovery period, the changes had completely reversed (Coggins *et al.*, 1992, 1993).

Male A/J and C57BL/6 mice were exposed for 6 h/day for up to 5 days to aged and diluted sidestream smoke (1 mg/m^3 TPM; 5.9 ppm CO; 549 µg/m^3 nicotine). Labelling indices in the epithelium of the large intrapulmonary airways and terminal bronchioles, but not in the alveoli, were significantly increased after 3 and 5 days of exposure in A/J mice. No signs of increased cell proliferation in the respiratory tract were seen in C57BL/6 mice (Rajini & Witschi, 1994).

Hamsters were exposed to aged and diluted sidestream smoke containing 1 mg/m^3 TPM for 6 h/day for 1–3 weeks, after which some subgroups were allowed a 1-week recovery period. Increased cell proliferation was observed in the respiratory epithelium of nasal septum after 1 week of exposure, but not at later time points. After 1 week of exposure and 1 week of recovery, cell proliferation in the terminal bronchioles was significantly increased when compared to concomitant controls and to the levels observed before recovery (Witschi & Rajini, 1994).

A similar initial increase in cell proliferation was seen in alveoli and terminal bronchioles in male A/J mice during the first 2 weeks of exposure to simulated environmental tobacco smoke (83.5 mg/m^3 TPM; 233 ppm CO; 18.9 mg/m^3 nicotine) (Witschi *et al.*, 1997a).

Wistar rats were exposed for 90 min/day, 5 days/week, for 3 months to sidestream smoke containing 35 ppm CO. Emphysematous changes (decreased number of distal airspaces and increase in alveolar chord) were observed in the lungs. These changes were accompanied by decreases in tissue density, internal alveolar perimeter, wall thickness and density and perimeter of elastic fibres (Escolar *et al.*, 1995).

Exposure of female rats to sidestream smoke (1 mg/m^3 TPM; 6.5 ppm CO) either on 1 day for 3 h or for 6 h/day on 4 days had no effect on dynamic compliance, lung resistance, lung weight/body weight, pulmonary artery pressure, or airway reactivity to methacholine (all $p > 0.4$) (Joad *et al.*, 1993).

(ii)   *Cardiovascular effects*

Cardiovascular changes resulting from exposure to sidestream smoke have been demonstrated in several animal models.

Male New Zealand rabbits, fed a cholesterol-rich diet, were exposed to low-dose or high-dose sidestream smoke (4 and 33 mg/m^3 TPM, respectively) for 6 h/day, 5 days/week for 10 weeks. A dose-dependent significant increase in the size of arteriosclerotic plaques was found in the aorta and the pulmonary artery when compared with control rabbits receiving the same diet but exposed to clean air (Zhu *et al.*, 1993).

Sprague-Dawley rats were exposed to sidestream smoke (60 mg/m³ TPM; 92 ppm CO; 1103 µg/m³ nicotine) 6 h/day, 5 days/week for 3 days, 3 weeks or 6 weeks. Infarct sizes increased in a time-dependent manner ($p = 0.023$) (Zhu et al., 1994).

Exposure of 6-week old cockerels for 6 h/day, 5 days/week to sidestream smoke containing 8 mg/m³ TPM (Penn & Snyder, 1993) or 2.5 mg/m³ TPM (Penn et al., 1994) resulted in a significant increase in the size of arteriosclerotic plaques in the aorta.

Roberts et al. (1996) developed a model to measure the rate of accumulation of low-density lipoproteins (LDL) in rat carotid arteries. First, rats were exposed to simulated environmental tobacco smoke for 4 h (3.3 mg/m³ TPM; 18 ppm CO; 615 µg/m³ nicotine) to obtain simulated tobacco smoke-plasma). Second, carotid arteries from unexposed rats were perfused with control plasma containing fluorescently labelled LDL and subsequently with tobacco smoke-plasma containing fluorescently labelled LDL. Photometric measurements were made during perfusion with labelled LDL. Perfusion with tobacco smoke-plasma increased the rate of LDL accumulation measured as fluorescence intensity (6.9 ± 1.8 mV/min (mean $\pm$ SEM)) when compared with control animals (1.6 ± 0.40 mV/min, $p < 0.01$). The maximal increase was observed after 40–60 min perfusion. LDL accumulation was primarily dependent on the interaction of tobacco smoke-plasma with LDL, which occurred before perfusion, rather than interaction with the artery wall. It was also noted that LDL accumulation resulted from its increased binding to artery wall rather than an increase in its permeability. Perfusion with tobacco smoke-plasma increased the lumen volume measured as fluorescence intensity (43.3 ± 5.1 mV versus 35.1 ± 4.4 mV; $p < 0.05$) in treated and untreated animals, respectively.

Rabbits receiving a 0.5% cholesterol diet and exposed for 6 h/day, 5 days/week for 10 weeks, to sidestream smoke (24 mg/m³ TPM; 45 ppm CO) were compared with control animals. There was no difference in serum lipids between cholesterol fed and control animals. Exposure to sidestream smoke significantly increased the percentage of surface lipid lesions in the aorta ($54 \pm 5\%$ versus $39 \pm 4\%$; $p = 0.049$) and in the pulmonary artery ($66 \pm 4\%$ versus $43 \pm 3\%$; $p < 0.001$). Exposure to nicotine-free cigarettes (35 mg/m³ TPM; 53 ppm CO) had the same effects as standard cigarettes. Vascular tension was measured in intact aortic rings. Endothelium-dependent and endothelium-independent relaxation were measured with acetylcholine and the calcium ionophore A23187, and nitroglycerin, respectively. There were no significant differences with any treatment between exposed and control animals (Sun et al., 2001).

Female ApoE-deficient mice, which are used as a mouse model of human atherosclerosis, were exposed to sidestream smoke (25 mg/m³ TPM) 6 h/day, 5 days/week for 7, 10 and 14 weeks. There were no consistent differences in serum concentrations of cholesterol between control mice and those exposed to sidestream smoke. In exposed mice, atherosclerotic lesions in the aorta covered a larger part of the intimal area at all time points than in non-exposed mice. Also the total affected area increased at a higher rate than in controls. The increase was most evident in the thoracic region. Lesions appeared thicker, as reflected by increased amounts of esterified and unesterified cholesterol in the aortic tissues of mice exposed to sidestream smoke (Gairola et al., 2001).

(iii) *Immunological effects*

BALB/c mice, sensitized with aluminium hydroxide-precipitated ovalbumin (OVA/AL) antigen, were exposed for 6 h/day, 5 days/week to simulated environmental tobacco smoke (1 mg/m³ TPM; 6.1 ppm CO; 269 µg/m³ nicotine), from days 15 to 58 after sensitization. Sensitized mice, with or without smoke exposure, had elevated levels of IgE. Exposure to simulated environmental tobacco smoke enhanced and prolonged the IgE response in sensitized mice, and the levels were significantly increased at all time points at which measurements were made (day 19 to day 58); the concentrations of OVA-specific IgG1 were elevated in the smoke-exposed group from days 34 to 54. For both IgE and IgG1 the increase was strongest at 54 days. The numbers of eosinophils were increased in the blood and lungs of smoke-exposed, pre-sensitized mice. The total number of bronchoalveolar lavage cells was increased ($p = 0.016$); about 90% of the increase was due to alveolar macrophages. The concentrations of cytokines IL-4 and IL-10 were significantly higher in the smoke-exposed group than in the control animals. The demonstration of an exaggerated inflammatory response in sensitized mice may have relevance to the early events in carcinogenesis where an inflammatory response often precedes mild hyperplasia (Seymour *et al.*, 1997).

(iv) *Effects on gastric ulceration*

A smoke chamber was designed to investigate the effects of exposure to secondhand smoke on gastric ulceration. Different concentrations of cigarette smoke (0%, 1%, 2% and 4%) were perfused during one hour into a chamber in which male Sprague-Dawley rats were placed. This exposure potentiated ethanol (70% v/v, oral administration)-induced gastric mucosal damage and increased serum nicotine concentrations, but did not affect the pH, pCO_2 or pO_2 and the concentration of HCO_3 in blood, or the systemic blood pressure and heart rate. Under these experimental conditions, exposure to cigarette smoke produced no significant changes in the blood acid/base balance or stress in the animals, but significantly potentiated ethanol-induced gastric mucosal damage. This experimental model is suitable for studying adverse interactions between passive smoking and alcohol drinking in gastric ulcer formation in rats (Chow *et al.*, 1996).

(b) *Effects of perinatal exposure*

(i) *Effects on lung development and lung function*

Exposure of Sprague-Dawley rats to aged and diluted sidestream smoke from birth (1 mg/m³ TPM; 6 h/day, 5 days/week) significantly reduced the labelling index of epithelial cells in distal airways at 7 and 14 days of age, but not at later times or in proximal bronchi (Ji *et al.*, 1994).

Gestating Sprague-Dawley rats were exposed to aged and diluted sidestream smoke (1 mg/m³ TPM; 4.9 ppm CO) from gestational day 5 until gestational day 14, 18 or 21. Maternal exposure to sidestream smoke significantly increased fetal expression of Clara cell secretory protein and mRNA in the terminal bronchioles at gestational day 21, but not at gestational day 14 or 18 (Ji *et al.*, 1998).

A series of studies was designed to determine the effects of perinatal exposure to side-stream smoke on airway reactivity in Sprague-Dawley rats. Female rats were exposed 6 h/day, 5 days/week from day 2 of life to week 8 or week 15 of age (1 mg/m³ TPM; 6.5 ppm CO). Exposure to sidestream smoke did not change the ratio of lung weight/body weight or the baseline values for lung resistance, dynamic compliance or pulmonary artery pressure. Airway reactivity to methacholine was also unaffected at either time-point (all $p > 0.2$). In animals exposed from day 2 of life to week 11 of age, sidestream smoke reduced airway ($p = 0.004$), but not pulmonary artery ($p = 0.63$) reactivity to serotonin (Joad et al., 1993). In a further study, Joad et al. (1999) exposed rats to aged and diluted sidestream smoke (1 mg/m³ TPM; 6.9 ppm CO) for 4–6 h/day from gestational day 3 until 21 days of age. The airway responsiveness of one female pup from each litter was assessed at 8 weeks of age. Perinatal exposure to sidestream smoke did not affect baseline lung function, but enhanced methacholine-induced changes in lung resistance (three-fold increase; $p = 0.02$), dynamic compliance ($p = 0.004$), and pulmonary pressure ($p = 0.007$). These changes occurred in the absence of any increase in pulmonary neuroendocrine cells, neuroepithelial bodies or mast cells. In another study, rats were exposed prenatally and/or postnatally to sidestream smoke (1 mg/m³ TPM; 4.9 ppm CO; 344 µg/m³ nicotine) for 4 h/day, 7 days/week from gestational day 3 until 7–10 weeks of age. Pulmonary pressure was not affected by any type of exposure. Prenatal or postnatal exposure alone did not affect baseline values or metacholine-induced changes in lung responsiveness. Prenatal followed by postnatal exposure to sidestream smoke reduced dynamic lung compliance at baseline ($p = 0.0006$) and increased lung responsiveness to methacholine ($p = 0.0001$). This reaction was accompanied by an increase in the number of neuro-endocrine cells and neuroepithelial bodies (Joad et al., 1995a).

Male guinea-pigs were exposed 6 h/day, 5 days/week from age 8 days to age 37–48 days (1 mg/m³ TPM; 5.6 ppm CO; 586 µg/m³ nicotine). Exposure to sidestream smoke did not change lung morphology, collagen or elastin deposition, lung volume, surface area or mean linear intercept length of alveolar airspace. Baseline dynamic lung compliance ($p = 0.05$), but not lung resistance ($p = 0.61$) was increased by exposure to sidestream smoke (see also Section 4.2.2(b)(iii)) (Joad et al., 1995b).

(ii)   Cardiovascular effects

Sprague-Dawley rats were exposed to filtered air or sidestream smoke (33 mg/m³ TPM; 60 ppm CO) for 6 h/day, 5 days/week, for 3 weeks before birth and/or for 12 weeks in the neonatal to adolescent period. Exposure to sidestream smoke postnatally increased endothelin-1 levels in plasma ($p = 0.001$) independently of in-utero exposure. Infarct size (infarct mass/risk area × 100) was greater in all animals exposed postnatally than in unexposed controls ($p = 0.005$), and was greater in males than in females ($p < 0.001$) (Zhu et al., 1997).

In rats exposed under the same conditions, aortic rings were excised and isometric force responses to phenylephrine, acetylcholine, the calcium ionophore A23187 and nitro-glycerin were studied in organ baths. In-utero exposure to sidestream smoke increased the sensitivity of aortic rings to phenylephrine ($p < 0.0005$) and reduced the half-maximal contraction (EC_{50}; $p = 0.04$). It reduced the maximal endothelium-dependent relaxation response to acetylcholine ($p = 0.04$) and increased its half-maximal contraction value ($p = 0.05$). Finally, in-utero exposure decreased the sensitivity to the endothelium-independent vasodilator nitroglycerin ($p = 0.003$). The sensitivity of aortic rings to phenylephrine was reduced after neonatal exposure ($p = 0.01$) (Hutchison et al., 1998).

(iii) *Neurological effects*

Female Sprague-Dawley rats were exposed to filtered air or sidestream smoke for 4 h/day, 7 days/week from day 3 of gestation until birth and/or for 9 weeks postnatally (1 mg/m³ TPM; 4.9 ppm CO; 344 µg/m³ nicotine). Postnatal exposure to sidestream smoke increased the mortality of the pups during the first 18 days of life ($p < 0.001$) and significantly reduced body weights at 9 weeks of age ($p = 0.016$). In-utero exposure had no effect on DNA, protein, or cholesterol concentration or on the weight of forebrain or hindbrain. Postnatal exposure reduced DNA concentration in the hindbrain, an indicator of cellular density, by 4.4% ($p < 0.001$) and increased the hindbrain protein/DNA ratio, an index of cell size, by 8.4% ($p = 0.001$). The weight of the hindbrain was not affected by exposure to sidestream smoke (Gospe et al., 1996).

Rhesus monkeys were exposed to aged and diluted sidestream smoke (1 mg/m³ TPM; 5.3 ppm CO; 190 µg/m³ nicotine) from gestational day 100 until 70–80 days after birth. Expression of beta-adrenergic and m2-muscarinic cholinergic receptors in heart and lungs of the offspring were not changed by exposure to smoke. Whereas there were no changes in the heart, a strong induction of adenylyl cyclase was observed in the lungs (Slotkin et al., 2000).

To mimic fetal and childhood exposure to secondhand smoke, gestating Sprague-Dawley rats were exposed to mainstream smoke (29 mg/m³ TPM; 94 ppm CO; 4600 µg/m³ nicotine) for 6 h/day, 7 days/week from gestational days 5 to 20. One to two days after delivery, dams and pups were exposed to sidestream smoke (1 mg/m³ TPM; 5.6 ppm CO; 117 µg/m³ nicotine) until postnatal day 21. Animals were exposed either prenatally, postnatally, or both. Prenatal and/or postnatal exposure significantly increased total adenylyl cyclase activity in brain and heart when monitored with the direct enzymatic stimulant forskolin (see Section 4.1.2(a)(iii) for details). In the brain, the specific coupling of beta-adrenergic receptors to adenylyl cyclase was inhibited in all exposed animals, despite normal expression of beta-receptors. In the heart, a decrease in m2-receptor expression was observed after postnatal or continuous exposure, but no inhibition of beta-adrenergic receptors was seen. In both tissues, and for all parameters, the effects of combined prenatal and postnatal exposure were equivalent to those seen in response to postnatal exposure alone (Slotkin et al., 2001).

In a series of studies, guinea-pigs were exposed to sidestream smoke (1 mg/m³ TPM; 6.2 ppm CO; 224 µg/m³ nicotine) for 6 h/day, 5 days/week from age 1 to 6 weeks (age equivalent of human childhood). Sidestream smoke reduced capsaicin-induced changes in lung resistance ($p = 0.02$) and lung dynamic compliance ($p = 0.04$), indicating a down-regulation of the lung C-fibre reflex response (Joad *et al.*, 1995b). Primary broncho-pulmonary C-fibres were tested for their responsiveness to chemical and mechanical stimuli. Exposure to sidestream smoke had no effect on baseline activity of C-fibres but augmented the responsiveness to left atrial injection of capsaicin ($p = 0.047$) and to lung hyperinflation ($p = 0.03$) (Mutoh *et al.*, 1999). A study on the impulse activity of broncho-pulmonary C-fibre-activated nucleus tractus solitarii neurons showed that exposure to sidestream smoke significantly augmented the peak ($p = 0.02$) and duration ($p = 0.01$) of the neuronal response to C-fibre activation, and prolonged the expiratory time (apnoea) ($p = 0.003$), at the higher dose of capsaicin ($2.0\ \mu g/kg$). Exposure to sidestream smoke did not alter baseline values or capsaicin-induced changes in tracheal pressure, arterial blood pressure or heart rate (Mutoh *et al.*, 2000). A recent study presented data to suggest that actions of the neuropeptide substance P in the nucleus tractus solitarius may contribute to these effects (Bonham *et al.*, 2001).

In summary, exposure of experimental animals to sidestream smoke can produce changes that are similar to those observed in response to exposure of humans to second-hand tobacco smoke, such as inflammatory changes in the airways and accelerated forma-tion of arteriosclerotic plaques. The results obtained from studies of perinatal exposure may provide a potential mechanism to explain the association between exposure to secondhand smoke and sudden infant death syndrome.

4.3   Reproductive, developmental and hormonal effects

4.3.1   *Humans*

(a)   *Reproductive effects*

There are inherent ambiguities in the interpretation of data on reproductive effects: if involuntary smoking in women is defined in terms of household exposure to secondhand smoke, reproductive effects could be due either to the exposure to secondhand smoke of the female or to a direct effect of active smoking on the fertility of the male partner. In most of the published studies, the effects of secondhand smoke have been estimated on the basis of paternal smoking. A possible direct effect of smoking on the father's sperm cannot be ruled out when the father has been the source of exposure to secondhand smoke (Lindbohm *et al.*, 2002).

(i)   *Fertility and fecundability*

The available data regarding the effects of passive smoking by women on fertility and fecundity are conflicting (US DHHS, 2001): some studies have reported an increased risk of delayed conception (Hull *et al.*, 2000), whereas others have found no association (US DHHS, 2001). The results of investigations of the association between passive smoking during the prenatal period or childhood and later fertility have also been inconsistent: in some studies such exposure has been associated with reduced fecundability (in the case of prenatal exposure) or an *increased* fecundability (in the case of childhood exposure), whereas others have reported no association (Weinberg *et al.*, 1989; Wilcox *et al.*, 1989; Jensen *et al.*, 1998; US DHHS, 2001; Lindbohm *et al.*, 2002). These investigations are particularly hampered by potential exposure measurement error, confounding factors and other biases.

(ii) *Pregnancy outcomes*

The data regarding the association between maternal exposure to secondhand smoke and preterm birth are not entirely consistent, but in aggregate they suggest a modestly increased risk associated with high exposure (Lindbohm *et al.*, 2002).

(iii) *Birth outcomes*

The adverse effect of cigarette smoking on birth weight is well-established; on average, women who smoke cigarettes deliver term infants that weigh about 150–250 g less than those of nonsmokers (Andres & Day, 2000; US DHHS, 2001). When expressed as relative risks, mothers who smoke have more than a doubled risk for having low-birth-weight babies (US DHHS, 2001). There is a similar association between maternal smoking and delivery of small-for-gestational-age infants (US DHHS, 2001). The association is characterized by a dose–response relationship that persists after adjustment for possible confounding factors, and seems to be more pronounced for older mothers (US DHHS, 2001).

Numerous studies have also investigated the association between fetal growth and maternal passive smoking (US DHHS, 2001). On average the birth weight of infants born to nonsmoking mothers exposed to secondhand smoke after adjustment for important potential confounders seems to be about 25–50 g lower than that of babies born to mothers who were not exposed (California EPA, 1997; Windham *et al.*, 1999a; US DHHS, 2001; Lindbohm *et al.*, 2002). However, some studies have not found such an adverse effect (Sadler *et al.*, 1999; US DHHS, 2001).

There has been little investigation of the association between maternal exposure to secondhand smoke and spontaneous abortion or stillbirth. The available data are inconsistent, although some studies have shown effects as large as those seen in investigations of the effects of active smoking (Windham *et al.*, 1999b; US DHHS, 2001; Lindbohm *et al.*, 2002).

The association between maternal smoking during pregnancy and the risk of birth defects has been extensively investigated (US DHHS, 2001). When the focus is on major defects as a single end-point, generally no association has been found. When separate classes of malformations are considered individually, there are indications that maternal smoking during pregnancy is associated with oral clefts, limb reductions, and perhaps malformations of the urinary tract (US DHHS, 2001).

(b) *Body weight*

In contrast to the extensive and consistent literature describing the effects of active smoking on body weight, findings on the effects of passive smoking on weight are sparse.

The available data suggest that women exposed to secondhand smoke weigh more than women who are not exposed. However, this association may be confounded by a more sedentary and less healthy lifestyle being adopted by nonsmokers exposed to secondhand smoke (Cress et al., 1994; Thornton et al., 1994; Bernstein, 1996).

(c)   Hormones

No data regarding involuntary exposure to tobacco smoke and levels of estrogens, androgens or vitamin D were available to the Working Group. In one study cord blood from mothers who smoke seemed to contain higher concentrations of insulin-like growth factor 1 (IGF-1) than specimens obtained from nonsmoking mothers (Beratis et al., 1994). In other studies, a decreased concentration of IGF-1 in cord blood has been reported (Heinz-Erian et al., 1998; Coutant et al., 2001).

(d)   Menopause

Three studies addressed the association between exposure to secondhand smoke and age at menopause. One study reported that passive smoking was associated with an advancement in the age at menopause similar to that reported for active smoking, but the study population was small (Everson et al., 1986). More recent investigations reported no association between exposure to secondhand smoke at home and age at menopause (Cramer et al., 1995; Cooper et al., 1999).

4.3.2   Experimental systems

A few studies have reported the effects of exposure of gestating female animals to sidestream smoke on embryo implantations, size of litters, mortality rate or body weight of pups in the first weeks of life.

Female hamsters were exposed to the smoke of 1, 2 or 3 cigarettes, twice a day, 7 days/week, from 14 days before mating until the third day of pregnancy. Transport of pre-implantation embryos through the hamster oviduct was retarded in exposed females at all three doses. In a study of exposure to a single dose of smoke, the rate of oviductal muscle contraction decreased significantly within 15 min of exposure and failed to return to baseline rates during a 25-min recovery period. Both pre-implantation embryo transport and muscle contraction were more sensitive to sidestream smoke than to mainstream smoke (see monograph on tobacco smoke, Section 4.3) (DiCarlantonio & Talbot, 1999).

Rats were exposed for 2 h/day, from days 1 to 20 of gestation, to the smoke of 10 king-size cigarettes/2 h [exposure concentrations not reported]. Exposure to smoke significantly reduced food consumption of gestating dams. The average fetal weight ($n = 8$) in the animals exposed to sidestream smoke was reduced to 91% of the pair-fed control values ($p < 0.05$). Litter size and proportion of resorptions were not significantly affected. Combination of smoke with alcohol had a synergistic effect that led to significantly smaller litter size and fetal weight than in pair-fed animals [no comparison was made with smoke exposure alone] (Leichter, 1989). In another study, gestating Sprague-Dawley rats were exposed to aged and diluted sidestream smoke (1 mg/m³ TPM; 5.5 ppm CO; 405 µg/m³ nicotine) for 6 h/day on days 3, 6–10 and 13–17 of pregnancy and killed on day 20. Maternal body weight gain, average daily food consumption and the number of fetuses and of implantation sites per litter were comparable between smoke-exposed and pair-fed controls. However, there was a small, but significant reduction in mean pup weight ($p < 0.05$). This was not accompanied by any significant decrease in fetal ossification, an index of gestational age (Rajini *et al.*, 1994). In a similar study, animals were exposed for 6 h/day to aged and diluted sidestream smoke (1 mg/m³ TPM) from day 3 to day 11 of gestation. Average pup weight per litter was not affected by exposure to smoke, but the average number of implantations and of live pups per litter were significantly lower ($p < 0.05$) in the smoke-exposed animals (Witschi *et al.*, 1994).

Gestating rats were exposed for 3 weeks before delivery to sidestream smoke, 4 cigarettes/15 min, 6 h/day, 5 days/week. Mortality at birth was higher in the exposed animals than in controls (11.9% versus 2.8%; $p < 0.001$), and body weights at 3 and 4 weeks of age were lower than those of controls ($p < 0.001$) (Zhu *et al.*, 1997). In a later study under the same conditions, mortality at birth was also greater in rats exposed *in utero* than in those not exposed (12% versus 3%, $p < 0.001$), but in-utero exposure did not reduce body weight at 4 weeks (Hutchison *et al.*, 1998). Other studies found that exposure of rats to aged and diluted sidestream smoke (1 mg/m³ TPM) *in utero* did not affect fetal body weight at any gestational age (Ji *et al.*, 1998) or at birth (Joad *et al.*, 1999).

4.4 Genetic and related effects

4.4.1 *Humans*

(*a*) *Mutagenicity, sister chromatid exchange and* HPRT *mutations*

(i) *Urinary mutagenicity*

Mutagenicity of urine from smokers has been detected by use of the *Salmonella* (Ames) mutagenicity test in a large number of studies ever since the first report by Yamasaki and Ames (1977). Urinary mutagenicity correlates significantly with the number of cigarettes smoked daily and with urinary nicotine and/or cotinine concentrations (e.g. Bartsch *et al.*, 1990; Vermeulen *et al.*, 2000).

Urine voided by nonsmokers exposed to secondhand tobacco smoke or to diluted sidestream smoke also shows bacterial mutagenicity (Bos *et al.*, 1983; Sorsa *et al.*, 1985; IARC, 1986; Kado *et al.*, 1987; Bartsch *et al.*, 1990; Smith, C.J. *et al.*, 2000; Vermeulen *et al.*, 2000). This is in accordance with the mutagenicity of sidestream smoke and samples of airborne particulate matter or the vapour-phase of the air collected from environments contaminated with secondhand tobacco smoke (see Section 4.4.2). However, the increase in urinary mutagenicity was small in many of the studies (Sorsa *et al.*, 1985; Husgafvel-Pursiainen *et al.*, 1987; Kado *et al.*, 1987; US Environmental Protection Agency, 1992; Smith C.J. *et al.*, 2000), and no increase in mutagenicity was found in the urine of volunteers (nonsmokers) after 8 h of exposure to the gaseous phase of secondhand tobacco smoke or to whole secondhand tobacco smoke under experimental conditions (Scherer *et al.*, 1990). The small increases in urinary mutagenicity that have been detected are subject to confounding from dietary, occupational and environmental exposures. Such confounding factors affect the sensitivity and specificity of the assay for secondhand tobacco smoke exposure in the same manner as they do in smokers (Sasson *et al.*, 1985; Malaveille *et al.*, 1989; US Environmental Protection Agency, 1992; Scherer *et al.*, 1996; Vermeulen *et al.*, 2000).

Increased urinary mutagenicity was clearly associated with exposure to secondhand tobacco smoke in two studies that used urinary cotinine concentrations to indicate exposure to tobacco smoke in smokers and nonsmokers (Bartsch *et al.*, 1990; Vermeulen *et al.*, 2000). Bartsch *et al.* (1990) found urinary mutagenicity to be a specific indicator of exposure to secondhand tobacco smoke. In the study by Vermeulen *et al.* (2000), an increase in urinary mutagenicity was found to follow an increase in urinary cotinine in a manner similar to that seen in smokers. In fact, cotinine-adjusted urinary mutagenicity levels showed an almost identical increase for both nonsmokers exposed to secondhand smoke and smokers (Vermeulen *et al.*, 2000).

(ii)   *Sister chromatid exchange*

Significantly higher levels of sister chromatid exchange, chromosomal aberrations and micronuclei have been found in cultured peripheral lymphocytes of smokers than in nonsmokers (IARC, 1986). However, studies on nonsmokers exposed to secondhand tobacco smoke in experimental or field conditions, where cotinine measurements were used as indicators of exposure and uptake, have shown predominantly negative results for sister chromatid exchange in cultured lymphocytes of peripheral blood (Sorsa *et al.*, 1985; Collman *et al.*, 1986; Husgafvel-Pursiainen, 1987; Husgafvel-Pursiainen *et al.*, 1987). A study of 106 adult nonsmokers who were divided into two groups according to whether they experienced high or low levels of exposure to secondhand tobacco smoke as determined from plasma cotinine levels, found no difference in sister chromatid exchange frequencies between the two groups (Gorgels *et al.*, 1992). More recently, sister chromatid exchange was investigated in 109 preschool children, aged 1–6 years, whose mothers or other persons living in the same household smoked. Exposure to secondhand tobacco smoke at home, based on interview data and plasma cotinine measurements, was found to be associated with an almost significant increase in sister chromatid exchange ($p = 0.076$) when compared with the level measured in children living in nonsmoking households. The increase paralleled statistically significant increases ($p < 0.05$) in 4-ABP-haemoglobin and PAH-albumin adducts in the children exposed to secondhand smoke (Tang *et al.*, 1999).

The frequencies of sister chromatid exchange in cord blood lymphocytes from mothers who smoked or who were exposed to secondhand tobacco smoke were not elevated when compared with those in non-exposed mothers (Sorsa & Husgafvel-Pursiainen, 1988). Chromosomal aberrations were not increased in nonsmoking waitresses and waiters exposed to secondhand tobacco smoke who had increased cotinine levels (Sorsa *et al.*, 1989).

In summary, studies on sister chromatid exchange have found marginal effects in non-smokers exposed to secondhand tobacco smoke. However, the lack of sensitivity of the assay for exposure to low doses of this complex mixture needs to be taken into account.

(iii) HPRT *gene mutations*

Smokers have been found to have higher frequencies of *HPRT* mutant lymphocytes than nonsmokers in most of the populations studied (Ammenheuser *et al.*, 1997; Curry *et al.*, 1999; see monograph on tobacco smoke). A set of studies has been conducted on *HPRT* mutations in the newborns of mothers who were exposed or not exposed to second-hand tobacco smoke. After an initial study that found no difference between *HPRT* mutant frequencies in T lymphocytes from the cord blood of infants born to mothers exposed to secondhand tobacco smoke and to non-exposed mothers (Finette *et al.*, 1997), the same authors carried out another study, in which the types of *HPRT* mutations were investigated (Finette *et al.*, 1998). Maternal exposure was based on self-reported smoking status, interview data on exposure to secondhand tobacco smoke at home or at work and on measured concentrations of cotinine in cord blood plasma. Analysis of 30 *HPRT* mutants from 12 infants whose mothers were classified as not exposed and 37 mutant isolates from 12 infants born to mothers who were exposed found a significant difference between the mutation spectra in these groups. The difference was attributed to *HPRT* exon 2–3 deletions, which are mutational events presumably mediated by illegitimate combinatorial rearrangement of multiple V (variable), D (diversity) and J (junctional) coding gene segments (V(D)J) recombinase activity (Finette *et al.*, 1998).

In another study, cord blood T lymphocytes from 60 newborns were investigated and were found not to show an independent effect of (self-reported) maternal exposure to secondhand tobacco smoke on *HPRT* mutant frequencies. However, the exon 2–3 deletions comprised 26.3 and 28.6% of all mutants in cord blood of infants of mothers who were not exposed or were passively exposed to secondhand smoke, respectively. In infants born to mothers who smoked, this percentage was 85.7% (Bigbee *et al.*, 1999).

(iv) *Other*

A study of lift workers conducted in China examined DNA damage in lymphocytes with the single-cell gel electrophoresis (comet) assay. It was found that in 255 never-smokers, the tail moment in the assay was significantly increased by any reported exposure to secondhand tobacco smoke at home or at work. Analysis of covariance showed a significant, independent effect of domestic, but not of occupational, exposure to second-hand tobacco smoke, measured by the number of smokers nearby, on the comet tail moment (Lam *et al.*, 2002).

(b)   Mutations in TP53, KRAS and related genes

(i)   TP53 gene mutations

The frequency of mutations of the TP53 gene is higher in lung tumours from smokers than in those from nonsmokers (as reviewed in Hussain & Harris, 1998; Hernandez-Boussard et al., 1999; see monograph on tobacco smoke) and this correlates with lifetime cigarette consumption or duration of smoking (Takeshima et al., 1993; Wang et al., 1995; Kondo et al., 1996; Husgafvel-Pursiainen et al., 1999). In addition, a significant difference has been observed between mutation spectra in smokers and nonsmokers (see monograph on tobacco smoke).

Frequencies of TP53 mutations found in lung cancer tissues from lifetime nonsmokers vary between 10 and 35% (Huang et al., 1998; Marchetti et al., 1998; Takagi et al., 1998; Gealy et al., 1999; Husgafvel-Pursiainen et al., 2000; Vähäkangas et al., 2001). A few studies have investigated lung tumours from patients who, as determined from interview data, were lifetime nonsmokers who had experienced long-term exposure to secondhand tobacco smoke at home and compared the mutation frequencies with those recorded in lifetime nonsmokers without exposure to secondhand smoke (Husgafvel-Pursiainen et al., 2000; Vähäkangas et al., 2001). Life-long nonsmokers studied as a single group (i.e. irrespective of exposure to secondhand tobacco smoke) were found to have a significantly lower prevalence of TP53 mutations than smokers (odds ratio, 2.9; 95% CI, 1.2–7.2; $n = 91$ for never-smokers) (Husgafvel-Pursiainen et al., 2000) or ex-smokers (odds ratio, 9.1; 95% CI, 2.1–40.0; $n = 117$ for never-smokers) (Vähäkangas et al., 2001). When the prevalence of mutations in the lifetime nonsmokers who reported exposure to secondhand tobacco smoke from spousal smoking was compared with that in cases who reported no exposure to secondhand tobacco smoke at home, mutations were more common in exposed cases who reported exposure from spousal smoking (odds ratio, 2.0; 95% CI, 0.5–8.7; based on six exposed cases with mutation and 42 exposed cases without mutation) (Husgafvel-Pursiainen et al., 2000). In addition, the predominant type of mutation detected in nonsmokers was GC→AT transition, but the number of mutations was too small to allow comparisons to be made between the exposure groups (Husgafvel-Pursiainen et al., 2000; Vähäkangas et al., 2001).

(ii)   KRAS mutations

Mutations of the KRAS gene (codons 12, 13 or 61) occur in approximately 30% of lung adenocarcinomas obtained from smokers (Rodenhuis et al., 1988; Slebos et al., 1991; Husgafvel-Pursiainen et al., 1993; Westra et al., 1993; Gealy et al., 1999). Studies that have looked for KRAS mutations in lung tumours from nonsmokers (typically codon 12) have found low frequencies of mutation: 0% (0/35) (Marchetti et al., 1998), 5% (2/40) (Rodenhuis & Slebos, 1992), 7% (2/27) (Westra et al., 1993), 9% (2/23) (Gealy et al., 1999) and 11% (13/117) (Vähäkangas et al., 2001). Only Vähäkangas et al. (2001) studied KRAS mutations in lifetime nonsmokers exposed to secondhand tobacco smoke: of the 13 nonsmokers with a KRAS mutation in codon 12, seven had been exposed to secondhand smoke and six had not.

(c) Polymorphisms in xenobiotic metabolizing genes

Many studies have investigated smokers for associations between polymorphisms of genes involved in xenobiotic metabolism, proposed as markers of susceptibility, and various end-points of genotoxicity and related effects (Vineis & Malats, 1999). However, many of the data from such studies are contradictory and were frequently based on small numbers. Few studies have addressed the influence of genetic polymorphisms on nonsmokers exposed to secondhand tobacco smoke, and no firm conclusion can be drawn regarding the influence of polymorphisms on smoking-associated biomarkers.

4.4.2 Experimental systems

(a) In-vitro studies on genotoxicity

The genotoxicity of whole sidestream smoke or fractions of sidestream smoke or secondhand tobacco smoke has been investigated in many studies. Sidestream smoke or secondhand tobacco smoke collected from indoor environments has been shown to be mutagenic in the *Salmonella* (Ames) mutagenicity assay (Husgafvel-Pursiainen *et al.*, 1986; Löfroth & Lazaridis, 1986; Ling *et al.*, 1987; Claxton *et al.*, 1989; Doolittle *et al.*, 1990) as reviewed by Sorsa and Löfroth (1989). Condensates of mainstream smoke and cigarette smoke were mutagenic in the presence of S9 activation systems (IARC, 1986; see monograph on tobacco smoke), and some studies found that sidestream smoke or secondhand tobacco smoke also induced bacterial mutagenicity in the absence of S9 (Ling *et al.*, 1987; Claxton *et al.*, 1989). One study that found that secondhand tobacco smoke condensate induced mutations in the *Salmonella* assay also observed a genotoxic response in the SOS chromotest with *Escherichia coli* (Chen & Lee, 1996). Another study investigated the particulate matter of secondhand tobacco smoke collected near the breathing zone of nonsmoking individuals and detected mutagenicity that correlated with the concentrations of nicotine in air (Kado *et al.*, 1991).

Several studies have shown sidestream smoke, secondhand tobacco smoke and their fractions to be potent inducers of sister chromatid exchange in Chinese hamster ovary cells in the presence and absence of metabolic activation (Husgafvel-Pursiainen *et al.*, 1986; Salomaa *et al.*, 1988; Doolittle *et al.*, 1990). Other studies have reported smaller effects (e.g. Chen & Lee, 1996). Sidestream smoke has also been found to induce chromosomal aberrations, but not *Hprt* gene mutations, in Chinese hamster ovary cells (Doolittle *et al.*, 1990).

(b) In-vivo studies on genotoxicity

Studies in rodents have indicated in-vivo genotoxicity of sidestream smoke, or of the combination of sidestream smoke and mainstream smoke, as reviewed by IARC (1986). Various studies have been conducted on the clastogenic effects of sidestream cigarette smoke in mice or rats under whole-body or nose-only exposure conditions. In mice exposed to sidestream smoke in an exposure chamber (whole-body exposure), a significant increase in the frequency of micronucleated polychromatic erythrocytes in the bone marrow was observed (Mohtashamipur *et al.*, 1987). Similarly, sidestream smoke and mainstream smoke condensates injected either separately or in a mixture increased the formation of micronuclei in polychromatic erythrocytes in treated mice in a dose-dependent manner (Mohtashamipur *et al.*, 1988). In agreement with chemical analyses showing that the concentrations of several genotoxic and carcinogenic substances are higher in sidestream smoke than in mainstream smoke, sidestream smoke condensate induced significantly more micronuclei than mainstream smoke condensate. This difference was more pronounced in animals pretreated with the enzyme inducer Arochlor 1254 (Mohtashamipur *et al.*, 1988).

Aged and diluted sidestream smoke was not found to induce chromosomal aberrations in alveolar macrophages in rats after nose-only exposure for 7 days (Lee *et al.*, 1992), or after 28 days or 90 days (Lee *et al.*, 1993). More recently, whole-body exposure of rats to a mixture of mainstream (11%) and sidestream (89%) cigarette smoke for 28 consecutive days was found to induce DNA adducts and cytogenetic damage in all tissues examined. The frequencies of micronucleated and polynucleated pulmonary alveolar macrophages as well as those of micronucleated polychromatic erythrocytes in bone marrow were significantly increased in animals exposed to sidestream smoke when compared with sham-exposed animals (Izzotti *et al.*, 2001).

4.5   Mechanistic considerations

Biological measurements have demonstrated uptake and metabolism of tobacco smoke constituents in nonsmokers who reported regular exposure to secondhand tobacco smoke. In particular, cotinine concentrations measured in the body fluids of nonsmokers have provided both qualitative and quantitative evidence of exposure to secondhand tobacco smoke. In addition, the presence of tobacco-specific nitrosamines and their metabolites in the urine of nonsmokers exposed to secondhand tobacco smoke, with a correlation between the metabolites and cotinine concentration in the urine, provides clear evidence of the exposure of nonsmokers to carcinogenic constituents of tobacco smoke. The results of current studies on individual variation due to environmental or genetic factors are insufficient to permit conclusions regarding the influence of these factors on the response of people to exposure to secondhand tobacco smoke.

Evidence is provided in this monograph for the genotoxicity of secondhand tobacco smoke in humans. Exposure of nonsmokers to secondhand tobacco smoke has often been demonstrated by measurements of both cotinine and protein adducts. Studies analysing somatic mutations in the *TP53* and *KRAS* genes in lung tumours from life-long non-smokers have suggested that the mutation burden in nonsmokers who are exposed to secondhand tobacco smoke may be higher than that in nonsmokers who have not been exposed. These observations in humans are supported by the findings from animal studies and other experimental systems that have demonstrated the genotoxicity of sidestream smoke (a major component of secondhand tobacco smoke), of a mixture of mainstream and sidestream smoke, and of secondhand tobacco smoke collected in indoor environments.

The evidence from studies of nonsmokers exposed to secondhand tobacco smoke, supported by other data from experimental systems, is compatible with the current concept of tobacco-related carcinogenesis. According to this concept, tobacco smoke carcinogens, regardless of the type of smoke in which they occur, are associated with genetic effects that disrupt crucial biological processes of normal cellular growth and differentiation in smokers as well as in nonsmokers (see monograph on tobacco smoke).

References

Al-Delaimy, W.K., Crane, J. & Woodward, A. (2000) Questionnaire and hair measurement of exposure to tobacco smoke. *J. Expo. anal. environ. Epidemiol.*, **10**, 378–384

Al-Delaimy, W.K., Crane, J. & Woodward, A. (2002) Is the hair nicotine level a more accurate bio-marker of environmental tobacco smoke exposure than urine cotinine? *J. Epidemiol. Community Health*, **56**, 66–71

Alpha-Tocopherol, Beta Carotene Cancer Prevention Study Group (1994) The effect of vitamin E and beta carotene on the incidence of lung cancer and other cancers in male smokers. *New Engl. J. Med.*, **330**, 1029–1035

Ammenheuser, M.M., Hastings, D.A., Whorton, E.B., Jr & Ward, J.B., Jr (1997) Frequencies of *Hprt* mutant lymphocytes in smokers, non-smokers, and former smokers. *Environ. mol. Mutag.*, **30**, 131–138

Anderson, R., Theron, A.J., Richards, G.A., Myer, M.S. & van Rensburg, A.J. (1991) Passive smoking by humans sensitizes circulating neutrophils. *Am. Rev. respir. Dis.*, **144**, 570–574

Anderson, K.E., Carmella, S.G., Ye, M., Bliss, R.L., Le, C., Murphy, L. & Hecht, S.S. (2001) Meta-bolites of a tobacco-specific lung carcinogen in nonsmoking women exposed to environ-mental tobacco smoke. *J. natl Cancer Inst.*, **93**, 378–381

Andres, R.L. & Day, M.C. (2000) Perinatal complications associated with maternal tobacco use. *Semin. Neonatol.*, **5**, 231–241

Arif, J.M., Gairola, C.G., Kelloff, G.J., Lubet, R.A. & Gupta, R.C. (2000) Inhibition of cigarette smoke-related DNA adducts in rat tissues by indole-3-carbinol. *Mutat. Res.*, **452**, 11–18

Arnould, J.P., Verhoest, P., Bach, V., Libert, J.P. & Belegaud, J. (1997) Detection of benzo[*a*]-pyrene–DNA adducts in human placenta and umbilical cord blood. *Hum. exp. Toxicol.*, **16**, 716–721

Ayer, H.E. & Yeager, D.W. (1982) Irritants in cigarette smoke plumes. *Am. J. public Health*, **72**, 1283–1285

Barad, C.B. (1979) Smoking on the job: The controversy heats up. *Occup. Health Saf.*, **48**, 21–24

Bartsch, H., Caporaso, N., Coda, M., Kadlubar, F., Malaveille, C., Skipper, P., Talaska, G., Tannenbaum, S.R. & Vineis, P. (1990) Carcinogen hemoglobin adducts, urinary mutagenicity, and metabolic phenotype in active and passive cigarette smokers. *J. natl. Cancer Inst.*, **82**, 1826–1831

Bascom, R., Kulle, T., Kagey-Sobotka, A. & Proud, D. (1991) Upper respiratory tract environ-mental tobacco smoke sensitivity. *Am. Rev. respir. Dis.*, **143**, 1304–1311

Basu, P.K., Pimm, P.E., Shephard, R.J. & Silverman, F. (1978) The effect of cigarette smoke on the human tear film. *Can. J. Ophthalmol.*, **13**, 22–26

Benowitz, N.L. (1996) Cotinine as a biomarker of environmental tobacco smoke exposure. *Epidemiol. Rev.*, **18**, 188–204

Benowitz, N.L. (1999) Biomarkers of environmental tobacco smoke exposure. *Environ. Health Perspect.*, **107** (Suppl. 2), 349–355

Beratis, N.G., Varvarigou, A., Makri, M. & Vagenakis, A.G. (1994) Prolactin, growth hormone and insulin-like growth factor-I in newborn children of smoking mothers. *Clin. Endocrinol.*, **40**, 179–185

Bernstein, M., Morabia, A., Héritier, S. & Katchatrian, N. (1996) Passive smoking, active smoking, and education: Their relationship to weight history in women in Geneva. *Am. J. public Health*, **86**, 1267–1272

Bianchini, F., Donato, F., Faure, H., Ravanat, J.-L., Hall, J. & Cadet, J. (1998) Urinary excretion of 5-(hydroxymethyl)uracil in healthy volunteers: Effect of active and passive tobacco smoke. *Int. J. Cancer*, **77**, 40–46

Bigbee, W.L., Day, R.D., Grant, S.G., Keohavong, P., Xi, L., Zhang, L. & Ness, R.B. (1999) Impact of maternal lifestyle factors on newborn *HPRT* mutant frequencies and molecular spectrum — Initial results from the Prenatal Exposures and Preeclampsia Prevention (PEPP) Study. *Mutat. Res.*, **431**, 279–289

Blache, D., Bouthillier, D. & Davignon, J. (1992) Acute influence of smoking on platelet behaviour, endothelium and plasma lipids and normalization by aspirin. *Atherosclerosis*, **93**, 179–188

Bolton-Smith, C., Woodward, M., Brown, C.A. & Tunstall-Pedoe, H. (1993) Nutrient intake by duration of ex-smoking in the Scottish Heart Health Study. *Br. J. Nutr.*, **69**, 315–332

Bonham, A.C., Chen, C.Y., Mutoh, T. & Joad, J.P. (2001) Lung C-fiber CNS reflex: Role in the respiratory consequences of extended environmental tobacco smoke exposure in young guinea pigs. *Environ. Health Perspect.*, **109** (Suppl. 4), 573–578

Bono, R., Vincenti, M., Meineri, V., Pignata, C., Saglia, U., Giachino, O. & Scursatone, E. (1999) Formation of *N*-(2-hydroxyethyl)valine due to exposure to ethylene oxide via tobacco smoke: A risk factor for onset of cancer. *Environ. Res.*, **81**, 62–71

Bos, R.P., Theuws, J.L.G. & Henderson, P.T. (1983) Excretion of mutagens in human urine after passive smoking. *Cancer Lett.*, **19**, 85–90

Branner, B., Kutzer, C., Zwickenpflug, W., Scherer, G., Heller, W.-D. & Richter, E. (1998) Haemoglobin adducts from aromatic amines and tobacco-specific nitrosamines in pregnant smoking and non-smoking women. *Biomarkers*, **3**, 35–47

Brunekreef, B., Fischer, P., Remijn, B., van der Lende, R., Schouten, J. & Quanjer, P. (1985) Indoor air pollution and its effect on pulmonary function of adult non-smoking women: III. Passive smoking and pulmonary function. *Int. J. Epidemiol.*, **14**, 227–230

Butler, T.L. (1988) *The Relationship of Passive Smoking to Various Health Outcomes Among Seventh-Day Adventists in California*, Doctor of Public Health Dissertation, Los Angeles, University of California

Cade, J.E. & Margetts, B.M. (1991) Relationship between diet and smoking — Is the diet of smokers different? *J. Epidemiol. Community Health*, **45**, 270–272

California Environmental Protection Agency (1997) *Health Effects of Exposure to Environmental Tobacco Smoke*, Sacramento, CA

Carey, I.M., Cook, D.G. & Strachan, D.P. (1999) The effects of environmental tobacco smoke exposure on lung function in a longitudinal study of British adults. *Epidemiology*, **10**, 319–326

Carmichael, P.L., Hewer, A., Jacob, J., Grimmer, G. & Phillips, D.H. (1993) Comparison of total DNA adduct levels induced in mouse tissues and human skin by mainstream and sidestream cigarette smoke condensates. In: Phillips, D.H., Castegnaro, M. & Bartsch, H., *Postlabelling Methods for Detection of DNA Adducts* (IARC Scientific Publications No. 124), Lyon, IARC*Press*, pp. 321–326

Carrer, P., Maroni, M., Alcini, D., Cavallo, D., Fustinoni, S., Lovato, L. & Visigalli, F. (2000) Assessment through environmental and biological measurements of total daily exposure to volatile organic compounds of office workers in Milan, Italy. *Indoor Air*, **10**, 258–268

Casto, D.T., Schnapf, B.M. & Clotz, M.A. (1990) Lack of effect of short-term passive smoking on the metabolic disposition of theophylline. *Eur. J. clin. Pharmacol.*, **39**, 399–402

Castro, A. & Monji, N. (1986) Dietary nicotine and its significance in studies on tobacco smoking. *Biochem. Arch.*, **2**, 91–97

Chen, C.-C. & Lee, H. (1996) Genotoxicity and DNA adduct formation of incense smoke condensates: Comparison with environmental tobacco smoke condensates. *Mutat. Res.*, **367**, 105–114

Chen, R., Tunstall-Pedoe, H. & Tavendale, R. (2001) Environmental tobacco smoke and lung function in employees who never smoked: The Scottish MONICA study. *Occup. environ. Med.*, **58**, 563–568

Chow, J.Y., Ma, L. & Cho, C.H. (1996) An experimental model for studying passive cigarette smoking effects on gastric ulceration. *Life Sci.*, **58**, 2415–2422

Ciruzzi, M., Pramparo, P., Esteban, O., Rozlosnik, J., Tartaglione, J., Abecasis, B., César, J. , De Rosa, J., Paterno, C. & Schargrodsky, H. (1998) Case–control study of passive smoking at home and risk of acute myocardial infarction. *J. Am. Coll. Cardiol.*, **31**, 797–803

Claxton, L.D., Morin, R.S., Hughes, T.J. & Lewtas, J. (1989) A genotoxic assessment of environmental tobacco smoke using bacterial bioassays. *Mutat. Res.*, **222**, 81–99

Cockcroft, D.W. (1988) Cigarette smoking, airway hyperresponsiveness, and asthma. *Chest*, **94**, 675–676

Coggins, C.R.E., Ayres, P.H., Mosberg, A.T., Ogden, M.W., Sagartz, J.W. & Hayes, A.W. (1992) Fourteen-day inhalation study in rats, using aged and diluted sidestream smoke from a reference cigarette. I. Inhalation toxicology and histopathology. *Fundam. appl. Toxicol.*, **19**, 133–140

Coggins, C.R.E., Ayres, P.H., Mosberg, A.T., Sagartz, J.W.& Hayes, A.W. (1993) Subchronic inhalation study in rats using aged and diluted sidestream smoke from a reference cigarette. *Inhal. Toxicol.*, **5**, 77–96

Coghlin, J., Gann, P.H., Hammond, S.K., Skipper, P.L., Taghizadeh, K., Paul, M. & Tannenbaum, S.R. (1991) 4-Aminobiphenyl hemoglobin adducts in fetuses exposed to the tobacco smoke carcinogen *in utero*. *J. natl Cancer Inst.*, **83**, 274–280

Collman, G.W., Lundgren, K., Shore, D., Thompson, C.L. & Lucier, G.W. (1986) Effects of α-naphthoflavone on levels of sister chromatid exchanges in lymphocytes from active and passive cigarette smokers: Dose–response relationships. *Cancer Res.*, **46**, 6452–6455

Comstock, G.W., Meyer, M.B., Helsing, K.J. & Tockman, M.S. (1981) Respiratory effects on household exposures to tobacco smoke and gas cooking. *Am. Rev. respir. Dis.*, **124**, 143–148

Cooper, G.S., Sandler, D.P. & Bohlig, M. (1999) Active and passive smoking and the occurrence of natural menopause. *Epidemiology*, **10**, 771–773

Coultas, D.B. (1998) Health effects of passive smoking. 8. Passive smoking and risk of adult asthma and COPD: An update. *Thorax*, **53**, 381–387

Coultas, D.B., Howard, C.A., Peake, G.T., Skipper, B.J. & Samet, J.M. (1987) Salivary cotinine levels and involuntary tobacco smoke exposure in children and adults in New Mexico. *Am. Rev. respir. Dis.*, **136**, 305–309

Coutant, R., Boux de Casson, F., Douay, O., Mathieu, E., Rouleau, S., Beringue, F., Gillard, P., Limal, J.M. & Descamps, P. (2001) Relationships between placental GH concentration and maternal smoking, newborn gender, and maternal leptin: Possible implications for birth weight. *J. clin. Endocrinol.*, **86**, 4854–4859

Cramer, D.W., Harlow, B.L., Xu, H., Fraer, C. & Barbieri, R. (1995) Cross-sectional and case-controlled analyses of the association between smoking and early menopause. *Maturitas*, **22**, 79–87

Crawford, W.A. (1988) On the health effects of environmental tobacco smoke. *Arch. environ. Health*, **43**, 34–37

Crawford, F.G., Mayer, J., Santella, R.M., Cooper, T.B., Ottman, R., Tsai, W.-Y., Simon-Cereijido, G., Wang, M., Tang, D. & Perera, F.P. (1994) Biomarkers of environmental tobacco smoke in preschool children and their mothers. *J. natl Cancer Inst.*, **86**, 1398–1402

Cress, R.D., Holly, E.A., Aston, D.A., Ahn, D.K. & Kristiansen, J.J. (1994) Characteristics of women nonsmokers exposed to passive smoke. *Prev. Med.*, **23**, 40–47

Cummings, K.M., Markello, S.J., Mahoney, M., Bhargava, A.K., McElroy, P.D. & Marshall, J.R. (1990) Measurement of current exposure to environmental tobacco smoke. *Arch. environ. Health*, **45**, 74–79

Curry, J., Karnaoukhova, L., Guenette, G.C. & Glickman, B.W. (1999) Influence of sex, smoking and age on human *hprt* mutation frequencies and spectra. *Genetics*, **152**, 1065–1077

Dahms, T.E., Bolin, J.F. & Slavin, R.G. (1981) Passive smoking. Effects on bronchial asthma. *Chest*, **80**, 530–534

Dales, R.E., Kerr, P.E., Schweitzer, I., Reesor, K., Gougeon, L. & Dickinson, G. (1992) Asthma management preceding an emergency department visit. *Arch. intern. Med.*, **152**, 2041–2044

Danuser, B., Weber, A., Hartmann, A.L. & Krueger, H. (1993) Effects of a bronchoprovocation challenge test with cigarette sidestream smoke on sensitive and healthy adults. *Chest*, **103**, 353–358

Daube, H., Scherer, G., Riedel, K., Ruppert, T., Tricker, A.R., Rosenbaum, P. & Adlkofer, F. (1997) DNA adducts in human placenta in relation to tobacco smoke exposure and plasma antioxidant status. *J. Cancer Res. clin. Oncol.*, **123**, 141–151

Davis, J.W. & Davis, R.F. (1981) Prevention of cigarette smoking-induced platelet aggregate formation by aspirin. *Arch. intern. Med.*, **141**, 206–207

Davis, J.W., Davis, R.F. & Hassanein, K.M. (1982) In healthy habitual smokers acetylsalicylic acid abolishes the effects of tobacco smoke on the platelet aggregate ratio. *Can. med. Assoc. J.*, **126**, 637–639

Davis, J.W., Hartman, C.R., Lewis, H.D., Jr, Shelton, L., Eigenberg, D.A., Hassanein, K.M., Hignite, C.E. & Ruttinger, H.A. (1985a) Cigarette smoking-induced enhancement of platelet function: Lack of prevention by aspirin in men with coronary artery disease. *J. Lab. clin. Med.*, **105**, 479–483

Davis, J.W., Shelton, L., Eigenberg, D.A., Hignite, C.E. & Watanabe, I.S. (1985b) Effects of tobacco and non-tobacco cigarette smoking on endothelium and platelets. *Clin. Pharmacol. Ther.*, **37**, 529–533

Davis, J.W., Shelton, L., Hartman, C.R., Eigenberg, D.A. & Ruttinger, H.A. (1986) Smoking-induced changes in endothelium and platelets are not affected by hydroxyethylrutosides. *Br. J. exp. Pathol.*, **67**, 765–771

Davis, J.W., Shelton, L., Watanabe, I.S. & Arnold, J. (1989) Passive smoking affects endothelium and platelets. *Arch. intern. Med.*, **149**, 386–389

Davis, R.A., Stiles, M.F., deBethizy, J.D. & Reynolds, J.H. (1991) Dietary nicotine: A source of urinary cotinine. *Food chem. Toxicol.*, **29**, 821–827

Dayal, H.H., Khuder, S., Sharrar, R. & Trieff, N. (1994) Passive smoking in obstructive respiratory diseases in an industrialized urban population. *Environ. Res.*, **65**, 161–171

De Flora, S., D'Agostini, F., Balansky, R., Camoirano, A., Bennicelli, C., Bagnasco, M., Cartiglia, C., Tampa, E., Longobardi, M.G., Lubet, R.A., & Izzotti, A. (2003) Modulation of cigarette smoke-related end-points in mutagenesis and carcinogenesis. *Mutat. Res.*, **523–524**, 237–252

Dempsey, D., Jacob, P., III & Benowitz, N.L. (2000) Nicotine metabolism and elimination kinetics in newborns. *Clin. Pharmacol. Ther.*, **67**, 458–465

DiCarlantonio, G. & Talbot, P. (1999) Inhalation of mainstream and sidestream cigarette smoke retards embryo transport and slows muscle contraction in oviducts of hamsters (*Mesocricetus auratus*). *Biol. Reprod.*, **61**, 651–656

Dimich-Ward, H., Gee, H., Brauer, M. & Leung, V. (1997) Analysis of nicotine and cotinine in the hair of hospitality workers exposed to environmental tobacco smoke. *J. occup. environ. Med.*, **39**, 946–948

Dobson, A.J., Alexander, H.M., Heller, R.F. & Lloyd, D.M. (1991) Passive smoking and the risk of heart attack or coronary death. *Med. J. Aust.*, **154**, 793–797

Doll, R. & Hill, A.B. (1964) Mortality in relation to smoking: Ten years' observations of British doctors. *Br. med. J.*, **i**, 1399–1410

Doll, R. & Hill, A.B. (1966) Mortality of British doctors in relation to smoking: Observations on coronary thrombosis. *Natl Cancer Inst. Monogr.*, **19**, 205–268

Doll, R. & Peto, R. (1976) Mortality in relation to smoking: 20 years' observations on male British doctors. *Br. med. J.*, **ii**, 1525–1536

Domino, E.F., Hornbach, E. & Demana, T. (1993) The nicotine content of common vegetables. *New Engl. J. Med.*, **329**, 437

Doolittle, D.J., Lee, C.K., Ivett, J.L., Mirsalis, J.C., Riccio, E., Rudd, C.J., Burger, G.T. & Hayes, A.W. (1990) Genetic toxicology studies comparing the activity of sidestream smoke from cigarettes which burn or only heat tobacco. *Mutat. Res.*, **240**, 59–72

Ece, A., Gürkan, F., Haspolat, K., Derman, O. & Kirbas, G. (2000) Passive smoking and expired carbon monoxide concentrations in healthy and asthmatic children. *Allergol. Immunopathol.*, **28**, 255–260

Emmons, K.M., Thompson, B., Feng, Z., Hebert, J.R., Heimendinger, J. & Linnan, L. (1995) Dietary intake and exposure to environmental tobacco smoke in a worksite population. *Eur. J. clin. Nutr.*, **49**, 336–345

Eriksen, M.P., LeMaistre, C.A. & Newell, G.R. (1988) Health hazards of passive smoking. *Ann. Rev. public Health*, **9**, 47–70

Escolar, J.D., Martínez, M.N., Rodríguez, F.J., Gonzalo, C., Escolar, M.A. & Roche, P.A. (1995) Emphysema as a result of involuntary exposure to tobacco smoke: Morphometrical study of the rat. *Exp. Lung Res.*, **21**, 255–273

Etter, J.-F., Duc, T.V. & Perneger, T.V. (2000) Saliva cotinine levels in smokers and nonsmokers. *Am. J. Epidemiol.*, **151**, 251–258

Etzel, R.A. (1990) A review of the use of saliva cotinine as a marker of tobacco smoke exposure. *Prev. Med.*, **19**, 190–197

Etzel, R.A., Greenberg, R.A., Haley, N.J. & Loda, F.A. (1985) Urine cotinine excretion in neonates exposed to tobacco smoke products in utero. *J. Pediatr.*, **107**, 146–148

Euler, G.L., Abbey, D.E., Magie, A.R. & Hodgkin, J.E. (1987) Chronic obstructive pulmonary disease symptom effects of long-term cumulative exposure to ambient levels of total suspended particulates and sulfur dioxide in California Seventh-Day Adventist residents. *Arch. environ. Health*, **42**, 213–222

Everson, R.B., Sandler, D.P., Wilcox, A.J., Schreinemachers, D., Shore, D.L. & Weinberg, C. (1986) Effect of passive exposure to smoking on age at natural menopause. *Br. med. J.*, **293**, 792

Fehily, A.M., Phillips, K.M. & Yarnell, J.W.G. (1984) Diet, smoking, social class, and body mass index in the Caerphilly Heart Disease Study. *Am. J. clin. Nutr.*, **40**, 827–833

Feldman, J., Shenker, I.R., Etzel, R.A., Spierto, F.W., Lilienfield, D.E., Nussbaum, M. & Jacobson, M.S. (1991) Passive smoking alters lipid profiles in adolescents. *Pediatrics*, **88**, 259–264

Finette, B.A., Poseno, T., Vacek, P.M. & Albertini, R.J. (1997) The effects of maternal cigarette smoke exposure on somatic mutant frequencies at the *hprt* locus in healthy newborns. *Mutat. Res.*, **377**, 115–123

Finette, B.A., O'Neill, J.P., Vacek, P.M. & Albertini, R.J. (1998) Gene mutations with characteristic deletions in cord blood T lymphocytes associated with passive maternal exposure to tobacco smoke. *Nat. Med.*, **4**, 1144–1151

Fontham, E.T.H., Correa, P., Reynolds, P., Wu-Williams, A., Buffler, P.A., Greenberg, R.S., Chen, V.W., Alterman, T., Boyd, P., Austin, D.F. & Liff, J. (1994) Environmental tobacco smoke and lung cancer in nonsmoking women. A multicenter study. *J. Am. med. Assoc.*, **271**, 1752–1759

Frette, C., Barrett-Connor, E. & Clausen, J.L. (1996) Effect of active and passive smoking on ventilatory function in elderly men and women. *Am. J. Epidemiol.*, **143**, 757–765

Gairola, C.G. (1987) Pulmonary aryl hydrocarbon hydroxylase activity of mice, rats and guinea pigs following long term exposure to mainstream and sidestream cigarette smoke. *Toxicology*, **45**, 177–184

Gairola, C.G., Wu, H., Gupta, R.C. & Diana, J.N. (1993) Mainstream and sidestream cigarette smoke-induced DNA adducts in C57B1 and DBA mice. *Environ. Health Perspect.*, **99**, 253–255

Gairola, C.G., Drawdy, M.L., Block, A.E. & Daugherty, A. (2001) Sidestream cigarette smoke accelerates atherogenesis in apolipoprotein E$^{-/-}$ mice. *Atherosclerosis*, **156**, 49–55

Garland, C., Barrett-Connor, E., Suarez, L., Criqui, M.H. & Wingard, D.L. (1985) Effects of passive smoking on ischemic heart disease mortality of nonsmokers. A prospective study. *Am. J. Epidemiol.*, **121**, 645–650

Gealy, R., Zhang, L., Siegfried, J.M., Luketich, J.D. & Keohavong, P. (1999) Comparison of mutations in the p53 and K-ras genes in lung carcinomas from smoking and nonsmoking women. *Cancer Epidemiol. Biomarkers Prev.*, **8**, 297–302

Gebremichael, A., Chang, A.M., Buckpitt, A.R., Plopper, C.G. & Pinkerton, K.E. (1995) Postnatal development of cytochrome P4501A1 and 2B1 in rat lung and liver: Effect of aged and diluted sidestream cigarette smoke. *Toxicol. appl. Pharmacol.*, **135**, 246–253

Gebremichael, A., Tullis, K., Denison, M.S., Cheek, J.M. & Pinkerton, K.E. (1996) Ah-receptor-dependent modulation of gene expression by aged and diluted sidestream cigarette smoke. *Toxicol. appl. Pharmacol.*, **141**, 76–83

Georgiadis, P., Topinka, J., Stoikidou, M., Kaila, S., Gioka, M., Katsouyanni, K., Sram, R., Autrup, H. & Kyrtopoulos, S.A. on behalf of the AULIS Network (2001) Biomarkers of genotoxicity of air pollution (the AULIS project): Bulky DNA adducts in subjects with moderate to low exposures to airborne polycyclic aromatic hydrocarbons and their relationship to environmental tobacco smoke and other parameters. *Carcinogenesis*, **22**, 1447–1457

Gillis, C.R., Hole, D.J., Hawthorne, V.M. & Boyle, P. (1984) The effect of environmental tobacco smoke in two urban communities in the west of Scotland. *Eur. J. respir. Dis.*, **133** (Suppl.), 121–126

Glantz, S.A. & Parmley, W.W. (1991) Passive smoking and heart disease. Epidemiology, physiology, and biochemistry. *Circulation*, **83**, 1–12

Glantz, S.A. & Parmley, W.W. (1995) Passive smoking and heart disease. Mechanisms and risk. *J. Am. med. Assoc.*, **273**, 1047–1053

Gorgels, W.J.M.J., van Poppel, G., Jarvis, M.J., Stenhuis, W. & Kok, F.J. (1992) Passive smoking and sister-chromatid exchanges in lymphocytes. *Mutat. Res.*, **279**, 233–238

Gospe, S.M., Jr, Zhou, S.S. & Pinkerton, K.E. (1996) Effects of environmental tobacco smoke exposure in utero and/or postnatally on brain development. *Pediatr. Res.*, **39**, 494–498

Greer, J.R., Abbey, D.E. & Burchette, R.J. (1993) Asthma related to occupational and ambient air pollutants in nonsmokers. *J. occup. Med.*, **35**, 909–915

Grimmer, G., Dettbarn, G., Seidel, A. & Jacob, J. (2000) Detection of carcinogenic aromatic amines in the urine of non-smokers. *Sci. total Environ.*, **247**, 81–90

Haley, N.J., Colosimo, S.G., Axelrad, C.M., Harris, R. & Sepkovic, D.W. (1989) Biochemical validation of self-reported exposure to environmental tobacco smoke. *Environ. Res.*, **49**, 127–135

Hall, G.L., Reinmann, B., Wildhaber, J.H. & Frey, U. (2002) Tidal exhaled nitric oxide in healthy, unsedated newborn infants with prenatal tobacco exposure. *J. appl. Physiol.*, **92**, 59–66

Hammer, D.I., Hasselblad, V., Portnoy, B. & Wehrle, P.F. (1974) Los Angeles Student Nurse study. Daily symptom reporting and photochemical oxidants. *Arch. environ. Health*, **28**, 255–260

Hammond, E.C. (1966) Smoking in relation to the death rates of one million men and women. *Natl Cancer Inst. Monogr.*, **19**, 127–204

Hammond, E.C. & Garfinkel, L. (1969) Coronary heart disease, stroke, and aortic aneurysm. *Arch. environ. Health*, **19**, 167–182

Hammond, E.C. & Horn, D. (1958) Smoking and death rates — Report on forty-four months of follow-up of 187,783 men. *J. Am. med. Assoc.*, **166**, 2840–2853

Hammond, S.K., Coghlin, J., Gann, P.H., Paul, M., Taghizadeh, K., Skipper, P.L. & Tannenbaum, S.R. (1993) Relationship between environmental tobacco smoke exposure and carcinogen–hemoglobin adduct levels in nonsmokers. *J. natl Cancer Inst.*, **85**, 474–478

Hansen, C., Sørensen, L.D., Asmussen, I. & Autrup, H. (1992) Transplacental exposure to tobacco smoke in human-adduct formation in placenta and umbilical cord blood vessels. *Teratog. Carcinog. Mutag.*, **12**, 51–60

Hansen, C., Asmussen, I. & Autrup, H. (1993) Detection of carcinogen–DNA adducts in human fetal tissues by the ³²P-postlabeling procedure. *Environ. Health Perspect.*, **99**, 229–231

Hatch, M.C., Warburton, D. & Santella, R.M. (1990) Polycyclic aromatic hydrocarbon–DNA adducts in spontaneously aborted fetal tissue. *Carcinogenesis*, **11**, 1673–1675

He, Y. (1989) [Women's passive smoking and coronary heart disease.] *Zhonghua Yu Fang Yi Xue Za Zhi*, **23**, 19–22 (in Chinese)

He, Y., Lam, T.H., Li, L.S., Li, L.S., Du, R.Y., Jia, G.L., Huang, J.Y. & Zheng, J.S. (1994) Passive smoking at work as a risk factor for coronary heart disease in Chinese women who have never smoked. *Br. med. J.*, **308**, 380–384

He, J., Vupputuri, S., Allen, K., Prerost, M.R., Hughes, J. & Whelton, P.K. (1999) Passive smoking and the risk of coronary heart disease — A meta-analysis of epidemiologic studies. *New Engl. J. Med.*, **340**, 920–926

Hecht, S.S. (2002) Human urinary carcinogen metabolites: Biomarkers for investigating tobacco and cancer. *Carcinogenesis*, **23**, 907–922

Hecht, S.S., Carmella, S.G., Murphy, S.E., Akerkar, S., Brunnemann, K.D. & Hoffmann, D. (1993) A tobacco-specific lung carcinogen in the urine of men exposed to cigarette smoke. *New Engl. J. Med.*, **329**, 1543–1546

Hecht, S.S., Ye, M., Carmella, S.G., Fredrickson, A., Adgate, J.L., Greaves, I.A., Church, T.R., Ryan, A.D., Mongin, S.J. & Sexton, K. (2001) Metabolites of a tobacco-specific lung carcinogen in the urine of elementary school-aged children. *Cancer Epidemiol. Biomarkers Prev.*, **10**, 1109–1116

Heinz-Erian, P., Spitzmüller, A., Schröcksnadel, H. & Birnbacher, R. (1998) Maternal smoking and inhibition of fetal growth factor (Letter to the Editor). *J. Am. med. Assoc.*, **279**, 1954

Hennekens, C.H., Buring, J.E., Manson, J.E., Stampfer, M., Rosner, B., Cook, N.R., Belanger, C., LaMotte, F., Gaziano, J.M., Ridker, P.M., Willett, W. & Peto, R. (1996) Lack of effect of long-term supplementation with beta carotene on the incidence of malignant neoplasms and cardio-vascular disease. *New Engl. J. Med.*, **334**, 1145–1149

Henningfield, J.E. (1993) More on the nicotine content of vegetables. *New Engl. J. Med.*, **329**, 1581–1582

Hernandez-Boussard, T., Montesano, R. & Hainaut, P. (1999) Analysis of somatic mutations of the *p53* gene in human cancers: A tool to generate hypotheses about the natural history of cancer. In: McGregor, D.B., Rice, J.M. & Venitt, S., eds, *The Use of Short- and Medium-term Tests for Carcinogens and Data on Genetic Effects in Carcinogenic Hazard Evaluation* (IARC Scientific Publications No. 146), Lyon, IARCPress, pp. 43–53

Hirayama, T. (1981) Non-smoking wives of heavy smokers have a higher risk of lung cancer: A study from Japan. *Br. med. J.*, **282**, 183–185

Hirayama, T. (1984) Lung cancer in Japan: Effects of nutrition and passive smoking. In: Mizell, M. & Correa, P., eds, *Lung Cancer: Causes and Prevention*, New York, Verlag Chemie International, pp. 175–195

Hirayama, T. (1990) Passive smoking. *N.Z. med. J.*, **103**, 54

Hoepfner, I., Dettbarn, G., Scherer, G., Grimmer, G. & Adlkofer, F. (1987) Hydroxy-phenanthrenes in the urine of non-smokers and smokers. *Toxicol. Lett.*, **35**, 67–71

Hole, D.J., Gillis, C.R., Chopra, C. & Hawthorne, V.M. (1989) Passive smoking and cardio-respiratory health in a general population in the west of Scotland. *Br. med. J.*, **299**, 423–427

Holz, O., Krause, T., Scherer, G., Schmidt-Preuss, U. & Rüdiger, H.W. (1990) ^{32}P-postlabelling analysis of DNA adducts in monocytes of smokers and passive smokers. *Int. Arch. occup. environ. Health*, **62**, 299–303

Hong, Y.C., Kim, H., Im, M.W., Lee, K.H., Woo, B.H. & Christiani, D.C. (2001) Maternal genetic effects on neonatal susceptibility to oxidative damage from environmental tobacco smoke. *J. natl Cancer Inst.*, **93**, 645–647

Hovell, M.F., Zakarian, J.M., Wahlgren, D.R. & Matt, G.E. (2000a) Reported measures of environmental tobacco smoke exposure: Trials and tribulations. *Tob. Control*, **9** (Suppl. 3), 22–28

Hovell, M.F., Zakarian, J.M., Matt, G.E., Hofstetter, C.R., Bernert, J.T. & Pirkle, J. (2000b) Effect of counselling mothers on their children's exposure to environmental tobacco smoke: Randomised controlled trial. *Br. med. J.*, **321**, 337–342

Howard, D.J., Ota, R.B., Briggs, L.A., Hampton, M. & Pritsos, C.A. (1998a) Environmental tobacco smoke in the workplace induces oxidative stress in employees, including increased production of 8-hydroxy-2′-deoxyguanosine. *Cancer Epidemiol. Biomarkers Prev.*, **7**, 141–146

Howard, D.J., Briggs, L.A. & Pritsos, C.A. (1998b) Oxidative DNA damage in mouse heart, liver, and lung tissue due to acute side-stream tobacco smoke exposure. *Arch. Biochem. Biophys.*, **352**, 293–297

Hu, F.B., Persky, V., Flay, B.R. & Richardson, J. (1997) An epidemiological study of asthma prevalence and related factors among young adults. *J. Asthma*, **34**, 67–76

Huang, C., Taki, T., Adachi, M., Konishi, T., Higashiyama, M. & Miyake, M. (1998) Mutations in exon 7 and 8 of *p53* as poor prognostic factors in patients with non-small cell lung cancer. *Oncogene*, **16**, 2469–2477

Hugod, C., Hawkins, L.H. & Astrup, P. (1978) Exposure of passive smokers to tobacco smoke constituents. *Int. Arch. occup. environ. Health*, **42**, 21–29

Hull, M.G.R., North, K., Taylor, H., Farrow, A., Ford, W.C.L. & the Avon Longitudinal Study of Pregnancy and Childhood Study Team (2000) Delayed conception and active and passive smoking. *Fertil. Steril.*, **74**, 725–733

Humble, C., Croft, J., Gerber, A., Casper, M., Hames, C.G. & Tyroler, H.A. (1990) Passive smoking and 20-year cardiovascular disease mortality among nonsmoking wives, Evans County, Georgia. *Am. J. public Health*, **80**, 599–601

Husgafvel-Pursiainen, K. (1987) Sister-chromatid exchange and cell proliferation in cultured lymphocytes of passively and actively smoking restaurant personnel. *Mutat. Res.*, **190**, 211–215

Husgafvel-Pursiainen, K., Sorsa, M., Møller, M. & Benestad, C. (1986) Genotoxicity and polynuclear aromatic hydrocarbon analysis of environmental tobacco smoke samples from restaurants. *Mutagenesis*, **1**, 287–292

Husgafvel-Pursiainen, K., Sorsa, M., Engström, K. & Einistö, P. (1987) Passive smoking at work: Biochemical and biological measures of exposure to environmental tobacco smoke. *Int. Arch. occup. environ. Health*, **59**, 337–345

Husgafvel-Pursiainen, K., Hackman, P., Ridanpää, M., Anttila, S., Karjalainen, A., Partanen, T., Taikina-Aho, O., Heikkilä, L. & Vainio, H. (1993) K-*ras* mutations in human adenocarcinoma of the lung: Association with smoking and occupational exposure to asbestos. *Int. J. Cancer*, **53**, 250–256

Husgafvel-Pursiainen, K., Karjalainen, A., Kannio, A., Anttila, S., Partanen, T., Ojajärvi, A. & Vainio, H. (1999) Lung cancer and past occupational exposure to asbestos: Role of *p53* and *K-ras* mutations. *Am. J. respir. Cell mol. Biol.*, **20**, 667–674

Husgafvel-Pursiainen, K., Boffetta, P., Kannio, A., Nyberg, F., Pershagen, G., Mukeria, A., Constantinescu, V., Fortes, C. & Benhamou, S. (2000) *p53* Mutations and exposure to environmental tobacco smoke in a multicenter study on lung cancer. *Cancer Res.*, **60**, 2906–2911

Hussain, S.P. & Harris, C.C. (1998) Molecular epidemiology of human cancer: Contribution of mutation spectra studies of tumor suppressor genes. *Cancer Res.*, **58**, 4023–4037

Hutchison, S.J., Glantz, S.A., Zhu, B.Q., Sun, Y.P., Chou, T.M., Chatterjee, K., Deedwania, P.C., Parmley, W.W. & Sudhir, K. (1998) In-utero and neonatal exposure to secondhand smoke causes vascular dysfunction in newborn rats. *J. Am. Coll. Cardiol.*, **32**, 1463–1467

IARC (1986) *IARC Monographs on the Evaluation of the Carcinogenic Risk of Chemicals to Humans*,Vol. 38, *Tobacco Smoking*, Lyon, IARCPress

Izzotti, A., Bagnasco, M., D'Agostini, F., Cartiglia, C., Lubet, R.A., Kelloff, G.J. & De Flora, S. (1999) Formation and persistence of nucleotide alterations in rats exposed whole-body to environmental cigarette smoke. *Carcinogenesis*, **20**, 1499–1505

Izzotti, A., Balansky, R.M,. D'Agostini, F., Bennicelli, C., Myers, S.R., Grubbs, C.J., Lubet, R.A., Kelloff, G.J. & De Flora, S. (2001) Modulation of biomarkers by chemopreventive agents in smoke-exposed rats. *Cancer Res.*, **61**, 2472–2479

Jaakkola, M.S., Jaakkola, J.J.K., Becklake, M.R. & Ernst, P. (1995) Passive smoking and evolution of lung function in young adults. An 8-year longitudinal study. *J. clin. Epidemiol.*, **48**, 317–327

Jackson, R.T. (1989) *The Auckland Heart Study: A Case–Control Study of Coronary Heart Disease*, PhD Thesis, Auckland, University of Auckland

Jacob, P., III, Yu, L., Shulgin, A.T. & Benowitz, N.L. (1999) Minor tobacco alkaloids as biomarkers for tobacco use: Comparison of users of cigarettes, smokeless tobacco, cigars, and pipes. *Am. J. public Health*, **89**, 731–736

Janson, C., Chinn, S., Jarvis, D., Zock, J.-P., Torén, K. & Burney, P. (2001) Effect of passive smoking on respiratory symptoms, bronchial responsiveness, lung function, and total serum IgE in the European Community Respiratory Health Survey: A cross-sectional study. *Lancet*, **358**, 2103–2109

Järvinen, R., Knekt, P., Seppänen, R., Reunanen, A., Heliövaara, M., Maatela, J. & Aromaa, A. (1994) Antioxidant vitamins in the diet: Relationships with other personal characteristics in Finland. *J. Epidemiol. Community Health*, **48**, 549–554

Jarvis, M.J. (1994) Dietary nicotine. …unless subjects eat 90 kg tomatoes a day. *Br. med. J.*, **308**, 62

Jarvis, M.J., Russell, M.A.H. & Feyerabend, C. (1983) Absorption of nicotine and carbon monoxide from passive smoking under natural conditions of exposure. *Thorax*, **38**, 829–833

Jarvis, M.J., Russell, M.A.H., Feyerabend, C., Eiser, J.R., Morgan, M., Gammage, P. & Gray, E.M. (1985) Passive exposure to tobacco smoke: Saliva cotinine concentrations in a representative population sample of non-smoking schoolchildren. *Br. med J.*, **291**, 927–929

Jarvis, M.J., Phil, M., Tunstall-Pedoe, H., Feyerabend, C., Vesey, C. & Saloojee, Y. (1987) Comparison of tests used to distinguish smokers from nonsmokers. *Am. J. public Health*, **77**, 1435–1438

Jarvis, M.J., McNeill, A.D., Bryant, A. & Russell, M.A. (1991) Factors determining exposure to passive smoking in young adults living at home: Quantitative analysis using saliva cotinine concentrations. *Int. J. Epidemiol.*, **20**, 126–131

Jarvis, M.J., Foulds, J. & Feyerabend, C. (1992) Exposure to passive smoking among bar staff. *Br. J. Addict.*, **87**, 111–113

Jarvis, M.J., Goddard, E., Higgins, V., Feyerabend, C., Bryant, A. & Cook, D.G. (2000) Children's exposure to passive smoking in England since the 1980s: Cotinine evidence from population surveys. *Br. med. J.*, **321**, 343–345

Jarvis, M.J., Feyerabend, C., Bryant, A., Hedges, B. & Primatesta, P. (2001) Passive smoking in the home: Plasma cotinine concentrations in non-smokers with smoking partners. *Tob. Control*, **10**, 368–374

Jensen, T.K., Henriksen, T.B., Hjollund, N.H.I., Scheike, T., Kolstad, H., Giwercman, A., Ernst, E., Bonde, J.P., Skakkebaek, N.E. & Olsen, J. (1998) Adult and prenatal exposures to tobacco smoke as risk indicators of fertility among 430 Danish couples. *Am. J. Epidemiol.*, **148**, 992–997

Ji, C.M., Plopper, C.G., Witschi, H.P. & Pinkerton, K.E. (1994) Exposure to sidestream cigarette smoke alters bronchiolar epithelial cell differentiation in the postnatal rat lung. *Am. J. respir. Cell mol. Biol.*, **11**, 312–320

Ji, C.M., Royce, F.H., Truong, U., Plopper, C.G., Singh, G. & Pinkerton, K.E. (1998) Maternal exposure to environmental tobacco smoke alters Clara cell secretory protein expression in fetal rat lung. *Am. J. Physiol.*, **275** , L870–L876

Jindal, S.K., Gupta, D. & Singh, A. (1994) Indices of morbidity and control of asthma in adult patients exposed to environmental tobacco smoke. *Chest*, **106**, 746–749

Jinot, J. & Bayard, S. (1996) Respiratory health effects of exposure to environmental tobacco smoke. *Rev. environ. Health*, **11**, 89–100

Joad, J.P., Pinkerton, K.E. & Bric, J.M. (1993) Effects of sidestream smoke exposure and age on pulmonary function and airway reactivity in developing rats. *Pediatr. Pulmonol.*, **16**, 281–288

Joad, J.P., Ji, C., Kott, K.S., Bric, J.M. & Pinkerton, K.E. (1995a) In utero and postnatal effects of sidestream cigarette smoke exposure on lung function, hyperresponsiveness, and neuro-endocrine cells in rats. *Toxicol. appl. Pharmacol.*, **132**, 63–71

Joad, J.P., Bric, J.M. & Pinkerton, K.E. (1995b) Sidestream smoke effects on lung morphology and C-fibers in young guinea pigs. *Toxicol. appl. Pharmacol.*, **131**, 289–296

Joad, J.P., Bric, J.M., Peake, J.L. & Pinkerton, K.E. (1999) Perinatal exposure to aged and diluted sidestream cigarette smoke produces airway hyperresponsiveness in older rats. *Toxicol. appl. Pharmacol.*, **155**, 253–260

Jones, J.R., Higgins, I.T.T., Higgins, M.W. & Keller, J.B. (1983) Effects of cooking fuels on lung function in nonsmoking women. *Arch. environ. Health*, **38**, 219–222

Jordanov, J.S. (1990) Cotinine concentrations in amniotic fluid and urine of smoking, passive smoking and non-smoking pregnant women at term and in the urine of their neonates on 1st day of life. *Eur. J. Pediatr.*, **149**, 734–737

Jörres, R. & Magnussen, H. (1992) Influence of short-term passive smoking on symptoms, lung mechanics and airway responsiveness in asthmatic subjects and healthy controls. *Eur. respir. J.*, **5**, 936–944

Kado, N.Y., Tesluk, S.J., Hammond, S.K., Woskie, S.R., Samuels, S.J. & Schenker, M.B. (1987) Use of a Salmonella micro pre-incubation procedure for studying personal exposure to mutagens in environmental tobacco smoke: Pilot study of urine and airborne mutagenicity from passive smoking. In: Sandhu, S.S., DeMarini, D.M., Mass, M.J., Moore, M.M. & Mumford, J.L., eds, *Short-term Bioassays in the Analysis of Complex Environmental Mixtures V*, New York, Plenum Press, pp. 375–390

Kado, N.Y., McCurdy, S.A., Tesluk, S.J., Hammond, S.K., Hsieh, D.P.H., Jones, J. & Schenker, M.B. (1991) Measuring personal exposure to airborne mutagens and nicotine in environmental tobacco smoke. *Mutat. Res.*, **261**, 75–82

Kahn, H.A. (1966) The Dorn study of smoking and mortality among US veterans: Report on eight and one-half years of observation. *Natl Cancer Inst. Monogr.*, **19**, 1–125

Kalandidi, A., Trichopoulos, D., Hatzakis, A., Tzannes, S. & Saracci, R. (1987) Passive smoking and chronic obstructive lung disease. *Lancet*, **ii**, 1325–1326

Kalandidi, A., Trichopoulos, D., Hatzakis, A., Tzannes, S. & Saracci, R. (1990) The effect of involuntary smoking on the occurrence of chronic obstructive pulmonary disease. *Soz. Präventivmed.*, **35**, 12–16

Kauffmann, F. & Perdrizet, S. (1981) Effect of passive smoking on respiratory function. *Eur. J. respir. Dis.*, **62** (Suppl. 113), 109–110

Kauffmann, F., Tessier, J.-F. & Oriol, P. (1983) Adult passive smoking in the home environment: A risk factor for chronic airflow limitation. *Am. J. Epidemiol.*, **117**, 269–280

Kauffmann, F., Dockery, D.W., Speizer, F.E. & Ferris, B.G., Jr (1989) Respiratory symptoms and lung function in relation to passive smoking: A comparative study of American and French women. *Int. J. Epidemiol.*, **18**, 334–344

Kawachi, I., Colditz, G.A., Speizer, F.E., Manson, J.E., Stampfer, M.J., Willett, W.C. & Hennekens, C.H. (1997) A prospective study of passive smoking and coronary heart disease. *Circulation*, **95**, 2374–2379

Kawamoto, T., Yoshikawa, M., Matsuno, K., Kayama, F., Oyama, T., Arashidani, K. & Kodama, Y. (1993) Effect of side-stream cigarette smoke on the hepatic cytochrome P450. *Arch. environ. Contam. Toxicol.*, **25**, 255–259

Keith, R.E. & Driskell, J.A. (1980) Effects of chronic cigarette smoking on vitamin C status, lung function, and resting and exercise cardiovascular metabolism in humans. *Nutr. Rep. int.*, **21**, 907–912

Kentner, M., Triebig, G. & Weltle, D. (1984) The influence of passive smoking on pulmonary function — A study of 1351 office workers. *Prev. Med.*, **13**, 656–669

Knight, A. & Breslin, A.B.X. (1985) Passive cigarette smoking and patients with asthma. *Med. J. Aust.*, **142**, 194–195

Köhler, E., Bretschneider, D., Rabsilber, A., Weise, W. & Jorch, G. (2001) Assessment of prenatal smoke exposure by determining nicotine and its metabolites in maternal and neonatal urine. *Hum. exp. Toxicol.*, **20**, 1–7

Kondo, K., Tsuzuki, H., Sasa, M., Sumitomo, M., Uyama, T. & Monden, Y. (1996) A dose–response relationship between the frequency of p53 mutations and tobacco consumption in lung cancer patients. *J. surg. Oncol.*, **61**, 20–26

Kopplin, A., Eberle-Adamkiewicz, G., Glüsenkamp, K.-H., Nehls, P. & Kirstein, U. (1995) Urinary excretion of 3-methyladenine and 3-ethyladenine after controlled exposure to tobacco smoke. *Carcinogenesis*, **16**, 2637–2641

Kritz, H., Schmid, P. & Sinzinger, H. (1995) Passive smoking and cardiovascular risk. *Arch. intern. Med.*, **155**, 1942–1948

Künzli, N., Schwartz, J., Stutz, E.Z., Ackermann-Liebrich, U. & Leuenberger, P. (2000) Association of environmental tobacco smoke at work and forced expiratory lung function among never smoking asthmatics and non-asthmatics. (The SAPALDIA-Team, Swiss Study on Air Pollution and Lung Disease in Adults). *Soz. Präventivmed.*, **45**, 208–217

Kurata, T., Suzuki, E., Hayashi, M. & Kaminao, M. (1998) Physiological role of L-ascorbic acid in rats exposed to cigarette smoke. *Biosci. Biotechnol. Biochem.*, **62**, 842–845

La Vecchia, C., D'Avanzo, B., Franzosi, M.G. & Tognoni, G. (1993) Passive smoking and the risk of acute myocardial infarction. *Lancet*, **341**, 505–506

Lackmann, G.M., Salzberger, U., Töllner, U., Chen, M., Carmella, S.G. & Hecht, S.S. (1999) Metabolites of a tobacco-specific carcinogen in urine from newborns. *J. natl Cancer Inst.*, **91**, 459–465

Lam, T.H., Zhu, C.Q. & Jiang, C.Q. (2002) Lymphocyte DNA damage in elevator manufacturing workers in Guangzhou, China. *Mutat. Res.*, **515**, 147–157

Laranjeira, R., Pillon, S. & Dunn, J. (2000) Environmental tobacco smoke exposure among non-smoking waiters: Measurement of expired carbon monoxide levels. *Sao Paulo med. J.*, **118**, 89–92

Larkin, F.A., Basiotis, P.P., Riddick, H.A., Sykes, K.E. & Pao, E.M. (1990) Dietary patterns of women smokers and non-smokers. *J. Am. Diet. Assoc.*, **90**, 230–237

Laurent, A.M., Bevan, A., Chakroun, N., Courtois, Y., Valois, B., Roussel, M., Festy, B. & Pretet, S. (1992) [Effects of chronic exposure to tobacco smoke on the health of non-smokers]. *Rev. Pneumol. clin.*, **48**, 65–70 (in French)

La Vecchia, C., D'Avanzo, B., Franzosi, M.G. & Tognoni, G. (1993) Passive smoking and the risk of acute myocardial infarction. *Lancet*, **341**, 505–506

Law, M.R., Morris, J.K. & Wald, N.J. (1997) Environmental tobacco smoke exposure and ischaemic heart disease: An evaluation of the evidence. *Br. med. J.*, **315**, 973–980

Layard, M.W. (1995) Ischemic heart disease and spousal smoking in the National Mortality Followback Survey. *Regul. Toxicol. Pharmacol.*, **21**, 180–183

Lebowitz, M.D. (1984a) Influence of passive smoking on pulmonary function: A survey. *Prev. Med.*, **13**, 645–655

Lebowitz, M.D. (1984b) The effects of environmental tobacco smoke exposure and gas stoves on daily peak flow rates in asthmatic and non-asthmatic families. *Eur. J. respir. Dis.*, **65** (Suppl. 133), 90–97

Lebowitz, M.D. & Burrows, B. (1976) Respiratory symptoms related to smoking habits of family adults. *Chest*, **69**, 48–50

Lebowitz, M.D., Quackenboss, J.J., Krzyzanowski, M., O'Rourke, M.K. & Hayes, C. (1992) Multipollutant exposures and health responses to particulate matter. *Arch. environ. Health*, **47**, 71–75

Lee, P.N. (1992) *Environmental Tobacco Smoke and Mortality*, Basel, Karger

Lee, P.N., Chamberlain, J. & Alderson, M.R. (1986) Relationship of passive smoking to risk of lung cancer and other smoking-associated diseases. *Br. J. Cancer*, **54**, 97–105

Lee, C.K., Brown, B.G., Reed, E.A., Rahn, C.A., Coggins, C.R.E., Doolittle, D.J. & Hayes, A.W. (1992) Fourteen-day inhalation study in rats, using aged and diluted sidestream smoke from a reference cigarette. II. DNA adducts and alveolar macrophage cytogenetics. *Fundam. appl. Toxicol.*, **19**, 141–146

Lee, C.K., Brown, B.G., Reed, E.A., Coggins, C.R.E., Doolittle, D.J. & Hayes, A.W. (1993) Ninety-day inhalation study in rats, using aged and diluted sidestream smoke from a reference cigarette: DNA adducts and alveolar macrophage cytogenetics. *Fundam. appl. Toxicol.*, **20**, 393–401

Lee, C.Z., Royce, F.H., Denison, M.S. & Pinkerton, K.E. (2000) Effect of in utero and postnatal exposure to environmental tobacco smoke on the developmental expression of pulmonary cytochrome P450 monooxygenases. *J. biochem. Toxicol.*, **14**, 121–130

Leichter, J. (1989) Growth of fetuses of rats exposed to ethanol and cigarette smoke during gestation. *Growth Dev. Aging*, **53**, 129–134

Le Marchand, L., Wilkens, L.R., Hankin, J.H. & Haley, N.J. (1991) Dietary patterns of female non-smokers with and without exposure to environmental tobacco smoke. *Cancer Causes Control*, **2**, 11–16

Leuenberger, P., Schwartz, J., Ackermann-Liebrich, U., Blaser, K., Bolognini, G., Bongard, J.P., Brandli, O., Braun, P., Bron, C., Brutsche, M., Domenighetti, G., Elsasser, S., Guldimann, P., Hollenstein, C., Hufschmid, P., Karrer, W., Keller, R., Keller-Wossidlo, H., Kunzli, N., Luthi, J.C., Martin, B.W., Medici, T., Perruchoud, A.P., Radaelli, A., Schindler, C., Schoeni, M.H., Solari, G., Tschopp, J.M., Villiger, B., Wuthrich, B., Zellweger, J.P. & Zemp, E. (Swiss Study on Air Pollution and Lung Diseases in Adults, SAPALDIA Team) (1994) Passive smoking exposure in adults and chronic respiratory symptoms (SAPALDIA Study). *Am. J. respir. crit. Care Med.*, **150**, 1222–1228

LeVois, M.E. & Layard, M.W. (1995) Publication bias in the environmental tobacco smoke/coronary heart disease epidemiologic literature. *Regul. Toxicol. Pharmacol.*, **21**, 184–191

Leyden, D.E., Leitner, E. & Siegmund, B. (1999) Determination of nicotine in pharmaceutical products and dietary sources. In: Gorrod, J.W. & Jacob, P., III, *Analytical Determination of Nicotine and Related Compounds and their Metabolites*, Amsterdam, Elsevier, pp. 393–421

Lindbohm, M.-L., Sallmén, M. & Taskinen, H. (2002) Effects of exposure to environmental tobacco smoke on reproductive health. *Scand. J. Work Environ. Health*, **28** (Suppl. 2), 84–96

Ling, P.I., Löfroth, G. & Lewtas, J. (1987) Mutagenic determination of passive smoking. *Toxicol. Lett.*, **35**, 147–151

Löfroth, G. & Lazaridis, G. (1986) Environmental tobacco smoke: Comparative characterization by mutagenicity assays of sidestream and mainstream cigarette smoke. *Environ. Mutag.*, **8**, 693–704

Maclure, M., Katz, R.B.-A., Bryant, M.S., Skipper, P.L. & Tannenbaum, S.R. (1989) Elevated blood levels of carcinogens in passive smokers. *Am. J. public Health*, **79**, 1381–1384

Maehira, F., Miyagi, I., Asato, T., Eguchi, Y., Takei, H., Nakatsuki, K., Fukuoka, M. & Zaha, F. (1999) Alterations of protein kinase C, 8-hydroxydeoxyguanosine, and K-ras oncogene in rat lungs exposed to passive smoking. *Clin. chim. Acta*, **289**, 133–144

Magnussen, H., Jörres, R. & Oldigs, M. (1992) Effect of one hour of passive cigarette smoking on lung function and airway responsiveness in adults and children with asthma. *Clin. Invest.*, **70**, 368–371

Malaveille, C., Vineis, P., Estève, J., Ohshima, H., Brun, G., Hautefeuille, A., Gallet, P., Ronco, G., Terracini, B. & Bartsch, H. (1989) Levels of mutagens in the urine of smokers of black and blond tobacco correlate with their risk of bladder cancer. *Carcinogenesis*, **10**, 577–586

Manchester, D.K. & Jacoby, E.H. (1981) Sensitivity of human placental monooxygenase activity to maternal smoking. *Clin. Pharmacol. Ther.*, **30**, 687–692

Marchetti, A., Pellegrini, S., Sozzi, G., Bertacca, G., Gaeta, P., Buttitta, F., Carnicelli, V., Griseri, P., Chella, A., Angeletti, C.A., Pierotti, M. & Bevilacqua, G. (1998) Genetic analysis of lung tumours of non-smoking subjects: p53 Gene mutations are constantly associated with loss of heterozygosity at the FHIT locus. *Br. J. Cancer*, **78**, 73–78

Margetts, B.M. & Jackson, A.A. (1993) Interactions between people's diet and their smoking habits: The dietary and nutritional survey of British adults. *Br. med. J.*, **307**, 1381–1384

Masi, M.A., Hanley, J.A., Ernst, P. & Becklake, M.R. (1988) Environmental exposure to tobacco smoke and lung function in young adults. *Am. Rev. respir. Dis.*, **138**, 296–299

Masjedi, M.-R., Kazemi, H. & Johnson, D.C. (1990) Effects of passive smoking on the pulmonary function of adults. *Thorax*, **45**, 27–31

Maskarinec, M.P., Jenkins, R.A., Counts, R.W. & Dindal, A.B. (2000) Determination of exposure to environmental tobacco smoke in restaurant and tavern workers in one US city. *J. Expo. anal. environ. Epidemiol.*, **10**, 36–49

Matsunga, S.K., Plezia, P.M., Karol, M.D., Katz, M.D., Camilli, A.E. & Benowitz, N.L. (1989) Effects of passive smoking on theophylline clearance. *Clin. Pharmacol. Ther.*, **46**, 399–407

Matthews, S.J., Hecht, S.S., Picton, H.M., Ye, M., Carmella, S.G., Shires, S., Wild, C.P. & Hay, A.W.M. (2002) No association between smoking and the presence of tobacco-specific nitrosamine metabolites in ovarian follicular fluid. *Cancer Epidemiol. Biomarkers Prev.*, **11**, 321–322

Mattson, M.E., Boyd, G., Byar, D., Brown, C., Callahan, J.F., Corle, D., Cullen, J.W., Greenblatt, J., Haley, N.J., Hammond, S.K., Lewtas, J. & Reeves, W. (1989) Passive smoking on commercial airline flights. *J. Am. med. Assoc.*, **261**, 867–872

McPhillips, J.B., Eaton, C.B., Gans, K.M., Derby, C.A., Lasater, T.M., McKenney, J.L. & Carleton, R.A. (1994) Dietary differences in smokers and nonsmokers from two southeastern New England communities. *J. Am. Diet. Assoc.*, **94**, 287–292

Meger, M., Meger-Kossien, I., Riedel, K. & Scherer, G. (2000) Biomonitoring of environmental tobacco smoke (ETS)-related exposure to 4-(methylnitrosamino)-1-(3-pyridyl)-1-butanone (NNK). *Biomarkers*, **5**, 33–45

Menon, P.K., Stankus, R.P., Rando, R.J., Salvaggio, J.E. & Lehrer, S.B. (1991) Asthmatic responses to passive cigarette smoke: Persistence of reactivity and effect of medications. *J. Allergy clin. Immunol.*, **88**, 861–869

Menon, P.K., Rando, R.J., Stankus, R.P., Salvaggio, J.E. & Lehrer, S.B. (1992) Passive cigarette smoke-challenge studies: Increase in bronchial hyperreactivity. *J. Allergy clin. Immunol.*, **89**, 560–566

von Meyerinck, L., Scherer, G., Adlkofer, F., Wenzel-Hartung, R., Brune, H. & Thomas, C. (1989) Exposure of rats and hamsters to sidestream smoke from cigarettes in a subchronic inhalation study. *Exp. Pathol.*, **37**, 186–189

Midgette, A.S., Baron, J.A. & Rohan, T.E. (1993) Do cigarette smokers have diets that increase their risks of coronary heart disease and cancer? *Am. J. Epidemiol.*, **137**, 521–529

Milunsky, A., Carmella, S.G., Ye, M. & Hecht, S.S. (2000) A tobacco-specific carcinogen in the fetus. *Prenat. Diagn.*, **20**, 307–310

Mohtashamipur, E., Norpoth, K. & Straeter, H. (1987) Clastogenic effect of passive smoking on bone marrow polychromatic erythrocytes of NMRI mice. *Toxicol. Lett.*, **35**, 153–156

Mohtashamipur, E., Steinforth, T. & Norpoth, K. (1988) Comparative bone marrow clastogenicity of cigarette sidestream, mainstream and recombined smoke condensates in mice. *Mutagenesis*, **3**, 419–422

Mooney, L.A., Santella, R.M., Covey, L., Jeffrey, A.M., Bigbee, W., Randall, M.C., Cooper, T.B., Ottman, R., Tsai, W.-Y., Wazneh, L., Glassman, A.H., Young, T.-L. & Perera, F.P. (1995) Decline of DNA damage and other biomarkers in peripheral blood following smoking cessation. *Cancer Epidemiol. Biomarkers Prev.*, **4**, 627–634

Morawska, L., Barron, W. & Hitchins, J. (1999) Experimental deposition of environmental tobacco smoke submicrometer particulate matter in the human respiratory tract. *Am. ind. Hyg. Assoc. J.*, **60**, 334–339

Morimoto, Y., Tsuda, T., Hori, H., Yamato, H., Ohgami, A., Hagashi, T., Nagata, N., Kido, M. & Tanaka, I. (1999) Combined effect of cigarette smoke and mineral fibers on the gene expression of cytokine mRNA. *Environ. Health Perspect.*, **107**, 495–500

Muramatsu, T., Weber, A., Muramatsu, S. & Akermann, F. (1983) An experimental study on irritation and annoyance due to passive smoking. *Int. Arch. occup. environ. Health*, **51**, 305–317

Muscat, J.E. & Wynder, E.L. (1995) Exposure to environmental tobacco smoke and the risk of heart attack. *Int. J. Epidemiol.*, **24**, 715–719

Mutoh, T., Bonham, A.C., Kott, K.S. & Joad, J.P. (1999) Chronic exposure to sidestream tobacco smoke augments lung C-fiber responsiveness in young guinea pigs. *J. appl. Physiol.*, **87**, 757–768

Mutoh, T., Joad, J.P. & Bonham, A.C. (2000) Chronic passive cigarette smoke exposure augments bronchopulmonary C-fibre inputs to nucleus tractus solitarii neurones and reflex output in young guinea-pigs. *J. Physiol.*, **523**, 223–233

Myers, S.R., Spinnato, J.A. & Pinorini-Godly, M.T. (1996) Characterization of 4-aminobiphenyl–hemoglobin adducts in maternal and fetal blood samples. *J. Toxicol. environ. Health*, **47**, 553–566

Nadadur, S.S., Pinkerton, K.E. & Kodavanti, U.P. (2002) Pulmonary gene expression profiles of spontaneously hypertensive rats exposed to environmental tobacco smoke. *Chest*, **121**, 83S–84S

Nafstad, P., Jaakkola, J.J.K., Hagen, J.A., Zahlsen, K. & Magnus, P. (1997) Hair nicotine concentrations in mothers and children in relation to parental smoking. *J. Expo. anal. environ. Epidemiol.*, **7**, 235–239

Ng, T.P., Hui, K.P. & Tan, W.C. (1993) Respiratory symptoms and lung function effects of domestic exposure to tobacco smoke and cooking by gas in non-smoking women in Singapore. *J. Epidemiol. Community Health*, **47**, 454–458

Nowak, D., Jörres, R., Schmidt, A. & Magnussen, H. (1997) Effect of 3 hours' passive smoke exposure in the evening on airway tone and responsiveness until next morning. *Int. Arch. occup. environ. Health*, **69**, 125–133

Nuttens, M.C., Romon, M., Ruidavets, J.B., Arveiler, D., Ducimetiere, P., Lecerf, J.M., Richard, J.L., Cambou, J.P., Simon, C. & Salomez, J.L. (1992) Relationship between smoking and diet: The MONICA-France project. *J. intern. Med.*, **231**, 349–356

Oberdörster, G. & Pott, F. (1986) Extrapolation from rat studies with environmental tobacco smoke (ETS) to humans: Comparison of particle mass deposition and of clearance behavior of ETS compounds. *Toxicol. Lett.*, **35**, 107–112

Oddoze, C., Pauli, A.M. & Pastor, J. (1998) Rapid and sensitive high-performance liquid chromatographic determination of nicotine and cotinine in nonsmoker human and rat urines. *J. Chromatogr.*, **B708**, 95–101

Olson, J.W. (1985) Chronic cigarette sidestream smoke exposure increases rat trachea ornithine decarboxylase activity. *Life Sci.*, **37**, 2165–2171

Ostro, B.D., Lipsett, M.J., Mann, J.K., Wiener, M.B. & Selner, J. (1994) Indoor air pollution and asthma. Results from a panel study. *Am. J. respir. crit. Care Med.*, **149**, 1400–1406

Otsuka, R., Watanabe, H., Hirata, K., Tokai, K., Muro, T., Yoshiyama, M., Takeuchi, K. & Yoshikawa, J. (2001) Acute effects of passive smoking on the coronary circulation in healthy young adults. *J. Am. med. Assoc.*, **286**, 436–441

Parsons, W.D., Carmella, S.G., Akerkar, S., Bonilla, L.E. & Hecht, S.S. (1998) A metabolite of the tobacco-specific lung carcinogen 4-(methylnitrosamino)-1-(3-pyridyl)-1-butanone in the urine of hospital workers exposed to environmental tobacco smoke. *Cancer Epidemiol. Biomarkers Prev.*, **7**, 257–260

Pastrakuljic, A., Schwartz, R., Simone, C., Derewlany, L.O., Knie, B. & Koren, G. (1998) Transplacental transfer and biotransformation studies of nicotine in the human placental cotyledon perfused in vitro. *Life Sci.*, **63**, 2333–2342

Penn, A. & Snyder, C.A. (1993) Inhalation of sidestream cigarette smoke accelerates development of arteriosclerotic plaques. *Circulation*, **88**, 1820–1825

Penn, A., Chen, L.-C. & Snyder, C.A. (1994) Inhalation of steady-state sidestream smoke from one cigarette promotes arteriosclerotic plaque development. *Circulation*, **90**, 1363–1367

Pérez-Stable, E.J,. Marín, G., Marín, B.V. & Benowitz, N.L. (1992) Misclassification of smoking status by self-reported cigarette consumption. *Am. Rev. respir. Dis.*, **145**, 53–57

Petruzzelli, S., Celi, A., Pulerà, N., Baliva, F., Viegi, G., Carrozzi, L., Ciacchini, G., Bottai, M., Di Pede, F., Paoletti, P. & Giuntini, C. (1998) Serum antibodies to benzo(*a*)pyrene diol epoxide–DNA adducts in the general population: Effects of air pollution, tobacco smoking, and family history of lung diseases. *Cancer Res.*, **58**, 4122–4126

Pichini, S., Basagaña, X., Pacifici, R., Garcia, O., Puig, C., Vall, O., Harris, J., Zuccaro, P., Segura, J. & Sunyer, J. (2000) Cord serum cotinine as a biomarker of fetal exposure to cigarette smoke at the end of pregnancy. *Environ. Health Perspect.*, **108**, 1079–1083

Pignatelli, B., Li, C.-Q., Boffetta, P., Chen, Q., Ahrens, W., Nyberg, F., Mukeria, A., Bruske-Hohlfeld, I., Fortes, C., Constantinescu, V., Ischiropoulos, H. & Ohshima, H. (2001) Nitrated and oxidized plasma proteins in smokers and lung cancer patients. *Cancer Res.*, **61**, 778–784

Pilger, A., Germadnik, D., Riedel, K., Meger-Kossien, I., Scherer, G. & Rüdiger, H.W. (2001) Longitudinal study of urinary 8-hydroxy-2′-deoxyguanosine excretion in healthy adults. *Free Radic. Res.*, **35**, 273–280

Pimm, P.E., Shephard, R.J. & Silverman, F. (1978) Physiological effects of acute passive exposure to cigarette smoke. *Arch. environ. Health*, **33**, 201–213

Pirkle, J.L., Flegal, K.M., Bernert, J.T., Brody, D.J., Etzel, R.A. & Maurer, K.R. (1996) Exposure of the US population to environmental tobacco smoke: The Third National Health and Nutrition Examination Survey, 1988 to 1991. *J. Am. med. Assoc.*, **275**, 1233–1240

Pooling Project Research Group (1978) Relationship of blood pressure, serum cholesterol, smoking habit, relative weight and ECG abnormalities to incidence of major coronary events: Final report of the pooling project. *J. chron. Dis.*, **31**, 201–306

Pope, C.A., III, Eatough, D.J., Gold, D.R., Pang, Y., Nielsen, K.R., Nath, P., Verrier, R.L. & Kanner, R.E. (2001) Acute exposure to environmental tobacco smoke and heart rate variability. *Environ. Health Perspect.*, **109**, 711–716

Rajini, P. & Witschi, H. (1994) Short-term effects of sidestream smoke on respiratory epithelium in mice: Cell kinetics. *Fundam. appl. Toxicol.*, **22**, 405–410

Rajini, P., Last, J.A., Pinkerton, K.E., Hendrickx, A.G. & Witschi, H. (1994) Decreased fetal weights in rats exposed to sidestream cigarette smoke. *Fundam. appl. Toxicology*, **22**, 400–404

Repace, J.L. (1994) Dietary nicotine. Won't mislead on passive smoking… *Br. med. J.*, **308**, 61–62

Riboli, E., Preston-Martin, S., Saracci, R., Haley, N.J., Trichopoulos, D., Becher, H., Burch, J.D., Fontham, E.T.H., Gao, Y.-T., Jindal, S.K., Koo, L.C., Le Marchand, L., Segnan, N., Shimizu, H., Stanta, G., Wu-Williams, A.H. & Zatonski, W. (1990) Exposure of nonsmoking women to environmental tobacco smoke: A 10-country collaborative study. *Cancer Causes Control*, **1**, 243–252

Riboli, E., Haley, N.J., Trédaniel, J., Saracci, R., Preston-Martin, S. & Trichopoulos, D. (1995) Misclassification of smoking status among women in relation to exposure to environmental tobacco smoke. *Eur. respir. J.*, **8**, 285–290

Richter, E., Rösler, S., Scherer, G., Gostomzyk, J.G., Grübl, A., Krämer, U. & Behrendt, H. (2001) Haemoglobin adducts from aromatic amines in children in relation to area of residence and exposure to environmental tobacco smoke. *Int. Arch. occup. environ. Health*, **74**, 421–428

Robbins, A.S., Abbey, D.E. & Lebowitz, M.D. (1993) Passive smoking and chronic respiratory disease symptoms in non-smoking adults. *Int. J. Epidemiol.*, **22**, 809–817

Roberts, K.A., Rezai, A.A., Pinkerton, K.E. & Rutledge, J.C. (1996) Effect of environmental tobacco smoke on LDL accumulation in the artery wall. *Circulation*, **94**, 2248–2253

Robertson, A.S., Burge, P.S. & Cockrill, B.L. (1987) A study of serum thiocyanate concentrations in office workers as a means of validating smoking histories and assessing passive exposure to cigarette smoke. *Br. J. ind. Med.*, **44**, 351–354

Rodenhuis, S. & Slebos, R.J.C. (1992) Clinical significance of *ras* oncogene activation in human lung cancer. *Cancer Res.*, **52** (Suppl.), 2665s–2669s

Rodenhuis, S., Slebos, R.J.C., Boot, A.J.M., Evers, S.G., Mooi, W.J., Wagenaar, S.S., van Bodegom, P.C. & Bos, J.L. (1988) Incidence and possible clinical significance of K-*ras* onco-gene activation in adenocarcinoma of the human lung. *Cancer Res.*, **48**, 5738–5741

Rogot, E. & Murray, J.L. (1980) Smoking and causes of death among US veterans: 16 years of observation. *Public Health Rep.*, **95**, 213–222

Ruppert, T., Scherer, G., Tricker, A.R. & Adlkofer, F. (1997) *trans,trans*-Muconic acid as a bio-marker of non-occupational environmental exposure to benzene. *Int. Arch. occup. environ. Health*, **69**, 247–251

Russell, M.A.H., Cole, P.V. & Brown, E. (1973) Absorption by non-smokers of carbon monoxide from room air polluted by tobacco smoke. *Lancet*, **i**, 576–579

Sadler, L., Belanger, K., Saftlas, A., Leaderer, B., Hellenbrand, K., McSharry, J.-E. & Bracken, M.B. (1999) Environmental tobacco smoke exposure and small-for-gestational-age birth. *Am. J. Epidemiol.*, **150**, 695–705

Salem, E.S., El Zahby, M., Senna, G.A. & Malek, A. (1984) [Pulmonary manifestations among 'passive smokers'.] *Bull. Union int. Tubercul.*, **59**, 52–56 (in French)

Salomaa, S., Tuominen, J. & Skyttä, E. (1988) Genotoxicity and PAC analysis of particulate and vapour phases of environmental tobacco smoke. *Mutat. Res.*, **204**, 173–183

Sandler, D.P., Comstock, G.W., Helsing, K.J. & Shore, D.L. (1989) Deaths from all causes in non-smokers who lived with smokers. *Am. J. public Health*, **79**, 163–167

Sasson, I.M., Coleman, D.T., LaVoie, E.J., Hoffmann, D. & Wynder, E.L. (1985) Mutagens in human urine: Effects of cigarette smoking and diet. *Mutat. Res.*, **158**, 149–157

Sastry, B.V.R., Chance, M.B., Hemontolor, M.E. & Goddijn-Wessel, T.A.W. (1998) Formation and retention of cotinine during placental transfer of nicotine in human placental cotyledon. *Pharmacology*, **57**, 104–116

Scherer, G. & Richter, E. (1997) Biomonitoring exposure to environmental tobacco smoke (ETS): A critical reappraisal. *Hum. exp. Toxicol.*, **16**, 449–459

Scherer, G., Conze, C., von Meyerinck, L., Sorsa, M. & Adlkofer, F. (1990) Importance of exposure to gaseous and particulate phase components of tobacco smoke in active and passive smokers. *Int. Arch. occup. environ. Health*, **62**, 459–466

Scherer, G., Conze, C., Tricker, A.R. & Adlkofer, F. (1992) Uptake of tobacco smoke constituents on exposure to environmental tobacco smoke (ETS). *Clin. Invest.*, **70**, 352–367

Scherer, G., Ruppert, T., Daube, H., Kossien, I., Riedel, K., Tricker, A.R. & Adlkofer, F. (1995) Contribution of tobacco smoke to environmental benzene exposure in Germany. *Environ. int.*, **21**, 779–789

Scherer, G., Doolittle, D.J., Ruppert, T., Meger-Kossien, I., Riedel, K., Tricker, A.R. & Adlkofer, F. (1996) Urinary mutagenicity and thioethers in nonsmokers: Role of environmental tobacco smoke (ETS) and diet. *Mutat. Res.*, **368**, 195–204

Scherer, G., Meger-Kossien, I., Riedel, K., Renner, T. & Meger, M. (1999) Assessment of the exposure of children to environmental tobacco smoke (ETS) by different methods. *Hum. exp. Toxicol.*, **18**, 297–301

Scherer, G., Frank, S., Riedel, K., Meger-Kossien, I. & Renner, T. (2000) Biomonitoring of exposure to polycyclic aromatic hydrocarbons of nonoccupationally exposed persons. *Cancer Epidemiol. Biomarkers Prevent.*, **9**, 373–380

Schilling, R.S.F., Letai, A.D., Hui, S.L., Beck, G.J., Schoenberg, J.B. & Bouhuys, A. (1977) Lung function, respiratory disease, and smoking in families. *Am. J. Epidemiol.*, **106**, 274–283

Schmidt, K.G. & Rasmussen, J.W. (1984) Acute platelet activation induced by smoking. *In vivo* and *ex vivo* studies in humans. *Thromb. Haemostas.*, **51**, 279–282

Schwartz, J. & Zeger, S. (1990) Passive smoking, air pollution, and acute respiratory symptoms in a diary study of student nurses. *Am. Rev. respir. Dis.*, **141**, 62–67

Seidman, D.S., Paz, I., Merlet-Aharoni, I., Vreman, H., Stevenson, D.K. & Gale, R. (1999) Non-invasive validation of tobacco smoke exposure in late pregnancy using end-tidal carbon monoxide measurements. *J. Perinatol.*, **19**, 358–361

Seymour, B.W.P., Pinkerton, K.E., Friebertshauser, K.E., Coffman, R.L. & Gershwin, L.J. (1997) Second-hand smoke is an adjuvant for T helper-2 responses in a murine model of allergy. *J. Immunol.*, **159**, 6169–6175

Sheen, S.J. (1988) Detection of nicotine in foods and plant materials. *J. Food Sci.*, **53**, 1572–1573

Shephard, R.J., Collins, R. & Silverman, F. (1979a) Responses of exercising subjects to acute 'passive' cigarette smoke exposure. *Environ. Res.*, **19**, 279–291

Shephard, R.J., Collins, R. & Silverman, F. (1979b) 'Passive' exposure of asthmatic subjects to cigarette smoke. *Environ. Res.*, **20**, 392–402

Shephard, R.J., Ponsford, E., LaBarre, R. & Basu, P.K. (1979c) Effect of cigarette smoke on the eyes and airway. *Int. Arch. occup. environ. Health*, **43**, 135–144

Shinozaki, R., Inoue, S., Choi, K.-S. & Tatsuno, T. (1999) Association of benzo[*a*]pyrene-diol-epoxide–deoxyribonucleic acid (BPDE–DNA) adduct level with aging in male smokers and nonsmokers. *Arch. environ. Health*, **54**, 79–85

Sidney, S., Caan, B.J. & Friedman, G.D. (1989) Dietary intake of carotene in nonsmokers with and without passive smoking at home. *Am. J. Epidemiol.*, **129**, 1305–1309

Siegel, M. (1993) Involuntary smoking in the restaurant workplace. A review of employee exposure and health effects. *J. Am. med. Assoc.*, **270**, 490–493

Sindhu, R.K., Rasmussen, R.E., Yamamoto, R., Fujita, I. & Kikkawa, Y. (1995) Depression of hepatic cytochrome P450 monooxygenases after chronic environmental tobacco smoke exposure of young ferrets. *Toxicol. Lett.*, **76**, 227–238

Siwinska, E., Mielzynska, D., Bubak, A. & Smolik, E. (1999) The effect of coal stoves and environmental tobacco smoke on the level of urinary 1-hydroxypyrene. *Mutat. Res.*, **445**, 147–153

Slebos, R.J.C., Hruban, R.H., Dalesio, O., Mooi, W.J., Offerhaus, G.J.A. & Rodenhuis, S. (1991) Relationship between K-ras oncogene activation and smoking in adenocarcinoma of the human lung. *J. natl Cancer Inst.*, **83**, 1024–1027

Slotkin, T.A., Pinkerton, K.E. & Seidler, F.J. (2000) Perinatal exposure to environmental tobacco smoke alters cell signaling in a primate model: Autonomic receptors and the control of adenylyl cyclase activity in heart and lung. *Dev. Brain Res.*, **124**, 53–58

Slotkin, T.A., Pinkerton, K.E., Garofolo, M.C., Auman, J.T., McCook, E.C. & Seidler, F.J. (2001) Perinatal exposure to environmental tobacco smoke induces adenylyl cyclase and alters receptor-mediated cell signaling in brain and heart of neonatal rats. *Brain Res.*, **898**, 73–81

Smith, C.J., Bombick, D.W., Ryan, B.A., Morgan, W.T. & Doolittle, D.J. (2000) Urinary mutagenicity in nonsmokers following exposure to fresh diluted sidestream cigarette smoke. *Mutat. Res.*, **470**, 53–70

Smith, C.J., Bombick, D.W., Ryan, B.A., Morton, M.J. & Doolittle, D.J. (2001) Pulmonary function in nonsmokers following exposure to sidestream cigarette smoke. *Toxicol. Pathol.*, **29**, 260–264

Sorsa, M. & Husgafvel-Pursiainen, K. (1988) Assessment of passive and transplacental exposure to tobacco smoke. In: Bartsch, H., Hemminki, K. & O'Neill, I.K., eds, *Methods for Detecting DNA Damaging Agents in Humans: Applications in Cancer Epidemiology and Prevention* (IARC Scientific Publications No. 89), Lyon, IARC*Press*, pp. 129–132

Sorsa, M. & Löfroth, G., eds (1989) *Environmental Tobacco Smoke and Passive Smoking*, Amsterdam, Elsevier Science

Sorsa, M., Einistö, P., Husgafvel-Pursiainen, K., Järventaus, H., Kivistö, H., Peltonen, Y., Tuomi, T., Valkonen, S. & Pelkonen, O. (1985) Passive and active exposure to cigarette smoke in a smoking experiment. *J. Toxicol. environ. Health*, **16**, 523–534

Sorsa, M., Husgafvel-Pursiainen, K., Järventaus, H., Koskimies, K., Salo, H. & Vainio, H. (1989) Cytogenetic effects of tobacco smoke exposure among involuntary smokers. *Mutat. Res.*, **222**, 111–116

Spector, S., Luparello, T.J., Kopetzky, M.T., Souhrada, J. & Kinsman, R.A. (1976) Response of asthmatics to methacholine and suggestion. *Am. Rev. respir. Dis.*, **113**, 43–50

Speer, F. (1968) Tobacco and the nonsmoker. A study of subjective symptoms. *Arch. environ. Health*, **16**, 443–446

Spitzer, W.O., Lawrence, V., Dales, R., Hill, G., Archer, M.C., Clark, P., Abenhaim, L., Hardy, J., Sampalis, J., Pinfold, S.P. & Morgan, P.P. (1990) Links between passive smoking and disease:

A best-evidence synthesis. A report of the Working Group on Passive Smoking. *Clin. invest. Med.*, **13**, 17–42

Stankus, R.P., Menon, P.K., Rando, R.J., Glindmeyer, H., Salvaggio, J.E. & Lehrer, S.B. (1988) Cigarette smoke-sensitive asthma: Challenge studies. *J. Allergy clin. Immunol.*, **82**, 331–338

Steenland, K. (1992) Passive smoking and the risk of heart disease. *J. Am. med. Assoc.*, **267**, 94–99

Steenland, K., Thun, M., Lally, C. & Heath, C., Jr (1996) Environmental tobacco smoke and coronary heart disease in the American Cancer Society CPS-II cohort. *Circulation*, **94**, 622–628

Stryker, W.S., Kaplan, L.A., Stein, E.A., Stampfer, M.J., Sober, A. & Willett, W.C. (1988) The relation of diet, cigarette smoking, and alcohol consumption to plasma beta-carotene and alpha-tocopherol levels. *Am. J. Epidemiol.*, **127**, 283–296

Subar, A.F., Harlan, L.C. & Mattson, M.E. (1990) Food and nutrient intake differences between smokers and non-smokers in the US. *Am. J. public Health*, **80**, 1323–1329

Sun, Y.P., Zhu, B.Q., Browne, A.E., Sievers, R.E., Bekker, J.M., Chatterjee, K., Parmley, W.W. & Glantz, S.A. (2001) Nicotine does not influence arterial lipid deposits in rabbits exposed to second-hand smoke. *Circulation*, **104**, 810–814

Svendsen, K.H., Kuller, L.H., Martin, M.J. & Ockene, J.K. (1987) Effects of passive smoking in the Multiple Risk Factor Intervention Trial. *Am. J. Epidemiol.*, **126**, 783–795

Takagi, Y., Osada, H., Kuroishi, T., Mitsudomi, T., Kondo, M., Niimi, T., Saji, S., Gazdar, A.F., Takahashi, T., Minna, J.D. & Takahashi, T. (1998) p53 Mutations in non-small-cell lung cancers occurring in individuals without a past history of active smoking. *Br. J. Cancer*, **77**, 1568–1572

Takenawa, J., Kaneko, Y., Okumura, K., Nakayama, H., Fujita, J. & Yoshida, O. (1994) Urinary excretion of mutagens and covalent DNA damage induced in the bladder and kidney after passive smoking in rats. *Urol. Res.*, **22**, 93–97

Takeshima, Y., Seyama, T., Bennett, W.P., Akiyama, M., Tokuoka, S., Inai, K., Mabuchi, K., Land, C.E. & Harris, C.C. (1993) p53 Mutations in lung cancers from non-smoking atomic-bomb survivors. *Lancet*, **342**, 1520–1521

Tang, D., Warburton, D., Tannenbaum, S.R., Skipper, P., Santella, R.M., Cereijido, G.S., Crawford, F.G. & Perera, F.P. (1999) Molecular and genetic damage from environmental tobacco smoke in young children. *Cancer Epidemiol. Biomarkers Prev.*, **8**, 427–431

Taniguchi, S., Niitsuya, M., Inoue, Y., Katagiri, H., Kadowaki, T. & Aizawa, Y. (1999) Evaluation of passive smoking by measuring urinary trans,trans-muconic acid and exhaled carbon monoxide levels. *Ind. Health*, **37**, 88–94

Tavares, R., Ramos, P., Palminha, J., Bispo, M.A., Paz, I., Bras, A., Rueff, J., Farmer, P.B. & Bailey, E. (1994) Transplacental exposure to genotoxins. Evaluation in haemoglobin of hydroxyethylvaline adduct levels in smoking and non-smoking mothers and their newborns. *Carcinogenesis*, **15**, 1271–1274

Tavares, R., Borba, H., Monteiro, M., Proença, M.J., Lynce, N., Rueff, J., Bailey, E., Sweetman, G.M.A., Lawrence, R.M. & Farmer, P.B. (1996) Monitoring of exposure to acrylonitrile by determination of *N*-(2-cyanoethyl)valine at the N-terminal position of haemoglobin. *Carcinogenesis*, **17**, 2655–2660

Thompson, S.G., Stone, R., Nanchahal, K. & Wald, N.J. (1990) Relation of urinary cotinine concentrations to cigarette smoking and to exposure to other people's smoke. *Thorax*, **45**, 356–361

Thorn, J., Brisman, J. & Torén, K. (2001) Adult-onset asthma is associated with self-reported mold or environmental tobacco smoke exposures in the home. *Allergy*, **56**, 287–292

Thornton, A., Lee, P. & Fry, J. (1994) Differences between smokers, ex-smokers, passive smokers and non-smokers. *J. clin. Epidemiol.*, **47**, 1143–1162

Thun, M., Henley, J. & Apicella, L. (1999) Epidemiologic studies of fatal and nonfatal cardiovascular disease and ETS exposure from spousal smoking. *Environ. Health Perspect.*, **107** (Suppl. 6), 841–846

Trédaniel, J., Boffetta, P., Saracci, R. & Hirsch, A. (1994) Exposure to environmental tobacco smoke and adult non-neoplastic respiratory diseases. *Eur. respir. J.*, **7**, 173–185

Tribble, D.L., Giuliano, L.J. & Fortmann, S.P. (1993) Reduced plasma ascorbic acid concentrations in nonsmokers regularly exposed to environmental tobacco smoke. *Am. J. clin. Nutr.*, **58**, 886–890

Triebig, G. & Zober, M.A. (1984) Indoor air pollution by smoke constituents — A survey. *Prev. Med.*, **13**, 570–581

Trout, D., Decker, J., Mueller, C., Bernert, J.T. & Pirkle, J. (1998) Exposure of casino employees to environmental tobacco smoke. *J. occup. environ. Med.*, **40**, 270–276

Tunstall-Pedoe, H., Woodward, M. & Brown, C.A. (1991) The drinking, passive smoking, smoking deception and serum cotinine in the Scottish Heart Health Study. *J. clin. Epidemiol.*, **44**, 1411–1414

Tunstall-Pedoe, H., Brown, C.A., Woodward, M. & Tavendale, R. (1995) Passive smoking by self report and serum cotinine and the prevalence of respiratory and coronary heart disease in the Scottish Heart Health Study. *J. Epidemiol. Community Health*, **49**, 139–143

Urch, R.B., Silverman, F., Corey, P., Shephard, R.J., Cole, P. & Goldsmith, L.J. (1988) Does suggestibility modify acute reactions to passive cigarette smoke exposure? *Environ. Res.*, **47**, 34–47

US Department of Health, Education and Welfare (DHEW) (1972) *The Health Consequences of Smoking. A Report of the Surgeon General* (DHEW Publ. No. (PHS) 72-7516), Washington DC

US Department of Health and Human Services (DHHS) (1983) *The Health Consequences of Smoking. Cardiovascular Disease. A Report of the Surgeon General* (DHHS Publ. No. (CDC) 84-50204), Rockville, MD

US Department of Health and Human Services (DHHS) (1984) *The Health Consequences of Smoking. Chronic Obstructive Disease. A Report of the Surgeon General* (DHHS Publ. No. (PHS) 84-50205), Rockville, MD

US Department of Health and Human Services (DHHS) (1986) *The Health Consequences of Involuntary Smoking. A Report of the Surgeon General* (DHHS Publ. No. (CDC) 86-8398), Rockville, MD

US Department of Health and Human Services (DHHS) (1990) *The Health Benefits of Smoking Cessation. A Report of the Surgeon General* (DHHS Publ. No. (CDC) 90-8416), Rockville, MD

US Department of Health and Human Services (DHHS) (2001) *Women and Smoking. A Report of the Surgeon General*, Rockville, MD [available at http://www.cdc.gov/tobacco/sgr/sgr_for-women/index]

US Environmental Protection Agency (EPA, 1992) *Respiratory Health Effects of Passive Smoking: Lung Cancer and Other Disorders. The Report of the US Environmental Protection Agency*

(Smoking and Tobacco Control Monograph No. 4; NIH Publ. No. 93-3605), Washington DC [available at http://cfpub.epa.gov/ncea/cfm/ets/etsindex.cfm]

US National Academy of Sciences (1986) *The Airliner Cabin Environment — Air Quality and Safety*, Washington DC, National Academy Press

US National Academy of Sciences (2000) *Clearing the Air: Asthma and Indoor Air Exposures*, Washington DC, National Academy Press

US National Institute for Occupational Safety and Health (NIOSH) (1971) *Health Aspects of Smoking in Transports Aircrafts*, Washington DC, US Government Printing Office

US National Research Council (1986) *Environmental Tobacco Smoke: Measuring Exposures and Assessing Health Effects*, Washington DC, National Academy Press

Vähäkangas, K.H., Bennett, W.P., Castrén, K., Welsh, J.A., Khan, M.A., Blömeke, B., Alavanja, M.C.-R. & Harris, C.C. (2001) *p53* and K-*ras* Mutations in lung cancers from former and never-smoking women. *Cancer Res.*, **61**, 4350–4356

Van Rooij, J.G.M., Veeger, M.M.S., Bodelier-Bade, M.M., Scheepers, P.T.J. & Jongeneelen, F.J. (1994) Smoking and dietary intake of polycyclic aromatic hydrocarbons as sources of inter-individual variability in the baseline excretion of 1-hydroxypyrene in urine. *Int. Arch. occup. environ. Health*, **66**, 55–65

Vermeulen, R., Wegh, H., Bos, R.P. & Kromhout, H. (2000) Weekly patterns in smoking habits and influence on urinary cotinine and mutagenicity levels: Confounding effect of nonsmoking policies in the workplace. *Cancer Epidemiol. Biomarkers Prev.*, **9**, 1205–1209

Vineis, P. & Malats, N. (1999) Strategic issues in the design and interpretation of studies on metabolic polymorphisms and cancer. In: Vineis, P., Malats, N., Lang, M., d'Errico, A., Caporaso, N., Cuzick, J. & Boffetta, P., eds, *Metabolic Polymorphisms and Susceptibility to Cancer* (IARC Scientific Publication No. 148), Lyon, IARC*Press*, pp. 51–61

Visioli, F., Galli, C., Plasmati, E., Viappiani, S., Hernandez, A., Colombo, C. & Sala, A. (2000) Olive phenol hydroxytyrosol prevents passive smoking-induced oxidative stress. *Circulation*, **102**, 2169–2171

Wagenknecht, L.E., Manolio, T.A., Sidney, S., Burke, G.L. & Haley, N.J. (1993) Environmental tobacco smoke exposure as determined by cotinine in black and white young adults: The CARDIA study. *Environ. Res.*, **63**, 39–46

Wallace, L., Pellizzari, E., Hartwell, T.D., Perritt, R. & Ziegenfus, R. (1987) Exposures to benzene and other volatile compounds from active and passive smoking. *Arch. environ. Health*, **42**, 272–279

Wang, X., Christiani, D.C., Wiencke, J.K., Fischbein, M., Xu, X., Cheng, T.J., Mark, E., Wain, J.C. & Kelsey, K.T. (1995) Mutations in the *p53* gene in lung cancer are associated with cigarette smoking and asbestos exposure. *Cancer Epidemiol. Biomarkers Prev.*, **4**, 543–548

Weaver, V.M., Davoli, C.T., Heller, P.J., Fitzwilliam, A., Peters, H.L., Sunyer, J., Murphy, S.E., Goldstein, G.W. & Groopman, J.D. (1996) Benzene exposure, assessed by urinary *trans,trans*-muconic acid, in urban children with elevated blood lead levels. *Environ. Health Perspect.*, **104**, 318–323

Weber, A. (1984a) Annoyance and irritation by passive smoking. *Prev. Med.*, **13**, 618-625

Weber, A. (1984b) Acute effects of environmental tobacco smoke. *Eur. J. respir. Dis.*, **Suppl. 133**, 98–108

Weber, A. & Fischer, T. (1980) Passive smoking at work. *Int. Arch. occup. environ. Health*, **47**, 209–221

Weber, A. & Grandjean, E. (1987) Acute effects of environmental tobacco smoke. In: O'Neill, I.K., Brunnemann, K.D., Dodet, B. & Hoffmann, D., eds, *Environmental Carcinogens: Methods of Analysis and Exposure Measurement* (IARC Scientific Publications No. 81), Lyon, IARC*Press*, pp. 59–68

Weber, A., Jermini, C. & Grandjean, E. (1976) Irritating effects on man of air pollution due to cigarette smoke. *Am. J. public Health*, **66**, 672–676

Weinberg, C.R., Wilcox, A.J. & Baird, D.B. (1989) Reduced fecundability in women with prenatal exposure to cigarette smoking. *Am. J. Epidemiol.*, **129**, 1072–1078

Weiss, S.T., Tager, I.B., Schenker, M. & Speizer, F.E. (1983) The health effects of involuntary smoking. *Am. Rev. respir. Dis.*, **128**, 933–942

Weiss, S.T., Utell, M.J. & Samet, J.M. (1999) Environmental tobacco smoke exposure and asthma in adults. *Environ. Health Perspect.*, **107** (Suppl. 6), 891–895

Wells, A.J. (1988) An estimate of adult mortality in the United States from passive smoking. *Environ. int.*, **14**, 249–265

Wells, A.J. (1994) Passive smoking as a cause of heart disease. *J. Am. Coll. Cardiol.*, **24**, 546–554

Wells, A.J. (1998) Heart disease from passive smoking in the workplace. *J. Am. Coll. Cardiol.*, **31**, 1–9

Westra, W.H., Slebos, R.J.C., Offerhaus, G.J.A., Goodman, S.N., Evers, S.G., Kensler, T.W., Askin, F.B., Rodenhuis, S. & Hruban, R.H. (1993) K-*ras* oncogen activation in lung adenocarcinoma from former smokers. *Cancer*, **72**, 432–438

White, J.R. & Froeb, H.F. (1980) Small-airways dysfunction in nonsmokers chronically exposed to tobacco smoke. *New Engl. J. Med.*, **302**, 720–723

White, J.R., Froeb, H.F. & Kulik, J.A. (1991) Respiratory illness in nonsmokers chronically exposed to tobacco smoke in the work place. *Chest*, **100**, 39–43

Wiedemann, H.P., Mahler, D.A., Loke, J., Virgulto, J.A., Snyder, P. & Matthay, R.A. (1986) Acute effects of passive smoking on lung function and airway reactivity in asthmatic subjects. *Chest*, **89**, 180–185

Wilcox, A.J., Baird, D.D. & Weinberg, C.R. (1989) Do women with childhood exposure to cigarette smoking have increased fecundability? *Am. J. Epidemiol.*, **129**, 1079–1083

Willes, S.R., Fitzgerald, T.K. & Bascom, R. (1992) Nasal inhalation challenge studies with sidestream tobacco smoke. *Arch. environ. Health*, **47**, 223–230

Willes, S.R., Fitzgerald, T.K., Permutt, T., Proud, D., Haley, N.J. & Bascom, R. (1998) Acute respiratory response to prolonged, moderate levels of sidestream tobacco smoke. *J. Toxicol. environ. Health*, **A53**, 193–209

Windham, G.C., Eaton, A. & Hopkins, B. (1999a) Evidence for an association between environmental tobacco smoke exposure and birthweight: A meta-analysis and new data. *Paediatr. perinat. Epidemiol.*, **13**, 35–57

Windham, G.C., Von Behren, J., Waller, K. & Fenster, L. (1999b) Exposure to environmental and mainstream tobacco smoke and risk of spontaneous abortion. *Am. J. Epidemiol.*, **149**, 243–247

Witorsch, P. (1992) Does environmental tobacco smoke (ETS) cause adverse health effects in susceptible individuals? A critical review of the scientific literature: I. Respiratory disorders, atopic allergy and related conditions. *Environ. Technol.*, **13**, 323–340

Witschi, H. & Rajini, P. (1994) Cell kinetics in the respiratory tract of hamsters exposed to cigarette sidestream smoke. *Inhal. Toxicol.*, **6**, 321–333

Witschi, H., Lundgaard, S.M., Rajini, P., Hendrickx, A.G. & Last, J.A. (1994) Effects of exposure to nicotine and to sidestream smoke on pregnancy outcome in rats. *Toxicol. Lett.*, **71**, 279–286

Witschi, H., Espiritu, I., Maronpot, R.R., Pinkerton, K.E. & Jones, A.D. (1997a) The carcinogenic potential of the gas phase of environmental tobacco smoke. *Carcinogenesis*, **18**, 2035–2042

Witschi, H., Espiritu, I., Peake, J.L., Wu, K., Maronpot, R.R. & Pinkerton, K.E. (1997b) The carcinogenicity of environmental tobacco smoke. *Carcinogenesis*, **18**, 575–586

Witschi, H., Joad, J.P. & Pinkerton, K.E. (1997c) The toxicology of environmental tobacco smoke. *Ann. Rev. Pharmacol. Toxicol.*, **37**, 29–52

Wu-Williams, A.H. & Samet, J.M. (1990) Environmental tobacco smoke: Exposure–response relationships in epidemiologic studies. *Risk Anal.*, **10**, 39–48

Xu, X. & Li, B. (1995) Exposure–response relationship between passive smoking and adult pulmonary function. *Am. J. respir. crit. Care Med.*, **151**, 41–46

Yamasaki, E. & Ames, B.N. (1977) Concentration of mutagens from urine by absorption with the nonpolar resin XAD-2: Cigarette smokers have mutagenic urine. *Proc. natl Acad. Sci. USA*, **74**, 3555–3559

Yates, D.H., Breen, H. & Thomas, P.S. (2001) Passive smoke inhalation decreases exhaled nitric oxide in normal subjects. *Am. J. respir. crit. Care Med.*, **164**, 1043–1046

Yu, R. & Weisel, C.P. (1996) Measurement of the urinary benzene metabolite *trans,trans*-muconic acid from benzene exposure in humans. *J. Toxicol. environ. Health*, **48**, 453–477

Zahlsen, K., Nilsen, T. & Nilsen, O.G. (1996) Interindividual differences in hair uptake of air nicotine and significance of cigarette counting for estimation of environmental tobacco smoke exposure. *Pharmacol. Toxicol.*, **79**, 183–190

van Zeeland, A.A., de Groot, A.J.L., Hall, J. & Donato, F. (1999) 8-Hydroxydeoxyguanosine in DNA from leukocytes of healthy adults: Relationship with cigarette smoking, environmental tobacco smoke, alcohol and coffee consumption. *Mutat. Res.*, **439**, 249–257

Zenzes, M.T., Puy, L.A. & Bielecki, R. (1998) Immunodetection of benzo[*a*]pyrene adducts in ovarian cells of women exposed to cigarette smoke. *Mol. hum. Reprod.*, **4**, 159–165

Zhu, B.-Q., Sun, Y.-P., Sievers, R.E., Isenberg, W.M., Glantz, S.A. & Parmley, W.W. (1993) Passive smoking increases experimental atherosclerosis in cholesterol-fed rabbits. *J. Am. Coll. Cardiol.*, **21**, 225–232

Zhu, B.Q., Sun, Y.P., Sievers, R.E., Glantz, S.A., Parmley, W.W. & Wolfe, C.L. (1994) Exposure to environmental tobacco smoke increases myocardial infarct size in rats. *Circulation*, **89**, 1282–1290

Zhu, B.Q., Sun, Y.P., Sudhir, K., Sievers, R.E., Browne, A.E., Gao, L., Hutchison, S.J., Chou, T.M., Deedwania, P.C., Chatterjee, K., Glantz, S.A. & Parmley, W.W. (1997) Effects of second-hand smoke and gender on infarct size of young rats exposed in utero and in the neonatal to adolescent period. *J. Am. Coll. Cardiol.*, **30**, 1878–1885

Zondervan, K.T., Ocké, M.C., Smit, H.A. & Seidell, J.C. (1996) Do dietary and supplementary intakes of antioxidants differ with smoking status? *Int. J. Epidemiol.*, **25**, 70–79

5. Summary of Data Reported and Evaluation

5.1   Exposure data

Involuntary (or passive) smoking is exposure to secondhand tobacco smoke, which is a mixture of exhaled mainstream smoke and sidestream smoke released from the smouldering cigarette or other smoking device (cigars, pipes, bidis, etc.) and diluted with ambient air. Involuntary smoking involves inhaling carcinogens, as well as other toxic components, that are present in secondhand tobacco smoke. Secondhand tobacco smoke is sometimes referred to as 'environmental' tobacco smoke. Carcinogens that occur in secondhand tobacco smoke include benzene, 1,3-butadiene, benzo[a]pyrene, 4-(methyl-nitrosamino)-1-(3-pyridyl)-1-butanone and many others.

Secondhand tobacco smoke consists of a gas phase and a particulate phase; it changes during its dilution and distribution in the environment and upon ageing. The concentrations of respirable particles may be elevated substantially in enclosed spaces containing secondhand tobacco smoke. The composition of tobacco smoke inhaled involuntarily is variable quantitatively and depends on the smoking patterns of the smokers who are producing the smoke as well as the composition and design of the cigarettes or other smoking devices. The secondhand tobacco smoke produced by smoking cigarettes has been most intensively studied.

Secondhand tobacco smoke contains nicotine as well as carcinogens and toxins. Nicotine concentrations in the air in homes of smokers and in workplaces where smoking is permitted typically range on average from 2 to 10 $\mu g/m^3$.

5.2   Human carcinogenicity data

Lung cancer

Involuntary smoking involves exposure to the same numerous carcinogens and toxic substances that are present in tobacco smoke produced by active smoking, which is the principal cause of lung cancer. As noted in the previous *IARC Monograph* on tobacco smoking, this implies that there will be some risk of lung cancer from exposure to secondhand tobacco smoke.

More than 50 studies of involuntary smoking and lung cancer risk in never-smokers, especially spouses of smokers, have been published during the last 25 years. These studies have been carried out in many countries. Most showed an increased risk, especially for persons with higher exposures. To evaluate the information collectively, in particular from those studies with a limited number of cases, meta-analyses have been conducted in which the relative risk estimates from the individual studies are pooled together. These meta-analyses show that there is a statistically significant and consistent association between lung cancer risk in spouses of smokers and exposure to secondhand tobacco smoke from the spouse who smokes. The excess risk is of the order of 20% for women and 30% for men and remains after controlling for some potential sources of bias and confounding. The excess risk increases with increasing exposure. Furthermore, other published meta-analyses of lung cancer in never-smokers exposed to secondhand tobacco smoke at the workplace have found a statistically significant increase in risk of 12–19%. This evidence is sufficient to conclude that involuntary smoking is a cause of lung cancer in never-smokers. The magnitudes of the observed risks are reasonably consistent with predictions based on studies of active smoking in many populations.

Breast cancer

The collective evidence on breast cancer risk associated with involuntary exposure of never-smokers to tobacco smoke is inconsistent. Although four of the 10 case–control studies found statistically significant increases in risks, prospective cohort studies as a whole and, particularly, the two large cohort studies in the USA of nurses and of volunteers in the Cancer Prevention Study II provided no support for a causal relation between involuntary exposure to tobacco smoke and breast cancer in never-smokers. The lack of a positive dose–response also argues against a causal interpretation of these findings. Finally, the lack of an association of breast cancer with active smoking weighs heavily against the possibility that involuntary smoking increases the risk for breast cancer, as no data are available to establish that different mechanisms of carcinogenic action operate at the different dose levels of active and of involuntary smoking.

Childhood cancer

Overall, the findings from studies of childhood cancer and exposure to parental smoking are inconsistent and are likely to be affected by bias. There is a suggestion of a modest association between exposure to maternal tobacco smoke during pregnancy and childhood cancer for all cancer sites combined; however, this is in contrast with the null findings for individual sites. Studies on paternal tobacco smoking suggest a small increased risk for lymphomas, but bias and confounding cannot be ruled out.

Other cancer sites

Data are conflicting and sparse for associations between involuntary smoking and cancers of the nasopharynx, nasal cavity, paranasal sinuses, cervix, gastrointestinal tract and cancers at all sites combined. It is unlikely that any effects are produced in passive smokers that are not produced to a greater extent in active smokers or that types of effects that are not seen in active smokers will be seen in passive smokers.

5.3   Animal carcinogenicity data

Secondhand tobacco smoke for carcinogenicity studies in animals is produced by machines that simulate human active smoking patterns and combine mainstream and sidestream smoke in various proportions. Such mixtures have been tested for carcinogenicity by inhalation studies in rodents. The experimental model systems for exposure to secondhand tobacco smoke do not fully simulate human exposures, and the tumours that develop in animals are not completely representative of human cancer. Nevertheless, the animal data provide valuable insights regarding the carcinogenic potential of secondhand tobacco smoke.

A mixture of 89% sidestream smoke and 11% mainstream smoke has been tested for carcinogenic activity in mouse strains that are highly susceptible to lung tumours (strains A/J and Swiss). In strain A/J mice, this mixture consistently produces a significant, modest increase in lung tumour incidence and lung tumour multiplicity when the mice are exposed for 5 months followed by a 4-month recovery period. These lung tumours are predominantly adenomas. Continuous exposure of strain A/J mice to the above mixture of mainstream and sidestream tobacco smoke for 9 months with no recovery period did not increase the incidence of lung tumours. In Swiss strain mice, the same mixture induced lung tumours by both protocols, i.e. when the animals were exposed for 5 months followed by a 4-month recovery period and when they were exposed continuously for 9 months with no recovery period. In addition, exposure of Swiss mice to the tobacco smoke mixture for a shorter period was sufficient to induce lung tumours.

Condensates of sidestream and of mainstream cigarette smoke have been tested for carcinogenicity. Both kinds of condensates produced a spectrum of benign and malignant skin tumours in mice following topical application, and the sidestream condensate exhibited higher carcinogenic activity. Sidestream smoke condensate was shown to produce a dose–dependent increase in lung tumours in rats following implantation into the lungs.

Increased relative risks for lung and sinonasal cancer have been reported in companion animals (dogs) exposed to secondhand tobacco smoke in homes.

5.4   Other relevant data

Involuntary smoking has been associated with a number of non-neoplastic diseases and adverse effects in never-smokers, including both children and adults. Epidemiological studies have demonstrated that exposure to secondhand tobacco smoke is causally associated with coronary heart disease. From the available meta-analyses, it has been estimated that involuntary smoking increases the risk of an acute coronary heart disease event by 25–35%. Adverse effects of involuntary smoking on the respiratory system have also been detected. In adults, the strongest evidence for a causal relation exists for chronic respiratory symptoms. Some effects on lung function have been detected, but their medical relevance is uncertain.

Data on the hormonal and metabolic effects of involuntary smoking are sparse. However, female involuntary smokers do not appear to weigh less than women who are not exposed to secondhand tobacco smoke, a pattern that contrasts with the findings for active smoking. No consistent association of maternal exposure to secondhand smoke with fertility or fecundity has been identified. There is no clear association of passive smoking with age at menopause.

Maternal cigarette smoking has repeatedly been associated with adverse effects on fetal growth; full-term infants born to women who smoke weigh about 200 g less than those born to nonsmokers. A smaller adverse effect has been attributed to maternal passive smoking.

Cotinine, and its parent compound nicotine, are highly specific for exposure to secondhand smoke. Because of its favourable biological half-life and the sensitivity of techniques for quantifying it, cotinine is currently the most suitable biomarker for assessing recent exposure to secondhand tobacco smoke uptake and metabolism in adults, children and newborns.

Several studies in humans have shown that concentrations of adducts of carcinogens to biological macromolecules, including haemoglobin adducts of aromatic amines and albumin adducts of polycyclic aromatic hydrocarbons, are higher in adult involuntary smokers and in the children of smoking mothers than in individuals not exposed to secondhand tobacco smoke. Protein adduct concentrations in fetal cord blood correlate with those in maternal blood but are lower. Fewer studies have investigated DNA adduct levels in white blood cells of exposed and unexposed nonsmokers, and most studies have not shown clear differences.

In studies of urinary biomarkers, metabolites of the tobacco-specific carcinogen, 4-(methylnitrosamino)-1-(3-pyridyl)-1-butanone, have been found to be consistently elevated in involuntary smokers. Levels of these metabolites are 1–5% as great as those found in smokers. The data demonstrating uptake of 4-(methylnitrosamino)-1-(3-pyridyl)-1-butanone, a lung carcinogen in rodents, by nonsmokers are supportive of a causal link between exposure to secondhand tobacco smoke and development of lung cancer.

The exposure of experimental animals, primarily rodents, to secondhand tobacco smoke has several biological effects that include (i) increases or decreases in the activity of phase I enzymes involved in carcinogen metabolism; (ii) increased expression of nitric oxide synthase, xanthine oxidase and various protein kinases; (iii) the formation of smoke-related DNA adducts in several tissues; and (iv) the presence of urinary biomarkers of exposure to tobacco smoke.

In adult experimental animals, sidestream tobacco smoke has been found to produce changes that are similar to those observed with exposure of humans to secondhand tobacco smoke. These include inflammatory changes in the airways and accelerated formation of arteriosclerotic plaques. Although the changes are often comparatively minor and require exposure to rather elevated concentrations of sidestream smoke, they support the results of human epidemiological studies. During pre- and postnatal exposure, side-stream smoke produces intrauterine growth retardation, changes the pattern of metabolic enzymes in the developing lung, and gives rise to hyperplasia of the pulmonary neuro-endocrine cell population. In addition, it adversely affects pulmonary compliance and airway responsiveness to pharmacological challenges.

In humans, involuntary smoking is associated with increased concentrations of muta-gens in urine. Some studies have shown a correlation of urinary mutagenicity with concentrations of urinary cotinine. Increased levels of sister chromatid exchange have not been observed in involuntary smokers; however, there is some indication of elevated levels in exposed children. Lung tumours from nonsmokers exposed to tobacco smoke contain *TP53* and *KRAS* mutations that are similar to those found in tumours from smokers. The genotoxicity of sidestream smoke, 'environmental' tobacco smoke, side-stream smoke condensate or a mixture of sidestream and mainstream smoke condensates has been demonstrated in experimental systems *in vitro* and *in vivo*.

5.5   Evaluation

There is *sufficient evidence* that involuntary smoking (exposure to secondhand or 'environmental' tobacco smoke) causes lung cancer in humans.

There is *limited evidence* in experimental animals for the carcinogenicity of mixtures of mainstream and sidestream tobacco smoke.

There is *sufficient evidence* in experimental animals for the carcinogenicity of side-stream smoke condensates.

In addition, the Working Group noted that there are published reports on possible carcinogenic effects of secondhand tobacco smoke in household pet dogs.

Overall evaluation

Involuntary smoking (exposure to secondhand or 'environmental' tobacco smoke) is *carcinogenic to humans (Group 1)*.

LIST OF ABBREVIATIONS USED IN THIS VOLUME

3-ABP: 3-aminobiphenyl
4-ABP: 4-aminobiphenyl
AC: adenylyl cyclase
AH: acetylhydrolase
AHH: aryl hydrocarbon hydroxylase
ALDH: aldehyde dehydrogenase
AMI: acute myocardial infarction
ApoE: apolipoprotein E
BaP: benzo[*a*]pyrene
BPDE: benzo[*a*]pyrene diolepoxide
CDK: cyclin-dependent kinase
CEVal: *N*-(2-cyanoethyl)valine
ChAT: choline acetyltransferase
CHD: coronary heart disease
CO: carbon monoxide
COHb: carboxyhaemoglobin
COPD: chronic obstructive pulmonary disease
COTAC: cotinine acid 4-(methylamino)-4-(3-pyridyl)butyric acid
COX: cyclooxygenase
CSC: cigarette smoke condensate
DDD: dichlorodiphenyldichloroethane
DDE: 1,1-dichloro-2,2-bis(p-chlorophenyl)ethylene
DDT: 1,1,1-trichloro-2,2-di-(4-chlorophenyl)ethane
DHEAS: dihydroepiandrosterone sulfate
DMBA: 7,12-dimethylbenz[*a*]anthracene
DRZ: diagonal radioactive zone
EH: epoxide hydrolase
ELISA: enzyme-linked immunosorbent assay
ERK: extracellular signal-regulated protein kinase
FAL: fractional allelic loss
FCTC: Framework Convention on Tobacco Control
FEF: forced expiratory flow

FEV₁: forced expiratory volume in 1 second

FEV_1: forced expiratory volume in 1 second

FGF-2: fibroblast growth factor-2

***FHIT* gene**: a gene coding for a dinucleoside 5′,5‴-P¹,P³-triphosphate hydrolase, a putative tumour suppressor protein

FHIT gene: a gene coding for a dinucleoside $5',5'''-P^1,P^3$-triphosphate hydrolase, a putative tumour suppressor protein

FID: flame ionizing detection

FISH: fluorescence in-situ hybridization

FPM: fluorescent particular matter

FTC: Federal Trade Commission

FVC: forced vital capacity

GC–MS: gas chromatography–mass spectrometry

gluc: glucuronide

GSH: glutathione

GST: glutathione-*S*-transferase

HCAs: heterocyclic amines

HC-3: [³H]hemicholinium-3

HOEtVal: *N*-(2-hydroxyethyl)valine

1-HOP: 1-hydroxypyrene

HPB: 4-hydroxy-1-(3-pyridyl)-1-butanone

HPLC: high-performance liquid chromatography

ICCSS: International Committee for Cigar Smoke Study

IgE: immunoglobulin E

IGF1: insulin-like growth factor 1

IgG: immunoglobulin G

IHD: ischaemic heart disease

IL: interleukin

iNOS: inducible nitric oxide synthase

ISO: International Standardization Organization

***iso*-NNAC**: 4-(*N*-nitrosomethylamino)-4-(3-pyridyl)butyric acid

KRAS oncogene: Kirsten-*ras* oncogene

LALN: lung-associated lymph nodes

LDL: low-density lipoproteins

LOH: loss of heterozygosity

MAPK: mitogen-activated protein kinase

7-MedG: 7-methyldeoxyriboguanosine

MEF: maximal expiratory flow

MEH: mitochondriol epoxyde hydrolase

MEK1: mitogen-activated extracellular kinase 1

MeP: methylpurine

MF: mutant frequency

MT: myocardial infarction

NAC: *N*-acetyl-L-cysteine

nAChRs: nicotinic acetylcholine receptors

NADPH: nicotinamide-adenine dinucleotide phosphate

NAT: *N*-acetyltransferase

NBOPA: *N*-nitrosobis(2-oxopropyl)amine

NDEA: *N*-nitrosodiethylamine

NDELA: *N*-nitrosodiethanolamine

NDMA: *N*-nitrosodimethylamine

NEMA: *N*-nitroethylmethylamine

NF: nuclear factor

nic: nicotine

NMBA: 4-(*N*-nitroso-*N*-methylamino)butyric acid

NMPA: 3-(*N*-nitroso-*N*-methylamino)propionic acid

NMTCA: *N*-nitroso-2-methylthiazolidine 4-carboxylic acid

iso-NNAC: see under *iso*

NNAL: 4-(*N*-nitrosomethylamino)-1-(3-pyridyl)-1-butanol

NNAL-*O*-gluc: [4-(methylnitrosamino)-1-(3-pyridyl)but-1-yl]-β-*O*-D-glucosiduronic acid

NNK: 4-(*N*-nitrosomethylamino)-1-(3-pyridyl)-1-butanone

NNN: *N*′-nitrosonornicotine

NO: nitric oxide

NO$_2$: nitrogen dioxide, also called nitrous oxide

NOx: nitrogen oxides

NOS: NO synthase

NPIC: *N*-nitrosopipecolic acid

NPIP: *N*-nitropiperidine

NPRO: *N*-nitrosoproline

NPYR: *N*-nitrosopyrrolidine

NSAR: *N*-nitrososarcosine

NTCA: *N*-nitrosothiazolidine 4-carboxylic acid

O^6-MedG: O^6-methyldeoxyriboguanosine

25-OH vitamin D: 25-hydroxyvitamin D

8-OHdG: 8-hydroxy-2′-deoxyguanosine

OVA/AL: aluminium hydroxide-precipitated ovalbumin

8-oxodG: 8-oxo-7,8-dihydro-2′-deoxyguanosine

P450: cytochrome P450

PAF: platelet-activating factor

PAH: polycyclic aromatic hydrocarbons

PCDD: polychlorodibenzodioxins

PCDF: polychlorodibenzofurans

PEF: peak expiratory flow

PhIP: 2-amino-1-methyl-6-phenylimidazo[4,5-*b*]pyridine

PKC: protein kinase C

RB gene: retinoblastoma gene

ROS: reactive oxygen species
RSP: respirable suspended particles
RYO: roll-your-own
SCN: serum thiocyanate
SFS: synchronous fluorescence spectroscopy
SH: spontaneously hypertensive
S-PMA: *S*-phenylmercapturic acid
S9: supernatant of 9000 g centrifugation
tar: particulate phase
TCDD: 2,3,7,8-tetrachloro-*para*-dibenzodioxin
TPM: total particulate matter
TSNA: tobacco-specific nitrosamines
***tt*-MA**: *trans,trans*-muconic acid
UDP: uridine-5′-diphosphate
UGT: uridine-5′-diphosphate glucuronosyltransferase
UVPM: ultraviolet particulate matter
V(D)J recombination: combinatorial rearrangement of multiple V (variable),
D (diversity) and J (junctional) coding gene segments
VOC: volatile organic compounds
WBC: white blood cell

CUMULATIVE CROSS INDEX TO *IARC MONOGRAPHS ON THE EVALUATION OF CARCINOGENIC RISKS TO HUMANS*

The volume, page and year of publication are given. References to corrigenda are given in parentheses.

A

A-α-C	*40*, 245 (1986); *Suppl. 7*, 56 (1987)
Acetaldehyde	*36*, 101 (1985) (*corr. 42*, 263); *Suppl. 7*, 77 (1987); *71*, 319 (1999)
Acetaldehyde formylmethylhydrazone (*see* Gyromitrin)	
Acetamide	*7*, 197 (1974); *Suppl. 7*, 56, 389 (1987); *71*, 1211 (1999)
Acetaminophen (*see* Paracetamol)	
Aciclovir	*76*, 47 (2000)
Acid mists (*see* Sulfuric acid and other strong inorganic acids, occupational exposures to mists and vapours from)	
Acridine orange	*16*, 145 (1978); *Suppl. 7*, 56 (1987)
Acriflavinium chloride	*13*, 31 (1977); *Suppl. 7*, 56 (1987)
Acrolein	*19*, 479 (1979); *36*, 133 (1985); *Suppl. 7*, 78 (1987); *63*, 337 (1995) (*corr. 65*, 549)
Acrylamide	*39*, 41 (1986); *Suppl. 7*, 56 (1987); *60*, 389 (1994)
Acrylic acid	*19*, 47 (1979); *Suppl. 7*, 56 (1987); *71*, 1223 (1999)
Acrylic fibres	*19*, 86 (1979); *Suppl. 7*, 56 (1987)
Acrylonitrile	*19*, 73 (1979); *Suppl. 7*, 79 (1987); *71*, 43 (1999)
Acrylonitrile-butadiene-styrene copolymers	*19*, 91 (1979); *Suppl. 7*, 56 (1987)
Actinolite (*see* Asbestos)	
Actinomycin D (*see also* Actinomycins)	*Suppl. 7*, 80 (1987)
Actinomycins	*10*, 29 (1976) (*corr. 42*, 255)
Adriamycin	*10*, 43 (1976); *Suppl. 7*, 82 (1987)
AF-2	*31*, 47 (1983); *Suppl. 7*, 56 (1987)
Aflatoxins	*1*, 145 (1972) (*corr. 42*, 251); *10*, 51 (1976); *Suppl. 7*, 83 (1987); *56*, 245 (1993); *82*, 171 (2002)
Aflatoxin B₁ (*see* Aflatoxins)	
Aflatoxin B₂ (*see* Aflatoxins)	
Aflatoxin G₁ (*see* Aflatoxins)	
Aflatoxin G₂ (*see* Aflatoxins)	
Aflatoxin M₁ (*see* Aflatoxins)	
Agaritine	*31*, 63 (1983); *Suppl. 7*, 56 (1987)
Alcohol drinking	*44* (1988)
Aldicarb	*53*, 93 (1991)

Benz[*c*]acridine — 3, 241 (1973); 32, 129 (1983); *Suppl. 7*, 58 (1987)

Benzal chloride (*see also* α-Chlorinated toluenes and benzoyl chloride) — 29, 65 (1982); *Suppl. 7*, 148 (1987); 71, 453 (1999)

Benz[*a*]anthracene — 3, 45 (1973); 32, 135 (1983); *Suppl. 7*, 58 (1987)

Benzene — 7, 203 (1974) (*corr. 42*, 254); 29, 93, 391 (1982); *Suppl. 7*, 120 (1987)

Benzidine — 1, 80 (1972); 29, 149, 391 (1982); *Suppl. 7*, 123 (1987)

Benzidine-based dyes — *Suppl. 7*, 125 (1987)

Benzo[*b*]fluoranthene — 3, 69 (1973); 32, 147 (1983); *Suppl. 7*, 58 (1987)

Benzo[*j*]fluoranthene — 3, 82 (1973); 32, 155 (1983); *Suppl. 7*, 58 (1987)

Benzo[*k*]fluoranthene — 32, 163 (1983); *Suppl. 7*, 58 (1987)

Benzo[*ghi*]fluoranthene — 32, 171 (1983); *Suppl. 7*, 58 (1987)

Benzo[*a*]fluorene — 32, 177 (1983); *Suppl. 7*, 58 (1987)

Benzo[*b*]fluorene — 32, 183 (1983); *Suppl. 7*, 58 (1987)

Benzo[*c*]fluorene — 32, 189 (1983); *Suppl. 7*, 58 (1987)

Benzofuran — 63, 431 (1995)

Benzo[*ghi*]perylene — 32, 195 (1983); *Suppl. 7*, 58 (1987)

Benzo[*c*]phenanthrene — 32, 205 (1983); *Suppl. 7*, 58 (1987)

Benzo[*a*]pyrene — 3, 91 (1973); 32, 211 (1983) (*corr. 68*, 477); *Suppl. 7*, 58 (1987)

Benzo[*e*]pyrene — 3, 137 (1973); 32, 225 (1983); *Suppl. 7*, 58 (1987)

1,4-Benzoquinone (see *para*-Quinone)

1,4-Benzoquinone dioxime — 29, 185 (1982); *Suppl. 7*, 58 (1987); 71, 1251 (1999)

Benzotrichloride (*see also* α-Chlorinated toluenes and benzoyl chloride) — 29, 73 (1982); *Suppl. 7*, 148 (1987); 71, 453 (1999)

Benzoyl chloride (*see also* α-Chlorinated toluenes and benzoyl chloride) — 29, 83 (1982) (*corr. 42*, 261); *Suppl. 7*, 126 (1987); 71, 453 (1999)

Benzoyl peroxide — 36, 267 (1985); *Suppl. 7*, 58 (1987); 71, 345 (1999)

Benzyl acetate — 40, 109 (1986); *Suppl. 7*, 58 (1987); 71, 1255 (1999)

Benzyl chloride (*see also* α-Chlorinated toluenes and benzoyl chloride) — 11, 217 (1976) (*corr. 42*, 256); 29, 49 (1982); *Suppl. 7*, 148 (1987); 71, 453 (1999)

Benzyl violet 4B — 16, 153 (1978); *Suppl. 7*, 58 (1987)

Bertrandite (*see* Beryllium and beryllium compounds)

Beryllium and beryllium compounds — 1, 17 (1972); 23, 143 (1980) (*corr. 42*, 260); *Suppl. 7*, 127 (1987); 58, 41 (1993)

Beryllium acetate (*see* Beryllium and beryllium compounds)

Beryllium acetate, basic (*see* Beryllium and beryllium compounds)

Beryllium-aluminium alloy (*see* Beryllium and beryllium compounds)

Beryllium carbonate (*see* Beryllium and beryllium compounds)

Beryllium chloride (*see* Beryllium and beryllium compounds)

Beryllium-copper alloy (*see* Beryllium and beryllium compounds)

Beryllium-copper-cobalt alloy (*see* Beryllium and beryllium compounds)

β-Butyrolactone   *11*, 225 (1976); *Suppl. 7*, 59
                                            (1987); *71*, 1317 (1999)
γ-Butyrolactone   *11*, 231 (1976); *Suppl. 7*, 59
                                            (1987); *71*, 367 (1999)

C

Cabinet-making (*see* Furniture and cabinet-making)
Cadmium acetate (*see* Cadmium and cadmium compounds)
Cadmium and cadmium compounds   *2*, 74 (1973); *11*, 39 (1976)
                                            (*corr. 42*, 255); *Suppl. 7*, 139
                                            (1987); *58*, 119 (1993)

Cadmium chloride (*see* Cadmium and cadmium compounds)
Cadmium oxide (*see* Cadmium and cadmium compounds)
Cadmium sulfate (*see* Cadmium and cadmium compounds)
Cadmium sulfide (*see* Cadmium and cadmium compounds)
Caffeic acid   *56*, 115 (1993)
Caffeine   *51*, 291 (1991)
Calcium arsenate (*see* Arsenic and arsenic compounds)
Calcium chromate (see Chromium and chromium compounds)
Calcium cyclamate (*see* Cyclamates)
Calcium saccharin (*see* Saccharin)
Cantharidin   *10*, 79 (1976); *Suppl. 7*, 59 (1987)
Caprolactam   *19*, 115 (1979) (*corr. 42*, 258);
                                            39, 247 (1986) (*corr. 42*, 264);
                                            Suppl. 7, 59, 390 (1987); *71*, 383
                                            (1999)
Captafol   *53*, 353 (1991)
Captan   *30*, 295 (1983); *Suppl. 7*, 59 (1987)
Carbaryl   *12*, 37 (1976); *Suppl. 7*, 59 (1987)
Carbazole   *32*, 239 (1983); *Suppl. 7*, 59
                                            (1987); *71*, 1319 (1999)
3-Carbethoxypsoralen   *40*, 317 (1986); *Suppl. 7*, 59 (1987)
Carbon black   *3*, 22 (1973); *33*, 35 (1984);
                                            Suppl. 7, 142 (1987); *65*, 149
                                            (1996)
Carbon tetrachloride   *1*, 53 (1972); *20*, 371 (1979);
                                            Suppl. 7, 143 (1987); *71*, 401
                                            (1999)
Carmoisine   *8*, 83 (1975); *Suppl. 7*, 59 (1987)
Carpentry and joinery   *25*, 139 (1981); *Suppl. 7*, 378
                                            (1987)
Carrageenan   *10*, 181 (1976) (*corr. 42*, 255); *31*,
                                            79 (1983); *Suppl. 7*, 59 (1987)
Cassia occidentalis (*see* Traditional herbal medicines)
Catechol   *15*, 155 (1977); *Suppl. 7*, 59
                                            (1987); *71*, 433 (1999)

CCNU (*see* 1-(2-Chloroethyl)-3-cyclohexyl-1-nitrosourea)
Ceramic fibres (*see* Man-made vitreous fibres)
Chemotherapy, combined, including alkylating agents (*see* MOPP and
     other combined chemotherapy including alkylating agents)
Chloral   *63*, 245 (1995)
Chloral hydrate   *63*, 245 (1995)

Chloroprene   *19*, 131 (1979); *Suppl. 7*, 160
                                               (1987); *71*, 227 (1999)

Chloropropham   *12*, 55 (1976); *Suppl. 7*, 60 (1987)
Chloroquine   *13*, 47 (1977); *Suppl. 7*, 60 (1987)
Chlorothalonil   *30*, 319 (1983); *Suppl. 7*, 60 (1987);
                                               73, 183 (1999)

para-Chloro-*ortho*-toluidine and its strong acid salts   *16*, 277 (1978); *30*, 65 (1983);
   (*see also* Chlordimeform)   *Suppl. 7*, 60 (1987); *48*, 123
                                               (1990); *77*, 323 (2000)

4-Chloro-*ortho*-toluidine (see *para*-chloro-*ortho*-toluidine)
5-Chloro-*ortho*-toluidine   *77*, 341 (2000)
Chlorotrianisene (*see also* Nonsteroidal oestrogens)   *21*, 139 (1979); *Suppl. 7*, 280
                                               (1987)

2-Chloro-1,1,1-trifluoroethane   *41*, 253 (1986); *Suppl. 7*, 60
                                               (1987); *71*, 1355 (1999)

Chlorozotocin   *50*, 65 (1990)
Cholesterol   *10*, 99 (1976); *31*, 95 (1983);
                                               Suppl. 7, 161 (1987)

Chromic acetate (*see* Chromium and chromium compounds)
Chromic chloride (*see* Chromium and chromium compounds)
Chromic oxide (*see* Chromium and chromium compounds)
Chromic phosphate (*see* Chromium and chromium compounds)
Chromite ore (*see* Chromium and chromium compounds)
Chromium and chromium compounds (*see also* Implants, surgical)   *2*, 100 (1973); *23*, 205 (1980);
                                               Suppl. 7, 165 (1987); *49*, 49 (1990)
                                               (*corr. 51*, 483)

Chromium carbonyl (*see* Chromium and chromium compounds)
Chromium potassium sulfate (*see* Chromium and chromium compounds)
Chromium sulfate (*see* Chromium and chromium compounds)
Chromium trioxide (*see* Chromium and chromium compounds)
Chrysazin (*see* Dantron)
Chrysene   *3*, 159 (1973); *32*, 247 (1983);
                                               Suppl. 7, 60 (1987)

Chrysoidine   *8*, 91 (1975); *Suppl. 7*, 169 (1987)
Chrysotile (*see* Asbestos)
CI Acid Orange 3   *57*, 121 (1993)
CI Acid Red 114   *57*, 247 (1993)
CI Basic Red 9 (*see also* Magenta)   *57*, 215 (1993)
Ciclosporin   *50*, 77 (1990)
CI Direct Blue 15   *57*, 235 (1993)
CI Disperse Yellow 3 (see Disperse Yellow 3)
Cimetidine   *50*, 235 (1990)
Cinnamyl anthranilate   *16*, 287 (1978); *31*, 133 (1983);
                                               Suppl. 7, 60 (1987); *77*, 177 (2000)
CI Pigment Red 3   *57*, 259 (1993)
CI Pigment Red 53:1 (*see* D&C Red No. 9)
Cisplatin (*see also* Etoposide)   *26*, 151 (1981); *Suppl. 7*, 170
                                               (1987)

Citrinin   *40*, 67 (1986); *Suppl. 7*, 60 (1987)
Citrus Red No. 2   *8*, 101 (1975) (*corr. 42*, 254);
                                               Suppl. 7, 60 (1987)

Clinoptilolite (*see* Zeolites)
Clofibrate   *24*, 39 (1980); *Suppl. 7*, 171
                                               (1987); *66*, 391 (1996)

Cyproterone acetate   *72*, 49 (1999)

D

2,4-D (*see also* Chlorophenoxy herbicides; Chlorophenoxy   *15*, 111 (1977)
  herbicides, occupational exposures to)
Dacarbazine   *26*, 203 (1981); *Suppl. 7*, 184
                                                                 (1987)
Dantron   *50*, 265 (1990) (*corr. 59*, 257)
D&C Red No. 9   *8*, 107 (1975); *Suppl. 7*, 61 (1987);
                                                                 57, 203 (1993)
Dapsone   *24*, 59 (1980); *Suppl. 7*, 185 (1987)
Daunomycin   *10*, 145 (1976); *Suppl. 7*, 61 (1987)
DDD (*see* DDT)
DDE (*see* DDT)
DDT   *5*, 83 (1974) (*corr. 42*, 253);
                                                                 Suppl. 7, 186 (1987); *53*, 179
                                                                 (1991)
Decabromodiphenyl oxide   *48*, 73 (1990); *71*, 1365 (1999)
Deltamethrin   *53*, 251 (1991)
Deoxynivalenol (*see* Toxins derived from *Fusarium graminearum*,
  F. culmorum and *F. crookwellense*)
Diacetylaminoazotoluene   *8*, 113 (1975); *Suppl. 7*, 61 (1987)
N,N'-Diacetylbenzidine   *16*, 293 (1978); *Suppl. 7*, 61 (1987)
Diallate   *12*, 69 (1976); *30*, 235 (1983);
                                                                 Suppl. 7, 61 (1987)
2,4-Diaminoanisole and its salts   *16*, 51 (1978); *27*, 103 (1982);
                                                                 Suppl. 7, 61 (1987); *79*, 619 (2001)
4,4'-Diaminodiphenyl ether   *16*, 301 (1978); *29*, 203 (1982);
                                                                 Suppl. 7, 61 (1987)
1,2-Diamino-4-nitrobenzene   *16*, 63 (1978); *Suppl. 7*, 61 (1987)
1,4-Diamino-2-nitrobenzene   *16*, 73 (1978); *Suppl. 7*, 61 (1987);
                                                                 57, 185 (1993)
2,6-Diamino-3-(phenylazo)pyridine (*see* Phenazopyridine hydrochloride)
2,4-Diaminotoluene (*see also* Toluene diisocyanates)   *16*, 83 (1978); *Suppl. 7*, 61 (1987)
2,5-Diaminotoluene (*see also* Toluene diisocyanates)   *16*, 97 (1978); *Suppl. 7*, 61 (1987)
ortho-Dianisidine (*see* 3,3'-Dimethoxybenzidine)
Diatomaceous earth, uncalcined (*see* Amorphous silica)
Diazepam   *13*, 57 (1977); *Suppl. 7*, 189
                                                                 (1987); *66*, 37 (1996)
Diazomethane   *7*, 223 (1974); *Suppl. 7*, 61 (1987)
Dibenz[*a,h*]acridine   *3*, 247 (1973); *32*, 277 (1983);
                                                                 Suppl. 7, 61 (1987)
Dibenz[*a,j*]acridine   *3*, 254 (1973); *32*, 283 (1983);
                                                                 Suppl. 7, 61 (1987)
Dibenz[*a,c*]anthracene   *32*, 289 (1983) (*corr. 42*, 262);
                                                                 Suppl. 7, 61 (1987)
Dibenz[*a,h*]anthracene   *3*, 178 (1973) (*corr. 43*, 261);
                                                                 32, 299 (1983); *Suppl. 7*, 61 (1987)
Dibenz[*a,j*]anthracene   *32*, 309 (1983); *Suppl. 7*, 61 (1987)
7*H*-Dibenzo[*c,g*]carbazole   *3*, 260 (1973); *32*, 315 (1983);
                                                                 Suppl. 7, 61 (1987)

Ethionamide   *13*, 83 (1977); *Suppl. 7*, 63 (1987)
Ethyl acrylate   *19*, 57 (1979); *39*, 81 (1986);
                                                         Suppl. 7, 63 (1987); *71*, 1447
                                                         (1999)
Ethylbenzene   *77*, 227 (2000)
Ethylene   *19*, 157 (1979); *Suppl. 7*, 63
                                                         (1987); *60*, 45 (1994); *71*, 1447
                                                         (1999)
Ethylene dibromide   *15*, 195 (1977); *Suppl. 7*, 204
                                                         (1987); *71*, 641 (1999)
Ethylene oxide   *11*, 157 (1976); *36*, 189 (1985)
                                                         (*corr. 42*, 263); *Suppl. 7*, 205
                                                         (1987); *60*, 73 (1994)
Ethylene sulfide   *11*, 257 (1976); *Suppl. 7*, 63 (1987)
Ethylenethiourea   *7*, 45 (1974); *Suppl. 7*, 207 (1987);
                                                         79, 659 (2001)
2-Ethylhexyl acrylate   *60*, 475 (1994)
Ethyl methanesulfonate   *7*, 245 (1974); *Suppl. 7*, 63 (1987)
N-Ethyl-*N*-nitrosourea   *1*, 135 (1972); *17*, 191 (1978);
                                                         Suppl. 7, 63 (1987)
Ethyl selenac (*see also* Selenium and selenium compounds)   *12*, 107 (1976); *Suppl. 7*, 63 (1987)
Ethyl tellurac   *12*, 115 (1976); *Suppl. 7*, 63 (1987)
Ethynodiol diacetate   *6*, 173 (1974); *21*, 387 (1979);
                                                         Suppl. 7, 292 (1987); *72*, 49
                                                         (1999)
Etoposide   *76*, 177 (2000)
Eugenol   *36*, 75 (1985); *Suppl. 7*, 63 (1987)
Evans blue   *8*, 151 (1975); *Suppl. 7*, 63 (1987)
Extremely low-frequency electric fields   *80* (2002)
Extremely low-frequency magnetic fields   *80* (2002)

F

Fast Green FCF   *16*, 187 (1978); *Suppl. 7*, 63 (1987)
Fenvalerate   *53*, 309 (1991)
Ferbam   *12*, 121 (1976) (*corr. 42*, 256);
                                                         Suppl. 7, 63 (1987)
Ferric oxide   *1*, 29 (1972); *Suppl. 7*, 216 (1987)
Ferrochromium (*see* Chromium and chromium compounds)
Fluometuron   *30*, 245 (1983); *Suppl. 7*, 63 (1987)
Fluoranthene   *32*, 355 (1983); *Suppl. 7*, 63 (1987)
Fluorene   *32*, 365 (1983); *Suppl. 7*, 63 (1987)
Fluorescent lighting (exposure to) (*see* Ultraviolet radiation)
Fluorides (inorganic, used in drinking-water)   *27*, 237 (1982); *Suppl. 7*, 208
                                                         (1987)
5-Fluorouracil   *26*, 217 (1981); *Suppl. 7*, 210
                                                         (1987)
Fluorspar (*see* Fluorides)
Fluosilicic acid (*see* Fluorides)
Fluroxene (*see* Anaesthetics, volatile)
Foreign bodies   *74* (1999)

L

Lasiocarpine	*10*, 281 (1976); *Suppl. 7*, 65 (1987)
Lauroyl peroxide	*36*, 315 (1985); *Suppl. 7*, 65 (1987); *71*, 1485 (1999)
Lead acetate (*see* Lead and lead compounds)	
Lead and lead compounds (*see also* Foreign bodies)	*1*, 40 (1972) (*corr. 42*, 251); *2*, 52, 150 (1973); *12*, 131 (1976); *23*, 40, 208, 209, 325 (1980); *Suppl. 7*, 230 (1987)
Lead arsenate (*see* Arsenic and arsenic compounds)	
Lead carbonate (*see* Lead and lead compounds)	
Lead chloride (*see* Lead and lead compounds)	
Lead chromate (*see* Chromium and chromium compounds)	
Lead chromate oxide (*see* Chromium and chromium compounds)	
Lead naphthenate (*see* Lead and lead compounds)	
Lead nitrate (*see* Lead and lead compounds)	
Lead oxide (*see* Lead and lead compounds)	
Lead phosphate (*see* Lead and lead compounds)	
Lead subacetate (*see* Lead and lead compounds)	
Lead tetroxide (*see* Lead and lead compounds)	
Leather goods manufacture	*25*, 279 (1981); *Suppl. 7*, 235 (1987)
Leather industries	*25*, 199 (1981); *Suppl. 7*, 232 (1987)
Leather tanning and processing	*25*, 201 (1981); *Suppl. 7*, 236 (1987)
Ledate (*see also* Lead and lead compounds)	*12*, 131 (1976)
Levonorgestrel	*72*, 49 (1999)
Light Green SF	*16*, 209 (1978); *Suppl. 7*, 65 (1987)
d-Limonene	*56*, 135 (1993); *73*, 307 (1999)
Lindane (*see* Hexachlorocyclohexanes)	
Liver flukes (*see Clonorchis sinensis*, *Opisthorchis felineus* and *Opisthorchis viverrini*)	
Lucidin (*see* 1,3-Dihydro-2-hydroxymethylanthraquinone)	
Lumber and sawmill industries (including logging)	*25*, 49 (1981); *Suppl. 7*, 383 (1987)
Luteoskyrin	*10*, 163 (1976); *Suppl. 7*, 65 (1987)
Lynoestrenol	*21*, 407 (1979); *Suppl. 7*, 293 (1987); *72*, 49 (1999)

M

Madder root (*see also Rubia tinctorum*)	*82*, 129 (2002)
Magenta	*4*, 57 (1974) (*corr. 42*, 252); *Suppl. 7*, 238 (1987); *57*, 215 (1993)
Magenta, manufacture of (*see also* Magenta)	*Suppl. 7*, 238 (1987); *57*, 215 (1993)
Malathion	*30*, 103 (1983); *Suppl. 7*, 65 (1987)
Maleic hydrazide	*4*, 173 (1974) (*corr. 42*, 253); *Suppl. 7*, 65 (1987)
Malonaldehyde	*36*, 163 (1985); *Suppl. 7*, 65 (1987); *71*, 1037 (1999)

Malondialdehyde (*see* Malonaldehyde)

Maneb   *12*, 137 (1976); *Suppl. 7*, 65 (1987)

Man-made mineral fibres (*see* Man-made vitreous fibres)

Man-made vitreous fibres   *43*, 39 (1988); *81* (2002)

Mannomustine   *9*, 157 (1975); *Suppl. 7*, 65 (1987)

Mate   *51*, 273 (1991)

MCPA (*see also* Chlorophenoxy herbicides; Chlorophenoxy   *30*, 255 (1983)
    herbicides, occupational exposures to)

MeA-α-C   *40*, 253 (1986); *Suppl. 7*, 65 (1987)

Medphalan   *9*, 168 (1975); *Suppl. 7*, 65 (1987)

Medroxyprogesterone acetate   *6*, 157 (1974); *21*, 417 (1979)
     (*corr. 42*, 259); *Suppl. 7*, 289
     (1987); *72*, 339 (1999)

Megestrol acetate   *Suppl. 7*, 293 (1987); *72*, 49 (1999)

MeIQ   *40*, 275 (1986); *Suppl. 7*, 65
     (1987); *56*, 197 (1993)

MeIQx   *40*, 283 (1986); *Suppl. 7*, 65 (1987)
     56, 211 (1993)

Melamine   *39*, 333 (1986); *Suppl. 7*, 65
     (1987); *73*, 329 (1999)

Melphalan   *9*, 167 (1975); *Suppl. 7*, 239 (1987)

6-Mercaptopurine   *26*, 249 (1981); *Suppl. 7*, 240
     (1987)

Mercuric chloride (*see* Mercury and mercury compounds)

Mercury and mercury compounds   *58*, 239 (1993)

Merphalan   *9*, 169 (1975); *Suppl. 7*, 65 (1987)

Mestranol   *6*, 87 (1974); *21*, 257 (1979)
     (*corr. 42*, 259); *Suppl. 7*, 288
     (1987); *72*, 49 (1999)

Metabisulfites (*see* Sulfur dioxide and some sulfites, bisulfites
    and metabisulfites)

Metallic mercury (*see* Mercury and mercury compounds)

Methanearsonic acid, disodium salt (*see* Arsenic and arsenic compounds)

Methanearsonic acid, monosodium salt (*see* Arsenic and arsenic
    compounds)

Methimazole   *79*, 53 (2001)

Methotrexate   *26*, 267 (1981); *Suppl. 7*, 241
     (1987)

Methoxsalen (*see* 8-Methoxypsoralen)

Methoxychlor   *5*, 193 (1974); *20*, 259 (1979);
     Suppl. 7, 66 (1987)

Methoxyflurane (*see* Anaesthetics, volatile)

5-Methoxypsoralen   *40*, 327 (1986); *Suppl. 7*, 242
     (1987)

8-Methoxypsoralen (*see also* 8-Methoxypsoralen plus ultraviolet   *24*, 101 (1980)
    radiation)

8-Methoxypsoralen plus ultraviolet radiation   *Suppl. 7*, 243 (1987)

Methyl acrylate   *19*, 52 (1979); *39*, 99 (1986);
     Suppl. 7, 66 (1987); *71*, 1489
     (1999)

5-Methylangelicin plus ultraviolet radiation (*see also* Angelicin   *Suppl. 7*, 57 (1987)
    and some synthetic derivatives)

2-Methylaziridine   *9*, 61 (1975); *Suppl. 7*, 66 (1987);
     71, 1497 (1999)

Methylazoxymethanol acetate (*see also* Cycasin)   *1*, 164 (1972); *10*, 131 (1976); *Suppl. 7*, 66 (1987)

Methyl bromide   *41*, 187 (1986) (*corr. 45*, 283); *Suppl. 7*, 245 (1987); *71*, 721 (1999)

Methyl *tert*-butyl ether   *73*, 339 (1999)
Methyl carbamate   *12*, 151 (1976); *Suppl. 7*, 66 (1987)
Methyl-CCNU (*see* 1-(2-Chloroethyl)-3-(4-methylcyclohexyl)-
   1-nitrosourea)
Methyl chloride   *41*, 161 (1986); *Suppl. 7*, 246 (1987); *71*, 737 (1999)

1-, 2-, 3-, 4-, 5- and 6-Methylchrysenes   *32*, 379 (1983); *Suppl. 7*, 66 (1987)
N-Methyl-*N*,4-dinitrosoaniline   *1*, 141 (1972); *Suppl. 7*, 66 (1987)
4,4'-Methylene bis(2-chloroaniline)   *4*, 65 (1974) (*corr. 42*, 252); *Suppl. 7*, 246 (1987); *57*, 271 (1993)

4,4'-Methylene bis(*N,N*-dimethyl)benzenamine   *27*, 119 (1982); *Suppl. 7*, 66 (1987)
4,4'-Methylene bis(2-methylaniline)   *4*, 73 (1974); *Suppl. 7*, 248 (1987)
4,4'-Methylenedianiline   *4*, 79 (1974) (*corr. 42*, 252); *39*, 347 (1986); *Suppl. 7*, 66 (1987)
4,4'-Methylenediphenyl diisocyanate   *19*, 314 (1979); *Suppl. 7*, 66 (1987); *71*, 1049 (1999)

2-Methylfluoranthene   *32*, 399 (1983); *Suppl. 7*, 66 (1987)
3-Methylfluoranthene   *32*, 399 (1983); *Suppl. 7*, 66 (1987)
Methylglyoxal   *51*, 443 (1991)
Methyl iodide   *15*, 245 (1977); *41*, 213 (1986); *Suppl. 7*, 66 (1987); *71*, 1503 (1999)

Methylmercury chloride (*see* Mercury and mercury compounds)
Methylmercury compounds (*see* Mercury and mercury compounds)
Methyl methacrylate   *19*, 187 (1979); *Suppl. 7*, 66 (1987); *60*, 445 (1994)

Methyl methanesulfonate   *7*, 253 (1974); *Suppl. 7*, 66 (1987); *71*, 1059 (1999)

2-Methyl-1-nitroanthraquinone   *27*, 205 (1982); *Suppl. 7*, 66 (1987)
N-Methyl-*N'*-nitro-*N*-nitrosoguanidine   *4*, 183 (1974); *Suppl. 7*, 248 (1987)
3-Methylnitrosaminopropionaldehyde [*see* 3-(*N*-Nitrosomethylamino)-
   propionaldehyde]
3-Methylnitrosaminopropionitrile [*see* 3-(*N*-Nitrosomethylamino)-
   propionitrile]
4-(Methylnitrosamino)-4-(3-pyridyl)-1-butanal [*see* 4-(*N*-Nitrosomethyl-
   amino)-4-(3-pyridyl)-1-butanal]
4-(Methylnitrosamino)-1-(3-pyridyl)-1-butanone [*see* 4-(-Nitrosomethyl-
   amino)-1-(3-pyridyl)-1-butanone]
N-Methyl-*N*-nitrosourea   *1*, 125 (1972); *17*, 227 (1978); *Suppl. 7*, 66 (1987)

N-Methyl-*N*-nitrosourethane   *4*, 211 (1974); *Suppl. 7*, 66 (1987)
N-Methylolacrylamide   *60*, 435 (1994)
Methyl parathion   *30*, 131 (1983); *Suppl. 7*, 66, 392 (1987)

1-Methylphenanthrene   *32*, 405 (1983); *Suppl. 7*, 66 (1987)
7-Methylpyrido[3,4-*c*]psoralen   *40*, 349 (1986); *Suppl. 7*, 71 (1987)
Methyl red   *8*, 161 (1975); *Suppl. 7*, 66 (1987)
Methyl selenac (*see also* Selenium and selenium compounds)   *12*, 161 (1976); *Suppl. 7*, 66 (1987)

Nickel-gallium alloy (*see* Nickel and nickel compounds)
Nickel hydroxide (*see* Nickel and nickel compounds)
Nickelocene (*see* Nickel and nickel compounds)
Nickel oxide (*see* Nickel and nickel compounds)
Nickel subsulfide (*see* Nickel and nickel compounds)
Nickel sulfate (*see* Nickel and nickel compounds)

Niridazole	*13*, 123 (1977); *Suppl. 7*, 67 (1987)
Nithiazide	*31*, 179 (1983); *Suppl. 7*, 67 (1987)
Nitrilotriacetic acid and its salts	*48*, 181 (1990); *73*, 385 (1999)
5-Nitroacenaphthene	*16*, 319 (1978); *Suppl. 7*, 67 (1987)
5-Nitro-*ortho*-anisidine	*27*, 133 (1982); *Suppl. 7*, 67 (1987)
2-Nitroanisole	*65*, 369 (1996)
9-Nitroanthracene	*33*, 179 (1984); *Suppl. 7*, 67 (1987)
7-Nitrobenz[*a*]anthracene	*46*, 247 (1989)
Nitrobenzene	*65*, 381 (1996)
6-Nitrobenzo[*a*]pyrene	*33*, 187 (1984); *Suppl. 7*, 67 (1987); *46*, 255 (1989)
4-Nitrobiphenyl	*4*, 113 (1974); *Suppl. 7*, 67 (1987)
6-Nitrochrysene	*33*, 195 (1984); *Suppl. 7*, 67 (1987); *46*, 267 (1989)
Nitrofen (technical-grade)	*30*, 271 (1983); *Suppl. 7*, 67 (1987)
3-Nitrofluoranthene	*33*, 201 (1984); *Suppl. 7*, 67 (1987)
2-Nitrofluorene	*46*, 277 (1989)
Nitrofural	*7*, 171 (1974); *Suppl. 7*, 67 (1987); *50*, 195 (1990)
5-Nitro-2-furaldehyde semicarbazone (*see* Nitrofural)	
Nitrofurantoin	*50*, 211 (1990)
Nitrofurazone (*see* Nitrofural)	
1-[(5-Nitrofurfurylidene)amino]-2-imidazolidinone	*7*, 181 (1974); *Suppl. 7*, 67 (1987)
N-[4-(5-Nitro-2-furyl)-2-thiazolyl]acetamide	*1*, 181 (1972); *7*, 185 (1974); *Suppl. 7*, 67 (1987)
Nitrogen mustard	*9*, 193 (1975); *Suppl. 7*, 269 (1987)
Nitrogen mustard *N*-oxide	*9*, 209 (1975); *Suppl. 7*, 67 (1987)
Nitromethane	*77*, 487 (2000)
1-Nitronaphthalene	*46*, 291 (1989)
2-Nitronaphthalene	*46*, 303 (1989)
3-Nitroperylene	*46*, 313 (1989)
2-Nitro-*para*-phenylenediamine (*see* 1,4-Diamino-2-nitrobenzene)	
2-Nitropropane	*29*, 331 (1982); *Suppl. 7*, 67 (1987); *71*, 1079 (1999)
1-Nitropyrene	*33*, 209 (1984); *Suppl. 7*, 67 (1987); *46*, 321 (1989)
2-Nitropyrene	*46*, 359 (1989)
4-Nitropyrene	*46*, 367 (1989)
N-Nitrosatable drugs	*24*, 297 (1980) (*corr. 42*, 260)
N-Nitrosatable pesticides	*30*, 359 (1983)
N'-Nitrosoanabasine	*37*, 225 (1985); *Suppl. 7*, 67 (1987)
N'-Nitrosoanatabine	*37*, 233 (1985); *Suppl. 7*, 67 (1987)
N-Nitrosodi-*n*-butylamine	*4*, 197 (1974); *17*, 51 (1978); *Suppl. 7*, 67 (1987)
N-Nitrosodiethanolamine	*17*, 77 (1978); *Suppl. 7*, 67 (1987); *77*, 403 (2000)

O

P

Q

R

Rhodamine 6G   *16*, 233 (1978); *Suppl. 7*, 71 (1987)
Riddelliine   *10*, 313 (1976); *Suppl. 7*, 71
                                                               (1987); *82*, 153 (2002)
Rifampicin   *24*, 243 (1980); *Suppl. 7*, 71 (1987)
Ripazepam   *66*, 157 (1996)
Rock (stone) wool (*see* Man-made vitreous fibres)
Rubber industry   *28* (1982) (*corr. 42*, 261); *Suppl. 7*,
                                                               332 (1987)
Rubia tinctorum (*see also* Madder root, Traditional herbal medicines)   *82*, 129 (2002)
Rugulosin   *40*, 99 (1986); *Suppl. 7*, 71 (1987)

S

Saccharated iron oxide   *2*, 161 (1973); *Suppl. 7*, 71 (1987)
Saccharin and its salts   *22*, 111 (1980) (*corr. 42*, 259);
                                                               Suppl. 7, 334 (1987); *73*, 517 (1999)
Safrole   *1*, 169 (1972); *10*, 231 (1976);
                                                               Suppl. 7, 71 (1987)
Salted fish   *56*, 41 (1993)
Sawmill industry (including logging) (*see* Lumber and
    sawmill industry (including logging))
Scarlet Red   *8*, 217 (1975); *Suppl. 7*, 71 (1987)
Schistosoma haematobium (infection with)   *61*, 45 (1994)
Schistosoma japonicum (infection with)   *61*, 45 (1994)
Schistosoma mansoni (infection with)   *61*, 45 (1994)
Selenium and selenium compounds   *9*, 245 (1975) (*corr. 42*, 255);
                                                               Suppl. 7, 71 (1987)
Selenium dioxide (*see* Selenium and selenium compounds)
Selenium oxide (*see* Selenium and selenium compounds)
Semicarbazide hydrochloride   *12*, 209 (1976) (*corr. 42*, 256);
                                                               Suppl. 7, 71 (1987)
Senecio jacobaea L. (*see also* Pyrrolizidine alkaloids) *10*, 333 (1976)
Senecio longilobus (*see also* Pyrrolizidine alkaloids, Traditional)   *10*, 334 (1976); *82*, ?? (2002)
    herbal medicines)
Senecio riddellii (*see also* Traditional herbal medicines)   *82*, 153 (1982)
Seneciphylline   *10*, 319, 335 (1976); *Suppl. 7*, 71
                                                               (1987)
Senkirkine   *10*, 327 (1976); *31*, 231 (1983);
                                                               Suppl. 7, 71 (1987)
Sepiolite   *42*, 175 (1987); *Suppl. 7*, 71
                                                               (1987); *68*, 267 (1997)
Sequential oral contraceptives (*see also* Oestrogens, progestins   *Suppl. 7*, 296 (1987)
    and combinations)
Shale-oils   *35*, 161 (1985); *Suppl. 7*, 339
                                                               (1987)
Shikimic acid (*see also* Bracken fern)   *40*, 55 (1986); *Suppl. 7*, 71 (1987)
Shoe manufacture and repair (*see* Boot and shoe manufacture
    and repair)
Silica (*see also* Amorphous silica; Crystalline silica)   *42*, 39 (1987)
Silicone (*see* Implants, surgical)
Simazine   *53*, 495 (1991); *73*, 625 (1999)
Slag wool (*see* Man-made vitreous fibres)
Sodium arsenate (*see* Arsenic and arsenic compounds)

Sulfafurazole	*24*, 275 (1980); *Suppl. 7*, 347 (1987)
Sulfallate	*30*, 283 (1983); *Suppl. 7*, 72 (1987)
Sulfamethazine and its sodium salt	*79*, 341 (2001)
Sulfamethoxazole	*24*, 285 (1980); *Suppl. 7*, 348 (1987); *79*, 361 (2001)

Sulfites (*see* Sulfur dioxide and some sulfites, bisulfites and metabisulfites)

Sulfur dioxide and some sulfites, bisulfites and metabisulfites	*54*, 131 (1992)

Sulfur mustard (*see* Mustard gas)

Sulfuric acid and other strong inorganic acids, occupational exposures to mists and vapours from	*54*, 41 (1992)
Sulfur trioxide	*54*, 121 (1992)

Sulphisoxazole (*see* Sulfafurazole)

Sunset Yellow FCF	*8*, 257 (1975); *Suppl. 7*, 72 (1987)
Symphytine	*31*, 239 (1983); *Suppl. 7*, 72 (1987)

T

2,4,5-T (*see also* Chlorophenoxy herbicides; Chlorophenoxy herbicides, occupational exposures to)	*15*, 273 (1977)
Talc	*42*, 185 (1987); *Suppl. 7*, 349 (1987)
Tamoxifen	*66*, 253 (1996)
Tannic acid	*10*, 253 (1976) (*corr. 42*, 255); *Suppl. 7*, 72 (1987)
Tannins (*see* also Tannic acid)	*10*, 254 (1976); *Suppl. 7*, 72 (1987)

TCDD (*see* 2,3,7,8-Tetrachlorodibenzo-*para*-dioxin)
TDE (*see* DDT)

Tea	*51*, 207 (1991)
Temazepam	*66*, 161 (1996)
Teniposide	*76*, 259 (2000)
Terpene polychlorinates	*5*, 219 (1974); *Suppl. 7*, 72 (1987)
Testosterone (*see also* Androgenic (anabolic) steroids)	*6*, 209 (1974); *21*, 519 (1979)

Testosterone oenanthate (*see* Testosterone)
Testosterone propionate (*see* Testosterone)

2,2′,5,5′-Tetrachlorobenzidine	*27*, 141 (1982); *Suppl. 7*, 72 (1987)
2,3,7,8-Tetrachlorodibenzo-*para*-dioxin	*15*, 41 (1977); *Suppl. 7*, 350 (1987); *69*, 33 (1997)
1,1,1,2-Tetrachloroethane	*41*, 87 (1986); *Suppl. 7*, 72 (1987); *71*, 1133 (1999)
1,1,2,2-Tetrachloroethane	*20*, 477 (1979); *Suppl. 7*, 354 (1987); *71*, 817 (1999)
Tetrachloroethylene	*20*, 491 (1979); *Suppl. 7*, 355 (1987); *63*, 159 (1995) (*corr. 65*, 549)

2,3,4,6-Tetrachlorophenol (*see* Chlorophenols; Chlorophenols, occupational exposures to; Polychlorophenols and their sodium salts)

Tetrachlorvinphos	*30*, 197 (1983); *Suppl. 7*, 72 (1987)

Tetraethyllead (*see* Lead and lead compounds)

Tetrafluoroethylene	*19*, 285 (1979); *Suppl. 7*, 72 (1987); *71*, 1143 (1999)
Tetrakis(hydroxymethyl)phosphonium salts	*48*, 95 (1990); *71*, 1529 (1999)

Tetramethyllead (*see* Lead and lead compounds)

U

Y

Yellow AB	8, 279 (1975); *Suppl. 7*, 74 (1987)
Yellow OB	8, 287 (1975); *Suppl. 7*, 74 (1987)

Z

Zalcitabine	76, 129 (2000)
Zearalenone (*see* Toxins derived from *Fusarium graminearum*, F. culmorum and F. crookwellense*)	
Zectran	12, 237 (1976); *Suppl. 7*, 74 (1987)
Zeolites other than erionite	68, 307 (1997)
Zidovudine	76, 73 (2000)
Zinc beryllium silicate (*see* Beryllium and beryllium compounds)	
Zinc chromate (*see* Chromium and chromium compounds)	
Zinc chromate hydroxide (*see* Chromium and chromium compounds)	
Zinc potassium chromate (*see* Chromium and chromium compounds)	
Zinc yellow (*see* Chromium and chromium compounds)	
Zineb	12, 245 (1976); *Suppl. 7*, 74 (1987)
Ziram	12, 259 (1976); *Suppl. 7*, 74 (1987); *53, 423* (1991)

List of IARC Monographs on the Evaluation of Carcinogenic Risks to Humans*

Volume 1
Some Inorganic Substances, Chlorinated Hydrocarbons, Aromatic Amines, *N*-Nitroso Compounds, and Natural Products
1972; 184 pages (out-of-print)

Volume 2
Some Inorganic and Organo-metallic Compounds
1973; 181 pages (out-of-print)

Volume 3
Certain Polycyclic Aromatic Hydrocarbons and Heterocyclic Compounds
1973; 271 pages (out-of-print)

Volume 4
Some Aromatic Amines, Hydra-zine and Related Substances, *N*-Nitroso Compounds and Miscellaneous Alkylating Agents
1974; 286 pages (out-of-print)

Volume 5
Some Organochlorine Pesticides
1974; 241 pages (out-of-print)

Volume 6
Sex Hormones
1974; 243 pages (out-of-print)

Volume 7
Some Anti-Thyroid and Related Substances, Nitrofurans and Industrial Chemicals
1974; 326 pages (out-of-print)

Volume 8
Some Aromatic Azo Compounds
1975; 357 pages

Volume 9
Some Aziridines, *N*-, *S*- and *O*-Mustards and Selenium
1975; 268 pages

Volume 10
Some Naturally Occurring Substances
1976; 353 pages (out-of-print)

Volume 11
Cadmium, Nickel, Some Epoxides, Miscellaneous Industrial Chemicals and General Considerations on Volatile Anaesthetics
1976; 306 pages (out-of-print)

Volume 12
Some Carbamates, Thio-carbamates and Carbazides
1976; 282 pages (out-of-print)

Volume 13
Some Miscellaneous Pharmaceutical Substances
1977; 255 pages

Volume 14
Asbestos
1977; 106 pages (out-of-print)

Volume 15
Some Fumigants, the Herbicides 2,4-D and 2,4,5-T, Chlorinated Dibenzodioxins and Miscella-neous Industrial Chemicals
1977; 354 pages (out-of-print)

Volume 16
Some Aromatic Amines and Related Nitro Compounds—Hair Dyes, Colouring Agents and Miscellaneous Industrial Chemicals
1978; 400 pages

Volume 17
Some *N*-Nitroso Compounds
1978; 365 pages

Volume 18
Polychlorinated Biphenyls and Polybrominated Biphenyls
1978; 140 pages (out-of-print)

Volume 19
Some Monomers, Plastics and Synthetic Elastomers, and Acrolein
1979; 513 pages (out-of-print)

Volume 20
Some Halogenated Hydrocarbons
1979; 609 pages (out-of-print)

Volume 21
Sex Hormones (II)
1979; 583 pages

Volume 22
Some Non-Nutritive Sweetening Agents
1980; 208 pages

Volume 23
Some Metals and Metallic Compounds
1980; 438 pages (out-of-print)

Volume 24
Some Pharmaceutical Drugs
1980; 337 pages

Volume 25
Wood, Leather and Some Associated Industries
1981; 412 pages

Volume 26
Some Antineoplastic and Immunosuppressive Agents
1981; 411 pages

Volume 27
Some Aromatic Amines, Anthraquinones and Nitroso Compounds, and Inorganic Fluorides Used in Drinking-water and Dental Preparations
1982; 341 pages

Volume 28
The Rubber Industry
1982; 486 pages

Volume 29
Some Industrial Chemicals and Dyestuffs
1982; 416 pages

Volume 30
Miscellaneous Pesticides
1983; 424 pages

---

*Certain older volumes, marked out-of-print, are still available directly from IARCPress. Further, high-quality photo-copies of all out-of-print volumes may be purchased from University Microfilms International, 300 North Zeeb Road, Ann Arbor, MI 48106-1346, USA (Tel.: 313-761-4700, 800-521-0600).

Achevé d'imprimer sur rotative
par l'imprimerie Darantiere à Dijon-Quetigny
en mai 2004

Dépôt légal : mai 2004
N° d'impression : 24-0491

Imprimé en France